D0926400

Complications in
ANESTHESIOLOGY

SECOND EDITION

Complications in ANESTHESIOLOGY

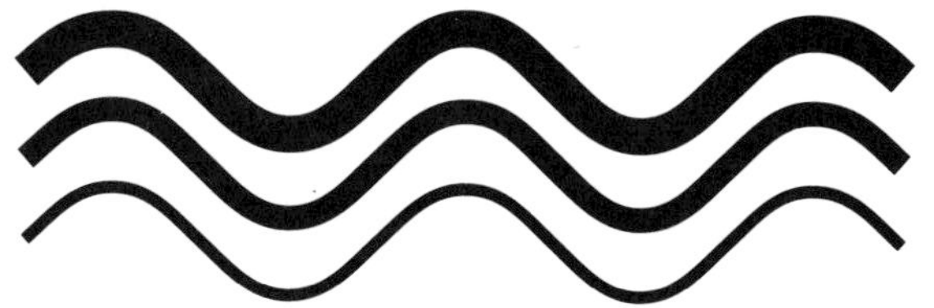

EDITED BY

Nikolaus Gravenstein, MD
Professor of Anesthesiology
and Neurosurgery
University of Florida College of Medicine
Gainesville, Florida

Robert R. Kirby, MD
Professor of Anesthesiology
University of Florida College of Medicine
Gainesville, Florida

With 70 Contributors

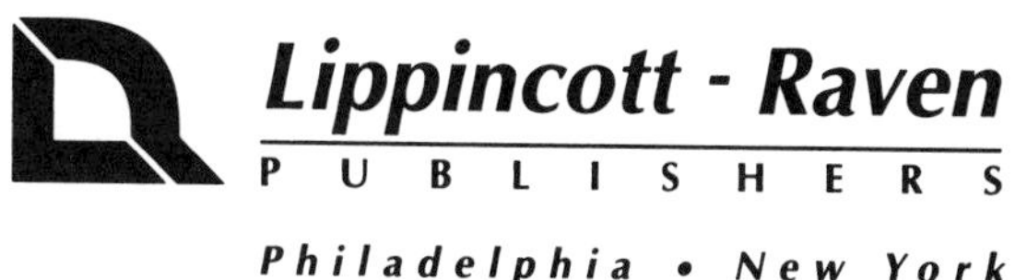

Developmental Editor: Melissa J. James
Associate Managing Editor: Elizabeth A. Durand
Production Manager: Caren Erlichman
Senior Production Coordinator: Kevin P. Johnson
Design Coordinator: Doug Smock
Indexer: Maria Coughlin
Compositor: Tapsco, Incorporated
Printer: Courier Book Company/Westford

2nd edition

Library of Congress Cataloging-in-Publication Data

Complications in anesthesiology/edited by Nikolaus Gravenstein,
Robert R. Kirby; with 70 contributors.—2nd ed.
p. cm.
Includes bibliographical references and index.
ISBN 0-397-51299-6 (alk. paper)
1. Anesthesia—Complications. I. Gravenstein, Nikolaus.
II. Kirby, Robert R.
[DNLM: 1. Anesthesia—adverse effects. 2. Postoperative
Complications. WO 245 C737 1995]
RD82.5.C64 1995
617.9′6041—dc20
DNLM/DLC
for Library of Congress 95-19472
CIP

9 8 7 6 5 4 3 2 1

Credits
Chapters 33, 34, 35, and 36 were originally submitted by the authors in 1988, and were revised in 1994 by Drs. Gravenstein and Kirby.

Contributors

John L. Atlee III, MD
Professor of Anesthesiology
Medical College of Wisconsin
Staff Anesthesiologist
Doyne Hospital
Froedtert Memorial Lutheran Hospital
Veterans Affairs Medical Center
Milwaukee, Wisconsin

Jeffrey M. Baden, MD
Professor of Anesthesiology
Stanford University School of Medicine
Chief
Anesthesiology Service
Palo Alto Veterans Affairs Medical Center
Palo Alto, California

Richard R. Bartkowski, MD, PhD
Professor of Anesthesiology
Jefferson Medical College
Thomas Jefferson University
Thomas Jefferson University Hospital
Philadelphia, Pennsylvania

Robert F. Bedford, MD
Clinical Professor of Anesthesiology
University of Virginia
School of Medicine
Attending Anesthesiologist
University of Virginia Health Sciences Center
Charlottesville, Virginia

Walter C. Bernards, MD
Clinical Assistant Professor
Department of Anesthesiology
The University of Texas Medical Branch
Galveston, Texas
Staff Anesthesiologist
St. Vincent Hospital
Portland, Oregon

Burton A. Briggs, MD
Professor of Anesthesiology
Loma Linda University
Medical Director
Operating Room Services
Loma Linda University Medical Center
Loma Linda, California

Beverley A. Britt, MD, FRCP(C)
Professor
Department of Anaesthesia and Pharmacology
University of Toronto
Senior Staff Anaesthetist
The Toronto Hospital (General Division)
Toronto, Ontario
Canada

Burnell R. Brown, Jr., MD, PhD, FRCA†
Professor Emeritus
University of Arizona
College of Medicine
Tucson, Arizona

Theodore G. Cheek, MD
Associate Professor
Anesthesia and Obstetrics and Gynecology
University of Pennsylvania School of Medicine
Director, Obstetric Anesthesia
Hospital of the University of Pennsylvania
Philadelphia, Pennsylvania

Charles J. Coté, MD
Vice Chairman
Director of Research
Department of Pediatric Anesthesia
Professor of Anesthesia and Pediatrics
Northwestern University Medical School
Chicago, Illinois

Benjamin G. Covino, PhD, MD†
Professor Emeritus
Department of Anaesthesia
Brigham and Women's Hospital
Harvard Medical School
Boston, Massachusetts

David J. Cullen, MD, MS
Professor of Anaesthesia
Harvard Medical School
Anesthetist
Massachusetts General Hospital
Boston, Massachusetts

† *Deceased*

J. Kenneth Denlinger, MD
Chairman
Department of Anesthesiology
Lancaster General Hospital
Lancaster, Pennsylvania

Donn M. Dennis, MD
Assistant Professor of Anesthesiology and Pharmacology
University of Florida College of Medicine
Staff Physician
Shands Hospital
Veterans Affairs Medical Center
Gainesville, Florida

Richard C. Dennis, MD
Associate Professor of Surgery and Anesthesiology
Boston University
Director
Critical Care Medicine
Boston University Medical Center
Boston, Massachusetts

Jules L. Dienstag, MD
Associate Professor of Medicine
Harvard Medical School
Physician
Massachusetts General Hospital
Boston, Massachusetts

Hillary F. Don, MD, FRCP(C)
Professor
Department of Anesthesia
University of California San Francisco
Physician
Veterans Affairs Medical Center
San Francisco, California

James R. Dooley, MD
Staff Anesthesiologist
Seton Medical Center
Daly City, California

Christopher W. Dueker, MD
Clinical Associate Professor of Anesthesia
Stanford University School of Medicine
Partner
Palo Alto Medical Foundation
Palo Alto, California

Marcel E. Durieux, MD
Assistant Professor of Anesthesiology
University of Virginia Health Sciences Center
Charlottesville, Virginia

John H. Eichhorn, MD
Professor and Chairman
Department of Anesthesiology
University of Mississippi
School of Medicine
Chairman
Department of Anesthesiology
University of Mississippi Medical Center
Jackson, Mississippi

Joan W. Flacke, MD
Professor Emeritus of Anesthesiology
University of California Los Angeles
Anesthesia Faculty
UCLA Medical Center
Los Angeles, California

Werner E. Flacke, MD
Professor Emeritus of Anesthesiology and Pharmacology
University of California Los Angeles School of Medicine
Los Angeles, California

David C. Flemming, MB
Clinical Assistant Professor
University of Chicago
Director, Medical Services
The Pain Institute in Chicago
Chicago, Illinois

H. Jerrel Fontenot, MD, PhD
Associate Professor of Anesthesiology and Pharmacology
University of Arkansas for Medical Sciences
Vice Chairman
Department of Anesthesiology
Medical Director of Operating Room and Clinical Services
University Hospital
Little Rock, Arkansas

William W. Fox, MD
Professor of Pediatrics
University of Pennsylvania School of Medicine
Neonatologist
Director of the Infant Breathing Disorders Center
Children's Hospital of Philadelphia
Philadelphia, Pennsylvania

Masahiko Fujinaga, MD
Research Assistant Professor of Biology in Anesthesia
Stanford University School of Medicine
Stanford, California
Research Assistant Professor of Biology in Anesthesia
Palo Alto Veterans Affairs Medical Center
Palo Alto, California

Thomas J. Gal, MD
Professor of Anesthesiology
University of Virginia Health Sciences Center
Charlottesville, Virginia

Jeffrey G. Garber, DMD
Private Practice
Former Chairman
Department of Dental Medicine
Graduate Hospital
Philadelphia, Pennsylvania

Marc Goldberg, MD
Chairman, Anesthesia Department
Wills Eye Hospital
Philadelphia, Pennsylvania
Chairman, Anesthesia Department
Rancocas Hospital
Willingboro, New Jersey

Michael L. Good, MD
Associate Professor of Anesthesiology
Chief, Anesthesiology Service
Veterans Affairs Medical Center
Gainesville, Florida

Nikolaus Gravenstein, MD
Professor of Anesthesiology and Neurosurgery
Executive Associate Chairman of Anesthesiology
University of Florida College of Medicine
Gainesville, Florida

Andrew Herlich, DMD, MD
Associate Professor of Anesthesiology and Critical Care Medicine
The University of Pittsburgh School of Medicine
Associate Professor and Medical Director
Nurse Anesthesia Program
University of Pittsburgh School of Nursing
Associate Professor of Oromaxillofacial Surgery
University of Pittsburgh School of Dental Medicine
Associate Chief Anesthesiologist
Eye and Ear Institute Pavilion
Department of Anesthesiology
The University of Pittsburgh Medical Center
Pittsburgh, Pennsylvania

Jan Charles Horrow, MD
Professor and Vice Chair, Anesthesiology
Medical College of Pennsylvania/Hahnemann University
Philadelphia, Pennsylvania

Marcia Jean Howton, MD
Chairman
Department of Anesthesiology
Mad River Hospital
McKinleyville, California

Catherine O. Hunt, MD
Anesthesiologist
Department of Anesthesia
Beverly Hospital
Beverly, Massachusetts

Ronald J. Hurley, MD
Assistant Professor of Anaesthesia
Harvard Medical School
Associate Director of Obstetric Anesthesia
Brigham and Women's Hospital
Boston, Massachusetts

Christopher F. James, MD
Associate Professor of Anesthesiology
University of Florida College of Medicine
Staff Physician
Shands Hospital
Veterans Affairs Medical Center
Gainesville, Florida

Donald E. Jones, MD, DABA
Vice President
Maryville Anesthesiologist PC
Vice Chief of Anesthesia
Blount Memorial Hospital
Maryville, Tennessee

Nancy Joy, AOCA
Professor Emeritus
Division of Biomedical Communications
Department of Surgery
University of Toronto
Faculty of Medicine
Toronto, Ontario
Canada

Arthur S. Keats, MD
Clinical Professor of Anesthesiology
University of Texas Health Science Center at Houston
Chief of Cardiovascular Anesthesiology
Texas Heart Institute
St. Luke's Episcopal Hospital
Houston, Texas

Robert R. Kirby, MD
Professor of Anesthesiology
University of Florida College of Medicine
Gainesville, Florida

G. Guy Knickerbocker, PhD
Chief Scientist
ECRI
Plymouth Meeting, Pennsylvania

A. Joseph Layon, MD
Associate Professor
Department of Anesthesiology and Medicine
University of Florida College of Medicine
Director
Preoperative Clinic
Shands Hospital
Gainesville, Florida

John H. Lecky, MD
Professor of Anesthesia
University of Washington
University of Washington Medical Center
Seattle, Washington

Jerry D. Levitt, MD
Associate Professor
Department of Anesthesiology
Medical College of Pennsylvania/Hahnemann University
Associate Vice Chairman
Department of Anesthesiology
Hahnemann University Hospital
Philadelphia, Pennsylvania

Letty M. P. Liu, MD
Associate Professor of Anaesthesia
Harvard Medical School
Anesthetist
Massachusetts General Hospital
Boston, Massachusetts

David E. Longnecker, MD
Robert Dunning Dripps Professor
Chair, Department of Anesthesia
Hospital of the University of Pennsylvania
Philadelphia, Pennsylvania

Margot B. Mackay, BSc, AAM
Associate Professor
Division of Biomedical Communications
Department of Surgery
University of Toronto
Faculty of Medicine
Toronto, Ontario
Canada

Richard I. Mazze, MD
Professor of Anesthesia
Associate Dean for Veterans Affairs
Stanford University
Stanford, California
Chief of Staff
Palo Alto Veterans Affairs Medical Center
Palo Alto, California

Kathryn E. McGoldrick, MD
Professor of Anesthesiology
Yale University School of Medicine
Medical Director
Ambulatory Surgery
Yale-New Haven Hospital
New Haven, Connecticut

Bucknam McPeek, MD
Associate Professor of Anaesthesia
Harvard University
Anesthetist to the Massachusetts General Hospital
Boston, Massachusetts

Terence M. Murphy, MB, ChB, FRCA
Professor
Department of Anesthesia and Clinical Pain Service
University of Washington Medical School
Attending Physician
University Hospital and Pain Center
Seattle, Washington

Gordon R. Neufeld, MD
Associate Professor of Anesthesia
University of Pennsylvania
School of Medicine
Staff Anesthesiologist
Veterans Affairs Medical Center
Philadelphia, Pennsylvania

Fredrick K. Orkin, MD, MBA
Professor of Anesthesiology, Community, and Family Medicine (Epidemiology)
Dartmouth Medical School
Mary Hitchcock Memorial Hospital
Lebanon, New Hampshire
Veterans Affairs Medical Center
White River Junction, Vermont

Gerard W. Ostheimer, MD
Professor of Anaesthesia
Harvard Medical School
Vice Chairman
Department of Anaesthesia
Brigham and Women's Hospital
Boston, Massachusetts

Orah S. Platt, MD
Associate Professor of Pediatrics
Harvard Medical School
Director, Department of Laboratory Medicine
Children's Hospital
Boston, Massachusetts

Allen K. Ream, MD, SB, MS
Clinical Associate Professor of Anesthesia
Stanford University
Stanford, California

Sandra L. Roberts, MD
Anesthesiologist
St. Joseph Hospital
Lexington, Kentucky

Henrietta Kotlus Rosenberg, MD
Professor of Diagnostic Imaging
Temple University School of Medicine
Chairman, Department of Radiology
Albert Einstein Medical Center
Philadelphia, Pennsylvania

Henry Rosenberg, MD
Professor and Chairman
Department of Anesthesiology
Medical College of Pennsylvania/Hahnemann University
Chairman of Anesthesiology
Hahnemann University Hospital
Philadelphia, Pennsylvania

John F. Ryan, MD
Associate Professor of Anaesthesia
Harvard Medical School
Anesthetist
Massachusetts General Hospital
Boston, Massachusetts

James C. Scott, MD
Associate Professor
Department of Anesthesiology and Critical Care Medicine
University of New Mexico
School of Medicine
University of New Mexico
Health Sciences Center
Albuquerque, New Mexico

John G. Shutack, DO
Associate Professor of Anesthesiology
Medical College of Pennsylvania/Hahnemann University
Hahnemann University Hospital
Philadelphia, Pennsylvania

Bradley E. Smith, MD
Professor
Department of Anesthesiology
Vanderbilt University
School of Medicine
Nashville, Tennessee

Cheri A. Sulek, MD
Assistant Professor of Anesthesiology
University of Florida College of Medicine
Shands Teaching Hospital
Gainesville, Florida

John H. Tinker, MD
Professor and Head
Department of Anesthesia
University of Iowa College of Medicine
Iowa City, Iowa

Leroy D. Vandam, MD, PhD, MA (Hon)
Professor Emeritus of Anaesthesia
Harvard Medical School
Anesthesiologist
Brigham and Women's Hospital
Boston, Massachusetts

R. Lee Wagner, MD
Assistant Clinical Professor
Department of Anesthesiology
University of California San Diego School of Medicine
San Diego, California
Staff Anesthesiologist
Green Hospital of the Scripps Clinic
La Jolla, California

Robert S. Wharton, MD
Staff Anesthesiologist
St. Peter's Hospital
Olympia, Washington

Margaret Wood, MB, ChB, FRCA
Professor of Anesthesiology
Associate Professor of Pharmacology
Department of Anesthesiology
Vanderbilt University Medical School
Attending Anesthesiologist
Vanderbilt University Medical Center
Nashville, Tennessee

Neil S. Yeston, MD
Professor of Surgery
University of Connecticut
School of Medicine
Director, Critical Care Medicine
Hartford Hospital
Hartford, Connecticut

Preface

The continued occurrence of complications in anesthesiology remains on every practitioner's mind. These complications have been the focus of several books, numerous articles, and countless case reports. Over the last decade, our largest professional society—The American Society of Anesthesiologists—has broadened our understanding of complications through reports of closed malpractice claims. This second edition of *Complications in Anesthesiology* is written by more than 60 contributing authors. Their goals and ours are to further describe, update, and refine our understanding of why complications occur, how to deal with them, how to prevent or minimize them, and how to understand their associated pathophysiology. Some material in this second edition will be familiar to readers of the first. However, much of the contained material is new, revised, or updated, reflecting the continued evolution of our approach to, and understanding of, what we hope is an ever-diminishing aspect of anesthesiology practice.

This book represents the work of many people in addition to the contributing authors. Most notable is the contribution of Fred Orkin, who edited the first edition and laid the groundwork for the second. Hope Olivo in our office edited, corrected, and managed every step along the way. We also extend our appreciation to Rich Lampert and Mary K. Smith, who encouraged, facilitated, cajoled, and *made* it happen. Finally, Galey, Liebe Tante, Niko, Kleiner Mann, Karling, Margie, and Robbie, thanks! Your patience and forbearance *let* it happen.

Nikolaus Gravenstein, MD
Robert R. Kirby, MD

Preface to the First Edition

Rarely are the services of the anesthesiologist an end in themselves. Rather, our principal effort is to enable another therapy, surgery, to be undertaken. This fact is so obvious that it is seldom even acknowledged, but because of it anesthesiology compels considerable attention. With an aging population and advances in surgical care and technology, we find ourselves treating increasingly sicker patients who are undergoing increasingly more complex procedures. It should not be forgotten that our anesthetic agents and adjuvants are among the most potent and rapidly acting drugs used in medicine. The anesthetics and technics that we have recourse to have the power to impair or abolish a variety of essential bodily functions, in addition to bearing potentially serious risks to the major organ systems. Thus, these medications and practices leave the patient open to the risk of anesthetic-related complications before the successful completion of surgery can be contemplated.

Complications noted after surgery and anesthesia may be categorized epidemiologically into those related to the surgical procedure, to the patient's medical condition, and to the anesthetic. Texts dealing with surgical complications abound. A number of excellent articles and books in the genre of medical management of the surgical patient have appeared in the past 5 years. Unfortunately, there has not been an equivalent comprehensive work covering anesthetic-related complications.

To fill this void, we, with acknowledged authorities, have put together a sourcebook of anesthetic-related complications that both the practitioner and academician should find helpful. Although it is often difficult to ascribe a given complication to anesthetic administration, as opposed to the surgical procedure, the patient's disease, or other factors, we have tried to include any topic that may be related to the anesthetic.

We have been fortunate to have enlisted the enthusiastic assistance of some five dozen colleagues from throughout North America who share our interest. Without their commitment, this book could not exist. Each has presented a specific complication or a set of related problems in his own way. Yet, each has written with three objectives in mind: to present a foundation of information accounting for the development of the complications; to provide the practicing anesthesiologist with guidance for the clinical management; and to set forth what is known about the prevention of the complications. Finally, each chapter includes an extensive reference list and suggestions for further reading.

In addition to our contributors, we are indebted to several persons whose efforts enabled publication of this volume: Lewis Reines, former Editor-in-Chief of Medical Books at J. B. Lippincott Company, launched this project; his successor, Stuart Freeman, spurred us to completion with unfailing vigor. Richard Winters, Lisa A. Biello, Kenneth Cotton, and Helen Ewan spared us much editorial detail. Joan Meranze, Librarian of the Dripps Memorial Library at the University of Pennsylvania, provided bibliographic assistance for a number of chapters. Drs. Harry Wollman and Henry Rosenberg provided advice. Lastly, we are grateful for the understanding and support of our families.

Novices in the practice of anesthesia encounter many complications. Experience enables them to recognize and treat complications and, later, to avoid them altogether. We hope that this sourcebook will aid all anesthesiologists in reaching the third and final stage sooner.

Fredrick K. Orkin, MD
Lee H. Cooperman, MD

Contents

Complications in Anesthesiology, second edition,
edited by Nikolaus Gravenstein and Robert R. Kirby.
Lippincott-Raven Publishers, Philadelphia © 1996.

CHAPTER 1

Risk Management, Quality Assurance, and Patient Safety

John H. Eichhorn

Risk management, quality assurance, and patient safety (RM/QA/PS) in anesthesia are receiving ever-increasing attention. Among the reasons are (1) the so-called "malpractice crisis" of the mid-1980s, which heightened awareness of these concerns among anesthesia practitioners; (2) the major emphasis on containment of the cost of medical care, which has caused thorough critical review of many traditionally accepted practices, with particular attention to outcome of care; and (3) the emphasis on the quality of medical care and, again, particularly on outcome, which has led to analysis of events at the most basic level in the medical care delivery system.

ADVERSE OUTCOMES

Incidence

Adverse outcome of anesthesia care spans a wide spectrum. The most severe untoward results are rivaled in effect only by those in obstetrics. In recent years, anesthesiologists accounted for about 3.5% of American physicians and correspondingly generate about 4% of the malpractice claims filed. These claims, however, represented about 11% of the total indemnity (dollars paid or set aside) for medical malpractice cases. While these statistics have improved recently, serious untoward results in anesthesia tend to have lasting and very expensive effects (death or permanent injury).

The incidence of anesthesia accidents has decreased[1] (particularly compared with that in other medical specialties), at least in terms of the frequency of malpractice claims if not in the severity of the accidents.[2] In some states and insurance companies, the "risk classification" for anesthesiologists has been reduced. However, major anesthesia accidents continue to occur, and malpractice premiums may again be showing a trend toward increases as of 1995.

Sources of Information

Exact current statistics are impossible to obtain because no central mechanism, organization, or agency compiles them. In the past, efforts to compile them were hampered because medical malpractice insurance companies almost always refused to reveal data (either statistical summaries or detailed case studies) about claims. In recent years, however, a number of investigators as well as the American Society of Anesthesiologists (ASA) Closed Claims studies, in collaboration with many malpractice insurers, have begun just such analyses, providing insight into the reasons why anesthesia providers are sued, the outcomes of the suits, and ways the outcomes might be improved.[3–10]

Hospital risk managers and involved anesthesiologists usually are reluctant to discuss untoward results of anesthesia care. Legal counsel often advises that no information about a questionable case be divulged, for fear that it could be misunderstood and provoke an actual or potential plaintiff. However, though lacking precise information, we do know that major anesthesia accidents continue to occur, as attested to by off-the-record discussions with anesthesia practitioners and their medical malpractice insurers and especially by the number of cases for which attorneys on both sides are seeking anesthesiologists as reviewers and expert witnesses.

Prevention

A comprehensive review of the causes of untoward outcome from anesthesia is beyond the scope of this chapter and is discussed elsewhere.[11–17] Prominent in these discussions is the issue of preventability. Debate focuses on the fraction of adverse incidents that might be prevented. An inescapable conclusion from study of the literature and from knowledge of current cases is that a significant majority of major anesthesia accidents are preventable.

QUALITY ASSURANCE IN ANESTHESIA CARE

Definitions of risk management, quality assurance, and patient safety as well as background information are provided in an "Addendum on Language" at the end of this chapter (Appendix I). Because of the complex interrelation of these three areas and their combined relevance to this chapter, the designation "RM/QA/PS" is used to refer to the broad effort toward the obvious but difficult-to-describe goal of the best possible anesthesia care.

Credentialing

Applications

The vast majority of medical practitioners are scrupulously honest. Unfortunately, rare exceptions occur. In documented cases, physicians, nurses, or even untrained lay people have forged credentials and lied on applications and in interviews and thus, inappropriately, obtained full medical licenses and privileges. In a few extraordinary instances patient injury has resulted. Such cases have received widespread, often sensational, publicity.

Probably less rarely, applicants for professional positions may have stretched the truth, either by exaggerating past status and experience or by omitting key details such as license suspensions or major malpractice judgments. Because of these individuals and their notoriety, the health care profession has tightened its credentialing procedures. To the vast majority, who are completely honest, the additional requirements for application may seem annoying and unwieldy. Transfer of certified copies of academic or training records from the distant past, for instance, is inconvenient and difficult. However, the honest majority must recognize that such efforts are directed at protecting patients and the integrity of the profession. The procedures are analogous to the use of the metal detectors and baggage screening at airports: the annoyance is tolerated in the interest of the safety of all concerned.

Reference Letters

Because of another type of legal problem, some examples of which have been highly publicized, medical practitioners may hesitate to give an honest evaluation (or any evaluation) of persons who are now seeking a professional position elsewhere. Of course, someone writing a reference letter for a current or former coworker should be honest. The subject of the reference should not object to inclusion of a fact that is in the public record (such as a malpractice case lost at trial); whether omission of such a fact is dishonest on the part of the letter writer is more debatable. Positive opinions and enthusiastic recommendation are no problem. Inclusion of facts that may be perceived as negative (such as a history of treatment for substance abuse) and negative opinions are what some writers fear will provoke retaliatory lawsuits, for libel or defamation of character, from the subject. As a result, some writers in these situations confine their letters to simple facts such as dates employed and position held.

Telephone Verification

Because an employer should not hesitate to state a positive opinion, receipt of a letter of reference that includes nothing more than dates worked and position held should suggest a potential problem. A telephone call to the writer is warranted in this instance and is advisable in all cases, independent of whatever information the letter contains. Frequently, pertinent questions over the telephone can elicit answers more candid than might otherwise be given. In rare instances, dishonesty by omission may occur even in conversation, particularly if the group or department wants to see a member leave.

This type of "sand-bagging" is, fortunately, infrequent. The best way to avoid it is to telephone an independent observer or source, perhaps a former employer or associate, when any question exists. Because the ultimate goal is optimal patient care, subjects applying for positions usually should not object to such calls. Discovery of a history of unsafe practices or of association with preventable anesthesia morbidity or mortality should prompt careful evaluation as to whether the applicant can be trained and supervised to be maximally safe in the proposed new environment.

Without exception, new personnel in an anesthesia practice environment must be given a thorough orientation and equipment check. Institutional policies, procedures, and equipment may be unfamiliar to even the most thoroughly trained, experienced, and safe practitioner. A crisis situation caused by unfamiliarity with a new setting is not the optimal method of orientation.

Granting of Privileges

Checklists are available for the granting of medical staff privileges by hospitals.[18,19] Verification of a valid license, medical school and residency training, board certification status, and previous disciplinary action is the responsibility of the hospital administration or medical staff executive department. Usually included, where applicable, is verification of previous hospital privileges and malpractice insurance. Even though the state licensing mechanism theoretically should detect any major discrepancies, the institution and representatives should verify these basic credentials. Court decisions in which the hospital was found negligent for failing to discover false statements on a negligent physician's application for privileges illustrate the key role in patient protection expected of the hospital.[19]

Renewal

Periodic renewal of privileges also involves an obligation to evaluate and verify the competence of the staff. Again, judicious checking of information on applications for renewal and of any relevant peer review activities is required. Groups of physicians or administrators responsible for evaluating the performance of hospital staff members and reviewing their privileges can be appropriately concerned about retaliatory legal action if a staff member is denied renewal.

Evaluating groups must be objective to eliminate any hint of political or financial motive and must be as close to certain as possible, with documentation, that the practice of the staff person whose privileges are being revoked is below standard and is a danger to patients. Believing this, groups within hospitals not only are justified in revoking privileges but also must do so or run the serious risk of being named codefendants in any subsequent malpractice action against the staff member in question. Court decisions demonstrate that the hospital can be found liable if the incompetence of a staff member was known or should have been known and was not addressed.[19] The ultimate ethical obligation, however difficult to carry out, is to protect the patients' best interests in such situations.

State Licensing

Specific requirements for medical licensing vary from state to state, but all states focus on education, postgraduate training, and personal qualifications. A widespread tendency recently is for more thorough verification of claimed credentials. As noted previously, inconvenience must be accepted as the cost of increased concern about the potential for harm from incompetent or dishonest practitioners.

Continuing Medical Education

A major involvement of state medical licensing authorities is in mandated continuing medical education (CME).[20] Many states specify the number of hours and distribution among categories of CME credits that must be obtained. Documented CME credits within one's declared specialty, as well as study of risk management and patient safety and of acquired immune deficiency syndrome and other blood-borne pathogens, may specifically be mandated.[21] The effectiveness of these programs, especially as they relate to objective indexes of patient care outcome, has yet to be thoroughly evaluated.

Disciplinary Action

Currently, the area of state involvement in RM/QA/PS issues receiving the most attention is discipline of incompetent, substance-dependent, and criminal physicians. Some states have reporting requirements specifying that any action taken against a practitioner (such as the restriction or suspension of privileges) by a group, department, or hospital be communicated to the state licensing or disciplining authority. In some circumstances, this requirement includes discovery of or treatment for substance dependency. State boards often believe that an independent investigation away from the subject's work place can yield the most objective evaluation of fitness to practice. The effectiveness of these efforts toward the laudable goal of reducing preventable patient morbidity is very difficult to evaluate. Partly in response to the general emphasis on quality of care and to public pressure, state authorities likely will continue to increase activity in this area.

Specialty Boards and Societies

Recertification

Of the recognized medical specialty boards, increasing numbers require periodic recertification of their diplomates. This number accounts for about half of the more than 350,000 certified medical specialists in the country. Many of the recertification programs are relatively recent (for instance, the American College of Surgery conducted its first examination in 1987), and some time will pass before any attempt can be made to assess their effect on the quality of care delivered or on patient care outcome. The American Board of Anesthesiology administered its first voluntary recertification examination in 1993. Of note is that although the recertification pass rate is very high, it is not 100%.

Continuing Medical Education

Several specialty societies require relevant CME participation.[20] Although the ASA offers a large number of CME activities (some directly concerning RM/QA/PS), there is no requirement for participation as a condition of membership.

Peer Review

One extremely valuable program available through many state societies of anesthesiology and, if necessary, through the ASA is peer review of an anesthesia group or department. When significant RM/QA/PS questions arise, a group or department may seek or be advised to seek external input and advice from an objective team of volunteer peer reviewers sponsored by the appropriate professional society. In such cases, the suggestions from the team, offered in a noncritical, nonthreatening manner, can help to initiate or enhance RM/QA/PS activities intended to maximize the quality of anesthesia care.

PEER REVIEW ORGANIZATIONS

Professional standards review organizations (PSRO) were established in 1972 as quality assurance overseers of the care of federally subsidized (Medicare and Medicaid) patients. Despite their efforts to address quality of care, these groups largely were seen as primarily interested in cost containment. A variety of negative factors led to the professional standards review organizations' replacement in 1984 with peer review organizations.[19]

Each state has a peer review organization (PRO), and most are associated with a state medical association. The objectives of the PRO are related to hospital admissions (including increased emphasis on outpatient care) and specifically to necessity, appropriateness, documentation, and quality of care (including reduction of avoidable deaths and postoperative or other complications). These organizations employ full-time support staff and pay physician reviewers as consultants or directors.

Goals

Ideally, PRO monitoring discovers suboptimal care and makes specific recommendations for improvement. However, a perception persists that quality-of-care efforts are hampered by a lack of realistic objectives and that the PROs, like other groups before them, function largely or entirely to limit the cost of health care services.[22]

Inpatient Admission for Outpatient Surgery

Aside from the as-yet-unrealized potential for quality improvement, the most likely interaction between an anesthesia provider and the local PRO involves a request for preoperative or postoperative admission of a patient whose care is scheduled to be outpatient surgery. This issue can involve RM/QA/PS. If the anesthesiologist believes, for example, that preoperative admission for treatment to optimize cardiac, pulmonary, diabetic, or other medical status will diminish anesthetic risk to the patient, an application to the PRO for approval of admission must be made and vigorously supported. Often, however, such issues are decided in a preanesthesia screening clinic or even in a preoperative holding area outside the operating room on the day of surgery.

This problem will continue to occur until anesthesiologists educate their constituent surgeons as to the types of associated medical conditions that may disqualify a proposed patient from the outpatient (ambulatory) surgical schedule. If adequate notice is given by the surgeon, such as at the time a case is booked for the operating room, the patient can be seen far enough in advance by an anesthesiologist to allow appropriate planning.

When the first awareness of a questionable case is 1 or 2 days before surgery, the anesthesiologist can try to have the procedure postponed, if possible and reasonable, or can undertake the time-consuming task of multiple telephone calls to get the surgeon's agreement, get PRO approval, and make the necessary arrangements. Because neither alternative is particularly attractive, the temptation may be strong to "let it slide" and to deal with the case on an outpatient basis, even though such an approach may be questionable from the RM/QA/PS viewpoint. Because anesthesia-related untoward outcome is very rare, the likelihood of an adverse result is small. Yet the patient will be exposed to an avoidable risk, and sooner or later in a long series of such circumstances, an unfavorable outcome or a probably preventable morbidity or mortality will occur.

The situation is even more difficult when the first contact with the patient in a questionable ambulatory case takes place immediately before surgery. Intense pressure often is initiated by the patient, the surgeon, and even the operating room staff to proceed with a case for which the anesthesiologist believes the patient is poorly prepared. The arguments made regarding patient inconvenience and anxiety are valid. However, they should not outweigh the patient's best medical interests. The anesthesiologist who faces this situation should state clearly to all concerned the reasons for postponing the surgery. The issue of avoidable risk must be stressed, and help with alternative arrangements, including if necessary dealing with the PRO, should be provided. Avoidance of such situations is enhanced by screening all outpatients before the day of surgery.

POLICIES, PROCEDURES, AND STANDARDS OF PRACTICE

Development of written policies and procedures often is perceived by medical practitioners as simply more bureaucratic drudgery. This task is much less likely to be so, however, for a practitioner who during an actual or impending emergency was able to turn to a detailed, carefully thought-out procedure manual and find the necessary information to deal with a problem or even prevent an untoward outcome. The Joint Commission on Accreditation of Healthcare Organizations (JCAHO) does require a policy and procedure manual for anesthesia services within a hospital.[23] This requirement, however, should not be the sole driving force behind this potentially very useful compendium.

Policy and Procedure Manuals

The major purpose of a written manual in any environment where anesthesia services are provided is to provide an instantly available source of suggestions, guidelines, recommendations, and standards for professional conduct. Necessary caveats state that specific circumstances differ and that the involved practitioners will apply their judgment at any given time along with the outlines provided in the manual.

An initial benefit of creating or updating a policy and procedure manual is that it forces those doing so to think about the topics being covered. Numerous examples are possible, but all anesthesiologists probably are aware of at least one instance in which some long-standing routine in a hospital ("that's the way we've always done it") has finally been reviewed as a manual is being updated for an impending JCAHO visit. The routine is found sadly out of date, possibly inappropriate, and potentially dangerous. After the routine is changed, all involved note the improvement and state that the old way was "an accident waiting to happen." Such reviews should be performed whenever needed but should be done annually and then particularly thoroughly every 3 years.

Organizational Component

PRIVILEGES AND RESPONSIBILITIES. Included is the delineation of privileges, responsibilities, and expectations for all involved personnel: the chief or director of anesthesia or the clinical director; deputy or division directors if any; attending staff physicians; resident and fellow physicians; other trainees; certified registered nurse anesthetists; physician assistants; monitoring technicians; equipment engineers and technicians; perfusionists, respiratory therapists, and chest therapists; and any others. Accompanying this list should be a communications section with verified addresses and telephone and pager numbers and details of how to reach all personnel. The intent is to minimize difficulty when help is being sought.

CALL RESPONSIBILITIES. Critically important is the delineation of call responsibilities (not a call schedule): a detailed list of what is expected of a staff member when on call, with regard to hours required at the institution, telephone availability, pager availability, and maximum permissible distance from the institution. Included also are expectations of each level of call; for instance, the "third-call" staff member covers obstetrics within the hospital from 3 p.m. until 8 a.m. unless he or she is allowed to take telephone calls at home from the "second-call" anesthesiologist staying in the hospital. All such duties must be spelled out clearly and prospectively. Unfortunately, this organization often becomes a key element in the aftermath of an accident in which, it is charged, the appropriate personnel were not available or could not be found.

ORIENTATION OF NEW PERSONNEL. The manual should include a clear explanation of orientation and check-out procedure for new personnel; CME requirements and opportunities; the mechanisms of evaluation of personnel and communication of the evaluation to them; disaster plans (or reference to a separate disaster manual or protocol); quality assurance activities of the department, including membership of any standing committees responsible; and the format for statistical record-keeping (including number of procedures, types of anesthetics given, characteristics of patients anesthetized, number and types of invasive monitoring techniques, and number of responses to emergency calls).

Procedural Component

The procedural component outlines specific courses of action for particular circumstances. Frequently, reference is made to the guidelines and standards appearing in the back of the ASA Directory of Members, which is published each year.[24] Also included are the standards mentioned in the JCAHO manual[23]: preanesthetic evaluation; immediate preinduction reevaluation; safety of the patient during anesthesia; recording of all pertinent events during anesthesia; release of the patient from the postanesthesia care unit; recording of postanesthesia visits; definition of the role of anesthesia services in hospital infection control; and safe use of general anesthetic agents. A partial list of other appropriate topics is provided in Table 1-1.

TABLE 1-1
Additional Procedural Topics for the Anesthesiology Policy and Procedure Manual

- Recommendation for preanesthesia apparatus check-out, such as from the Food and Drug Administration
- Guidelines for minimal monitoring: infant, child, and adult; in recovery room
- Procedure for transport of patients: to operating room, to postanesthesia care unit, and to ICU
- Policy on ambulatory surgical patients: screening, use of regional anesthesia, and discharge home
- Policy on same-day admissions
- Policy on recovery room admission and discharge
- Policy on ICU admission and discharge
- Policy on physicians responsible for writing orders in recovery room and ICU
- Policy on informed consent
- Policy on the participation of patients in clinical research
- Guidelines for the support of cadaver organ donors and its termination
- Guidelines on environmental safety, including pollution with trace gases and inspection, maintenance, and hazard prevention for electrical equipment
- Procedure for exchanging personnel during an anesthetic
- Procedure for the introduction of new equipment, drugs, or clinical practices
- Procedure for epidural and spinal narcotic administration and subsequent patient monitoring
- Procedure for initial treatment of cardiac or respiratory arrest
- Policy on a patient's refusal of blood or blood products, including the mechanism to obtain a court order to treat
- Procedure for the management of malignant hyperthermia (MH)
- Procedure for the induction and maintenance of barbiturate coma
- Procedure for anesthesia for electroconvulsive therapy
- Procedure for evaluation of possible pseudocholinesterase deficiency

ICU, intensive care unit.

Individual departments or groups can add to these suggestions as dictated by their specific needs. The importance of a thorough, carefully conceived policy and procedure manual to RM/QA/PS is clear. Many of the components are intended to mandate or encourage practices that will prevent untoward events, such as unfamiliarity with a new anesthesia machine when one is called "stat" for an emergency case; help in the management of crisis, such as malignant hyperthermia; and facilitate communication in difficult situations, such as the refusal of blood products. Ideally, each staff member of a group or department should review the manual at least annually and sign off in a log indicating current familiarity.

Standards of Practice

Many elements of policy and procedure could be labeled "standards" and are in some institutions.[17] Others have avoided the term "standards" because of the potential medicolegal implications, especially if an untoward outcome occurs when practice is carried out in a manner other than that published. The medicolegal importance of the term "standard of care" tends to reinforce the perception that once promulgated, standards dictate mandatory practice. Accordingly, individual groups or departments may or may not choose to label components of their policy and procedure as standards. An alternative is to label descriptions of certain policies or procedures as "guidelines." Guidelines serve to identify a responsible option rather than dictate an approach, as do standards.

Monitoring

After retrospective study suggested that better patient monitoring would have prevented several major anesthesia accidents, the Harvard Medical School developed "Standards of Practice" for minimal intraoperative monitoring for its nine component hospital departments[25] and called them "standards" specifically to emphasize that the practices are important enough to be mandatory.

The same type of thinking was involved when the ASA, in

October 1986, adopted as national policy "Standards for Basic Anesthetic Monitoring," which included standards for the presence of personnel during an anesthetic and for continual evaluation of oxygenation, ventilation, circulation, and temperature. The original standards have since been updated and amended, most recently on October 13, 1993 (Appendix II).[26]

The minimal monitoring standards are "process" standards in that they prescribe actions and are met by carrying out these actions. At various levels (hospital, local, state, and national), additional efforts at improving patient safety likely will lead to promulgation of other standards intended to be mandatory. Of note is that an occasional deviation from many of the written standards is anticipated in their description and thus does not necessarily represent a violation, as long as the reasons for the deviation are explained in the patient's chart or on the anesthesia record.[26]

Outcome

The other type of standard pertains to outcome. Outcome standards might state, for example, that "the number of patients experiencing myocardial infarction intraoperatively or within 24 h of operation should not exceed 0.5% of those anesthetized" or "the number of ambulatory surgical patients experiencing unplanned admission to the hospital for reasons related to the anesthesia should not exceed 1.0% of those anesthetized."

Continuous Quality Improvement

During the 1980s the JCAHO focused on quality assurance theory, particularly structure, process, and outcome. However, beginning in 1992 major effort encouraged the application of continuous quality improvement (CQI) as a part of the "Agenda for Change."[27] Of perhaps major importance is a decrease in the total number of the standards and transfer of some of the anesthesia standards to the medical staff and quality assurance sections of the current Accreditation Manual for Hospitals.[23]

EQUIPMENT

Failure

Compared with human error, overt equipment failure is relatively rare as a cause of critical incidents during anesthesia[11] or anesthesia-associated deaths.[28] Anesthesia apparatus problems have been well studied.[29] The large majority of equipment-related problems, aside from clear human error such as misuse or unfamiliarity, probably can be prevented by correct maintenance and servicing.

When a major equipment failure occurs that, if undetected, would lead to patient harm, the monitoring guidelines outlined in the preceding section should detect development of an untoward situation. Assuming an appropriate response from the anesthesiologist (which may even mean detaching the anesthesia delivery system and ventilator from the patient and ventilating with a hand resuscitator bag until a new anesthesia machine can be secured), no adverse event should result. Because occasional damage to a patient does result from equipment failure, efforts to minimize such failures must continue.

Maintenance and Service

An excellent published summary of a complete program for anesthesia equipment maintenance and service is available.[30] A distinction is made between failure due to progressive deterioration of equipment, which should be preventable because it is observable and prompts appropriate action, and catastrophic failure, which often is not predictable.

Emphasis is placed on preventive maintenance for mechanical parts and involves performance checks every 4 to 6 months. A detailed example for the handling of an oxygen monitor is provided. Also, an annual safety inspection of each anesthetizing location covers 49 points and includes the surrounding area and the immediate location as well as the equipment itself. For equipment service, a description of a cross-reference system to identify the piece needing service and the mechanism to secure the needed repair is provided.

Handling and Purchase

The general principles of equipment purchase and handling are straightforward.[31] Before purchase, it should be verified that the proposed piece of equipment meets all applicable standards (as usually it does if produced by a recognized major manufacturer). On arrival, electrical equipment must be checked for absence of hazard and for compliance with applicable electrical standards. Complex equipment such as anesthesia machines and ventilators should be assembled and checked by a representative from the manufacturer or manufacturer's agent. Mishaps leading to potential adverse medicolegal implications may occur when relatively untrained personnel certify a particular piece of equipment as functioning within specification. The manufacturer's representative, if necessary, should be involved in preservice and inservice training for those who will use the new equipment.

In addition, a sheet or section in the master equipment log must be created with the make, model, serial number, and in-house identification for each new piece of equipment. This procedure not only allows immediate identification of any equipment involved in a future recall or product alert, but also serves as a permanent record of every problem, problem resolution, maintenance, and servicing until that particular piece is discarded. This log must be kept up to date at all times. Rare but frightening examples of potentially lethal problems with anesthesia machines have led to product-alert notices requiring immediate identification of certain equipment and its service status.

Service Personnel

The question of who should maintain and service anesthesia equipment has been widely debated. After the initial setup and check-out some groups or departments rely on "factory" service representatives for all attention to equipment, whereas others engage independent service contractors. Still others (usually large departments) have access to engineers or technicians in their institution, their department, or a separate bioengineering or medical engineering department within the facility.

Needs and resources differ. The single underlying tenet is simple: the person providing preventive maintenance and service must be qualified. Anesthesia practitioners may wonder how they can assess qualifications. The best way is to ask, unhesitatingly, pertinent questions about the education, training, and experience of those involved and to request references and speak to supervisors and managers responsible for those doing the work. Whether an engineering technician who spent a week at a course at a factory can perform the most complex repairs depends on a variety of factors that can be investigated by the practitioners ultimately using the equipment.

Day-to-day Maintenance

Aside from preventive maintenance and servicing, adequate day-to-day clinical maintenance of equipment must be available. In this era of great emphasis on cost containment, it seems anesthesia technicians are a popular target for budget cutters. Reduction of these personnel to below the number genuinely needed to retrieve, clean, sort, disassemble, sterilize, reassemble, store, and distribute the equipment and supplies used in daily anesthesia practice represents false economy. Inadequate service in this area truly creates "an accident waiting to happen." An improperly installed canister of carbon dioxide absorbent is only one example of the numerous sources of potential danger from inadequate technical support.

Replacement of Obsolete Equipment

The period after which anesthesia equipment becomes obsolete and should be replaced is another question difficult to answer. Replacement of obsolete anesthesia machines and monitoring equipment is a key element of risk-modification programs.[16] Ten years is cited as an estimated useful life for an anesthesia machine: anesthesia machines currently more than 10 years old often do not meet the safety standards now in force for new machines and do not incorporate the new technology that has advanced very rapidly during the 1980s and 1990s. Yet the practice of arbitrary replacement based on age alone has been challenged.[30,32]

Procedure in Case of Failure

Last, should equipment fail, it must be removed from service and a replacement substituted. Groups or departments are obligated to have sufficient backup equipment to cover any reasonable incidence of failure. The equipment removed from service must be marked with a prominent label (so that it is not returned to service by a well-meaning technician or practitioner). The label should include the date, time, name of the person discovering the problem, and details of the problem.

Responsible personnel must be notified so that they can remove the equipment, make an entry in the log, and initiate the repair. In the event that a piece of equipment is involved or suspected in an anesthesia accident, it must be immediately sequestered and not touched by anybody, particularly not by service personnel. If a severe accident occurs, the equipment in question should be inspected jointly at a later time by a group consisting of qualified representatives of the manufacturer, the service personnel, the insurance companies involved, and the plaintiff and defense attorneys if litigation is in progress. When accident, injury, or death occurs it must be reported to the Food and Drug Administration.[33]

INFORMED CONSENT

General Considerations

The patient has the right to exercise control over his or her own body, and therefore the patient's consent to proposed treatments or procedures must be sought.[18] The absence of any consent (for whatever reason but usually gross misunderstanding) may result in claims for assault and battery. This event is relatively rare and much less likely to involve the provision of anesthesia than the issue of informed consent. Informed consent is obtained by discussing the potential risks and benefits of a proposed treatment or procedure and any available alternatives and ascertaining that the patient (or the patient's agent in the cases of a child or an incompetent person) agrees to what is being proposed.

Whether a separate informed consent is necessary for the anesthetic for a planned operation is unclear: many argue that consent for the operation implies consent for anesthesia. Nevertheless, most anesthesia providers obtain separate informed consent because of the "material risks" associated with the anesthetic, independent of surgery. To expect that the surgeon will fully discuss anesthesia and, particularly, any special considerations pertaining to the use of anesthesia given the patient's medical condition is unrealistic.

Disclosure

In seeking informed consent for anesthesia, what should be disclosed to the patient during the discussion? Enough information must be given to allow a reasoned decision; frightening the patient with a long list of potential severe, but extremely rare, complications—thus making a trusting, friendly doctor–patient relationship very difficult—is counterproductive. In times past, the policy seemed to be that disclosure should include the risks that any "reasonable physician" would think appropriate. This doctrine has been altered over time to involve the "reasonable person" (patient) and now centers on the concept of "material risk."

Material Risk

A material risk "is one which the physician knows or ought to know would be significant to a reasonable person in the patient's position of deciding whether or not to submit to a particular medical treatment or procedure."[18] The landmark Harnish decision[34] stated that all material risks must be disclosed to the patient to obtain informed consent. An equally important subsequent decision added the qualification that disclosure of every conceivable, remotely possible complication the incidence of which is "negligible" need not be made.[35] The latter decision stressed balancing the patient's right to know with fairness to physicians to avoid "unrealistic and unnecessary burdens on practitioners."

BRAIN DAMAGE OR DEATH. When the issue of informed consent for anesthesia arises, it usually involves the occurrence of a rare, devastating complication, such as severe neurologic damage or death. Whether the risk of these complications is "negligible" in a legal context remains to be determined. Therefore, no firm guideline can be advanced as to whether all patients should be told that general anesthesia might lead to anoxic brain damage or death or that regional anesthesia could cause permanent paralysis.

All anesthesia procedures carry some risks, including injury and death, just as riding in a car or crossing the street involves risk. The majority of patients can identify with this analogy and are not threatened by it. Questions as to specific complications prompted by this statement, of course, should be answered. Statistics can be cited to give perspective. Any special risks attendant to the patient's medical or surgical condition should be discussed in more detail.

Liability

Many anesthesia practitioners ask patients to sign a consent form that has on it a long list of potential complications and any specific additional risks for that patient. Both the practitioner and the patient must understand that no matter what the form says, it does not release the anesthesiologist from liability. The form is one way to document that an informed consent discussion took place, but it does not limit the patient's right to make a claim later in the event of an accident. Whether or not the form is used, a note should be written in the patient's chart stating that a discussion took place and that informed consent was obtained. Verbal consent alone is not enough when a later question arises.

In certain life-threatening, emergency circumstances, anesthesia may have to be administered without consent. Case law recognizes this situation, and consent requirements necessarily are modified. In such an event, a note should be written in the chart as soon as possible about the necessity to proceed, and hospital legal counsel should be notified.

RECORD-KEEPING

Indications

The number of malpractice cases involving anesthesia providers that have been lost because of inadequate, incomplete, or illegible anesthesia records is unknown. The anesthesia chart is the cornerstone of all information about an anesthetic case, both for risk management and quality assurance purposes. The old dictum "if you didn't write it down, it didn't happen" is still used in the medicolegal sense. Even the very best anesthetic care cannot be defended, or even referenced, if no clear record shows that such care took place. "If the record hardly exists, . . . it is tantamount to an outright confession, in the eyes of the law, to careless practice."[34]

Content

A helpful review of the reasoning behind and the elements of the anesthesia record[36] cites a 1976 study in which 95% of respondent anesthetists thought it important to keep anesthetic records and 74% included medicolegal concerns among the reasons for doing so. An excellent approach to the record is to try to (1) create a legible record of "all pertinent events" as required by the JCAHO[23] and description of the anesthetic procedure and (2) have a compendium of all salient features (history, allergies, chronic medications, acute medications, positioning, monitoring used, reasons for special monitoring, events, and the patient's responses).

These items should be as complete as the practitioner would like to see them if he or she (1) were to be the next person to provide anesthesia care for the patient or (2) were asked to defend the care in the event of a complication. The majority of facilities in which anesthesia is given have a preprinted form that allows accomplishment of these goals. The form should be as easy as possible to use, should encourage completeness, and should be reviewed frequently by those using it to see if it can be improved.

Basic Requirements

Medications and vital signs should be recorded together and should be recorded first, when many events must be recorded, such as the period immediately after induction. Descriptive information, important as it is, can wait a moment. Should an adverse event occur, with or even without patient injury, a complete account of facts and, when appropriate, impressions and opinions should be entered into the chart as soon as possible. One important caution, however, is that the entry made must not be influenced by the heat of the moment, by guilt, by the desire to imply blame or innocence on the part of any individual, or by the general disorganization that may accompany a significant event. The advice of an objective person, perhaps a coworker not involved in the case, should be sought while an account of the event is recorded.

The single most important admonition in all such cases is never to change the existing record.[37] No matter what is on it, the actual record is better than an altered one. However excellent the anesthetic care may have been, alteration of the record almost guarantees inability to defend against any charges, however unjustified they might be.[38] If explanation, elaboration, or filling in of gaps is necessary, do so as soon as practical with a dated and timed amendment note in the chart.

Additional benefits in quality assurance efforts accrue from complete and legible anesthetic records. Certain necessary and desirable activities described subsequently depend on the ability to retrieve and compile data about the anesthetic practice of a group or department. In summary, all components of RM/QA/PS are aided by good anesthetic record-keeping.

Automated Records

Electronic, computer-assisted, or computer-driven devices are now available to maintain intraoperative anesthesia records.[39] Noninvasive or invasive monitors may be connected to these computers so that vital signs, delivered oxygen and expired volume, oxygen saturation, and end-tidal carbon dioxide tension are automatically recorded (with no possibility to edit) at preset intervals. Entries as to gas flow, agents used, drugs and fluids given, blood lost, and events noted can be keyed in by the anesthesiologist. Alternatives such as light-pen or voice entry of data may be options available in the future. The instrument automatically records the time of the entry, even if its operator states in the entry that an event or action took place at some previous time.

Large-scale studies on the efficacy or desirability of these automated records are unavailable. Proponents state that the technology allows more time to focus on the patient's care and that a genuinely complete record of data such as vital signs gives a truer picture of events and trends and thus aids in evaluation of poor outcome, usually by demonstrating the absence of untoward intraoperative events. Detractors state that automatic sampling may miss trends by picking up and recording transient major variations and even may record erroneous or grossly incorrect values caused by mechanical or electrical artifact, thus exposing the anesthesiologist to unjustified charges later in the event of a poor outcome. Acceptance of this technology will depend on the resolution of ease-of-use issues, the cost of implementation, and the perceived risk-to-benefit ratio.

QUALITY REVIEW, REPORTING OF CRITICAL EVENTS, AND GENERIC SCREENING

Mechanisms of Review

A designated committee or person within an organized anesthesia service or department should be responsible for quality assurance and CQI. Solo practitioners can be just as aware of the quality assurance principles and apply them, perhaps less formally, to their practice. The quality assurance appointees periodically should review the state of the anesthesia organization along the lines described in this chapter. Are the licenses, privileges, and CME status of all anesthetists current? Are the departmental policy, procedures, and standards up to date? Is a well-functioning mechanism for equipment acquisition, tracking, maintenance, and repair in place? Are consents and records appropriate? Are meaningful case discussions presented within the group? Is the opportunity for CME adequate and appropriate? Once these key elements have been confirmed, the committee can turn to its other functions.

Problem Definition

Quality assurance includes looking for problems.[40] Because debate may center on what constitutes a problem, criteria for expected outcomes need to be established, usually by the committee with input from the remainder of the department. Many of the criteria may be difficult to articulate. The acceptable frequency for many adverse patient outcomes is not universally agreed upon, and thus national standards are lacking.[41] However, problems frequently can be identified in a straightforward manner (Table 1-2).

TABLE 1-2
Criteria for Assessment of Untoward Events

UNAVOIDABLE EVENTS

A. Preexisting disease that
   1. Makes event(s) inevitable (eg, caries associated with chipped tooth; cardiac arrest in unstable ASA physical status 5 patient; uncontrolled hypertension requiring emergency operation during which hypertension occurs; or hypoxemia after chest contusion)
   2. Was adequately treated preoperatively but nevertheless presents intraoperative problems (eg, asthma that was well controlled with bronchodilators)
   3. Despite good control intraoperatively, develops a problem from causes that cannot be explained by failure of anesthetic management (eg, MI in a patient who was well monitored and otherwise stable, MH in a patient with no historical indicators of MH)

B. Conditions that develop as a result of the operative procedure and that could not have been anticipated or ameliorated by the anesthetic management (eg, properly checked but mismatched blood; improperly sterilized devices; or failure of equipment despite proper maintenance and pre-use checkout)

AVOIDABLE EVENTS

Events that could have been avoided or significantly ameliorated by pre-, intra-, or postoperative anesthetic management, whether or not these events were caused directly by the anesthesiologist (eg, failure to replace blood loss)

APPROPRIATE TREATMENT

Treatment within the standards of practice that would be expected of a typical anesthesiologist trained in an approved residency training program

INAPPROPRIATE TREATMENT

Treatment that does not meet current standards of practice where time and logistical constraints did not prevent meeting the standards of practice

Cohen JA: Quality assurance and risk management. In Gravenstein N (ed): Manual of complications during anesthesia. Philadelphia: JB Lippincott, 1991: 26.

Individual overt accidents, of course, are reviewed. Trends over large numbers of cases may be clear. For example, a perioperative myocardial infarction rate of 20% in patients receiving spinal anesthesia for transurethral resection of the prostate exceeds reasonable expectation for this complication. Input from the reporting of critical events, postanesthesia visit records, anesthesia morbidity and mortality rounds, the urology service, and the personal knowledge of the committee members should rapidly reveal such a situation. Another approach is to compare the frequency of an adverse event from one year to the next. This method will show a trend, if present, but will not define acceptable limits for frequency of occurrence.

Problem Assessment and Resolution

Once a problem is identified, it must be assessed: for instance, are the myocardial infarctions occurring intra- or postoperatively, and why, in either case? Problem resolution and CQI require change, such as significantly greater attention to prehydration and rapid treatment of incipient hypotension, perhaps even prophylactically, or closer and longer observation in a postanesthesia care unit. Follow-up involves verification that the resolution was effective and that the problem does not recur. This process can be effectively accomplished, in the example of myocardial infarction, for instance, by a concurrent monitoring program (discussed below).

Identification of Potential Problems

Possibly even more important, the quality assurance mechanism can identify potential problems before complications occur. Committee-initiated audits in which care is examined for specific indicators and criteria may reveal habits or recurrent situations (such as the failure to use minimal basic monitoring for a certain type of case) that have the potential to lead to avoidable complications.[17,40,41] The same mechanism of assessment, resolution, and follow-up can then be used in a preventive manner, with the aim of avoiding as-yet unrealized morbidity or mortality.

Reporting of Critical Events

Purposes

Overt accidents in anesthesia should always be examined and discussed. As noted, these accidents are relatively rare. "Near misses" and "near accidents" probably occur much more frequently.[11,42] These near misses have also been termed "critical events," "critical incidents," "impact events," and anesthetic "occurrences." Frequently in the past, such events have been unrecorded, never studied, and almost never discussed.

Practitioners naturally are reluctant to admit, whether a mistake was involved or not, that they came close to an accident. Perhaps this attitude is a carry-over of the "no harm, no foul" mentality from basketball: no "real" event or damage occurred, so why report it? The obvious answer is the potential to reduce the occurrence of similar events in the future. Classic studies of critical incidents spotlighted breathing-circuit disconnection as the most common near miss.[42] Not only did this emphasis significantly enhance anesthesiologists' awareness of this frequent problem, but it also led to modifications of designs and practices to reduce its likelihood.

Prevention

The same principle can apply within an anesthesia department or group. Reporting of critical events to the quality assurance committee can lead to early intervention in problems regarding equipment, routine, case mix, environment, or personnel. Of 38 "critical incidents" associated with relief of one anesthesiologist by another, 28 reflected existing adverse conditions, and 10 were created by the reliever.[43] Appropriate steps to heighten awareness of this vulnerable interval were taken.

Cooperation must exist between the anesthesiologists and the committee. If hesitation occurs for fear of embarrassment or recrimination, reports can be made anonymously. Anonymity, however, eliminates an element of quality assurance—identification of involved personnel, who might be evaluated and possibly directly influenced. However, an anonymous program is better than none at all.

Concurrent Monitoring

Looking through each patient's medical record for a specific, well-defined process, outcome, or event reflects concurrent monitoring (generic or "occurrence" screening).[40,41] In an example of interest to anesthesia providers, the chart of a patient who had both a surgical procedure and a myocardial infarction may be flagged for review and determination of the time and probable cause of the myocardial infarction. The result from this continual (not selective) examination of every discharged patient's chart can be an excellent source of problem identification for the quality assurance committee. Large, hospital-wide screening programs have been proposed. Ongoing review on this scale is typically a function of a full-time administrator or risk manager rather than a function of a specific clinical department, service, or group.

Concurrent monitoring of the office copy of the anesthesia chart from every case can be practical if the involved staff members are interested and cooperative. This is a major undertaking and must be thought out carefully in advance. Detailed outlines of criteria and indicators that can be screened and methods for carrying out the process are available.[17] Areas of interest include equipment malfunction, drug-associated problems, airway or ventilation incidents, fluid or circulation incidents, and neurologic problems. Within these and other areas, more specific complications may be listed.

The results of such a screen provide clear guidance to a quality assurance or CQI committee as to the aspects of the department's or group's anesthetic practice that need to be fine-tuned; appropriate action, including continuing education, should ensue. Evidence of the beneficial results of the intervention should be expected in subsequent summaries from the concurrent monitoring process. Alternatively, a special screen can be constructed to evaluate the target issue. Absence of improvement in either case should start the cycle again and lead to remedial efforts.

CONFERENCES AND CONTINUING EDUCATION

Format

Most anesthesia departments, services, and groups have staff meetings or departmental conferences or rounds at least monthly. Presentation of cases of unusual interest, or in which a problem occurred, followed by a thorough group review and discussion of the popular question, "What would you do differently next time?" is a reasonable avenue to pursue. Likewise, staff meetings at which policy, procedure, equipment, and any associated problems are discussed are useful. Inclusion of an open review of departmental statistics, including all complications, however trivial, with thorough presentation and discussion of quality assurance activities such as audits, reviews, screens, and the resultant recommendations for action round out an ideal, by JCAHO standards, meeting.

Purpose

Requirements aside, all of the suggestions for meetings (whether called "case conferences," "case presentations," or "morbidity and mortality rounds") are intended to encourage anesthesiologists to combine their thoughts and efforts for the common good: minimization of untoward outcome in their anesthesia practice. Pro forma meetings hurried through by a small fraction of the staff benefit no one and waste time. A meaningful case presentation needs interactive discussion.

Continuing Medical Education

Formal CME needs the same thoughtfulness to be worthwhile. Larger groups and departments usually run their own programs, at which staff members speak about areas of their interest and expertise. They also bring in outside speakers to present reviews of basic material, news of recent developments, or ongoing research. By no means should all of the presentations deal directly with anesthesia—a format that would become tedious for even the most committed audience. Awareness of current critical topics such as the acquired immune deficiency syndrome is equally important and in many states is mandated for licensing.

Smaller departments or groups need to make deliberate efforts to ensure adequate opportunity for continuing education. Access to an accredited CME program conducted by a large hospital or medical school department with guaranteed time for the staff to participate is one approach. Another method involves providing time, and in some circumstances, financial support for staff to attend local, regional, or national CME programs: specific workshops, symposia, and theme meetings or the CME components of professional society meetings. Most CME requirements for licensing or certification include some acknowledgment of individual reading. Every department, service, or group, regardless of size, needs a library containing as many textbooks, manuals, and journals as is practical.

RESPONSE TO AN ANESTHESIA ACCIDENT

Despite rigorous application of all of the RM/QA/PS and CQI principles outlined, every anesthesiologist probably will be involved in at least one major anesthesia accident. Precisely because such an event is so rare, few practitioners are prepared for it. The involved personnel often have no relevant past experience regarding what to do and, perhaps as importantly, what not to do.[44] Fortunately, a thoughtful, comprehensive, and very valuable guideline exists that every anesthesia provider should be familiar with.[44]

The appropriate immediate response to an accident is straightforward and logical. However, the personnel involved in a significant untoward event may react with such surprise or shock that logic is in short supply. Major accidents have occurred in which the responsible anesthesiologist was so stunned on realizing what had happened that he or she was unable to respond or, worse, left the room before help arrived.

Call for Help

At the moment anyone recognizes that a major anesthetic complication has occurred or is occurring, a sufficient number of people to deal with the situation must be secured as quickly as possible. For example, in the event an esophageal intubation goes unrecognized long enough during the induction of general anesthesia to cause a cardiac arrest, the immediate need is for enough skilled personnel to conduct the resuscitative efforts (including making the correct diagnosis and replacing the tube into the trachea).

Whether the person apparently responsible for the complication should direct the immediate remedial efforts depends on the person and the situation. In such a circumstance, a senior or supervising anesthesiologist should quickly evaluate the appropriateness of the behavior and actions of those involved. A decision can then be made as to who should be in charge. Even in the heat of the moment, tact must be exercised.

Recognition of an evolving or impending major complication followed by failure to call for help is foolish and not in the patient's best interest. However strong the feelings of pride and fear, they could impair judgment and so must be put aside. Delay in "fixing" a problem so that no one will know could turn an embarrassing but remediable situation into one that is more serious or even fatal.

Evaluation and Care

Immediately after a nonfatal accident, comprehensive evaluation and care of the patient should be carried out quickly and efficiently. Consultants should be called without hesitation. Often a cardiologist, neurologist, neurosurgeon, or nephrologist can offer constructive suggestions that might improve the prognosis. When such requests are delayed and the consultant is later forced to state, "You might have had a better chance to save the patient if only you had acted immediately after the incident, 4 days ago," this point becomes clear.

Damage Control

Once comprehensive care is underway, notify the facility administrator, risk manager, or both.[38] This person may in turn choose to notify the facility's malpractice insurance carrier. The anesthesiologist's insurer also should be called. The risk manager and the insurers may become involved after their first contact with the family. If a surgeon of record is involved, he or she probably will first notify the family, but the anesthesiologist and others (risk manager, insurance loss-control officer, or even legal counsel) might appropriately be included at the outset.

Full disclosure of facts as they are best known, with no confessions, opinions, speculation, or placing of blame, is the best approach throughout all interaction with the family and, when possible, the patient. Any attempt to conceal, withhold, or shade the truth will only confound an already difficult situation. Obviously, comfort and support should be offered, including, if appropriate, the services of facility personnel such as clergy, social workers, and counselors. All discussions with the patient or family should be carefully documented in the chart.

INDIVIDUAL PRACTICE

The RM/QA/PS area in anesthesia is large and somewhat diffuse; in addition, the field has suffered from an unappealing image. However, awareness and interest are increasing. The

TABLE 1-3
Harvard Data on Adverse Outcomes

DATES	ASA PHYSICAL STATUS 1 AND 2 PATIENTS	INTRAOPERATIVE ACCIDENTS	ASSOCIATED DEATHS
January 1976 to June 1985	757, 000	10 (1/75,700)	5 (1/151,400)
July 1985 to June 1990 (Standards July 1985)[25]	392,000	1 (1/392,000)	0 (0)
		$p = .08$	$p = .12$

Eichhorn JH: Risk reduction in anesthesia. In Duncan PG (ed): Anesthetic risk and complications. Problems in Anesthesia 6:278–294, 1992.

founding of the Anesthesia Patient Safety Foundation in 1986 was greeted with enthusiasm. This event likely would not have happened only a few years previously. Still, anesthesiologists often ask, "I am only one person; what can I do?" The answer is multifaceted.

Anesthesiologists in individual practice can strive to make their work as safe as humanly possible. They should stay current in their knowledge and practices without embracing potentially dangerous fads. They should incorporate formally issued policies, procedures, and standards into their practice; consider risk–benefit ratios for all actions; be scrupulous about consent; keep clear and complete records; and generally try to have a good time in their work.

Specific Efforts

As a Member of a Department or Group

Anesthesiologists can and should be involved in influencing policy (including credentialing), procedures, and standards in their practice environment. Closely allied is cooperation with and genuine support of quality assurance and CQI activities as well as encouragement of and participation in departmental conferences, rounds, and meetings.

As a Member of Professional Organizations

Organized groups and, particularly, professional societies influence general policy, procedure recommendations, and standards. Members often grumble about the finished products and claim that a "select few" prescribe for the large group. Usually the select few are the only ones interested enough to make the effort to speak out. Anesthesiologists can and should get involved and should not hesitate to make their opinions known, loud and clear.

General Efforts

Outcome in anesthesia practice is improving,[45] as is evident from the updated Harvard data on adverse outcomes (Table 1-3). Continued application of the outlined principles will further the effort to eliminate preventable anesthesia-related morbidity and mortality and to minimize adverse anesthesia outcome for patient and provider alike.[46]

REFERENCES

1. Unpublished data. Boston: The Risk Management Foundation of the Harvard Medical Institutions, 1991
2. Wood M: Anesthesia claims decrease. Anesthesia Patient Safety Foundation Newsletter 1:21, 1986
3. Caplan RA, Ward RJ, Posner K, et al: Unexpected cardiac arrest during spinal anesthesia: a closed claims analysis of predisposing factors. Anesthesiology 68:5, 1988
4. Tinker JH, Dull DL, Caplan RA, et al: Role of monitoring devices in prevention of anesthetic mishaps: a closed claims analysis. Anesthesiology 71:535, 1989
5. Caplan RA, Posner KL, Ward RJ, et al: Adverse respiratory events in anesthesia: a closed claims analysis. Anesthesiology 72:828, 1990
6. Kroll DA, Caplan RA, Posner K, et al: Nerve injury associated with anesthesia. Anesthesiology 73:202, 1990
7. Cheney FW, Posner KL, Caplan RA: Low incidence adverse respiratory events in anesthesia: a closed claims analysis. Anesthesiology 75:932, 1991
8. Gild W, Posner KL, Caplan RA, et al: Eye injuries associated with anesthesia: a closed claims analysis. Anesthesiology 76: 204, 1992
9. Carpenter RL, Caplan RA, Brown DL, et al: Incidence and risk factors for side effects of spinal anesthesia. Anesthesiology 76: 906, 1992
10. Morray JP, Geiduschek JM, Caplan RA, et al: A comparison of pediatric and adult closed claims. Anesthesiology 78:461, 1993
11. Keats AS: Anesthesia mortality in perspective. Anesth Analg 71: 113, 1991
12. Cooper JB, Newbower RS, Long CD, et al: Preventable anesthesia mishaps: a study of human factors. Anesthesiology 49: 399, 1978
13. Hamilton WK: Unexpected deaths during anesthesia: wherein lies the cause? Anesthesiology 50:381, 1979
14. Keenan RL, Boyan CP: Cardiac arrest due to anesthesia. JAMA 253:2373, 1985
15. Keenan RL: Anesthesia disasters: incidence, causes, preventability. Seminars in Anesthesia 5:175, 1986
16. Pierce EC: Risk modification in anesthesiology. In Chapman-Cliburn G (ed): Risk management and quality assurance: issues and interactions. A special publication of the Quality Review Bulletin. Chicago: Joint Commission on Accreditation of Hospitals, 1986: 20
17. Duberman SM: Quality assurance in the practice of anesthesiology 1986. Park Ridge, IL: American Society of Anesthesiologists, 1986
18. Peters JD, Fineberg KS, Kroll DA, et al: Anesthesiology and the Law. Ann Arbor, MI: Health Administration Press, 1983
19. Gilbert B: Relating quality assurance to credentials and privileges. In Chapman-Cliburn G (ed): Risk management and quality assurance: issues and interactions. A special publication of the Quality Review Bulletin. Chicago: Joint Commission on Accreditation of Hospitals, 1986: 79
20. Osteen A, Gannon MI: Continuing medical education. JAMA 256:1601, 1986
21. Department of Labor (Occupational Safety and Health Administration): Part II: occupational exposure to bloodborne pathogens. Final rule (29 CFR 1910.1030). Federal Register 56(235): 64176, December 6, 1991
22. Dans PE, Weiner JP, Otter SE: Peer review organizations: promises and potential pitfalls. N Engl J Med 313:1131, 1985; see also Peer review organizations (letters). N Engl J Med 314: 1121, 1986

23. Joint Commission on Accreditation of Healthcare Organizations manual for hospitals. Chicago: Joint Commission on Accreditation of Healthcare Organizations, 1994
24. 1995 Directory of Members. 60th ed. Park Ridge, IL: American Society of Anesthesiologists, 1995: 384
25. Eichhorn JH, Cooper JB, Cullen DJ, et al: Standards for patient monitoring during anesthesia at Harvard Medical School. JAMA 256:1017, 1986
26. 1994 Directory of members. American Society of Anesthesiologists standards for basic anesthetic monitoring. Approved by House of Delegates Oct 21, 1986; last amended Oct 13, 1993, pp. 735–736.
27. Joint Commission on Accreditation of Healthcare Organizations: Task forces lay groundwork for new survey process. In Agenda for Change Update 1(1):1, 1987
28. Lunn JN, Mushin WW: Mortality associated with anaesthesia. London: Nuffield Provincial Hospitals Trust, 1982
29. Spooner RB, Kirby RR: Equipment-related anesthetic incidents. In Pierce EC, Cooper JB (eds): Analysis of anesthetic mishaps. International Anesthesiology Clinics 22(2):133, 1984
30. Duberman Sm, Wald A: An integrated quality control program for anesthesia equipment. In Chapman-Cliburn G (ed): Risk management and quality assurance: issues and interactions. A special publication of the Quality Review Bulletin. Chicago: Joint Commission on Accreditation of Hospitals, 1986: 105
31. Paulus DA: Medicine and anesthesia: the costs, financial and otherwise. In Kirby RR, Gravenstein N (eds): Clinical anesthesia practice. Philadelphia: WB Saunders, 1994: 109
32. Good M: The anesthesia machine, anesthesia ventilators, breathing circuits, scavenging system. In Kirby RR, Gravenstein N (eds): Clinical anesthesia practice. Philadelphia: WB Saunders, 1994: 276
33. Health and Human Services Publication (FDA) 85-4196. Rockville, MD: Food and Drug Administration, Center for Devices and Radiologic Health, 1990
34. Harnish v Children's Hospital Medical Center, 387 MA 152, 1982
35. Curran WJ: Informed consent in malpractice cases: a turn toward reality. N Engl J Med 314:429, 1986
36. Lunn JN: The role of the anaesthetic record. In Lunn JN (ed): Epidemiology in anaesthesia. London: Edward Arnold, 1986: 136
37. Seed RGFL: Documentation. In Lunn JN (ed): Epidemiology in anaesthesia. London: Edward Arnold, 1986: 144
38. Lichtiger M, Eckhart J: Medicolegal issues and concerns. In: Kirby RR, Gravenstein N (eds): Clinical anesthetic practice. Philadelphia: WB Saunders, 1994: 53
39. Gravenstein JS: The role of the automated anesthesia record. In Eichhorn JH (ed): Improving anesthesia outcome. Problems in Anesthesia 5:241, 1991
40. Cohen JA: Quality assurance initiatives. In Eichhorn JH (ed): Improving anesthesia outcome. Problems in Anesthesia 5:277, 1991
41. Cohen JA: Quality assurance and risk management. In Gravenstein N (ed): Manual of complications during anesthesia. Philadelphia: JB Lippincott, 1991
42. Cooper JB, Newbower RS, Kitz RJ: An analysis of major errors and equipment failure in anesthesia management: considerations for prevention and detection. Anesthesiology 60:34, 1984
43. Cooper JB, Long CD, Newbower RS, et al: Critical incidents associated with intraoperative exchanges of anesthesia personnel. Anesthesiology 56:456, 1982
44. Cooper JB, Cullen DG, Eichhorn JH, et al: Administrative guidelines for response to an adverse anesthesia event. J Clin Anesth 5:79, 1993
45. Eichhorn JH: Risk reduction in anesthesia. In Duncan PG (ed): Anesthetic risk and complications. Problems in Anesthesia 6: 278, 1992
46. Holzer JF: Current concepts in risk management. In Pierce EC, Cooper JB (eds): Analysis of anesthetic mishaps. International Anesthesiology Clinics 22(2):91, 1984

FURTHER READING

Eichhorn JH (ed): Improving anesthesia outcome. Problems in Anesthesia 5:179, 1991

APPENDIX I
Addendum on Language

The terminology used in risk management and quality assurance has been borrowed by the medical profession from business, industry, and other professions. Medical practitioners may understand these terms enough to communicate among themselves but not always to communicate with others, such as hospital administrators, insurance company personnel, and regulatory or accrediting inspectors.

Many medical practitioners associate "risk management" and "quality assurance" with endless reams of apparently irrelevant paperwork demanded as fuel by a self-sustaining bureaucracy. Early in the development of this still-young field, overzealous emphasis on compiling statistics, doing "audits," and filling out forms created a legacy of reluctance regarding involvement by anesthesia practitioners, who are more used to hands-on activity with rapid feedback.

Nonetheless, in the late 1990s all concerned must realize that this type of activity not only is here to stay but also has the potential, when properly used, to be beneficial to the practice of anesthesia. The field has advanced significantly and will continue to do so with the unhesitating, thoughtful involvement of those most interested in the elimination of preventable anesthesia morbidity and mortality.

RISK MANAGEMENT

The concept of "risk management" traditionally has been associated with the financial or economic side of business or professional activity. It started with the insurance industry recognizing "risk": certain activities predictably lead to a degree of loss. This risk then became the subject of efforts to (1) plan to pay for the loss and (2) try to reduce the likelihood of loss (and consequent cost) and to control or "manage" the known risk.

Regarding anesthesia, it was clear that data "demonstrate that anesthetic mishaps, although relatively few in number, present considerable risk of loss in the areas of hospital cost, human suffering, and the integrity of the medical profession"; as a result, providers "have developed formal programs to systematically identify and control risks that may lead to patient injury or financial loss."[46] "Financial loss" usually means settlements and judgments associated with malpractice claims and suits. The emphasis of medical risk management is, correctly, on the prevention of any loss-generating untoward incident or outcome. However, a key traditional component also is the effort to limit financial loss once an incident has occurred. A common impression is that the hospital or insurance company risk manager is the person to call as soon as an accident or injury is identified. However, a necessary shift in perception is that prevention is primary and damage control (financial or otherwise), when needed, is secondary.

Types of Problems

Classic risk management involves four steps: (1) identification of a problem (actual or potential injury or loss); (2) assessment and evaluation of the problem (determining the cause of injury or loss); (3) resolution of the problem (modification or elimination of the cause, by change of practice, procedures, equipment, or behavior, and enforcement, with sanctions if necessary); and (4) follow-up on the resolution (to verify the desired result and to ensure continued effectiveness). A detailed application of this process to anesthesia practice has been published.[46]

Minor Injuries

An example of minor injury but no financial loss involves a major medical center performing a large number of cases of facial surgery. Through a combined mechanism of anesthesiologists' postoperative visits (and reports back to the clinical director of anesthesia), incident reports filed by floor nurses from the postoperative ward, and a call from the surgeon doing most of these cases, a disproportionately large number of corneal abrasions were noted to occur during one type of operation. Investigative evaluation revealed that all anesthesia practitioners had put lubricating ointment in the patients' eyes, which were then shut with paper tape. Some had used gauze pads, and some had not. The patients with corneal abrasions had not had gauze pads over their eyes.

Resolution of the problem involved discussion and distribution of a written guideline, which was put in the procedure manual, stating that gauze pads should be used to cover the eyes of patients having that operation. After several months, the surgeon was asked to confirm the impression that not one identified corneal abrasion associated with the procedure had occurred since the new guideline had been implemented.

Large-scale Problems

The Risk Management Committee of the Harvard Medical School Department of Anaesthesia reviewed the available literature and all anesthesia-related claims, files, and incidents for 1976 through 1986 from the department's malpractice insurer. Considering substantive identifiable problems, the committee generated a list of "areas of attention" into which problems and incidents were categorized. In order of perceived magnitude, the list included (1) minimal monitoring during an anesthetic and in the postanesthetic recovery period (by far the most frequent); (2) anesthetizing locations outside traditional operating rooms; (3) equipment standards, including preanesthetic equipment checkout; (4) equipment maintenance and servicing; (5) record-keeping; and (6) pre- and postoperative visits by personnel.[1]

This list formed the basis of a program to attempt to devise strategies to improve each of the identified areas of attention. This example shows the application of risk management techniques that include but go beyond the traditional emphasis on financial loss.

QUALITY ASSURANCE/CONTINUOUS QUALITY IMPROVEMENT

The concept of quality assurance can be viewed as growing out of "quality control," a process commonly used in business and industry to guarantee the production of a uniform product that meets an established standard for performance. In the health professions, the "product" is medical care. The idea of uniformity is not as important as the degree of quality, which should be measurable. Because the highest realistic quality of medical care is the desired goal, "quality assurance" has evolved to mean "the evaluation of the level of care provided (quality assessment) and the establishment of mechanisms for improvement, when necessary."[17]

Quality assurance depends on assessing the structure involved in medical care (resources, including personnel, facilities, equipment, and administration); the process involved (the actual activities of patient care), and the resultant outcome (eg, wellness, length of stay, dysfunction, morbidity, or mortality).[17] These assessments require standards or criteria against which the feature being assessed can be measured.

Establishment of these criteria involves major effort, because legitimate disagreement exists as to exactly what constitutes desirable features for structure, process, and outcome of medical care. These criteria can be established by an individual for his or her own practice; by a group or department at a hospital; by a governing or regulatory agency (such as local or state department of health); by a professional society; or by an accrediting body such as the JCAHO, which has assumed a major role in the development of these measurement criteria as applied to anesthesia. Detailed suggestions for quality assurance criteria in anesthesia are available, as are plans for various programs (some of which are similar in scope to those for risk management) to improve care.[17]

CQI activities have as their goal the delivery of the highest quality care practical. This approach, in turn, implies minimization of untoward outcome. Elimination of preventable morbidity and mortality is one of many goals of a successful program. Many other quality-related issues do not involve medically adverse results. Patients left minimally attended on stretchers in a dimly lit, cold corridor for more than an hour immediately preoperatively represent a quality-of-care issue appropriately addressed by a hospital quality assurance committee. They are at the opposite end of the spectrum from a series of intraoperative cardiac arrests associated with a specific procedure, anesthetic technique, anesthetic drug, anesthetist, or other common factor.

PATIENT SAFETY

Anesthesia appears to be the medical specialty with the most emphasis on "patient safety." This concept is narrower and more focused than quality assurance. The specific target is the elimination of injuries resulting from untoward incidents related to anesthesia care. Quite likely, some irreducible minimum number of cases will have adverse results that cannot be foreseen or prevented. However, the majority of major, untoward incidents are believed to be overt accidents that cause injuries leading to morbidity and mortality. This type of accident is amenable to mitigation or prevention by many of the methods inherent in risk management and quality assurance. What differs is focus and emphasis. Proponents of patient safety stress that in some circumstances, patients clearly are not safe and are hurt by preventable anesthesia-related complications.

Because anesthesia practice is procedure-oriented, technology-dependent, fast-moving, and increasingly complex, it is one of the medical specialties most prone to potentially devastating accident. Even the most skilled, experienced, and thoughtful anesthesiologist can have a momentary lapse and cause or overlook an unrecognized development that may lead to an injury. The same characteristics of practice, however, make anesthesiology probably the medical specialty most amenable to specific efforts at accident prevention. Debate and attention focus on exactly what is preventable. To this end, drawing from risk management and quality assurance techniques, workers in anesthesia patient safety have the specific immediate and long-term goal of minimizing anesthesia-related morbidity and mortality and improving outcome through CQI.

REFERENCE

1. Eichhorn JH, Cooper JB, Cullen DJ, et al: Standards for patient monitoring during anesthesia at Harvard Medical School. JAMA 256: 1017, 1986

APPENDIX II

Standards for Basic Intraoperative Monitoring

(Approved by House of Delegates on October 21, 1986 and last amended on October 13, 1993)

These standards apply to all anesthesia care although, in emergency circumstances, appropriate life support measures take precedence. These standards may be exceeded at any time based on the judgment of the responsible anesthesiologist. They are intended to encourage quality patient care, but observing them cannot guarantee any specific patient outcome. They are subject to revision from time to time, as warranted by the evolution of technology and practice. They apply to all general anesthetics, regional anesthetics, and monitored anesthesia care. This set of standards addresses only the issue of basic anesthetic monitoring, which is one component of anesthesia care. In certain rare or unusual circumstances, (1) some of these methods of monitoring may be clinically impractical, and (2) appropriate use of the described monitoring methods may fail to detect untoward clinical developments. Brief interruptions of continual† monitoring may be unavoidable. Under extenuating circumstances, the responsible anesthesiologist may waive the requirements marked with an asterisk (*); it is recommended that when this is done, it should be so stated (including the reasons) in a note in the patient's medical record. These standards are not intended for application to the care of the obstetric patient in labor or in the conduct of pain management.

STANDARD I

Qualified anesthesia personnel shall be present in the room throughout the conduct of all general anesthetics, regional anesthetics, and monitored anesthesia care.

Objective. Because of the rapid changes in patient status during anesthesia, qualified anesthesia personnel shall be continuously present to monitor the patient and provide anesthesia care. In the event there is a direct known hazard, eg, radiation, to the anesthesia personnel that might require intermittent remote observation of the patient, some provision for monitoring the patient must be made. In the event that an emergency requires the temporary absence of the person primarily responsible for the anesthetic, the best judgment of the anesthesiologist will be exercised in comparing the emergency with the anesthetized patient's condition and in the selection of the person left responsible for the anesthetic during the temporary absence.

(1995 Directory of Members, 60th ed. Park Ridge, IL: American Society of Anesthesiologists, 1995, 384–385.)

† *Note that "continual" is defined as "repeated regularly and frequently in steady rapid succession" whereas "continuous" means "prolonged without any interruption at any time."*

STANDARD II

During all anesthetics, the patient's oxygenation, ventilation circulation, and temperature shall be continually evaluated.

Oxygenation

Objective. To ensure adequate oxygen concentration in the inspired gas and the blood during all anesthetics.

Methods

1. Inspired gas: During every administration of general anesthesia using an anesthesia machine, the concentration of oxygen in the patient breathing system shall be measured by an oxygen analyzer with a low oxygen concentration limit alarm in use.*
2. Blood oxygenation: During all anesthetics, a quantitative method of assessing oxygenation such as pulse oximetry shall be employed.* Adequate illumination and exposure of the patient is necessary to assess color.*

Ventilation

Objective. To ensure adequate ventilation of the patient during all anesthetics.

Methods

1. Every patient receiving general anesthesia shall have the adequacy of ventilation continually evaluated. While qualitative clinical signs such as chest excursion, observation of the reservoir breathing bag, and auscultation of breath sounds may be adequate, quantitative monitoring of the CO_2 content and/or volume of expired gas is encouraged.
2. When an endotracheal tube is inserted, its correct positioning in the trachea must be verified by clinical assessment and by identification of carbon dioxide in the expired gas.* End-tidal carbon dioxide analysis, in use from the time of endotracheal tube placement, is strongly encouraged.
3. When ventilation is controlled by a mechanical ventilator, there shall be in continuous use a device that is capable of detecting disconnection of components of the breathing system. The device must give an audible signal when its alarm threshold is exceeded.
4. During regional anesthesia and monitored anesthesia care, the adequacy of ventilation shall be evaluated, at least by continual observation of qualitative clinical signs.

Circulation

Objective. To ensure the adequacy of the patient's circulatory function during all anesthetics.

Methods

1. Every patient receiving anesthesia shall have the electrocardiogram continuously displayed from the beginning of anesthesia until preparing to leave the anesthetizing location.*
2. Every patient receiving anesthesia shall have arterial blood pressure and heart rate determined and evaluated at least every 5 min.*
3. Every patient receiving general anesthesia shall have, in addition to the above, circulatory function continually evaluated by at least one of the following: palpation of a pulse, auscultation of heart sounds, monitoring of a tracing of intra-arterial pressure, ultrasound peripheral pulse monitoring, or pulse plethysmography or oximetry.

Body Temperature

Objective. To aid in the maintenance of appropriate body temperature during all anesthetics.

Methods. There shall be readily available a means to continuously measure the patient's temperature. When changes in body temperature are intended, anticipated, or suspected, the temperature shall be measured.

Complications in Anesthesiology, second edition,
edited by Nikolaus Gravenstein and Robert R. Kirby.
Lippincott-Raven Publishers, Philadelphia © 1996.

CHAPTER 2

Epidemiologic Methods in Anesthesia

Bucknam McPeek

Epidemiologists have developed specialized methods to study the extent and cause of disease. As practicing physicians, anesthesiologists use these data and benefit from their results, often without much understanding of the methods themselves. Nonetheless, if one wishes to use or interpret epidemiologic studies, a working knowledge of the underlying concepts, potentials, and limitations of the various methods involved is necessary.

Epidemiology is the study of the distribution and cause of disease or injury in human populations. It differs from clinical medicine because it is concerned with the health of groups or populations of people rather than of a single patient.

CASE REPORTS

A clinical case report details the disease-related experiences of a single patient. A hospital record room contains shelf upon shelf of individual clinical case reports. A magnificent array of medical information may be available concerning each patient.

Anesthesiologists are constantly challenged with clinical case reports that suggest anesthetic problems. Often, a clinical case report is the anesthesiologist's first signal of a complication. A physician, observing one or more unexpected events after exposure to an anesthetic agent, may write such a report. The report alerts the anesthesiologist to the possibility of undesirable therapy, thus forming the first line of defense against continued use of the therapy. Anesthesiologists depend on the sensitivity of physicians to detect unexpected events and to record them accurately for publication.[1]

Drawbacks

Despite its wealth of carefully documented detail, an individual clinical case report has a major defect. Usually one cannot determine the number of cases in the group from which a single case is drawn. Thus, regardless of the care and energy with which a clinical case report is investigated, it tells us nothing about the incidence of similar cases in a population. In other words, the numerator (observed case) is always "1," and the denominator (population) is unknown. If a case of jaundice occurred after an exposure to an anesthetic drug or a case of paraplegia after administration of a spinal anesthetic, knowledge of the incidence of these complications would be of great value. A significant difference clearly exists between one case of jaundice that occurs after 10 exposures to anesthetics and one case that occurs after 10,000 exposures. Similarly, three cases of paraplegia drawn from an experience of 300 spinal anesthetic administrations carries greater significance than a single case from a hospital's experience of 300,000 administrations.

Thus, even if a relatively large number of individual clinical cases of a specific complication after exposure to a drug are reported in the literature, nothing can be said about the incidence of the complication without some knowledge of the size of the population at risk. Therefore, the probability of similar cases occurring in the future cannot be estimated. Increasing numbers of clinical case reports of a specific complication may suggest that it is a more common occurrence than if only one such report had been made. Yet even as new reports come to our attention, the prediction of the likelihood of the complication cannot be made, nor can the probability of occurrence of a specific event be estimated; certainly, nothing can be determined about any causal relation to a particular treatment or practice.

Value

Isolated case reports or uncontrolled series alert us to potential complications and are indispensable precursors to good clinical research. Such studies help principally to generate research questions or hypotheses. However, such hypotheses can be accepted only with rigorous study and scientific logic. They should be tested only after they have been set forth in advance, not post hoc by means of "fishing expeditions" into existing data or by dredging of information we gather ourselves. Characteristically, advances in the clinical sciences are small, and progress is gradual.

POPULATION STUDIES

The ability to identify a particular complication or to diagnose a specific disease with reasonable reliability is vital to its epidemiologic study. If it cannot be identified, it cannot be included in cases that constitute a numerator.[1] For instance, this problem has been largely responsible for the inability to study the halothane–hepatitis question adequately.

Epidemiologists are interested in population studies because such studies enable them to discuss the incidence or probability of an observed event. These studies, as mentioned, require a denominator, which is the defined population serving as a comparison group for the persons who are experiencing the event or undergoing the treatment. Individual case histories frequently are triggered by knowledge gained through published case reports. The denominator distinguishes the two and facilitates an epidemiologic study from a collection of case histories.

Individual Details

Many individual details are often available from a clinical case report. Yet in a population study, if the denominator is very large, only a few details are available about every case. Ordinarily, financial considerations preclude use both of many cases and of a large number of facts per case. In the National Halothane Study, an elaborate design allowed reference to a denominator of 856,000 patients.[2] Yet the analysis was based on 8 to 10 individual items of information about each of the surveyed patients. In outcome studies at the Massachusetts General Hospital, 40 to 50 items of information were recorded for each of the 80,000 patients surveyed.[3,4] Thus, an inverse relation usually is found between the size of a study's population and the number of facts available for each case.

Sampling

An investigator ordinarily has available for study a specific group of patients, such as those treated in a particular hospital or practice. Frequently, study of all the patients involved in the treatment in question is impractical. A representative number of subjects may be selected from the larger population. This process is called sampling, and the extent to which information obtained may be extrapolated to the total population depends in large measure on the skill with which the sampling was performed. Sometimes a process called stratification is used. Stratified samples are drawn to ensure that specified proportions of selected groups are included. For example, a study may necessitate that a sample consist of two groups of pregnant women: one group of those pregnant for the first time and a second group consisting of an equal number of those who have been pregnant before.

Methods

Within specified subgroups, selection may be either random or systematic. A random sample is one that is drawn so that every subject in the total population has an equal chance of being represented in the sample. A systematic sample in one in which subjects are selected by a system; for example, every 10th person or every 100th person may be included in a sample. If the organization of the population before drawing the sample is random, or at least not highly structured with respect to some confounding variable, systematic sampling works. Sometimes, however, it is disastrous. A number of years ago, the popularity of noncommissioned officers in the Army was studied by using a systematic sample of every 30th man from the post list. Imagine the investigator's surprise when he found that sergeants were almost universally respected. Further investigation revealed that the post list consisted of hundreds of barrack lists; each barrack housed 27 privates, two corporals, and a sergeant. The sergeant was the 30th name on each list.

EPIDEMIOLOGIC STUDIES

Epidemiologic studies customarily are separated into two broad categories: descriptive and analytic.

Descriptive

Descriptive epidemiology focuses on the causes of disease or the factors influencing its extent. Descriptive studies are important because they take a first step toward uncovering the causes of disease or injury by identifying groups with a high or low rate of specific illness.

Once such an identification has been made, the next step is an attempt to understand why the rate is high or low in a particular population. The results of these studies aid the formulation of hypotheses that can be tested by analytic studies to determine the underlying causes of the disease and explain its distribution.

Analytic

In their purest form, analytic studies are executed to test a hypothesis that a specific factor or cause is related to a particular effect. This goal is accomplished by measuring both the exposure to the cause and the presence or absence of the effect for each person in the study. That is, the study is designed to test the following general hypothesis: if the frequency of illness or injury within two groups is dependent on the presence of an identified factor, that particular factor should appear more frequently in the group with the illness or injury than in the group without it.

The majority of analytic epidemiologic studies survey the individual members of each group. Some studies examine the experience of the group as a whole, but this approach is not very common. Analytic studies of individual members of the group are either of the cross-sectional, case–control, or cohort variety.

Cross-sectional Studies

In a cross-sectional study, the cause and the effect are measured at the same time. A study of the relation between body build and difficulty in passing an endotracheal tube is an example.

Case-control Studies

A case–control study is retrospective. It starts with the effect and determines the frequency of the hypothesized cause. Persons with the illness or injury are compared with a control group free of the illness, and an attempt is made to determine whether the two groups differ in their previous exposure to the causative factor.

Cohort Studies

Cohort studies are prospective. The investigator starts with the cause and looks for the development of the effect. Subjects who are exposed to the hypothesized causal factor are observed and compared with a control group composed of subjects not exposed to the causal factor. Both groups are carefully observed to determine the incidence of the subsequent development of the effect.

Each of these methods attempts to relate cause and effect. The cross-sectional study examines cause and effect by a single measurement in time. The case–control study involves two groups that differ in the presence of the effect; the investigator looks back in time to compare their exposure to a hypothesized cause. The cohort study involves two groups, or cohorts, that differ in their exposure to a possible cause; the investigator observes them over time to determine the rates at which the effect may occur.

CAUSATION HYPOTHESES

Two approaches are used to investigate hypotheses about causation: nonexperimental and experimental.

Nonexperimental

In the nonexperimental (sometimes called observational) approach, the investigator observes the occurrence of the disease in persons who are already separated into groups on the basis of exposure to a factor, such as a particular anesthetic agent. An example of this type of investigation was the National Halothane Study.[2] The allocation of individual subjects into groups on the basis of exposure to specific anesthetic agents was not done by the investigators but instead depended on the person's previous anesthetic experience. This classification may raise questions about the comparability of the groups.

In a nonexperimental study, the differences between study groups are observed but are not experimentally manipulated by the investigator. Because these groups are not created experimentally, they must be accepted as the investigator finds them. They ordinarily differ in other ways, in addition to the specific causal factor under study. One group may be older; another may have more men than women; or the participants may show different states of general health. Thus, the role of the factor under investigation can be obscured by many variables. Nonexperimental studies continue to provide much useful knowledge for medical research. Yet physicians have come to rely more and more on the experimental approach.

Experimental

In the experimental approach, which is always a cohort study, the investigator examines the effect of deliberately varying some causative factor under his or her control. Experimental studies can establish causation with more surety than can nonexperimental studies, primarily because of the increased control with which experimental studies may be conducted. The degree of control usually can be determined from the fundamental structure of a study.

Gilbert and colleagues studied evaluations of various treatments given to patients undergoing surgery and anesthesia.[5,6] Using the National Library of Medicine medical literature analysis and retrieval system, they drew a sample of 107 reports from the surgery and anesthesia literature published between 1964 and 1972. The sample reports used three kinds of studies, described in the following paragraphs.

Randomized Controlled Trials

In a randomized controlled trial, the investigator compares two or more treatment groups, and patients are assigned to the groups by a formal randomization process.

Nonrandomized Controlled Trials

Nonrandomized controlled trials are not formally randomized. Patients treated concurrently in the same institution are compared, and patients treated previously by one method are compared with patients treated currently by another.

Series

A series consists of reports of patients treated in a particular manner, but with no specific reference for comparison, aside from other published reports describing similar patients. A series, like other nonexperimental methods, ordinarily tells the anesthesiologist little about causation, although much can be learned about the results of a particular treatment or the effects of a disease.

The strength of an epidemiologic study and thus the surety with which its results can be accepted depends on a variety of factors, but primarily on the degree of control. Sometimes a series consists simply of a collection of selected case reports and thereby suffers from the same limitations as do individual case reports. We have more confidence in a series if it is a census, consisting of all cases of a given complication over a specified period, or if an *unbiased* sample of observed cases of the complication is drawn to form the reported series.

Association or Causation

As clinicians, we constantly remind ourselves that association does not necessarily mean causation. Ordinarily, we develop truly convincing evidence for causation through only the most careful of experimental approaches. The strongest, most reliable evidence for cause and effect is a well-conducted randomized controlled trial. Because a series is not a controlled trial, the results cannot be used with much certainty to form conclusions about causation. However, exceptions to this general statement do occur.

Bradford-Hill suggests factors to consider in the examination of associations when the evidence is derived from a series or other nonexperimental method (Table 2-1).[7]

Strength of the Association

If the exposed subjects show the outcome variable to a marked degree, we can infer causation more comfortably. Nevertheless, we can be misled. A very strong association may be just that: a strong association, and not a cause-and-effect relation at all.

Consistency of the Observed Causation

The connection between smoking and lung cancer has been observed repeatedly by investigators using different methods over many years. Similar results from different studies are much more convincing than are results from a collection of similarly designed studies. Weakly designed studies pointing in the same direction frequently have misled us in the past into concluding that causation exists, when in fact each group of investigators simply repeated the others' mistakes.

Specificity of the Association

If the association is unusual or if unusual outcomes develop in specifically exposed subjects, we have a strong argument for causation. The deformity phocomelia, which followed the exposure of pregnant women to thalidomide, is an example.

Temporal Relation of the Observed Association

An argument for causation is severely undermined if the effect appears before the postulated cause.

TABLE 2-1
Factors to Consider in the Evaluation of Associations Derived From Series or Other Nonexperimental Studies

- Strength of the association
- Consistency of the observed causation
- Specificity of the association
- Temporal relation of the observed association
- Dose–response curve
- Biologic plausibility
- Coherence of evidence
- Reversibility of the association
- Analogous situations

Modified from Bradford-Hill A: Principles of medical statistics. 9th ed. New York: Oxford University Press, 1971.

Dose–Response Curve

Persons who smoke many cigarettes per day have a much higher death rate from cancer of the lungs than do those who smoke little; the latter, in turn, have a higher rate of death from lung cancer than do nonsmokers. This is an example of a dose–response curve, in which the degree of the effect parallels the degree of the cause.

Biologic Plausibility

If the association makes no sense at all, we are cautious in suggesting causation. At the same time, we continue to learn more about human biology. Perhaps 20 years from now, associations that currently seem to make no sense will have biologic plausibility.

Coherence of the Evidence

The evidence ought to fit and should not seriously conflict with generally accepted facts of the natural history and biologic features of the disease studied.

Reversibility of the Association

Reversibility is illustrated by the decrease in the number of reported cases of phocomelia when thalidomide was taken off the market.

Analogous Situation

When we find a specific complication resulting from one drug, we are much more ready to accept similar evidence with the use of another similar or related drug that the second drug could cause the same complication.

Therefore, a series can supply information about causation as well as information about levels of performance, outcome, and the natural history of disease. Nevertheless, the controlled study provides the primary support for theories of cause, and its credibility rests mainly on the strength of the control. Only to the extent that the control group is truly similar to the exposed group will differences in outcome illustrate the role of the casual factor. On very rare occasions, natural groups may be found that seem to be similar in all respects except for the degree of exposure to a hypothesized causal factor. This relation is called a natural experiment, and in these unusual circumstances a nonexperimental study may establish causal association.

CONTROLLED STUDIES

General Characteristics

In a controlled study, assignment of patients to the exposed group or to the control group is an important issue. The principal aim is to achieve similarity between the groups. A number of factors must be considered in the pursuit of this goal. For instance, the known information about the disease or complication under study should be examined. Any potentially confounding variables that might have a large effect must be identified. In a study of anesthetic drugs, the exposed and control groups should be similar with respect to age, physical status, and the operation performed. In a study of heart disease, the groups might be matched with respect to risk factors such as hypertension, smoking, diabetes, and history of cardiac illness.

Unfortunately, the investigator frequently does not know enough about the specific disease or complication to guarantee that even the most careful matching has eliminated all possible confounding factors. Consequently, elimination of the effect of previously unknown factors is difficult. To a very limited extent, this problem can be addressed by ensuring general similarity between the exposed and control groups: the groups may be drawn from the same general population, from patients seen at the same clinic or hospital, or from the same ethnic or socioeconomic group.

Finally, one must ensure that information required in the study can be obtained from both groups in the same fashion. In other words, the same information should be available from both the control group and the exposed group. Any difference in response rates between the groups raises serious questions about a study's validity.

Clinical Trials

A well-designed, properly conducted, controlled clinical trial provides the only reliable basis for evaluating the efficacy and safety of treatment. It is a planned experiment involving patients or volunteers. The results, which are based on a limited sample of subjects, are used to make inferences about future treatment policy for the general population of patients. Thus, in a clinical trial, we are concerned not only with the logic and the strength of inference but also with the ability to generalize the derived information.

Efficacy

Efficacy is the benefit that we expect to confer to patients after the intervention is provided and after they have complied with the required regimen of care. In the real world, just as anesthesiologists vary in skill and their techniques for a given treatment differ, patients and actual benefits also vary.

Effectiveness

Effectiveness is the outcome of treatment achieved when an intervention is introduced into widespread clinical practice. In general, the benefits actually achieved in widespread practice are less than those obtained in a controlled trial. Similarly, complication rates derived from careful clinical trials or even reported series from prestigious institutions may not be applicable to widespread clinical practice, because actual skills and techniques are likely to vary.

Omitted Information

Reports of clinical trials often omit information about study design, implementation, and analysis. Yet such information is essential for accurate evaluation of research reports. In DerSimonian and coworkers' survey of 67 clinical trials for 11 important aspects of design and analysis (Table 2-2), only 56% of the items were reported clearly; 10% were mentioned ambiguously; and 34% were not reported (see Table 2-2).[8] They selected the 11 items on the basis of importance to a reader in determining the confidence that should be placed in the authors' conclusions, their applicability across a variety of medical specialty areas, and their ability to be identified by the scientific, literate, general reader. Similar results have been found by Emerson and colleagues for surgical literature.[9]

Allocation to Treatment Groups

As in population sampling, two methods of allocation, random and systematic, commonly are used. A random allocation is one that is drawn so that every subject of the population to be studied has an equal chance of being represented in each

TABLE 2-2
Important Features of Study Design and Analysis

ELIGIBILITY CRITERIA	Criteria for admission of patients to the trial
ADMISSION BEFORE ALLOCATION	Information used to determine whether eligibility criteria were applied before knowledge of the specific treatment assignment had been obtained
RANDOM ALLOCATION	Random allocation to treatment
METHOD OF RANDOMIZATION	Mechanism used to generate the random assignment
PATIENT'S BLINDNESS TO TREATMENT	Information about whether patients knew which treatment they were receiving
BLIND ASSESSMENT OF OUTCOME	Information about whether the person assessing the outcome knew which treatment had been given
TREATMENT COMPLICATIONS	Presence or absence of side effects or complications after treatment
UNAVAILABILITY FOR FOLLOW-UP	Numbers of patients unavailable for follow-up and the reasons why they were unavailable
STATISTICAL ANALYSES	Analyses beyond the computation of means, percentages, or standard deviations
STATISTICAL METHODS	Specific tests, techniques, or computer programs used for statistical analyses
POWER	Determination of sample size or the size of detectable differences

Data from DerSimonian R, Charette LJ, McPeek B, et al: Reporting on methods in clinical trials. N Engl J Med 306:1332, 1982.

group. Random allocation has great theoretical and practical advantages. A systematic allocation is one in which individual subjects are selected systematically to form the groups. For example, every second person may be assigned to the experimental group. If the organization of the study population before the allocation to groups is random or at least not highly structured with respect to some confounding variable, systematic allocation produces satisfactory results.

BIAS. The method of allocation is important. It deserves careful thought, and once the procedure is selected it must be followed exactly. Little confidence can be placed in data acquired from treatment groups that have been selected haphazardly. Often investigators report so briefly on their method of allocation that the reader cannot determine how the allocation was done. In other studies, investigators use methods that readily lead to bias. For example, when someone conducting the trial personally chooses the patients who are to receive a specific treatment, the allocation is no longer unbiased.[10]

NONRANDOM ALLOCATION. Knowing who is to receive the treatment next may influence decisions about eligibility and thus create bias. All schemes designed to balance allocation have this weakness. Eligibility must always be decided before allocation. Furthermore, when investigators alternate cases to assign patients to two treatments, they may encounter two or more candidates appearing almost simultaneously. In this case, some preference or prejudice of the person who assigns the treatment can affect the trial. If that person prefers that the treatment be administered to women or young people, more women and young people will receive it.

Sometimes patients present in a nearly random order; if picking and choosing did not occur, this method of assigning treatments would suffice. Yet "bunching" usually occurs: someone will probably influence the assignments, either consciously or subconsciously. For example, one recent study that allegedly used alternate cases for assignments resulted in two groups of about 150 and 250, respectively, instead of groups that differed by, at most, 1 or 2 members.

Another method predisposed to nonrandom allocation involves the assignment of treatment by birth date, depending, for example, on whether the date is odd or even. An investigator who knows in advance the subject's birth date and the treatment that would be associated with it can decide that the subject is not eligible for the study and thereby introduce selection effect. The same objection applies to the use of patients' hospital numbers in prospective studies, though not in retrospective studies.

The objection here is not to rules that disallow entrance into the study. Rules for exclusion often are essential, but these rules must be strictly insulated from the choice of treatment once the patient's eligibility has been established. Although informal methods of random allocation can be used rather effectively, they are subject to abuse: "Let's flip the coin again since we've already had four heads in a row." Informal methods, such as coin-tossing, are usually difficult to document, and therefore they cannot be checked later if questions arise, as they often do.

RANDOMIZATION. The use of a published table of random digits makes it easy to keep a written record of which numbers were chosen and how they were used to make the assignments. Tables of random numbers are widely available and inexpensive to use. Still, the application of any randomization technique must be examined for possible bias.

As randomizing devices, slips of paper marked with a treatment in a sealed envelope appear to be efficient. However, sometimes the envelopes are not opaque, especially when held against bright light, and the assigner can shuffle envelopes, knowing the characteristics of the participant and the possible treatments. Even the use of a random number table may introduce bias, depending on the method by which numbers are assigned. If an investigator is responsible for entering each patient in the order of arrival on a list of random numbers, nonrandom assignment could occur when two patients appear at the same time and the investigator must choose the order in which to place them. As a protection against this possibility, the investigator should not be told how the numbers correspond to the treatments.

Although these precautions may seem elaborate, one should assume that if something can go wrong in an investigation, it usually will. When the quality of randomization is questionable, the guarantee of lack of bias disappears, and therefore the uncertainty of the conclusions increases. Of course, randomization alone does not ensure that an experiment has been carried out properly or that valid results will be obtained. Therefore, when expensive and delicate studies such as randomized clinical trials are performed, their component parts, like the steps of randomization and the degree of blindness, must be thoroughly inspected and secured. When quality control measures have been applied in a study, they should be reported in detail. The amount of care taken in the design and execution of an investigation is a major indicator of its quality. When such care is not reported, some readers may assume that these steps have not been taken.

BLINDNESS. One of the methodologic lessons that researchers learned from medical trials at the beginning of this century was the extreme difficulty of obtaining objective and reproducible data from human subjects. Because few people view their own death with equanimity, only with the greatest difficulty can patients admit to themselves and to their physicians that a long-desired treatment has failed. In less dramatic circumstances, patients' respect for physician-researchers, as well as their own personal hopes, may exert a similar inhibiting effect. Humans communicate with each other in many different ways, some completely subconscious. As a result, the hopes of the research team can often be communicated to patients without the awareness of either, much like an infection.

Blind evaluation, in which neither physicians nor patients know which treatment has been received, is a way of preventing contamination of this sort. The requirement of a double-blind design, when it is possible, is no more an aspersion on the honesty and integrity of the investigator than the use of latex gloves is an aspersion on the personal hygiene of a surgeon. In both cases, experience has taught that failure to follow the best possible practices often leads to disastrous results.

Whether bias has affected the observed results is often impossible to tell. A randomized double- or triple-blind trial carries weight because it provides the researcher with the maximum protection against these subtle sources of error. When the treatment cannot be concealed from the physician because of the type of therapy being investigated, bias may be avoided safely by the use of an unbiased or blind evaluator. These considerations do not mean that nonblinded studies are always wrong or that blind studies are always right; rather, nonblinded studies are more likely to be biased, and the absence of such effects is virtually impossible to document. When the possibility of bias cannot be dismissed, our confidence in these studies is weakened. Thus, nonblinded studies are inherently less useful for decision-making, even when their findings are correct.

Power and Generalization

SAMPLE SIZES. When generalization follows the results of a clinical trial, two dangers are present. One is that a true difference will be overlooked. This is referred to as a type II error: concluding that there is no difference when one does exist.[11] The other danger is that a difference will be reported erroneously. This is called a type I error: reporting a difference when there is none. Because the sizes of experimental groups are limited, there is always some risk that the data will suggest a false conclusion because of sampling fluctuation. Large differences tend to be more easily detected than small ones, and in any particular study larger samples are more likely to lead to the correct conclusions than smaller ones. Because the level of significance is affected by the degree of the true but unknown difference in effectiveness of the treatments, as well as by the strength of the evidence as determined by the sample size, it is easier to obtain significant results when the true differences are large than when they are small. The capability of a trial to detect small effects is called its power and depends primarily on the unknown difference between the treatment effects, the design of the trial, and the sizes of the groups.

Power Analysis

Consider a 5% change in a death rate. (Five percent is about four times the average death rate from all operations in the United States.) Reduction of a death rate from 35% to 30% may represent an important improvement in patient care, but this finding does not mean that it will be easily identified in the everyday setting of clinical practice. Indeed, statistical theory shows that a well-run, randomized, controlled trial must have 1000 patients in each group for 80% confidence in the detection of such a difference. Without a large formal study, uncontrolled effects of patient selection, concurrent treatments, and other factors make the reliable detection of such differences almost impossible.

A power analysis is a statistical test, ideally performed before a study is begun, that is used to determine the appropriate sample size necessary to avoid a type I or type II error at whatever level of difference is considered clinically meaningful. It is intuitive, therefore, that studies looking for small improvements with a high probability of validity, such as the effect of pulse oximetry on perioperative mortality,[12] require extremely large study populations.

EXTRAPOLATION TO DIFFERENT POPULATIONS. The results of a carefully designed study in anesthesiology may represent the true situation for the particular institution involved. Yet how do these results apply to anesthesia care nationally? Essentially, they relate only to a sample of patients having anesthesia in one institution. Therefore, applicability elsewhere requires considerable argument beyond direct conclusions from the empirical data. The patient population in a large city charity hospital differs from that of an affluent suburban practice. Patients seen in a Veterans Affairs hospital differ from those of an obstetric or a pediatric hospital. Edinburgh is not Boston. Each physician must consider such differences and evaluate how reports of studies performed by others in other settings can be applied locally. This is one reason that physicians prefer more than one clinical trial and multi-institutional studies; they want to broaden the base of the inference.

Comparisons of Clinical Measurements

With the continuing evolution of technology in the operating room, we are increasingly confronted with new or different ways to measure clinical parameters. Traditionally, these sorts of comparisons (eg, invasive versus noninvasive blood pressure or brand A versus brand B devices) were analyzed by regression analysis and correlation coefficients. We have learned that these tests usually are not appropriate because they do not measure agreement and so may be misleading.[13] Instead, Bland and Altman[14] convincingly propose that bias and precision be used as the preferred statistical test for comparative measurements. Bias, or accuracy, is the mean of the error and reflects the proximity of the reported value to the true or reference value. Precision is the standard deviation of the errors and describes the reproducibility of an observation.

Meta-analysis

Meta-analysis is a retrospective technique whereby the results of previously, it is hoped compatible, studies are combined.[15] This approach is useful to increase statistical power, provide a majority opinion, enhance estimates of effects, and answer questions not posed at the start of individual trials.[16] These studies are gaining in popularity, but the reader must be cautioned that they are vulnerable to design flaws as much as any other study as well as to flaws unique to this combined-studies approach. As meta-analysis techniques are refined, the pooling of data is becoming more acceptable. Meta-analysis is best applied when definitive randomized studies are impossible, inconclusive, or conflicting. In these circumstances it provides an excellent quantitative estimate of the weight of available evidence.[16]

FUTURE PROGRESS IN ANESTHESIA

Experience with research on treatments in anesthesia indicates that relatively small gains or losses are to be expected from most studies.[4,6] Clinical trials must be designed routinely to detect these small differences accurately and reliably. When a systematic study of a new anesthetic treatment is first considered, it is frequently viewed with great optimism. The investigators may believe that the new procedure will prove to be greatly superior, and preliminary and informal experience may seem to support their position. However, this initial optimism is frequently unwarranted. Careful trials usually show only modest gains, and sometimes the new treatment is demonstrated to be inferior to the standard.

A necessary part of the design of any clinical study is to ensure sufficient power to detect effects of clinical importance. Just as individual innovations are likely to produce relatively small gains, much of the progress made in any area of anesthesia or any large-scale research program consists of a number of modest gains, each adding to previous results rather than providing one or two revolutionary breakthroughs. Because small gains can easily be negated by small losses if new treatments or modified practices are adopted uncritically,[17,18] careful unbiased evaluation plays an important role both in guiding research programs and in documenting their progress. Appreciation of this gradual development can result in greater understanding of the time and effort required for progress in anesthesia and hence to more realistic expectations; critical reading of published studies can yield greater confidence in the observations made and conclusions drawn.

REFERENCES

1. Riesenberg DE: Case reports in the medical literature. JAMA 255:2067, 1986
2. Bunker JP, Forrest WH Jr, Mosteller F, et al: The National Halothane Study. Bethesda: National Institute of General Medical Sciences, 1969
3. Owens WD, Dykes MHM, Gilbert JP, et al: Development of two indices of postoperative morbidity. Surgery 77:586, 1975
4. McPeek B, Gasko M, Mosteller F: Measuring outcome from anesthesia and operation. Theoretical Surgery 1:2, 1986
5. Gilbert JP, McPeek B, Mosteller F: Progress in surgery and anesthesia: benefits and risks of innovative therapy. In Bunker JP, Barnes BA, Mosteller F (eds): Costs, risks and benefits of surgery. New York: Oxford University Press, 1977:124
6. Gilbert JP, McPeek B, Mosteller F: Statistics and ethics in surgery and anesthesia. Science 198:684, 1977
7. Bradford-Hill A: Principles of medical statistics. 9th ed. New York: Oxford University Press, 1971
8. DerSimonian R, Charette LJ, McPeek B, et al: Reporting on methods in clinical trials. N Engl J Med 306:1332, 1982
9. Emerson JD, McPeek B, Mosteller F: Reporting clinical trials in general surgical journals. Surgery 95:572, 1984
10. Student: The Lanarkshire milk experiment. Biometrika 23:398, 1931
11. Freiman JA, Chalmers TC, Smith H Jr, et al: The importance of beta, the type II error and sample size in the design and interpretation of the randomized control trial: survey of 71 negative trials. N Engl J Med 299:690, 1978
12. Möller JT, Pederson T, Rasmussen L, et al: Randomized evaluation of pulse oximetry in 20,802 patients (I and II). Anesthesiology 69:106, 1993
13. Altman DG, Bland JM: Measurement in medicine: the analysis of method comparison studies. Statistician 32:307, 1983
14. Bland JM, Altman DG: Statistical methods for assessing agreement between two methods of clinical measurement. Lancet 1: 307, 1986
15. Valonovich V: Crystalloid versus colloid fluid resuscitation: A meta-analysis of mortality. Surgery 105:70, 1989
16. Sacks HS, Berrier J, Reitman D, et al: Meta-analysis of randomized controlled trials. N Engl J Med 316:450, 1987
17. Issacs H, Badenhorst M: False-negative results with muscle caffeine halothane contracture testing for malignant hyperthermia. Anesthesiology 79:5, 1993
18. Larach MG: Should we use muscle biopsy to diagnose malignant hyperthermia susceptibility? (editiorial). Anesthesiology 79:1, 1993

FURTHER READING

Cotton T, Civetta JM: A primer for understanding the medical literature. In Civetta JM, Taylor RW, Kirby RR (eds): Critical care. 2nd ed. Philadelphia: JB Lippincott, 1992:1835

Fletcher RH, Fletcher SW, Wagner EH: Clinical epidemiology: the essentials. Baltimore: Williams & Wilkins, 1982

Friedman GD: Primer of epidemiology. 2nd ed. New York: McGraw-Hill, 1980

Gehlbach SH: Interpreting the medical literature. Lexington, MA: DC Heath, 1982

Gilbert JP, McPeek B, Mosteller F: The clinician's responsibility for helping to improve the treatment of tomorrow's patient. N Engl J Med 302:630, 1980

Hoaglin D, Light R, McPeek B, et al: Data for decisions: information strategies for policy makers. Cambridge, MA: Abt Books, 1982

Louis T, Shapiro SW (eds): Clinical trials: issues and approaches. New York: Marcel Dekker, 1983

Lowrance WW: Of acceptable risk: science and the determination of safety. Los Altos, CA: William Kaufman, 1976

Lunn JN: Epidemiology in anaesthesia: the techniques of epidemiology applied to anaesthetic practice. Baltimore: Edward Arnold, 1986

MacMahon B, Pugh TF: Epidemiology principles and methods. Boston: Little, Brown, 1970

Troidl H, Spitzer WO, McPeek B, et al (eds): Principles and practice of research: strategies for surgical investigators. New York: Springer-Verlag, 1986

Complications in Anesthesiology, second edition,
edited by Nikolaus Gravenstein and Robert R. Kirby.
Lippincott-Raven Publishers, Philadelphia © 1996.

CHAPTER 3

The Role of Anesthesia in Surgical Mortality

Arthur S. Keats

On previous occasions I wrote about mortality resulting from anesthesia from the perspective of "anesthetic risk."[1,2] To do so required a review of studies specifically addressing anesthetic and surgical mortality as well as a review of collateral data necessary to document the tenuous basis for risk estimates. The following conclusions were drawn:

> The poor predictability of anesthetic mortality should be expected, since a significant portion of this mortality is due to human error, which cannot be predicted, and to other factors that never have been quantified. To a small degree physical status and the operation contemplated provide some predictive basis. To a large degree, unknown factors related to the skill of the personnel and the environment of therapy contribute to anesthetic risk. Estimates of anesthetic risk for individual patients remain, therefore, almost entirely intuitive, and one cannot deny an anesthetic to any patient who urgently requires operation.[2]

Since 1970, little has happened to alter this general conclusion, which—applied to risk—is a concept whose essential element is ability to predict.

In contrast, the subject of the current chapter ignores predictability and asks instead, "What do we in fact know about deaths caused by anesthesia?" The data previously reviewed apply equally here; in addition, new data now are available. We can assume, reasonably, that today few patients who urgently require surgery are denied an anesthetic. To what degree, then, can the role of anesthesia in surgical mortality be quantified?

EARLY STUDIES

Basic to the answer to the forgoing question is the definition of the term "anesthetic death." Today this term is still largely undefined, except in guidelines put forth by individual reporters (or select committees) who have rendered opinions of the role of anesthesia in a surgical death. The bias of those who have made these judgments has tainted all published estimates of death rates from anesthesia and probably has stifled alternate approaches to the question as well.

When anesthesiology emerged from its status as a subspecialty of surgery, it retained much of the format of training for general surgery, including systematic review of all postoperative deaths, a practice that continues in all anesthesia training programs. In conferences on morbidity and mortality, the relative roles of the patient's disease, errors in surgical management, and errors in anesthetic management in mortality were discussed and assigned. In the earliest of these conferences surgeons tended to ascribe complications that were not clearly surgery- or disease-related to the anesthetic. Anesthesiologists tended to be defensive and to deny the charge. Not surprisingly, the first systematic study of the death rate from anesthesia in the post–World War II era reviewed data on surgical deaths to approximate the role of anesthesia in overall surgical mortality.

Death Rate: The Study by Beecher and Todd

Beecher and Todd's study of death rate[3] is a landmark in clinical investigation. Ten institutions participated; the method was prospective, reflecting current anesthesia practice (records of surgical deaths were reviewed shortly after the event); the approach was multidisciplinary (in each institution both surgeons and anesthesiologists examined all surgical death records); and it included large numbers of patients (almost 600,000 anesthetic administrations from 1948 to 1952).[3] "Anesthesia deaths" were not defined for the institutional committees that made the judgments. Instead, a series of examples was provided as a guide to the types of situations to be classified this way.

The data from this study, published in 1954, provided estimates of the incidence of primary anesthesia deaths and the incidence of deaths in which anesthesia was secondary or contributory, based on a total of 384 anesthesia deaths. However, neither a description of the circumstances surrounding these deaths nor a tabulation by cause was ever made available. The investigators chose to interpret their data in terms of death rates for specific anesthetic agents and concluded that the death rate associated with the use of muscle relaxants was several times that of any other agent.

Although they attributed this high death rate to the "inherent toxicity of curare," the authors classified 79% of the "curare deaths" as caused by errors of anesthetic technique, choice, or management. Charges of bias in the interpretation of the "curare deaths" and in the presentation of data promptly followed, as did a rebuttal.[4] The influence of these data on the clinical use of muscle relaxants was profound but rapidly diminished during the next few years as the use of succinylcholine gained wide acceptance. Compared with traditional muscle relaxants, succinylcholine's facilitation of tracheal intubation was so dramatic and obvious that the stigma of "curare deaths" was ignored (but not forgotten). No prospective study of anesthesia deaths of this magnitude has since been undertaken, although the same study design was used subsequently in the National Halothane Study.[5]

Self-Examination: The Study by Dripps and Colleagues

In response to the general unhappiness with Beecher and Todd's report, Dripps and colleagues reviewed deaths of patients who received a total of 33,000 administrations of anesthetics over a 10-year period in the investigators' own institution.[6] However, the study included only patients who received a spinal anesthetic or a general anesthetic and a muscle relaxant during the procedure. Regarding their own bias in reviewing death records, they wrote:

> There is nothing to be gained in a mortality study by omitting a particular death merely to lower a statistical death rate. Avoiding responsibility or taking refuge in the fact that a patient was desperately ill prior to anesthesia and operation may improve one's mortality figures, but it will not advance general knowledge or change one's own practices. On the other hand, one should not resort to self-flagellation, assuming responsibility for a fatality merely because an anesthetic was administered and death occurred.[6]

The last sentence is a moderate expression of the bias then prevailing in the review of postoperative death records. Improvement in anesthesia practices was thought sure to follow if anesthesiologists would substitute for denial a generous acceptance of responsibility for the unfavorable outcomes of surgical procedures. Dripps and colleagues also noted the most serious defect common to every study of anesthesia mortality: "We cannot provide individual protocols because of lack of space. This we realize is a serious omission, because it prevents others from gauging our material by their own standards." Instead of providing individual protocols, they tabulated the contribution of anesthesia to surgical mortality in broad categories such as inadequate preoperative preparation, hypotension, inexperience in anesthetic management, and inadequate postoperative ventilation. In only 10 of 80 patients in whom anesthesia definitely or probably contributed to death did they find "no anesthetic or surgical error in light of present knowledge." From records of the remaining 70 patients, they tallied 160 errors. With regard to Beecher and Todd's report, they concluded, "When deaths were related to the use of muscle relaxants, errors of omission or commission were always apparent. A plea is made for the preparation of detailed written death reports."[6]

Written Death Reports

To some degree, written death reports had in fact been implemented as early as 1945, by Ruth, with the establishment of a community-wide anesthesia study commission.[7] During the next 2 decades, many community- or state-wide commissions were established. These usually relied on voluntary submission of surgical death reports from a group of participating hospitals. Alternatively, some commissions, such as the well-known Baltimore Anesthesia Study Committee, obtained all death certificates filed with the Department of Health to collect data on all deaths within 36 hours of anesthetic administration.[8] Detailed reports of these deaths were solicited from the participating hospitals and were reviewed by the Committee. A similar voluntary reporting system with committee review existed in Great Britain.[9]

The study of anesthesia deaths by retrospective review of death records was of course the classic approach to the study of all disease. The expectation was that careful analysis of a large number of deaths would identify patterns or common denominators that would then clarify the role of anesthesia in surgical deaths and, as a consequence, improve anesthetic care. None of the studies could arrive at an incidence or rate, however, because the population from which the voluntarily submitted sample was drawn was never known.

Criteria for Anesthetic-related Deaths

An operative death was considered to be related to anesthesia by the opinion of a committee or, in some institutional studies, by the opinion of one reviewer. In view of the previously described bias, review of a death record actually consisted of a search for errors in surgical or anesthetic management; if neither was found, death was usually ascribed to the inexorable course of disease. The proportion of errors to patients varied with the study but was always greater than 1. "Errors" were departures from whatever was considered optimal anesthetic management at the time of review, and a causal relation between error and death was not required to categorize a death as anesthetic-related.

For example, the Baltimore Anesthesia Study Committee asked the following questions of each submitted death report.[8] Did the anesthetic management contribute to the death of this patient? If yes, was it primary or contributory? Which phase of the anesthetic management was principally at fault? Five choices were given for classifying the error, and all anesthetic deaths were included in some error category. Without an error, anesthesia management was considered not to have contributed to death. Details of these judgments were not recorded, and no allowance was made for a subsequent review based on changing concepts or knowledge. In their study of operating and recovery room deaths, Boba and Landmesser did not include deaths unless "anesthetic error contributed to or caused the collapse."[10]

"Preventable" Deaths

Given this bias in the review of death records, not surprisingly, published studies of anesthetic mortality generally report a predominance of "errors" and classify most anesthetic deaths as preventable. For example, regarding the almost 1600 records of anesthetic-related deaths collected on a voluntary basis in Great Britain over a 15-year period,[11] the investigators noted that "in the great majority of the reports there were departures from accepted practices." In a survey of anesthetic-contributory death in Groote Schuur Hospital, Harrison considered 54% to 93% as probably to possibly preventable.[12] Memery classified all anesthetic deaths collected from records at a large private practice as "errors."[13]

Inconsistencies

The patient population from whom these "errors" were collected showed some annoying inconsistencies. Most studies recognized cases in which surgery had been undertaken in desperation and in which a fatal outcome had been expected. Dripps and associates included patients with an American Society of Anesthesiologists (ASA) physical status of 5 (a moribund patient not expected to survive 24 hours with or without operation) in their anesthetic-related mortality,[6] whereas others excluded "inevitable deaths."[12,14] Deaths considered fortuitous, such as those attributable to pulmonary embolism and coronary thrombosis, were included inconsistently[11] or were excluded.[12] Finally, some studies identified a group of deaths that "cannot at present be fully explained and for which countermeasures are either lacking or largely empirical" but were still considered anesthetic-contributory deaths.[6,12]

In view of the bias in all these studies, their most serious defect is their failure to describe even briefly the circumstances of the deaths leading to the judgments so meticulously tabulated. Considering the vast changes in surgical practice, the advancement in the understanding of diseases, and the rapid growth of knowledge of anesthetics even in the past decade, these generally uninterpretable data are of little direct value today.

STUDIES OF ANESTHESIA IN SURGICAL MORTALITY

Since 1970, data from several additional studies directly relating to the epidemiology of anesthetic deaths have become available.[2] Though improved in some aspects of design and reporting compared with earlier studies, none has answered any critical questions, and none is immune to the criticisms expressed above.

New South Wales: 1960 to 1968

In 1970, a special committee that investigated anesthetic deaths in New South Wales from 1960 to 1968 published its accumulated findings.[15] Relying on voluntary reporting of deaths and coroners' reports, the committee classified deaths by three degrees of relation to the anesthetic: "reasonably certain," "some elements of doubt," and "caused by both the anesthetic and the surgical techniques." These categories were considered "true" anesthetic deaths, of which 286 reports were collected. Five other categories included surgical deaths, inevitable deaths, fortuitous deaths, deaths that could not be assessed despite considerable data, and deaths not assessed because of inadequate data. The number of "committee-defined" deaths (all eight categories) was 745, of which 151 were attributable entirely to the surgical technique and 234 were considered inevitable deaths. Of their bias, they state the following:

> In those cases classified in categories 1, 2, and 3, the Committee held that the anesthetic was in part or wholly responsible for the patient's death. This implies that there has been some error of judgement, management, or technique on the part of the anaesthetist, and these cases have been analyzed according to the error thought to have been involved.

They then identified 1215 errors in the 286 anesthetic-related deaths and classified them in 12 categories, such as inadequate preoperative preparation, inadequate resuscitation, incorrect choice of anesthetic technique, hypoxic gas mixture, overdose, or inadequate ventilation. The remainder of the report discussed each of these types of errors in a tutorial manner without further analysis of the specific event in each category.

Of special interest is that the committee's opinion with regard to errors in each death report was made available to the reporting anesthetist. In 141 (49%) of the 286 deaths, the responsible anesthetist disagreed with the committee's judgment of error. Of additional special interest is one conclusion of the report that states "anaesthetic agents themselves are not lethal except when they are misused."

1965 to 1969: The Study by Marx and Colleagues

Marx and colleagues reviewed all postanesthetic deaths in their institution over the 5-year period from 1965 to 1969.[16] The review was facilitated by computer storage of anesthetic records. Of all deaths, 83% were attributed to the patient's preexisting disease, 10% to the operation, 4% to anesthesia, and 3% to the postoperative management. Their report was unique in providing reasonably descriptive, though brief, details of the deaths related to anesthesia.

Of the 27 deaths primarily related to the anesthetic, 20 (74%) were considered preventable. The single most common cause was aspiration of vomitus, which occurred in 6 patients. The 7 unpreventable deaths "primarily related to anesthetic management" involved 3 patients with obstruction of a Carlen's tube by blood clot or tumor; 1 premature infant with hypothermia during laparotomy despite vigorous warming efforts; and 3 elderly patients on the fifth or sixth postoperative day who died of "bilateral bronchopneumonia following endotracheal intubation." These events are not further detailed, and the basis for judging those primarily related to the anesthetic was not recorded. Five of the 20 deaths attributed to errors in postoperative management were the result of pulmonary aspiration in nonanesthetized patients.

Postanesthetic Death

Bodlander[17] continued for a second decade the study of postanesthetic deaths first reported by Clifton and Hotten[14] from the same institution. Despite a large increase in the incidence of all postoperative deaths, those ascribed solely to anesthesia decreased from 29.9% to 3.7%—an enviable statistic, which they ascribed to improvement in numbers of senior anesthetic staff and the use of regional anesthesia for obstetric procedures. Primary anesthetic deaths were not described but were classified by cause in broad categories.

Cardiac Arrest

In a retrospective study of cardiac arrests in infants and children, Salem and colleagues reviewed 73 instances in which anesthesia was primarily responsible or importantly contributory to the arrest.[18] However, records of cardiac arrests not attributable to the anesthetic were not also collected, and no information on their incidence could be obtained. These investigators classified causes of arrest according to cardiovascular and respiratory factors and described some well-known patterns leading to cardiac arrest. One third of these patients died after arrest, and the investigators considered "most of these accidents preventable."

In a unique study, Taylor and associates reviewed 41 instances of cardiac arrest during operation from records supplied by a professional liability insurance company.[19] Presumably, all instances were the subject of litigation and represented a highly selective sample. More than half of the patients were healthy and of ASA physical status 1; none was categorized as physical status 4 or 5. Sixteen of the operations were minor, and 32 were elective.

The probable causes of cardiac arrest, according to the single reviewer who judged them, were anesthetic mismanagement in 9, cardiovascular abnormality in 9, hypoxia caused by hypoventilation in 18, and miscellaneous causes in 5 patients. Judgments as to causes of arrest were listed only very briefly, and no details of events leading to cardiac arrest in this group of healthy patients were given. The most surprising finding, but one that recurred in later studies, was the apparent failure to recognize arrest and institute resuscitation; only 3 of the 41 patients survived without neurologic deficit. These conclusions are in large part echoed in the 1988 closed-claims analysis of unexpected cardiac arrest during spinal anesthesia in another group of otherwise healthy young patients.[20]

The pattern of studies in the 1970s was not greatly different from that of earlier studies. Analyses continued to focus on "errors" that were barely described, and these judgments the investigators did not believe required documentation. In all early and many recent studies, no reporter believed it necessary to assure the reader that the cause ("error") led to the death.

ERROR AS A CAUSE OF ANESTHETIC DEATH

In 1948, Macintosh wrote, "I hold there should be no deaths due to anesthesia."[21] He is also claimed to have said, "The causes of anesthetic death are all too often mundane and obvious and rarely require much, if any, scientific investigation to establish them, provided a truthful account of the facts can be obtained."[22] Considering Macintosh's stature in the decades encompassing the modern anesthetic era, this statement more than likely represented the prevailing and enlightened view of anesthetic deaths during this period. Studies devised to discover the role of anesthesia in surgical mortality were actually designed to discover errors only. They were indeed successful in discovering an extraordinary number of "errors," most of which remain undescribed. What is surprising is the persistence and pervasiveness of this error bias to the present time.

The Error Bias

Clearly, human errors do play a role in the contribution of anesthesia to surgical mortality. Although certainly any error constitutes too large a role, it is of special importance in today's litigious medical climate to know if the term "large" means 10% or 90% of anesthetic deaths. High estimates of error have resulted from the deliberate search for errors; failure to seek out anesthetic causes other than error; lack of knowledge, until recently, of mechanisms of anesthetic death other than by error; and, particularly, the loose equating of "departure from current practice" with death. The failure to publish sufficient details of death so that the quality of judgments can be reviewed by others is a serious limitation to any reasonable estimate of error frequency. Because of the brevity of the details of some judgments in published reports, the relation of an identified error with a death strains one's cause–effect imagination.

Despite this general criticism, the generous reporting of errors clearly pointed to some patterns of anesthetic-associated deaths. When these patterns were sufficiently specific—such as aspiration of vomitus, circulatory collapse on change of position, failure of oxygen supply, or delay in institution of appropriate resuscitative measures—recognition was made of clinical situations that merit precaution, prevention, or other special attention. When identified patterns were not specific—such as inadequate preparation for anesthesia, incorrect choice of anesthetic technique, hypoventilation, or hypotension—little of educational value and nothing of value in identifying mechanisms or methods of prevention was gained.

Specific Problems

Two categories of anesthetic death by error, overdose and aspiration of vomitus, merit special comment.

Anesthetic Overdose

In almost every study reviewed, "overdose" is prominent as a cause of anesthesia mortality. Most reports identify overdose specifically with sodium thiopental, whereas others do not specify the agent and still others include overdose with inhalation agents as well. Amazingly, in no report is there a definition of what constitutes the toxic dose or "overdose" of thiopental or of any other agent. Regarding thiopental, Edwards and coworkers stated that "as little as 0.15 or 0.2 g caused sudden death."[9] If this observation is indeed true, the hemodynamic effects of thiopental urgently need reappraisal, considering its wide use even in seriously ill patients. Either the toxicity of thiopental is unappreciated, or "overdose" was not the cause of death. One can only speculate why this presumably common cause of anesthetic death was never investigated by experimentation.

Aspiration of Vomitus

Aspiration of vomitus continues to be a cause of mortality.[16,23] Anesthesiologists now generally agree that no method will prevent aspiration of vomitus with absolute certainty in a patient with a full stomach. Whether in an awake or anesthetized person, however, this event still is considered a cause of death related solely to the anesthetic and always preventable. A reappraisal of this position, however, is necessary. In patients with a full stomach who urgently require surgery, for whom no choice other than general anesthesia is appropriate and who then aspirate despite all proper precautions, death cannot be considered to have resulted from an error or to have been preventable. The proper alternative view is that aspiration constitutes a known risk of anesthesia in these patients, a risk they accept as part of the informed consent process.

Preventable Errors

Other patterns of anesthetic death clearly pointed to errors that are preventable and do not strain the cause–effect relation. Among these are death resulting from high spinal or epidural anesthesia in conventional doses; excessive doses of local anesthetics or of neostigmine; obstructed endotracheal tubes; intubation of the esophagus; failure of the oxygen supply; disconnection of a ventilator; air embolism as a result of infusion; bilateral pneumothorax unrelated to the operation; and administration of the wrong drug.

Remedial Measures

The preceding list only provides examples of clearly preventable errors that can lead to death and that require little judgment to establish a mechanism. Knowledge of these errors has led to the invention or use of devices or methods to decrease the likelihood of error and death: wide availability of resuscitation drugs and equipment; improved nonkinking endotracheal tubes with better cuffs; fail-safe oxygen delivery systems; pulse oximeters and capnographs to assess oxygenation and ventilation; low-pressure and low–minute volume alarms to indicate disconnection of a ventilator; plastic infusion containers that can be vented before pressurization; and improved labeling of drug containers (still to be achieved in some cases). The now famous study of cardiac arrest during spinal anesthesia provides a model of error patterns that can promptly lead to remedial measures or may at least stimulate a search for them.[24]

Critical Incidents

Another promising approach to the detection of error patterns and direction of preventive measures has been described by Cooper and associates.[25] Their approach does not require a death to identify an error. Using a nonspecific interview technique, investigators asked anesthesiologists and trainees to describe "near misses" experienced or observed at any time in the past during administration of anesthesia. These critical incidents were categorized as attributable to human error (82%) or equipment failure (14%). Such studies, it is hoped, will describe specific error patterns, which can then be eliminated.

Potential Role in Anesthetic Mortality

Certainly the critical incident approach is a fruitful approach to identifying the potential role of errors in anesthesia mortality. Although it will not define the actual role of errors, the data obtained can significantly strengthen any cause–effect relations between error and postanesthetic death. For example, how long can a ventilator be disconnected without death? How often were X mL of drug Y mistakenly injected for drug Z without ill effects? How often did air embolism not lead to mortality? With such data supporting or not supporting cause–effect relations, the true role of error in anesthesia mortality may one day be approximated.

ANESTHETIC DEATHS THAT ARE NOT THE RESULT OF ERROR

The pervasive bias of error in all considerations of anesthetic death probably impeded progress in the discovery of causes of anesthetic death by other means, because the effects of this bias are so profound.

Adverse Drug Reactions

This bias leads to the assumption that drugs used during anesthesia are different from all other drugs, that they exhibit no idiosyncrasies, that patients do not show hypersensitivity, and that interactions with other drugs and disease do not occur. Adverse responses to these drugs are thought to result only when they are misused. Perhaps this view is derived secondarily from the concepts, once widely held as fundamental, that inhalation agents were inert and were not metabolized and that blood and brain levels of anesthetics could be controlled at will.

The naiveté of assuming that anesthetics are innocuous is equivalent to that of believing, for instance, that antibiotic toxicity is always caused by an overdose error and is unrelated to the severity of infection or that digitalis toxicity is caused by an error unrelated to the degree of heart failure. The same naiveté characterizes drug surveillance studies that ascribe all untoward events in patients with disease treated by medication to adverse drug reactions, regardless of whether a cause–effect relation can be demonstrated and independent of the stage of disease treated. These attitudes completely ignore well-established concepts of clinical pharmacology, such as the interpatient variability in response to a drug dose, influence of specific diseases on drug responses, drug interactions, enzyme induction, active drug metabolites, and pharmacogenetics.

Anesthetic Agents

Until recently, these pharmacologic principles were not conceived as applying to anesthetic drugs in humans. The opinion has been that anesthetic agents themselves are not lethal except when misused. Drugs used in clinical anesthesia are potent and potentially lethal, and, like all drugs, anesthetics have primary desired actions and unwanted side effects. At times side effects become unintentionally severe and noxious and constitute an adverse drug reaction, which may be fatal.

Fatalities from drug administration, anesthetic or otherwise, even when cause and effect can be demonstrated, are not tantamount to error. For example, suppose 0.2 mg atropine is given to treat sudden mesenteric traction–related bradycardia and hypotension in a patient with mitral stenosis who has received digitalis and who is undergoing vaginal hysterectomy with epidural anesthesia. Instead of the anticipated result of this logical action, severe tachycardia and pulmonary edema develop, resulting in death. Clearly this is an adverse drug reaction during anesthesia. It is not an error, but it is related to the hazard of administration of atropine to patients with mitral stenosis.

Similar examples include the consequences of excessive hypertension from an average dose of vasopressor or profound respiratory depression from a conventional dose of narcotic. Drugs, like all therapeutic modalities, are prescribed in anticipation of benefits and at the risk of adverse responses. Never have drugs used during anesthesia been excluded from this basic therapeutic principle with justification.

Anesthetic Techniques

This dictum applies equally to anesthetic techniques, as in the following example. Profound muscle relaxation is required to permit a surgeon to accomplish a therapeutic operation to relieve severe intestinal obstruction in a seriously ill patient. This relaxation is best achieved by large but conventional doses of muscle relaxants. Failure of the patient to breathe after surgery is an accepted risk; its consequence is prolongation of tracheal intubation and the need for mechanical ventilation. When bilateral bronchopneumonia develops and the patient dies several days later, the previous use of large doses of muscle relaxants does not constitute an error or adverse drug reaction; it is simply a risk necessarily taken to effect a lifesaving therapy.

Knowledge Concerning Mechanisms of Anesthetic Death

Previously Unknown Factors

A second implication of the bias of ever-present errors in anesthesia mortality is that it explicitly precludes any new knowledge concerning mechanisms of death attributable to anesthesia.[24] I have indicated the few instances in which deaths that are not obviously attributable to any error are even mentioned. It is precisely in this group that one should explore for undescribed and subtle mechanisms by which anesthetics contribute to mortality.[26] Discovery of major new mechanisms of anesthetic death during the past 20 years did not follow from any study directed to anesthesia mortality by review of death reports. Succinylcholine-induced hyperkalemia, malignant hyperthermia, genetic variants in plasma cholinesterase, post-halothane hepatitis, and methoxyflurane nephrotoxicity were discovered by alert clinicians investigating adverse effects not attributable to error. Current studies of the immunosuppressant properties of general anesthetics may yet reveal even more subtle mechanisms.[26] One can properly wonder how deaths from these causes were classified by omniscient committees before these new mechanisms were described.

Confounding Variables

Delineation of the role of anesthesia in surgical mortality still requires a definition of anesthetic deaths that are not the result of error. Elements of this definition are described elsewhere in this book. Difficulties in identifying other elements have been considered.[2] The most obvious difficulty is that, with rare exception, anesthesia is not therapeutic and is administered only to facilitate some other goal. No controlled study of the hazards of operation without anesthesia will ever be performed. The hazards of anesthesia therefore can never be considered independent of a second procedure. Risks and benefits of anesthesia are confounded with a disease state, with an operation or manipulation by a second set of persons who act primarily independently, and, finally, with a third set of persons who care for patients while they are still vulnerable to the adverse effects of anesthesia.

In this complex interaction of procedures and personnel, differentiation of the adverse effects of anesthetics from surgically induced effects, nonanesthetic drug–induced effects, and adverse responses induced by nursing procedures is difficult if not impossible. This complexity applies particularly to patients with serious systemic disease undergoing hazardous operations and requiring maximum postoperative care. In these patients an anesthetic may contribute importantly to overall surgical mortality, but complexity and ignorance of what to look for impede progress.

Factors Contributing to Overall Surgical Mortality

Interhospital Variability

The challenge seems almost overwhelming in view of the difficulties now recognized in attempting to identify factors contributing to overall surgical mortality, of which anesthesia mortality is only a part. A by-product of the National Halothane Study[5] was the discovery of the large differences in surgical mortality for specific operations among the participating hospitals.[27] These could not be explained by any readily identifiable differences in patient populations and led to a larger study undertaken by the Stanford Center for Health Care Research.[28,29] The outcomes after 15 categories of surgical operations in 17 hospitals were adjusted for physical status, stage of surgical disease, age, sex, stress level, and insurance coverage. When so standardized, substantial and significant differences among hospitals in mortality and severe morbidity measures still existed. These differences correlated poorly with the qualifications of the medical and nursing staffs.

The investigators[28] postulated that postoperative adjusted mortality and morbidity rates are most likely to correlate with hospital features related to organizational and sociologic structure rather than measurable characteristics of the patient population. Anesthesia mortality as a subset of surgical mortality incorporates most of these same variables. Identification of its role in overall surgical mortality is not readily forthcoming.

Future Studies Involving Healthy Patients

Discovery of other mechanisms in anesthesia mortality may be more feasible in a less complex milieu. For example, a study of anesthesia limited to patients not expected to die might reveal new mechanisms, although these mechanisms would not be subtle or applicable to the critically ill. Patients of ASA physical status 1 or 2 (healthy or with mild systemic disease producing no limitation of activity, respectively) who are undergoing operations that are not life-threatening might exhibit adverse anesthetic effects that become more visible in relation to the smaller distortions resulting from operation. Detailed reports of deaths in these patients now have been published, although they are few.[20] In such a group at least the frequency of error as a cause of death could be identified more easily. Among the rest, a search for new mechanisms could realistically begin.

Analysis of Death Reports

Those of us who have participated regularly in mortality conferences for a sufficiently long period remember at least one reasonably healthy patient who underwent a non–life-threatening operation and who died unexpectedly during or shortly after operation. As an example, suppose a 50-year-old man undergoing subtotal gastrectomy for peptic ulcer disease cannot be resuscitated after cardiac arrest during operation. According to the death record, a summary prepared by the anesthesiologist, preoperative anesthetic and surgical management were impeccable. Autopsy reveals diffuse mild coronary disease without occlusion, lung changes consistent with chronic bronchitis, and duodenal ulcer. None of these changes can account for death. How can such an event be explained?

Three mechanisms are possible: Death was fortuitous and was part of the obligatory mortality of hospitalized patients; death was caused by a mechanism as yet undiscovered; or (if Macintosh's view[22] is accepted), the anesthesiologist who prepared the death report lied, and no further investigation is necessary. This last possibility is no longer tenable intellectually in view of increasing knowledge of the clinical pharmacologic characteristics of anesthetic drugs.[24] The image of the guilt-laden anesthesiologist accepting all unanticipated and unexplained outcomes of surgical therapy as a consequence of error has become counterproductive.

Further progress requires that reports be accepted as true accounts, that they be collected in a repository or registry, that cause–effect relations be sought according to rigorous scientific standards, and that admission of ignorance is acceptable when no causes can be found. These steps are now being taken with closed-claims studies. The ASA will soon enter its second decade of these analyses.[20,30–33]

Sudden Death

Incidence

Study of the healthy population also may quantify the role of the obligatory death rate of hospitalization in surgical mortality, described in one of my earlier publications.[2] More than 350,000 Americans annually are expected to die of sudden death syndrome, defined as unexpected natural death occurring within 1 hour after collapse of an individual in apparent good health.[34] Assuming that 16 to 20 million operations are performed annually, with a mean hospitalization of 5 days per patient, there are 80 to 100 million person-days during which any death would be part of surgical mortality. If the day of and day after operation are assumed to be the vulnerable period for anesthetic-associated mortality, 32 to 40 million person-days are available during which any of the 350,000 occurrences of sudden death syndrome could be considered anesthetic mortality.

Causes

Although almost all of these deaths are assumed to be the result of a fatal dysrhythmia resulting from coronary artery disease, increasing recent interest in sudden death reveals a disconcerting number of cases that cannot be accounted for by autopsy findings. Not surprisingly, in many patients with occult or even clinically identified coronary artery disease, autopsy does not show an anatomic cause for the fatal event. Mitral valve prolapse syndrome, coronary artery spasm (Prinzmetal's angina), prolonged QT interval, and silent ischemia can lead to sudden death without evidence at autopsy.

Relation to Anesthetic Mortality

Sudden deaths that are not the result of heat stroke occur every fall among college football players and other students. Autopsies often show cardiovascular abnormalities, but they are usually insufficient to account for death. Unexplained sudden death is well known among healthy soldiers. Crib death (sudden infant death syndrome) is a similar enigma in infants; cardiovascular abnormalities may be revealed at autopsy, but they are not severe enough to have been diagnosed ante mortem or to have caused death. By no reasonable approximation can sudden death syndrome account for a large portion of deaths associated with anesthesia. Of great significance, however, is its existence and its potential to cause death during anesthesia or in the early postoperative period. A diagnosis of anesthetic death should never be made by exclusion. The possibility of sudden death syndrome requires that anesthetic causes be reasonably related to death before a judgment of anesthetic death is accepted.

KNOWLEDGE ABOUT ANESTHESIA AND SURGICAL MORTALITY

Little is known about the role of anesthesia in surgical mortality. Forty years of self-flagellation in anesthesia mortality studies has generated an abundance of anesthetic "errors." Some of these "errors" survive the test of the cause–effect relation. Some anesthetic deaths have been caused by human error or equipment failure. We have no idea of their frequency. All other generated "errors" now exist only in the vague memory of the omniscient committees that equated deviation from accepted practice, as perceived during the particular year of review, with "error," and "error" with anesthetic death. The need for evidence of a causal relation was waived in the belief that inclusion of even the most remote relations would improve standards of practice. Knowing the bias that generated the data, we should consider as unacceptable all published estimates of the incidence of anesthetic deaths; for all practical purposes this incidence is unknown. Potential mechanisms of anesthetic death are the subject of this book. Their frequency as a contribution to overall surgical mortality is yet to be determined.

Presumption of Innocence

A fresh approach is needed in this determination. Anesthesiology consists of the administration of a variety of potent drugs, engages in numerous maneuvers requiring technical skill and the use of mechanical equipment, and necessitates knowledge of equipment function and malfunction. In every aspect of this activity, something is actively done to a patient; during any phase of it, any untoward event may be attributed to an immediately preceding action by simple post hoc reasoning.

Whereas untoward events in specialties of medicine in which there is less interaction with the patient are readily ascribed to the patient's disease or an unrelated fortuitous event, the almost continuous ministrations of the anesthesiologist leave him or her vulnerable to the easy post hoc hypothesis. Demonstration of a cause–effect relation is absolutely essential if any secure knowledge of mechanisms of anesthetic death is to be achieved. In consideration of deaths during anesthesia, a presumption of innocence must be substituted for one of guilt until cause and effect are demonstrated.

Risk–Benefit Computation

The anesthesiologist's application of drugs, maneuvers, techniques, and machines to patients must be viewed on the same risk–benefit scale as all forms of medical therapy. Each is designed to benefit total surgical care. However, each also carries risk in terms of adverse drug reactions, unwanted outcomes of technical maneuvers, and malfunction of machines, including erroneous information from monitors actually designed to increase safety. Risks exist because they are not completely preventable by the most skilled and knowledgeable human. Patients react to drugs individually in a spectrum of responses not usually predictable and at times adverse.

Individual humans are not anatomically the same, and all technical maneuvers cannot be consistently successful.[35,36] Machines do not perform optimally at all times. Risks may occur in the hands of the most competent anesthesiologist using techniques and drugs faultlessly and conscientiously while caring for the patient. These risks, alone or in combination, may lead to anesthetic death. Death during anesthesia is possible without error or agent toxicity, which are precisely the risks that need to be quantified to determine the role of anesthesia in surgical mortality. With respect to prevention, if no actions are taken, no risks are assumed, and all untoward events are prevented.

Finally, more attention needs to be given to the sudden death syndrome in the hospital population, both in adults and children. Active specialties of medical practice, such as anesthesiology and surgery, are absorbing responsibility for these deaths as related to their therapy. Doing so not only confounds estimates of risk and mortality, but also leads to malpractice litigation and costly defensive anesthesia practices that do not represent optimal patient care.

MORTALITY IN THE PAST TEN YEARS

Suggested Incidence

We remain without an accurate estimate of anesthetic-related mortality. Studies that attempted to derive an incidence have largely followed the format of earlier studies and perpetuate many of their deficiencies. Particularly deficient is the continued lack of reasonable descriptions of the events that have been judged to represent anesthetic mortality. The lack of accurate data indicates the overwhelming need for some expression of the magnitude of the problem in the United States. To satisfy this need while acknowledging the intuitive nature of the estimate, experts[37] commonly cite 200 to 10,000 deaths related to anesthesia, or 1 to 5 deaths per 10,000 anesthetics annually in the United States.

Descriptive Terminology

In the absence of descriptions of events considered to represent anesthetic-related mortality, the lack of common terminology for classification of these events ("taxonomy") has been recognized as a serious impediment to communication and progress in this area. Generalizations such as "failure of airway management" or "circulatory collapse" simply do not describe the events sufficiently and do not provide a basis for comparing data from several sources or for remedying any identified causes. Systems for classification of adverse outcomes based on process or organ affected, anesthesia management area, or simply an extended list have now been established.[38–40]

Classification

An earlier sign of progress was the classification system used in summarizing anesthetic accidents reported to the Medical Defense Union of the United Kingdom.[39] The reviewers combined deaths and severe cerebral damage in a single category and divided them into those "apparently due to misadventure" and "apparently due to error." "Misadventure" was defined as an unlucky chance or accident, an event "one is not able to protect oneself adequately against" and included "coexisting disease, drug sensitivity, halothane hepatic failure, hyperthermia, blood loss, and embolism." However, most significantly, it included the category "unknown." Accidents apparently due to error were not meaningfully classified. Of the 348 events summarized, 35% were attributed mainly to misadventure and 65% to error.

Continued Critical Incident Studies

Cooper and associates continued their innovative studies of critical incidents by using a technique designed specifically to discover the frequency and causes of errors and to suggest remedial measures.[40] Critical to the validity of this technique is the demonstration of some relation between errors discovered and negative outcome. They were successful in doing so when "substantive negative outcomes" were defined as death, cardiac arrest, canceled procedure, or increased stay in recovery room, intensive care unit, or hospital.

However, the process by which a critical incident led to a negative outcome was not described, and the quality of the judgment used in establishing the relation was not available for review by others. The primary strength of critical-incident studies is that human errors and equipment failure can continue to be observed and documented and remedial action can be taken without knowledge of incidence or adverse outcome. Based on critical-incidence studies and reviews of malpractice claims, measures to prevent breathing-circuit disconnections and undetected esophageal intubation have been vigorously explored, even though the frequencies of their occurrence are unknown. This method in part forms the basis for modern quality assurance and risk management.[41]

Sudden Death Revisited

Sudden cardiac death in young, ostensibly healthy children and adults occurs during exercise and during rest and continues to be an enigma. Although in many victims a cardiovascular abnormality can be found at autopsy, the abnormality is not always severe enough to account for death and in many cases would not have been diagnosed during life.[42] In 10% of one group of young children and adults who died suddenly, no cardiac or other abnormality was found.[43] An abnormal cardiac conduction mechanism probably accounts for some of these cases.[44]

To add to the mystery, sudden death during sleep has been described among young, healthy Southeast Asian refugees,[45] and sinus arrest for as long as 9 seconds has been observed in healthy young adults during rapid–eye-movement sleep.[46] The extent to which these unusual and rare deaths may occur in young, healthy patients during general anesthesia remains worthy of consideration.

Newer Observations

Regarding mechanisms of death related to anesthesia, some new observations are provocative. The prolonged QT interval that may follow right radical neck dissection can lead to tachyrhythmia and circulatory failure in the postoperative period.[47] Malignant dysrhythmias in the absence of pyrexia appeared in four nonanesthetized patients with malignant hyperthermia susceptibility, suggesting a myocardial muscle abnormality as a genetic variant of the malignant hyperthermia syndrome.[48]

Anaphylactic and anaphylactoid reactions to intravenous drugs administered or even latex gloves used during anesthesia or surgery do not appear to be as rare as once supposed.[49–50] Finally, reviewers are now putting into print what I long have contended would be the case: some adverse events occur for which no explanation based on current knowledge is possible, yet no negligence, error, or fault is demonstrable. Although it relates to morbidity rather than mortality, the recently published ASA closed-claims reports on peripheral nerve injury associated with anesthesia are prime examples.[51,52]

REFERENCES

1. Keats AS: The estimate of the anesthetic risk in medical evaluations. Am J Cardiol 12:330, 1963
2. Goldstein A Jr, Keats AS: The risk of anesthesia. Anesthesiology 33:130, 1970
3. Beecher HK, Todd DP: A study of the deaths associated with anesthesia and surgery. Ann Surg 140:2, 1954
4. Abajian J Jr, Arrowwood JG, Barrett RH, et al: Critique of 'A study of the deaths associated with anesthesia and surgery.' Ann Surg 142:138, 1955
5. Bunker JP, Forest WH, Mosteller F, et al. The National Halothane Study. Bethesda, MD: National Institute of General Medical Sciences, 1969
6. Dripps RD, Lamont A, Eckenhoff JE: The role of anesthesia in surgical mortality. JAMA 178:261, 1961
7. Ruth HS: Anesthesia study commissions. JAMA 127:514, 1945
8. Phillips OC, Frazier TM, Graff TD, et al: The Baltimore Anesthesia Study Committee: review of 1024 postoperative deaths. JAMA 174:2015, 1960
9. Edwards G, Morton HJV, Pask EA, et al: Deaths associated with anaesthesia: Report on 1000 cases. Anaesthesia 11:194, 1956
10. Boba A, Landmesser CM: Total cardiorespiratory collapse (cardiac arrest). New York State Journal of Medicine 61:2928, 1961
11. Dinnick OP: Deaths associated with anaesthesia. Anaesthesia 19:536, 1964
12. Harrison GG: Anesthetic contributory death: its incidence and causes—I. incidence; II. causes. S Afr Med J 42:514, 1968
13. Memery HN: Anesthesia mortality in private practice: a ten year study. JAMA 194:1185, 1965
14. Clifton BS, Hotten WIT: Deaths associated with anaesthesia. Br J Anaesth 35:250, 1963
15. Special Committee Investigating Deaths Under Anaesthesia: Report on 745 classified cases, 1960-1968. Med J Aust 1:573, 1970
16. Marx GF, Mateo CV, Orkin LR: Computer analysis of postanesthetic deaths. Anesthesiology 39:54, 1973
17. Bodlander FM: Deaths associated with anaesthesia. Br J Anaesth 47:35, 1975
18. Salem MR, Bennett EJ, Schweiss JF, et al: Cardiac arrest related to anesthesia: contributing factors in infants and children. JAMA 233:238, 1975
19. Taylor G, Larson CP Jr, Prestwich R: Unexpected cardiac arrest during anesthesia and surgery: an environmental study. JAMA 236:2758, 1976
20. Caplan RA, Ward RN, Posner K, et al: Unexpected cardiac arrest during spinal anesthesia: a closed claims analysis of predisposing factors. Anesthesiology 68:5, 1988
21. Macintosh R: Deaths under anaesthetics. Br J Anaesth 21:107, 1948
22. Macintosh R: Quoted by Wylie WD: 'There, but for the grace of God . . .' Ann R Coll Surg Engl 56:171, 1975
23. Chadwick HS, Posner KL, Caplan RA, et al: A comparison of obstetric and nonobstetric anesthesia malpractice claims. Anesthesiology 74:242, 1991
24. Keats AS: Anesthesia mortality: a new mechanism. Anesthesiology 68:2, 1988
25. Cooper JB, Newbower RS, Long CB, et al: Preventable anesthesia mishaps: a human factors study. Anesthesiology 49:399, 1978
26. Aleixo LL, Layon AJ, Peck AB, et al: Effects of halothane anesthesia on immune function and outcome from a septic challenge in healthy mice (abstract). Crit Care Med 20:S77, 1992
27. Moses LE, Mosteller F: Institutional differences in postoperative death rates. JAMA 203:492, 1968
28. Scott WR, Forrest WH Jr, Brown BW Jr: Hospital structure and

postoperative mortality and morbidity. In Shortell SM, Brown M (eds): Organizational research in hospitals. Chicago: Blue Cross Association, 1976: 72

29. Stanford Center for Health Care Research: Comparison of hospitals with regard to outcomes of surgery. Health Serv Res 11: 112, 1976
30. Davis DA: An analysis of anesthetic mishaps from medical liability claims. Int Anesthesiol Clin 22:31, 1984
31. Caplan RA, Posner KL, Ward RJ, et al: Adverse respiratory events in anesthesia: a closed-claims analysis. Anesthesiology 72:828, 1990
32. Tinker JH, Dull DL, Caplan RA, et al: Role of monitoring devices in prevention of anesthesia mishaps. Anesthesiology 71:541, 1989
33. Cheney FW, Posner KL, Caplan RA: Adverse respiratory events infrequently leading to malpractice suits. Anesthesiology 75: 932, 1991
34. Doyle JT: Mechanisms and prevention of sudden death. Modern Concepts in Cardiovascular Disease 45:111, 1976
35. Van Gessel EF, Forster A, Gamulin Z: Continuous spinal anesthesia: where do spinal catheters go? Anesth Analg 76:1004, 1993
36. Hogan QH: Tuffier's line: the normal distribution of anatomic parameters. Anesth Analg 78:194, 1994
37. Davies JM, Strunin L: Anaesthesia in 1984: how safe is it? Can Med Assoc J 131:437, 1984
38. Harrison GG: Anaesthetic accidents. Clinics in Anaesthesiology 1:415, 1983
39. Utting JE, Gray TC, Shelley FC: Human misadventures in anaesthesia. Can Anaesth Soc J 26:472, 1979
40. Cooper JB, Newbower RS, Kitz RJ: An analysis of major errors and equipment failures in anesthetic management: considerations for prevention and detection. Anesthesiology 60:218, 1984
41. Cohen JA: Quality assurance and risk management. In Gravenstein N (ed): Manual of complications during anesthesia. Philadelphia: JB Lippincott, 1991: 1
42. Maron BJ, Roberts WC, McAllister HA, et al: Sudden death in young athletes. Circulation 62:218, 1980
43. Topaz O, Edwards JE: Pathologic features of sudden death in children, adolescents, and young adults. Chest 87:476, 1985
44. Benson DW, Benditt DG, Anderson RW, et al: Cardiac arrest in young, ostensibly healthy patients: clinical, hemodynamic, and electrophysiologic findings. Am J Cardiol 52:65, 1983
45. Baron RC, Thacker SB, Gorelkin L, et al: Sudden death among southeast Asian refugees: an unexplained nocturnal phenomenon. JAMA 250:2947, 1983
46. Guilleminault C, Pool P, Motta J, et al: Sinus arrest during REM sleep in young adults. N Engl J Med 311:1006, 1984
47. Otteni JC, Pottecher T, Bronner G, et at: Prolongation of the QT interval and sudden cardiac arrest following right radical neck dissection. Anesthesiology 59:358, 1983
48. Huckell VF, Staniloff HM, Britt BA, et al: Cardiac manifestations of malignant hyperthermia susceptibility. Circulation 58:916, 1978
49. Fisher M McD, More DG: The epidemiology and clinical features of anaphylactic reactions in anaesthesia. Anaesth Intensive Care 9:226, 1981
50. Gold M, Swartz JS, Braude BM, et al: Intraoperative anaphylaxis: an association with latex sensitivity. J Allergy Clin Immunol 87: 662, 1991
51. Kroll DA, Caplan RA, Posner K, et al: Nerve injury associated with anesthesia. Anesthesiology 73:202, 1990
52. Stoelting RK: Postoperative ulnar nerve palsy: is it a preventable complication? Anesth Analg 76:7, 1993

FURTHER READING

Brown DL: Risk and outcome in anesthesia. Philadelphia: JB Lippincott, 1992: 1

Pierce EC Jr, Cooper JB (eds): Analysis of anesthetic mishaps. Int Anesthesiol Clin 22:1, 1984

Complications in Anesthesiology, second edition,
edited by Nikolaus Gravenstein and Robert R. Kirby.
Lippincott-Raven Publishers, Philadelphia © 1996.

CHAPTER 4

The Hazards of Viral Hepatitis and Acquired Immunodeficiency Syndrome

Jules L. Dienstag
A. J. Layon

Hepatitis and human immunodeficiency virus (HIV) are perhaps the two most significant infectious occupational hazards for those of us who work in the operating room. Despite failure to cultivate most of the strains of these viruses in vitro, rapid progress has been made in our understanding of them. Although both diseases have been recognized as an occupational hazard in the health care professions for many years, recent discoveries have increased our awareness of and sensitivity to the problem of transmission from patients to health care personnel and have provided us some methods for prevention.

The risk of hepatitis exposure among hospital workers increases as a function of contact with patients' blood. Often more difficult to control and much less publicized is the exposure of operating room staff to hepatitis viruses in saliva and other secretions. Hepatitis B virus (HBV) is approximately 100 times more infectious than is the human immunodeficiency virus (HIV) when blood-borne and is 10 times more prevalent among health care workers than is HIV.[1]

In 1988, approximately 56,773 cases of hepatitis were reported. Of this total, 28,507 were hepatitis A; 23,177 were hepatitis B; 2600 were non-A, non-B hepatitis; and 2500 nonspecific cases were recorded.[1] The decreasing percentage of nonspecified cases by 1992–310 of 21,452–presumably reflects improved serologic testing for non-A, non-B hepatitis.[2]

CLASSIFICATION OF HEPATITIS

The terms "infectious hepatitis" and "serum hepatitis" have been used to describe what we call today "viral hepatitis type A" and "viral hepatitis type B," respectively. We know, however, that epidemiologic and clinical patterns of infection with these viruses often overlap and that the older, descriptive terms are both inadequate and misleading. Viral hepatitis is now classified by etiologic agent when serologic testing can implicate one of the following viruses.

Hepatitis A Virus

Hepatitis A virus (HAV) is a ribonucleic acid (RNA) virus of unusual stability to heat, acid, and ether inactivation; it has been classified as enterovirus type 72. Infection with HAV results in a relatively mild acute hepatitis after an incubation period of 15 to 50 days (Fig. 4-1). After its short incubation period and mild acute stage, HAV illness rarely lasts more than 2 to 4 weeks. The subclinical attack rate far exceeds the frequency of overt clinical illness.

Until recently, much of our information about this virus had been generated by epidemiologic studies and transmission experiments in volunteers. Accelerated progress followed the identification of the virus by immune electron microscopy and the development of animal models using marmoset monkeys and chimpanzees. The virus has now been cultivated in vitro, and its entire genome has been characterized.[3–5]

Hepatitis B Virus

Much has been learned about HBV in the years since the discovery of the "Australia antigen." What was originally called the Australia antigen is actually an element of the coat protein of HBV. The coat protein antigen appears in great abundance in the serum of infected persons. HBV is a deoxyribonucleic

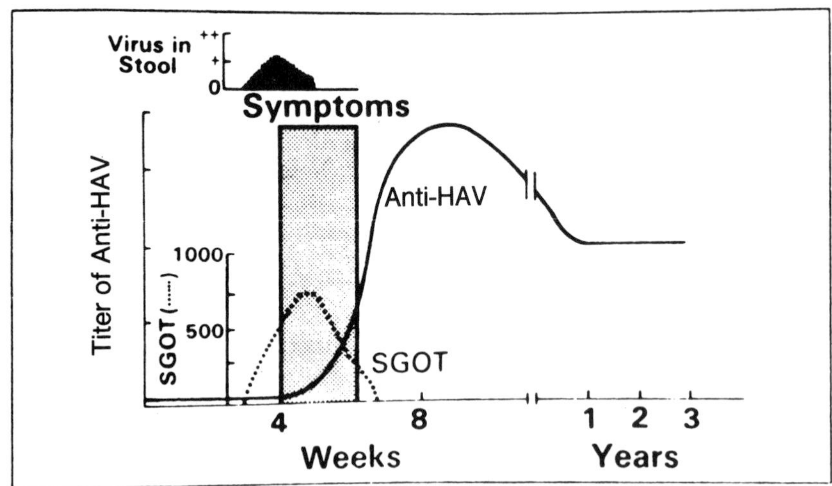

FIGURE 4-1. The sequence of events of HAV infection. Virus excretion in stool predates any symptom. The aspartate aminotransferase (serum glutamic-oxaloacetic transaminase [*SGOT*]) is elevated before and anti-HAV is elevated after onset of symptoms. (Lamont JT: Viral hepatitis. In Stein JH (ed): Internal medicine. Boston: Little, Brown, 1983.)

acid (DNA) virus containing a circular, partially double-stranded DNA genome and an endogenous DNA polymerase.

Viral hepatitis B accounts for a large proportion of cases initially described as serum hepatitis. It also is implicated in approximately half of the hepatitis cases unrelated to percutaneous exposure to contaminated blood products. Asymptomatic chronic carriers serve as the major reservoir of infection and constitute approximately 0.1% of the population in the United States and Western Europe. Frequencies as high as 5% to 20% are found in tropical and economically underdeveloped areas. Illness occurs after a long incubation period of 30 to 180 days and is commonly heralded by a serum-sickness–like prodrome of arthritis or rash and fever. The incubation period is modified by the size and portal of the inoculum; for instance, infusion of 50 mL of infected blood may result in surface antigenemia in only a few weeks, whereas a 50-μL inoculation usually results in surface antigenemia after 3 to 4 months (Fig. 4-2).

Duration of the illness is quite variable, but most infected persons recover within approximately 3 to 4 months. On the other hand, fulminant hepatitis, persistent hepatitis, and chronic active hepatitis, as well as a protracted carrier state, follow acute HBV in a small percentage of cases. Several subtypes of HBV have been identified, but the subtype does not determine severity or chronicity of the illness.[6,7]

δ Hepatitis

The δ agent, which produces δ hepatitis, contains defective RNA and requires the presence of hepatitis B for its own replication. HBV and the δ virus can infect a susceptible person simultaneously (coinfection), or the δ agent can superinfect someone who is already chronically infected with hepatitis B.

Its epidemiologic properties are similar to those of HBV; however, geographic differences exist in the predominant modes of transmission. In Mediterranean countries, δ hepatitis is transmitted by person-to-person spread, whereas in North America and northern Europe it is spread primarily by percutaneous inoculation such as transfusion or intravenous drug abuse. The clinical importance of δ hepatitis is its tendency to be associated with a poorer outcome than is hepatitis B:

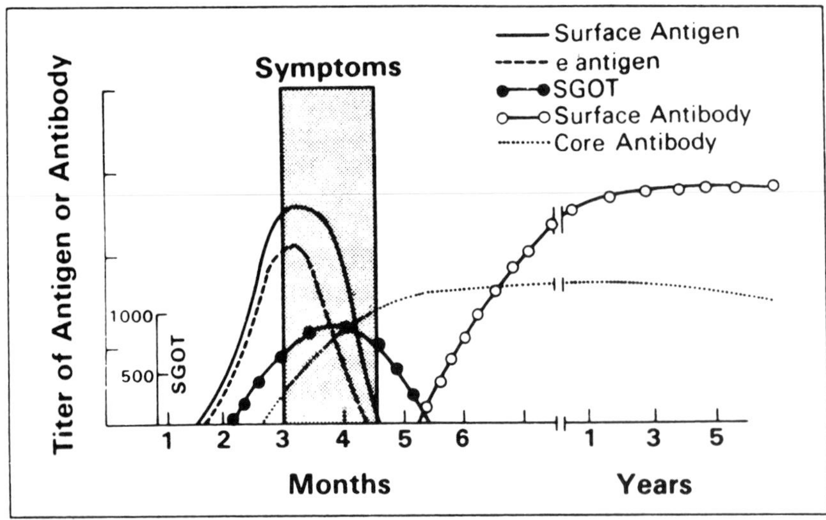

FIGURE 4-2. The sequence of events of infection with HBV. Both hepatitis B surface antigen and hepatitis B e antigen (which correlate with infectivity) are in relatively high concentration before the onset of symptoms. The late appearance of the surface antigen usually implies a successful host response to HBV. [*SGOT*, serum glutamic-oxaloacetic transaminase. (LaMont JT: Viral hepatitis. In Stein JH (ed): Internal Medicine. Boston: Little, Brown, 1983.)

fulminant hepatitis and severe, progressive, chronic active hepatitis are seen more frequently.[8,9]

Non-A, Non-B Hepatitis

Until recently, only HAV and HBV had been recognized; however, in many patients with hepatitis, failure of sensitive serologic tests to detect either of these two viruses, cytomegalovirus (CMV), or Epstein-Barr virus (EBV), suggested that one or more other pathogens exist. The diagnosis of non-A, non-B viral hepatitis requires a negative result on HAV and HBV serologic tests; also, hepatotoxic drug exposure must be ruled out, and an incubation period and mode of transmission epidemiologically associated with viral hepatitis must be identified.

To date, non-A, non-B hepatitis has been found to contribute to transfusion-associated hepatitis, multiple bouts of hepatitis in illicit-drug users, and hepatitis after renal transplantation.[10,11] In addition, cases of non-A, non-B hepatitis have appeared in hemodialysis units, within families and institutions, and in occupationally exposed medical personnel. Both short (2 to 4 weeks) and long (1 to 3 months) incubation periods have been recorded for cases occurring after percutaneous exposure. This observation as well as the occasional occurrence of two bouts of non-A, non-B hepatitis in a single patient and the results of cross-challenge experiments in chimpanzees demonstrate that more than one viral agent is responsible. Differences in biochemical properties and ultrastructural hepatocyte alterations provide additional clinical and epidemiologic support for at least two distinct viruses.

Clinically and epidemiologically, non-A, non-B hepatitis resembles HBV infection: it occurs after parenteral exposure and is highly endemic in some groups but is not readily spread from person to person. It appears to perpetuate itself through human carriers and contributes to chronic hepatitis. In approximately 50% of patients with transfusion-related non-A, non-B hepatitis, chronic hepatitis develops. In about 20% of these patients progression to cirrhosis occurs within 10 years. All of these observations have been derived from epidemiologic investigation because until recently, no viral agents or serologic marker for any of these agents had been identified.[12,13]

Hepatitis C

Recently, one agent responsible for non-A, non-B hepatitis has been cloned and is called hepatitis C virus (HCV).[14] A serologic test to detect antibodies to this agent has been developed.[15] HCV appears to be a member of the Togaviridae family. HCV is most commonly transmitted through needle sticks and transfusion.

Epidemic Non-A, Non-B Hepatitis

Another agent of viral hepatitis, serologically unrelated to HAV and HBV but similar in epidemiologic and clinical features to those of HAV, has been identified in Asia and India. Transmitted by exposure to contaminated water, it is spread primarily by the fecal–oral route. It has a mean incubation period of 40 days and is associated with a 10% fatality rate but is not linked to chronic hepatitis.[16]

Other Viruses Affecting the Liver

Both EBV and CMV can produce hepatitis in humans as part of a generalized systemic illness. Occasionally these agents are implicated serologically in an isolated case or in small outbreaks of hepatitis.[17] CMV may be an important pathogen in liver disease after renal transplantation but is rarely implicated in posttransfusion hepatitis, despite its frequent transmission in blood.[18] Still, these viral agents should be kept in mind when etiologic agents for hepatitis are considered. Other viruses occasionally implicated in hepatitis, such as herpes simplex, contribute even less than CMV and EBV and can be discounted, except in very unusual circumstances.

IMMUNOLOGIC FEATURES AND DIAGNOSTIC TESTS

Hepatitis A Virus

Only one antigen, HAV antigen, has been associated with the surface of the 27-nm virion. No serologic subtypes have been described. HAV is excreted in the feces during the late incubation period, but after the development of jaundice, fecal excretion becomes insignificant. HAV antigen is not readily detected in blood, even though it may be infectious; no asymptomatic chronic carrier state exists.

Antibody to HAV (anti-HAV) is detected shortly after acute illness (see Fig. 4-1) and persists for many years; the prevalence of previous exposure to HAV increases as a function of age, rendering immune more than 70% of urban adults older than 50 years. During acute hepatitis A infection, the anti-HAV detected is primarily an M class immunoglobulin (IgM); after 3 months, most anti-HAV is of the immunoglobulin G (IgG) class. Therefore, a simple serologic diagnosis can be made by demonstrating IgM anti-HAV in a single serum sample obtained during acute illness (Table 4-1).[3,4,19]

Hepatitis B Virus

The presence of immunologic markers for HBV constitutes the basis of diagnostic tests used to identify acute or chronic infection. Hepatitis B surface antigen (HBsAg) is associated with three morphologic forms: 20-nm spheres, tubules of the same diameter but of variable length, and the surface of the 42-nm virion. Within the virion is a 27-nm nucleocapsid core expressing hepatitis B core antigen, which is immunologically distinct from HBsAg and to which the host mounts a specific immune response. A third antigen associated with HBV is hepatitis B e antigen, a soluble, nonparticulate protein that is an internal component of the core of HBV. Its presence correlates with high-level replication and high infectivity. Antibody to hepatitis B e antigen appears as levels of HBV replication and infectivity decrease. HBV DNA also correlates with a high level of virus replication but is not detectable with routinely available assays.

TABLE 4-1
Viruses Associated With Hepatitis in Humans

TYPE	NOMENCLATURE	ANTIGENS	CORRESPONDING ANTIBODIES	INCUBATION PERIOD	TRANSMISSION	ROUTINE SEROLOGIC TESTS
A	Hepatitis A	Hepatitis A antigen	Anti-HAV	15–50 days	Predominantly fecal–oral	Anti-HAV and IgM anti-HAV: radioimmunoassay, enzyme immunoassay
B	Hepatitis B	HBsAg	Anti-HBs	30–180 days	Percutaneous inoculation, intimate contact	HBsAg: radioimmunoassay, enzyme immunoassay Anti-HBs: radioimmunoassay, enzyme immunoassay
		HBcAg	Anti-HBc		Blood and blood products	Anti-HBc: radioimmunoassay, enzyme immunoassay
		Hepatitis B e antigen	Antibody to B e antigen		Perinatal (maternal–fetal)	
D	δ Hepatitis	δ Hepatitis antigen	Anti-δ	Similar to hepatitis B	Similar to hepatitis B	Anti-δ: radioimmunoassay, enzyme immunoassay
	Non-A, non-B (hepatitis C)	None identified	Anti-HCV	2–22 weeks	Similar to hepatitis B	Anti-HCV

Detection

For the detection of these viral antigens and their corresponding antibodies, commercial radioimmunoassays and enzyme immunoassays are available (see Table 4-1 and Fig. 4-2). These are the methods used most commonly to screen donated blood before transfusion. Despite its sensitivity, however, radioimmunoassay does not detect HBsAg in blood at a particle concentration of less than 10^6 per milliliter and therefore fails to identify all HBsAg-positive serum. Free hepatitis B core antigen is not found circulating in the blood of acutely or chronically infected persons, but antibody to hepatitis B core antigen (anti-HBc) can be detected (see Table 4-1).

With the diagnostic techniques available, the following sequence of serologic events can be detected during a typical case of acute HBV infection. Approximately 1 month after exposure, HBsAg is detectable in the blood, predating clinical and biochemical evidence of the illness by several weeks. During HBsAg antigenemia, around the time of clinically apparent illness, anti-HBc becomes detectable, but not until HBsAg disappears (several months after it is first detectable) can antibody to HBsAg (anti-HBs) be detected.

Although anti-HBs is produced earlier during illness and can circulate complexed to HBsAg, it cannot be detected by standard serologic techniques until antibody excess is achieved. For practical purposes, then, detectable anti-HBs is a serologic marker of previous infection with HBV and has been shown to correlate with immunity to reinfection.

Anti-HBc can be detected during acute illness, as mentioned previously, but also persists as an indicator of past infection. The class of anti-HBc discriminates between acute and previous infection. IgM anti-HBc predominates during the first 6 months (approximately) after acute infection, whereas a predominance of IgG anti-HBc is thought to reflect high levels of HBV replication and therefore the replicative stage of infection. It usually disappears as the acute illness (nonreplicative phase of infection) resolves. Its persistence beyond early infection suggests ongoing high-level virus replication.[6,7]

Variations

Several variations on this theme of typical serologic events are noteworthy. First, the time course may be protracted or contracted. Second, occasionally a patient does not acquire detectable HBsAg antigenemia; the HBV illness can be identified by the detection of IgM anti-HBc or an anti-HBs response during convalescence.

The third and most important variation involves the patient who does not clear HBsAg but becomes a chronic HBsAg carrier. In approximately 5% to 10% of acutely infected persons, HBsAg persists in the circulation for several months to 1 year. A small percentage of these persons become chronic HBsAg carriers and indefinitely infectious. In these cases HBsAg remains detectable, and anti-HBc of the IgG class is present; anti-HBs, however, the antibody that correlates with immunity, is not detectable, or just barely so.

A fourth serologic pattern worth mentioning is a secondary anti-HBs response. An example is an anamnestic antibody response that occurs when an anti-HBs–positive person is reexposed to HBV. Acute illness, HBsAg antigenemia, and an increase in anti-HBc titer do not occur, but a boost in serum anti-HBs does.[6,7] To reiterate the significance of detectable HBsAg: HBsAg antigenemia can be seen in several clinical settings. In patients with acute or chronic liver disease, the presence of HBsAg indicates HBV infection; asymptomatic HBsAg-positive persons may be carrying the virus during the prodromal period of an evolving acute illness, during early convalescence after a symptomatic illness before antigen clearance, during an acute asymptomatic illness, or as chronic HBsAg carriers.

Among carriers, a clinical spectrum ranging from normal liver function, to minimal hepatocellular abnormalities, to chronic active liver disease, and to cirrhosis occurs. Although infectivity is linked with the severity of liver disease in chronic carriers, these correlations have not been confirmed. Indeed, asymptomatic HBsAg-positive patients who are undergoing hemodialysis and who have normal liver function and histologic specimens of normal morphologic appearance are often highly infectious. For practical purposes, contact with all HBsAg-positive patients and their secretions should be considered potentially infectious. Relative infectivity can be measured by testing for hepatitis B e antigen.

δ Hepatitis

δ Antigen can be detected in hepatocyte nuclei but is difficult to detect in serum by conventional immunoassays. During acute δ infection, anti-δ antibody for the IgM immunoglobulin class predominates; in chronic δ infection, both IgM and IgG anti-δ antibodies can be detected. Commercial assays are available for total (not class-specific) anti-δ. In the future, assays may become available to detect δ RNA in serum as an indicator of active virus replication.[8,9]

Epstein-Barr Virus and Cytomegalovirus

Unlike the hepatitis viruses, infection with these herpesviruses can be diagnosed by virus isolation in cell culture. Like hepatitis viruses, EBV and CMV can be identified serologically. Although several isolated strains of CMV do not show complete antigenic homology, serologic tests are available for the detection of anti-CMV. For EBV, a complex array of antigens has been identified in various lymphoblastoid lines. Four major categories exist: (1) viral capsid antigens; (2) cell membrane antigens, both early and late; (3) early antigens, both diffuse and restricted; and (4) nuclear antigen, the reactive component in soluble complement-fixing antigens. During acute EBV infection, the titers of antibody to the first three antigens appear, whereas antibody to nuclear antigen does not appear for weeks to months after acute illness.

Non-A, Non-B Hepatitis

Until recently the diagnosis of non-A, non-B hepatitis was one of exclusion. With the development of an antibody assay for HCV, this is no longer the case. The prevalence of anti-HCV in inner-city populations is estimated at 18%.[18,20]

TRANSMISSION OF VIRAL HEPATITIS

Traditional distinctions between fecal–oral transmission of "infectious" hepatitis A and parenterally spread "serum" hepatitis B have come under question with the application of new serologic techniques to epidemiologic investigation. Most striking is the finding that in approximately 50% of cases without antecedent overt percutaneous inoculation, HBV can be implicated serologically.[21] Because of the high HBsAg serum titers achieved in HBV infection, the development of sensitive serologic tests for detection of HBV infection, and the wide availability of these tests, an enormous amount of new information about the natural history of this virus now exists. Many inferences can be drawn about HBV transmission.

Nosocomial Implications

HBsAg has been detected in virtually every body secretion, including saliva, urine, semen, cerebrospinal fluid, pleural fluid, blood, sweat, and tears; several nonpercutaneous modes of spread have been suggested. The most important of these are perinatal spread from mother to offspring at the time of birth or shortly thereafter and spread via intimate contact, such as breast-feeding. The epidemiologic evidence supporting the potential risk from body fluids and nonpercutaneous modes of spread is convincing. Moreover, HBV is so stable that it can be recovered from contaminated environmental surfaces long after HbsAg-positive blood or body fluid has dried.[22]

Alternate Sources of Transmission

Aside from overt percutaneous inoculation with an HBsAg-contaminated needle or scalpel, many other avenues exist for infection of operating room staff exposed frequently to blood and body fluids. In support of this increased risk are anecdotal and published reports of hepatitis B among surgical teams and a high prevalence of anti-HBs immunoglobulin (indicative of previous HBV infection) in operating room personnel.[23,24] In many serologic surveys of hospital personnel, surgeons and operating room staff ranked highest in serologic evidence of exposure. Pattison and colleagues found the highest anti-HBs immunoglobulin prevalence (29%) in operating room personnel.[25] The prevalence of HBV exposure has been found by others as well to be much higher in surgical specialists than in other medical specialists.[26]

The Risk to Anesthesiologists

Hepatitis B Virus Infection

Among 267 anesthesia residents in seven training programs, 12.7% had detectable anti-HBs or anti-HBc or both; of those who had more than 12 months of nonanesthesia postgraduate clinical training before entering anesthesia, 17.8% demonstrated seropositivity.[24]

These results are not surprising if possible modes of exposure are considered. Anesthesiologists often insert intravenous catheters, administer injections, obtain arterial blood samples, handle urine specimens, administer spinal anesthesia, and insert their hands into patients' mouths during intubation, and they are present in the operating room where blood contaminates the environment. The Centers for Disease Control and Prevention considers anesthesiologists to be at intermediate risk for hepatitis infection.[27]

Transmission of HBV is a risk not only when the patient undergoing surgery is a known HBsAg carrier but also (and even more so) when the patient is an unidentified HBsAg carrier. In the latter situation, no special precautions are instituted. In studies of HBsAg among routine hospital admissions, investigators have reported prevalences of 0.8% to 1.5%, far in excess of the 0.1% to 0.2% found in the general population.[28,29] Furthermore, 90% of these HBsAg-positive patients were admitted for reasons unrelated to hepatitis, and the risk to hospital personnel would have remained undetected if these HBsAg screening surveys had not been done.

In addition, the risk of HBV to health care personnel has been shown to increase with the duration of occupational exposure. The risk is greatest, however, during the first few years of exposure.[24,30]

TABLE 4-2
Universal Precautions

Barriers: Gloves, masks, and eyewear as appropriate
Decontamination: Wash hands
Needles: Do not bend, break, or resheath
Ventilation devices: use for cardiopulmonary resuscitation
Dermatologic considerations: cover weeping, exudative lesions
Pregnant health care workers: Be extra careful: fetus is at risk

Layon AJ, Kilroy RA: Occupational hazards. In Gravenstein N (ed): Complications during anesthesia. Philadelphia: JB Lippincott, 1991: 51.

Based on these data, anesthesiologists should treat every patient's blood and secretions as potentially infectious for HBV and adhere to "universal precautions" (Table 4-2). In addition, the possible presence of non-A, non-B hepatitis agents or, less commonly but just as importantly, HIV, make scrupulous avoidance of unprotected contact with body fluids of critical significance.[11,31]

Non-A, Non-B Virus Infection

Non-A, non-B hepatitis, as mentioned, appears to have modes of transmission and epidemiologic features in common with those of HBV. Most importantly, these agents are transmitted readily by blood transfusion (90% of transfusion-associated hepatitis is non-A, non-B), and epidemiologic evidence suggests an asymptomatic chronic carrier state.[9] Given the correlation between blood contact and HBV exposure among health care personnel and given the similarities between type B hepatitis and non-A, non-B hepatitis, it is clear that anesthesiologists and other hospital employees are exposed to the agents of both.[11]

Hepatitis A Virus, Epstein-Barr Virus, and Cytomegalovirus Infection

With HAV, transmission by the fecal–oral route predominates. Because no asymptomatic chronic carrier state appears to exist and because natural transmission (except in experimental inoculation studies) by way of blood or percutaneous routes is extraordinarily rare, the risk of HAV infection to operating room personnel is inconsequential. Both EBV and CMV are transmitted by intimate contact and by blood transfusion and theoretically therefore can be a threat; in practice, such occurrences are not common. For hospital personnel, then, the major identified risk is from HBV hepatitis and non-A, non-B hepatitis. Susceptibility correlates directly with the extent of exposure to patients' body fluids, most notably blood.

PREVENTIVE MEASURES

Although all body fluids should be handled with caution routinely, identification of the HBsAg carrier state should be attempted (Table 4-3). When known HBsAg-positive patients are treated in surgical suites, the measures listed in Table 4-4 are thought to minimize potential infection of staff and other patients.

Ideally, HBsAg and anti-HBs screening among operating room staff should be done at regular intervals to identify increases in exposure or lack of immune prophylaxis and then to proceed with investigation and intervention as required. Prophylaxis with hepatitis B vaccine should command high priority.

TABLE 4-3
Prevalence of Hepatitis B Serologic Markers in Various Populations

		PREVALENCE OF SEROLOGIC MARKERS OF HBV INFECTION	
RISK	POPULATION	*HB_s Ag (%)*	*All Markers (%)*
High	Immigrants or refugees from areas of high HBV endemicity	13	70–85
	Clients in institutions for the mentally retarded	10–20	35–80
	Users of illicit parenteral drugs	7	60–80
	Homosexually active men	6	35–80
	Household contacts of HBV carriers	3–6	30–60
	Patients in hemodialysis units	3–10	20–80
Intermediate	Healthcare workers with frequent blood contact	1–2	15–30
	Men in prisons	1–8	10–80
	Staff of institutions for the mentally retarded	1	10–25
Low	Healthcare workers with no or infrequent blood contact	0.3	3–10
	Healthy adults (first-time volunteer blood donors)	0.3	3–5

HBV, hepatitis B virus; *HB_sAG*, hepatitis B surface antigen

Centers for Disease Control: Recommendations for protection against viral hepatitis. Ann Int Med 103: 395, 1985.

TABLE 4-4
Measures to Minimize Risks of Caring for High-risk Patients in the Operating Room

- Strict adherence to universal precautions should be maintained
- Gowns, gloves, caps, and plastic overshoes should be worn by anyone in contact with the patient
- Materials, such as syringes, sheets, pillows, and endotracheal tubes, should be disposable whenever possible
- Presence of unnecessary personnel in the room should be discouraged
- Buckets containing hypochlorite should be used for all disposable and contaminated material; hypochlorite should be added to trap bottle on suction line
- HBsAg-positive patients should be scheduled last to minimize exposure to other patients
- All disposable surgical and anesthetic items should be incinerated
- Special caution should be exercised when handling or disposing contaminated sharp objects
- Surgical specimens should be carefully wrapped and labeled as biohazardous
- Reusable contaminated instruments (eg, laryngoscopes or airways) and linens should be autoclaved or gas-sterilized (with ethylene oxide)
- Contaminated surfaces and equipment that cannot be sterilized (eg, walls, floors, anesthesia machine, or ventilator) should be washed with hypochlorite, formalin, or glutaraldehyde

Immunoprophylaxis of Viral Hepatitis

For health personnel and others at risk of infection with HBV, active immunization with hepatitis B vaccine is strongly recommended. Since 1982, a vaccine consisting of noninfectious, 20-nm spherical HBsAg particles purified from the plasma of chronic carriers has been available.[32–34] It is subjected to three chemical inactivation steps (pepsin, urea, and formalin) that cumulatively destroy all viruses, including HIV.[35] Studies in high-risk groups have shown that the vaccine is safe, immunogenic, and protective. More than a decade of clinical use has confirmed its safety and value.[36] Now a second-generation hepatitis B vaccine, prepared by recombinant-DNA technology, has been released. It appears to be interchangeable with the plasma-derived vaccine.[37] Recommendations for HBV postexposure treatment are summarized in Tables 4-5 and 4-6.

For preexposure prophylaxis of immunocompetent adults, three 1-mL injections of hepatitis B vaccine are given intramuscularly in the deltoid (not gluteal) region initially and at 1 and 6 months. This regimen produces protective antibody in about 90% of healthy adults. For nonvaccinated persons who are exposed accidentally to HBV (eg, by needle-stick contamination of an open cut or mucous membrane exposure), a combination of passive immunoprophylaxis with hepatitis B immunoglobulin, 0.06 mL/kg intramuscularly, and a complete three-injection course of hepatitis B vaccine is recommended.[38–40] Hepatitis B immunoglobulin is about 75% effective in preventing acute HBV infection after two hepatitis B immunoglobulin doses, one immediately after exposure and one 1 month later.

Although exposure to HAV is unlikely to occur in the operating room, should such exposure become apparent, immunoprophylaxis consists of standard immune serum globulin with an intramuscular dose of 0.02 mL/kg.[40] Prevention of δ hepatitis in persons susceptible to hepatitis B is achieved by vaccinating against hepatitis B. Hepatitis B carriers, however, present a more difficult challenge. No vaccine is available to protect them from δ superinfection; only rigid adherence to the universal precautions can be recommended.

Immunoprophylaxis against hepatitis C is not yet available. However, treatment of chronic HCV infection with interferon alpha has been shown to improve liver function and to decrease lobular and periportal inflammation.[41,42]

TABLE 4-5
Recommendations for Hepatitis B Prophylaxis After Percutaneous Exposure

	TREATMENT OF EXPOSED PERSON	
SOURCE	*Not vaccinated*	*Vaccinated*
HBsAg-positive	Give one dose of HBIG immediately Initiate hepatits B vaccine series*	Test exposed person for anti-HBs If antibody inadequate (<10 sample ratio units by radioimmunoassay or negative by enzyme immunoassay), give one dose of HBIG immediately plus hepatitis B vaccine booster dose
Known source High risk of being HBsAg-positive	Initiate hepatitis B vaccine series†	Test source of HBsAg only if exposed person is vaccine nonresponder; if source is HBsAg positive, give one dose of HBIG immediately plus hepatitis B vaccine booster dose
Low risk of being HBsAg-positive	Initiate hepatitis B vaccine series	Nothing required
Unknown source	Initiate hepatitis B vaccine series	Nothing required

* The first dose can be given at the same time as the dose of hepatitis B immmune globulin (*HBIG*) but at a different site.

† Vaccine is recommended for homosexual men and for regular sexual contacts of HBV carriers and is optional in the initial treatment of heterosexual contacts of persons with acute hepatitis B.

Centers for Disease Control: Recommendations for protection against viral hepatitis. Ann Intern Med 103: 399, 1985, and Facts and comparisons. Philadelphia: JB Lippincott 1990: 467.

TABLE 4-6
Hepatitis B Virus Postexposure Recommendations

	HBIG		INACTIVATED VACCINE DOSE (μg IM)		
			Plasma-derived	*Recombinant*	
EXPOSURE	DOSE	RECOMMENDED TIMING	HEPATAVAX-B	RECOMBIVAX	ENGERIX-B
Perinatal	0.5 mL IM	Within 12 h	10*	5*	10*
Sexual	0.06 mL/kg IM	Single dose within 14 days of sexual contact	20†	10†	20†
Percutaneous	NA	NA	20	10	20
Dialysis and immunocompromise	NA	NA	40 (20 μg in each of two sites)	—	40

IM, intramuscular; *NA*, not applicable.

* The first dose can be given at the same time as the dose of hepatitis B immune globulin (*HBIG*) but at a different site.

† Vaccine is recommended for homosexual men and for regular sexual contacts of HBV carriers and is optional in the initial treatment of heterosexual contacts of persons with acute hepatitis B.

Centers for Disease Control: Recommendations for protection against viral hepatitis. Ann Intern Med 103: 399, 1985, and Facts and comparisons. Philadelphia, JB Lippincott, 1990: 467.

ACQUIRED IMMUNODEFICIENCY SYNDROME

AIDS is caused by infection with HIV. In 1995, unlike hepatitis infection, HIV infection is essentially uniformly fatal. As of 1995, over 400,000 cumulative cases of AIDS had been reported in the United States. Approximately, 60% of those patients have died.

Terminology

Although the terms AIDS and HIV are often used interchangeably, "HIV infection" is more correctly reserved for cases in which seroconversion has occurred in the absence of symptoms. Once someone is symptomatic, for example with an opportunistic infection, it is more appropriate to speak of the HIV-positive patient as having AIDS. Several reported systems are available for use in disease classification and progression[43–46]; we prefer the Walter Reed staging classification.[47]

Human Immunodeficiency Virus

HIV is a retrovirus that binds to the CD4 molecule on helper/inducer ($T4^+$) lymphocytes and macrophages and in the central nervous system. After binding, the virus enters the host cell, where its genomic RNA is transcribed into DNA; most of this genetic material is integrated into the host cell DNA, although some unincorporated pieces of viral DNA remain free in the cytoplasm. An important feature is that as a result of this integration of the viral genome into the hosts, the cell infection and infectiousness persist throughout the life of the host cell. Most infected patients have circulating levels of the infectious agent.

The $T4^+$ cell is a central functionary in the immune system, where it facilitates macrophage, monocyte, cytotoxic T-cell, natural killer, and B-cell function (Table 4-7). The $T4^+$ cell is involved directly or indirectly in the induction of most immunologic responses. Thus, even a functional defect in the $T4^+$ subset of lymphocytes could lead to a global immunologic defect as a result of loss of inductive signals to various limbs of the immune system. Because as many as 1 in 100 $T4^+$ cells is infected with HIV, it comes as no surprise that as progressive and selective quantitative, as well as qualitative, depletion of this cell line occurs, severe and recurrent infections result.[48] The infected $T4^+$ cell eventually dies, but the HIV-infected monocyte or macrophage is relatively resistant to cytolysis and, at least in the central nervous system, may be the viral reservoir.

Epidemiology

As of November 27, 1993, 93,282 new cases of AIDS had been reported in the United States for that year.[49] Each week between 200 and 600 cases of AIDS are reported to the Centers for Disease Control and Prevention.[50,51] The distribution of cases is shown in Table 4-8.

TABLE 4-7
T4 Lymphocyte Functions

ACTIVATES
Macrophages
INDUCES
Cytotoxic T-cell function
Natural killer cell function
Suppressor cell function
B-cell function
SECRETES
Lymph cell growth and differentiation factors
Hematopoietic colony-stimulating factors
Factors to induce nonlymphoid cell function

TABLE 4-8
Distribution of AIDS Cases (%)

Gay or bisexual activity	55
Intravenous drug abuse (heterosexual)	24
Heterosexual transmission	7
Perinatal transmission, transfusion-related, or indeterminate	14

HIV infection is now the fourth leading cause of death in women 25 to 44 years of age and the leading cause of death in men of the same age.[52] Furthermore, and perhaps of most concern, in 1989 AIDS became the sixth leading cause of death among adolescents and young adults (aged 15 to 24 years) of both sexes.[53] Estimates of HIV prevalence and projected AIDS cases are of great concern.[54] Today, there are thought to be approximately 1 million HIV-infected people in the United States (with a plausible range of 850,000 to 1,250,000, the differences due to differences in statistical method).[55] The HIV-infected persons who receive medical care today were likely infected 8 to 10 years ago.[55] Estimates were that by the end of 1994, the cumulative total of AIDS cases would range between 415,000 and 535,000 with between 330,000 and 385,000 deaths.[55] By the end of 1993, medical care was required by 139,000 to 200,000 AIDS patients, and the number of AIDS-related deaths probably was in excess of 50,000.

Diagnosis

Infection with and seroconversion to HIV may be associated with a nonspecific viral-like syndrome. Initial symptoms include fever, sore throat, and lymphadenopathy. In some patients rash, myalgias, diarrhea, and central nervous system dysfunction are the initial symptoms. A routine blood test may show evidence of leukopenia or thrombocytopenia. The time from exposure to symptoms is usually 2 weeks, and the antibody response occurs 4 weeks after exposure. Of note is that in some cases, seroconversion may take as long as several years.[56]

A variety of serologic tests are available. The enzyme-linked immunosorbent assay (ELISA) has a positive predictive value of 93% for persons who engage in high-risk activity.[57] In low-risk persons, however, the positive predictive value for a positive test may be only 67%.[58] The importance of a confirmatory study in either case is obvious. The most commonly used confirmatory test is the Western blot. In this assay, viral antigen is dispersed by electrophoresis, and the serum is evaluated for specific viral antibodies. A positive test requires that at least two of the following bands be identified: p24 (core antigen), gp41 (envelope antigen), or gp 120/gp160 (envelope antigen).[59] A negative test is absence of any of the above, whereas an intermediate result would be, for example, the detection of one band. An indeterminate result that persists for 6 months or longer may, in the absence of risk factors, be considered negative for HIV. Newer tests[60,61] being evaluated use polymerase chain reaction techniques to identify viral DNA; another test using the antigen-capture technique measures the p24 antigen (core antigen) concentration, which confirms infection and also gives an indication of the progression of the disease.[62]

Risk of Human Immunodeficiency Virus Infection to Anesthesia Providers

Transmission of HIV to the health care worker is a risk not only when the patient is known to be HIV-seropositive but also when HIV status is seropositive but unknown.

Seroconversion of health care workers after a puncture wound with a blood- or secretion-contaminated instrument is less than 1%.[63,64] Current data show that there is no excess prevalence of HIV among health care workers, as there is for hepatitis. These data may, of course, change, but at this time they support the notion that HIV is less infectious than hepatitis B.[65,66]

The following epidemiologic calculation, however, provides a more somber perspective. If we assume an HIV seroprevalence of 1% (the current range is 0.02% to 5.2%), a frequency of puncture wounds of 1% (conservative), and an overall risk of seroconversion of 1% (currently approximately 0.5%) after a needle-stick injury from a patient who is HIV positive, then

$$0.01 \times 0.01 \times 0.01 = 0.000001 = 10^{-6}$$

Hence, the risk of HIV infection after one needle-stick injury is 1 in 1 million. However, an anesthesiologist cares for approximately four patients per day for 250 workdays per year. Thus,

$$4 \times 250 = 1{,}000 = 10^3$$

$$10^{-6} \times 10^3 = 10^{-3}$$

Over a 1-year period, then, the risk increases to 1 in 1000. Over a 40-year career, it increases by

$$40 \times 10^{-3} = 0.04$$

Thus, the risk of HIV disease during a lifetime may actually be closer to 1 in 25.[67]

Protection Against Human Immunodeficiency Virus Infection

It appears that many, but not all, exposures to HIV are preventable if adequate precautions are taken. It has been shown conclusively that depending on geography, age, and likely economic class, there is an apparently asymptomatic[68–70] HIV-positive pool that ranges from 16% to 18% of the populations studied.[71] This information should make us more attentive to prevention of contamination by HIV-positive material, especially in the emergency and operating rooms.

The precautions that should be taken to prevent transmission of HIV are of several categories. If there is any single message to be taken from the precautions described below, it is that all patients and all blood and body fluid specimens must be considered infective at all times. We can prevent transmission of HIV in the health care setting only if the recommendations for prevention of HIV-infection are followed consistently and carefully.

Universal Precautions

Universal precautions are those that should be taken with all patients because it is not always possible to identify HIV in-

TABLE 4-9
Invasive Procedure Precautions

TAKE UNIVERSAL PRECAUTIONS AND
• Wear gown, mask, and gloves
• Watch for glove tears

Layon AJ, Kilroy RA: Occupational hazards. In Gravenstein N (ed): Complications during anesthesia. Philadelphia, JB Lippincott, 1991: 52.

fection from the history or medical examination. These precautions are of particular importance in emergency-care settings, where exposure to blood and body fluids is likely and infectious status is unknown (see Table 4-2).

Invasive Precautions

Invasive precautions (Table 4-9) are those that should be taken in addition to the Universal Precautions when any invasive procedure is performed. As defined by the Centers for Disease Control and Prevention, an invasive procedure is a surgical entry into tissues, cavities, or an organ, or any repair of traumatically induced lesions. These include lesions treated in the physician's office as well as in the emergency room. In addition, cardiac catheterization and other angiographic procedures, vaginal or cesarean delivery, intravenous catheter placement, or dental surgical procedures are included under the rubric of invasive procedures. We also consider nasogastric and airway intubation as procedures requiring invasive precautions.

Laboratory Precautions

Laboratory precautions (Table 4-10) are those recommended for health workers in clinical laboratories. Blood (eg, a blood gas specimen) and body fluids (eg, saliva, nasogastric drainage, or urine) from all patients, regardless of HIV status, must be considered infective.

Although there are many therapeutic possibilities for HIV infection, to date the most effective deterrent is prevention. Recent data suggest that all too frequently, preventive measures, such as the universal precautions, are ignored by health workers.[72]

TABLE 4-10
Laboratory AIDS Precautions

UNIVERSAL PRECAUTIONS AND
• Use well-constructed containers with tops
• Wear gloves, masks, and eyewear
• Use biologic safety cabinet if droplets are generated
• Do not pipette by mouth; use mechanical pipettes
• Use needles or syringes only if no alternative; follow precautions
• Decontaminate work surfaces after spills
• Wash hands and remove contaminated clothing

Layon AJ, Kilroy RA: Occupational hazards. In Gravenstein N (ed): Complications during anesthesia. Philadelphia: JB Lippincott, 1991: 52.

Further precautions that may be taken, albeit without substantial support from the literature, include careful cleaning (with surgical scrub brushes and povidone-iodine soap) of laryngoscope blades, and elimination of all used syringes after each case. We consider it appropriate to use multidose vials as long as penetration of the rubberized barrier is always carried out with a new needle and a new syringe. Of course, gloves should always be worn when the risk of contamination with blood or body fluids exists. We are unaware of data suggesting any differences between latex or vinyl gloves. Finally, needles should never be resheathed, because doing so may lead to punctures. All sharp objects should be discarded in puncture-proof containers, which should be placed as close to the site of the procedure as possible.

REFERENCES

1. Centers for Disease Control: Summary of notifiable diseases: United States, 1988. MMWR 3:37, 1988
2. Centers for Disease Control: Summary of selected notifiable diseases: United States week ending June 27, 1992 (26th week). MMWR 41:471, 1992
3. Lemon SM: Type A viral hepatitis: new developments in an old disease. N Engl J Med 313:1059, 1985
4. Mijch AM, Gust ID: Clinical, serologic, and epidemiologic aspects of hepatitis A virus infection. Semin Liver Dis 6:42, 1986
5. Ticehurst JR: Hepatitis A virus: clones, culture, and vaccines. Semin Liver Dis 6:46, 1986
6. Krugman S, Overby LR, Mushahwar IK, et al: Viral hepatitis, type B: studies on natural history and prevention re-examined. N Engl J Med 300:101, 1979
7. Hoofnagle JH, Schafer DF: Serologic markers of hepatitis B virus infection. Semin Liver Dis 6:1, 1986
8. Rizzetto M, Verme G: Delta hepatitis: present status. J Hepatol 1:187, 1985
9. Jacobson IM, Dienstag JL, Werner BG, et al: Epidemiology and clinical impact of hepatitis D virus (delta) infection. Hepatology 5:188, 1985
10. Lettau LA, McCarthy JG, Smith MH, et al: Outbreak of severe hepatitis due to delta and hepatitis B viruses in parenteral drug abusers and their contacts. N Engl J Med 317:1256, 1987
11. Aach RD, Stevens CE, Hollinger FB, et al: Hepatitis C virus infection in post-transfusion hepatitis: an analysis with first and second generation assays. N Engl J Med 325:1325, 1991
12. Alter JH, Purcell RH, Reinstone SM, et al: Non-A, non-B hepatitis: its relationship to cytomegalovirus, to chronic hepatitis, and to direct and indirect test methods. In Szmuness W, Alter JH, Maynard JE (eds): Viral hepatitis: 1981 International Symposium. 1982: 279
13. Feinstone SM, Kapakian AZ, Purcell RH, et al: Transfusion associated hepatitis not due to viral hepatitis A or B. N Engl J Med 292:767, 1975
14. Choo QL, Davis GL, Weiner AS, et al: Isolation of a cDNA clone derived from a blood-borne non-A, non-B viral hepatitis genome. Science 244:359, 1989
15. Aach RD, Stevens CE, Hollinger FB, et al: Hepatitis C virus infection in post-transfusion hepatitis—an analysis with first- and second-generation assays. N Engl J Med 325:1325, 1991
16. Maynard JE: Epidemic non-A, non-B hepatitis. Semin Liver Dis 4:336, 1984
17. Weller TH: The cytomegaloviruses—ubiquitous agents with protean clinical manifestations. N Engl J Med 285:267, 1971
18. Lang DJ: Cytomegaloviruses infection. In Wyngarten JB, Smith LH (eds): Cecil's Textbook of Medicine, 18th ed. Philadelphia: JB Lippincott, 1988:1784
19. Dienstag JL, Sznuness W, Stevens CE, et al: Hepatitis A virus

infection: new insights from seroepidemiologic studies. J Infect Dis 137:328, 1978
20. Kelen GD, Green GB, Purcell RH, et al: Hepatitis B and hepatitis C in emergency department patients. N Engl J Med 326:1399, 1992
21. Prince AM, Hargrove RL, Sznuness W, et al: Immunologic distinction between infectious and serum hepatitis. N Engl J Med 282:987, 1970
22. Favero MS, Bond WW, Petersen JF, et al: Detection methods for study of the stability of hepatitis B antigen on surfaces. J Infect Dis 129:210
23. Jovanovich JF, Saravolatz LD, Arking LM: The risk of hepatitis B among select employee groups in an urban hospital. JAMA 250:1893, 1983
24. Berry AJ, Isaacson IJ, Kane MA, et al: A multicenter study of the epidemiology of hepatitis B in anesthesia residents. Anesth Analg 64:672, 1985
25. Pattison CP, Maynard JE, Berquist KR, et al: Epidemiology of hepatitis B in hospital personnel. Am J Epidemiol 101:59, 1975
26. Smith JL, Maynard JE, Berquist DR, et al: Comparative risk of hepatitis B among physicians and dentists. J Infect Dis 133:705, 1976
27. Centers for Disease Control: Recommendations for protection against viral hepatitis. Ann Intern Med 103:391, 1985
28. Linneman CC, Hegg ME, Ramundo N, et al: Screening hospital patients for hepatitis B surface antigen. Am J Clin Pathol 67: 257, 1977
29. Feinman SV, Krassnitzky O, Sinclair JC, et al: Prevalence and significance of hepatitis B surface antigen in a general hospital. Can Med Assoc J 112:43, 1973
30. Snydman DR, Nunoz A, Werner BG, et al: A multivariate analysis of risk factors for hepatitis B virus infection among hospital employees screened for vaccination. Am J Epidemiol 120:684, 1984
31. Stevens CE, Taylor PE, Pindyck J, et al: Epidemiology of hepatitis C virus: a preliminary study in volunteer blood donors. JAMA 263:49, 1990
32. Szmuness W, Stevens CE, Zang EA, et al: A controlled clinical trial of the efficacy of the hepatitis B vaccine (Hepatavax B): a final report. Hepatology 1:377, 1981
33. Jacobson IM, Dienstag JL: Viral hepatitis vaccines. Annu Rev Med 36:241, 1985
34. Stevens CD: Hepatitis B vaccines: clinical experience, indications and recommendations. Semin Liver Dis 6:23, 1986
35. Francis DP, Feorino PM, McDougal S, et al: The safety of the hepatitis B vaccine: inactivation of the AIDS virus during routine vaccine manufacture. JAMA 256:869, 1986
36. Hadler SC, Francis DP, Maynard JE, et al: Long-term immunogenicity and efficacy of hepatitis B vaccine in homosexual men. N Engl J Med 315:209, 1986
37. Scolnick EM, McLean AA, West DJ, et al: Clinical evaluation in healthy adults of a hepatitis B vaccine made by recombinant DNA. JAMA 251:2812, 1984
38. Seeff LB, Hoofnagle JH: Immunoprophylaxis of viral hepatitis. Gastroenterology 77:161, 1979
39. Seeff LB, Koff R: Passive and active immunoprophylaxis of hepatitis B. Gastroenterology 86:958, 1984
40. Centers for Disease Control and Department of Health and Human Services recommendations for protection against viral hepatitis: recommendations of the Immunization Practices Advisory Committee. Ann Intern Med 103:391, 1985
41. Davis GL, Balart LA, Schiff ER, et al: Treatment of chronic hepatitis C with recombinant interferon alpha. N Engl J Med 321:1501, 1989
42. DiBisceglie AM, Martin P, Kassianides C, et al: Recombinant interferon alpha therapy for chronic hepatitis C. N Engl J Med 321:1506, 1989
43. Centers for Disease Control: Classification system for the human T-lymphotropic virus type III/lymphadenopathy-associated virus infections. Ann Intern Med 105:234, 1986
44. Centers for Disease Control: Classification for human immunodeficiency virus (HIV) infection in children under 13 years of age. MMWR 36:226, 1987
45. Turner BJ, Kelly JV, Ball JK: A severity classification system for AIDS hospitalizations. Med Care 27:423, 1989
46. Justice AC, Feinstein AR, Wells CK: A new prognostic staging system for the acquired immunodeficiency syndrome. N Engl J Med 320:1388, 1989
47. Redfield RR, Wright DC, Tramont EC: The Walter Reed staging classification for HTLV-III/LAV infection. N Engl J Med 314: 131, 1986
48. Witt DJ, Craven DE, McCabe WR: Bacterial infections in adult patients with the acquired immunodeficiency syndrome (AIDS) and AIDS-related complex. Am J Med 82:900, 1987
49. Centers for Disease Control and Prevention: Cases of specified notifiable diseases, United States, cumulative, week ending December 25, 1993. MMWR 42:997, 1994
50. Centers for Disease Control: Cases of specified notifiable diseases, United States, cumulative, week ending May 16, 1992. MMWR 41:356, 1992
51. Centers for Disease Control: Cases of specified notifiable diseases, United States, cumulative, week ending May 30, 1992. MMWR 41:392, 1992
52. Centers for Disease Control: Update: mortality attributable to HIV infection among persons aged 25-44 years—United States, 1991 and 1992. MMWR 42:868, 1993
53. Centers for Disease Control: Selected behaviors that increase risk for HIV infection among high school students: United States, 1990. MMWR 41:231, 1992
54. Centers for Disease Control: HIV prevalence estimates and AIDS case projections for the United States: report based upon a workshop. MMWR 39(RR-16):1, 1990
55. Centers for Disease Control and Prevention: Projections of the number of persons diagnosed with AIDS and the number of immunosuppressed HIV-infected persons, United States, 1992-1994. MMWR 41(RR-18):1, 1992
56. Imagawa DT, Lee MH, Wolinsky SM, et al: Human immunodeficiency virus type 1 infection in homosexual men who remain seronegative for prolonged periods. N Engl J Med 320:1458, 1989
57. Weiss R, Thier SO: HIV testing is the answer: what's the question? (editorial). N Engl J Med 319:1010, 1988
58. Meyer KB, Pauker SG: Screening for HIV: can we afford the false positive rate? N Engl J Med 317:238, 1987
59. Centers for Disease Control: Interpretation and use of Western Blot assay for serodiagnosis of human immunodeficiency virus type 1 infection. MMWR 38(S-7):1, 1989
60. Sloand EM, Pitt E, Chiarello RJ, Nemo GJ: HIV testing: state of the art. JAMA 266:2861, 1991
61. Arpadi S, Caspe WB: HIV testing. J Pediatr 119:S8, 1991
62. Merigan TC, Skowron G, Bozzette SA, et al: Circulating p24 antigen levels and responses to dideoxycytidine in human immunodeficiency virus (HIV) infections. Ann Intern Med 110: 189, 1989
63. Lifson AR, Castro KG, McCray E, et al: National surveillance of AIDS in health care workers. JAMA 256:3231, 1986
64. McCray E: Occupational risk of the acquired immunodeficiency syndrome among health care workers. N Engl J Med 314:1127, 1986
65. Centers for Disease Control: Update: acquired immunodeficiency syndrome and human immunodeficiency virus infection among health care workers. MMWR 37:229, 1988
66. Henderson DK, Fahey BJ, Willy M, et al: Risk for occupational transmission of human immunodeficiency virus type 1 (HIV-1) associated with clinical exposures: a prospective evaluation. Ann Intern Med 113:740, 1990
67. Lopalo S, Layon AJ: Occupational hazards in the operating room. In Kirby RR, Gravenstein N (eds): Clinical anesthesia practice. Philadelphia: WB Saunders, 1994: 855
68. Wolinsky SM, Rinaldo CR, Kwok S, et al: Human immunodeficiency virus type 1 (HIV 1) infection median of 18 months before a diagnostic western blot. Ann Intern Med 111:961, 1989
69. Merigan TC, Skowron G, Bozzette SA, et al: Circulating P24 antigen levels and responses to dideoxycytidine in human immunodeficiency virus (HIV) infections. Ann Intern Med 110: 189, 1989

70. Imagawa DT, Lee MH, Wolinsky SM, et al: Human immunodeficiency virus type 1 infection in homosexual men who remain seronegative for prolonged periods. N Engl J Med 320:1458, 1989
71. Baker JL, Kelen GD, Sivertson KT, et al: Unsuspected human immunodeficiency virus in critically ill emergency patients. JAMA 257:2609, 1987
72. Hammond JS, Eckes J, Gomez C, et al: HIV, trauma and infection control: universal precautions are universally ignored. J Trauma 30:555, 1990

FURTHER READING

Alter HJ (ed): Hepatitis. Semin Liver Dis 6:1, 1986

Berry AJ, Greene ES: The risk of needlestick injuries and needlestick-transmitted diseases in the practice of anesthesiology. Anesthesiology 77:1007, 1992

Gerety RJ (ed): Hepatitis A. Orlando, FL: Academic Press, 1984

Gerety RJ (ed): Hepatitis B. Orlando, FL: Academic Press, 1985

Hollinger FB, Melnick JL, Robinson WS: Viral hepatitis. New York: Raven Press, 1985

Layon AJ, Kilroy RA: Occupational hazards. In Gravenstein N (ed): Manual of complications in anesthesia. Philadelphia: JB Lippincott, 1991: 53

LoPalo S, Layon AJ: Occupational hazards in the operating room. In Kirby RR, Gravenstein N (eds): Clinical anesthesia practice. Philadelphia: WB Saunders, 1994: 853

Wormser GP, Rabkin CS, Joline C: Frequency of nosocomial transmission of HIV infection among health care workers (letter). N Engl J Med 319:307, 1988

Complications in Anesthesiology, second edition, edited by Nikolaus Gravenstein and Robert R. Kirby. Lippincott-Raven Publishers, Philadelphia © 1996.

CHAPTER 5

Herpes Simplex Virus and Herpetic Whitlow

Fredrick K. Orkin

Herpetic whitlow is an uncommon but painful and temporarily disabling finger infection caused by the herpes simplex virus (HSV). Among the many curious facets of this infection is its occurrence almost exclusively among anesthesia and other health-care personnel whose work exposes them to upper respiratory tract secretions. The lesion resembles a pyogenic infection so closely that it is usually subjected to unwarranted surgical intervention. This approach only compounds the severity of what otherwise is a benign, self-limiting disease. The epidemiologic characteristics, clinical features, management, and prevention of this occupational hazard to anesthesia personnel are presented in this chapter.

THE PATHOGEN

Structure

A virus has been characterized as "the ultimate form of intracellular parasite, stripped to the barest essentials necessary for its own propagation."[1] Lacking metabolic systems, it is wholly dependent on the host cell that it infects for the means to carry on activities characterizing living organisms, such as replication. The HSV is essentially a small package of double-stranded deoxyribonucleic acid (DNA) of a specific composition, designed to program the host cell's metabolic systems for viral replication. Hence, it is an obligatory intracellular parasite.

The genetic material constitutes the dense "core" of the virus. The core is surrounded by a protective coat composed of protein arranged in hexagonal clusters that collectively resemble a geodesic sphere; this coat is termed the "capsid." It in turn is surrounded by a lipid-containing protein "envelope." Small differences in DNA composition differentiate HSV type 1 from type 2.

Replication

On contact with a susceptible cell, the virus undergoes phagocytosis (viropexis); once it is inside the cell, digestion of the capsid and envelope occurs. The free viral DNA then enters the cell's nucleus, where it is replicated by the host's enzyme systems. The newly synthesized DNA is covered with viral protein synthesized in the cytoplasm from scavenged host protein. Within 10 hours, an infected cell lyses, releasing as many as 100 infectious virus particles, which then repeat the process.

PATHOGENESIS OF HERPETIC INFECTIONS

HSV has a predilection for cells of ectodermal origin (eg, skin, mucous membrane, and eye). The portal of entry and host factors determine the particular manifestation of the *primary* illness. True to its ancient Greek name, which means "to creep," herpes spreads locally and usually superficially from cell to cell. When the infected cells lyse, host white cells arrive to remove debris, and an inflammatory response results. In the midst of the debris, the lesion characteristic of superficial HSV infection appears: a thin-walled vesicle on an inflammatory base.

Immune Response

As infection proceeds, the lymphatics drain infectious material and debris to regional lymph nodes. Protective antibodies, interferon, and sensitized "killer" lymphocytes are produced to check the spread of infection. In the absence of competent immune mechanisms, viremia soon disseminates the infection throughout the body. Among the many disease states characterized by impaired immune mechanisms and susceptibility to disseminated HSV infection are malignancy (especially hematologic); malnutrition (eg, kwashiorkor); associated infectious disease (eg, measles or infection with *Haemophilus influenzae*); thermal burns; defective cell-mediated immunity (eg, acquired immunodeficiency syndrome,[2,3] Wiskott-Aldrich syndrome, and thymic dysplasia), drug-induced immunosuppression (eg, transplantation and asthma); prematurity; and pregnancy. Without vigorous supportive measures and specific antiviral chemotherapy, disseminated HSV infection is usually fatal. Mild immune deficiency can result in chronic herpetic infection.[4]

Latent Phase

Under normal circumstances, this primary infection subsides and HSV cannot be detected. However, HSV persists in a *latent* state within the ganglion associated with the sensory nerves innervating the site of infection.[5–7] Within the ganglion the only identifiable portion of the virus is its DNA, which, given an appropriate stimulus, migrates peripherally along the sensory nerve. Although various mechanisms have been advanced to explain HSV latency and reactivation, none has been proven.

Reactivation

Among the diverse factors associated with reactivation of latent HSV are fever, menstruation, corticosteroid or foreign protein administration, emotional stress, and sunlight, and in obstetric patients, possibly epidural morphine administration.[8–11] Reactivation of HSV results in a *recurrent* infection in the vicinity of the primary infection. In general, the symptoms accompanying a recurrence are milder than those associated with the primary infection.

Figure 5-1 summarizes the possible courses of infection with HSV.

EPIDEMIOLOGIC CHARACTERISTICS OF HERPETIC INFECTIONS

Herpes simplex virus is ubiquitous and worldwide in distribution. Although animals in experimental models can be infected, humans are the only known reservoirs. The principal

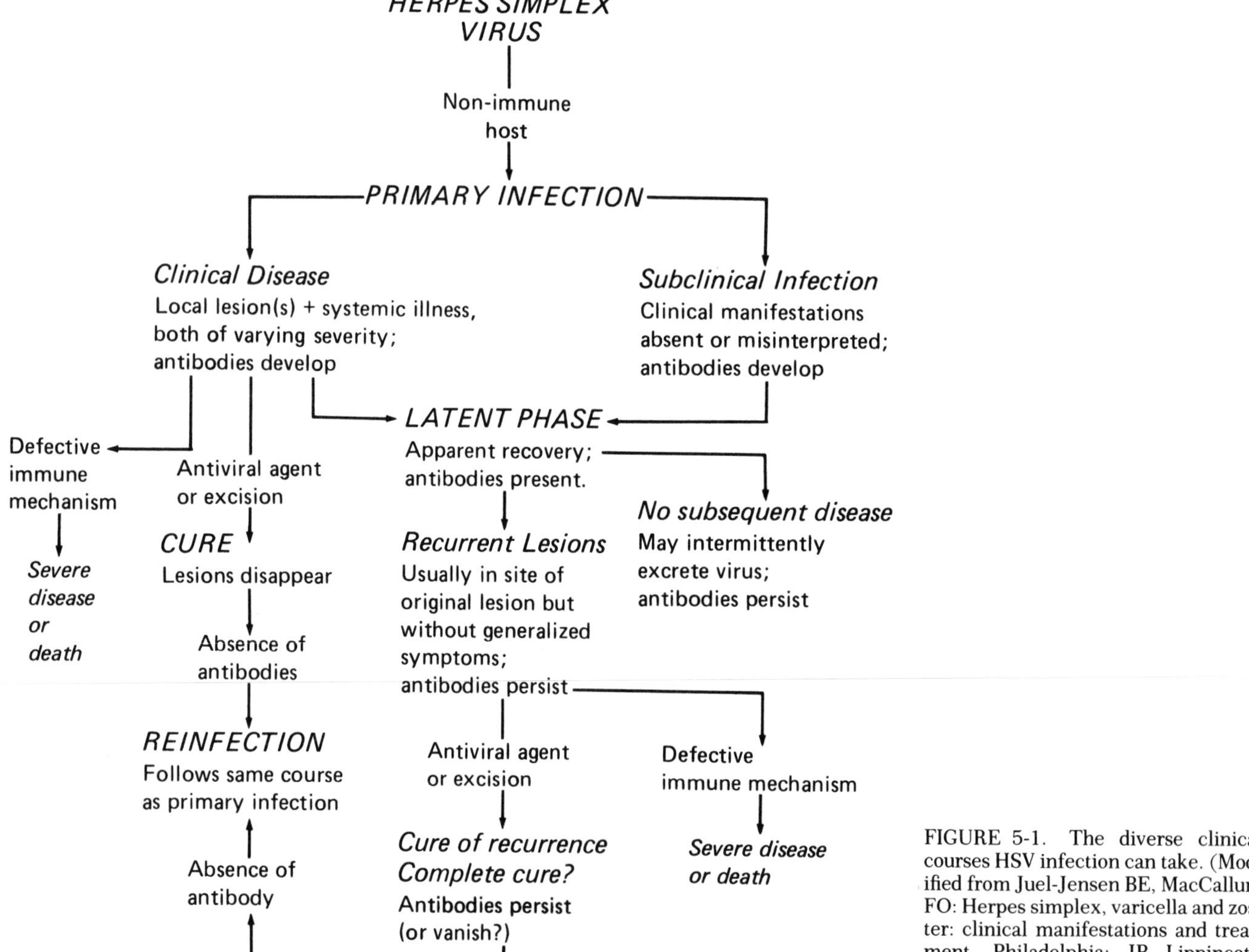

FIGURE 5-1. The diverse clinical courses HSV infection can take. (Modified from Juel-Jensen BE, MacCallum FO: Herpes simplex, varicella and zoster: clinical manifestations and treatment. Philadelphia; JB Lippincott, 1972: 32.)

mode of spread is direct contact with infected secretions. Type 1 HSV is spread primarily by contact with oral secretions, whereas type 2 is spread by contact with genital secretions. Until recently the teaching was that HSV type 1 causes infections "above the belt" and type 2, "below the belt"; however, we now know that no strict boundaries exist.[12,13] HSV infections of the hand are associated with either type.[13,14] The incubation period for both types ranges from 2 to 12 days; illness usually appears 3 to 9 days after infection.

Herpes Simplex Virus Type 1

The fetus and infant until about 6 months of age are protected by transplacental maternal antibodies. Between 6 months and 5 years of age, infections with and antibody response to HSV type 1 are frequent. By the age of 15 years, as much as 96% of the population possesses type-specific antibody.[15] Whereas 80% to 100% of adults in lower socioeconomic groups possess antibodies to type 1, only 30% to 50% of those in higher socioeconomic groups exhibit seroconversion.[16]

Herpes Simplex Virus Type 2

Infection with HSV type 2 also is related to age and socioeconomic status. Infection and seroconversion increase rapidly after age 14 years. Among adults of upper socioeconomic groups, type-specific antibody is found in 10%, whereas it is present in 20% to 60% of those in lower socioeconomic groups.[16] Only 10% to 15% of infected persons have experienced clinical illness as a result of the *primary* infection.[8]

Because most primary infections lead to *subclinical* disease, the susceptibility of a given person to HSV infection is impossible to assess without antibody testing. Similarly, because virus continues to be shed for several months after recovery from infection, it cannot be verified that a given person is not a reservoir of HSV.

HERPETIC WHITLOW

Historical Aspects

Herpetic infection of the finger is probably not rare, although it is likely to be misdiagnosed. Recognized only during the past 30 years as an occupational hazard among certain health-care personnel, it had been described decades earlier. Typically, the patient sustained an apparent or overt injury to the finger that was then contaminated by oral secretions.

Children

One of the earliest reports described four children who had pinhead-sized vesicles resembling those usually seen with herpes febrilis ("cold sores") near the tip of a finger. Two of the children also had similar lesions on the lower lip, suggesting self-contamination, and another had repeated eruptions at the fingertip.[17]

Subsequent case reports highlighted other clinical aspects. The coalescence of several similar vesicles on the finger of a hairdresser, who probably traumatized it on a curling iron, resulted in a painful bullous lesion resembling bacterial infection; on incision, however, no pus was found. The lesion recurred several times, sometimes with a prodromal neuralgia of the arm, and virus was isolated.[18]

A similar lesion occurred in a child who had sucked her finger when she had gingivostomatitis.[19] Another report suggested that an eruption on an infant's hand after trauma resulted from contamination with the child's own saliva or that of one of her parents, who had "kissed the hurt."[20]

Adults

In contrast, the finger infection occurring in adults has been reported almost exclusively among health-care personnel who sustained trivial or inapparent injury and whose occupation exposed them to oral secretions.

MEDICAL PERSONNEL. Stern and colleagues were the first to identify the lesion as an occupational hazard after reviewing 54 such infections in nurses between the ages of 18 and 29 years.[21] In a reflection of their origin among the upper socioeconomic classes, half of the nurses had no antibody to HSV before beginning work, and in one third of this group, lesions (primary illness) developed within 1 year. Lesions (recurrence) also developed in other nurses with moderate antibody titers. Most of the lesions developed during the care of patients lacking clinical evidence of HSV infection. Stern and colleagues isolated HSV from 1.2% of asymptomatic adults and 6.5% of postoperative neurosurgical patients, many of whom were comatose and required frequent oropharyngeal suctioning. Seven nurses had recurrences.

Stern's group termed the lesion a "whitlow" (synonym, "felon") to emphasize its resemblance to pyogenic infection such as the familiar paronychia. With or without surgical intervention, secondary bacterial infection was common but resistant to antibiotic agents even when isolates demonstrated sensitivity in vitro. Although most of their patients had vesicles that permitted a clinical diagnosis, others had large bullous lesions when first seen. Constitutional symptoms such as fever and lymphadenopathy were uncommon. Pain and the natural course of the illness resulted in a loss of an average of 3 weeks work per nurse.

More recently, others have reported this lesion in surgeons,[22] nurses,[23] dentists,[24] and anesthesiologists,[25–27] all personnel whose work exposed them to oral secretions. Usually the constitutional symptoms are more prominent than those in Stern and colleagues' report and include fever, lymphangitis, lymphadenopathy, and malaise. This difference in symptoms is probably more apparent than real, because these reports described persons who sought care, whereas Stern's group's report included all cases. It is important to remember that the finger lesion can serve as the reservoir for self-inoculation of the eye and oropharynx. In as many as 37% of infected persons, symptomatic HSV pharyngitis develops from contact with secretions from the infected finger.[28]

Symptoms

Although the development of the lesion can be insidious, a progression of symptoms is often evident. Intense itching and

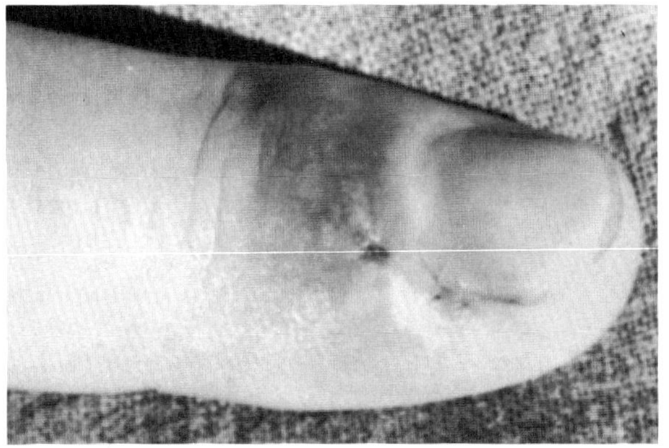

FIGURE 5-2. Appearance of herpetic whitlow on an index finger of an intensive care nurse on day 5, when a periungual blister surrounded by erythema had formed from the coalescence of vesicles. Note the proximity of the lesion to the minor trauma in the cuticle.

pain are followed within 1 day by the appearance of a vesicle with surrounding erythema at the site of minor injury on the fingertip (Fig. 5-2). Satellite vesicles appear during the next 7 to 10 days and often coalesce to form a yellow, honeycombed structure. Although the contained fluid is clear and yellowish at first, within 1 week it becomes cloudy, and the lesion becomes a grayish blister (Fig. 5-3).

Throbbing pain becomes considerable as the distal portion of the involved finger, now erythematous or violaceous, swells. During the third week, the pain abates and the lesions become encrusted. Desquamation of superficial layers of the skin occurs, with complete healing after 3 weeks. Many reports emphasize that needless surgical intervention only ensures bacterial superinfection and prolongs the clinical course.

Diagnosis

Usually the lesion can be identified on clinical grounds alone, such as its appearance. Though often absent, a history of trauma at the site of infection and an exposure to a source of HSV are important in diagnosis. Definitive diagnosis is established by HSV isolation and identification with virus-specific antiserum, demonstration of multinucleated giant epithelial cells or nuclear inclusion bodies in smears taken from the base of a vesicle (Tzanck smear), and a fourfold increase in HSV antibody titers in serum from the convalescent patient. If the presumed diagnosis of herpetic whitlow is not supported, then one must consider paronychia caused by bacteria (eg, *Staphylococcus* or *Streptococcus* species) or fungus (eg, *Candida albicans*) as well as deep fungal infections such as histoplasmosis, blastomycosis, or coccidioidomycosis.

Treatment

General Considerations

Therapy should be conservative and consist of immobilization, elevation, and analgesia. Although particularly tense and

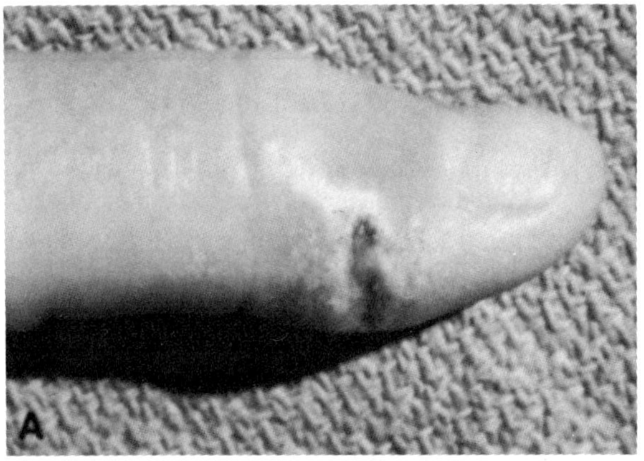

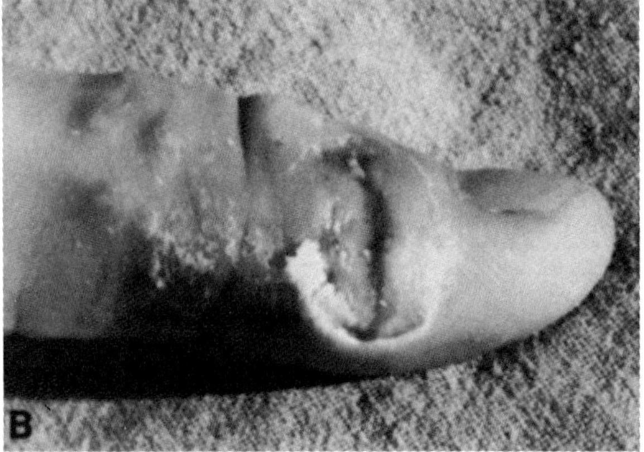

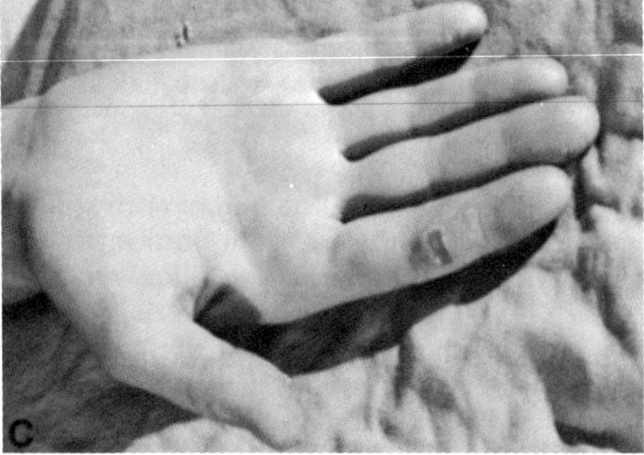

FIGURE 5-3. An early lesion on the thumb of an anesthesiology resident. It has been subjected to incision and drainage (**A**), with subsequent bacterial infection and ulceration of the lesion 1 week later (**B**), at which time satellite vesicles appeared proximal to the superinfected lesion. After 2 weeks, satellite lesions appeared over both the thumb and adjacent finger (**C**). Note also the numerous sites of trauma on other fingers.

painful vesicles may be incised, deep incision is contraindicated. Should lymphangitis appear, penicillin administration is indicated.

Specific Measures

Much of what is known about specific therapy for herpetic whitlow has been gleaned from clinical experience and investigation with the more common and serious HSV infections, such as keratitis, meningoencephalitis, and visceral herpetic infection. Although controlled clinical trials have been conducted with specific therapy in these diseases, no rigorous studies of the clinical efficacy of the potential specific therapies for herpetic whitlow have been performed. In addition, patients often do not seek treatment at the onset of the illness, when it is possible to alter and possibly abort the progression of symptoms.[29]

Antiviral Chemotherapy

Antiviral agents include nucleoside derivatives that interfere with HSV DNA replication. These nucleoside analogues are activated by a virus-specific enzyme (thymidine kinase); poor substrate for healthy cells, these substances are more selective for virus-infected cells and thus less toxic to normal cells.

ACYCLOVIR. 9-2[2-Hydroxyethoxymethyl]guanine (acyclovir) is currently the agent most effective against HSV.[29,30] Available in topical, oral, and intravenous preparations, this purine analogue can be administered topically, as a 5% ointment, to vesicles when they first appear; alternatively, oral administration should be begun if the therapy is to influence the duration of the illness. The need for prompt institution of therapy means that this (and most other) treatment is reserved for recurrent rather than initial lesions. Typically, the affected person experiences premonitory symptoms of itching and burning pain before vesicles appear; thus, he or she is advised to begin applying acyclovir or to begin taking the oral formulation. Though probably not a relevant clinical problem in healthy persons, acyclovir-resistant HSV has emerged in association with acquired immunodeficiency syndrome.[3]

IDOXURIDINE. 5-Iodo-2′-Deoxyuridine (idoxuridine) has proven effective in the treatment of HSV keratitis,[31] but, without a suitable carrier substance, it is not effective against herpetic whitlow. It seems to be effective when applied as a solution of 5% idoxuridine in dimethyl sulfoxide.[32] However, dimethyl sulfoxide is not approved for this application, and the use of idoxuridine as an antiviral agent is giving way to the use of acyclovir.

VIDARABINE. 9-β-D-Arabinofuranosyladenine (vidarabine), like idoxuridine, is effective in the treatment of other herpetic infections (keratitis and meningoencephalitis) but, possibly because of poor solubility in the solvent, is not effective in the treatment of herpetic whitlow.[33,34]

2-DEOXY-D-GLUCOSE. 2-Deoxy-D-glucose is effective in the treatment of genital skin lesions when applied as a cream, but its efficacy in the treatment of herpetic whitlow is unknown.

Interferon

Interferon, a protein produced by stimulated white cells, induces an antiviral state. It has been found effective in the topical therapy of herpetic keratitis and, when administered intramuscularly, in the prevention of recurrence of skin lesions after surgery on the trigeminal root. The limited supply of interferon has precluded its use in herpetic whitlow.

Surgery

Superficial epidermal excision of recurrent herpetic whitlow within 36 hours of its appearance appears to prevent recurrence at the given site in almost all cases.[35]

Other Approaches

In recent years a variety of other potential therapies have been found to be ineffective. These include topical application of diethyl ether and chloroform, presumably to dissolve the lipid-containing viral envelope; parenteral administration of nonspecific immunoenhancers such as bacille Calmette-Guérin (BCG) vaccine and levamisole; and the application of heterotricyclic dyes with exposure to ultraviolet light (photodynamic inactivation).

PREVENTION

The ubiquity and infectivity of HSV, the frequency with which minor finger trauma occurs, the uncertain immunity of anesthesia (and other health care) personnel, and the morbidity and time lost to herpetic whitlow all argue for the importance of prevention.

Identification of Potential HSV Carriers

In addition to persons with obvious herpetic lesions, potential carriers include young children, patients recently recovered from HSV infection, and a wide variety of patients with impaired immune defenses (Table 5-1). Anesthesia and other personnel with active and recent herpetic infections should refrain from treating immunocompromised patients.

TABLE 5-1
Clinical Reservoir States for Herpes Simplex Virus

- Malignant disease (especially hematologic)
- Malnutrition (eg, kwashiorkor)
- Infectious disease (eg, measles, *Haemophilus influenzae*)
- Defective cell-mediated immunity (eg, acquired immunodeficiency syndrome)
- Thermal burns
- Drug-induced immunosuppression (eg, transplantation or asthma)
- Overt HSV infection
- Convalescence from recent HSV infection
- Young age (children)

Avoidance of Unprotected Contact With Oral Secretions

The virus has been found in oral, oropharyngeal, and tracheobronchial secretions. Consistent adherence to universal precautions—especially the wearing of gloves, adopted as protection against more severe infections (eg, hepatitis or acquired immunodeficiency syndrome)—suffices.

Now that an effective antiviral agent, acyclovir, is available, the lesion should be treated at the earliest time to prevent or shorten its natural course, including the possibility of recurrence. In addition, because unwarranted surgical intervention (ie, incision and drainage as opposed to excision) prolongs the course of this lesion, considerable morbidity can be avoided by resisting the urge to incise and drain it.

REFERENCES

1. Fenwick ML: Viruses and viral infection: I. the nature of viruses and their growth. In Florey L (ed): General pathology. 4th ed. Philadelphia, WB Saunders, 1970: 898.
2. Siegal FP, Lopez C, Hammer GS, et al: Severe acquired immunodeficiency in male homosexuals manifested by chronic perianal ulcerative herpes simplex lesions. N Engl J Med 305: 1439, 1981
3. Erlich KS, Mills J, Chatis P, et al: Acyclovir-resistant herpes simplex virus infections in patients with the acquired immunodeficiency syndrome. N Engl J Med 320:293, 1989
4. Shneidman DW, Barr RJ, Graham JH: Chronic cutaneous herpes simplex. JAMA 241:592, 1979
5. Baringer JR, Swoveland P: Recovery of herpes simplex virus from human trigeminal ganglions. N Engl J Med 288:648, 1973
6. Cook ML, Bastone VB, Stevens JG: Evidence that neurons harbor latent herpes simplex virus. Infect Immun 9:946, 1974
7. Warren KG, Brown SM, Wroblewska Z, et al: Isolation of latent herpes simplex virus from the superior cervical and vagus ganglions of human beings. N Engl J Med 298:1068, 1978
8. Warren SL, Carpenter CM, Boak RA: Symptomatic herpes, a sequela of artificially induced fever: incidence and clinical aspects; recovery of virus from herpetic vesicles; and comparison with a known strain of herpes virus. J Exp Med 71:155, 1940
9. Douglas MJ, McMorland GH: Possible association of herpes simplex type I reactivation with epidural morphine administration. Can J Anaesth 34:426, 1987
10. Crone L-A L, Conly JM, Clark KM, et al: Recurrent herpes simplex virus labialis and the use of epidural morphine in obstetric patients. Anesth Analg 67:318, 1988
11. Gieraerts R, Vaes L, Navalgund A, et al: Recurrent HSVL and the use of epidural morphine in obstetrics. Anesth Analg 68: 413, 1989
12. Young EJ, Vainrub B, Musher DM, et al: Acute pharyngotonsillitis caused by herpesvirus type 2. JAMA 239:1885, 1978
13. Wolontis S, Jeanson SS: Correlation of herpes simplex virus types 1 and 2 with clinical features of infection. J Infect Dis 135:28, 1977
14. Giacobetti R: Herpetic whitlow. Dermatology 18:55, 1979
15. Buddingh GJ, Schrum DI, Lanier JC, et al: Studies of the natural history of herpes simplex infections. Pediatrics 11:595, 1952
16. Nahmias AJ, Roizman B: Infection with herpes simplex virus types 1 and 2. N Engl J Med 289:667, 719, 781, 1973
17. Adamson HG: Herpes febrilis attacking the fingers. Br J Dermatol 21:323, 1909
18. Nicolau S, Poincloux P: Etude clinique et experimentale d'un cas d'herpes recidivant du doigt. Ann Inst Pasteur 38:977, 1924
19. Burnet FM, Williams SW: Herpes simplex: a new point of view. Med J Aust 1:;637, 1939
20. Findlay GM, MacCallum FO: Recurrent traumatic herpes. Lancet 1:249, 1940
21. Stern H, Elek SD, Millar DM, et al: Herpetic whitlow: a form of cross-infection in hospitals. Lancet 2:871, 1959
22. Greaves WL: The problem of herpetic whitlow among hospital personnel. Infect Control 1:381, 1980
23. Chang T-W, Gorbach SL: Primary and recurrent herpetic whitlow. Int J Dermatol 16:752, 1977
24. Brightman VJ, Guggenheimer JG: Herpetic paronychia: primary herpes simplex infection of the finger. JAMA 80:112, 1970
25. DeYoung GG, Harrison AW, Shapley JM: Herpes simplex cross infection in the operating room. Can Anaesth Soc J 15:394, 1968
26. Orkin FK: Herpetic whitlow: occupational hazard to the anesthesiologist. Anesthesiology 33:671, 1970
27. Goldberg ME, Brajer J, Seltzer JL: Herpetic whitlow: hazard for the anesthesiologist and an unusual complication. Anesthesiology Review 12:26, 1985
28. Grey L, Spear PG: Infections with herpes simplex viruses. N Engl J Med 314:686, 1986
29. Spruance SL, Hamill ML, Hoge WS, et al: Acyclovir prevents reactivation of herpes simplex labialis in skiers. JAMA 260:1597, 1988
30. Dorsky DI, Crumpacker CS: Drugs five years later: acyclovir. Ann Intern Med 107:859, 1987
31. Kaufman HE: Ocular antiviral therapy in perspective. J Infect Dis 133(suppl):96, 1976
32. MacCallum FO, Juel-Juenson BE: Herpes simplex virus skin infection in man treated with idoxuridine in dimethyl sulfoxide: results of double-blind controlled trial. Br Med J 2:805, 1966
33. Goodman EL, Luby JP, Johnson MT: Prospective double-blind evaluation of topical adenine arabinoside in male herpes progenitalis. Antimicrob Agents Chemother 8:693, 1975
34. Adams HG, Benson EA, Alexander ER: Genital herpetic infection in men and women: clinical course and effect of topical application of adenine arabinoside. J Infect Dis 133(suppl):151, 1976
35. Shelley WB: Surgical treatment for recurrent herpes simplex. Lancet 2:1021, 1978

FURTHER READING

Hirsch MS: Herpes simplex virus. In Mandell GL, Douglas RG Jr, Bennett JE (eds): Principles and practice of infectious disease. 3rd ed. New York: John Wiley & Sons, 1990: 1144

Complications in Anesthesiology, second edition,
edited by Nikolaus Gravenstein and Robert R. Kirby.
Lippincott-Raven Publishers, Philadelphia © 1996.

CHAPTER 6

Anesthesia Equipment

Michael L. Good
Nikolaus Gravenstein

Anesthesia equipment may be implicated in complications occurring during anesthesia. Cooper and Newbower reported on an analysis of critical incidents in anesthesia—situations that did or could have resulted in undesirable patient outcomes—and found nearly one third attributable to equipment failure or disconnection.[1] Gilron, in a review of medical device problems reported to the Health Protection Branch of Health and Welfare Canada from 1987 to 1992, reports that although only 2.3% of newly marketed devices are anesthesia devices, 8.6% of all problem reports or recalls and 37.5% of all alerts originate from anesthesia devices.[2] He further observes that this may underrepresent actual problems, as only 19% of reports were received from anesthetists. Whether anesthetic equipment constitutes a greater risk of failure than other medical equipment is debatable.[3] However, it is clear from both Cooper and Gilron's data that the user equipment interface can still be improved. Although anesthesia equipment failure is inevitable, patient injury from equipment failure should be preventable.

When confronted with untoward clinical situations, the clinician must rapidly determine whether the difficulty lies with the patient or the equipment and have a plan to systematically identify and then correct or compensate for equipment failure before it causes injury to the patient.

HYPOXEMIA

Equipment problems causing hypoxemia can be grouped into three general categories: (1) those producing a hypoxic inspired gas mixture; (2) those that render the patient apneic or severely hypoventilated; and (3) those that cause mismatching of pulmonary ventilation and perfusion.

Hypoxic Inspired Gas Mixture

A hypoxic inspired gas mixture contains less than 21% oxygen (O_2) and can be diagnosed only by measuring the O_2 concentration in the breathing circuit. Thus, the American Society of Anesthesiologists (ASA) Standards for Basic Intraoperative Monitoring[4] stipulate the use of a low oxygen concentration alarm during the administration of every general anesthetic. The cause of a hypoxic gas mixture is determined by tracing the "path of O_2" in a retrograde fashion from the breathing circuit back to the pressurized O_2 source (Fig. 6-1). Possible causes are listed in Table 6-1.

Obstructed Fresh Gas Hose

An obstructed fresh gas hose prevents O_2 from flowing into the breathing circuit (see Fig. 6-1, label *A*). Because the patient continues to consume O_2 at approximately 4 mL/kg/min, the O_2 concentration in the breathing circuit decreases, eventually reaching hypoxic levels. Inspection of the hose will usually reveal obvious kinks such as when the fresh gas hose is inadvertently closed in a drawer of the anesthesia machine. Verification of fresh gas flow can be made by momentarily disconnecting the distal end of the fresh gas hose and feeling or listening for the movement of gas from the open end.

Hypoxic Gas Flow Settings

Older anesthesia machines may not have O_2-nitrous oxide interlock or proportioning systems that prevent the user from setting hypoxic fresh gas flows. Alternatively, machines with proportioning systems may have been modified for additional gases, such as helium or carbon dioxide. If the additional gas flow controls are not incorporated into the interlock or proportioning system, the potential for hypoxic gas flow settings remains (see Fig. 6-1, label *B*). Other factors that contribute to the potential for hypoxic gas flow settings include (1) the lack of international agreement on the standard position for the O_2 flow control (positioned to the right of the other flow controls in the United States and Canada, but positioned to the left of the other flow controls in many other countries); (2) draping wires or hoses around the flow control knobs

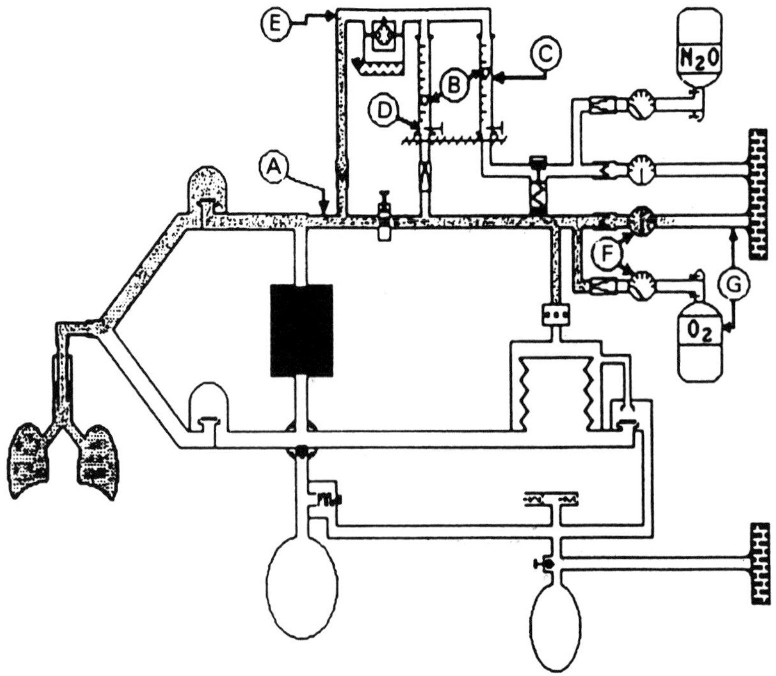

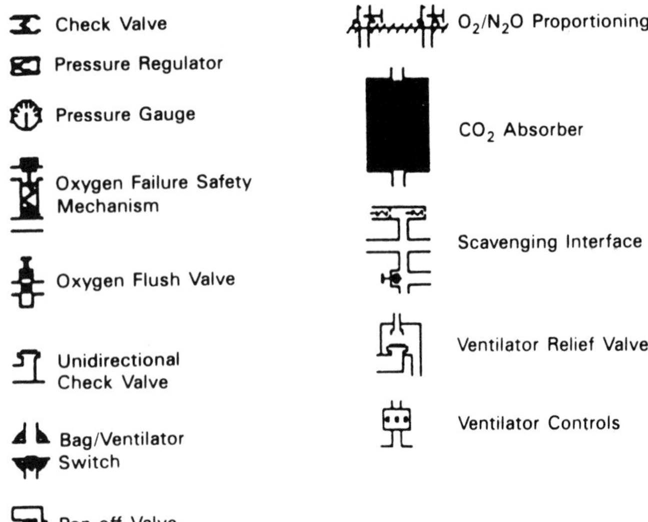

FIGURE 6-1. The differential diagnosis of hypoxic inspired gas mixture is evaluated by tracing the path of oxygen (*shaded*) through the anesthesia machine. Potential causes of a hypoxic inspired gas mixture are identified in this machine schematic (schematic courtesy of J.S. Gravenstein, MD). *A*, obstructed fresh gas hose; *B*, hypoxic fresh gas flow setting; *C*, inaccurate flowmeters; *D*, inadequate oxygen flow; *E*, low pressure circuit leak; *F*, loss of oxygen supply pressure; *G*, contaminated oxygen supply. (Good ML, Paulus DA: Equipment. In Gravenstein N (ed). Manual of complications during anesthesia, p 85. Philadelphia, JB Lippincott, 1991)

(which may alter the settings); and (3) dual O_2 flow controls (separate high and low) making it easy to misread which control is actually being set.

Inaccurate Flowmeters

Flowmeters are gas-specific; they should not be interchanged. Each flowmeter tube and its bobbin is individually calibrated. The bobbin from one flowmeter tube should not be used with a different flowmeter tube. Dirt, grease, oil, static electricity, misalignment, improper calibration, and cracks all lead to inaccurate flow readings, and, consequently, may cause hypoxic gas flows (see Fig. 6-1, label *C*). Flowmeter accuracy decreases at low flows.

Inadequate O_2 Flow Rate

Oxygen must enter the breathing circuit at a rate that equals or exceeds the patient's O_2 consumption and other sources of oxygen loss from the circuit (see Fig. 6-1, label *D*). Generally the most prominent source of oxygen loss is that into a sidestream gas analyzer—unless the sampled gas is then

TABLE 6-1
Hypoxic Gas Etiologies

- Obstructed fresh gas hose
- Hypoxic fresh gas flow settings
- Inaccurate flowmeters
- Inadequate O_2 flow
- Leak in the low-pressure system
- Loss of O_2 supply pressure
- Contaminated O_2 supply

reinfused into the expiratory limb of the breathing circuit. Many gas analyzers sample circuit gas at 250 mL/min. If the circuit contains a FIO_2 of 0.4, the gas analyzer sampling 250 mL/min consumes 100 mL O_2/min. A 70-kg patient consuming 4 mL O_2/kg/min then requires an O_2 flow of at least 380 mL/min plus that attributable to any other leaks in the breathing system.

If the minimum O_2 flow rate (patient consumption plus loss to leaks) is not met, the O_2 concentration in the breathing circuit will fall. This fall will be hastened if a breathing circuit leak is present and a "hanging bellows" type of ventilator is in use. The negative pressure generated by the falling bellows during expiration will draw air into the breathing circuit, which dilutes the O_2 concentration. This effect is most significant at low fresh gas flow rates.

Leak in the Low Pressure System

The low pressure system (LPS) of the anesthesia machine encompasses all components of the anesthesia machine between the flow control valves and the common fresh gas outlet (see Fig. 6-1, label *E*). This includes the gas flow control valves, flowmeters, vaporizers, and all piping and connectors. A leak in any of these components will cause fresh gas, including O_2, to escape from the anesthesia machine and, therefore, not be delivered to the breathing circuit. Clinically, "light anesthesia" and hypoxemia may develop. Leaks in the LPS can develop with cracked, loose, or misaligned flowmeter tubes, loose connections between system components, or misaligned or defective vaporizers. A loose cap on the vaporizing filling port is perhaps the most common site for this type of leak.

On anesthesia machines that have a common gas outlet check valve (eg, Ohmeda), the pre-use positive pressure leak check of the breathing circuit will not detect leaks in the LPS as the common gas outlet check valve prevents retrograde gas flow from the breathing circuit into the anesthesia machine. On machines with an outlet check valve, leaks in the LPS are detected reliably only by the negative pressure leak test (Fig. 6-2) performed during pre-use machine checkout. With the anesthesia machine turned off (to exclude the minimum O_2 flow), a vacuum bulb is attached to the fresh gas outlet and squeezed to generate negative pressure within the LPS. If the LPS is leak-free, the bulb will remain collapsed for at least 10 seconds (Fig. 6-2*A*). If the bulb expands to its normal shape in less than 10 seconds, a leak is present in the LPS (Fig. 6-2*B*). The test must be repeated with each vaporizer individually turned on; otherwise, a leak in the vaporizer such as from a loose filler cap will not be detected.

An alternative and very practical test that can be performed during machine use is to observe the flowmeters during mechanical ventilation for ventilator cycling-related bobbin oscillation. Similarly, the fresh gas hose can be *momentarily* kinked and released. If the LPS is leak free, back pressure will rapidly develop and cause the flowmeter bobbins to oscillate down and up as the fresh gas hose is kinked and released, respectively. If a large leak is present in the LPS, back pressure will not develop, and the bobbins will remain stationary. Occlusion of the fresh gas hose should be brief (<1 second), as prolonged occlusion in a leak-free system results in excessive pressure, which can damage the anesthesia machine. The occlusion test is not as sensitive as the negative pressure test, and may not detect small LPS leaks. Thus, the negative pressure test should be performed each day before the anesthesia machine is used.

Manufacturers of some anesthesia machines that do not have a common gas outlet check valve (eg, Drager Narkomed), recommend a positive pressure leak check (Fig. 6-3). A single breathing hose is connected to the inspiratory and expiratory ports of the absorber canister and, with a sphygmomanometer bulb attached to the breathing bag mount, 50 cm H_2O pressure is generated. If the pressure remains greater than 30 cm H_2O for 30 seconds, a significant LPC leak is not present. If pressure falls below 30 cm H_2O within 30 seconds, a leak exists in the LPC, the breathing hose, or the absorber canister.

The negative pressure test or the occlusion test described previously can be used to differentiate a canister or breathing hose leak from a LPC leak. We recently compared the sensitivity of the various leak check procedures for detecting LPS leaks on anesthesia machines with and without common outlet check valves.[5] Only the negative pressure leak check detected all leaks on all machines. Other leak check procedures, including the positive-pressure leak check and the fresh gas hose occlusion test, failed to detect many of the smaller LPS leaks. Thus, the negative pressure leak check is recommended during pre-use machine checkout. The fresh gas hose occlusion test, despite its insensitivity to small leaks, remains the only leak check that can be performed during an anesthetic with the anesthesia machine turned on.

Loss of O_2 Supply Pressure

Contemporary anesthesia machines include an O_2 pressure failure safety mechanism—or "fail-safe" device—that interrupts the flow of all gases when O_2 supply pressure is lost and a "low O_2 pressure" alarm (see Fig. 6-1, label *F*). Failure of these safety devices or their absence on older anesthesia machines will allow other gases to continue flowing when O_2 supply pressure has been lost. Hypoxic-inspired gas mixtures may then develop. Separate gauges on the front of the anesthesia machine report the O_2 supply pressure from the central hospital O_2 pipeline and also from the reserve O_2 cylinders on the anesthesia machine. The stem valve of the O_2 cylinder must be open before the pressure gauge will indicate the cylinder pressure. Because these cylinders are located in the high

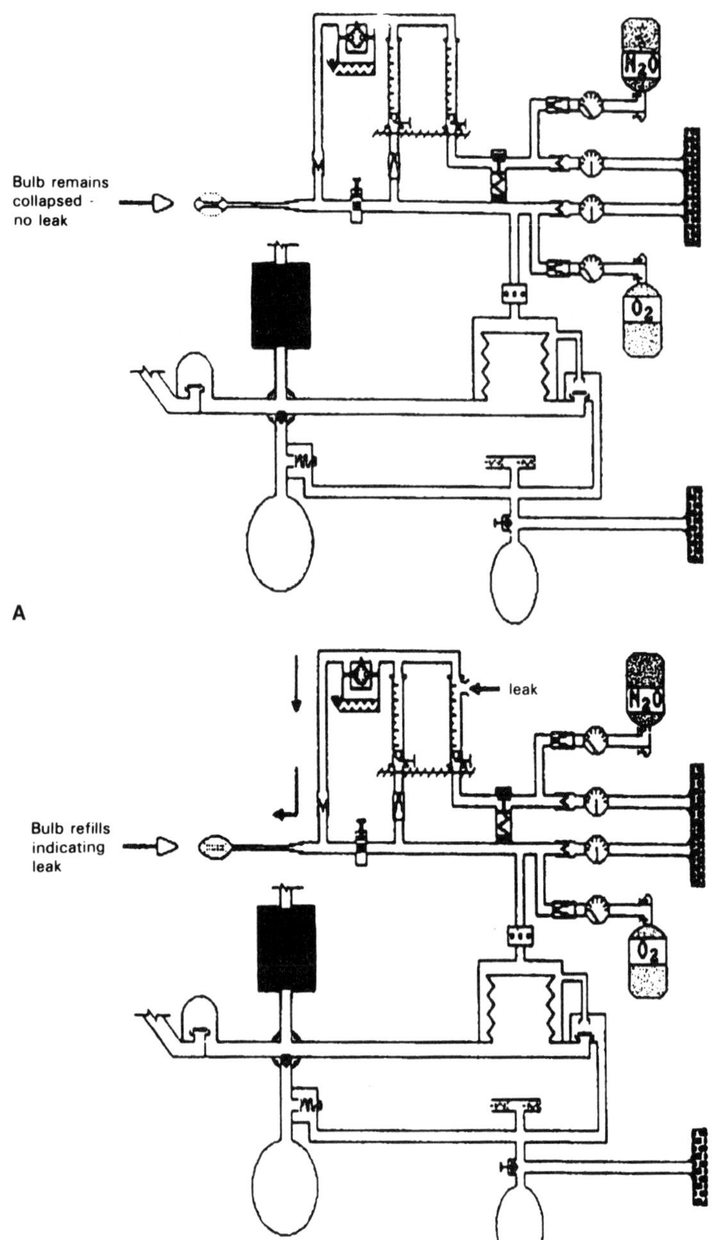

FIGURE 6-2. (**A**) Low pressure circuit leak check–negative pressure test. With the anesthesia machine turned off, a vacuum bulb is attached to the common gas outlet and squeezed until it collapses. This generates negative pressure in the low pressure circuit. If the low pressure circuit is leak free, the bulb remains collapsed for 10 seconds or longer. (**B**) If the bulb expands to its original shape in less than 10 seconds, a significant leak is present in the low pressure circuit. (See Figure 6-1 for schematic legend.) (Good ML, Paulus DA: Equipment. In Gravenstein N (ed). Manual of complications during anesthesia, p 88. Philadelphia, JB Lippincott, 1991)

pressure system of the anesthesia machine and frequently have slow leaks at their connections, they should be kept closed except during testing or while in use to avoid their inadvertent depletion.

Contaminated O_2 Supply

Hypoxic-inspired gas mixtures rapidly develop when a non-O_2–containing gas is substituted for O_2 in the anesthesia machine (see Fig. 6-1, label *G*). Such errors occur when the hospital's central O_2 pipeline is either misfilled or misconnected at a site remote to the anesthetizing location, or if the diameter index system is defeated and hoses are misconnected between the pipeline wall outlet box and the anesthesia machine inlet. Similarly, gas cylinders can be misfilled, mislabeled, or have their pin-indexing system defeated in a number of ways. The diagnosis of a contaminated O_2 supply is made by excluding the other causes of a hypoxic-inspired gas mixture. It is important to remember that the fail-safe mechanism and the "low O_2 pressure" alarm are pressure-driven safety devices—they do not identify, prevent, or warn the anesthetist of a contaminated oxygen supply. Importantly, if a pipeline contamination or crossover is present, the reserve O_2 cylinder will not be effective until the O_2 supply hose has been disconnected from the wall outlet (Fig. 6-4). Cylinder pressure is reduced inside the anesthesia machine to approximately 45 psi, while the pipeline pressure is typically 50 to 55 psi. If both the pipeline source and cylinder source are connected

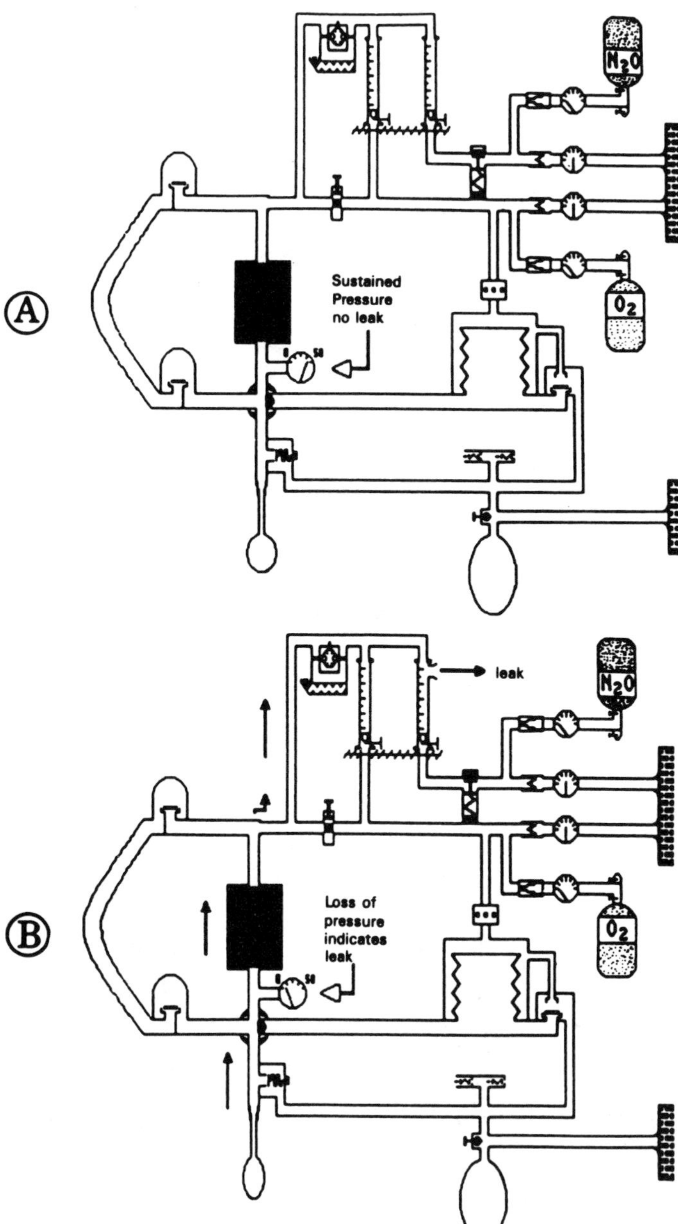

FIGURE 6-3. (**A**) Low pressure circuit leak check–positive pressure test. This test is for anesthesia machines *without* a common gas outlet check valve or a vaporizer check valve. With the anesthesia machine turned off, a single hose connecting the inspiratory and expiratory parts of the absorber canister, and the "pop-off" valve closed, a sphygmomanometer bulb is attached to the bag mount and squeezed until 50 cm H_2O of pressure is registered on the absorber pressure gauge. If the pressure remains at least 30 cm H_2O for 30 seconds, the low pressure circuit (and O_2 canister) is without significant leaks. (**B**) If the pressure drops below 30 cm H_2O in less than 30 seconds, a significant leak is present in the low pressure circuit, breathing hose, or CO_2 canister. (See Figure 6-1 for schematic legend). (Good ML, Paulus DA: Equipment. In Gravenstein N (ed). Manual of Complications During Anesthesia, p 90. Philadelphia, JB Lippincott, 1991)

to the anesthesia machine, the pipeline source, regardless of the gas contained, will be preferentially used if its pressure exceeds the regulated cylinder pressure.

Hypoventilation

The O_2 in the breathing circuit must be delivered to the patient's lungs for oxygenation to occur. Equipment-related problems that prevent this delivery include esophageal intubation, apnea, and alveolar hypoventilation. Patient examination (inspection, palpation, auscultation) and measurements of airway pressure, gas flow, and CO_2 are used to differentiate among the three (Table 6-2).

Esophageal Intubation

With an esophageal intubation, there is no exhaled CO_2, but airway pressure and gas flow are present during gastric ventilation. If the stomach has been distended with CO_2-containing gas during mask ventilation, or as a consequence of ingestion of a carbonated beverage, a capnogram may be obtained initially, but the capnogram will likely have an abnormal shape, will not be sustained for more than the first minute of ventilation, and will quickly decrease with each ventilatory cycle.[6] When CO_2 is absent in the exhaled gas, one must suspect an esophageal intubation until proven otherwise. The comprehensive review by Birmingham and coworkers discusses the various methods of detecting an esoph-

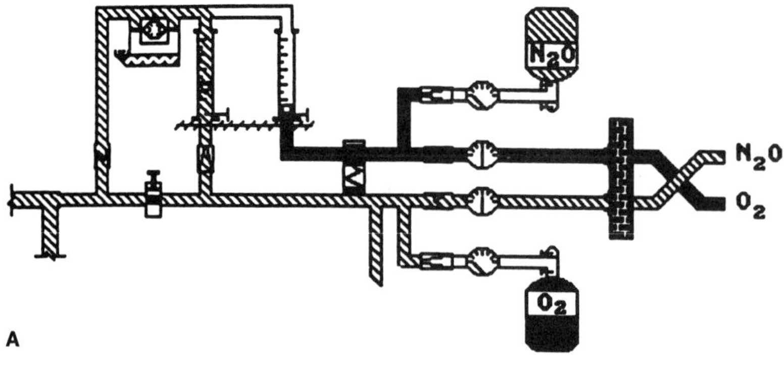

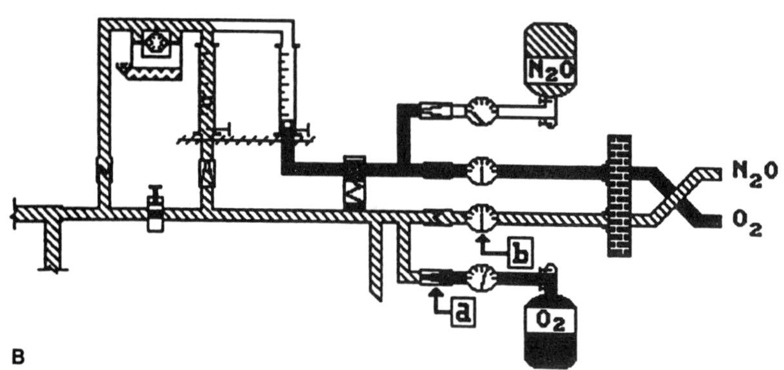

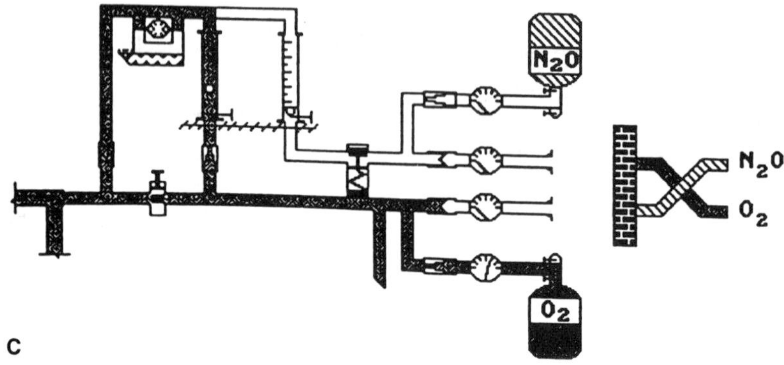

FIGURE 6-4. Contaminated O_2 supply. (**A**) Oxygen and nitrous oxide pipelines are crossed at site remote from operating room. When the fresh gas flow is set at 100% oxygen, nitrous oxide (*striped*) rather than oxygen is actually delivered to the patient. (**B**) When the reserve oxygen cylinder is opened, gas from the pipeline supply (ie, 100% nitrous oxide) continues to be delivered to the patient. This occurs because the pipeline pressure is 50–55 psi (*a*) while the cylinder pressure is regulated to approximately 45 psi by the cylinder pressure regulator (*b*). (**C**) Once the supply hoses (which connect the anesthesia machine to the wall outlets) have been disconnected, oxygen from the reserve oxygen cylinder (*shaded*) enters the anesthesia machine, and corrects the hypoxic inspired gas mixture. (See Figure 6-1 for schematic legend.) (Good ML, Paulus DA: Equipment. In Gravenstein N (ed). Manual of complications during anesthesia, p 92. Philadelphia, JB Lippincott, 1991)

TABLE 6-2
Hypoxemia Caused by Hypoventilation

	ESOPHAGEAL INTUBATION	APNEA	ALVEOLAR HYPOVENTILATION
Exhaled CO_2	No*	No	Yes
Airway pressure fluctuations	Yes	No	Yes
Gas flow at the airway	Yes	No	Yes

* CO_2 may be present for several breaths but rapidly declines as any CO_2 in the stomach is rapidly washed out.

Good ML, Paulus DA: Equipment. In Gravenstein N (ed): Manual of complications during anesthesia. Philadelphia; JB Lippincott, 1991:89.

ageal intubation and highlights the utility of capnography in identifying this complication.[7]

Apnea

Apnea is defined as the absence of exhaled CO_2, airway pressure fluctuations, and gas flow (see Table 6-1). There are neither breath sounds nor chest excursions. Causes of apnea in an intubated, mechanically ventilated patient include a disconnect at any site in the breathing circuit, an open adjustable pressure-limiting (APL or pop-off) valve, or failure of the mechanical ventilator. Apnea also occurs if the mechanical ventilator is not turned on, or if the bag–ventilator selector switch is left in the bag position. Equipment failures that cause apnea are shown in Figure 6-5.

Alveolar Hypoventilation

If supplemental O_2 is in use, only severe alveolar hypoventilation will cause hypoxemia.[8] Nonetheless, alveolar hypoventilation is included in the differential diagnosis of hypoxemia. During hypoventilation, exhaled CO_2, airway pressure fluctuations, and gas flow are all present (see Table 6-2). Causes of hypoventilation include leaks in the breathing circuit or around the endotracheal tube (eg, no cuff, deflated cuff) in which the peak airway pressure is decreased, breathing circuit obstructions in which the peak airway pressure is increased, and mechanical ventilator failures in which the set ventilator parameters are not actually delivered. This type of failure highlights the benefit of actually measuring the patient's exhaled tidal volume rather than simply relying on the ventilator control setting. Leaks, obstructions, and ventilator failures typically cause hypercapnia before they cause hypoxemia, and are discussed under the heading Hypercapnia.

VENTILATION/PERFUSION MISMATCH

Inadvertent endobronchial intubation creates a large intrapulmonary shunt, as an entire nonventilated lung continues to be partially perfused. This is the most likely equipment related cause of ventilation/perfusion mismatch. Diagnosis is

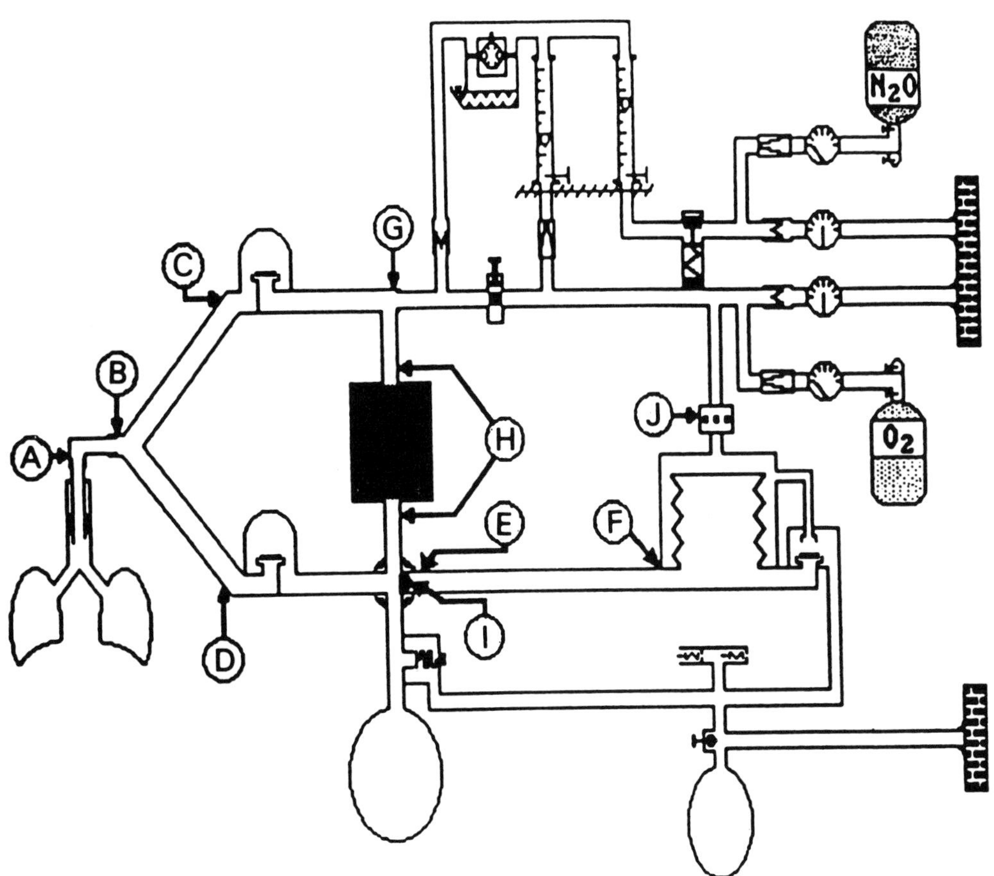

FIGURE 6-5. Equipment problems that cause apnea: disconnection between endotracheal tube and elbow connector (*A*); elbow connector and breathing circuit Y-piece (*B*); breathing circuit attachments to the inspiratory (*C*) and expiratory (*D*) ports of the CO_2 canister; ventilator hose attachments to the CO_2 canister (*E*) and ventilator (*F*) and fresh gas hose attachment to the CO_2 canister (*G*); an open CO_2 canister (*H*); a bag/ventilator selector switch in the bag position during mechanical ventilation (*I*); and a mechanical ventilator that is malfunctioning or not turned on (*J*). (Good ML, Paulus DA: Equipment. In Gravenstein N (ed). Manual of complications during anesthesia, p 95. Philadelphia, JB Lippincott, 1991)

made by inspecting, auscultating, and palpating the chest for symmetric chest and lung expansion. High and sustained airway pressure decreases pulmonary blood flow, increasing ventilation/perfusion mismatch, and causing arterial hypoxemia if severe. Excessively high airway pressures may lead to pulmonary barotrauma (eg, pneumothorax), and hypoxemia. Because the elevated airway pressure precedes the desaturation, these complications are discussed in the section on increased airway pressure.

HYPERCAPNIA

Hypercapnia is defined as an elevated end-tidal or peak expired partial pressure of carbon dioxide ($P_{ET}CO_2$) concentration. In most instances, the equipment malfunctions described also result in hypercarbia, which is defined as an elevated arterial CO_2 partial pressure. Causes of hypercapnia are grouped into three categories: (1) decreased CO_2 removal, (2) CO_2 rebreathing, and (3) increased CO_2 production. Equipment-related causes of hypercapnia fall into categories 1 and 2.

Decreased CO_2 Removal

Decreased CO_2 removal is synonymous with alveolar hypoventilation. The primary equipment-related problems that cause inadequate alveolar ventilation are leaks (including disconnects), obstructions, compliant and large volume breathing hoses, and ventilator misuse and malfunction.

Breathing Circuit Leaks

During positive-pressure ventilation with a leak present in the breathing circuit, a portion of the ventilator-delivered tidal volume escapes. The larger the leak, the smaller the tidal volume received by the patient. Higher peak inspiratory pressures and longer inspiratory times increase leak volume. Leaks can occur anywhere in the breathing circuit. Common leak sites are similar to the disconnect sites shown in Figure 6-5 and include the following:

1. Connection sites
   a. Endotracheal tube (ETT) at elbow connector
   b. Elbow connector at Y-piece
   c. Breathing hose attachments at absorber canister
   d. Breathing hose attachment at Y-piece
   e. Attachment sites of breathing circuit "add-ons" (eg, gas analyzers and humidifiers)
2. Breathing circuit hoses, especially the reusable type
3. Adjustable pressure-limiting (APL or "pop-off") valve
   a. Partially open valve
   b. Defective valve
4. Absorbent canister
   a. Misaligned canisters
   b. Defective seals
   c. Cracked canister casing
   d. Inadequately tightened casing

Endotracheal Tube

If the ETT cuff is not properly inflated, is defective, or is disrupted by the surgeon, gas will leak around the ETT during positive-pressure inflation of the lungs, and alveolar ventilation will be reduced. An ETT cuff leak can be detected by placing a stethoscope over the patient's larynx or mouth, and simultaneously delivering a positive pressure breath. A gurgling noise will be heard if gas is escaping around the endotracheal tube. If the cuff is underinflated, adding several mL of air to the pilot tube may inflate the cuff enough to seal the leak.

Persistence of the leak despite attempts to further inflate the ETT cuff indicates the cuff or pilot tube assembly is probably defective or damaged. It is possible to compensate for a defective pilot valve by using a three-way stopcock to occlude the pilot tube after the cuff has been inflated. Continued leakage may reflect a cracked pilot valve casing. This requires that the pilot tube itself be clamped following cuff inflation.

The leak may persist despite these maneuvers, in which case a clinical decision is made as to whether or not adequate alveolar ventilation can be maintained in this situation. Factors that are helpful in determining whether to proceed with the cuff leak or to exchange the defective ETT for one with an intact cuff include:

- Inspection and palpation of chest excursions
- Auscultation of breath sounds
- Measurement of the peak inspiratory pressure that can be achieved with the leak present
- The end-tidal CO_2 concentration
- The type and progress of the operative procedure
- Position of the patient
- Degree of difficulty of initial intubation.

If ventilation is significantly compromised but tube exchange is deemed difficult, a trial of packing the larynx with moistened gauze to seal the airway or changing to a ventilation pattern with lower inspiratory pressures (small tidal volumes at an increased respiratory rate) is an option.

In the case of an uncuffed endotracheal tube, an unacceptable leak around the ETT may occur with (1) an undersized ETT; (2) decreased lung-thorax compliance; or (3) tube displacement to a level such that the ETT tip is above the level of the cricoid ring.

Leaks in the Anesthesia Machine

Because anesthesia machines with a common gas outlet check valve (see Fig. 6-2) prevent the retrograde flow of gas from the breathing circuit to the anesthesia machine, positive-pressure ventilation of the patient will proceed normally even if a leak is present in the LPS of the anesthesia machine. However, because the tidal volume delivered by the ventilator includes the volume of fresh gas that flows in from the anesthesia machine during the inspiratory time, loss of the fresh gas flow through a LPC leak will decrease the tidal volume delivered to the patient.[9] When a circle breathing circuit is used, mild hypercapnia may develop, depending on the tidal volume and fresh gas flow setting. When a Mapleson D, Bain, or Jackson-Reese circuit is used, loss of fresh gas flow through a LPS leak may result in significant CO_2 rebreathing and significant hypercapnia.

Compliant Breathing Circuit Hoses

Although the patient's lung–thorax compliance is greater than the compliance of the breathing circuit hoses, a portion of the tidal volume delivered during a positive-pressure ventilation remains trapped within the breathing circuit (Table 6-3).[10] The higher the peak inspiratory pressure and the larger the breathing circuit compliance, the greater the effect. For example, if a breathing circuit has a total compliance ($C_{circuit}$) of 10 mL/cm H_2O (includes the distensibility of the breathing circuit and the compressibility of gas within the CO_2 absorber, breathing, and ventilator hoses), and the peak inspiratory pressure (PIP) is 20 cm H_2O, then approximately 200 mL of each positive pressure breath remains within the apparatus and is not delivered to the patient's lungs.

$$\text{Portion of } V_T \text{ lost to system compliance and gas compression} = C_{circuit} \times PIP$$
$$= 10 \text{ mL/cm } H_2O \times 20 \text{ cm } H_2O$$
$$= 200 \text{ mL}$$

In an adult patient with the ventilator set to deliver an 800 mL tidal volume (V_{Tset}), this results in a 25% loss of effective ventilation. The significance of this effect is even more pronounced in the pediatric patient, where the set tidal volume may only be 30 to 400 mL per breath. A 200 mL loss of effective tidal volume due to breathing circuit compliance and gas compression now represents a 50% to 66% decrease in effective ventilation. Knowing (calculating) the loss of delivered tidal volume allows the clinician to compensate by increasing V_{Tset}. The effect of breathing circuit compliance and gas compression on delivered tidal volume is clinically most significant at low fresh gas flows and low set tidal volumes.

Note that a spirometer positioned in the expiratory limb measures both patient-exhaled and breathing system-decompressed gas. During exhalation, the breathing hoses decompress, and the trapped gas exits with gas from the patient's lungs through the expiratory hose. This may mislead the anesthesiologist into thinking that the *patient's* tidal volume is appropriate when it is actually low.

The magnitude of breathing system compliance and gas compression can be *estimated* by occluding the Y-piece, pressurizing the circuit by cycling the ventilator, and observing the exhaled volume measured by a spirometer positioned in the expiratory limb. The compliance (expressed as milliliters exhaled volume per centimeter of H_2O inspiratory pressure) is determined from this value and the measured peak pressure. This maneuver is especially helpful when pediatric patients are being mechanically ventilated.

TABLE 6-3
Compression Volume Versus Pressure*

	PEAK INFLATION PRESSURE (cm H_2O)				
CIRCUIT	*10*	*20*	*30*	*40*	*50*
MAPLESON D CIRCUITS					
Bain (H)	20	60	100	120	167
Piggyback (H)	27	67	127	147	180
Our own (H)	27	53	94	120	160
CIRCLE CIRCUITS					
Adult rubber	127	240	353	487	600
Adult rubber (H)	147	267	380	547	687
Adult plastic	74	147	220	294	347
Adult plastic (H)	100	187	274	360	447
Adult wire (H)	74	147	220	280	353
Pediatric rubber	53	107	167	207	260
Pediatric rubber (H)	67	133	200	267	320
Pediatric plastic	53	113	174	233	267
Pediatric plastic (H)	67	140	200	274	333

* This table presents the mean volume of compressed oxygen (in mL) of six determinations at each peak inflation pressure (in cm H_2O). The letter H indicates that the study was carried out with a heated humidifier.

Coté CJ, Petkau AJ, Ryan JF, et al: Wasted ventilation in vitro with eight anesthetic circuits with and without inline humidification. Anesthesiology 59:442, 1983.

Obstructed Gas Flow

Breathing Circuit Hoses

Kinks or foreign bodies in the breathing circuit hoses can result in increased airway pressures. A PEEP valve which allows unidirectional gas flow will cause a complete obstruction of the breathing system if inadvertently inserted in the inspiratory limb. Patency of the breathing circuit must be confirmed during pre-use machine checkout. A simple positive-pressure leak test does not accomplish this. Breathing system patency is confirmed by attaching a breathing bag to the Y-piece to serve as a test lung, which is then ventilated by cycling the mechanical ventilator. Partial obstructions in the expiratory limb initially result in elevated end-expiratory pressure, but as air trapping develops, peak inspiratory pressure increases as well. It is important to recognize that with older anesthesia machines, the airway pressure gauge on the CO_2 absorbent canister measures pressure inside the canister and *not* distal (Y-piece) breathing circuit pressure. In this case, end-expiratory pressure elevations are not evident on the pressure gauge. On newer absorbent canisters, the gauge is similarly positioned on the canister, but the pressure sensing line is tunneled to sense airway pressure on the patient side of the inspiratory valve. With this configuration, true airway pressure is displayed throughout the respiratory cycle, including any positive end-expiratory pressure.

Endotracheal Tube

Typical causes of gas flow obstruction includes kinking of the ETT, blood or secretions in the ETT, cuff herniation, or expiratory valve malfunction.

Although it is semirigid at room temperature, the ETT's polyvinylchloride polymer softens as it warms inside the patient's airway. The weight of the attached breathing circuit may be sufficient to kink the ETT. The tube may kink where it enters the mouth and be visible, or it may kink in the posterior pharynx where it is not visible. In either case, the effective diameter of the ETT is markedly reduced and elevated inspiratory airway pressure results. Because an ETT kink increases the time it takes to complete an exhalation, an upsloping (nonhorizontal) expiratory plateau will be evident on the capnogram (Fig. 6-6).

Airway secretions and blood may hinder gas movement within the ETT. The result is an increased resistance to gas flow, a prolonged expiratory phase, and elevated inspiratory airway pressure.

If a high-volume, low-pressure ETT cuff is overinflated, the cuff may herniate over the end of the ETT. This may result in a partial or complete obstruction, or may create a ball-valve mechanism. A ball-valve mechanism minimally restricts inspiratory flow but completely obstructs expiratory flow, resulting in progressive air trapping. Because the ball-valve closes during expiration, the elevated pressure is not transmitted to the airway pressure gauge, and expiratory pressures initially (if measured) remain normal. However, peak inspiratory pressure will rise significantly as progressively greater pressures are needed to open the ball-valve and ventilate the distended lungs.

If the expiratory valve does not open at all, gas will enter the patient's lungs during inspiration, but will have no way to escape during expiration. Air trapping will occur, airway pressure will rapidly increase, and pneumothoraces may develop. Similarly, if a PEEP valve that only allows unidirectional flow is improperly oriented by insertion into the expiratory limb, complete obstruction to exhalation occurs.

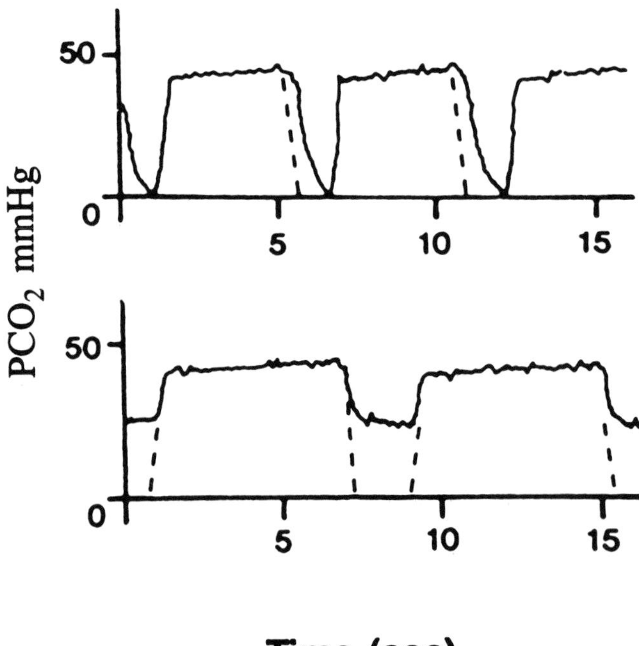

FIGURE 6-7. Capnograms demonstrate CO_2 rebreathing (*continuous lines*) with superimposed normal waveforms (*dotted lines*). The upper capnogram is recorded when the inspiratory valve is incompetent and a portion of the exhaled tidal volume flows back into the inspiratory limb, where it will be reinspired during the next inhalation. A waveform resembling the lower capnogram is recorded during expiratory valve incompetence, partial exhaustion, or channeling through the CO_2 absorbent, or if a CO_2 rebreathing (absorbent bypass) valve is open. (van Genderingen HR, Gravenstein N, Gravenstein JS, et al: Computer-assisted capnogram analysis. J Clin Monit 3:198, 1987)

Rebreathing

Capnography is an excellent monitor for detecting CO_2 rebreathing and in identifying its cause. Equipment faults causing CO_2 rebreathing tend to have characteristic capnograms (Fig. 6-7). For those faults with similar capnograms, quick and simple diagnostic checks can be used to differentiate them (Table 6-4).

Open Rebreathing Valve

Some anesthesia machines have a CO_2 bypass valve located on the CO_2 absorbent canister. When open, the bypass valve allows a portion of the exhaled gas containing CO_2 to pass directly into the inspiratory limb of the breathing circuit without passing through the CO_2 absorbent. The capnogram associated with an open CO_2 rebreathing valve is demonstrated in Figure 6-7 (*lower*), and is similar to that associated with exhausted CO_2 absorbent, gas channeling through the absorber, and an incompetent expiratory valve. If unintended CO_2 rebreathing is detected, one should verify that the CO_2 bypass valve, if present, is closed.

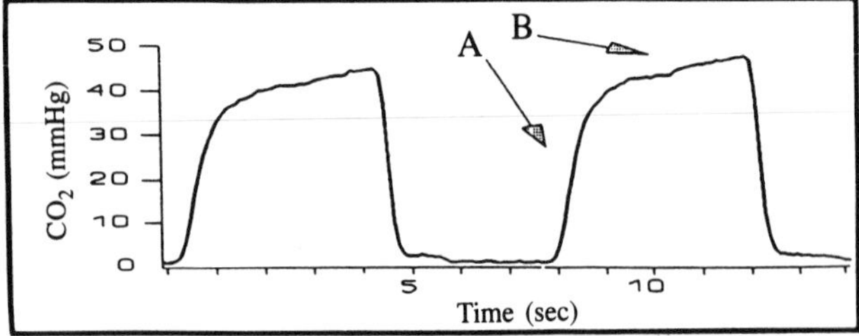

FIGURE 6-6. Capnogram associated with a kinked endotracheal tube. Note the prolonged expiratory upstroke (*A*) and slanted expiratory plateau (*B*). Slower gas flow rate occurs during each of these phases of the capnogram. (Good ML, Paulus DA: Equipment. In Gravenstein N (ed). Manual of complications during anesthesia, p 98. Philadelphia, JB Lippincott, 1991)

Exhausted CO_2 Absorbent

While the dye indicator reaction designed to identify exhausted CO_2 absorbent may fail outright or be hidden from view (eg, channeling of the expired gas through the inner portion of the canister), a characteristic CO_2 rebreathing capnogram (Fig. 6-7, *lower*) is observed when the CO_2 absorbent begins to fail. To differentiate this capnogram from the similar capnogram of an incompetent expiratory valve, the clinician increases (doubles or triples) the total fresh gas flow being delivered into the breathing circuit so that it is in excess of the minute ventilation. With exhausted CO_2 absorbent, the high fresh gas flow rate will decrease the amount of rebreathing and will eliminate the inspiratory CO_2 (see Table 6-4). In distinction, increasing the fresh gas flow (FGF) will minimally affect the amount of inspired CO_2 observed with an incompetent expiratory valve.

TABLE 6-4
Differential Diagnosis of CO_2 Rebreathing

FAULT	END-INSPIRATORY CO_2	DECREASED $PICO_2$ WITH INCREASED FGF	CHANGE IN V_T
Open rebreathing valve	+	+	0
Exhausted CO_2 absorbent (including channeling)	+	+	0
Incompetent expiratory valve	+	−	0
Incompetent inspiratory valve	±	−	↓

$PICO_2$, partial pressure of inspired CO_2; *FGF*, fresh gas flow; *V_T*, tidal volume measured in expiratory limb.
Good ML, Paulus DA: Equipment. In Gravenstein N (ed): Manual of complications during anesthesia. Philadelphia; JB Lippincott, 1991, 101.

Incompetent Expiratory Valve

A characteristic CO_2-rebreathing capnogram is observed (see Fig. 6-7, *lower*). In this circumstance, however, increasing the total fresh gas flow does not significantly reduce the inspired CO_2 (see Table 6-4). Because an incompetent expiratory valve causes retrograde gas flow in the expiratory limb during inspiration, a respirometer that can detect retrograde flow will identify the expiratory valve incompetence. Incompetent expiratory valves develop when humidity prevents the valve from properly sealing during inspiration, or when valves are damaged or left out after cleaning or servicing of the anesthesia machine.

Incompetent Inspiratory Valve

The shape of the capnogram associated with an incompetent inspiratory valve is much different from that of the previously discussed capnograms. Instead of the sharp downstroke normally observed in the capnogram at the beginning of inspiration, an incompetent inspiratory valve will manifest as a prolonged or sloping downstroke (see Fig. 6-7, *upper*). If the delivered tidal volume is much greater than the volume of the inspiratory hose, fresh gas (without CO_2) will reach the patient's airway, and the capnometer will incorrectly report the inspired CO_2 as "0". The capnometer does not measure flow; it merely reports the minimum CO_2 during a respiratory cycle and not the presence of CO_2 during the inspiratory phase of ventilation.

When the inspiratory valve is incompetent, approximately equal portions of the delivered tidal volume return through the inspiratory and expiratory breathing hoses. Thus, tidal volume measured in the expiratory limb will be approximately one half of the actual tidal volume delivered to the breathing circuit. This "apparent leak" may be the first abnormal signal noticed. Without consideration of the capnogram, this results in a fruitless search for what otherwise appears to be a large breathing circuit leak or spirometer error.

Nonrebreathing Circuits

Nonrebreathing anesthesia circuits (eg, Bain, Mapleson D) do not include a CO_2 absorber. In spite of their classification, partial rebreathing regularly occurs with these circuits. If the amount is excessive (ie, interferes with adequate ventilation, causing hypercapnia and hypercarbia), increasing the FGF has the greatest effect in reducing the amount of rebreathing and thereby improving effective alveolar ventilation.[11]

INCREASED AIRWAY PRESSURE

Airway pressure in the breathing circuit is measured by a manometer (also called the breathing system pressure gauge). Ideally, the sensing port of the manometer is positioned in such a way that it senses pressure on the patient side of the inspiratory and expiratory valves. In this position, it measures pressure as close to the patient's airway as possible. A simple test to determine whether the airway pressure gauge is measuring canister or breathing circuit pressure is to insert a PEEP valve in the expiratory limb. If the pressure gauge does not reflect the PEEP, it is measuring canister and not circuit pressure. Many anesthesia ventilators incorporate a high pressure alarm.

A variety of equipment problems can result in excessive airway pressure. This can lead to cardiovascular compromise by interfering with venous return and may also cause barotrauma. Increased airway pressure can develop whenever an equipment malfunction causes excessive pressure delivery, obstruction to expired gas flow, or inadequate pressure relief.

Excessive Pressure Delivery

Faulty Pressure Regulators

A faulty pressure regulator can allow the high pressures of the gas source (pipeline or cylinder) to be transmitted directly to the breathing circuit and to the patient's lungs.

Open Oxygen Flush Valve

The O_2 flush valve, when held open, exposes the breathing circuit and the patient's lungs to high gas flows (35 to 75 L/min), and excessive airway pressures can rapidly develop. This is prevented by opening the O_2 flush valve in short intermittent bursts, never during mechanical inspiration, and observing the breathing circuit pressure manometer while the flush valve is activated.

Obstructed Gas Flow

Obstructions of the breathing circuit are discussed in the section on hypercapnia.

Inadequate Pressure Relief

Fresh gas is typically delivered to the breathing circuit at a total flow between 0.05 and 10 liters per minute. If gas is not consumed or vented from the breathing circuit at a similar rate, pressure will build in the breathing circuit and be transmitted to the patient's lungs. A number of pressure relief valves are included in the contemporary anesthesia machine. Failures of these valves can result in elevated airway pressures.

Adjustable Pressure-Limiting Valve

Located on or near the CO_2 absorber, the adjustable pressure-limiting (APL, or pop-off) valve can be adjusted to control the pressure at which the valve will open and vent gas from the breathing circuit into the scavenging system. During manual or spontaneous ventilation, if this valve is completely closed, gas will not be able to exit from the breathing circuit. The breathing bag will distend, and breathing circuit pressures will rise. Anesthesia breathing bags are designed so that, regardless of the volume of gas put into them, pressure should not exceed 50 to 60 mm Hg.[12]

Ventilator Pressure Relief Valve

A pressure relief (spill) valve is also part of each anesthesia mechanical ventilator. This valve is closed during the inspiratory phase of a positive pressure breath, and opens to vent gas after the bellows has refilled. Failure of this valve (ie, stuck in the closed position) will result in increased airway pressures.

Scavenging System Pressure Relief Valve

Gas vented through either the breathing circuit pop-off or ventilator spill valve enters the scavenging system. If gas removal by the scavenging system is inadequate, its reservoir begins to fill. When the reservoir bag distends and begins to develop pressure, a pressure relief valve opens in the scavenging system to vent pressure to atmosphere. If this valve fails in the presence of inadequate scavenger flow (eg, anesthesia machine wheel occluding vacuum hose), the increased pressure will be transmitted back to the breathing circuit and will result in elevated airway pressures.

DECREASED AIRWAY PRESSURE

Airway pressure in the breathing circuit decreases (1) when there is inadequate gas flow into the breathing circuit, (2) when there is leakage of gas from the breathing circuit, or (3) if a negative pressure source is attached to the breathing circuit.

When a mechanical ventilator is used to administer anesthesia, the anesthesia system must include a device to detect disconnection.[4] An audible breathing circuit low pressure alarm is one method for detecting disconnection. The alarm sounds when airway pressure fails to exceed a threshold value within a specified number of seconds during mechanical ventilation. Some systems allow the user to set the threshold pressure value, in which case it should ideally be set to a value just slightly less than the peak inspiratory pressure. The pressure-sensing line should be connected as close to the patient's airway as possible (ie, at the Y-piece or patient-side of the unidirectional valves, *not* in the ventilator or at the ventilator hose cannister connection). The low pressure alarm may not sound during a partial disconnection if the inspiratory pressure exceeds its threshold and if the fresh gas flow is equal to or greater than the leak.

INADEQUATE GAS SUPPLY

A pressurized gas supply is necessary to provide fresh gas flow to the patient and to drive the mechanical ventilator. Loss of O_2 supply pressure should sound a "low O_2 pressure" alarm. Pressure gauges on the front of the anesthesia machine indicate the current hospital pipeline and reserve cylinder (if the cylinder stem valve is open) gas supply pressures. An O_2 failure safety mechanism (fail-safe) should interrupt the flow of all gases if the O_2 supply pressure is lost. When that occurs, the reserve oxygen cylinder should be opened and the pipeline hose disconnected from the wall to prevent retrograde flow from the reserve cylinders into the hospital pipeline. To minimize O_2 usage, the mechanical ventilator, which is often completely or partially oxygen-powered, should be turned off and replaced by manual or spontaneous ventilation. Ventilator oxygen use is often several times the set minute ventilation.[13]

A portion of the inspiratory tidal volume delivered by a mechanical ventilator is made up from the fresh gas flow into the breathing circuit during the inspiratory phase.[9] Loss of the fresh gas inflow will, therefore, decrease the delivered tidal volume, and will result in small to moderate decreases in airway pressure. Fresh gas is not delivered to the breathing circuit if the common fresh gas hose is obstructed. A leak in the low pressure system of the anesthesia machine will also decrease fresh gas delivery to the breathing circuit.

Breathing Circuit Leaks

A decrease in airway pressure is most often caused by leaks or disconnects in the breathing circuit or endotracheal tube (see Hypercapnia).

Negative Pressure Source

Gas vented from the adjustable pressure-limiting (or pop-off) valve in the breathing circuit and the pressure relief (or spill) valve in the ventilator is removed by the hospital's waste vacuum system. A scavenging system interface or manifold is interposed between the pressure relief valves and the vacuum source. If the interface is bypassed or malfunctions (due to an obstructed inlet valve or inlet port), negative pressure may be transmitted to the patient's breathing circuit. Negative pressure applied to the airway will decrease effective ventilation, decrease functional residual capacity, and may cause negative pressure pulmonary edema. Nasogastric tubes that are inadvertently passed into the trachea and placed on suction will also introduce a negative pressure source to the patient's airway and result in decreased airway pressures.

DEEP ANESTHESIA

Deep anesthesia presents clinically as hypotension, bradycardia, or in extreme cases, even cardiac arrest. Deep anesthesia is the result of a relative or gross anesthetic overdose. Although deep anesthesia may be caused by improper titration of the anesthetic concentration to the patient's response, it may also represent an equipment-related (delivery system) complication that results in an excessive delivery of anesthetic agent.

Back Pressure and the Pumping Effect

The anesthesia machine, or preferably the vaporizer itself, should have a mechanism that negates the effect of retrograde gas flow into the vaporizer. If such a device is absent or malfunctioning, pressure fluctuations generated during positive pressure ventilation or with the activation of the O_2 flush valve will increase the pressure in both the vaporizing and bypass chambers of the vaporizer. If the vaporizing chamber has a greater volume, more gas will be compressed within it. When the positive (back) pressure is released, the low resistance bypass chamber decompresses more quickly than the vaporizing chamber. Vapor saturated gas from the not yet decompressed vaporizing chamber passes into the decompressed bypass chamber, and the fresh gas intermittently receives a higher concentration of anesthetic than that set on the vaporizer concentration control[14] (Fig. 6-8).

Spillage of Liquid Anesthetic

If a vaporizer is overfilled or tipped, as may occur with a free-standing vaporizer, liquid anesthetic may spill into the internal plumbing of the anesthesia machine, the inspiratory hose, or into chambers within the vaporizer that are not intended to contain anesthetic. When fresh gas flows through these areas, the anesthetic agent vaporizes, and the patient receives a higher concentration of anesthetic than that set on the vaporizer concentration control. Free-standing vaporizers should never be tipped and any vaporizer that has been shipped or has been remounted should be purged by flowing gas through it or have its calibration checked prior to patient use.

Misfilled Vaporizer

Contemporary vaporizers are agent-specific and, therefore, calibrated for only one anesthetic agent. If an agent-specific

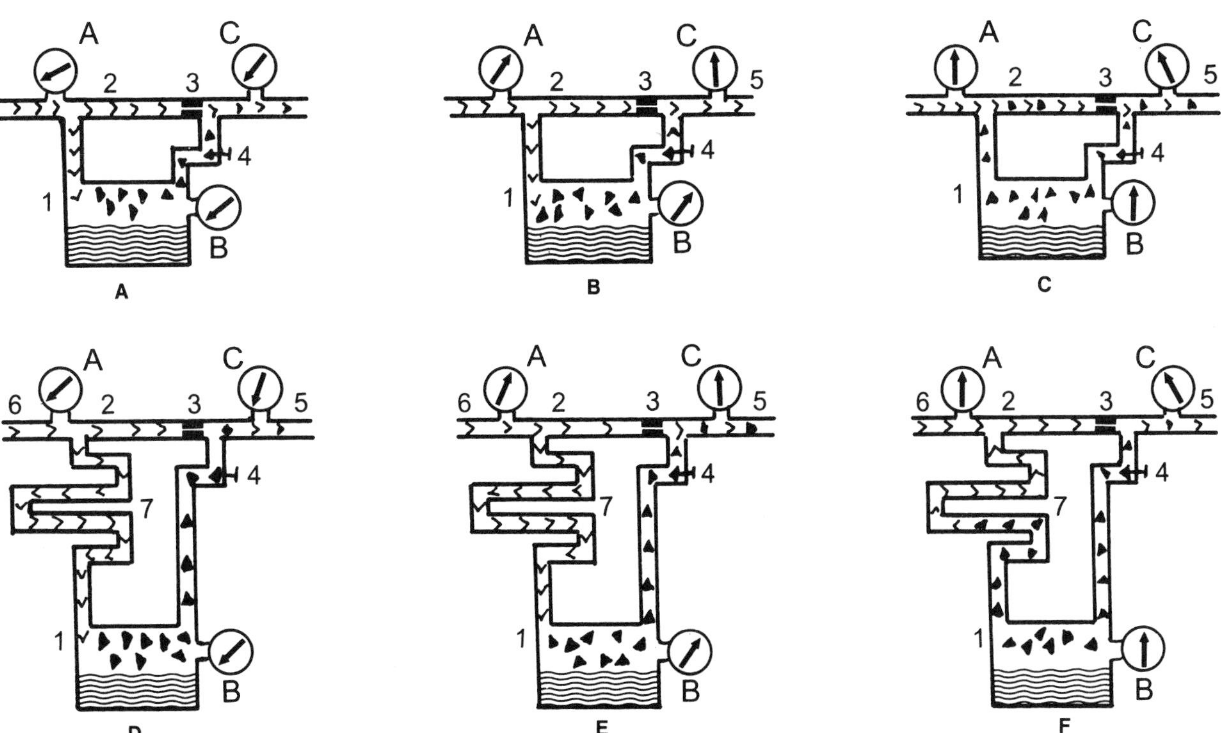

FIGURE 6-8. The pumping effect in a variable bypass vaporizer. (**A**, **B**, and **C**) During exhalation, gas containing anesthetic vapor flows into the bypass, increasing the vaporizer output. (**D**, **E**, and **F**) The long spiral tube prevents vapor-laden gas from reaching the bypass. (Hill DW: The design and calibration of vaporizers for volatile anaesthetic agents. Br J Anaesth 40:656, 1968)

vaporizer is filled with the wrong anesthetic agent, the anesthetic concentration delivered to the patient may be significantly higher or lower than the concentration set on the vaporizer concentration dial (Table 6-5). The actual delivered concentration depends on the anesthetic potency (ie, MAC value) and the difference in vapor pressure between the anesthetic agent for which the vaporizer is intended and the one with which it is misfilled. Because halothane and isoflurane have virtually identical vapor pressures, their delivery is relatively unaffected by misfilling; however, the difference in MAC results in approximately a 50% over- or 30% underdosage error (see Table 6-5).

Miscalibrated Vaporizer

Agent-specific vaporizers require calibration checks. A vaporizer out of calibration or miscalibrated will deliver an anesthetic concentration different from that set on the concentration control. Prevention consists of routine maintenance per manufacturer specifications.

Monitoring Instruments

Monitoring instruments used during anesthetic administration may also contribute to patient morbidity or mortality if they (1) fail to provide data or (2) provide inaccurate but physiologically conceivable data.

FAILURE TO PROVIDE DATA

The basics of patient monitoring are inspection, auscultation, palpation, and percussion. Electronic monitoring instruments greatly enhance these basic skills, allowing the clinician to quantitate more frequently, precisely, and objectively physiologic parameters (eg, oxyhemoglobin saturation). Because of their dependability, it is tempting to omit basic monitoring skills and rely solely on monitoring instruments. This practice is unacceptable, for when the monitoring instruments fail, which they will, the instrument-dependent clinician is left with unpolished clinical skills.

Examples of situations in which monitoring instruments fail to provide data include the electrocardiograph and pulse oximeter during electrocautery, electrically powered instruments without battery backup during power failure, noninvasive blood pressure monitors during bradycardia or dysrhythmia, and the electrocardiograph with disconnected leads.

Inaccurate Data

Perhaps more worrisome is the situation in which monitoring instruments provide incorrect but physiologically conceivable data. Inappropriate clinical management is likely when decision-making is based on inaccurate data. Specific examples are discussed in the following paragraphs.

Artifactual ST Depression

Electronic filtering intended to minimize baseline drift may cause artifactual depression or normalization of the ST segment on the electrocardiographic oscilloscope.[15] Clinicians must appreciate the difference between the *monitoring* mode and *diagnostic* mode of electrocardiographic monitors. ST segment depression evident in the monitoring mode should be verified in the diagnostic mode, ideally with a calibrated strip chart recording.

Noninvasive Blood Pressure Monitors

Most automatic noninvasive blood pressure monitors (NIBPMs) use the oscillometric technique. Motion of the cuff or tubing often results in inaccurate blood pressure determination, as does the application of an incorrectly sized (especially undersized) cuff. Many NIBPMs have difficulty accurately determining blood pressure in patients with slow heart rates and cardiac dysrhythmias. A back-up manual sphygmomanometer can be used to verify the patient's blood pressure when data from the NIBPM is suspect. Another approach is to palpate the radial artery to obtain a systolic (return to flow) pressure as the NIBPM is bleeding down the cuff pressure by reading the cuff pressure displayed on the monitor during deflation. The pulse oximeter signal loss or reacquisition can be used in analogous fashion.

Pulse Oximeter

Measurement errors for the pulse oximeter have been reported due to electrocautery interference, venous congestion, synthetic fingernails, dirt, adhesives, dye indicators (methylene blue, indocyanine green), and surgical lights.[16] The al-

TABLE 6-5
Resultant Anesthetic Delivery From a Misfilled Vaporizer

ANESTHETIC AGENT	VAPOR PRESSURE AT 20°C (mm Hg)	VAPORIZER TYPE—SET AT 1 MAC		
		Enflurane	*Isoflurane*	*Halothane*
Enflurane	184	1 MAC	<1 MAC	<1 MAC
Isoflurane	239	>1 MAC	1 MAC	<1 MAC
Halothane	243	>1 MAC	>1 MAC	1 MAC

Good ML, Paulus DA: Equipment. In Gravenstein N (ed): Manual of complications during anesthesia. Philadelphia; JB Lippincott, 1991:107.

gorithms used in converting the red and infrared light absorption into oxyhemoglobin saturation have been found to be inaccurate for some pulse oximeters, especially during significant hypoxemia.[17] Because carboxyhemoglobin and oxyhemoglobin absorb infrared light at 660 nm, the pulse oximeter considers carboxyhemoglobin to be oxyhemoglobin and overestimates the true oxygen saturation of hemoglobin in patients with carboxyhemoglobin.[18] Methemoglobin absorbs both the red and infrared wavelength used by the pulse oximeter, which causes the pulse oximeter to report an oxyhemoglobin saturation near 85%.[19] Motion of the sensor or of the a digit to which it is attached disrupts the pulse oximeter's ability to sense the arterial pulsation. When the heart rate reported by the pulse oximeter differs from that counted by the ECG, or if the plethysmographic pulse waveform is erratic, the oxyhemoglobin saturation reported by the pulse oximeter should be viewed with suspicion.

Capnometer

Airway carbon dioxide concentration may be measured by sidestream sampling devices or in-line CO_2 sensors. Units that sample gas from the breathing circuit are subject to error when cracks and leaks occur in the sampling line,[20] or if the sampling line becomes disconnected or occluded. Some units require calibration with a calibration gas of known carbon dioxide concentration. If the unit is not properly calibrated, the carbon dioxide measurements will also be inaccurate.

Airway Pressure Manometers

Pressure gauges may give inaccurate readings if they are dropped or otherwise damaged. On older anesthesia machines, the pressure gauge measures pressure in the CO_2 canister, not in the breathing circuit. In this case, positive end-expiratory pressure will not register on the airway pressure gauge.

Transfer of Energy to the Patient

Monitoring instruments may injure the patient if they transfer energy (force, heat, electricity) directly to the patient. This type of injury is reviewed in Chapter 8.

PREVENTING ANESTHESIA EQUIPMENT COMPLICATIONS

It must be assumed that even the most safely designed and durable anesthesia equipment will fail, and will do so in an unpredictable or previously undescribed fashion. Patient injury from anesthesia equipment failure, then, is prevented by a plan that includes the following:

1. Preparation for equipment failure with backup ventilation equipment
2. Performance of a thorough pre-use checkout of the anesthesia equipment in a systematic fashion before each use (Table 6-6)
3. Maintenance of anesthesia equipment in optimum operating condition
4. Ongoing user education to better understand the equipment, its normal behavior, and its known and potential shortcomings.[21]

Backup Ventilation Equipment

Each anesthetizing location should include a backup means for ventilating an anesthetized and often chemically paralyzed patient. The device should require neither electrical nor pneumatic power. We keep a self-inflating resuscitation bag on each anesthesia cart. If a Mapleson circuit is used, a separate reserve cylinder of O_2 should be available, and the cylinder's supply pressure checked before each anesthetic. Having backup ventilation equipment means that, even in a worst-case situation (ie, complete loss of electricity and pressurized gas supplies including O_2), the patient can be adequately ventilated with room air or O_2, clinically monitored (inspection, auscultation, palpation), and anesthetized with intravenous anesthetic agents.

Pre-use Checkout

Most equipment faults can be identified with a systematic inspection and pre-use check of the anesthesia equipment. As anesthesia equipment becomes more and more complex, unfortunately so does the checkout procedure. The importance of a thorough pre-use check of the anesthesia equipment cannot be emphasized enough (see Table 6-6). Each component system of the anesthesia machine (high pressure system, low pressure system, breathing circuit, and scavenging circuit) and each safety device or alarm (low O_2 pressure, fail-safe, disconnect) must be individually tested and its proper function verified before a patient is anesthetized. The procedure is akin to that conducted by pilots before flying an airplane.

The FDA first published in 1986 a recommended protocol to be followed when conducting a pre-use checkout of the anesthesia equipment. In 1994, an updated and revised protocol was released (see Table 6-6). The protocol is generic; it can be applied to any type or brand of anesthesia machine and related equipment. Local modifications of the protocol to specific types of equipment (eg, anesthesia machines with check valves at the common gas outlet) are appropriate and encouraged but should undergo peer review. The protocol should be completed in its entirety daily, and in abbreviated form before each anesthetic administration. In addition, the proper performance of backup ventilation equipment should be verified each day. A notation in the anesthesia record should reflect the performance of the checkout procedure.

Maintenance

Each anesthesia department should have an organized equipment inspection and maintenance program encompassing all anesthesia equipment. Routine checks by trained personnel often identify equipment that is beginning to fail (eg, calibration drift of a vaporizer) before the failure is overt and potentially dangerous to the anesthetized patient. Proper documentation of inspections and repairs is important, and may have medicolegal implications in the event of an equipment

TABLE 6-6
Anesthesia Apparatus Checkout Recommendations, 1994

This checkout, or a reasonable equivalent, should be conducted before administration of anesthesia. These recommendations are valid only for an anesthesia system that conforms to current and relevant standards and includes an ascending bellows ventilator and at least the following monitors: capnograph, pulse oximeter, oxygen analyzer, respiratory volume monitor (spirometer) and breathing system pressure monitor with high and low pressure alarms. This is a guideline that users are encouraged to modify to accommodate differences in equipment design and variations in local clinical practice. Such local modifications should have appropriate peer review. Users should refer to the operator manual for specific procedures and precautions.

Emergency Ventilation Equipment

*1. Verify backup ventilation equipment is available & functioning.

High Pressure System

*2. Check O_2 cylinder supply
   a. Open O_2 cylinder and verify at least half full (about 1000 psi).
   b. Close cylinder.

*3. Check central pipeline supplies
   a. Check that hoses are connected and pipeline gauges read about 50 psi.

Low Pressure System

*4. Check initial status of low pressure system
   a. Close flow control valves and turn vaporizers off.
   b. Check fill level and tighten vaporizers' filler caps.

*5. Perform leak check of machine low pressure system
   a. Verify that the machine master switch and flow control valves are OFF.
   b. Attach "Suction Bulb" to common (fresh) gas outlet.
   c. Squeeze bulb repeatedly until fully collapsed.
   d. Verify bulb stays *fully* collapsed for at least 10 seconds.
   e. Open one vaporizer at a time and repeat "c" and "d" as above.
   f. Remove suction bulb, and reconnect fresh gas hose.

*6. Turn on machine master switch and all other necessary electrical equipment.

*7. Test flowmeters
   a. Adjust flow of all gases through their full range, checking for smooth operation of floats and undamaged flowtubes.
   b. Attempt to create a hypoxic O_2/N_2O mixture and verify correct changes in flow and/or alarm.

Scavenging System

*8. Adjust and check scavenging system
   a. Ensure proper connections between the scavenging system and both APL (pop-off) valve and ventilator relief valve.
   b. Adjust waste gas vacuum (if possible).
   c. Fully open APL valve and occlude Y-piece.
   d. With minimum O_2 flow, allow scavenger reservoir bag to collapse completely and verify that absorber pressure gauge reads about zero.
   e. With the O_2 flush activated, allow the scavenger reservoir bag to distend fully, and then verify that absorber pressure gauge reads < 10 cm H_2O.

Breathing System

*9. Calibrate O_2 monitor
   a. Ensure monitor reads 21% in room air.
   b. Verify low O_2 alarm is enabled and functioning.
   c. Reinstall sensor in circuit and flush breathing system with O_2.
   d. Verify that monitor now reads greater than 90%.

10. Check initial status of breathing system
   a. Set selector switch to "Bag" mode.
   b. Check that breathing circuit is complete, undamaged and unobstructed.
   c. Verify that CO_2 absorbent is adequate.
   d. Install breathing circuit accessory equipment (eg, humidifier, PEEP valve) to be used during the case.

11. Perform leak check of the breathing system
   a. Set all gas flows to zero (or minimum).
   b. Close APL (pop-off) valve and occlude Y-piece.
   c. Pressurize breathing system to about 30 cm H_2O with O_2 flush.
   d. Ensure that pressure remains fixed for at least 10 seconds.
   e. Open APL (pop-off) valve and ensure that pressure decreases.

Manual and Automatic Ventilation Systems

12. Test ventilation systems and unidirectional valves
   a. Place a second breathing bag on Y-piece.
   b. Set appropriate ventilator parameters for next patient.
   c. Switch to automatic ventilation (Ventilator) mode.
   d. Turn ventilator ON and fill bellows and breathing bag with O_2 flush.
   e. Set O_2 flow to minimum, other gas flows to zero.
   f. Verify that during inspiration bellows delivers appropriate tidal volume and that during expiration bellows fills completely.
   g. Set fresh gas flow to about 5 L/min.
   h. Verify that the ventilator bellows and simulated lungs fill and empty appropriately without sustained pressure at end expiration.
   i. *Check for proper action of unidirectional valves.*
   j. Exercise breathing circuit accessories to ensure proper function.
   k. Turn ventilator OFF and switch to manual ventilation (Bag/APL) mode.
   l. Ventilate manually and assure inflation and deflation of artificial lungs and appropriate feel of system resistance and compliance.
   m. Remove second breathing bag from Y-piece.

Monitors

13. Check, calibrate and/or set alarm limits of all monitors: Capnograph, pulse oximeter, O_2 analyzer, respiratory volume monitor (spirometer), pressure monitor with high and low airway pressure alarms

Final Position

14. Check final status of machine
   a. Vaporizers off
   b. APL valve open
   c. Selector switch to "Bag"
   d. All flowmeters to zero (or minimum)
   e. Patient suction level adequate
   f. Breathing system ready to use

* If an anesthesia provider uses the same machine in successive cases, these steps need not be repeated or may be abbreviated after the initial checkout.

Anesthesia Patient Safety Foundation Newsletter 9:35, 1994 failure causing patient injury. Repair of the anesthesia equipment should be made only by manufacturer-approved service representative. "Home" or "custom" repairs by the anesthesiologist or anesthesia technician (typically involving some type of adhesive tape) often create more hazards than they correct. This practice is actively discouraged.

Efforts should be made to replace obsolete anesthesia equipment. Older anesthesia machines do not contain many important safety features (eg, O_2–nitrous oxide rationing, agent-specific vaporizers, O_2 failure-safety mechanisms, disconnect and low O_2 supply pressure alarms) that have been developed in recent years. Similarly, efforts should be made to standardize the anesthesia equipment as much as possible within a department (ie, same brand of anesthesia machine) to minimize the risk of an equipment-related injury related to unfamiliarity with different types of equipment.

User Education

Owner's Manual

The source that contains the most information about a specific type of anesthesia machine or other piece of anesthesia equipment—the owner's manual—usually remains unread by the anesthetist. Indeed, many such manuals are wordy and not well written. Still, they contain vital information for understanding and proper operation of the equipment and should be read by all who use the equipment.

Study of Anesthesia Equipment

Just as we continue to study pharmacology and human pathophysiology, our formal continuing medical education program should also include the study of anesthesia equipment. Structure, function, safety features, and potential failures of the equipment should be known, and each clinician should have a plan for diagnosing different types of complications due to equipment failure (eg, those causing hypoxemia, hypercarbia).

Disaster Drills

Anesthesia simulators have been developed that allow the anesthetist to "practice" administering anesthesia, either interacting with a computer or in a realistic environment using actual anesthesia equipment, but with a simulated patient.[22] With these simulators, potentially fatal equipment complications and other critical events can be repeatedly experienced. The anesthetist is able to rehearse a systematic approach to detect and correct critical incidents. With simulation, one learns by hands-on experience, and thus from one's own mistakes. Because many equipment failures occur infrequently in actual practice, simulation is particularly well suited for helping the clinician maintain the necessary cognitive and psychomotor skills required to respond efficiently and correctly to an equipment-related disaster. Although training with simulators is still relatively new to the field of anesthesiology and requires further study, its track record in other industries, such as aviation, is excellent, and its use in anesthesia education, particularly in the area of anesthesia equipment failure, is equally promising.[22]

REFERENCES

1. Cooper JB, Newbower RS, Kitz RJ: An analysis of major errors and equipment failures in anesthesia management: considerations for prevention and detection. Anesthesiology 60:34, 1984
2. Gilron I: Anaesthesia equipment safety in Canada: the role of government regulation. Can J Anaesth 140:987, 1993
3. Webb RK, Davies JM: Adverse events in anaesthesia: the role of equipment (editorial). Can J Anaesth 140:911, 1993.
4. American Society of Anesthesiologists. Standards for Basic Intraoperative Monitoring. Directory of Members, 1995;384
5. Myers JA, Good ML, Andrews JJ: Relative sensitivity of different check procedures for detecting low pressure circuit leaks in anesthesia gas machines. In preparation, 1995
6. Sum Ping ST, Mehta MP, Symreng T: Reliability of capnography in identifying esophageal intubation with carbonated beverage or antacid in the stomach. Anesth Analg 73:333, 1991
7. Birmingham PK, Cheney FW, Ward RJ: Esophageal intubation: A review of detection techniques. Anesth Analg 65:886, 1986
8. Frumin MJ, Epstein RM, Cohen G: Apneic oxygenation in man. Anesthesiology 20:789, 1959
9. Gravenstein N, Banner MJ, McLaughin G: Tidal volume changes due to the interaction of anesthesia machine and anesthesia ventilator. J Clin Monit 3:187, 1987
10. Coté CJ, Petkau AJ, Ryan JF, et al: Wasted ventilation measured in vitro with eight anesthetic circuits with and without inline humidification. Anesthesiology 59:442, 1983
11. Jaeger MJ, Schultetus RR: The effect of the Bain circuit on gas exchange. Can J Anaesth 34:26, 1987
12. Johnstone RE, Smith TC: Rebreathing bags as pressure-limiting devices. Anesthesiology 38:192, 1973
13. Raesller KL, Kretzman WE, Gravenstein N: Oxygen consumption by anesthesia ventilators. Anesthesiology 69:A271, 1988
14. Eisenkraft JB: Anesthesia vaporizers. In Ehrenwerth J, Eisenkraft JB (eds). Anesthesia Equipment: Principles and Applications. St. Louis: CV Mosby, 1993: 89
15. Taylor D, Vincent RV: Artifactual ST segment abnormalities due to electrocardiograph design. Br Heart J 54:121, 1985
16. Alexander CM, Teller LE, Gross JB: Principles of pulse oximetry: Theoretical and practical considerations. Anesth Analg 68:368, 1989
17. Severinghaus JW, Naifeh KH: Accuracy of response of six pulse oximeters to profound hypoxia. Anesthesiology 67:551, 1987
18. Barker SJ, Tremper KK: The effect of carbon monoxide on pulse oximetry and transcutaneous PO_2. Anesthesiology 66:677, 1987
19. Eisenkraft JB: Pulse oximeter desaturation due to methemoglobinemia. Anesthesiology 68:279, 1988
20. Martin M, Zupan J, Benumof JL: Unusual end-tidal CO_2 waveform. Anesthesiology 66:712, 1987
21. Symposium-The Australian Incident Monitoring Study. Anaesthesia and Intensive Care Oct 21(5), 1993 tire issue]
22. Good ML, Gravenstein JS: Training for safety in an anesthesia simulator. Seminars in Anesthesia XII:235, 1993

SUGGESTED READING

Dorsch JA, Dorsch SE: Understanding anesthesia equipment, 3rd ed. Baltimore: Williams & Wilkins, 1994

Ehrenwerth J, Eisenkraft JB (eds): Anesthesia Equipment—Principles and Applications. St. Louis: CV Mosby, 1993

Good ML, Cooper JB: Monitoring the anesthesia machine. In Saidman LJ, Smith NT (eds): Monitoring in anesthesia. Boston, Butterworth-Heinemann, 1993: 387

Complications in Anesthesiology, second edition,
edited by Nikolaus Gravenstein and Robert R. Kirby.
Lippincott-Raven Publishers, Philadelphia © 1996.

CHAPTER 7

Fires and Explosions

Gordon R. Neufeld

Of the complications encountered in the practice of anesthesia, a fire or an explosion is among the most devastating. The development of nonflammable anesthetic gases and vapors has reduced the occurrence of this complication. This chapter reviews the epidemiology, underlying fundamental physical processes, and methods for the control and prevention of fires and explosions in the operating room.

CAUSES

Review of the literature reveals interesting features of this complication, including the changing role of anesthetics.[1-3] For example, a survey published in 1941 reported the causes of 230 operating room fires and explosions.[1] Of 91% of these, the fuel was a flammable anesthetic, and of 70%, the source of ignition was something other than a static spark. The incidence reported by the Ministry of Health in Britain was approximately 4.2 per 100,000 administrations in the 7-year period ending in 1956.[3]

Flammable Anesthetic Agents

Over the past 4 decades, considerable effort and expense have been directed toward the development of systems for the control of fires and explosions in operating rooms. Most of this effort, including the development of nonflammable anesthetics, has been based on the concept that flammable anesthetics serve as the fuel in the majority (80%) of cases. This observation was indeed true before 1955. However, it no longer is.

Other Fuels

In the 15-year period from 1959 to 1974, 36 fires or explosions in operating room settings were reported. Fewer than one third (31%) of these were related to the use of a flammable anesthetic, although flammable agents were still the single most common fuel. Second (28%) were plastic, rubber, paper, and fabric components of apparatuses and disposable products. Third (22%) was enteric gas, most commonly ignited by electrosurgical apparatus. Fourth (8%) were volatile preparatory solutions. The remaining materials included cleaning compounds, electric apparatus and components, and oxygen-line contaminants such as oil and dust.

During this period 11 fires or explosions resulted from flammable anesthetics. However, by 1975 the use of flammable anesthetics had dropped to an estimated 5% or less of all anesthetic administrations[4] in fewer than 8% of United States hospitals,[5] compared with approximately 31% of anesthetics in Great Britain in 1956.[3] In 1980, the abandonment of explosive anesthetics was recommended because of concern about safety risks and the high cost of maintaining a safe environment for their use.[5] The incidence of operating room fires and explosions subsequently was reduced by the decline in use of the formerly common fuel sources and other preventive measures.

Ignition Sources

An examination of the sources of ignition is also revealing. Electrocautery devices were the source of ignition in 53% of operating room fires and explosions. Rapid compression of high-pressure gases accounted for 17% and electric devices for 17%. The remaining 13% were caused by static sparks (6%), open flames (6%), and unknown sources (1%). During the past decade the laser has emerged as a new and increasingly frequent source of ignition.

OXIDATION, COMBUSTION, AND FLAMES

Energy Release

In the strict chemical sense, "oxidation" is the loss of electrons from one molecular species to another. The species that gains electrons is "reduced." In general, oxidative processes are associated with a release of energy resulting from the difference in the bond energies between the compounds that are oxidized and the new compounds that are formed. For example, a water molecule contains two hydroxyl (oxygen–hydrogen) bonds, each with a bond energy of 109 kcal. The bond energy of water thus is 218 kcal/mol. The bond energy between the two hydrogen atoms of the hydrogen molecule is 103 kcal/mol hydrogen. Similarly, the oxygen–oxygen bond represents 117 kcal/mol. From these bond energies, one can calculate the energy released from the oxidation of hydrogen to form water:

$$2\ H_2 + O_2 \rightarrow 2\ H_2O$$

$$(2 \times 103) + 117 \rightarrow (2 \times 218)$$

$$\downarrow$$

$$\text{Energy excess} = 113\ \text{kcal}$$

$$= 57\ \text{kcal/mol}\ H_2O\ \text{formed}$$

Enhancement

Oxidation may occur at ambient room temperatures, but in general the reaction rates at these temperatures are extremely slow because they depend on the random occurrence of collisions between the reactants. Not all such collisions cause oxidation to occur. Only those that involve sufficient energy of impact to disrupt the existing molecular bonds and allow the formation of the product molecule result in oxidation and the release of energy. The probability of these collisions between a flammable material and oxygen can be enhanced by the factors listed in Table 7-1.

Heat Dissipation

As oxidation proceeds, the heat of reaction must be dissipated, or the temperature of the mixture rises. If the heat is rapidly conducted or convected away, the reaction temperature may drop to a point at which the oxidation stops (as when a match is blown out). If the heat is dissipated at a rate equal to the rate of combustion, combustion proceeds at a steady level (as it does in a gas burner). If, on the other hand, conditions are such that heat is not dissipated as quickly as it is given off, the temperature of the reaction rises. This sequence increases the probability of collision among the reactants, generating more heat and higher temperatures. The result is an accelerating flame or explosion.

TABLE 7-1
Enhancement of Collisions Between Flammable Material and Oxygen

OCCURRENCE OF REACTANTS (FUEL AND OXYGEN) IN GAS PHASE

- Permits complete mixing of fuel
- Molecular oxygen enhances probability of collision

ABSENCE OF NONREACTIVE COMPONENTS IN MIXTURE

- Nonreactive components (eg, nitrogen dilute mixture) and decreased probability of reactional collisions

INCREASING VELOCITY OF MOLECULES IN MIXTURES

- Increases probability of collisions with sufficient energy to react
- Velocities are directly proportional to temperature

FUEL–OXYGEN MIXTURES

Stoichiometric Mixtures

When the proportions of a fuel–oxygen mixture are such that all of the fuel is oxidized by all of the oxygen present, leaving only oxidized products, the mixture is said to be "stoichiometric." For example, a mixture of 2 mol hydrogen and 1 mol oxygen is stoichiometric, because oxidation yields 1 mol water vapor and no excess of either hydrogen or oxygen. Mixtures containing an excess of oxygen, such that oxygen remains in the mixture after oxidation of the fuel, are "lean." Mixtures with an excess of fuel, such that fuel remains among the combustion products after oxidation, are "rich."

Limits of Flammability

As a fuel–oxygen mixture becomes increasingly lean, a proportion is reached at which the heat of combustion of the mixture is dissipated faster than it can be generated by the available fuel, and the mixture becomes nonflammable. This proportion is the lower limit of flammability. Similarly, as a mixture is made richer, the reaction products formed dilute the available oxygen, and the heat is dissipated to a point at which combustion ceases and the mixture becomes nonflammable, defining the upper limit of flammability.

FLAMES AND EXPLOSIONS

A combustion that proceeds with the generation of light is a flame. Depending on the conditions, a flame may remain static and continue to burn at the source of fuel and oxygen (such as a gas burner), or it may spread along the fuel–oxygen supply and cause a deflagration. Smith described an accident involving a copper kettle vaporizer that was being cleaned with liquid ether.[6] The ether vapor passed from the cleaning area to an adjacent room, where it was ignited by a cigarette, and deflagration was initiated; the flame traveled back to the cleaning room and ultimately caused an explosion in the copper kettle. Fortunately, the technician sustained only slight injuries, although the kettle was damaged extensively.

Conditions Necessary for Explosion

The conditions necessary to cause an explosion must include those that favor the retention of heat. Explosions occur when the heat energy of combustion is retained by the mixture, causing a temperature rise sufficient to accelerate the combustion process. The rising temperature and accelerating combustion cause a rapid expansion of gas, resulting in a shock wave, compression traveling at supersonic speeds. The shock wave contains the mechanical energy necessary to cause damage (as illustrated by the aforementioned vaporizer).

Just as fuel–oxygen mixtures have a range of flammability,

they also have a range of explosivity or detonability. The range of detonability is narrower than the range of flammability.

NITROUS OXIDE IN FIRES AND EXPLOSIONS

The ranges of flammability and detonability of fuel–air mixtures are much narrower than those of fuel–oxygen mixtures. The nitrogen in air acts as a diluent, absorbing energy without entering the reaction, and as a medium for conducting heat. Nitrous oxide, on the other hand, not only supports the combustion process but also enhances it.

Ranges of Flammability and Detonability

Detonability, like flammability, is enhanced by nitrous oxide. The chemical formation of nitrous oxide requires the input of energy (19 kcal/mol); it is an endothermic chemical reaction. This energy of formation is released when nitrous oxide is broken down or enters a combustion process. As shown earlier, the combustion of hydrogen and oxygen yields 57 kcal for each mol of water formed. The same reaction using nitrous oxide in place of oxygen yields 76 kcal/mol of water produced, an increase of 33%; the extra 19 kcal results from the breakdown of nitrous oxide. Consequently, the ranges of flammability and detonability of fuel–nitrous oxide mixtures are wider than those of fuel–oxygen mixtures.

These ranges can be extended still further by oxygen enrichment of fuel–nitrous oxide mixtures, as in clinical practice. Under hyperbaric conditions considerable caution must be taken because materials that may be deemed nonflammable at 1 atm absolute may become flammable at higher pressures. However, halothane and enflurane are nonflammable to pressures as high as 3 atm absolute.[7,8]

TYPES AND SOURCES OF IGNITION

Chemical Ignition

The presence of ether, oxygen, and light in storage containers is conducive to the formation of ether peroxides, which are very labile oxidizers and resemble chemical detonators. Although peroxide formation was at one time a source of ignition, it has been eliminated by the use of antioxidants (eg, a copper lining) in light-proof ether containers.

Spontaneous Ignition

Mixtures of fuel and air or oxygen will ignite spontaneously if their temperature is raised to a certain minimum at which the temperature is high enough to start an oxidation reaction. The locally produced heat raises the temperature and accelerates the oxidation process until ignition occurs. This is the mechanism of spontaneous ignition operative in haystacks and oil-saturated rags. The temperature required to start the process of spontaneous ignition is considerably lower than the temperature required for local ignition by an open flame or spark. For example, mixtures of some volatile anesthetics and oxygen have temperatures of spontaneous ignition that range from 350°C to 400°C. Rich mixtures of diethyl ether and air can ignite spontaneously at temperatures as low as 200°C.

Local Ignition

Local ignition requires that a small zone of the flammable mixture be heated to the ignition temperature. This is by far the most common type of ignition and requires the concentration of only small amounts of heat in a localized area.

Open Flames

Open flames are a source of local ignition. Examples include burners, matches, and cigarettes. Although these items are not found in the operating room, they may be found in adjacent lounges and laboratories.

Light and Heat Sources

Light and heat sources also cause local ignition. Examples include lasers and projection lamps used in fiberoptic light sources, drills and burrs, endoscopic bulbs, hot wire cautery units, lasers, and argon beam coagulators.

Sparks

Sparks are the most common source of ignition in operating room fires and explosions. A spark occurs when sufficient electric potential or voltage exists between two points separated by insulation to cause a breakdown of that insulation. Electrical energy flows between the points through the gap. High temperatures are generated when this energy flows through a material of high resistance (eg, air gap); this process is the basis of all electric heating devices.

MacIntosh and colleagues provide an example in which a spark develops 0.001 cal of heat.[9] If the spark passes through a volume of air equal to 1 mm^3 in 1 ms, the temperature within the air volume can reach 1000°C. This temperature is sufficient, in the presence of a flammable mixture, to cause ignition. The major sources of sparks in operating rooms are electrosurgical devices, other electric apparatus, and static electricity.

Static Electricity

Static electricity is generated when two dissimilar nonconducting materials are in motion and in contact with each other. One material tends to give up electrons in the frictional process to the other material. As a result, a negative charge builds up on the material that gains electrons, and a positive charge on the other material. The two materials then behave like the plates of a capacitor separated by an air gap. If the process continues, accumulation of charge and voltage increases until a spark jumps across the air gap. This is the mechanism by which the Van der Graaff generator operates. In the operating room, the equivalent of this device is a roller with a nonconductive cover for transporting patients between a stretcher and operating table.

Electrical Devices

Electrical devices are the most common source of electric sparks in the modern operating room. Sparks from electrical devices may be generated by the "making" or "breaking" of switch or relay contacts or by electric motor brushes, commutators, loose or faulty electric plugs and receptacles, electrosurgical units, and electrocautery units.

Mechanical Sources

Mechanical sources of ignition energy include rapid gas compression, hammers, drills, and saws. Garfield and colleagues reported a small explosion that occurred when an oxygen tank was opened into a pressure regulator contaminated with oil.[10] The rapid compression of gas within the regulator caused by oxygen release created sufficient heat to ignite the oil and explode the regulator.

TYPES OF FIRES

The types of fires that can occur from various combinations of ignition sources, fuels, and oxidizers include many that, on reflection, are intuitively obvious, as well as some that are not (Table 7-2). In most cases common sense, a basic understanding of the principles discussed in this chapter, and attention to detail can prevent them or minimize the associated damage, morbidity, and occasional mortality.[11]

CONTROL OF FIRE AND EXPLOSION HAZARDS

For fires and explosions to occur, the following must be present simultaneously: a source of fuel, a source of oxygen, and a source of ignition. Prevention is directed toward their control.

Control of Flammable Materials

Investigations and discussions of operating room fires and explosions usually focus on the use of flammable anesthetic drugs. The clinical issues that involve the use of flammable anesthetic agents have been discussed by Ngai.[4] However, other flammable materials are commonly used in the operating room (Table 7-3). These include alcohol, other organic volatile preparatory solutions (acetone, ether, tincture of iodine, aerosol adhesive sprays, ophthalmic ointment,[12] local anesthetic aerosol,[13] tincture of benzoin, plastic coating sprays, collodion, and surgical drapes[14]). Many of these materials are not labeled as flammable.

Disposable Products

In the past 2 decades the use of disposable products has increased and has brought large amounts of paper and plastic waste into the operating room. Although not explosive, these materials are readily flammable, and if ignited some can liberate dense smoke or toxic fumes. Volatile preparatory solutions and aerosols require adequate ventilation, as do the flammable anesthetics. These materials should be handled in such a way that pooling in or saturation of patient drapes is avoided. Alcohol-saturated drapes on patients undergoing electrocautery are a significant fire hazard. Although complete elimination of flammable materials is not practical, some thought should be given to their control.

Facilities Design

The National Fire Protection Association (NFPA) develops consensus standards for the design of health care facilities, including the locations where patient anesthesia will be performed. These are contained in a comprehensive document entitled *Standard for Health Care Facilities*,[15] which covers power distribution requirements for anesthetizing locations, as well as environmental specifications regarding conductive flooring, temperature and humidity maintenance, and air exchange. These requirements are used by most accreditation agencies as de facto standards for health care facility design and maintenance.

Control of Ignition Sources

Sources of chemical and spontaneous ignition are not common in operating room facilities, although sources of local ignition are. Common sense dictates that sources of open flame (eg,

TABLE 7-2
Operating Room Fires: Ignition, Fuels, and Oxidizers

LOCATION OF FIRE	IGNITION SOURCE	FUEL	OXIDIZER
Colon	ESU	Bowel gas	Air
Lung	ESU	Gauze	Oxygen (100%)
Eyelid	ECU	Ointment	Oxygen, nitrous oxide
Adjacent to sterile field	ESU, laser, ECU	Drapes	Air
Tracheostomy	ESU	Tube	Oxygen (100%)
Tonsillectomy	ESU, tissue ember	Gauze	Oxygen
Face	Burr spark	Moustache	Oxygen, nitrous oxide

ECU, electrocautery unit; *ESU*, electrosurgical unit.
ECRI: Surgical fire case summaries. Health Devices 21:31, 1992.

TABLE 7-3
Flammable Materials (Fuels) in the Operating Room

PATIENT
Hair, skin
Gastrointestinal gases (methane)

PREPARATORY AGENTS
Ether, acetone
Aerosol adhesives
Alcohol (bottled and cotton packets)
Antiseptic agents

LINENS
Drapes
Gowns, markers, caps, hoods, shoe covers
Egg-crate mattresses, padding
Mattresses, pillows
Blankets

DRESSING MATERIALS
Gauze, sponges
Tape
Stockinettes
Collodion

OINTMENTS
Benzoin
Petroleum jelly
Aerosols
Wax

EQUIPMENT AND SUPPLIES
Anesthesia machine components (circuits, tubes, catheters)
Endoscopes (flexible)
Wire coverings, insulators
Tourniquets, blood pressure cuffs
Stethoscope tubing
Disposable packing material
Boxes, cabinets
Hoses, connectors

cigarettes) should be kept well away from operating rooms, recovery rooms, equipment, and storage areas.

Humidification

An adequate relative humidity promotes the formation of a water film over surfaces and the dissipation of static charges. The relative humidity should be at least 50%. Because operating room humidities may vary greatly with the prevailing weather, spot checks are an inadequate safeguard. Sparks from an electrical device can be avoided by the use of equipment specifically labeled "for use in hazardous atmospheres."

Electrosurgical Units

Surgical personnel should be made aware that electrosurgical units are currently the most common source of ignition in operating room fires and explosions and that most fires and explosions now involve fuel other than anesthetics. Enteric gas is one of the most commonly reported. For this reason, the use of nitrous oxide as an insufflating gas for laparoscopy is hazardous[16,17]; thus, carbon dioxide is preferred not only because the consequences of an air embolus are minimized but also because it reduces the risk of fire or explosion, especially when electrocoagulation is used.[16,17]

The explosive properties of colonic gas have been described.[18–20] Explosive concentrations of methane, hydrogen, or both often are present in patients whose intestines have not been prepared for surgery. Patients undergoing laparoscopy rarely have bowel preparation. Both methane and hydrogen can diffuse into the abdominal cavity. Nitrous oxide can diffuse into the bowel cavity, as has been well documented in cases of intestinal obstruction.

Although carbon dioxide insufflation for laparoscopy may cause mild peritoneal irritation and slightly increased propensity for cardiac dysrhythmias, these disadvantages can be minimized by drugs and ventilatory support. In contrast, the consequences of an intra-abdominal fire or explosion are treated less easily. Although no case of this type has been reported during laparoscopy, the possibility has been discussed, and some preliminary measurements have been made.[15,16]

Lasers

High-powered carbon dioxide, neodymium-yttrium aluminum garnet (Nd:YAG), and argon lasers have become an increasingly common source of ignition in the modern operating room. When accidentally directed at conventional polyvinyl chloride endotracheal tubes containing nitrous oxide–oxygen mixtures, a "blow torch" can develop and result in severe burns to the adjacent tissues.[21,22] Ignition of the endotracheal tube also liberates gases that are noxious to distal respiratory surfaces. The use of aluminum foil–wrapped or special metal endotracheal tubes (laser-resistant endotracheal tubes) that are capable of reflecting the laser energy has been advocated when the laser is used near the tube.[23] However, such tubes also can redirect the laser energy, resulting in undesired burns to the tracheal or pharyngeal mucosa.[22] Available evidence shows that Nd:YAG lasers can damage all available laser-resistant tubes.[24]

Because of high thermal conductivity and inertness, it has been recommended that helium be used instead of nitrogen as the "balance" gas to prevent airway fires. However, studies have shown that fires propagate faster in helium–oxygen mixtures than in nitrogen–oxygen mixtures.[25,26] These helium–oxygen mixtures may therefore actually be more harmful if an airway fire starts during laser surgery.[24]

REFERENCES

1. Greene BA: The hazard of fire and explosion in anesthesia: report of a clinical investigation of 230 cases. Anesthesiology 2:144, 1941
2. Woodbridge PD: Incidence of anesthetic explosions. JAMA 113: 2308, 1939
3. Ministry of Health: Anaesthetic explosions: report of a working party. London: Her Majesty's Stationery Office, 1956
4. Ngai SH: Explosive agents: are they needed? Surg Clin North Am 55:975, 1975
5. Fineberg HV, Pearlman LA, Gabel RA: The case for abandonment of explosive anesthetic agents. N Engl J Med 303:613, 1980

6. Smith TC: Serious explosion during cleaning of a copper kettle. Anesthesiology 29:386, 1968
7. Slack WK: Hyperbaric oxygen. In Hewer CL (ed): Recent advances in anaesthesia and analgesia. London: Churchill-Livingstone, 1967: 212
8. Baker AB, Unsworth IP: No ignition risk with hyperbaric enflurane. Anaesthesia and Intensive Care 6:157, 1978
9. MacIntosh R, Mushin WW, Epstein HG: Sources of ignition and explosion hazards. In Physics for the anaesthetist. 3rd ed. Oxford: Blackwell Scientific Publications, 1963: 358
10. Garfield JM, Allen GW, Silverstein P, et al: Flash fire in a reducing valve. Anesthesiology 34:578, 1971
11. ECRI: Surgical fire case summaries. Health Devices 21:31, 1992
12. Miller R, Kruchek D: An explosive spray. Anaesthesia 38:1101, 1983
13. Datta TD: Flash fire hazard with eye ointment. Anesth Analg 63:700, 1984
14. Milliken RA, Bizzarri DV: Flammable surgical drapes: a patient and personnel hazard. Anesth Analg 64:54, 1985
15. National Fire Protection Association: Standard for health care facilities. Bulletin 99-93. Quincy, MA: National Fire Protection Association, 1993
16. Robinson JC, Thompson JM, Wood AW: Laparoscopy explosion hazards with nitrous oxide. Br Med J 3:764, 1975
17. Drummond GB, Scott DB: Laparoscopy hazards with nitrous oxide. Br Med J 1:586, 1976
18. Ragans H, Shinya H, Wolff W: The explosive potential of colonic gas during colonoscopic electrosurgical polypectomy. Surg Gynecol Obstet 138:554, 1974
19. Bigard MA, Gaucher P, Lassale C: Fatal colonic explosion during colonoscopic polypectomy. Gastroenterology 77:1307, 1979
20. Augerinos A, Kalantzis N, Rekoumis G, et al: Bowel preparation and the risk of explosion during colonoscopic polypectomy. Gut 25:361, 1984
21. Hirshman CA, Smith J: Indirect ignition of the endotracheal tube during carbon dioxide laser surgery. Arch Otolaryngol 106: 639, 1980
22. Assoff RH, Duncavage JA, Eisenman TS, et al: Comparison of tracheal damage from laser-ignited endotracheal tube fires. Ann Otol Rhinol Laryngol 92:333, 1983
23. Assoff RH, Karlan MS: Safe instrumentation in laser surgery. Otolaryngol Head Neck Surg 92:644, 1984
24. ECRI: Laser-resistant tracheal tubes. Health Devices 21:4, 1992
25. Bunker RL, Hirsch DB, Janoff D: Effects of oxygen concentration, diluents, and pressure on ignition and flame-spread rates of non-metals: a review paper. In McElroy K, Sloltzfuc JM (eds): Flammability and sensitivity of materials in oxygen-enriched atmosphere, vol. 5. Philadelphia: American Society for Testing and Materials, 1991: ASTM STP 1111
26. Sidebotham GW, Stern J, Wolf GL, et al: Endotracheal tube fires: a flame spread phenomenon. In McElroy K, Stoltyfus JM (eds)" Flammability and sensitivity of materials in oxygen-enriched atmosphere, vol. 5. Philadelphia: American Society for Testing and Materials, 1991: ASTM STP 1111

FURTHER READING

ECRI: Fighting airway fires. Health Devices 19:111, 1990

ECRI: OR fires: preventing them and putting them out. Health Devices 15:132, 1986

National Fire Protection Association: Fire protection handbook. 16th ed. Quincy, MA: National Fire Protection Association, 1986

National Fire Protection Association: Fire hazards in oxygen enriched atmospheres. National Fire Protection Association 53M, 1990

Sosis MB: Anesthesia for laser surgery. Problems in Anesthesia 1993: 7, 157

Complications in Anesthesiology, second edition,
edited by Nikolaus Gravenstein and Robert R. Kirby.
Lippincott-Raven Publishers, Philadelphia © 1996.

CHAPTER 8

Electrotrauma in the Operating Room: Shock, Electrocution, and Burns

Guy G. Knickerbocker
Gordon R. Neufeld

Many of the hazards discussed in a book of anesthesia complications arise from the use of devices and techniques that constitute the working armamentarium of the anesthesiologist. Electrotrauma occurs as a consequence of the increasingly widespread use of electrically powered devices in the conduct of anesthesia and modern surgery. Often, experience and training have not been adequate to enable the practitioner to place in perspective the various factors that may lead to an electrical injury. At times, electricity may seem to act at variance with the basic physical principles that the clinician understands.

In this chapter we provide an overview of the principles necessary to an understanding of the mechanism and risks of electrotrauma so that injury may be averted. In particular, we review the physical principles underlying the flow of electrical current, the cause of damage, and the factors that should be considered in the use and control of electrical equipment.

INCREASING EXPOSURE TO POTENTIAL ELECTROTRAUMA

Sources

In the operating room, many sources of electrical energy are focused on the patient. The control of this energy forms the basis of electrical safety. Complications arising from electrical sources include tissue lesions such as skin burns; altered organ function because of interruption of normal physiologic processes, such as neuromuscular excitation; reversible interference with processes such as cardiac function, which can lead to a cardiac arrest or ventricular fibrillation; and because of electric shock, a startle reaction in attending personnel, which can lead to patient injury. We include all of these under the general category "electrotrauma." We also include as electrotrauma complications the consequences of misinformation and interference with the performance of devices such as monitors as the result of malfunction of another device.

Electrical Apparatus

Over the past 3 decades, advances in technology have led to the increased use of electrical apparatuses in the operating room. These devices can be grouped into three categories: (1) labor savers, such as electric operating room tables, dermatomes, drills, saws, and pumps; (2) energy-conversion devices, including hypothermia units, blood warmers, humidifiers, heat exchangers, transducers, and electrosurgical units (ESUs); and (3) information-acquisition and information-display devices, such as electrocardiographs, other patient monitoring devices, cathode ray tubes, computers, meters, and imaging devices.

Progressive improvements in monitoring equipment have been substantial. Technology has provided the means to continuous, instant displays of information through the development of solid-state electronics, integrated circuits, and microprocessor techniques. As a result of technologic innovation, however, the increased role of electronics in patient care has brought more electrical devices (and their related hazards) into an already hazardous environment.

ELECTRICAL ENERGY DISSIPATION IN TISSUES

Voltage, Current, and Resistance

Occasionally, terms relating to electricity are confused or confusing. To facilitate the discussion of electrotrauma, below we review some of the important terms and concepts so that misunderstandings can be avoided. We begin with a familiar physiologic relation: a patient's blood pressure (BP) is a reflection of cardiac output (CO) and peripheral resistance (PR), in accordance with the following equation:

$$BP = CO \times PR$$

This is the equivalent of Ohm's law applied to the circulation. Ohm's electrical law is an equation that describes voltage (E) (electrical equivalent of blood pressure) as directly proportional to the product of current (I) (cardiac output or flow) and resistance (R). Voltage is expressed in terms of volts or its common fractions (millivolts or microvolts); current, in amperes (or milliamperes or microamperes); and resistance, in ohms. Hence, Ohm's law is usually written:

$$E = I \times R$$

Energy and Power

The universal concepts of work (energy) and power that may be applied to circulatory physiology are important to characterize system performance and are fundamental in electricity. The rate of expenditure of energy is power, expressed in watts or, equivalently, joules per second, and can be calculated as the product of voltage and current. Rearrangement of Ohm's law allows power to be calculated as the product of current squared and resistance, or as the voltage squared divided by resistance. The energy expended in an electrical circuit is the product of the power and the duration of power delivery (when power does not change with time) or the integral of power with respect to time (when power is time-varying). Energy is expressed in joules, watt-seconds, or in the case of utility bills, kilowatt-hours.

Current Density

Adverse effects of electricity on the human body usually can be attributed to the excitatory effect of the passage of the electrical current or the thermal response to the heating by the current. Virtually all tissues in the body are conductors of electricity to varying degrees; accidental contact with energized electrical sources results in current flow through tissues. Thus, one must understand concepts of current, power, and energy density to gain insight into electrical injuries. Again, a physiologic analogue is helpful. If a patient has a cardiac output of 6 L/min and the aorta has a cross-sectional area of 10 cm^2, the flow density through the aorta is 0.6 L/min/cm^2. In electrical flow, if 1 mA of current flows through a conducting medium with a cross-sectional area of 10 cm^2, the current density is 0.1 mA/cm^2. However, if 1 mA flows through a fine wire or catheter of 0.1 cm^2 cross-sectional area, the current density is 100-fold larger, or 10 mA/cm^2.

Power Density

Whereas current density is determined by the current through a cross-sectional area, energy and power density take into account the dissipation per unit volume. Hence, they are expressed in terms of watt-seconds (or joules) per cubic centimeter of tissue. Power density, for example, is calculated from the product of the current density squared and the resistivity (in ohm-centimeters) of the tissue through which the current flows. Total energy expended is the product of the power and the duration of application.

Effects of Electric Current in Tissue

The risk of electrotrauma is present whenever a portion of the body forms a part of an electrical circuit that is energized. Usually, points of a current's entry and exit can be identified. Virtually all of the components of the human body are conductors of electricity to some degree (Fig. 8-1). Muscle, blood, and vascular organs are among the better conductors.[1] Among the vascular organs, the lungs are the poorest conductors (ie, have the highest specific resistance) because of the very large volume of air in the alveoli. Fat and bone have high resistivities. Skin can provide high resistance to electric current, particularly if it is dry. The varying resistivities contribute to a heterogeneity of current density within the body as current flows. As a result, various organs and vessels may provide preferential pathways for current flow (Fig. 8-2).

Two levels of electric shock can be distinguished: macroshock and microshock. Both have the capacity to inflict clinically important morbidity or death, but they differ in magnitude and site of application.

MACROSHOCK

Physical Aspects

Macroshock results from contacts on the surface of the body (or just inside the skin) with energized conductors. Macro-

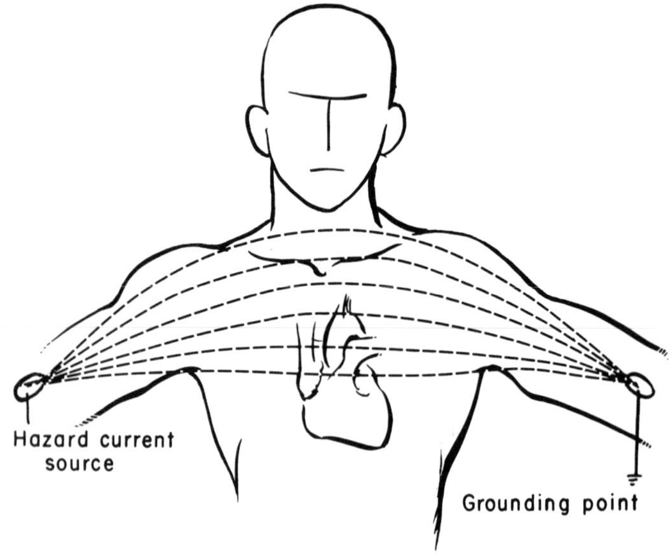

FIGURE 8-1. A very simplified view of electrical current flow in the human body, in which the body is considered to be a leather bag filled with a homogeneously conducting electrolyte solution.

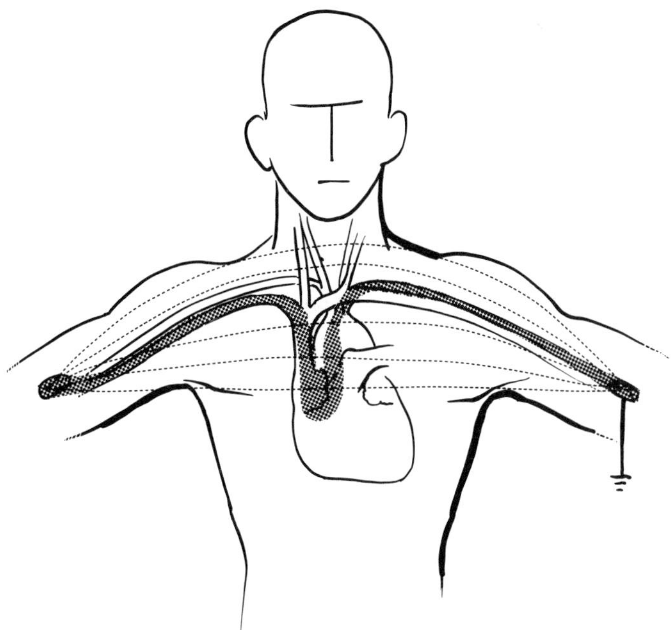

FIGURE 8-2. Electrical current flows through the human body in preferential pathways that reflect the relative conductivity of the tissues. The highly conductive components are the great vessels and the muscle masses of the shoulder girdle and chest wall.

shock currents are of sufficient magnitude to be perceived as an electric shock. Their magnitudes are greater than a few milliamperes and often result from a failure of insulation or components in an electrically operated device. The effect of the passage of current through the human body depends on several factors, which include the magnitude of the current density through the various tissues; the points of entry to and exit from (ie, the path through) the body; the frequency of the current; and the duration of application.

Awareness and Tetanus

At low levels of current and with 0.5- to 8-mA currents that result from contact with points on the surface of the body, the effect is limited to the sensation of shock. As current increases to 10 mA, tetanic muscular contraction occurs; if electrical contact is made with the hand, for instance, release of the grip is then impossible. At higher levels of current, the respiratory muscles may undergo tetanic contraction and breathing is interrupted if the current passes through the phrenic nerves or thorax.

Burns, Fibrillation, and Electrocution

For currents of 100 mA and greater, ventricular fibrillation may result as the current density in the myocardium reaches the fibrillation threshold. With a current of more than a few amperes, the risk of serious burns increases as current densities become high enough to raise the temperature of the tissues through which the current passes.[2] Macroshocks that lead to fatal dysrhythmias are termed "electrocutions."

Causes

Macroshock and electrocution result from exposure to currents that arise from the failure, unsafe design, or misuse of electrical devices.[3]

Exposure to Electric Current

Exposure to electric current with electrical devices (medical or other) generally occurs for one of three reasons.

INTENTIONAL APPLICATION. Exposure can result from the intentional application of electric currents to achieve some therapeutic or diagnostic purpose. Electrosurgery, impedance plethysmography, cardiac pacing, electrogalvanism, and defibrillation are but a few of many such techniques.

SHORT CIRCUITS. Exposure occurs when a fault ("short circuit") develops (for example, a component failure) or when a significant human error, oversight, or misconnection occurs. The outcome of the exposure again depends on the magnitude, frequency, and duration of the current; the points of contact with the body and current distribution between them; and the physical state or condition of the affected person.

LEAKAGE CURRENTS. Exposure may occur because of well-recognized leakage currents and other potentially hazardous currents inherent in the design of most electrically operated devices, particularly those that are powered from the electrical distribution system, in contrast to self-contained, battery-powered devices.

Enhancement and Prevention of Body Contact

Many electrotherapeutic currents, although relatively innocuous when used as intended, pose great risks for macroshock, electrocution, and burns to personnel and patients if they are not used properly (ie, enhanced, or raised above therapeutic levels). The defibrillator current is an excellent example. Unacceptable risks also may result if the choice or application of the electrotherapeutic current is inappropriate, as in an unsynchronized cardioversion that induces an R- on T-wave phenomenon.

The design of electrically powered equipment should preclude contact with any energized conductive parts, except of course those intended for contact to achieve their therapeutic purpose or ungrounded conductive surfaces on the enclosure that are likely to become energized. Usually this goal can be accomplished effectively by insulation, isolation of electric circuits from ground, and physical grounding of exposed metal surfaces.

Ground Faults

Macroshocks can occur when the line voltage makes contact with the main housing (chassis) of a device that is inadequately grounded. This problem may occur when a plug is inserted into an incorrect or improperly wired receptacle such that the grounding conductor mates with the "live" supply line. More commonly, it occurs through component failure—in particular, worn insulation on the power cord with a fractured ground lead or broken grounding pin.

The risk of macroshock is increased greatly with the abuse of power cords and plugs, as when a device is disconnected by simply pulling on the power cord. This unfortunate practice can loosen conductors in the plug from their terminals. If the grounding conductor becomes disconnected, the loose conductor can contact the energized plug terminal or its conductor, making the chassis of the device live with line voltage and putting anyone touching a conductive case of the device at risk of a severe shock. Similar hazards are present where heavy equipment is rolled over power cords lying on the floor.

MOISTURE. Moisture accelerates component degradation or leaves conductive salt deposits that promote electrical faults. Thus, every effort must be made to avoid spilling liquids on electrically operated devices. This hazard is becoming less likely as manufacturers improve equipment housings, making them more impermeable to fluid entry.

Failures attributable to moisture are, fortunately, rare. Nevertheless, they continue to occur because of inadequate preventive maintenance, abuse or misuse of equipment, or ignorance. They also may occur for reasons that are less easily controlled, such as an internal component failure.

Conventional Power Distribution

Hot and Neutral Wires

Normally, the power supplied to a wall receptacle in the home or at the hospital bedside involves three wires (Fig. 8-3). Two wires provide the power necessary to permit the device to operate. In a conventional grounded distribution system, one of them is "hot," is color-coded black (or red or blue), and operates at 120 V. The other one is "neutral," is color-coded white, and is maintained at ground potential (0 V). It serves to return current from the device to the distribution panel and ultimately to the utility company.

Ground Wire

The third wire is the grounding wire and is either uninsulated or covered with green insulation. The neutral and grounding conductors are bonded together at the distribution panel (or at the point of incoming power) and firmly grounded. Although both operate at ground potential, the grounding conductor does not normally carry any of the operating current from connected devices. It does provide an ensured pathway for fault currents, thereby minimizing the risk of shock and facilitating rapid tripping of the circuit breaker when a fault occurs. Thus, under most conditions, only the hot wire supplies potentially injurious electrical power.

Hospital Equipment

Hospital electrical equipment is supplied with a corresponding three-wire power cord and plug. The wires within the power cord also are color-coded. The black (or brown) and white wires carry the load current; the green wire is the grounding conductor. The plug, by design and with proper wiring, ensures that corresponding conductors in the device's power cord and in the system supplying the wall outlet are connected appropriately. The correspondence can be overridden through the use of "cheater" adapters (which enable a three-pronged plug to be used in a two-pronged outlet or extension cord) or improperly wired extension cords, neither of which should be used.

The green grounding wire in the power cord is connected

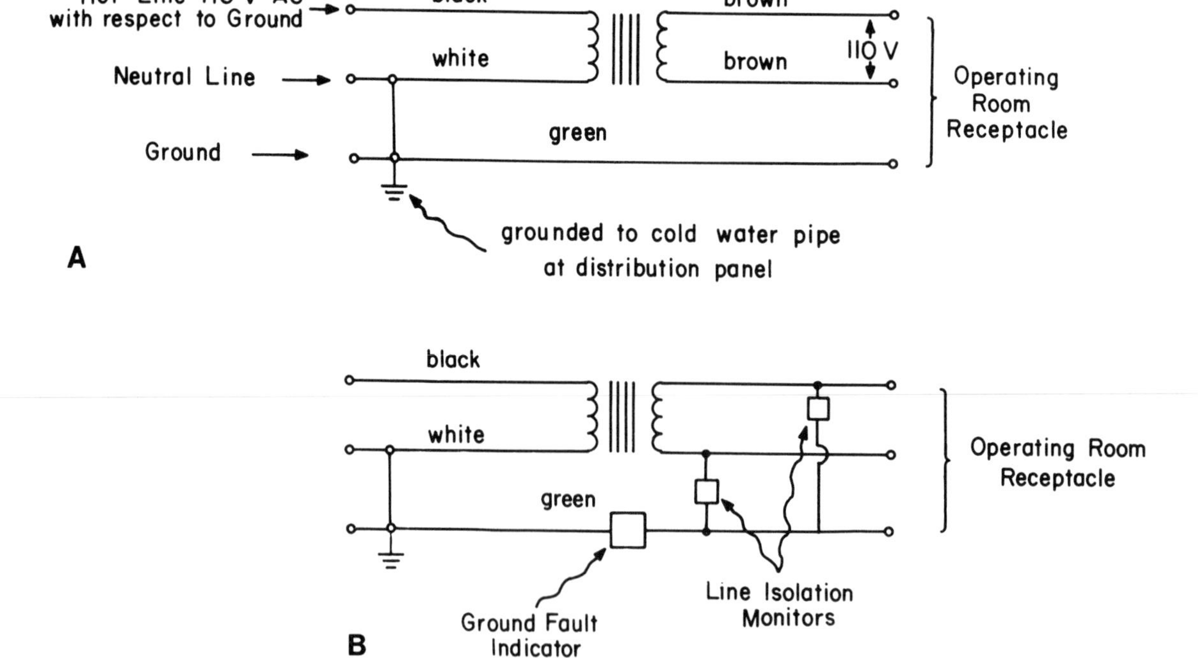

FIGURE 8-3. (**A**) Isolation transformer and (**B**) ground fault indicator and line isolation monitors built into the isolation transformer. In both, the electrical power source (*left*) consists of three wires, two supplying the power and the third furnishing a pathway for dissipation of fault currents to ground.

within the electrical device to the chassis and to any exposed metal parts that might otherwise become energized easily. If a fault develops in the equipment so that the hot lead comes into contact with the frame or metal case of the device, a short circuit develops, and a fuse or circuit breaker interrupts the supply of power, preventing a macroshock to the person in contact with the device.

Isolated Power Distribution

The power receptacles in most operating rooms are separated from the main hospital power by a transformer (see Fig. 8-3A). The isolated system includes a warning system (line isolation monitor or ground fault detector) (see Fig. 8-3B). This warning system indicates when an electrical fault from either of the power conductors to ground exists in the affected circuit. Such systems prevent a macroshock condition until two simultaneous electrical faults exist. Hence, short circuits to ground present less risk in an isolated power system.

Justifications

For many years, operating rooms have been designed with isolated electrical power distribution systems. These systems were provided originally to reduce fire and explosion hazards in locations where flammable anesthetics were used. A short circuit is a potential source of ignition for a fire or explosion if a spark occurs and increases the risk of macroshock. Flammable anesthetic agents have been eliminated from practice in the United States.[4] As the use of flammable agents declined, however, the use of electrical apparatuses has increased rapidly.

PROTECTION FROM MACROSHOCK. Although recent codes and standards no longer require the installation of isolated power in areas in which nonflammable anesthetics will be administered, some argue that isolated power distribution still is desirable in operating rooms because it offers protection from macroshock conditions.

In an operating room supplied with isolated power, energy from the electric utility company is coupled through a transformer to the secondary load supplying windings. Neither of the load-supplying conductors is intentionally connected ("referenced") to ground (see Fig. 8-3A). Under normal circumstances, only currents that are inconsequential (with regard to macroshock) can be made to flow to ground. A grounding wire is also provided in this system but of course is not connected to either load-carrying conductor. It is nevertheless bonded (connected) to the cold-water piping and other grounds in the area. As a consequence of the isolation of the power conductors from ground, simultaneously touching a single secondary power lead and ground will not complete a circuit that allows significant current to flow (see Fig. 8-3B).

Thus, an isolated power supply provides operating room personnel and the patient with protection from macroshock somewhat greater than that provided by a conventional grounded system. The isolated power supply also prevents a device in which a fault to the chassis or ground has developed from causing a circuit breaker to trip. A fault that causes one load conductor to become grounded simply leaves the other "hot" with respect to ground, as it would be if it were operating from a conventional grounded power-distribution system. However, because the isolated system is equipped with an alarm, the line isolation monitor or ground fault detector alerts personnel that degradation to a grounded system has occurred. The offending device can be removed as quickly as is convenient after the patient's needs have been met adequately. With prompt attention, and in the unlikely event of another fault, the second fault, which would lead to a macroshock hazard, usually can be averted.

FUTURE USE. Although they are no longer required in operating rooms and although their need is controversial, some isolated power systems continue to be installed. Protection against macroshock and continuity of operation of connected equipment under first-fault conditions are attractive features, particularly to the immediate health care staff.

On the other hand, the occurrence of line-to-ground faults has decreased because of more rugged power cords and improved plugs; receptacle and plug strain reliefs; and isolation of patient leads. This decrease in faults has prompted demonstration by statistical analysis that isolated power, compared with conventional grounded power, provides only a small incremental increase in safety.[5-7] Clearly, economics and practice will ultimately decide this issue.

Double Insulation

Double insulation is a second type of device design that enhances electrical safety, but it is implemented without the need for a three-conductor power cord. In many cases, hospital personnel have become so well indoctrinated in the importance of a three-pronged plug on devices that sometimes they object to the use of an appropriate double-insulated device with a two-wire power cord.

Design

A double-insulated device has two distinct layers of insulation between any conductor or surface that may be or is likely to become energized by supply-system voltage and surfaces accessible to contact or to patient connected leads. Strict adherence to current codes and standards suggests that hospitals should use only double-insulated devices that are recognized by qualified testing organizations, such as the Underwriters Laboratories. Unfortunately, only a few medical devices (eg, some infant apnea monitors, infusion pumps, and enteral feeding pumps) currently are qualified as double-insulated, although their number is sure to grow. In the meantime, hospital personnel should know that qualified two-wire devices are acceptable if they are labeled as being double-insulated.

MICROSHOCK

Physical Aspects

When a hazard current is delivered directly to the heart through an insulated conductor such as a pacing electrode on the epicardium, a significantly greater risk of ventricular fibrillation exists with minute currents. This risk occurs because the current density within a portion of the heart muscle can be high, although the total current is low (Fig. 8-4). Currents

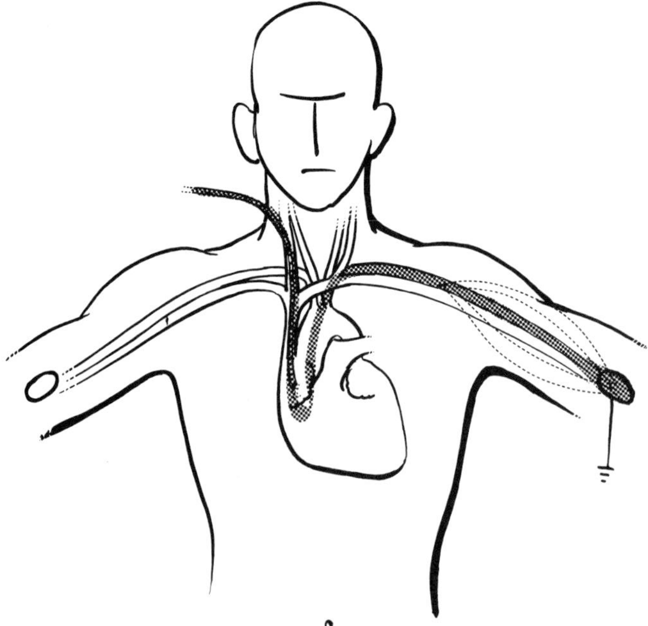

FIGURE 8-4. Microshock results when electric current, accidentally applied to the exposed end of an externalized conductor (saline-filled central venous catheter), is dissipated as a high-current density from the tip of the conductor through the great vessels, blood, and myocardium.

as low as 20 μA, well below perceptible levels, can cause fibrillation. Such currents are referred to as "microshock."

Starmer and coworkers reported fibrillatory currents ranging from 20 to 800 (mean 258) μA with intracardiac electrodes in anesthetized dogs.[8] Catheter position is an important factor in the current level required for fibrillation; the most sensitive area is the inner aspect of the right ventricular wall near the apex. At current levels well below the fibrillatory threshold, ventricular activity ceases while the current flows, but normal activity resumes when the current is turned off.[9] This type of current flow probably mimics more closely the clinical situation in which the combined leakage of current of several devices or a single faulty device through an intracardiac or central venous catheter can cause ventricular arrest.

Fibrillatory Thresholds

Few data on fibrillatory thresholds of the human myocardium exist, but those that do indicate a higher threshold in humans than in dogs. Starmer and coworkers found that the current necessary to induce ventricular fibrillation during open heart procedures was 180 to 1,500 (mean 583) μA.[8] No data exist on the levels of sustained current flow necessary for ventricular standstill in humans, but from data obtained from experiments in dogs it is inferred that they are much lower than those causing fibrillation.

Work by Roy and colleagues[9] helps to clarify the discrepancies in fibrillatory thresholds observed by different investigators and in different species. They examined the current density required to produce three phenomena. The first is disruption of cardiac rhythm while current is applied; it occurs at the lowest current densities. The second is pump failure, that is, cardiac standstill, which is reversible as defined by resumption of sinus rhythm when the current is turned off. The third is pump failure with fibrillation, which is not spontaneously reversible. Pump failure and pump failure with fibrillation are related directly to the current density. The investigators did not observe either effect at currents less than 10 μA, regardless of the contact area.

Leakage Current

Leakage currents, inherent in the operation of line-powered electrical equipment, can be minimized but never eliminated. They are due primarily to stray impedances within the equipment (and to a lesser extent the power cord), through which current from the ground-referenced power distribution system can pass to ground. The stray impedance occurs primarily between the primary winding of the power supply transformer and the chassis. The resulting leakage current is therefore at the frequency of the power distribution system, which is 60 Hz in North America and 50 or 60 Hz elsewhere.

GROUNDING. Because most devices are supplied with a grounding conductor in the power cord, leakage current from the chassis is diverted harmlessly to ground. If for some reason, however, the device is not grounded—as through an interruption of the grounding conductor by a mechanical break in the plug or cord, a wiring error in the outlet, or the inappropriate use of two- to three-pronged cheater adapter—the available leakage current will flow through any convenient alternate pathway to ground.

The current may flow through another grounded device with which the faulty device is connected, in which case the risk may be minimal. If, however, the device is not otherwise grounded, the convenient pathway may be through the individual (staff person or patient) who comes in contact with the chassis and simultaneously with ground through another device object or the floor (Fig. 8-5).

MAGNITUDE. Leakage currents are typically small (eg, 20 μA). As a result, normal contact with them is not perceived (no "shock" is felt) and does not pose a hazard unless the flow of current includes a direct conductive pathway to the myocardium via a monitoring catheter, invasive device, or pacing electrode. Leakage current poses a hazard to monitored patients in the intensive care unit, operating room, or radiology suite who have invasive conductive pathways. Additional stray impedances develop between the power input and patient-connected leads. As a general rule, leakage currents from patient leads to ground are significantly less when the grounding of the device is intact and are greater when device grounding is interrupted. However, the current leakage from patient-connected leads is not always as great as the chassis leakage.

Performance Standards

Guidelines and standards developed for design and performance of electrical devices and particularly medical devices ensure that the leakage current inherent in the device is kept sufficiently low that the risks of any leakage current are small even if grounding of the device is faulty.

ELECTRICAL BURNS

When electrical injury is mentioned, one is likely to think of electrical shock, but electrotrauma in the operating room is far more likely to cause a burn. Burns may result from a ma-

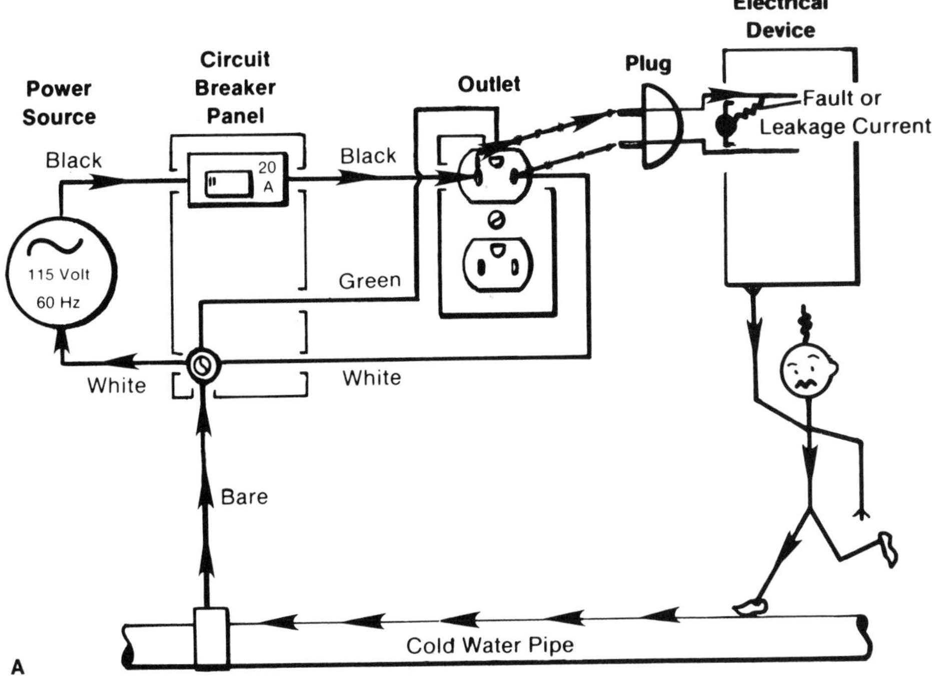

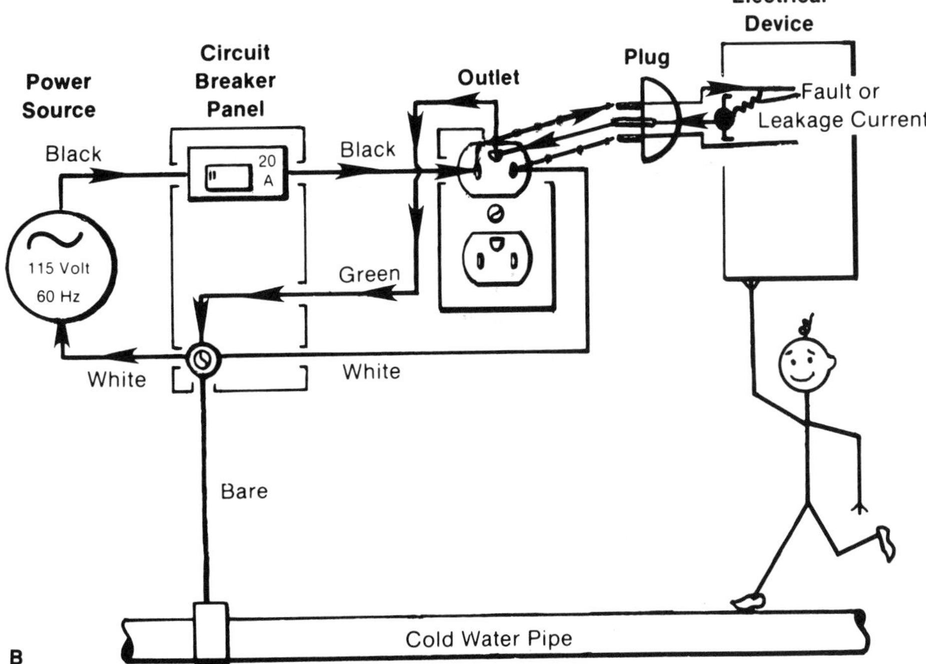

FIGURE 8-5. (**A**) An ungrounded device chassis (eg, two-pronged plug) does not protect against shock from line-to-chassis fault or leakage current. (**B**) Grounding the device chassis (three-pronged plug) minimizes the shock hazard by providing a pathway for fault and/or leakage current.

croshock but most commonly are associated with the use of ESUs. This discussion specifically addresses lesions arising from the heating or electrochemical effects of electric current flow in the tissue, and not thermal burns such as those resulting from a hyperthermia blanket or skin lesions resulting from chemical irritation or pressure necrosis.

Alternating Current

Thermal lesions from electric current occur when the current density in tissue is great enough that the resistive electric heating effect raises the tissue temperature high enough and long enough to cause damage.

Line-frequency Currents

Rarely do burns in the hospital result from line-frequency electric currents; currents lower than those necessary to cause burns cause a severe electrical shock. These of course are noticed, at least when they occur in health care personnel or nonanesthetized patients, before a significant burn lesion occurs. Anesthetized patients, however, may be burned when a particularly large macroshock occurs, the pathway of the current does not involve the heart, and electrocution is averted. Burns from line-frequency macroshocks are rare in the hospital but are common in severe electrical injuries in the home or in "high-tension" accidents involving utility company line-maintenance crews.

Electrosurgical Units

Unipolar Electrodes

The most frequent cause of electric current burns in the operating room is the ESU. Electrosurgery (the use of an electrically heated wire for therapy without the passage of an electric current through the body) accomplishes its effect by the application of radiofrequency (greater than approximately 300 kHz) electric current of high current density at the tip of a small electrode in contact with the target tissue. Radiofrequency current avoids electrical shock effects that would occur with low-frequency currents. The resistive electrical heating of the tissue either explosively destroys cells, thereby cutting through the tissue, or coagulates protein to control bleeding. These effects depend on the characteristics of the output current waveform (cutting or coagulation) of the ESU generator.

BURNS AT ALTERNATIVE SITES. Burns occur at a site other than the site of surgery when the former area receives unintended high current density. For example, if the dispersive electrode (grounding pad) becomes partially detached or another point on the body becomes the accidental site of ESU current passage, tissue heating will occur if the current density is sufficiently high. Three factors are involved in tissue burns. First, current density must be high enough to cause tissue heating. Virtually all ESUs designed for operating room use are capable of heating tissue under an improperly applied dispersive electrode at power settings of two-thirds maximum output. Second, the duration of current application must be sufficient. Heating of tissue is not instantaneous; the burn potential is proportional to the product of power density and duration of application. Third, the tissue or dispersive electrode must retain heat.

PHYSICAL FACTORS. Well-perfused tissue dissipates heat; poorly perfused tissue does not. The temperature increase required is not large. Heat of 44°C applied continuously for 4 to 6 hours will produce a first-degree burn (transcutaneous PO_2 electrodes do this routinely). Temperatures greater than 44°C cause burns in a much shorter period of time. Becker and colleagues reported that an ESU current density of 100 mA/cm^2 for 10 seconds is sufficient to cause a second-degree burn.[10] General ESU procedures often require 600 to 800 mA, suggesting that a contact area of less than 6 to 8 cm^2 (a circle $\leqslant$3 cm in diameter) would be prone to serious burn in the event of a technical error. Pearce and coworkers have examined many of these factors in detail.[11]

Besides partial detachment, burns may be caused by current concentration at the point of connection of the electrode cable or deformations of the dispersive electrode. In addition, burns may result from poor heat dissipation resulting from uneven pressure over the area of the electrode due to bony prominences or heat retention by the electrode itself.

Bipolar Electrodes

Thus far, we have discussed unipolar ESU systems, which use a single-pole active electrode with a large-area electrode (grounding pad) elsewhere on the body for return of the current to the generator. Bipolar electrosurgery uses a double electrode, one for source and one for return, both at the surgical site. Coagulation forceps for neurosurgery and tubal ligation are notable examples of bipolar electrosurgery that do not require a dispersive electrode.

BURNS AT ALTERNATIVE SITES. Burns at other sites occur when the active electrode is mistakenly energized while it is lying on the patient or on a wet drape covering the patient. Operator negligence plays a role in this type of injury, first in placing the active electrode in an unprotected place when it is not in use, and second in accidentally activating the pedal control. Even systems with hand-switched active electrodes have been prone to unexpected activation by fluids entering the switch mechanism.

Ground-Referenced Units

ESUs have outputs that are either isolated or ground-referenced (the dispersive electrode lead kept at ground potential, at least at the electrosurgical frequencies). In the event of a disconnection or break in the dispersive electrode cable or degraded performance of the dispersive electrode in a ground-referenced generator, burns can occur at an alternate site of patient contact with a grounded object (eg, metal leg rest, "iron intern," or headframe) if that site becomes the principal return pathway for electrosurgical current. When the area of contact is small, a burn is possible because insufficient area is available for effective dispersal of the current and heat. Alternate current pathways to ground include not only patient contact with grounded metal surfaces on the operating table but also electrodes placed on the patient's body for monitoring purposes.

Isolated Output

An ESU with an isolated output stage rather than a ground-referenced one will reduce but not eliminate the hazard of alternate-site burns. Radiofrequency currents are isolated with difficulty, and isolation is never complete. Moreover, the connection of the patient to the generator by the dispersive electrode provides some de facto grounding by capacitive coupling, and unintended grounding is always possible. Care must be exercised to keep as many alternate ground pathways as possible away from the patient, particularly those that might be close to the ESU site.

Summary

Most ESU burns occur because of failure to properly apply and maintain the dispersive electrode contact with the patient. This hazard cannot be overemphasized. Although burns under electrodes do occur, skin lesions often have been attributed to electrosurgery when in fact they were an early manifestation of pressure necrosis or an allergic reaction to the components of the electrode (notably the adhesive or gel). Some particularly aggressive adhesives may cause a stripping of the stratum corneum of the skin if removed too rapidly. This problem is critical in elderly, neonatal, and other patients with sensitive skin.

Direct Current

The accidental application of direct current may produce skin lesions. In these cases, the current may be low enough that no effects of electrical shock are perceived. As a general rule, a direct current must be two to three times greater than an alternating current to produce the sensation of electrical shock. At these low levels of current, however, electrochemical reactions can occur under electrodes or at contact points through which the current flows. In contrast to alternating current, direct current does not constantly reverse its polarity. As a result, electrode decomposition products, which can be caustic, may accumulate.

Electrochemical Reactions

Leeming and colleagues[6] have reported a case of a serious skin lesion with sustained contact with a 9-V source. They have described the likely reactions occurring under each electrode.

ANODE. Free chlorine is liberated under the anode (positive electrode) and hydrogen and other products are liberated under the cathode as body fluids are electrolyzed by the current. The difference in products accumulated under each electrode causes a remarkable distinction between the lesions. Thus, direct-current electrotrauma should be considered when two points of contact, with different types of skin lesions, are identified.

CATHODE. The cathode lesion is likely to be more severe, with evidence of crater formation. This finding is undoubtedly caused by the accumulation of caustic sodium hydroxide at the cathode, where the pH can be as high as 9.[12] Under the anode, the lesion may be discolored. Green, black, and hemorrhagic appearances have been described and may reflect by-products of corrosion of the metallic electrode at the site.[6]

REGULATORY INSTRUMENTS

Regulatory and quasiregulatory documents and procedures exist to reduce the risk of electrotrauma. They are discussed here to provide a better understanding of the requirements and their incorporation into hospital practice.

Accreditation

Accreditation is almost universally desired by hospitals, if for no other reason than to ensure that the institution will be more attractive to patients who look for these institutional credentials. More importantly, hospitals require accreditation because it is a prerequisite for reimbursement by third-party payors. Hospitals over the course of the past several years have responded to the evolving requirements of the Joint Commission on Accreditation of Healthcare Organizations (JCAHO)[13] that have incorporated several provisions intended to reduce the risk of electrotrauma. In the past, this agency has drawn on requirements promulgated by other groups, most notably the National Fire Protection Association.[14,15]

Surveillance and Maintenance Programs

While the requirements contained in the JCAHO's *Accreditation Manual for Hospitals*[13] have evolved to be less prescriptive, hospitals' programs for the surveillance and maintenance of equipment and installed systems to ensure the proper functioning of equipment and risk reduction, established on the basis of earlier JCAHO requirements, are generally considered to fulfill present requirements. Hence, physicians can expect that hospitals will require inspection not only of their own hospital-owned equipment, but of any equipment brought into the hospital, including physician-owned devices, before authorizing their use.

JCAHO-acceptable equipment management and patient safety programs generally call for regular inspection of equipment in the operating room (typically semiannually); restrictions in the use of equipment with spark hazards (such as ESUs) to procedures in which the agents and preparatory solutions used are nonflammable; readily available operator manuals for all electrically operated devices; and power distribution systems that are appropriate and regularly tested.

Electrical Codes of the National Fire Protection Association

The national consensus standards frequently cited by the JCAHO as well as local and state agencies are the publications of the NFPA. Two documents in particular, the "National Electrical Code" (NFPA Bulletin 70)[14] and the "Standard for Health Care Facilities" (NFPA Bulletin 99-1987),[15] are important to practitioners in anesthesia.

*Bulletin 70**

The NFPA Bulletin 70[14] is widely recognized as the basis for the safe installation of power distribution systems in residences, commercial, and industrial establishments. One subchapter (Article 517) is specifically devoted to the installation of power distribution systems in health care facilities, including locations in which anesthetics will be administered. The NEC (NFPA 70) is updated and published on a strict schedule triennially. The 1984 edition, paragraph 517-104 (a) (1), was published requiring isolated power systems in all anesthetizing locations, but bore a notation that this particular paragraph

* The use of the term "Bulletin" is, in the opinion of the ECRI, unusual and non-standard. We use—and we believe we see others use—the notation NFPA 70, NFPA 99, etc.

was derived material, based on requirements published elsewhere—in this case, NFPA56A (NFPA 99). During the period in which this edition was in effect, the requirements of NFPA 99 were altered to remove the requirement for isolated power systems in non-flammable anesthetizing locations. Hence, the Association was bound by their operating rules to announce the amendment of §517-104 (a) (1) in mid-edition—1985—a change that was incorporated in the next edition of the NEC (1987).

Bulletin 56A

The "Standard for the Use of Inhalation Anesthetics" (NFPA Bulletin 56A)[16] was from 1973 through 1984 the most widely recognized regulatory document for anesthesia personnel and the primary document used by state and local agencies regarding many aspects of anesthetic practice. The document includes requirements for the installation and maintenance of conductive floors, temperature, humidity control, air exchange, and power distribution systems in anesthetizing locations. This standard was incorporated into the first edition of "Standard for Health Care Facilities" (NFPA Bulletin 99), published in 1984.[15]

NFPA Bulletin 99-1987

NFPA standards differentiate between general and critical patient-care areas. Operating rooms are included among the critical areas. Several chapters and appendix items in the 1993 edition of NFPA 99-1993[15] are applicable to locations in which anesthetics are given and to operating rooms. These include Chapter 3, Electrical Systems, and Chapter 4, Gas and Vacuum Systems. Chapters 7, Electrical Equipment, and 12, Hospital Requirements, describe a comprehensive set of standards governing electrical safety in all patient-care areas of hospitals, including operating rooms. Topics discussed include installed power distribution and grounding systems, specifications for electrical equipment used in patient care (including leakage current requirements and grounding provisions), and administrative and testing procedures to be followed to achieve acceptable reduction of electrical risks. Although this document has not been widely codified in regulatory documents and ordinances, it has received such a wide degree of acceptance as to become de facto law and the standard of community practice.

Finally, Annex 2 in NFPA 99-1993, "Safe Use of High-frequency Electricity in Health Care Facilities," recommends practices for the use of high-frequency equipment, particularly electrosurgical devices.

State and Local Agencies

Whereas state and local municipalities' jurisdictions usually rely heavily on national codes and standards for their regulation of health care facilities, they may and often do impose requirements that go beyond national requirements. Frequently, these added requirements are apparent at the time of design and construction of an operating suite and have little effect on the day-to-day operation of the facility. State departments of labor and industry and state or municipal departments of health and related inspection authorities are usually responsible for imposing additional requirements.

Municipalities with strong local enforcement of electrical codes may be active in the inspection and use of electrical devices. Chicago is a notable example. Authorities there have been a strong force in calling for the extensive grounding of electrical equipment, metallic furniture, and nonelectrical equipment.

Regulations regarding the installation of isolated power, conductive flooring, or electrical outlets of prescribed configuration are examples of areas in which locally unique requirements may prevail. Awareness of these special considerations must be maintained, and new staff should acquaint themselves with local variations.

Independent Agencies

Several agencies, independent and governmental, contribute directly or indirectly to electrical safety in the operating room.

The Association for the Advancement of Medical Instrumentation

The Association for the Advancement of Medical Instrumentation is a voluntary, independent professional organization whose membership consists of manufacturers, clinical and biomedical engineers, and medical personnel who have a common interest in improving medical devices and the environment in which they are used. In addition to regular professional meetings and exhibits, the Association for the Advancement of Medical Instrumentation also has developed a series of voluntary consensus standards for the use of several medical devices, among them performance standards for electrocardiographs and defibrillators.

Of particular interest is their "Standard for Safe Current Limits for Electromedical Apparatus."[17] This document defines acceptable limits for leakage current from the chassis and patient-connected leads. Although it does not have the force of law, it is widely regarded as a reasonable standard, consistent with the standards of several other bodies. It serves as a guideline for manufacturers in the design and fabrication of devices, and hospitals refer to it for medical device specifications before the purchase of equipment. The Association for the Advancement of Medical Instrumentation also has developed a standard for high-frequency therapeutic devices, namely electrosurgical generators and accessories.

Independent Testing Laboratories

Underwriters Laboratories, ETL Testing Laboratories, MET Electrical Testing Company, and the Canadian Standards Association are noteworthy examples of independent testing laboratories. Each draws on various standards in the field or writes its own standards, against which voluntarily submitted devices are tested. If, in the opinion of the testing laboratory, the device meets its standard, the manufacturer is authorized to affix a label (commonly called a listing mark) of the testing laboratory on each device of the model tested. The manufacturer pays a fee for this testing. In the case of a medical device, the listing mark attests that, in the judgment of the testing laboratory, the device does not pose an undue risk with regard to fire, electrical shock, and burns. However, it does not attest to the expected performance of the device for its intended purpose nor does it imply that each listed device is inspected and meets safety requirements before it leaves the factory.

The listing mark is important to purchasers and signifies that a third party has tested the device for some practical safety aspects. In some municipalities, such as Los Angeles, a listing mark is a requirement for sale of devices within their jurisdiction. In the absence of a listing by a recognized testing laboratory, devices can be submitted to a testing laboratory operated by the city.

ECRI

ECRI, formerly known as the Emergency Care Research Institute, is an evaluation agency that performs safety and performance testing of medical devices. Its findings are available to members of its Health Devices System through its own journal, *Health Devices*. ECRI does not provide a listing or labeling service.

The Center for Devices and Radiological Health

The Center for Devices and Radiological Health, a division of the United States Food and Drug Administration, exercises some control over the safety of medical devices. Currently, they promulgate few mandatory standards but instead monitor the quality of devices and exercise regulatory control principally over manufacturers rather than users. Their mechanisms of regulation include registration of medical device producers; control of the introduction of new technologies into regular commerce; inspection for adherence to good manufacturing practices (specified by the Good Manufacturing Practices [GMP] regulations published by the agency); investigation of devices involved in incidents; and encouragement of manufacturers to conform to the existing voluntary consensus standards, largely by the threat of more agency-promulgated mandatory standards. Recently, the Food and Drug Administration has implemented a mandatory program requiring manufacturers to report information received about their products that suggest the risk of serious injury or death.[16]

Liability Insurance Companies

Not unexpectedly, hospital liability insurance carriers also actively promote safety. In this role, their influence may be felt in the operating room, because they require certain technical features and operating procedures to reduce the hospital's exposure to liability. On their inspection tours, they may question the unreasonable use of extension cords and other aspects of electrical safety. Thus, liability insurance carriers can be another good resource for safety information.

EQUIPMENT CONTROL PROGRAMS

An established equipment control program should be an important component of any hospital's efforts to ensure the highest level of patient and personnel safety. Most hospitals have one in place because it is required by JCAHO. Often, this program is centered in a clinical engineering department. Usually, members of that department also serve on the hospital's electrical safety committee, frequently with representatives from the operating room and anesthesiology staff.

All equipment placed in the hands of clinical staff, whether hospital- or physician-owned, borrowed, or rented, should be monitored by the equipment control program. In this way, the hospital can be sure that all appropriate documentation, incoming and periodic inspection, and investigation of incidents involving the device will be carried out. Also, the clinical engineering department should be given the opportunity to review requests for purchase and to participate in the formulation of purchase specifications for most devices, particularly electrically operated ones.

Inspection

An effective equipment program provides periodic inspection of all equipment on a regular basis. Equipment in the operating room usually is inspected on a quarterly to semiannual basis, with certain pieces of equipment (eg, defibrillators) inspected more frequently. Both safety and performance are likely to be tested, and inspection protocols often provide an option for major and minor inspections; the distinction is that certain aspects need not be tested as frequently as others. Thus, examination of the line cord and plug for evidence of abuse and measurement of chassis leakage current may be deemed appropriate at each inspection. However, measurement of certain performance characteristics, such as the frequency response of a cardiac monitor, may be checked only annually. Inspections must be documented, either by noting deviations from expected results (exception reporting) or by recording all data collected, and a report of significant findings should be available to hospital staff.

Operator Manuals

Every clinician should be thoroughly familiar with each device he or she uses. Equipment control programs (as required by JCAHO) must make operator manuals for all equipment readily available to all clinical users. Increasingly, manufacturers' manuals note precautions for use and recognized hazards. Clinicians must be familiar with these limitations, not only to protect themselves but also to afford the highest level of safety for their patients.

Investigation of Adverse Incidents

A thorough investigation of any adverse incident believed to be associated with the use of a device is prudent. Only in this way can repetitions be prevented. The clinical engineering department should be involved in these investigations. All devices and components, including disposable products, that are involved in the incident must be saved for the investigation.[18] All too often, a critical disposable item, such as an electrosurgical dispersive electrode, has been discarded at the conclusion of a surgical case, possibly even after an adverse effect has been noted.

Reporting of Adverse Incidents

In November 1991, the user reporting requirements of the Safe Medical Device Act were implemented.[19] This act requires that equipment-related accidents resulting in morbidity or mortality be reported to the Food and Drug Administration.

OPERATING ROOM EQUIPMENT AND SAFETY EDUCATION

As important as electrical safety is in the operating room, the demands on staff time do not facilitate regular attention to the issue, and formal periodic programs are hard to schedule with any expectation that all staff will participate. Historically, the nursing and anesthesiology staffs have been the most visible advocates for adherence to electrical-safety practices, although at times their perspectives may not have reflected sound principles. The years since 1980 have brought new focus on issues of electrical safety. Also, in that time, some concepts have been modified, and the emphasis on isolated power systems, conductive floors, and accessories has changed. Although comprehensive, periodic, formal instructional programs in electrical safety may not be possible, several things can and are being done.

Professional groups such as the Association of Operating Room Nurses[20] and the American Society of Anesthesiologists have published articles in their journals and routinely devote sessions in their national and regional meetings to these topics.[21] Clinical engineering personnel have done one-on-one teaching in fundamental principles as they go about their work in the operating suite or have been invited to present formal or informal lectures and demonstrations for small groups during in-service educational programs. Short film strips and video tapes are available for use during departmental meetings. Posters, such as the one shown in Figure 8-6, can be put on corridor walls or bulletin boards or can be placed on the back of toilet stall doors, where the captive occupant may have a few moments to read and contemplate the message. Some manufacturers, particularly those producing electrosurgical products, have excellent printed and audiovisual materials available on request.

Numerous educational approaches are available from which to choose. The important factor is to make use of any appropriate resources so that staff members recognize an institutional commitment to promoting electrical safety; personnel are also encouraged to make a personal commitment. Increases in awareness and understanding permit the beneficial application of electricity in patient care while minimizing or eliminating the adverse effects.

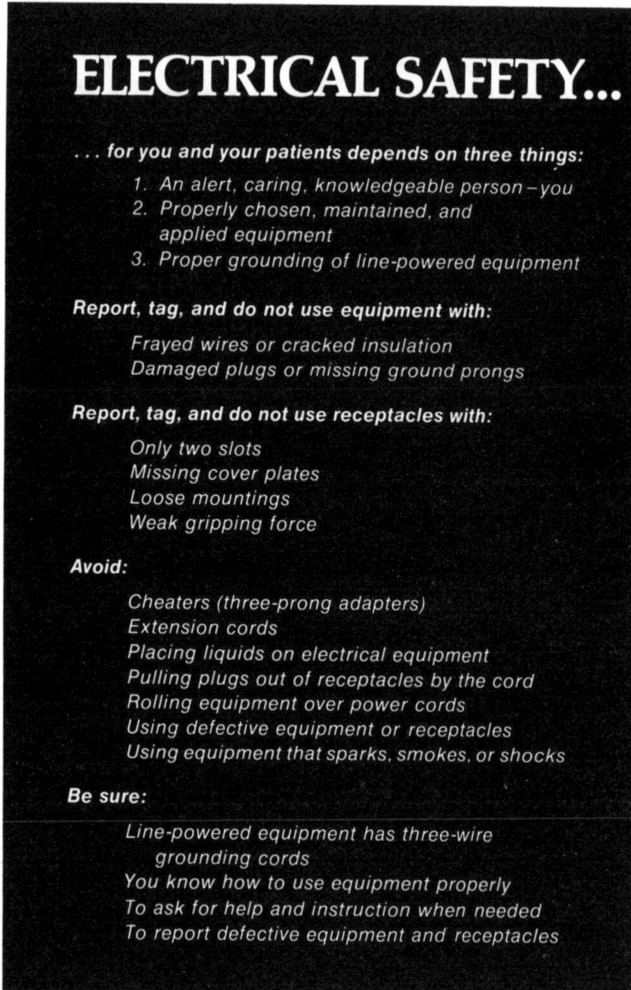

FIGURE 8-6. A poster promoting electrical safety. (Courtesy of ECRI, Plymouth Meeting, PA.)

REFERENCES

1. Geddes LA, Baker LE: The specific resistance of biological material: a compendium of data for the biomedical engineer and physiologists. Med Biol Eng 5:271, 1967
2. Dalziel CF: Deleterious effects of electric shock. In Steere NV (ed): Handbook of laboratory safety. 2nd ed. Cleveland: Chemical Rubber Company, 1971: 521
3. Katcher ML, Shapiro MM: Severe burns and death associated with electronic monitors (letter). New Engl J Med 317:56, 1987
4. Fineberg HV, Pearlman LA, Gabel RA: The case for abandonment of explosive anesthetic agents. N Engl J Med 303:613, 1980
5. Ridgway MG: Hospital environmental safety and the safety codes. Journal of Clinical Engineering 2:211, 1977
6. Leeming MN, Ray C, Howland WS: Low-voltage, direct-current burns. JAMA 214:1681, 1970
7. Scott RN, Paasche PE: Safety considerations in clinical engineering. Critical Reviews in Biomedical Engineering 13:201, 1986
8. Starmer CF, Whalen RE, McIntosh HD: Hazards of electric shock in cardiology. Am J Cardiol 14:537, 1964
9. Roy OZ, Scott JR, Park GC: 60 Hz ventricular fibrillation and pump failure thresholds versus electrode area. IEEE Trans Biomed Eng 23:45, 1976
10. Becker CM, Malhotra IV, Hedley-White J: The distribution of radio-frequency current and burns. Anesthesiology 38:106, 1973
11. Pearce JA, Geddes LA, VanVleet JF, et al: Skin burns from electrosurgical current. Medical Instrumentation 17:225, 1983
12. Orpin JA: Unexpected burns under skin electrodes. Can Med Assoc J 127:1106, 1982

13. JCAHO: 1995 Accreditation Manual for Hospitals. Vol. I: Standards. Oakbrook Terrace, IL, 1994
14. National Fire Protection Association: National electrical code, 1993 ed. Bulletin 70. Quincy, MA: National Fire Protection Association, 1984
15. National Fire Protection Association: Standard for health care facilities. Bulletin 99-1993. Quincy, MA: National Fire Protection Association, 1993
16. National Fire Protection Association: Standard for the use of inhalation anesthetics. Bulletin 56A. Quincy, MA: National Fire Protection Association, 1978
17. Association for the Advancement of Medical Instrumentation: American National Standard Safe Current Limits for Electromedical Apparatus. 3rd ed. ANSI/AAMI ES 1-1993. Arlington, VA, 1993
18. Spooner RB, Kirby RR: Equipment-related anesthetic mishaps. In Pierce EC Jr, Cooper JF (eds): Analysis of anesthetic mishaps. Int Anesthesiol Clin 22(2):133, 1984
19. Safe Medical Device Act (SMDA) of 1990. 1990 PL 101-629
20. Association of Operating Room Nurses, Inc. 1994 Standards and Recommended Practices. Denver, CO, 1994
21. Bruner JM: Electrical safety in the operating room. In ASA Refresher Course Lectures. Park Ridge, IL: American Society of Anesthesiologists, 1988: 11

FURTHER READING

Buczko GB, McKay WPS: Electrical safety in the operating room. Can J Anaesth 34:315, 1987

Pearce JA (ed): Electrosurgery. London, Chapman & Hall, 1986

Bruner JMR, Leonard PF: Electrical safety and the patient. Chicago: Year Book Medical Publishers, 1989

Health Devices. Plymouth Meeting, PA: ECRI, 1971–1995, Volumes 1–25. Monthly publication devoted exclusively to medical devices, safety standards, regulations, etc.

Horrow JC: Electrical safety. In: Kirby RR, Gravenstein N (eds): Clinical anesthesia practice. Philadelphia: EB Saunders, 1994: 885

Horrow JC, Seitman DT: Electrical safety and device calibration. Anesthesiol Clin North Am 6:699, 1988

Complications in Anesthesiology, second edition,
edited by Nikolaus Gravenstein and Robert R. Kirby.
Lippincott-Raven Publishers, Philadelphia © 1996.

CHAPTER 9

Complications of Invasive Cardiovascular Monitoring

Robert F. Bedford

Direct invasive vascular pressure monitoring is common in anesthesia practice. A poll of anesthesiologists inquiring as to the most valuable modalities in their armamentarium no doubt would show accurate blood pressure monitoring to be at or near the top of the list. Close behind would be monitoring of the central venous and pulmonary artery circulation. Nevertheless, despite the value of the information drawn from such technology, complications, many severe and some life threatening, occur and are the subject of this chapter.

ARTERIAL CATHETERS

Thromboembolic Phenomena

Radial Artery

The most feared complications of arterial cannulation are those related to thromboembolic phenomena induced by an indwelling catheter. The radial artery is the most popular site for arterial cannulation, as much because of the ease of determining collateral blood supply to the hand as because of the relative simplicity of cannulating the vessel. Although ischemic necrosis of the hand may occur spontaneously in patients who have sustained emboli from the heart,[1] the incidence of extremity necrosis related to uncomplicated radial artery cannulation (Fig. 9-1) is possibly as low as 0.01%.[2–6] Most of the reported cases are complicated by low-flow states due to hypovolemia or infusion of α-adrenergic agents,[7–13] situations in which distal vascular insufficiency may also occur in the absence of an arterial catheter.

COLLATERAL CIRCULATION. Because radial arterial cannulation may cause an immediate decrease in blood flow even without thrombus formation,[14] prior documentation of collateral flow to the hand seems prudent. Although not a foolproof guarantee against distal ischemic events, Allen's test[15] is widely recommended because it is simple to perform and because approximately 5% of patients have incomplete palmar arterial anastomoses between the radial and ulnar arteries.[16,17] Allen did not specify how rapidly a "return to color" should occur after release of digital pressure over the ulnar artery after hand exsanguination, but my experience is that 15 seconds is too long (resulting in a 10% incidence of cold white digits), whereas 5 seconds appears to be satisfactory.[18,19]

Because of the difficulty in interpreting Allen's test in unconscious or uncooperative patients, other measures of collateral circulation have been advocated, such as occlusion of the radial artery with digital pressure followed by detection of retrograde distal flow with a Doppler probe.[20] A pulse oximeter may give a qualitative assessment of pulsatile flow at the thumb while each vessel is occluded.[21] I attempt to feel a retrograde pulse from the palmar arches; if this pulse is absent, I move to the opposite hand or another artery. If collateral circulation to the hand is satisfactory bilaterally, cannulation of the nondominant hand seems reasonable when possible in case some untoward event occurs.

THROMBUS FORMATION. Radial artery cannulation predictably induces thrombosis, the incidence of which correlates with the duration of cannulation (Fig. 9-2)[18,22–25] and the percentage of the vessel lumen occupied by the catheter (Fig. 9-3).[19] Thus, women, who generally have smaller arteries than men,[19,26] also have a higher incidence of arterial occlusion associated with cannulation.[10,18,27,28] Weiss and Gattiker have postulated that the critical wrist circumference for a 20-G catheter is 15 cm; they recommend that for smaller wrists and therefore also smaller radial arteries a smaller-gauge catheter be used.[29] The plastic from which the catheter is manufactured also affects the incidence of thrombus formation; polytetrafluorethylene (Teflon) catheters induce signif-

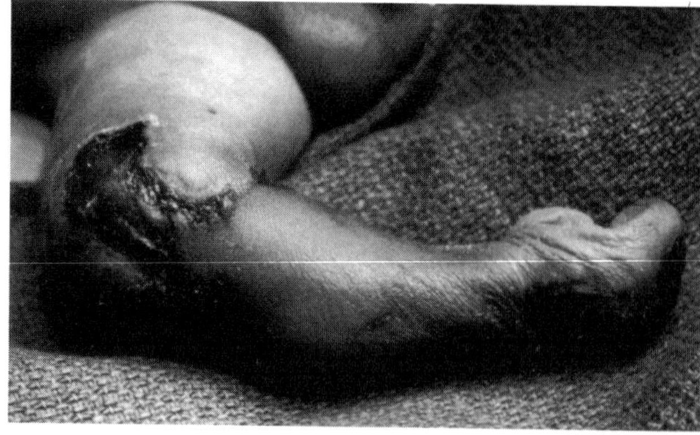

FIGURE 9-1. Necrosis of hand and forearm after radial artery cannulation in a child with Reye's syndrome.

icantly fewer thrombi than those made of polypropylene, polyvinylchloride, or polyethylene.[10,27,30,31] Factors of importance are listed in Table 9-1.

Considerable controversy surrounds the correlation between traumatic cannulation techniques and the likelihood of subsequent vascular compromise. A surgical cutdown significantly increases the risk of arterial occlusion,[10,12] and some investigators believe that multiple attempts at cannulation are responsible for a higher incidence of ischemic complications.[13,32,33] Others, however, have found no evidence to support traumatic cannulation as an etiologic factor in causing subsequent vascular occlusion.[18,27,34,35]

FLUSHING. Heparinized saline flush solution is required not only to maintain catheter patency, but also to prevent thrombosis of the radial artery while the catheter is in place.[36] Embolization of thrombotic material to the hand[37] or to the central circulation[38] has been reported with intermittent flushing of radial artery cannulas, whereas use of continuous-infusion flush devices reduces both the hazard of embolization and the incidence of radial artery thrombosis.[39] Because of the risk of retrograde embolization of clot to the cerebral circulation with as little as a 3-mL hand-injection of flush solution, radial artery cannulas should be flushed slowly and with small volumes (1 to 3 mL) of solution.[38] The risk of retrograde embolization to the central nervous system is greatest for catheters placed in the right arm and proximally (ie, brachial,

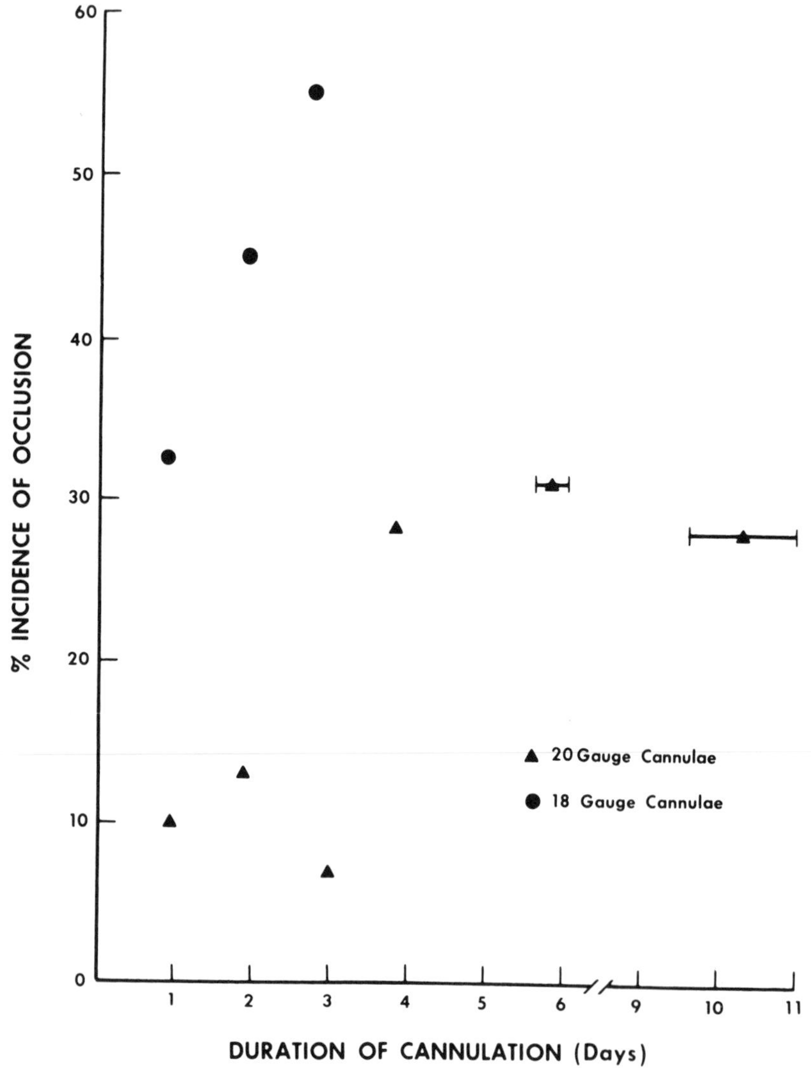

FIGURE 9-2. The incidence of radial arterial thrombosis tends to increase with greater duration of cannulation with both 18- and 20-G catheters. Unlike 18-G devices, the 20-G catheters retain a reasonably low incidence of arterial occlusion for the first 3 days after catheter insertion. (Bedford RF: Long-term radial artery cannulation: effects on subsequent vessel function. Crit Care Med 6:64, 1978.)

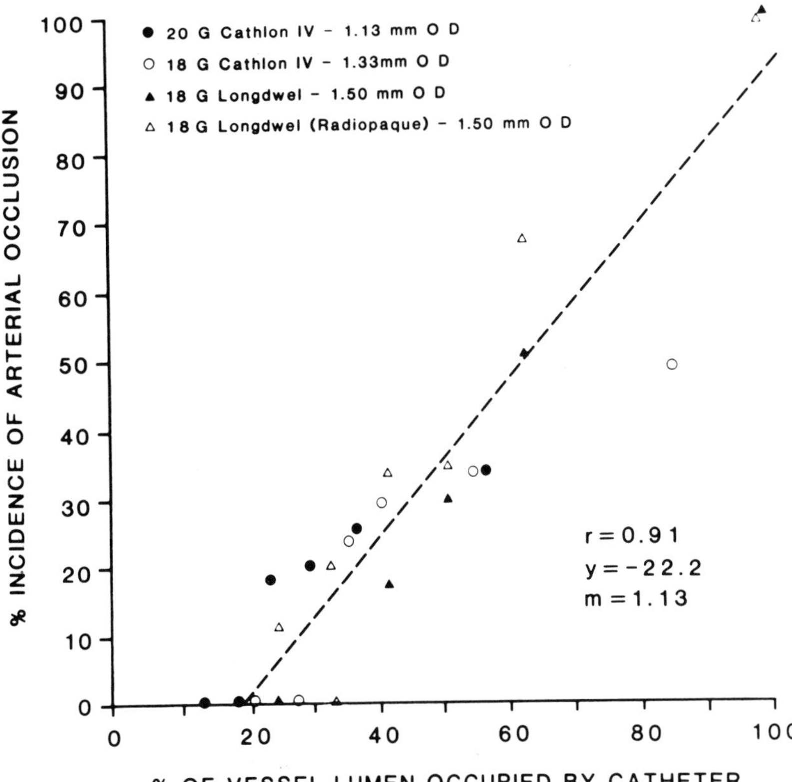

FIGURE 9-3. Radial artery thrombosis after 24 h of cannulation. The incidence of arterial occlusion increases linearly as more of the vessel lumen is occupied by the cannula. Small cannulas in large vessels generate very few occlusive lesions, whereas large cannulas almost always cause occlusion of small arteries. *IV*, intravenous; *OD*, outer diameter. *Cathlon:* Jelco Laboratories, Raritan, NJ 08869; *Longdwel:* Becton Dickinson, Rutherford, NJ 07070. (Bedford RF: Radial arterial function following percutaneous cannulation with 18- and 20-gauge catheters. Anesthesiology 47: 39, 1977.)

axillary, or temporal arteries). Right-sided catheters pose a higher risk because an air embolus or thromboembolus must traverse the origin of the carotid and vertebral arteries before reaching the descending thoracic aorta.

SKIN ISCHEMIA. Whereas ischemia of the hand is one of the most feared thromboembolic phenomena associated with radial artery cannulation, ischemia of the skin overlying the cannula is probably the most common form of morbidity associated with this procedure. Originally described as an incidental complication,[18,24,40] volar skin necrosis has been found in 0.5% to 3% of all radial artery cannulations,[41,42] and 10% of all thrombosed radial arteries.[22] Angiographic and postmortem studies have shown occlusion of the small cutaneous perforating branches of the radial artery supplying the skin over the cannula-induced thrombus.

TABLE 9-1
Factors Associated With Increased Incidence of Cannulation-related Arterial Thrombosis

- Cannulation >20 h
- Polyethylene rather than polytetrafluorethylene (Teflon) catheters
- Intermittent rather than continuous irrigation
- 18-G rather than 20-G catheters
- Female gender
- Tapered rather than straight catheters
- Abnormal results on Allen's test

Gravenstein N: Invasive vascular monitoring. In Gravenstein N (ed): Manual of complications during anesthesia. Philadelphia: JB Lippincott, 1991: 256.

Johnson suggested that patients who developed intense skin blanching over the catheter when flush solution was injected were particularly prone to develop this complication.[40] Although he believed it was the flush solution that caused the damage, such blanching may represent absent blood flow past the catheter, thus indicating a high probability that the vessel will occlude. The incidence of this complication is decreased with smaller-gauge catheters, presumably because they induce fewer arterial occlusions.[41]

MANAGEMENT. Cannula-induced radial artery thrombi recanalize with time, but Kim and coworkers[27] noted that the average duration of occlusion was 13 days; in my experience, some vessels have required as long as 75 days to reestablish flow.[18] Recanalization, then, cannot be relied upon to acutely reestablish flow distal to an occluded radial artery. If a patient shows evidence of distal vascular ischemia while a radial artery catheter is in place, an attempt should be made to remove the catheter and the offending thrombus. Occasionally this can be done simply by aspirating with a syringe through the catheter while it is withdrawn from the artery[43] (Fig. 9-4). After a catheter has been removed, however, thrombus removal requires a surgical cut-down on the artery and use of a 3-French embolectomy catheter to clear the vessel of clot.[32]

Ulnar Artery

The ulnar artery has been suggested as an alternate site for monitoring,[14,17,27] particularly because Husum and Palm[17]

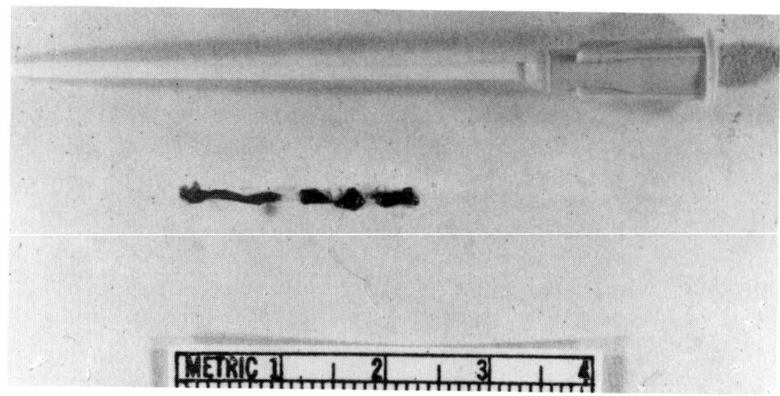

FIGURE 9-4. Specimen of thrombotic material successfully aspirated from a radial artery during decannulation. Arteriography demonstrated complete occlusion of the lumen by thrombus and catheter, yet vessel function was normal after decannulation. Scale in centimeters. (Bedford RF: Removal of radial artery thrombi following percutaneous cannulation for monitoring. Anesthesiology 46:431, 1977.)

found the ulnar artery was dominant in only 12% of 200 hands examined. Accordingly, ulnar artery occlusion might be less likely to cause hand ischemia. Although the nondominant vessel should be cannulated when possible, it may be so small or tortuous as to be not suitable. An additional consideration is that the ulnar artery, unlike the radial artery, is adjacent to a nerve (ulnar nerve) at the wrist and thus ulnar artery cannulation probably increases the risk of nerve injury by either direct injury or compression from a hematoma.

Brachial Artery

Brachial artery cannulation offers the advantage of a larger vessel that is less subject to the systolic pressure augmentation seen with more peripheral arterial sites. An abundance of collateral vessels usually is present about the elbow so that occluded brachial arteries rarely induce distal vascular ischemia[43]; thousands of brachial arterial cannulations have been performed safely.[33,44,45] Just as is the case in radial artery monitoring, the longer a brachial catheter remains in place, the higher the incidence of complications.

Comstock and colleagues[46] found a 41% incidence of brachial artery occlusion in 29 patients, with three radial and five ulnar occlusions, respectively, despite the use of only 20-G catheters. They concluded that radial artery cannulation caused fewer vascular lesions than brachial artery cannulation. This observation may be related to the fact that the elbow joint is more difficult to immobilize in a conscious patient than the wrist joint, with consequent catheter-induced trauma to the intima of the brachial artery.

Axillary Artery

The axillary artery is relatively large and has a low reported incidence of thrombotic complications.[47,48] The large size of the axillary artery makes thrombosis relatively unlikely, and its proximity to the aortic arch makes it easier to cannulate than more peripheral arteries during hypotensive states. This relation demands meticulous attention to avoid intraarterial injection of clot or air bubbles that could embolize to the cerebral circulation during catheter flushing. For this reason, the left axillary artery is preferred to the right side, because a catheter in the latter may have its tip in the brachiocephalic artery.

More common than thrombotic complications are neurovascular injuries due to extravasation of blood from the axillary artery into the surrounding neurovascular sheath. Clearly, the smallest feasible catheter (usually a 20-G pediatric central venous pressure [CVP] catheter) and an atraumatic cannulation technique will minimize extravasation, subsequent hematoma formation, and possible neural compromise.

Dorsalis Pedis Artery

The dorsalis pedis artery may be useful for monitoring when the upper extremities are unavailable because of trauma, previous cannulations or burns. Because it is relatively small, the vessel is subject to an 8% to 25% incidence of thrombotic occlusion,[49,50] that may result in ischemic damage to the toes and foot.[3,49] Husum and colleagues[50] found a 21% incidence of impaired perfusion to the great toe (systolic pressure <40 mm Hg) with compression of the dorsalis pedis artery. Collateral circulation probably should be documented before cannulation to avoid ischemic complications.

One method for doing so consists of occluding both the dorsalis pedis and posterior tibial pulses with digital pressure, then blanching the patient's great toe with direct pressure. If the toe color does not return to normal within 5 seconds when the posterior tibial artery pressure is released, another site should be selected for cannulation.[51]

Anterior Peroneal Artery

The anterior peroneal artery, just proximal to the lateral malleolus also can be used. It is a small vessel that may not be palpable in 12% of patients and is "less than prominent" in 43%. In experienced hands, however, Moorthy found it could be cannulated successfully 9 of 11 times.[52]

Femoral Artery

The femoral artery is controversial for arterial cannulation. When it is used for arteriographic studies, a high incidence of occlusive lesions and pseudoaneurysm formation occurs requiring surgical intervention to prevent distal vascular ischemia.[43,53] When it is used only for cardiovascular monitoring, however, the femoral artery appears to be remarkably free of major complications.[54,55] However, it is prone to develop atherosclerotic lesions that sometimes make cannulation difficult, promote vascular occlusion, or break off and embolize distally.

The incidence of ischemic events requiring embolectomy after femoral artery cannulation appears to be about 0.5%,[56–58] whereas transient, self-limited, vascular insufficiency develops in another 0.5%.[54,56,59] Catheter size in these studies ranged from 14- to 20-G with no clear difference in the incidence of ischemic lesions. This finding suggests that atheromata may be a more important factor in thrombosis during femoral artery cannulation than is the case with other peripheral arteries.

Infectious Complications

Local

Arterial monitoring catheters can be sources for both local and systemic infections, particularly when cardiovascular monitoring is required for more than just a few days. *Staphylococcus epidermidis* is the usual organism causing local infections at the cannulation site after several days of continuous monitoring.[22] Pinella and coworkers[60] found the rate of local infection to be 0% with only 1 day of cannulation; it increased to 14% when catheters were left in place between 5 and 7 days.[60] Another study of 536 patients found a 4% incidence of positive cultures with catheters left in place for an average of 6 days.[11] A surgical cutdown to the artery markedly increases the risk of local infection, however, with a 30% to 39% incidence reported when cannulation lasts longer than 4 days.[12,61]

TOPICAL ANTIBIOTIC AGENTS. The subject of topical antibiotic use to control local infection has received considerable attention, with few definitive answers. Iodophor and triple-antibiotic (polymyxin, bacitracin, and neomycin) ointments have been shown to reduce local infection rates from 6.5% in untreated patients to 3.6% and 2.2%, respectively.[62] Most infections occurring with iodophor ointment were relatively benign staphylococcal species, however, whereas infections with triple-antibiotic ointment tended to be from gram-negative pathogens. The recommendation from this study was to use iodophor ointment on intravascular cannulation sites.[62]

Systemic

Systemic infection is also a potential hazard of indwelling arterial catheters, usually as a result of bacteria entering through a nonsterile stopcock, but occasionally as a sequela to nonsterile techniques. An outbreak of *Serratia marscesens* in one intensive care unit was traced to a contaminated stock of heparinized saline flush solution,[63] and an epidemic of *flavobacterium* was caused by precooling sampling syringes in a contaminated ice machine.[64]

Bacteria may be transferred from the surface of a contaminated pressure-transducer diaphragm to the patient via a stopcock (Fig. 9-5) when disposable domes are attached.[65,66] One report[67] showed that 16% of flush solution line stopcocks became contaminated with arterial cannulation lasting 25 to 439 hours. Maki and Hassemer[68] found an 11% incidence of contaminated disposable transducers during long-term monitoring and proposed that all flush systems be changed every 48 hours.

Patients with infectious processes may contaminate their arterial catheters, which, in turn, act as a nidus for continued infection. Five of 37 patients in one intensive care unit had arterial catheters that grew out bacteria identical to the organisms infecting the patients.[69] Gas gangrene induced by *Clostridium* species[70]; sepsis caused by *Proteus mirabilis*; and *Staphylococcus aureus* arteritis with Osler's node, Janeway lesions, and splinter hemorrhages[71] have been reported as complications of infected catheter-induced arterial thrombi.

Recommendations to reduce infectious complications of arterial cannulation are shown in Table 9-2.[69]

Intraarterial Injection of Noxious Substances

The grave complications resulting from intraarterial injection of thiopental are well known to anesthesiologists; thiamylal likewise produces distal tissue necrosis when it is injected accidentally through an arterial catheter.[72] Similarly, injection of ketamine in the dorsalis pedis artery resulted in severe skin necrosis extending proximally over the anterior and lateral leg and foot.[73] The catheter probably was occluding the arterial lumen, forcing the ketamine retrograde before it entered the microvasculature. The lesion required 5 weeks to heal.

More serious retrograde injection may occur if thrombotic material is embolized from a peripheral arterial catheter into the central and cerebral circulations, causing distal vascular or cerebral ischemia.[37,38] Thus, not only should indwelling arterial catheters injections occur slowly and carefully, but also arterial stopcocks should be labeled clearly so no one mistakes them for an intravenous access site.

Problems of Pressure Data Interpretation

Etiology of Misinterpretation

Many clinicians believe that intraarterial pressure monitoring is the "gold standard" for accuracy of blood pressure measurement. The truth is that it is fraught with a variety of potential inaccuracies that may endanger patient well-being if the clinician does nothing to assure the validity of the displayed data. Constant repetition in the form of blinking diodes does not confer accuracy; the prudent physician should be alert to the possible sources of error that might lead to mismanagement. In short, "A needle in an artery does not guarantee a pressure or accuracy any more than an endotracheal tube guarantees a patent airway."*

More than a few clinicians hope that a small arterial catheter placed in a peripheral artery not only reveals accurate systolic, mean and diastolic pressures, but also provides a representation of stroke volume from computation of the area under the pulse-pressure curve; an estimate of myocardial contractility from the systolic upstroke; and a reflection of peripheral vascular resistance from the position of the dicrotic notch,

---

* N. Ty Smith: Guest discussion at the 46th Congress of the International Anesthesia Research Society. Anesth Analg 51:756, 1972.

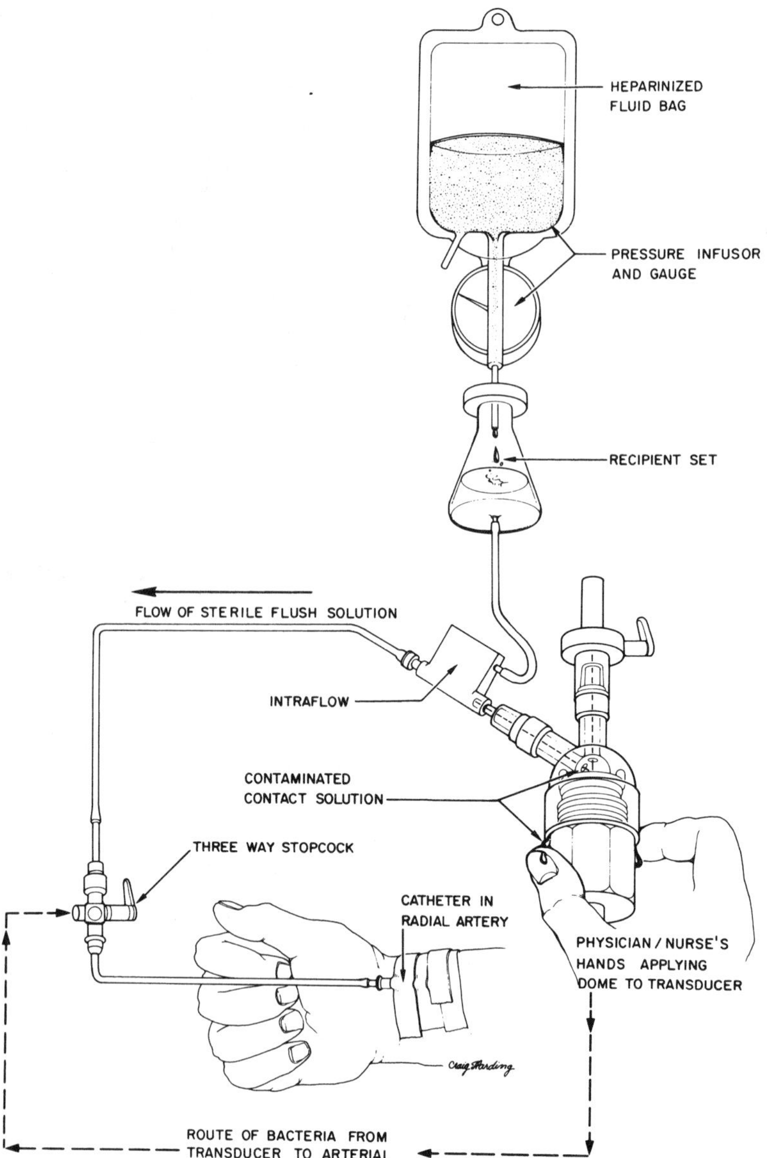

FIGURE 9-5. Route of transfer of bacteria from a nonsterile pressure transducer into a prepackaged sterile disposable plumbing system. (Bedford RF: Invasive blood pressure monitoring. In Blitt CD (ed): Monitoring in anesthesia and critical care medicine. New York: Churchill Livingstone, 1985:48.)

slope of the diastolic pressure runoff, or both. Whereas these parameters can be estimated accurately from a microtransducer placed in the aortic arch, the only parameter that can be determined reliably from a peripheral arterial cannula is the mean arterial pressure. The arterial pulse-pressure wave undergoes a series of transformations as it progresses from the arch of the aorta out into the more distal arterial tree where blood pressure is determined clinically (Fig. 9-6).

Determinants of Aortic Root Pulse Pressure

As blood is ejected from the left ventricle into the aortic root, the upper aorta functions as a "fixed-capacity, high-pressure reservoir"[6] that expands to produce a higher pressure than would occur if the entire aorta distended uniformly. The rounded aortic root pulse-pressure wave is the result of three phenomena: (1) the volume ejected by the left ventricle, (2) the distention of the aorta, and (3) the runoff of blood into the branches of the aorta. Aortic blood flow is not a function of the aortic pressure wave but, in fact, is the result of aortic elastic recoil after ventricular ejection. Thus, blood flow is much slower than the pulse-pressure wave (0.5 vs 10 m/s)[74]; the dorsalis pedis artery receives the pulse pressure wave even before ventricular systole is completed. A pulse-pressure wave observed in the periphery has relatively little to do with the stroke volume generated by the left ventricle; reliance upon the area under the curve of a peripheral pulse pressure wave may lead to serious errors in estimating ventricular performance.

Waveform Transition

As the pulse-pressure wave is transmitted away from the aortic root, it becomes narrowed, with a progressive increase in the

TABLE 9-2
Methods to Reduce Infectious Complications of Arterial Catheterization

- Use sterile gloves during cannulation
- Use iodine disinfectant and sterile drapes
- If possible, use a percutaneous cannulation technique
- Use iodophor ointment on cannulation site
- Keep stopcocks capped
- Inspect puncture site daily
- Discontinue catheter if
  - a. Local discoloration, pain, or pus develops
  - b. The patient becomes septic (culture the catheter)
  - c. The duration of cannulation exceeds 3 days

systolic pressure and decrement in the diastolic pressure. Realization of what is happening is critical, because most arterial pressure monitoring is done at peripheral sites where this phenomenon has its most profound effect.

SYSTOLIC AMPLIFICATION. The increase in pulse-pressure width is due partially to progressive tapering of vessel diameter as blood passes toward the periphery, amplifying the waveform much as a tapering ear trumpet amplifies sound waves. In addition, the walls of the more peripheral vessels have fewer elastic fibers and more muscle, resulting in less intravascular compliance and more pressure change per unit of volume change. The high-frequency early systolic components of the arterial pressure wave tend to travel faster than the later low-frequency components, such that they tend to summate into a higher systolic pressure peak. Finally, augmentation of the systolic component is due to reflection of the arterial pressure wave from both branch-points and from the main point of vascular impedance, the artery–arteriole junction.[6] This factor is particularly crucial when radial and dorsalis pedis arterial catheters are used, because the site of reflection is so close to the catheter tip that systolic augmentation is inevitable. The radial artery has been shown repeatedly to have higher systolic pressure values than the brachial artery for this reason.[6] Alternatively, when arterial vasodilators are used, a profound reduction in systolic pressure may be observed as the impedance at the artery–arteriole junction is reduced, and the pulse pressure wave is transmitted more peripherally instead of being reflected back to the arterial catheter.

In summary, remember that although the mean arterial pressure value determined from a peripheral arterial cannula may accurately indicate what is taking place in the aortic root, the same cannot be said for the systolic or diastolic value and derived parameters such as rate–pressure product.

Artifactual Changes

Artifactual changes in the blood pressure reading are caused by the plumbing devices that typically connect the peripheral arterial cannula with an external pressure transducer.

FREQUENCY RESPONSE. Modern pressure transducers are precision electronic instruments capable of responding to rapidly changing pressure values at rates in excess of 100

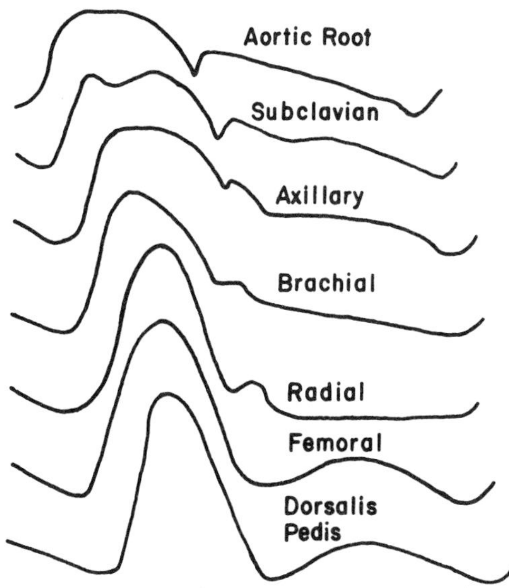

FIGURE 9-6. Transformation of the arterial pulse pressure wave as it travels from the aortic root to the sites commonly used for clinical arterial pressure monitoring. (Bedford RF: Invasive blood pressure monitoring. In Blitt CD (ed): Monitoring in anesthesia and critical care medicine. New York: Churchill Livingstone, 1985:50.)

cycles per second (hertz [Hz]). When plastic domes, extension tubes, stopcocks and flush devices are interfaced between the pressure transducer and the cannulated artery, however, the frequency response of the transducer-flush system is lowered to values similar to those seen in the arterial pulse-pressure wave.

The brachial artery pulse-pressure wave has peak frequencies of 15 to 19 Hz, whereas those of the radial and dorsalis pedis arteries probably are higher because of the sharper upstroke of the systolic pressure wave at these sites. Only 15.2 cm (6 inches) of extension tubing lower the frequency response of a transducer (Statham P50, Gould, Oxnard, CA) to 33 Hz; 1.5 m (5 feet) of tubing lower it to 6.45 Hz.[75]

RESONANCE. As the natural frequency of the monitoring system approaches the frequencies found in the arterial tree, the system begins to resonate, much as a diving board resonates when one repetitively jumps upon it. The result is a further amplification of the frequencies in the arterial pulse-pressure wave that tend to have the highest values, that is, the systolic component. A 16.3% systolic overshoot occurs in the brachial artery and even higher systolic artifact in the radial artery.[75] Shinozaki and colleagues[76] found a 7.2% systolic augmentation occurs with 0.9 m (3 feet) of extension tubing and a 31.3% systolic error with 2.4 m (8 feet) of tubing added.[76]

The natural frequency (fn) at which a catheter-tubing system begins to oscillate harmonically is given by the formula:

$$fn = \frac{1}{2}\pi \frac{\pi D^2}{4pL} \times \frac{dP}{dV}$$

where dP/dV = compliance; D = diameter; L = length; and p = density of the flush solution.

To maximize the natural frequency of the monitoring sys-

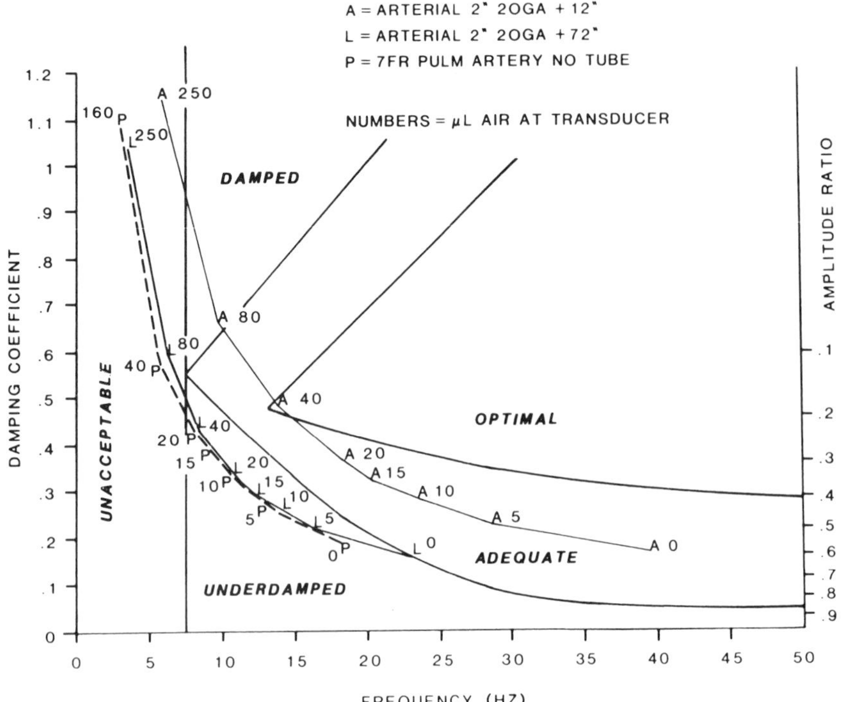

FIGURE 9-7. Natural frequency versus damping coefficient for two arterial and one pulmonary artery pressure monitoring system shows the effect of inserting small bubbles into the transducer dome. Results are presented for 2-inch radial artery catheters with 12 inches (*A*) and 72 inches (*L*) of pressure tubing. The pulmonary artery catheter results (*P*) are without extension tubing. For all situations, the operating point moves up and to the left with the addition of air into the system. (Gardner RM: System concepts for invasive pressure monitoring. In Civetta JM, Taylor RW, Kirby RR (eds): Critical care. Philadelphia: JB Lippincott, 1988:308.)

tem, and thus prevent it from "ringing," extension tubing should be as short as possible. Because compliance also should be minimal, all air bubbles must be eliminated from the system and very stiff tubing used. Air bubbles increase damping and thus appear to reduce ringing, but they also lower the natural frequency of the system and thus contribute to systolic pressure augmentation.

DAMPING. In contrast to resonance, damping is the tendency of a waveform to die down. A critically damped system (damping coefficient [β] = 1.0) displays a slowly oscillating mean pressure waveform. Optimal damping usually occurs at about β = 0.6 to 0.7; here, a waveform is reproduced accurately, yet with minimal overshoot. Unfortunately, most monitoring systems have a β of only 0.2. At β = 0.2, a system can reliably measure rapidly fluctuating pressures only up to one fifth of its natural frequency. Thus a system with a natural frequency of 30 Hz will begin to show systolic augmentation at frequencies above 6 Hz, the same as those found in the arterial tree. Again, the result is systolic overshoot and inaccuracy, both in pressure measurement and in the derived hemodynamic parameters that are calculated from systolic pressure.

Occasionally a clinician may be tempted to add air bubbles to the extension tubing or to the dome of the pressure transducer in an attempt to increase β and produce a more "socially acceptable" arterial pressure waveform (Fig. 9-7). However, the addition of only 0.05 to 0.25 mL of air to an arterial monitoring system raises the systolic pressure from 150 to 190 mm Hg, even though the diastolic and mean pressures are nearly unchanged.[76]

The guidelines to obtain accurate direct blood pressure measurements are listed in Table 9-3.

CONTINUOUS-INFUSION DEVICES. Continuous-infusion devices help to avoid complications such as damping by or distal embolization of thrombi that otherwise accumulate in the catheter tip[19,37,39] and also serve as a simple device to check the resonance and damping characteristics of an arterial pressure monitoring system (Figs. 9-8 and 9-9). Sudden pressure transients caused by a rapid-flush of a continuous-infusion device can be analyzed easily with conventional clinical recording paper, and otherwise unsuspected errors in pressure measurement can be minimized.

DISPOSABLE PLASTIC DOMES. Disposable plastic domes that cover pressure transducer membranes with a thin plastic diaphragm introduce their own peculiar opportunities for data misinterpretation. Probably the most obvious of these occurs when the dome is not seated tightly and becomes slightly dislodged during normal activities, resulting in an apparent sudden decrement in blood pressure even though the pulse-pressure configuration remains normal. This effect is similar to the decrement in pressure that occurs if the operating room table is suddenly lowered while the transducer remains affixed to its mounting pole.

TABLE 9-3
Guidelines to Enhance Accurate Direct Actual Pressure Monitoring

- Use as short and stiff an extension tube as possible
- Eliminate all air bubbles from the system
- Cannulate more central rather than peripheral arteries
- Use a continuous flush device to infuse heparinized saline

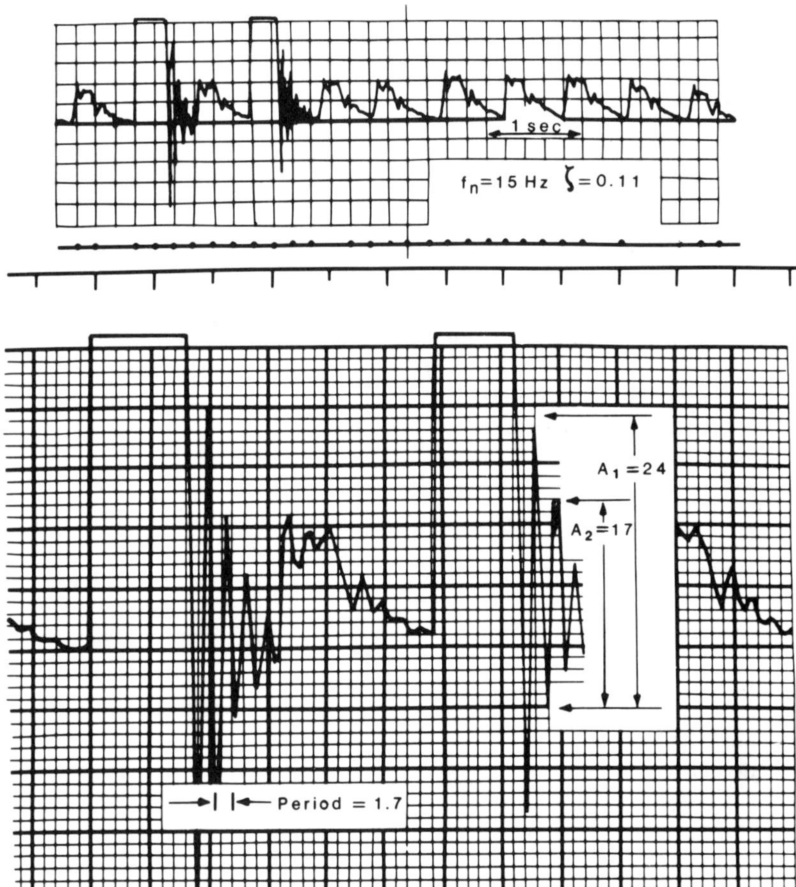

FIGURE 9-8. (*Top*) An arterial pulse waveform with two flushes. The natural frequency and damping coefficient can be determined from either flush. (*Bottom*) The flush segment enlarged to illustrate the method. The natural frequency (f_n) of the system is estimated by dividing period of one cycle (period)—in this case 1.7 mm—into the paper speed, 25 mm/s: $f_n = 25/1.7 = 15$ Hz. The damping coefficient is determined by taking the ratio of the amplitudes (A_1 and A_2) of successive peaks of the oscillations, in this case $A_2/A_1 = 17/24 = 0.71$. Then, by using the scale on Figure 9-9, the damping coefficient can be determined, in this case 0.11. A damping coefficient (ζ) less than 0.8 is usually adequate. (Legend modified from Gardner RM: Direct blood pressure measurements: dynamic response requirements. Anesthesiology 54:233, 1981.)

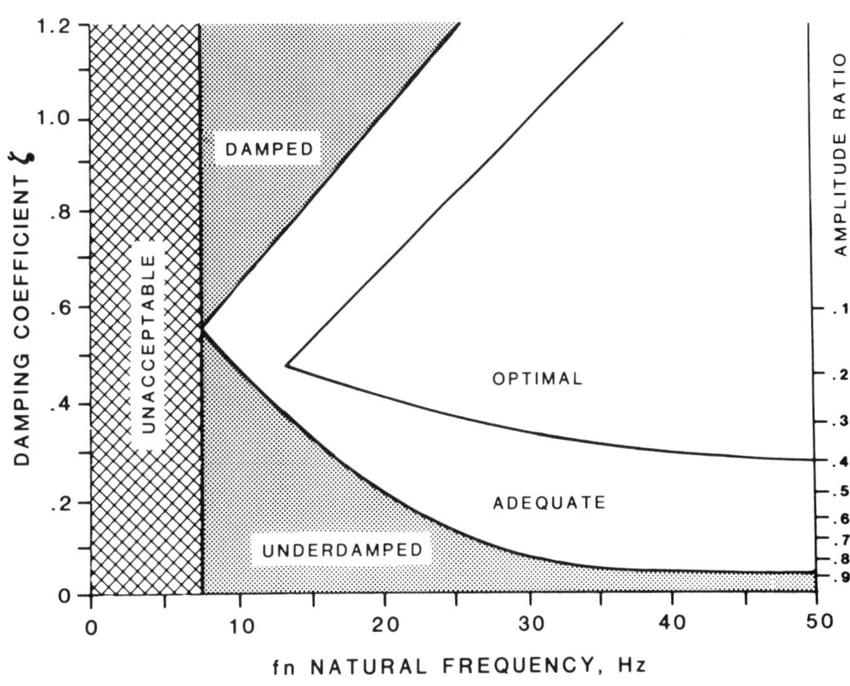

FIGURE 9-9. Frequency versus damping coefficient plot illustrating the five areas into which catheter tubing–transducer systems fall. Systems in the optimal area reproduce even the most demanding (fast heart rate and rapid systole upstroke) waveforms without distortion. Systems in the adequate area reproduce most typical patient waveforms with little or no distortion. All other areas cause serious and clinically important waveform distortion. (Gardner RM, Hollingsworth KW: Optimizing the electrocardiogram and pressure monitoring. Crit Care Med 14:656, 1986.)

Other sources of error occur if the contact solution is placed improperly between the membrane of the dome and the pressure-sensitive diaphragm of the transducer. Although properly applied contact solution allows a transducer to operate with only a 1% to 5% error, an insufficient amount of solution can lower the frequency response of a system by as much as 40%. If the dome is abruptly screwed onto the transducer with excess contact solution, a high pressure head can be generated. This artifact, in turn, is eliminated electronically when the transducer is "zeroed" or balanced to atmospheric pressure. Subsequently, the high pressure between the diaphragm and the membrane gradually escapes, producing a slow negative drift in pressure readings.[77]

This source of error is even more serious when one is attempting to interpret right atrial or pulmonary arterial pressure measurements. This problem can be avoided by electronically balancing the transducer to zero before the dome is applied. Then, if a positive pressure value appears after application of the dome, the dome should be alternately released and snugged until a value close to zero is achieved.

ELECTRONIC VERSUS STATIC CALIBRATION. Because of the ease of electronic calibration of modern blood pressure monitoring systems, many clinicians set themselves up for errors in judgment based on faulty information. All pressure transducers should ideally undergo static calibration with a mercury manometer on a daily basis, if not several times daily. This is the only means by which zero drift can be detected in a clinical monitoring system.

TRANSDUCER LEVEL. Meticulous attention also should be directed to the level of the pressure transducer. When a patient is supine, the midaxillary line usually reflects the position of the left atrium and serves as a useful reference point for zeroing. Blood pressure readings increase by 10 mm Hg for every 13 cm that the transducer is lowered below heart level and conversely decrease if the transducer is raised or zeroed above the heart.

Probably the most outrageous clinical error I ever observed was sodium nitroprusside administration to treat "hypertension" caused by a transducer that had fallen on the floor. I am also familiar with cases of cerebrovascular insufficiency that went undiagnosed during operations in the seated position because the pressure transducer was faithfully recording blood pressure at heart level instead of documenting what the more relevant blood pressure was in the head.

In another case, renal shutdown developed after massive rhabdomyolysis occurred in a patient's legs following prolonged use of the high stirrups, lithotomy position for radical prostatectomy. The blood pressure at heart level was normal, but it was clearly insufficient in the legs. Whenever a patient is placed in an extreme position, the blood pressure transducer is best placed at the highest level of circulatory concern to document adequate perfusion pressure to the site most at risk for vascular insufficiency.

CENTRAL VENOUS CATHETERS

Access to the central venous circulation is usually achieved by an external or internal jugular vein, a subclavian vein or an antecubital vein.

Subclavian Vein

Pneumothorax and Mediastinal Bleeding

The subclavian route is so fraught with the twin risks of pneumothorax and noncompressible arterial puncture that most anesthesiologists have eschewed its use for central venous cannulation, particularly because it is not as readily accessible from the head of the operating room table as is the internal jugular route.

As with any invasive procedure, the incidence of complications decreases with experience; even in the best of hands, however, pneumothorax occurs between 1.4% and 6% of the time after attempted subclavian venipuncture.[78] Because of this risk, a postcannulation chest radiograph is mandatory, particularly if bilateral attempts have been made. This procedure thus delays the beginning of surgery and risks development of a tension pneumothorax during positive-pressure ventilation, especially if nitrous oxide is administered. With these hazards well recognized, the reluctance of anesthesiologists to use this technique in the immediate preoperative period is understandable. Finally, because tamponade of a subclavian vessel is impossible, the threat of undiagnosed massive mediastinal hemorrhage occurring during surgery is always a potential problem.

Despite these problems, the subclavian route probably affords the best placement of a central venous catheter for long-term parenteral nutrition because it can be stabilized on the anterior chest. Furthermore, in extreme hypovolemia it may be the only site available for obtaining venous access because the surrounding connective tissues tend to keep the vessel patent even when other veins are severely collapsed.

Arterial and Thoracic Duct Injuries

As with the other techniques of venous cannulation, the basic principle for avoiding insertion complications is to make the vein as large as possible. Thus, institution of a head-down position and Valsalva's maneuver at the moment of venipuncture are mandatory. Although the subclavian vein and artery are separated by the anterior scalene muscle, arterial puncture and hematoma formations still occur with a 1% to 3% incidence.[79,80] Hemothorax or chylothorax (from injury to the thoracic duct) occurs in as many as 2% of subclavian catheterizations.[81,82] Other less frequent complications from misdirected introducing needles include brachial plexus palsy, mediastinal hemorrhage and arteriovenous fistula formation.[83,84]

Air Embolization

Subclavian catheters originally were placed with "needle over catheter" devices; two additional complications with this approach were air embolism[82] and catheter embolism.[83] Air embolism occurs when venous pressure is subatmospheric while the introducing needle tip is in the vessel lumen and air entry is not impeded by the presence of a catheter or syringe in the needle. As much air as 100 mL per second (which is greater than the the median lethal dose) could be sucked into the standard 14-G needles used at the time. Prevention involves placement of the patient in a steep head-down position and performance of Valsalva's maneuver while the aspirating syringe is removed until the catheter or a guide wire is placed. Patients in cardiac failure who are dyspneic present a significant risk because they may be unable to hold their breath long enough, tolerate a steep head-down position, or both.

Internal Jugular Vein

Internal jugular vein cannulation has achieved popularity among anesthesiologists because it is a reliable route to the right heart, is convenient to perform from the head of an operating table, and has a reasonably low incidence of complications. Because the internal jugular vein is located next to or occasionally even behind the carotid artery within the carotid sheath (Fig. 9-10), the most common complication of this technique is carotid artery puncture.

Carotid Artery Puncture

Puncture of the carotid artery with an 18- or 16-G central venous catheter–needle assembly is not nearly as serious as introduction of a 7-French pulmonary artery introducer, but it may lead to life-threatening hemorrhage[84] or upper-airway obstruction requiring surgical exploration.[85,86] In experienced hands carotid artery puncture occurs in approximately 4% to 7% of cannulation attempts.[86,87] Additional arterial injuries during internal jugular cannulation include aortic dissection[88] and cervical trunk, vertebral, or brachiocephalic artery injury.[89]

Because of the hazard of inadvertent arterial puncture, some investigators recommend identification of the course of the internal jugular vein and its relation to the carotid artery using a Doppler probe.[90–92] Mere palpation of the carotid artery may not be of assistance, because this maneuver compresses the internal jugular vein and, therefore, makes cannulation more difficult.[92]

Pneumothorax

Pneumothorax is relatively infrequent during internal jugular vein catheterization, occurring in approximately 0.3% of cases[93–95] when a relatively "low" approach (near the clavicle) is used. Although reports of fewer instances of pneumothorax with higher approaches (above the level of the cricoid cartilage, for instance), are not available, logic suggests this is the case. When a lateral approach to the internal jugular vein is taken, the possibility of the needle impinging on the trachea[97] or puncturing an endotracheal tube cuff should be kept in mind.[96]

Nerve Damage

Immediately deep to the carotid sheath are a variety of nerves, many of which have been injured by needle laceration or hematoma compression. Among these are the recurrent laryngeal,[97] sympathetic chain,[98] cervical plexus,[99] and phrenic nerves.[100] In general, these structures are at risk with repeated and traumatic attempts at internal jugular cannulation. Once again, the best means for avoidance is to make the vein as large as possible before attempting cannulation. The patient should be placed in as steep a head-down position as can be tolerated and Valsalva's maneuver performed just as cannulation is attempted.

Thoracic Duct Injury

Injury to the thoracic duct also has been reported after attempted low internal jugular vein cannulation on the left side. Because the thoracic duct enters the subclavian vein at the junction with the left internal jugular vein, a low approach may result in persistent chylothorax requiring surgical intervention. Some clinicians are of the opinion that a posterior approach to the internal jugular vein minimizes the incidence of thoracic duct injury during left internal jugular vein cannulation.

Venous Air Embolism

As is the case with cannulation of the subclavian vein, venous air embolism is also a threat during internal jugular cannulation.[101] Furthermore, if an internal jugular catheter becomes

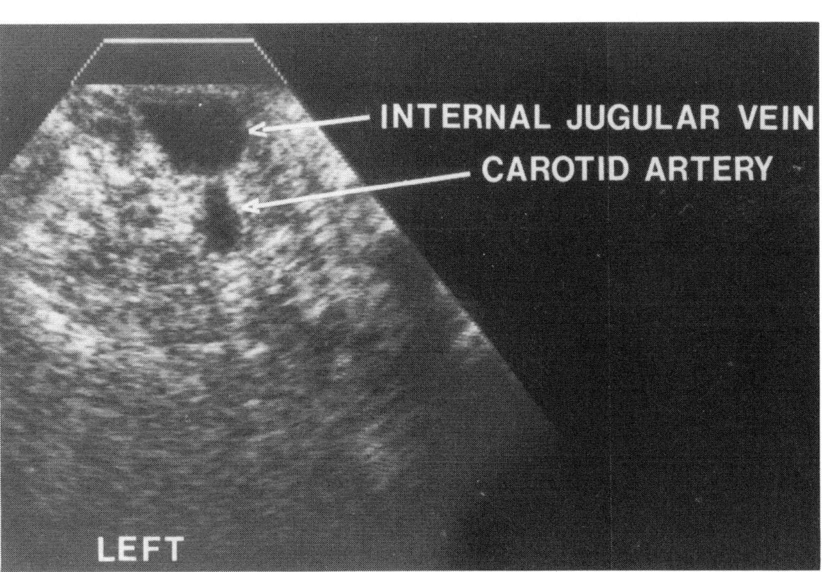

FIGURE 9-10. Sonogram of left side of patient's neck demonstrating relation of the internal jugular vein and carotid artery at the level of the cricoid cartilage. (Bedford RF: Limiting the complications of invasive monitoring. Current Reviews in Clinical Anesthesia 5:172, 1985.)

disconnected while the patient is upright, rapid air entrainment and sudden cardiac decompensation is possible at a time when the patient may not be under continuous observation.[102] Veins that collapse, such as the external jugular or antecubital, are far less likely to cause air embolism after accidental catheter removal. Luer-lock connectors, suture-secured connectors, or both are mandatory whenever a central venous catheter is placed.

External Jugular Vein

The flexible J-wire guide has facilitated external jugular central venous cannulation, with a success rate of approximately 90%.[103] Before the J-wire was introduced, the published success rate was only 50% to 70%.[104,105] Assuming that the vein is visible for cannulation, the venous valves and the acute angle formed by the junction of the external jugular and subclavian veins can usually be negotiated by alternately twisting and advancing the J-wire. A central venous catheter can then be threaded over the J-wire and placed in the superior vena cava.

Spring-tip J-wire guides are not altogether benign. If the J-wire is advanced too far (>20 cm), it may strike the right atrium or ventricle, inducing cardiac dysrhythmias. Coiling or knotting of a J-wire may occur if the operator persists in advancing the device despite encountering resistance and suggests passage into a non-central venous location. When resistance is encountered during passage of a flexible J-wire, the wire must be gently withdrawn and/or rotated and carefully readvanced.

If resistance to withdrawal occurs, a knot or coil in a J-wire may be undone by carefully advancing an 8-French vessel dilator over the wire while it is gently withdrawn.[106] When this approach is unsuccessful, proceed to a chest radiograph or fluoroscopy to identify the nature of the problem before continuing with additional maneuvers. Spring-tip guide wires should be handled gently because the soft tip may be fractured easily, resulting in exposure of the solid core of the wire. The latter portion may, in turn, perforate an intrathoracic vein.[107]

Safety

Because the external jugular vein is superficial and easy to visualize, it has a remarkable record of safety for central venous access. Because it is lodged in the cervical subcutaneous fat, it is far enough removed from other major structures to assure the safety of cannulation. To my knowledge, no fatalities have been reported during cannulation. I have seen one case of mediastinal and cervical hematoma in an anticoagulated patient who was positioned in such a way that the anesthesiologist could not see the cannulation site intraoperatively. This problem resolved spontaneously without evidence of airway or other compromise. In general, the external jugular vein appears to provide an excellent route to central venous cannulation for those with relatively little invasive cardiovascular monitoring experience.

Basilic Vein

The antecubital (basilic vein) route for central venous cannulation is probably the least traumatic of the techniques described. When a flexible J-wire is used, the success rate is 90% when the vein can be entered.[108] Without use of the J-wire, most series report a 50% to 60% success rate due to the catheter's "hanging up" in the axilla.[109,110] J-wire insertion before cannulation also permits passage of a relatively large catheter into a small antecubital vein.[111]

Because the basilic vein is in close proximity to the brachial artery and median nerve, neurovascular injury is possible, particularly if the vein is "palpable," but not visible. Palpation of arterial pulsations before attempted basilic vein cannulation probably is wise simply to avoid accidental cannulation of the brachial artery.

Catheter Complications

Once a central venous catheter is in place, its location should be determined to be satisfactory. If a catheter is used only briefly in the perioperative period, easy aspiration of venous blood and the presence of normal oscilloscopic venous waveforms probably are adequate signs of the tip's placement in the central venous circulation. However, when long-term cannulation is anticipated, if difficulty has been encountered during cannulation, and if resistance to aspiration of blood, abnormal (usually damped) waveforms, or both are present, a chest radiograph should be obtained. Ideally, the tip of the central venous catheter should be at the level of the inferior border of the clavicles on a standard posterior–anterior chest radiograph.[112]

Tip Erosion

MULTIPLE ORIFICE CATHETERS. Catheter tips impinging on the walls of central veins or the right atrium may erode through, resulting in hemothorax or pericardial tamponade. New, relatively stiff, multiorifice catheters tend to compound this problem because of their tapered tip configuration[113] and because the side-ports may permit aspiration of blood and transmission of waveforms despite tip perforation. In general, subclavian and internal jugular vein catheters should never be inserted more than 20 cm. In this regard, catheters placed from the antecubital veins may be more dangerous for long-term monitoring because the tips can migrate up to 10 cm with arm movement.[114] As a general rule, the softer and less pointed the tip of the catheter, the shallower the depth of insertion, and the fewer the lumina, the less likely it will cause perforation.

LEFT INTERNAL JUGULAR VEIN PLACEMENT. Central venous catheters placed via the left external jugular vein specifically have been identified as the cause of contralateral right hemothorax. As the catheter passes rightward from the left subclavian vein, the tip may impinge on the right lateral wall of the superior vena cava and perforate (Fig. 9-11).[115] Fifteen-centimeter (6-inch) catheters in particular are implicated because their length does not permit the catheter to make the turn toward the right atrium as occurs with a 20-cm (8-inch) catheter.[116] In vitro data show that the perforation potential of a catheter tip increases when its incident angle with the vessel wall increases to 40° or greater (Table 9-4).[117] If such findings are present on a chest radiograph the catheter should be repositioned or replaced.

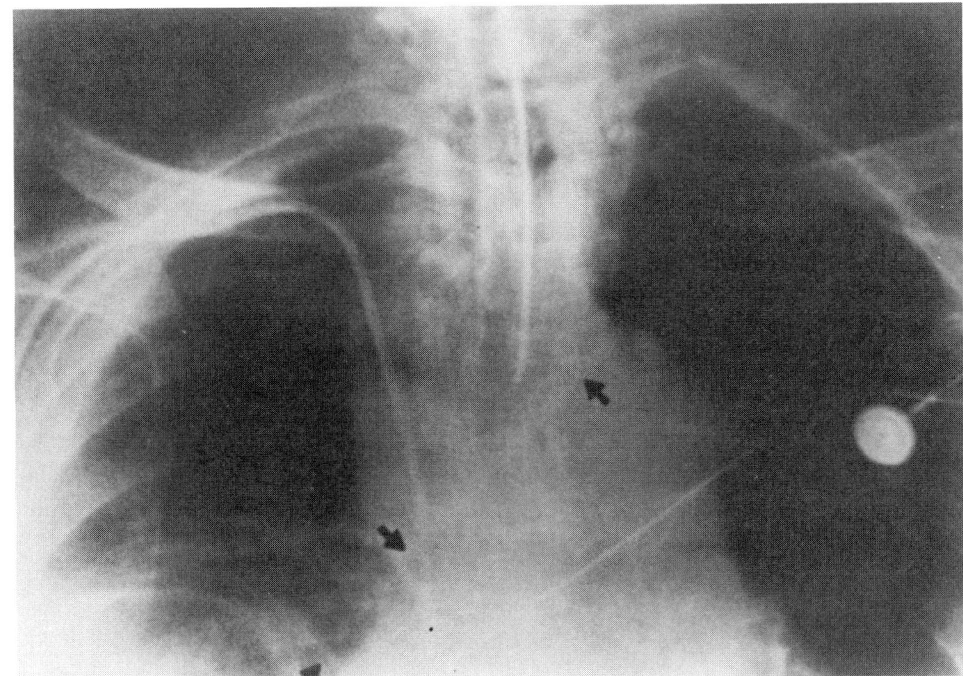

FIGURE 9-11. Chest radiograph showing a right subclavian PA catheter and a central venous catheter placed via the left external jugular vein. The left catheter tip has perforated the superior vena cava wall and entered the right pleural space. Arrows indicate catheter location. (Eichold BH, Berryman CR: Contralateral hydrothorax: an unusual complication of central venous catheter placement. Anesthesiology 62:673, 1985.)

VASCULAR PERFORATION AND PERICARDIAL TAMPONADE. Pericardial tamponade and extravasation into the pleural space are particularly dangerous conditions, with a mortality of as high as 80% to 95%.[113,114] The diagnosis sometimes is difficult because the condition frequently does not develop until more than 1 day after cannulation is performed. In general, however, easy aspiration of blood and normal readings of CVP and CVP waveforms from the distal lumen of the catheter indicate continued intravascular placement, whereas a rapidly increasing venous pressure and/or difficulty aspirating blood suggests extravascular migration. Central venous catheters that are converted from monitoring to long-term infusion afford less opportunity for the diagnosis of perforation. Treatment, of course, requires prompt intervention to drain either the pericardial sac or pleural compartment and withdrawal of the catheter. Most cases do not require surgical exploration.

Infection

Infectious complications are another major hazard of central venous catheters. Whereas these devices can be kept infection-free for long periods of time with strict aseptic techniques for parenteral nutrition, they can become a nidus for infection after 2 to 4 days in situ in 2% to 4% of critically ill patients.[118] Skin organisms, usually *S. aureus* or *S. epidermidis*, are the most common source of recognized catheter infections[119]; inevitably, these organisms come either from the patient or

TABLE 9-4
Effect on Vessel Perforation of Angle of Incidence Between Catheter Tip and Simulated Vessel Wall

NUMBER OF PULSATIONS UNTIL PERFORATION OF SIMULATED VESSEL	ANGLE OF INCIDENCE BETWEEN CATHETER TIP AND VESSEL WALL					
	40°	*50°*	*60°*	*70°*	*80°*	*90°*
Mean	30,583*	18,198†	1249*†	1434*†	5*†	7*†
SD	8862	13,367	1717	2564	2	3
Range	680–>33,600	427–>33,600	73–6,207	21–9,607	4–9	4–12

Results of in vitro perforation study with simulated vessel pulsating into catheter tip 80 times per minute.

* $P < 0.05$ compared with 50°.

† $P < 0.05$ compared with 40°.

Gravenstein N, Blackshear RH: In vitro evaluation of relative perforating potential of central venous catheters: comparison of materials, selected models, number of lumens, and angles of incidence to simulated membrane. J Clin Monit 7:1, 1991.

from the individual performing the cannulation. Because of this hazard, sterile technique should be observed during venipuncture and afterwards.

PRECAUTIONS. Most authorities recommend sterile gowns, gloves, and face masks, as well as aseptic skin preparation and draping, during cannulation. Once a central venous catheter is placed, povidone iodine ointment is applied to the puncture site and a sterile, nonwatertight dressing affixed. Daily dressing changes with strict attention to aseptic protocol are often advocated, with a maximum duration of cannulation of 2 to 4 days unless no other sites are available.[120] This period, however, may be too restrictive; as a practical matter, longer durations frequently are employed. Relative immobility is thought to be important for maintaining catheter sterility, because subclavian venous catheters generally have a lower incidence of infection than do jugular catheters. Antecubital catheters have the highest rate of infection of these three sites.

Central venous and pulmonary artery catheters can be contaminated from nonsterile stopcocks or from bacteria within intravenous solutions. In an effort to minimize this risk, lipid-containing solutions or blood products should not be infused through them if other sites are available. Injections into the tubing should be avoided, and flush solutions and tubing should be replaced every 24 hours.[121]

Catheter-Associated Sepsis

The diagnosis of catheter-associated sepsis should be suspected whenever a patient with a low risk for infection develops bacteremia. If discontinuation of an infusion promptly ends the episode, fluid contamination should be suspected, particularly if the offending organism is a *Klebsiella* species. These organisms have a particular affinity for dextrose-containing fluids.

Not infrequently, central venous catheters become secondarily infected with bacteria seeded from a remote site of infection such as the urinary tract. If bacteremia persists despite appropriate antibiotic therapy, the central venous and all other intravascular catheters should be removed and cultured by a quantitative technique. A gram stain of the distal catheter tip affords a rapid and accurate test for the diagnosis of catheter-related infection.[122]

Miscellaneous Problems

Other less frequent but occasionally dangerous complications of central venous catheterization include cardiac ectopy when a catheter is advanced into the right ventricle, or when a long-arm catheter migrates into the right ventricle with movement of the shoulder or elbow. Air embolism may occur with jugular or subclavian catheters as a result of disconnection from the flush infusion tubing. Universal use of Luer-lock connectors undoubtedly minimizes this hazard. Thrombosis of the cannulated vein is an additional complication, ranging in severity from antecubital discomfort to occlusion of the internal jugular vein or the superior vena cava. Because the latter is a time-related event, it provides yet another reason for removing central catheters as soon as the patient's condition warrants.

Data Interpretation

The historical, time-honored device for measurement of CVP was a water manometer with its zero level at the midaxillary line and a fluid-filled extension tube attached to the central venous catheter. Although this technique permits intermittent determinations of pressure at heart level, it permits neither a continuous read-out nor a continuous flush infusion to maintain catheter patency. Furthermore, it measures pressure in centimeters of water, not millimeters of mercury, thus making correlation with pulmonary and systemic hemodynamics more difficult than if the CVP was transduced electronically.

Finally, the absence of a discernible pressure waveform during water column measurement precludes the accurate diagnosis of complications such as catheter tip placement in the right ventricle, nodal rhythm producing an artifactually high CVP due to retrograde "V-waves," atrioventricular dissociation causing "Cannon A-waves," or extravascular migration of the catheter tip with incipient hemothorax or pericardial tamponade.

Transducer Position

Because venous pressure is normally low (3 ± 2 mm Hg), extreme precision is necessary to ensure that the transducer is at a proper and consistent zero reference point, and that no drift occurs in the values detected by the monitoring system. This problem can be excluded by periodically reverifying that when the system is opened to air at the level of the zero reference point, it still reads zero. A more obvious cause of a sudden change in CVP occurs when the operating room table is lowered or raised. The CVP will be increased or decreased by 7.4 mm Hg for every 10 cm of elevation or lowering, respectively, of the table unless the transducer (or water column) moves with the patient.

Airway Pressure

Changes in airway pressure also affect the pressure measured in the central venous circulation. Increases in mean airway pressure due to initiation of positive-pressure ventilation or positive end-expiratory pressure will be reflected as an increase in CVP, and should not be misinterpreted as a change in either intravascular volume status or myocardial performance. Conversely, when a patient initiates spontaneous ventilation at the end of an operation, an abrupt decrease in CVP is to be expected and should not be interpreted as sudden onset of hypovolemia.

Right and Left Ventricular Disparity

Perhaps the most serious problems in CVP interpretation relate to whether CVP truly reflects left ventricular performance. Clear-cut disparities in right and left ventricular function occur in conditions such as acute myocardial infarction and cor pulmonale. Concern that changes in CVP may not reflect intravascular volume status or left ventricular contractility, just at a time when a knowledge of them is of paramount importance in clinical management is understandable.[124,125]

Because CVP monitoring probably is intrinsically less hazardous than pulmonary artery catheterization (as discussed below), it remains the method of choice for documenting volume status in patients with normal myocardial performance who are undergoing a major surgical procedure. Ideally, it should be electronically transduced; traditionally, the value at end-expiration is used as the most accurate reflection of cardiovascular status, but proof that this value is the "true" one is questionable at best.

PULMONARY ARTERY CATHETERS

A significant advance in the care of critically ill patients during the past generation was achieved with flow-directed pulmonary artery catheters. These devices afford a reasonably safe and simple means to determine overall cardiovascular performance in a wide variety of disease states. They also facilitate the diagnosis of complex dysrhythmias and intracardiac pacing. However, a variety of complications are possible (Table 9-5).

Introducer Complications

Misplacement

Pulmonary artery catheterization has all of the hazards previously outlined for central venous catheterization plus the difficulties inherent in the passing of a larger catheter through a larger introducer. Although some catheters are introduced directly via a surgical cut-down, the majority are placed by using a modified Seldinger guide wire technique. The first priority is to place the guide wire safely in the desired peripheral vein. Most introducer kits contain guide wires to be placed through a steel needle, but the majority of errant catheter introductions I have observed have been related to the introducer needle's not being in the desired vein. An extreme example is that of a pulmonary artery catheter that was placed inadvertently into the subarachnoid space after the guide wire was passed through a steel needle whose tip was thought to be in the internal jugular vein.[126] Other errant sites include the carotid artery, mediastinum and pleural spaces.

TABLE 9-5
Pulmonary Artery Catheterization Complications

COMPLICATION	INCIDENCE (%)
Carotid artery puncture	2.00
Pneumothorax	0.50
Dysrhythmia (all)	72.00
Transient premature ventricular contractions	68.00
Premature ventricular contractions requiring therapy	3.00
Premature atrial contractions	1.30
Right bundle branch block	0.05
Left bundle branch block	0.02
Right ventricle perforation	0.02
Pulmonary artery perforation	0.06
Pulmonary infarct	0.06

Data from Shah KB, Rao TLK, Laughlin S, et al: A review of pulmonary artery catheterization in 6,245 patients. Anesthesiology 61:271, 1984.

CAROTID OR SUBCLAVIAN ARTERY PERFORATION. Because of the considerable hazard of passing an 8-French dilator/introducer into the wrong location, many authorities suggest that the guide wire should be advanced through a catheter that has been placed in the desired vein (verified by easy aspiration of dark blood). In addition, arterial cannulation should be ruled out by verification of venous pressures within the cannula before the guide wire is advanced.[127] Introduction of a dilator/introducer sheath into the carotid or subclavian artery is a major surgical emergency requiring prompt oversewing of the vascular defect before life-threatening hemorrhage occurs.[84,85] When simple external compression has been used to stop hematoma formation, arteriovenous fistulas between the carotid and the internal jugular vein have developed.

Assuming that the guide wire has been safely introduced, passage of the pointed dilator/introducer sheath may still cause perforation of the great veins or superior vena cava with subsequent hematoma formation. Errant placement of the catheter may be suspected by observation of equal distal and proximal port pressures despite having advanced the catheter far enough to place its tip in the right ventricle or pulmonary artery.[128]

Air Embolism

Air embolism is another major hazard associated with placement of a large bore dilator/introducer. Originally described only as a possible complication of pulmonary artery catheter insertion because of the large amount of air that theoretically could be entrained through an 8-French introducer,[129] life-threatening air embolism in fact has occurred with conventional venous cannulation.[130] It can best be prevented by head-down positioning and performance of Valsalva's maneuver at any time the central venous circulation is opened to the atmosphere.

Air embolism probably occurs more commonly during the postoperative period when the side-arm of the introducer is used for infusion of intravenous fluids. When patients are placed in the head-up position or when venous pressure is below atmospheric pressure, air is entrained through a defect in the supposedly air-tight occluding membrane that separates the introducer lumen from the atmosphere.[131,132] Some manufacturers have supplied obturators to help prevent embolization by occluding the opening created after the catheter has been removed.[133]

Although introducers provide excellent routes for intravenous access, I believe they should not be retained in situ merely for convenience. Because of the unexpected and catastrophic nature of postoperative venous air embolism or erosion of the rigid introducer through the wall of the superior vena cava, they should be removed at the earliest possible opportunity compatible with good patient care.

Cardiovascular Stress

Insertion of a catheter introducer is performed with some degree of patient anxiety and discomfort. Lunn and associates[134] noted marked increases in cardiac rate–pressure product in patients undergoing internal jugular cannulation and pulmonary artery catheter insertion, particularly in those not premedicated with propranolol. Fifty per cent of their inadequately pretreated patients developed angina pectoris or other manifestations of coronary ischemia. Other investigators, however, have found that more generous premedication and concomitant use of intravenous nitroglycerin results in satisfactory patient tolerance of percutaneous catheter introduction with no evident increase in myocardial oxygen demand.[135,136]

Catheter Passage

Dysrhythmias

The most frequent complications of catheter passage are cardiac dysrhythmias occurring as the catheter tip traverses the right ventricle. During continuous monitoring of the electrocardiogram, premature ventricular contractions have been noted during approximately half of pulmonary artery catheterizations; brief ventricular tachycardia occurs in approximately one third.[137] Ventricular fibrillation, though rare, also has been reported.[138]

CATHETER LOOPING. Looping of the catheter in the right ventricle may produce persistent ventricular ectopy, although this problem should be easily detected by observing that the catheter has been advanced farther than necessary to achieve a pulmonary artery occlusion pressure (PAOP) tracing.

LIDOCAINE PROPHYLAXIS. Because of the high incidence of dysrhythmias during passage of pulmonary artery catheters, prophylactic administration of an antidysrhythmic agent such as intravenous lidocaine has a logical appeal. When all patients are treated with lidocaine, however, no significant reduction in ventricular irritability ensues.[139] Mechanically induced dysrhythmias generally respond best and most predictably to removal (withdrawal) of the catheter or stimulus. One interesting observation is that the use of a 5° head-up position with a right lateral tilt markedly reduces the incidence of malignant dysrhythmias[140] (Table 9-6). This maneuver probably facilitates catheter flotation. Other measures advocated for reducing ventricular irritability include rapid passage of the catheter once the right ventricle has been reached and always advancing the catheter with the balloon inflated to minimize contact of the more rigid catheter tip with the right ventricle wall.

TABLE 9-6
Incidence of Dysrhythmias During Pulmonary Artery Catheter Insertion

POSITION	BENIGN	MALIGNANT
5° head-up position with right lateral tilt	18	8
5°–10° Trendelenburg position*	12	17

Number of insertions = 34.

* $P < 0.05$.

Modified from Keusch DJ, Winters S, Thys DM: The patient's position influences the incidence of dysrhythmias during pulmonary artery catheterization. Anesthesiology 70:582, 1989.

BUNDLE BRANCH BLOCK. Bundle branch block is another common dysrhythmia observed during catheter passage. Right bundle branch block develops in approximately 5% of patients, although it usually is of no clinical significance.[141] However, those with a preexisting left bundle branch block may develop complete heart block as the catheter contacts the right ventricular wall and stimulates the right bundle conducting system.[142] Left bundle branch block has been reported as well, apparently caused by impingement of the catheter on the bundle of His.[143]

COMPLETE HEART BLOCK. Clearly, patients with preexisting conduction defects are at risk for complete heart block during passage of pulmonary artery catheters. Placement of a pacing electrode, use of a pacing catheter, or ready access to a pacing wire should be considered before catheterization.[144] If a pacing wire is placed within 2 weeks before passage of the catheter, both procedures probably should be performed in the cardiac catheterization laboratory under fluoroscopic guidance to minimize the risk of dislodging the pacing wire.

Knotting

Knotting is a potential major complication of pulmonary artery catheterization. Most knots likely form in the right atrium or ventricle where catheters can loop around themselves during insertion.[145] If no cardiac structure is attached, knots usually can be removed with little more than a venotomy incision.[146] Conversely, if a chorda or papillary muscle is involved, the knot must be evaluated under fluoroscopy and, when possible, disentangled using guide wires and snares advanced cephalad via the femoral vein.[147,148] Operative intervention for this problem should be needed only rarely. However, withdrawal of a catheter should always be performed gently and with the balloon deflated to avoid tightening a knot or damaging an intracardiac structure. If resistance is detected during withdrawal, a chest radiograph is mandatory before deciding what course should be pursued.

Complications After Catheter Placement

Pulmonary Artery Perforation

Perforation of the pulmonary artery is the most devastating complication of pulmonary artery catheterization (Table 9-7). It usually is heralded by hemoptysis after balloon inflation or manipulation of the catheter.[149,150] Hemoptysis may be massive or relatively minute.[151] Approximately one third of the cases reported occurred shortly after patients were weaned from cardiopulmonary bypass (approximately 0.2% of patients undergoing open heart operations).[152] On a review of Table 9-7, it is clear that in general, patients undergoing cardiac surgery meet several criteria predisposing them to this complication.[153]

TABLE 9-7
Factors Predisposing to Pulmonary Artery Rupture

- Age > 60 yr
- Female gender
- Cardiopulmonary bypass
- Hypothermia
- Anticoagulation
- Pulmonary hypertension
- Catheter tip location peripheral (ie, >5 cm lateral to mediastinum)
- Multiple determinations of wedge pressure
- Atypical pulmonary artery pressure waveform (mitral valve disease)

Gravenstein N: Invasive vascular monitoring. In Gravenstein N (ed): Manual of complications during anesthesia. Phildelphia: JB Lippincott, 1991: 290.

CAUSES. Pulmonary artery rupture generally occurs when a flotation catheter balloon is placed or migrates too far distal in the pulmonary vasculature. One should expect every catheter to spontaneously migrate distally from its original position as it warms to body temperature and becomes more flexible. When the balloon is inflated, it may rupture the distal pulmonary artery wall[154]; alternatively, as the balloon is inflated in a small artery, it may force the tip of the catheter through the vessel wall (Fig. 9-12).[155]

PREVENTION. Because this problem occurs so frequently as patients are separated from cardiopulmonary bypass, distal migration of the catheter tip is thought to occur during the bypass period. Some clinicians routinely withdraw the catheter 5 to 7 cm on the initiation of cardiopulmonary bypass.[156]

Other common-sense precautions that reduce the likelihood of pulmonary artery rupture include: (1) minimizing the number of times the balloon is inflated for determination of PAOP, particularly if pulmonary diastolic pressure has been shown to correspond closely to values observed during PAOP measurements, (2) making sure the balloon never remains inflated longer than the time required to measure PAOP, and (3) only using 1.5 mL of air to inflate the balloon.

RISK FACTORS. Risk factors that correlate with pulmonary artery rupture are listed in Table 9-7 and include pulmonary hypertension, advanced age, and female gender.[153–155] Pulmonary hypertension may contribute by causing the cath-

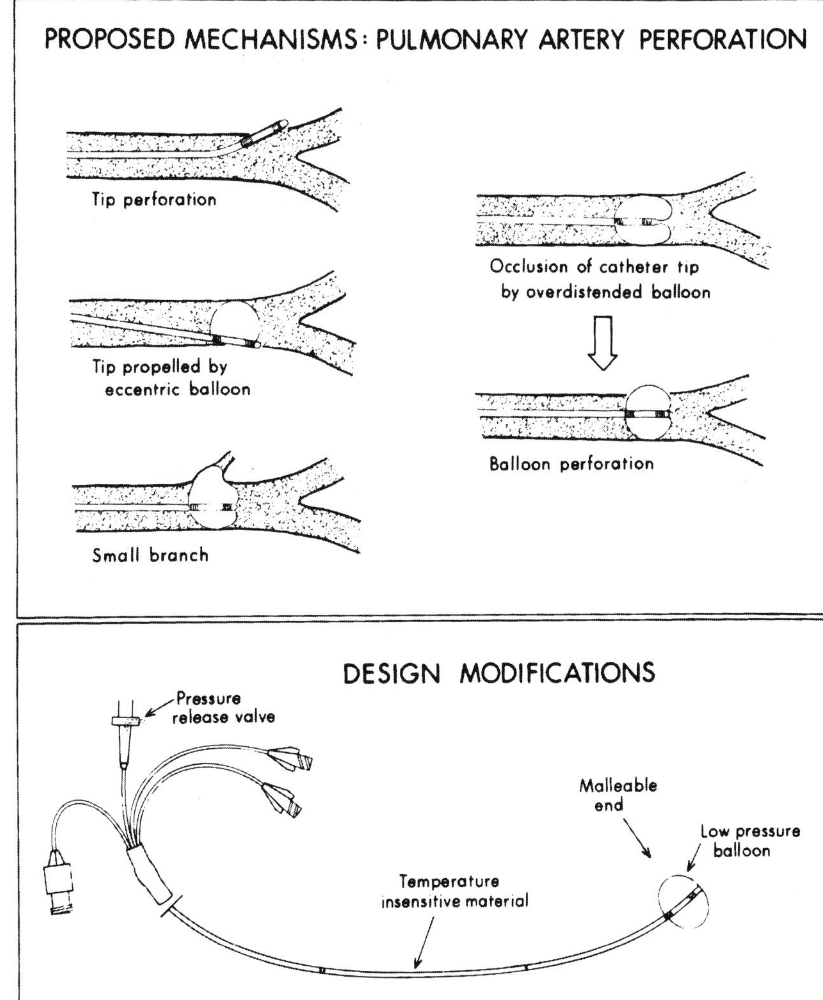

FIGURE 9-12. The possible pathophysiologic mechanisms of balloon-induced pulmonary artery rupture (*top*) and catheter modifications (*bottom*). (Barash PG, Nardi D, Hammond G, et al: Catheter-induced pulmonary artery perforation: mechanisms, management and modifications. J Thorac Cardiovasc Surg 82:7, 1981.)

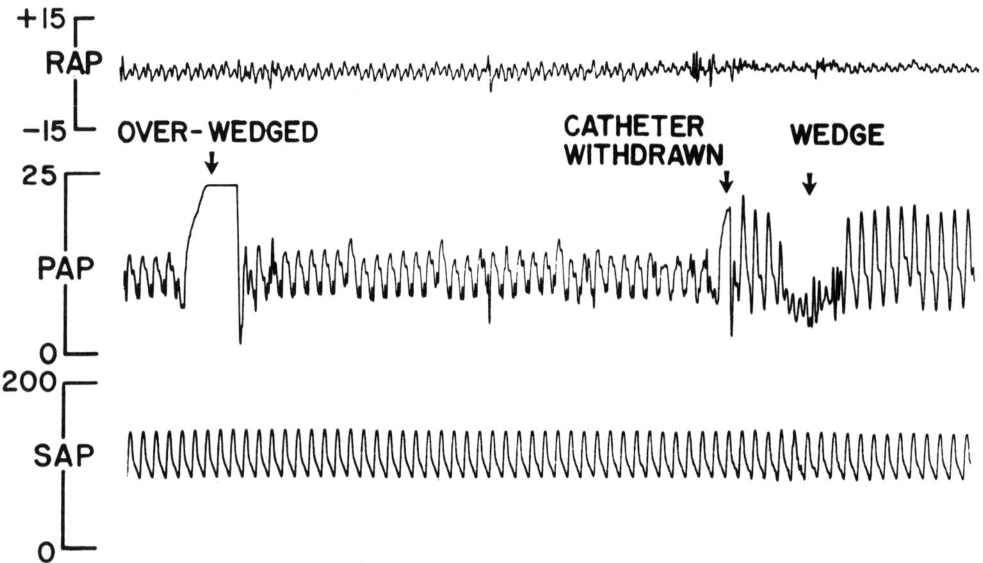

FIGURE 9-13. Pulmonary artery pressure record demonstrating an "over-wedged" trace due to distal tip migration, and subsequent correction after catheter withdrawal. (Bedford RF: Limiting the complications of invasive monitoring. Current Reviews in Clinical Anesthesia 5:170, 1985.)

eter to lodge in distal branches that are more distended than normal. Advanced age may cause degenerative sclerosis that makes the vessel less tolerant of distending pressure. Because women are smaller than men, the pulmonary artery catheters may simply have a shorter distance to migrate before they reach the critical distal location at which vessel rupture is most likely to occur.

The classic sign of distal migration of a catheter tip is the "over-wedge" pressure trace (Fig. 9-13), indicating impingement on the vessel wall or balloon herniation over the tip. In either event, withdrawal of the catheter several centimeters eliminates the over-wedge phenomenon. I normally expect to see a pulmonary artery catheter develop an over-wedge trace after it has been in place for 1 or 2 hours, presumably as a result of distal migration as the curve created by passage of the catheter through the right heart tightens with softening of the catheter and continued cardiac action.

A flotation catheter can be advanced too far into the pulmonary artery if the balloon is not inflated to its recommended 1.5 mL. Similarly, overdistending the balloon with more than 1.5 mL of air may cause rupture of the vessel wall even if the tip is in the proper position.[154] Many instances of pulmonary artery rupture have been shown to be the result of improper manipulation of the catheter or its balloon mechanism.[155]

TREATMENT. Treatment of pulmonary hemorrhage is outlined in Table 9-8.

Other Problems with Balloon Inflation

Other complications related to balloon inflation are relatively rare. Simple rupture of the balloon is not a serious problem as long as only small volumes of air are used in an attempt to inflate it. Usually this condition is suspected by failure to obtain a PAOP tracing and absence of resistance to balloon inflation; it is confirmed by aspiration of blood into the air syringe. Occasionally an over-wedge trace may herald balloon rupture.[153]

After pneumonectomy, inflation of the balloon in the remaining pulmonary artery may reduce left heart filling sufficiently to cause a sudden reduction in blood pressure.[157] In some patients, the "failure to occlude" may be taken as a sign of massive pulmonary embolism, and the catheter then can be used to deliver thrombolytic agents.[158]

Thromboembolic Events

Thromboembolic events resulting in pulmonary infarction are another set of complications related to catheterization. Clots form on the catheter within a few hours of insertion.[159,160] This thrombus may obstruct pulmonary perfusion when the catheter is placed too far distally[161] or when it embolizes from clots in the internal jugular[162] or subclavian[163] veins, superior

TABLE 9-8
Treatment of Internal Hemorrhages Resulting from Pulmonary Artery Catheterization

1. Administration of protamine if the patient's blood is anticoagulated
2. Prompt institution of positive end-expiratory pressure at levels as high as can be tolerated to tamponade the rupture
3. Fiberoptic bronchoscopy or pulmonary angiography to identify the bleeding site
4. Endobronchial intubation to isolate the bleeding lung if hemorrhage is massive
5. Supportive respiratory and cardiovascular support as needed
6. Consideration of surgical resection of the affected segment if the above measures are not adequate

vena cava, or right atrium.[164] In addition to pulmonary complications, thrombi on pulmonary artery catheters may also result in venous obstruction to the head and upper extremities, may impair the ability of the catheter to determine pressures and cardiac output accurately, and may be responsible for reductions in platelet counts after open-heart operations.[165]

Because of these problems, manufacturers bonded heparin to the surface of their catheters in an attempt to reduce thrombogenicity. Although these devices delay the appearance of clot on the catheter,[166] reports indicate no difference in the incidence of thromboembolic complications or in the decrease of platelet counts with heparin-bonded devices.[167] Possibly the reversal of systemic heparinization at the end of cardiopulmonary bypass causes the heparin-coated catheter to become thrombogenic again.

Infection

Infectious complications are another major problem of long-term pulmonary artery catheterization, just as they are with any other invasive cardiovascular catheter. Whereas the overall incidence of pulmonary artery catheter-related sepsis has been reported as between 2%[168] and 35%,[169] 3 days appears to be the point at which the risks of infectious complications begin to outweigh the benefits of continued use of the same catheter; many (but by no means all) authorities recommend removal or replacement of the catheter after this period of time.[170–172]

S. epidermidis is the predominant organism that infects these catheters, presumably as a result of skin contact or cannulation manipulation. Maki and Band[62] recommend antiseptic skin preparation, sterile insertion technique, and a povidone iodine dressing to minimize catheter contamination. A sterile sleeve over the portion of the catheter that enters the introducer may help to reduce infection related to catheter manipulation.[173]

The same sterility precautions applied to systemic arterial and CVP monitoring systems also apply to pulmonary artery catheters,[68,69] with daily changes of flush solutions and meticulous attention to the sterility of stopcocks, particularly those used for repeated thermodilution cardiac output determinations. If catheter-related sepsis is suspected, removal of the catheter and work-up similar to that for an infected central venous catheter is warranted.

Cardiac Trauma

A final group of complications involves cardiac trauma when the catheter is in place. Linear endocardial lesions have been observed involving the right atrium, tricuspid valve, chordae tendineae and pulmonic valves after prolonged catheterization. Hemorrhage into valve cusps and separation of valve tissue also has been observed. In general, these lesions are thought to be the result of direct cardiac trauma from prolonged catheterization, and are probably yet another reason why catheters should be removed just as soon as is practical.

Data Misinterpretation

Because the pulmonary artery catheter generates the greatest amount of data among the monitoring modalities discussed thus far, it is not surprising that these data are also subject to the greatest misinterpretation.[174–178] In the optimal situation using a standard thermistor tipped catheter, accurate determinations of pulmonary artery pressures (systolic, diastolic and mean), PAOP, cardiac output, mixed venous oxygen partial pressure and right atrial oxygen partial pressure should be possible. Continuous mixed venous oxygen saturation obtained by reflectance spectrophotometry is also available. All of these data, however, may be inaccurate if the clinician is not constantly wary of the sources of misinterpretation. The upshot is that a patient may be mismanaged based on faulty data generated by an inherently hazardous monitoring modality.

Inaccurate Pressure Measurements

As is the case with CVP monitoring, the pulmonary artery pressure transducer zero reference must be maintained at heart level (ie, the midaxillary line) and must be assiduously checked for evidence of zero drift. Small changes in PAOP or pulmonary artery diastolic pressure may suggest large shifts in intravascular volume status, or may simply indicate measurement error.[179]

CATHETER WHIP. As with systemic arterial pressure monitoring, all the problems of an underdamped pressure measurement system apply to the pulmonary artery catheter. In addition, is the problem of "catheter whip," created by a long, hyperresonant catheter that is repeatedly hit by the right ventricle. If pulmonary artery diastolic pressure is used to reflect left heart filling pressure, the values observed may actually be far below true pulmonary artery diastolic pressure simply because the monitor is picking off the pressure nadir rather than filtering out the artifactually depressed values created by catheter whip and hyperresonance. The clinician must be satisfied that measurement error has been minimized before embarking on a therapeutic intervention based on these data.

RESPIRATORY VARIATION. Alterations in respiratory status are a well-recognized source of confusion during catheterization. A change from spontaneous to assisted or controlled ventilation, for example, produces an apparent increase in pulmonary artery pressure or PAOP as airway pressures are transmitted to the right and left atria and pulmonary circulation. Because at end-expiration no air flow occurs and intrapleural pressure is thought to be static, this point is the most logical one at which to measure pressures with a pulmonary artery catheter.[174]

POSITIVE END-EXPIRATORY PRESSURE. Positive end-expiratory pressure creates even more opportunities for data misinterpretation. As raised airway pressure is transmitted to the intrathoracic contents, pulmonary arterial pressures are also increased, resulting in a discrepancy between PAOP and actual left atrial pressure.[175,176] Downs suggested monitoring intrapleural pressure in an attempt to determine transmural pressure across intrathoracic vessels.[177] However, most clinicians seem to rely on trends in PAOP at whatever level end-expiratory pressure is maintained. Sudden cessation of positive end-expiratory pressure for PAOP determination or other reasons has been associated with marked deterioration in cardiovascular parameters and arterial oxygenation.[178,180]

CATHETER TIP MALPOSITION. Malposition of the tip of the catheter can result in spurious assessments of hemodynamic performance. Placement in the pulmonary vasculature above the level of the left atrium may result in PAOP readings significantly in excess of left atrial pressure when positive end-expiratory pressure is used.[181,182] Cardiac output determinations performed when a catheter has migrated sufficiently distal to occlude a branch (wedge) may read spuriously high because the thermistor sees a relatively smaller amount of the pulmonary artery blood flow and the computer calculates this as a higher cardiac output. This problem is compounded if a "mixed venous" blood oxygen partial pressure is then measured, because contamination with pulmonary capillary blood will increase the oxygen partial pressure and lead the unwary clinician to interpret these findings as compatible with a high cardiac output. Continuous mixed venous oxygen saturation monitoring should reveal this trend. In summary, proper placement of the tip of the catheter in a major branch of the pulmonary artery must be verified to prevent mismanagement based on spurious data.

CARDIAC OUTPUT. Because cardiac output determination requires both electronic and human elements, this measurement too can result in bad data and pose a risk to proper patient management (Table 9-9). This hazard is compounded by iced injectate solution, which, while perhaps conferring more sensitivity, also increases the risk of errors. If the injectate temperature probe falls out of the ice bath, for instance, a low cardiac output measurement will result. If the syringe containing the injectate warms while being held in the hands too long, a higher cardiac output reading will be noted. A lower output will also be reported if repeat injections occur too quickly for the liquid in the catheter lumen to achieve body temperature. Use of iced injectate has also been associated with a high incidence of bradycardia, and a resultant decrease in cardiac output, apparently related to cooling of the sinus node.[183] For these reasons I prefer to use room temperature injectate because its accuracy appears to be very nearly equal to iced injectate when 10-mL injectate volumes are used,[184] and the sources of inaccuracy are reduced.

Finally, inaccurate cardiac output determinations may be the result of sheer inattention to detail. Injecting the wrong volume of solution or putting it into the wrong port, having the wrong calibrating factors in the microprocessor, and using a catheter that is too long (placing the right atrial port in the subclavian vein[185]) are just a few of the other possibilities.

TABLE 9-9
Common Sources of Errors in the Measurement of Cardiac Output by Thermodilution

- Incorrect computation constant
- Incorrect injectate volume
- Incorrect injectate temperature
- Inconsistent respiratory cycle
- Concurrent change in intravenous infusion
- Inconsistent injection technique

Modified from Gravenstein N: Invasive vascular monitoring. In Gravenstein N (ed): Manual of complications during anesthesia. Philadelphia: JB Lippincott, 1991: 296.

REFERENCES

1. Vender JS, Watts DR: Differential diagnosis of hand ischemia in the presence of an arterial cannula. Anesth Analg 61:465, 1982
2. Cartwright GW, Schreimer RL: Major complication secondary to percutaneous radial artery catheterization in the neonate. Pediatrics 65:139, 1980
3. Johnson FE, Summer DS, Shandness DE Jr: Extremity necrosis caused by indwelling arterial catheters. Am J Surg 131:375, 1976
4. Mangano DT, Hickey RF: Ischemic injury following uncomplicated radial artery catheterization. Anesth Analg 58:55, 1979
5. Mayer T, Matlak ME, Thompson JA: Necrosis of the forearm following radial artery catheterization in a patient with Reye's syndrome. Pediatrics 65:141, 1980
6. Bunner JMR: Handbook of blood pressure monitoring. Littleton, MA: PSG Publishing, 1978
7. Baker RJ, Shunpraph B, Nybrus LN: Severe ischemia of the hand following radial artery catheterization. Surgery 80:449, 1976
8. Cannon BW, Meshier TW: Extremity amputation following radial artery cannulation in a patient with hyperlipoproteinemia type V. Anesthesiology 56:222, 1983
9. Dalton B, Laver MB: Vasospasm with an indwelling radial artery cannula. Anesthesiology 34:194, 1971
10. Davis FM, Stewart JM: Radial artery cannulation: a prospective study of inpatients undergoing cardiothoracic surgery. Br J Anaesth 52:41, 1980
11. Gardner RM, Schwartz R, Wong KC, et al: Percutaneous indwelling radial artery catheters for monitoring cardiovascular function. N Engl J Med 290:1227, 1974
12. Hayes MF, Morello DC, Rosenbaum RW, et al: Radial artery catheterization by cut-down technique. Crit Care Med 1:151, 1973
13. Wilkins RG: Radial artery cannulation and ischaemic damage: a review. Anaesthesia 40:896, 1985
14. Ryan JF, Raines J, Dalton BC, et al: Arterial dynamics of radial artery cannulation. Anesth Analg 52:1017, 1973
15. Allen EV: Thromboangiitis obliterans: methods of diagnosis of chronic occlusive arterial lesions distal to the wrist with illustrative cases. Am J Med Sci 178:237, 1929
16. Coleman SS, Anson BJ: Arterial patterns in the hand based upon a study of 650 specimens. Surg Gynecol Obstet 113:409, 1961
17. Husum B, Palm T: Arterial dominance in the hand. Br J Anaesth 50:913, 1978
18. Bedford RF, Wollman H: Complications of percutaneous radial artery cannulation: an objective prospective study in man. Anesthesiology 38:228, 1971
19. Bedford RF: Radial arterial function following percutaneous cannulation with 18- and 20-gauge catheters. Anesthesiology 47:37, 1977
20. McSwain GR, Ameriks JA: Doppler-improved Allen's test. South Med J 72:1620, 1979
21. Cheng EY, Lauer KK, Stommel KA, et al: Evaluation of the palmar circulation by pulse oximetry. J Clin Monit 5:1, 1989
22. Bedford RF: Long-term radial artery cannulation: effects on subsequent vessel function. Crit Care Med 6:64, 1978
23. Downs JB, Chapman WL, Hawkins IF: Prolonged radial artery catheterization. Anesthesiology 38:283, 1973
24. Palm T: Evaluation of peripheral arterial pressure in the thumb following radial artery cannulation. Br J Anaesth 49:819, 1977
25. Shenoy PN, Leaman DM, Field JM: Safety of short-term percutaneous arterial cannulation. Anesth Analg 58:256, 1979
26. Bedford RF: Wrist circumference predicts the risk of radial arterial occlusion after cannulation. Anesthesiology 51:176, 1979
27. Kim JM, Arakawa K, Bliss J: Arterial cannulation: factors in the development of occlusion. Anesth Analg 54:836, 1975

28. Slogoff S, Keats AS, Arlund C: On the safety of radial artery cannulation. Anesthesiology 59:42, 1983
29. Weiss BM, Gattiker RI: Complications during and following radial artery cannulation: a prospective study. Intensive Care Med 12:424, 1986
30. Bedford RF: Percutaneous radial artery cannulation: increased safety using Teflon catheters. Anesthesiology 42:119, 1975
31. Brown AE, Sweeney DB, Lumley J: Percutaneous radial artery cannulation. Anaesthesia 24:532, 1969
32. Feeley TW: Reestablishment of radial artery patency. Anesthesiology 46:73, 1977
33. Prys-Roberts C: Measurement of intravascular pressure. In Saidman LJ, Smith NT (eds): Monitoring in anesthesia. New York: Wiley, 1978: 64
34. Davis FM: Methods of radial artery cannulation and subsequent arterial occlusion (letter). Anesthesiology 56:331, 1982
35. Jones RM, Hill AB, Nahrwold ML, et al: The effect of method of radial artery cannulation on postcannulation blood flow and thrombus formation. Anesthesiology 55:76, 1981
36. Bedford RF, O'Brien TE: Comparison of bovine lung and porcine intestinal heparin for arterial thrombosis in man. Am J Hosp Pharm 34:936, 1977
37. Downs JB, Rackstein AD, Klein EF, et al: Hazards of radial artery catheterization. Anesthesiology 38:283, 1973
38. Lowenstein E, Little JW III, Lo HH: Prevention of cerebral embolization from flushing radial artery cannulae. N Engl J Med 284:1414, 1971
39. Gardner RM, Bond EL, Clark JS: Safety and efficacy of continuous flush systems for arterial and pulmonary artery catheters. Ann Thorac Surg 23:534, 1977
40. Johnson FW: A complication of radial artery cannulation. Anesthesiology 40:598, 1974
41. Wyatt R, Glaves I, Cooper DJ: Proximal skin necrosis after radial artery cannulation. Lancet 2:1135, 1974
42. Bartlett RM, Munster HW: Brief recording: improved technique for prolonged arterial cannulation. N Engl J Med 279:92, 1968
43. Bedford RF: Removal of radial artery thrombi following percutaneous cannulation for monitoring. Anesthesiology 46:430, 1977
44. Barnes RW, Foster EJ, Janssen GA, et al: Safety of brachial artery catheters as monitors in the intensive care unit: prospective evaluation with the Doppler ultrasonic velocity detector. Anesthesiology 44:260, 1976
45. Moran F, Lorimer AR, Boyd G: Percutaneous arterial catheterization for multiple sampling. Thorax 22:253, 1967
46. Comstock MK, Ellis T, Carter JG, et al: Safety of brachial *versus* radial arterial catheters. Anesthesiology 51:S158, 1979
47. DeAngelis J: Axillary arterial monitoring. Crit Care Med 4: 205, 1976
48. Adler DC, Bryan-Brown CW: Use of the axillary artery for intravascular monitoring. Crit Care Med 1:148, 1973
49. Youngberg JA, Miller ED: Evaluation of percutaneous cannulations of the dorsalis pedis artery. Anesthesiology 44:80, 1976
50. Husum B, Palm T, Eriksen J: Percutaneous cannulation of the dorsalis pedis artery. Br J Anaesth 51:1055, 1979
51. Kaplan JA: Hemodynamic monitoring. In Kaplan JA (ed): Cardiac anesthesia. New York: Grune and Stratton, 1979: 183
52. Moorthy SS: Cannulation of the anterior peroneal artery in adults. Anesth Analg 60:360, 1981
53. Eriksson I, Jorulf H: Surgical complications associated with arterial catheterization. Scand J Thorac Cardiovasc Surg 4:69, 1970
54. Ersoz CJ, Hedden M, Lain L: Prolonged femoral arterial catheterization for intensive care. Anesth Analg 49:160, 1970
55. Soderstrom CA, Wasserman DH, Denham CM, et al: Superiority of the femoral artery for monitoring: a prospective study. Am J Surg 144:309, 1982
56. Colvin MP, Curran JP, Jarvis D, et al: Femoral artery pressure monitoring. Anaesthesia 32:451, 1977
57. Gurman G, Nebler R, Shachar J: The use of alpha-system set for arterial catheterization. Anaesthetist 29:494, 1980
58. Russell RA, Joel M, Hudson RJ, et al: A prospective evaluation of radial and femoral catheterization sites in critically ill patients (abstract). Crit Care Med 9:144, 1981
59. Puri VK, Carlson RW, Bander JJ, et al: Complications of vascular catheterization in the critically ill: a prospective study. Crit Care Med 8:495, 1980
60. Pinella JC, Ross DF, Martin T, et al: Study of the incidence of intravascular catheter infection and associated septicemia in critically ill patients. Crit Care Med 11:21, 1983
61. Davis FM: Bacterial contamination of radial artery catheters. N Z Med J 89:128, 1979
62. Maki DG, Band JD: A comparative study of polyantibiotic and iodophor ointments in prevention of vascular catheter-related infection. Am J Med 70:739, 1981
63. Walton JR, Shapiro BA, Harrison RA, et al: Serratia bacteremia from mean arterial pressure monitors. Anesthesiology 43:113, 1975
64. Stamm WE, Colella JJ, Anderson RL, et al: Indwelling arterial catheters as a source of nosocomial bacteremia: an outbreak caused by *Flavobacterium* species. N Engl J Med 292:1099, 1975
65. Hekker TA, van Overhagen W, Schneider AJ: Pressure transducers: Overlooked source of nosocomial infection. Intensive Care Med 16:511, 1990
66. Donowitz LG, Marsik FJ, Hoyt JW, et al: Serratia marcescens bacteremia from contaminated pressure transducers. JAMA 242:1749, 1979
67. Shinozaki T, Deane RS, Mazuzan JE Jr, et al: Bacterial contamination of arterial lines: a prospective study. JAMA 249: 223, 1983
68. Maki DG, Hassemer CA: Endemic rate of fluid contamination and related septicemia in arterial pressure monitoring. Am J Med 70:733, 1981
69. Band JD, Maki DG: Infections caused by arterial catheters used for hemodynamic monitoring. Am J Med 67:735, 1979
70. Rose HD: Gas gangrene and *Clostridium perfringens* septicemia associated with the use of an indwelling radial arterial catheter. Can Med Assoc J 121:1595, 1979
71. Michaelson ED, Walsh RE: Osler's node: a complication of prolonged arterial cannulation. N Engl J Med 283:472, 1970
72. Dohi S, Naito H: Intraarterial injection of 2.5% thiamylal does cause gangrene (letter). Anesthesiology 59:154, 1983
73. Zweibel FR, Monies-Chas I: Accidental intraarterial injection of ketamine. Anaesthesia 31:1084, 1976
74. Remington JW: Contour changes of the aortic pulse during propagation. Am J Physiol 199:331, 1960
75. Boutros A, Albert S: Effect of the dynamic response of transducer-tubing system on accuracy of direct blood pressure measurement in patients. Crit Care Med 11:124, 1983
76. Shinozaki T, Deane RS, Mazuzan JE, et al: The dynamic responses of liquid-filled catheter systems for direct measurement of blood pressure. Anesthesiology 53:498, 1980
77. Shipley RF, Maruschak GF, Mack S: Pressure measurement error with disposable domes for transducers: brief report. Crit Care Med 12:913, 1984
78. Herbst CA: Indications, management and complications of percutaneous subclavian catheters. Arch Surg 113:1421, 1978
79. Szradjer JI, Zveibil FR, Bitterman H, et al: Central vein catheterization: Failure and complication rates by three percutaneous approaches. Arch Intern Med 146:260, 1986
80. Davidson JT, Ben-Hur N, Nathen H: Subclavian venipuncture. Lancet 2:11349, 1963
81. Smith BE, Modell JH, Gaub ML, et al: Complications of subclavian vein catheterization. Arch Surg 90:228, 1965
82. James PM, Myers RT: Central venous pressure monitoring: complications and a new technique. Am J Surg 39:75, 1973
83. Ryan JA, Abel RM, Abbott WM, et al: Catheter complications in total parenteral nutrition. N Engl J Med 290:757, 1974
84. McEnany MT, Austen WG: Life-threatening hemorrhage from inadvertent cervical arteriotomy. Ann Thorac Surg 24:233, 1977
85. Knoblanche GE: Respiratory obstruction due to hematoma following internal jugular vein cannulation. Anaesthesia and Intensive Care 7:286, 1979
86. Goldfarab G, Lebrec D: Percutaneous cannulation of the internal jugular vein in patients with coagulopathies: an experience based on 1,000 attempts. Anesthesiology 56:321, 1982

87. Jobes DR, Schwartz AJ, Greenhow DE, et al: Safer jugular vein cannulation: recognition of arterial puncture and preferential use of the external jugular route. Anesthesiology 59:353, 1983
88. McDaniel MM, Grossman M: Aortic dissection complicating percutaneous jugular vein catheterization. Anesthesiology 49: 213, 1978
89. Shield CF, Richardson JD, Buckley CF, et al: Pseudoaneurysm of the brachiocephalic arteries: a complication of percutaneous internal jugular vein catheterization. Surgery 78:190, 1975
90. Ullman JI, Stoelting RK: Internal jugular vein location with the ultrasound doppler flow detector. Anesth Analg 57:118, 1978
91. Legler D, Nugent M: Doppler localization of the internal jugular vein facilitates central venous cannulation. Anesthesiology 60: 481, 1984
92. Mallory DL, McGee WT, Shewker TH, et al: Ultrasound guidance improves the success rate of internal jugular vein cannulation. Chest 98:157, 1990
93. English ICW, Frew RM, Pigott JF, et al: Percutaneous catheterization of the internal jugular vein. Anaesthesia 24:521, 1969
94. Rao TLK, Wong AY, Salem MR: A new approach to percutaneous catheterization of the internal jugular vein. Anesthesiology 46:362, 1977
95. Arnold S, Feathers RS, Gibbs E: Bilateral pneumothoraces and subcutaneous emphysema: a complication of internal jugular venipuncture. Br Med J 1:211, 1973
96. Blitt CD, Wright WA: An unusual complication of percutaneous internal jugular vein cannulation: puncture of an endotracheal tube cuff. Anesthesiology 40:306, 1974
97. Butsch JL, Butsch WL, DaRossa JFT: Bilateral vocal cord paralysis: a complication of percutaneous cannulation of the internal jugular veins. Arch Surg 111:828, 1976
98. Parikh RK: Horner's syndrome: a complication of percutaneous cannulation of the internal jugular vein. Anaesthesia 27:327, 1972
99. Briscoe CE, Bushman JA, McDonald WI: Extensive neurological damage after cannulation of internal jugular vein. Br Med J 1: 314, 1974
100. Stock CM, Downs JB: Transient phrenic nerve blockade during internal jugular vein cannulation using the anterolateral approach. Anesthesiology 57:230, 1982
101. Kashuk JL: Air embolism after central venous catheterization. Surg Gynecol Obstet 159:249, 1984
102. Durant TM, Oppenheimer MJ, Lynch PR, et al: Body position in relation to venous air embolism: a roentgenologic study. Am J Med Sci 227:509, 1954
103. Blitt CD, Wright WA, Petty WC, et al: Central venous catheterization via the external jugular vein: a technique employing the J-wire. JAMA 229:817, 1974
104. Dietel M, McIntyre JA: Radiographic confirmation of site of central venous pressure catheters. Can J Surg 14:42, 1971
105. Malatinsky J, Kadlic M, Majec M, et al: Misplacement and loop formation of central venous catheters. Acta Anaesthesiol Scand 20:237, 1976
106. Teba L, Zakaria M, Schiebel F: Guide wire complication during central vein catheterization (letter). Anesth Analg 64:460, 1985
107. Schwartz AJ, Horrow JC, Jobes DR, et al: Guide wires: a caution. Crit Care Med 9:347, 1981
108. Smith SL, Albin MS, Ritter RR, Bunegin L: CVP catheter guide. Anesthesiology 60:238, 1984
109. Webre DR, Arens JF: Use of cephalic and basilic veins for introduction of central venous catheters. Anesthesiology 38: 389, 1973
110. Burgess GE, Marino RJ, Peuler MJ: Effect of head position in the location of venous catheters inserted by basilic veins. Anesthesiology 46:212, 1977
111. Bowdle TA: Improved technique for placement of Sorenson CVP catheters (letter). Anesth Analg 63:1143, 1984
112. Greenall JM, Blewitt RW, McMahon MJ: Cardiac tamponade and central venous catheters. Br Med J 2:595, 1975
113. Maschke SP, Rogove HJ: Cardiac tamponade associated with a multilumen central venous catheter. Crit Care Med 12:611, 1984
114. Jay AWL, Aldridge HE: Perforation of the heart or vena cava by central venous catheters inserted for monitoring or infusion therapy. Can Med Assoc J 135:1143, 1986
115. Eichold BH, Berryman CR: Contralateral hydrothorax: an unusual complication of central venous catheter placement. Anesthesiology 62:673, 1985
116. Ghani GA, Berry AJ: Right hydrothorax after left external jugular vein catheterization. Anesthesiology 58:93, 1983
117. Gravenstein N, Blackshear RH: In vitro evaluation of relative perforating potential of central venous catheters: comparison of materials, selected models, number of lumens and angles of incidence to simulated membrane. J Clin Monit 7:1, 1991
118. Ponce de Leon S, Critchley S, Wenzel RP: Polymicrobial bloodstream infections related to prolonged vascular catheterization. Crit Care Med 12:856, 1984
119. Damen J, Verhoef J, Bolton DT, et al: Microbiologic risk of invasive hemodynamic monitoring in patients undergoing open-heart operations. Crit Care Med 13:548, 1985
120. Maki DG, Goldman DA, Rhame FS: Infection control in intravenous therapy. Ann Intern Med 79:867, 1973
121. Centers for Disease Control: Guidelines for the prevention of intravascular infections. In Farber B (ed): Infection control in intensive care. New York: Churchill Livingstone, 1987: 50
122. Cooper GL, Hopkins CC: Rapid diagnosis of intravascular catheter-associated infection by direct gram staining of catheter segments. N Engl J Med 312:1141, 1985
123. Civetta JM, Gabel JC, Laver MB: Disparate ventricular function in surgical patients. Surg Forum 22:522, 1971
124. Quinn K, Quebbeman EJ: Pulmonary artery pressure monitoring in the surgical intensive care unit. Arch Surg 116:872, 1981
125. Forrester JS, Diamond G, McHugh TJ, et al: Filling pressures in the right and left sides of the heart in acute myocardial infarction. N Engl J Med 285:190, 1971
126. Nagai K, Kemmotsu O: An inadvertent insertion of a Swan-Ganz catheter into the intrathecal space. Anesthesiology 62: 848, 1985
127. Ellison N, Jobes DR, Schwartz AJ: Cannulation of the internal jugular vein: a cautionary note. Anesthesiology 55:336, 1981
128. Carlon GC, Howland WS, Kahn RC, et al: Unusual complications during pulmonary artery catheterization. Crit Care Med 6:364, 1978
129. Conohan TJ III: Air embolization during percutaneous Swan-Ganz catheter placement. Anesthesiology 50:360, 1979
130. Horrow JC, Laucks SO: Coronary air embolism during venous cannulation. Anesthesiology 56:212, 1982
131. Doblar DD, Hinkle JC, Marshall LF, et al: Air embolism associated with pulmonary artery catheter introducer kit. Anesthesiology 56:307, 1982
132. Bristow A, Batjer H, Chow W, et al: Air embolism via a pulmonary artery catheter introducer (letter). Anesthesiology 63: 340, 1985
133. Frankhouser PL: Air embolism via a pulmonary artery catheter introducer (reply). Anesthesiology 63:341, 1985
134. Lunn JK, Stanley TH, Webster LR, et al: Arterial blood-pressure and pulse-rate responses to pulmonary and radial arterial catheterization prior to cardiac and major vascular operations. Anesthesiology 51:265, 1979
135. Barash PG, Kopriva CJ: Anesthesia for cardiac surgery. In Glenn WWL, Bave AE, Geha AS, et al (eds): Thoracic and cardiovascular surgery. 4th ed. New York: Appleton, 1982: 1076
136. Waller JL, Zaidan JR, Kaplan JA, et al: Hemodynamic responses to preoperative vascular cannulation in patients with coronary artery disease. Anesthesiology 56:219, 1982
137. Sprung CL, Pozen RG, Rozanski JJ, et al: Advanced ventricular arrhythmias during bedside pulmonary artery catheterization. Am J Med 72:203, 1982
138. Cairns JA, Holder D: Ventricular fibrillation due to passage of a Swan-Ganz catheter. Am J Cardiol 35:589, 1975
139. Salmenpera M, Petola K, Rosenberg P: Does prophylactic lidocaine control cardiac arrhythmias associated with pulmonary artery catheterization? Anesthesiology 56:212, 1982
140. Keusch DJ, Winters S, Thys DM: The patient's position influences the incidence of dysrhythmias during pulmonary artery catheterization. Anesthesiology 70:582, 1989

141. Luck JC, Engel TR: Transient right bundle branch block with Swan-Ganz catheterization. Am Heart J 92:263, 1976
142. Thompson IR, Dalton BC, Lappas DG, et al: Right bundle-branch block and complete heart block caused by Swan-Ganz catheter. Anesthesiology 51:359, 1979
143. Castellanos A, Ramirez AV, Mayorga-Cortes A, et al: Left fascicular blocks during right-heart catheterization using the Swan-Ganz catheter. Circulation 64:1271, 1981
144. Sprung CL, Elser B, Schein RMH, et al: Risk of right bundle branch block and complete heart block during pulmonary artery catheterization. Crit Care Med 17:1, 1989
145. Wilson SW, Moorthy SS, Mahomed Y, et al: Catheter doubling in left main pulmonary artery (letter). Anesthesiology 60:266, 1984
146. Daum S, Schapira M: Intracardiac knot formation in a Swan-Ganz catheter. Anesth Analg 52:862, 1973
147. Mond HG, Dwight WC, Nesbitt SJ, et al: A technique for unknotting an intracardiac flow-directed balloon catheter. Chest 67:731, 1975
148. Thomas HA: The knotted Swan-Ganz catheter: a safer solution (letter). Am J Radiol 138:986, 1982
149. Kelly TF Jr, Morris GC Jr, Crawford ES, et al: Perforation of the pulmonary artery with Swan-Ganz catheter. Ann Surg 193: 686, 1981
150. Paulson DM, Scott SM, Sethi GK: Pulmonary hemorrhage associated with balloon flotation catheters: a report of a case and review of the literature. J Thorac Cardiovasc Surg 80:453, 1980
151. Rosenbaum L, Rosenbaum SH, Askanazi J, et al: Small amounts of hemoptysis as an early warning sign of pulmonary artery rupture by a pulmonary arterial catheter. Crit Care Med 9:319, 1981
152. McDaniel DD, Stone JG, Faltas AN, et al: Catheter-induced pulmonary artery hemorrhage: diagnosis and management in cardiac operations. J Thorac Cardiovasc Surg 82:1, 1981
153. Hannan AT, Brown M, Bigman O: Pulmonary artery catheter-induced hemorrhage. Chest 85:128, 1984
154. Harady JF, Morisset M, Taillefer J, et al: Pathophysiology of rupture of the pulmonary artery by pulmonary artery balloon-tipped catheters. Anesth Analg 62:925, 1983
155. Barash PG, Nardi D, Hammond G, et al: Catheter-induced pulmonary artery perforation: mechanisms, management and modifications. J Thorac Cardiovasc Surg 82:5, 1981
156. Johnston WE, Royster RL, Choplin RH, et al: Pulmonary artery catheter migration during cardiac surgery. Anesthesiology 64: 258, 1986
157. Willis CW, Wight D, Zidulka A: Hypotension secondary to balloon inflation of a pulmonary artery catheter. Crit Care Med 12:915, 1984
158. Traeger SM: 'Failure to wedge' and pulmonary hypertension during pulmonary artery catheterization: a sign of totally occlusive pulmonary embolism. Crit Care Med 13:544, 1985
159. Hoar PF, Stone JG, Wicks AE, et al: Thrombogenesis associated with Swan-Ganz catheters. Anesthesiology 48:445, 1978
160. Yorra FH, Oblath R, Jaffe H, et al: Massive thrombosis associated with use of the Swan-Ganz catheter. Chest 65:682, 1974
161. Foote GA, Schabel SI, Hodges M: Pulmonary complications of the flow-directed balloon-tipped catheter. N Engl J Med 209: 927, 1974
162. Chastre J, Cornud F, Bouchama A, et al: Thrombosis as a complication of pulmonary-artery catheterization via the internal jugular vein. N Engl J Med 306:278, 1982
163. Dye LE, Segall PH, Russell RO Jr, et al: Deep venous thrombosis of the upper extremity associated with use of the Swan-Ganz catheter. Chest 73:673, 1978
164. Lange HW, Galliani CA, Edwards JE: Local complication associated with indwelling Swan-Ganz catheters: autopsy study of 36 cases. Am J Cardiol 52:1108, 1983
165. Kim YL, Richman KA, Marshall BE: Thrombocytopenia associated with Swan-Ganz catheterization in patients. Anesthesiology 53:262, 1980
166. Hoar, PF, Wilson RM, Mangano DT, et al: Heparin bonding reduces thrombogenicity of pulmonary artery catheters. N Engl J Med 305:993, 1981
167. Feinberg BI, LaMantia KR, Addonizio VP, et al: Swan-Ganz catheter associated thrombocytopenia: effects of heparin coating. Anesthesiology 61:A101, 1984
168. Boyd KD, Thomas SJ, Gold J, et al: A prospective study of complications of pulmonary artery catheterizations in 500 consecutive patients. Chest 84:245, 1983
169. Elliott CG, Zimmerman GA, Clemmer TP: Complications of pulmonary artery catheterization in the care of critically ill patients. Chest 76:647, 1979
170. Applefeld JJ, Caruthers TE, Reno DJ, et al: Assessment of the sterility of long-term cardiac catheterization using thermodilution Swan-Ganz catheter. Chest 74:377, 1978
171. Michel L, Marsh M, McMichan JC, et al: Infection of pulmonary artery catheters in critically ill patients. JAMA 245:1032, 1981
172. Sise MJ, Hollingsworth P, Brimm JE, et al: Complications of the flow-directed pulmonary artery catheter: a prospective analysis in 219 patients. Crit Care Med 9:315, 1981
173. Bessette MC, Quinton L, Whalley DG, et al: Swan-Ganz catheter contamination: a protective sleeve for repositioning. Can Anaesth Soc J 28:86, 1981
174. King EG: Influence of mechanical ventilation and pulmonary disease on pulmonary artery pressure monitoring. Can Med Assoc J 121:901, 1979
175. Hobelmann CF Jr, Smith DE, Vergilio RW, et al: Left atrial and pulmonary artery wedge pressure difference with positive end-expiratory pressure. Surg Forum 25:232, 1974
176. Kane PB, Askanazi J, Neville JF Jr, et al: Artifacts in the measurement of pulmonary artery wedge pressure. Crit Care Med 6:36, 1978
177. Downs JB: A technique for direct measurement of intrapleural pressure. Crit Care Med 4:207, 1976
178. DeCampo T, Civetta JM: The effect of short-term discontinuation of high-level PEEP in patients with acute respiratory failure. Crit Care Med 7:47, 1979
179. Schmitt EA, Brantigan CO: Common artifacts of pulmonary artery and pulmonary wedge pressure: recognition and interpretation. J Clin Monit 2:44, 1986
180. Robotham JL, Lixfeld W, Holland L, et al: The effects of positive end-expiratory pressure on right and left ventricular performance. Am Rev Respir Dis 121:677, 1980
181. Benumof JL, Saidman LJ, Arkin DB, et al: Where pulmonary artery catheters go: intrathoracic distribution. Anesthesiology 46:336, 1977
182. Shasby DW, Dauber IM, Pfister S, et al: Swan-Ganz catheter location and left atrial pressure determine the accuracy of the wedge pressure when positive end-expiratory pressure is used. Chest 80:666, 1981
183. Harris AP, Miller CF, Beattie C, et al: The slowing of sinus rhythm during thermodilution cardiac output determination and the effect of altering injectate temperature. Anesthesiology 63:540, 1985
184. Elkayam U, Berkley R, Azen S, et al: Cardiac output by thermodilution technique: effect of injectate's volume and temperature on accuracy and reproducibility in the critically ill patient. Chest 84:418, 1983
185. Badenhorst CC: Proximal port dysfunction in pulmonary artery catheters inserted from the right subclavian vein (letter). Anesthesiology 62:546, 1985

FURTHER READING

Bedford RF: Invasive blood pressure monitoring. In: Blitt CD (ed): Monitoring in anesthesia and critical care. 2nd ed. New York: Churchill Livingstone, 1990: 93

Gardner RM: System concepts for invasive pressure monitoring. In Civetta JM, Taylor RW, Kirby RR (eds): Critical care. 2nd ed. Philadelphia: JB Lippincott, 1992: 247

Gravenstein N: Invasive vascular monitoring. In Gravenstein N (ed): Manual of complications during anesthesia. Philadelphia: JB Lippincott, 1991: 253

Varon AJ: Hemodynamic monitoring: arterial and pulmonary artery catheters. In Civetta JM, Taylor RW, Kirby RR (eds): Critical care. 2nd ed. Philadelphia: JB Lippincott, 1992: 255

Venus B, Mallory DL: Vascular cannulation. In Civetta JM, Taylor RW, Kirby RR (eds): Critical care. 2nd ed. Philadelphia: JB Lippincott, 1992: 149

Complications in Anesthesiology, second edition,
edited by Nikolaus Gravenstein and Robert R. Kirby.
Lippincott-Raven Publishers, Philadelphia © 1996.

CHAPTER 10

Temperature: Homeostasis and Unintentional Hypothermia

Unlike other chapters in this book, Section 1 of this chapter deals not with specific complications but rather with normal physiology and serves as an introduction to abnormal temperature regulation, described in Section 2. Temperature regulation in mammals, including humans, involves two types of physiologic functions: behavioral or "voluntary," which is usually conscious, and autonomic or "involuntary," which is usually subconscious.[1,2]

Section 1:
NORMAL HOMEOSTASIS

Werner E. Flacke
Joan W. Flacke

BEHAVIORAL RESPONSES

Behavioral responses include changes of body posture, locomotion, nest-building by animals, and construction of houses by humans, including technological extensions such as heating and air conditioning. Behavioral activities are most important for temperature homeostasis, a fact that may surprise many readers, because, accustomed as we are to seeing them in everyday life, we usually do not consider their significance in thermoregulation.

Humans and beasts come in from the cold if they can, and many languages have expressions meaning that not to do so exemplifies lack of intelligence. Characteristic body postures take place for heat conservation and heat dissipation. A patient whose body temperature is below the "set point" curls up with knees flexed and extremities close to the body, in a fetal position. Conversely, a patient whose body temperature is higher than the set point stretches out, with extremities widely extended.

The purpose of these postures is to minimize or maximize surface area and thus heat dissipation. These postures do not indicate body temperature per se; they indicate only its relation to the set point.[2] If a patient has an elevated temperature, observation of posture permits recognition of whether the temperature already has reached a peak or whether it is still rising. Although these behavioral temperature-related activities are interesting to examine, such study may not be productive in the operating room because anesthetics obliterate patient volition.

INVOLUNTARY RESPONSES

Involuntary responses involve autonomic functions, such as cutaneous vasoconstriction, nonmuscular thermogenesis or skin vasodilation, and increased sweating. They also include some processes usually not considered to be autonomic, such as the use of skeletal muscles for heat production through increased muscle tone and shivering. Of course, this apparently voluntary use of muscle is not really voluntary and is often even subconscious. Heat generation by brown fat tissue plays the most important role in nonshivering thermogenesis in infants until 3 months of age.[3]

THE THERMOREGULATORY SYSTEM

The basic components of the thermoregulatory system are shown in Figure 10-1 and are summarized in Table 10-1.

Afferent Systems

Peripheral "Sensors"

Until relatively recently, peripheral temperature receptors were assumed not to play any significant role in the maintenance of constant body temperature. This assumption was based on studies in which the properties of these receptors were deduced only from subjective sensations of temperature described by human subjects. Of course, humans have no built-in "thermometer" calibrated on an absolute scale. Temperature sensation changes with time and is influenced by other factors (such as attention, experience, and emotions). These

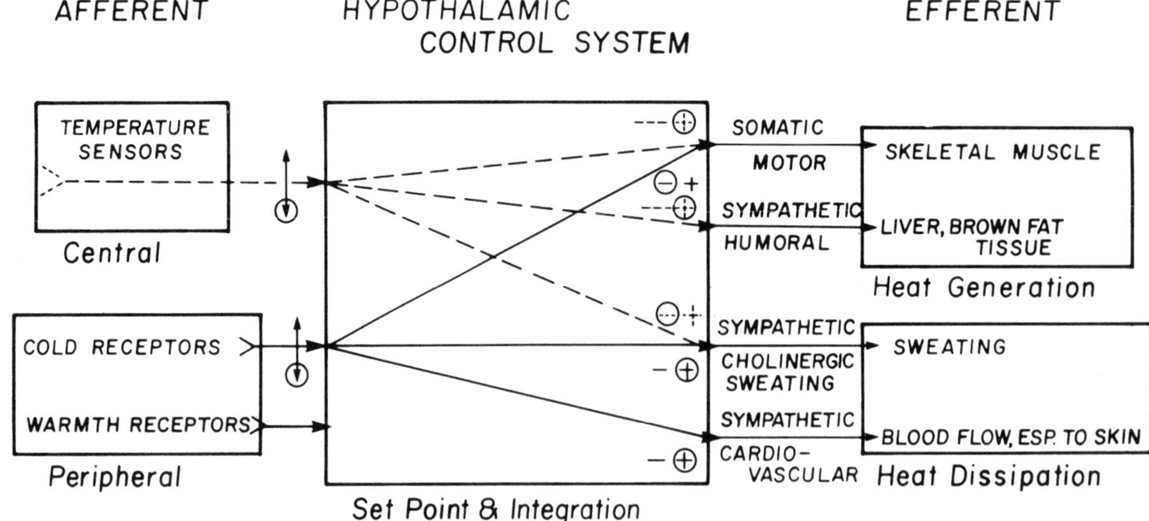

FIGURE 10-1. The 3 main components of the thermoregulatory systems: afferent, sensory input from the periphery (cold and warmth receptors) and from the anterior hypothalamus; the "integrating and regulating" central system, with its main neuronal networks located in the anterior and the posterior hypothalamus; and the efferent or motor systems, subserving heat generation and heat dissipation. No attempt is made to indicate details of the network that must possess feedback circuits and involve several neurohumoral systems; rather, the effects of changes in afferent inputs on various parts of the efferent system are shown. *Upward arrows*, increase or *downward arrows*, decrease in afferent input (downward arrows are circled for easier identification of changes on the efferent side brought about by afferent changes); *solid* and *dashed lines*, connections between inputs and outputs, to facilitate recognition of related changes. For clarity, no connections have been drawn between the input from warmth receptors and the efferent system.

subjective sensations do not directly reflect the magnitude of the signal coming from the sensors; they are likely to be modulated by central processing.

That peripheral reception is indeed important was proven first by Hensel and Zotterman in 1949, when they measured the frequency of firing of single afferent nerve fibers while controlling the temperature at the site where the corresponding receptor was located.[4] They found that temperature receptors are calibrated on an absolute scale, and that they "report" the local temperature without change, as long as this temperature remains constant. (That a transient "overshoot" occurs when local temperature is changed rapidly is unimportant in this context.) Cold and warm receptors were found; the former respond with increased frequency of discharge to decreasing temperature, and the latter respond in the reverse manner.

TABLE 10-1
Components of the Thermoregulatory System

AFFERENT OR "TEMPERATURE SENSORS"

- Peripheral (in skin, mucosa, and deep tissues)
- Central (located in the anterior hypothalamus and other CNS structures)

EFFERENT OR "MOTOR SYSTEMS"

- Heat-generating mechanisms
- Heat-dissipating mechanisms

CONTROL SYSTEM

- Neuronal network in the posterior hypothalamus

These observations, confirmed and greatly extended since 1949, have made possible (indeed, mandatory) the assignment of a role in body temperature homeostasis to these peripheral sensors. The density of temperature receptors varies among different parts of the body. Some skin areas (such as the fingertips and circumoral areas) are much more richly endowed than most, whereas others have less than the average. Assignment of weighting factors to the various peripheral areas has not been possible, but the weighted, integrated peripheral temperature input is postulated to be one of the most important inputs for temperature regulation.

Central "Sensors"

Since about 1885 certain areas of the brain have been known to play a prominent role in temperature regulation; for example, electric or mechanical stimulation of the corpus striatum caused marked increases in body temperature in many species. A distinct area in the anterior hypothalamus is temperature sensitive. Localized cooling of this area causes an increase in body temperature; heating has the opposite effect.

The electric activity of single neurons recorded in the same area changes systematically, either with only local temperature or with both local and peripheral temperatures.[5,6] Controversy continues over whether at least some of these neurons are indeed sensory end organs for temperature or whether they are simply interneurons with a high temperature coefficient. Temperature in the anterior hypothalamus is the dominant factor in the regulation of body temperature.

Efferent Systems

The efferent systems serve as effector mechanisms for temperature regulation and consist of heat-generating and heat-dissipating components, although none serves exclusively for thermoregulation.

Heat-generating Mechanisms

All chemical processes in the body release heat as a by-product. The magnitude of the chemical process is usually determined by factors other than thermoregulation. However, some chemical processes other than those in skeletal muscles can be activated specifically for thermoregulatory purposes. These processes involve mainly brown fat tissues and are probably mediated by β-adrenergic hormones.

Although nonshivering heat production has long been known, only more recently has detailed information been elucidated about the location, control mechanisms (central and peripheral), and importance (physiologic and pathophysiologic) of brown fat in nonshivering thermogenesis. Differences exist among species, and most current information has been derived from observations in animals. Yet the brown-fat mechanism probably plays an important role in human temperature regulation as well.

Even more interesting is the possibility that brown fat may play a major role in the regulation of energy balance. The mitochondria of brown-fat tissue are unique in their physiologic ability to uncouple electron transport from oxidative phosphorylation and thus uncouple energy production from energy utilization.[3,7] Nevertheless, the main "engine" for heat generation is the skeletal muscle, which can increase heat generation by four- to fivefold.

Heat-dissipating Mechanisms

Heat dissipation is accomplished by evaporation of water and by vasodilation of skin vessels, with resultant radiation and conductive heat loss to the environment (Fig. 10-2). Some water diffuses through the intact skin, but the major proportion is produced by sweat glands innervated by cholinergic nerves that belong, anatomically, to the sympathetic nervous system. Evaporation of moisture from the airways also plays a role, but humans are unique among primates in not using respiration to any recognizable extent for thermoregulatory purposes. Overall, total heat-dissipating capacity roughly equals heat-generating capacity.[8] This balance is not surprising; any engineer who designed a temperature control system suitable for a wide range of environmental temperatures, with unequal overall heating and cooling capacities, would not have a job for long.

The cardiovascular system plays a far greater role in temperature regulation than just that of regulating skin perfusion. It is responsible for heat distribution from sites of generation to other tissues and for transport from the body core to the surfaces, where dissipation takes place.

Control Systems

Occasionally, the term "center" is used to describe an anatomic location in the central nervous system (CNS) where mechanical, electric, or chemical interventions can affect the central thermoregulatory system. However, this term cannot be understood literally to mean the anatomic locations where nerve cells that are involved in thermoregulatory functions are concentrated. Actually, a center is simply a location at which contact can be made with these neurons.

In the case of biochemical or pharmacologic observations, the contact areas likely represent the location of synaptic junctions in the neuronal network that makes up the regulatory system. For electrophysiologic observations, especially single-unit recordings, the contact site may be in or near the neuronal cell body or close to axonal or dendritic extensions. Thus, all centers are only one part of a neuronal network, with connections reaching into many parts of the CNS that are never mentioned in conjunction with temperature regulation.

The operation of the temperature-regulating system is depicted in Figure 10-3.[8]

Heat Dissipation

Heat dissipation begins only when the central temperature rises above 37.1°C but increases very sharply with increasing

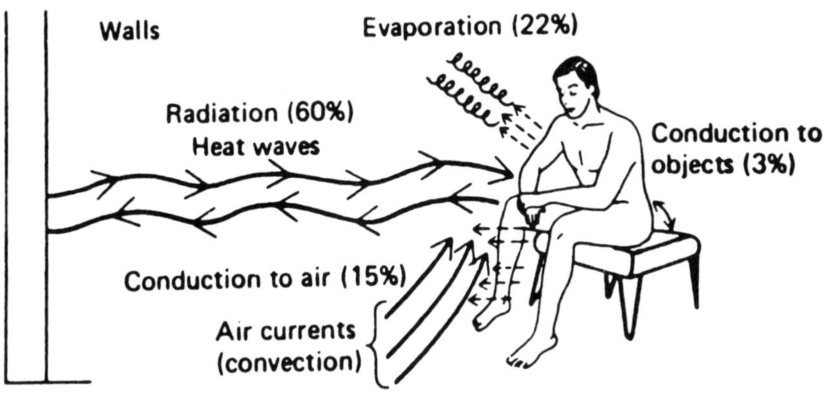

FIGURE 10-2. Mechanisms of heat loss from the body. (Guyton AC: Textbook of medical physiology. Philadelphia: WB Saunders, 1986: 850.)

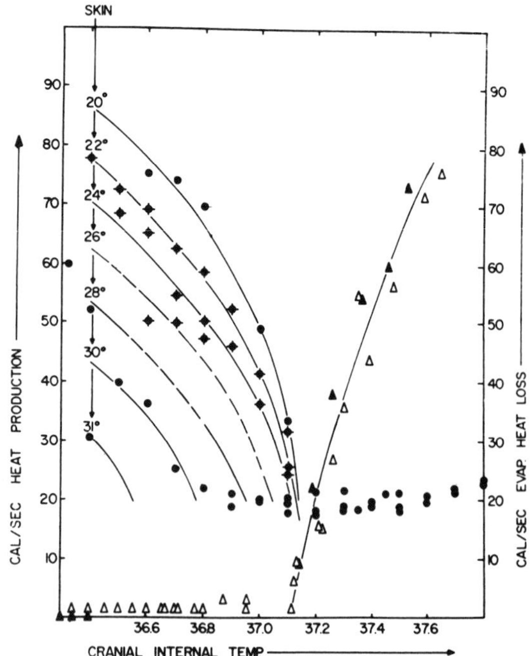

FIGURE 10-3. Influence of changes in central and peripheral temperature on heat production and evaporative heat dissipation: summary of the observations made in one volunteer. Central temperature was measured by a tympanic thermometer, and skin temperature and heat dissipation were measured by a rapidly responding calorimeter. Heat generation was calculated from continuously recorded oxygen uptake. Temperature "loads" consisted of ingestion of cold water and served to drive central and peripheral temperature apart. (Benzinger TH, et al: The thermostatic control of human metabolic heat production. Proc Natl Acad Sci U S A 47:730, 1961.)

central temperature and is apparently insensitive to skin temperature. For an increase of 0.5°C in central temperature, from 37.1° to 37.6°C, heat loss is quadrupled, from about 20 to nearly 80 calories per second. Throughout this range, heat generation remains at or near the lowest observed level, presumably at a basal level, with an increment due to the increased enzyme activity resulting from increased body temperature (van't Hoff's law). The increased metabolism required to support activation of the evaporative heat-dissipating system (eg, increased blood flow and sweat gland activity) also raises heat generation above the basal level.

Heat Generation

When central temperature falls or, rather, is forced by experimental measures below 37.1°C, heat generation rises nearly as sharply with falling central temperature as does heat dissipation with rising central temperature. Unlike heat dissipation, input from skin temperature clearly occurs and affects both the internal temperature at which heat generation begins and the magnitude of increase in heat generation per degree of decrease of central temperature. The value to which the central temperature is permitted to drop before the regulatory system begins counteracting the decrease is directly proportional to the level of the skin temperature. In other words, the integrated skin temperature determines the sensitivity of the central regulatory system. Thus, the critical central temperature for initiation of either heat generation or heat dissipation is the set-point temperature. A central temperature above the set point results in heat dissipation, whereas a lower central temperature results in heat generation.[1,2,8,9]

Humoral Agents

Several humoral agents have been implicated as central mediators in thermoregulation. However, two points should be kept in mind regarding research in this area. First, even localized application of these substances to specific areas often involves quantities and volumes that guarantee that a large number of synaptic junctions will be affected; very likely even closely spaced synapses mediate processes or events of opposite functional significance. Second, although the "wiring" of the temperature control system is likely to be similar in principle among species, the transmitters or mediators possibly differ from one species to another, both in the periphery and likely in the CNS as well. Thus, extrapolation of findings from one species to another, especially to humans, is risky.

Catecholamines.
High concentrations of norepinephrine and other catecholamines are found throughout the hypothalamus. Histochemical studies indicate that their location is predominantly presynaptic (ie, in axonal terminals or nerve endings). Local injection in the anterior hypothalamus causes hypothermia in a neutral or cold environment in several species, including monkeys. The action of drugs such as the tricyclic antidepressant agents that inhibit reuptake of norepinephrine into the nerve endings imitates injection of the amine. Thus, norepinephrine may play a role in activating heat-dissipating processes.[10,11]

5-Hydroxytryptamine.
The effects of norepinephrine are opposed by those of 5-hydroxytryptamine. Microinjection into the anterior hypothalamus causes increased body temperature in several species, including monkeys.[2,10] When unanesthetized animals are exposed to cold, as investigators try to increase their heat generation, increased concentrations of 5-hydroxytryptamine are found in fluid perfusing through the same CNS area in which 5-hydroxytryptamine injection is effective.

Acetylcholine.
Carbachol, the acetylcholine analogue that is not as rapidly hydrolyzed as acetylcholine, has been found to prompt thermoregulatory responses when microinjections were made in several sites in the hypothalamus. These effects are blocked by atropine and are thus "cholinergic–muscarinic" in nature. Atropine, given locally or injected into the ventricular system, causes hypothermia in a cold environment.[10,12] Acetylcholine is effective only when given with or after physostigmine, which decreases cholinesterase activity.

These findings suggest that acetylcholine is the transmitter at several synaptic junctions of neuronal pathways involved in temperature regulation. If all of these sites are blocked by atropine, hypothermia follows when the ambient temperature is low. Hyperthermia is often seen in atropine or scopolamine poisoning. Usually little information about ambient temperature is available in such cases, but because hyperthermia is not reported invariably, probably it is seen only when ambient temperature is high.

Prostaglandin E_1

When injected in minute amounts (20 to 30 μg) into the anterior hypothalamus, prostaglandin E_1 causes marked hyperthermia,[9,12] which has all of the hallmarks of a temperature increase caused by an increase in the set point. As a result, when ambient temperature is high enough to raise body temperature, vasoconstriction, rather than vasodilation and heat loss, occurs.

Shivering takes place when active heat generation is needed to raise body temperature in a cold environment. Also, thermal stimuli at the new elevated temperature, such as ingestion of cold water, elicit a thermoregulatory response, just as they would at normal temperature. In other words, the body is regulated with respect to the set point raised by prostaglandin E_1 with intact thermoregulation, a characteristic of the febrile state. Therefore, the suggestion has been made that prostaglandin E_1 is a mediator in the fever production elicited by exotoxins, endotoxins, or other pyrogens.[9,12]

This thesis, though very attractive because it accounts for the temperature-lowering effect of anti-inflammatory antipyretic agents such as acetylsalicylic acid (aspirin), which are known to inhibit formation of prostaglandins, has not been confirmed by all investigators. These humoral agents, with the exception of acetylcholine, act only when they make contact with sites in the anterior hypothalamus. They have been proposed therefore as "transmitters" in synaptic junctions between peripheral or central temperature sensors and the neuronal network subserving temperature regulation (eg, the set point).[5]

Sodium–Calcium Balance

Perfusion of the posterior hypothalamus near the mammillary bodies with an artificial cerebrospinal fluid that has high concentrations of sodium or calcium ions or that contains a calcium-chelating agent such as ethylenediamine tetraacetate effects a temperature change.[13] No temperature changes occur when the anterior hypothalamus is thus perfused.

A high concentration of calcium reduces body temperature while leaving thermoregulation intact, and a high concentration of sodium or reduction of ionized calcium by chelating agents increases body temperature in the same fashion. Thus, these conditions of the extracellular ionic environment may also be described as a resetting of the set point but in a different location in the CNS. Fever induced by toxins or pyrogens seems to be accompanied by appropriate ionic changes in the hypothalamic extracellular fluid.

Endogenous Opioids

Since their discovery, the possibility has been investigated that endogenous opioids, mainly β-endorphin and the enkephalins, are involved in the central thermoregulatory mechanisms. Evidence implicates their involvement; however, the question of species differences must be answered before any conclusions concerning humans can be drawn.[14]

Summary

Regardless of the many known details involved in temperature regulation (such as mediators and ion ratios), in fact we have no real understanding of the nature of the underlying biologic mechanisms. How is the set-point temperature defined? How are deviations of body temperatures from the set point detected? How are these differences translated into efferent signals to thermoregulatory "motor" systems that serve to return body temperature to the set point? Mechanisms can be suggested, but we do not even know if these mechanisms are mainly electrophysiologic or biochemical.

DRUG ACTIONS

The actions of drugs may be considered in the same sequence as the physiologic aspects of body temperature regulation are discussed: in terms of their actions on the afferent or sensory system, the efferent or motor system, and the central processing apparatus. Of course, any drug may have effects on more than one site, but in general, a drug's actions on body temperature are most prominent and important at a single site.

Afferent Effects

We do not know whether centrally acting drugs act on the temperature-sensitive structures in the anterior hypothalamus. With regard to the peripheral sensors, locally applied menthol increases ("sensitizes") the frequency of firing of cold receptors. Systemic administration of large doses of menthol also increases body temperature, as theory suggests. On the other hand, increased local carbon dioxide concentration reduces the activity of cold receptors; for some time carbon dioxide baths have been known to induce a sensation of warmth out of proportion to the bath temperature. We are not aware of any reliable studies of the effect of carbon dioxide baths on body temperature.

Much new information has become available concerning another substance that exerts powerful effects, mainly on afferent temperature receptors. This agent is capsaicin, the active ingredient of paprika, well known for its use in Hungarian cooking. Application of capsaicin to the skin or mucous membranes elicits a strong sensation of warmth and a lowering of body temperature. Local application of capsaicin affects both sodium and potassium currents; an injection into a peripheral sensory nerve blocks axonal transport mechanisms. Prolonged treatment of young animals destroys the afferent system in the areas where it has been applied and the entire sensory apparatus when it is given systemically. Intrathecal application causes profound depletion of substance P.[15]

Efferent Effects

Drugs acting on the efferent thermoregulatory mechanisms limit the range of temperature loads that the body can tolerate without recourse to behavioral actions. For example, neuromuscular blocking agents, so commonly used by anesthesiologists, block only muscle heat generation. Their quaternary ammonium structure prevents penetration of the blood–brain barrier; thus, these agents have no "central" effect. Not unexpectedly, these drugs do not alter body temperature unless heat generation by muscle is needed to maintain a normal value.

The peripheral effect of atropine, the inhibition of sweating, greatly decreases the body's capacity to dissipate heat and reduces toleration of high heat loads. This effect must be considered in locations with high ambient temperatures or when significant heat generation occurs. The thermal effects of most drugs can be derived similarly, once their general pharmacologic actions are known.

Central Effects

General anesthetic agents probably act centrally, although we are not aware of a single complete analysis of the mechanism and site of action of a specific agent. The action may be specific for thermoregulatory systems, affecting the sensor mechanisms in the anterior hypothalamus, the regulatory mechanisms in the posterior hypothalamus, or the central mechanisms subserving the efferent, thermoregulatory peripheral systems. General anesthetics induce neither hypothermia nor hyperthermia; they only depress the regulatory system. The direction of change in body temperature depends on the environment: in air-cooled operating rooms, hypothermia is, of course, the usual problem, but in tropical countries where modern air conditioning is not prevalent, hyperthermia is still the most common and most serious problem during general anesthesia.

Deliberate Hypothermia

A clinical example of the use of centrally acting drugs is deliberate hypothermia. The important point to be remembered during induction of hypothermia is the need to attenuate or block thermoregulation. If this process is not sufficient, activation of the powerful heat-generating mechanisms will result in increased oxygen consumption and therefore additional loads on the respiratory and circulatory systems. Because deliberate hypothermia is most commonly used in critically ill patients, this additional stress is hardly inconsequential. Thus, induction of hypothermia should not begin until the patient's central temperature regulation has been sufficiently blocked.

This process requires deep anesthesia, if only general anesthetic agents are used, or lighter levels of anesthesia, if more specific inhibitors of central thermoregulation are also used. One such specific inhibitor is chlorpromazine. From about 1950 to 1955, the French pioneers of *hibernation artificiel* used a mixture of agents, commonly referred to as *cocktail lytique*, consisting of promethazine, chlorpromazine, and meperidine. The central actions of the phenothiazines and the action of the narcotic analgesic agent probably were additive or perhaps synergistic in the thermoregulatory-blocking action of the mixture.

Antipyretic Agents

A few comments are pertinent regarding the mechanism of action of the antipyretic agents, the prototype of which is aspirin. These agents do not induce hypothermia but act only to reduce an elevated body temperature; they reset the set point.[16] In monkeys, high doses of salicylates also reduce the magnitude of the increase in body temperature brought about by exposure to a very high ambient temperature.[17] These observations demonstrate that antipyretic agents have an effect in the presence of a normal set point. However, the doses required are much larger (>25 mg/kg) than those clinically used. The appearance of a new type of effect at higher doses is very common in pharmacology and should not lead us to question the selectivity of action of a drug at lower doses.

Analeptic Agents

Of mainly theoretical interest is the action of several so-called analeptic agents, such as pentylenetetrazole and picrotoxin. These agents actively induce hypothermia, and their effect is blocked by small doses of barbiturates. The usual CNS stimulatory effects of these agents and the blocking effect of the hypnotic agents suggest that analeptic drugs stimulate heat-dissipating central mechanisms.

Section 2:

UNINTENTIONAL HYPOTHERMIA

John F. Ryan
Donald E. Jones

TEMPERATURE REGULATION

Although thermoregulation is a basic homeostatic mechanism, only in the last 30 to 40 years have these regulatory principles been demonstrated. From 1959 to 1969, Benzinger, working for the United States Navy, used the total body gradient calorimeter and measurements of direct oxygen consumption to explain the principles by which the human body maintains a given temperature.[18] In the course of his studies, he perfected tympanic thermometry. Many investigators have studied temperature homeostasis, but our understanding of temperature control is largely a result of Benzinger's meticulous efforts.

Homeostatic Mechanisms

The Hypothalamus

Benzinger identified two mechanisms that are activated by a decrease in body temperature and three mechanisms activated by an increase in body temperature (Table 10-2). He further noted that the body precisely maintains the temperature of blood that perfuses the posterior hypothalamus; any deviation activates the appropriate mechanisms to bring the temperature of the blood back to the set point. The set point, thus, is analogous to the temperature at which a room thermostat is set; the posterior hypothalamus acts as the thermostat, and

TABLE 10-2
Principal Mechanisms of Human Thermoregulation

RESPONSE TO TEMPERATURE DECREASE

1. The excitation of metabolic heat production by cold reception at thermal receptors throughout the body
2. The central release from inhibition of thermoregulatory heat production

RESPONSE TO TEMPERATURE INCREASE

1. The excitation of sweating by central warmth reception
2. Vasodilation elicited by central warmth reception
3. The inhibition of thermoregulatory sweating by cold reception at the skin and other sites.

Modified from Benzinger TH: Heat regulation: homeostasis of central temperature in man. Physiol Rev 49:67, 1969

the body temperature normally remains within about 0.5°C (thermoregulatory threshold) of the set point. The temperature that the central thermostat maintains is affected by several variables, such as local hypothalamic concentrations of sodium, calcium, norepinephrine, tryptophan, hormones, and pyrogens. Fever sets the thermostat at a higher level, and the body attempts to reach that new set point by increasing metabolism. Aspirin resets the thermostat to a lower level in the febrile state and thus decreases metabolic demand.

Skin Temperature

In accordance with this single-input thermoregulatory model, as body temperature falls below the set point of the hypothalamic center, heat production increases. However, this model was recognized as an oversimplification when it was noted that skin temperature constitutes about one third of thermal sensory input to the hypothalamus.[19] The increase in heat production is regulated by the integration of total body skin temperature and is weighted in favor of exposed areas. At a skin temperature greater than 33°C, heat production is minimal. As the integrated skin temperature decreases below 33°C, the heat production at a given hypothermic level increases in a stepwise manner to a maximum that is reached at 20°C; below 20°C, heat production decreases. These stepwise changes are caused by an increase in the frequency and amplitude of the firing of cold sensors in the skin as temperature decreases. The maximum response at 20°C defines critical ambient temperature.[20,21] An awake, undraped person will maintain body temperature at an ambient temperature of 20°C; below this level, central temperature falls.

The only situation in which the skin temperature cannot stimulate increased heat production occurs when the central, or core, temperature (the temperature of the blood perfusing the hypothalamus) is at or above the set point. Loss of skin temperature regulation has been observed in paraplegic patients with spinal cord section,[22] which interrupts the central ingress of information, and in severely burned patients,[23] in whom sensors have been destroyed. More recently, physiologists have reported active thermoregulation in response to isolated warming and cooling at sites other than the hypothalamus and skin. Indeed, thermoregulation is now viewed as a complex integration of multiple, redundant sensory inputs, with varying thermal sensitivities, from the brain, spinal cord, and abdominal organs, among other tissues.

Sweating

An increase in body temperature is followed by a change in blood flow from central to more peripheral distribution and the initiation of sweating.

Evaporation of sweat leads to cooling of the blood. An increase of 0.7°C above the set point leads to a fourfold increase in sweating. At or below the set point of the hypothalamic thermostat, sweating does not occur. Inhibition of sweating can occur at a low ambient temperature.[24] An athlete perspiring from exercise stops sweating when he or she steps out into the chill winter air. In this situation, evaporation does not occur, and the layer of perspiration acts as insulation to the raised blood temperature. Therefore, skin temperature, if decreased sufficiently (to 29°C), can shut off sweating.

THE EFFECT OF ANESTHESIA

Oxygen Consumption

Typically, oxygen consumption decreases slightly during normothermic general anesthesia. However, we have found a twofold increase in oxygen consumption during anesthesia and surgery in children during mild hypothermia (34.0°C to 36.5°C). Deep hypothermia has been well studied during anesthesia,[25] but until recently few data existed for mild hypothermia,[22] during which compensatory heat production may occur.[26] These studies parallel the work of Dawkins and Scopes in awake neonates.[27] As a result, body temperature should be maintained at 37°C for measurements of oxygen consumption during anesthesia.

Thermoregulation

Except for the absence of shivering, no evidence shows that thermoregulation ceases during anesthesia. However, the thermoregulatory threshold for response to hypothermia is altered. That is, instead of responding to a temperature decrease of 0.5°C, as in the normal, nonmedicated state, the anesthetized patient's thermoregulatory mechanisms are not activated until the temperature decreases by about 2.5°C (Fig. 10-4).[28] This effect has been observed both with inhalation anesthetics (eg, halothane and isoflurane) and with nitrous oxide–narcotic techniques. With isoflurane, the change in the thermoregulatory threshold is approximately proportional to the inhaled concentration.

Poikilothermic Range

Because the anesthetized patient exhibits a broader temperature range over which active thermoregulation is absent, within this range, the patient is poikilothermic: body temperature changes are determined by the difference between metabolic heat production (itseif reduced during general anesthesia) and heat loss to the environment. Once the ther-

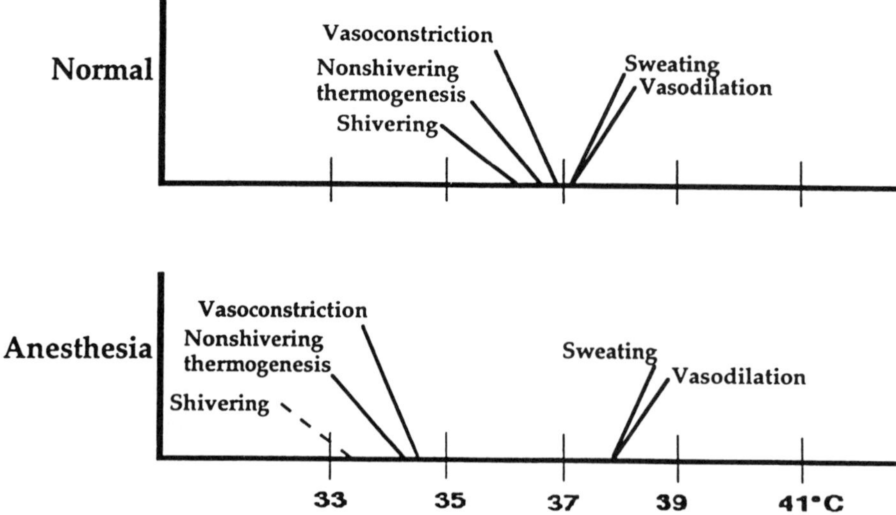

FIGURE 10-4. Thresholds and gains for common thermoregulatory responses in awake and anesthetized humans. *Vertical lines,* different regulatory responses; *horizontal lines,* mean body temperature. The intersection of each line with the temperature scale is the threshold, and the slope indicates the gain of that response. Thermoregulatory sensitivity is shown as the distance between the first cold response (vasoconstriction) and the first warm response (active vasodilation); temperatures within this range do not elicit thermoregulatory compensation. The slope of the line representing shivering is relatively small because there is a broad range of shivering intensity, and intensity increases in proportion to hypothermia. Nonshivering thermogenesis is not triggered until vasoconstriction is nearly complete. The slope of the line representing vasoconstriction is high because the response is an all-or-nothing phenomenon. Because each thermoregulatory response has its own threshold and gain, there is an orderly progression of responses, and response intensifies in proportion to need. During general anesthesia *(bottom)*, shivering *(dashed line)* is inhibited by muscle relaxants and local effects of inhaled anesthetics. The thresholds for vasoconstriction and nonshivering thermogenesis are shifted down to approximately 34.5°C (depending on anesthetic type and dose). Anesthetics increase the thresholds for active vasodilation and sweating by approximately 1°C. (Modified from Sessler DI: Temperature monitoring. In Miller RD (ed): Anesthesia, 4th ed. New York: Churchill Livingstone, 1994:1367.)

moregulatory threshold is reached, however, peripheral cutaneous vasoconstriction results.[29] This change requires sophisticated equipment to detect and is not associated with blood pressure changes.

Shivering

Shivering, the common heat-generating response, does not occur in the anesthetized patient presumably because of the CNS-depressant effects of general anesthetics as well as muscle relaxation, especially if neuromuscular blocking agents are used. Shivering, however, is not necessary for marked heat production and temperature elevation, as is apparent in malignant hyperthermia.

During emergence from anesthesia in the postanesthesia care unit, the hypothermic patient strives to return to normothermia, at a metabolic cost. Shivering patients commonly are observed to increase heat production at the end of anesthesia. Although studies suggest that much of this postanesthetic muscular activity represents anesthetic-enhanced spinal cord reflexes,[30] the result is a markedly increased utilization of oxygen (as much as 500% above normal).

Roe and colleagues demonstrated increased oxygen consumption in patients with temperature decreases of 0.3°C or more.[31] A broad range of increases in postoperative oxygen consumption in hypothermic patients was noted after various anesthetics (Fig. 10-5). Aged patients are not able to increase their oxygen consumption in response to decreased temperature and thus develop peripheral hypoxemia. Roe's group concluded that the sickest (often the oldest) patients are at greatest risk from mild hypothermia in the immediate postoperative period.

Especially vulnerable to postanesthetic shivering are patients rewarming from hypothermic extracorporeal circulation after coronary artery bypass procedures. One study documented that patients who shiver have an oxygen consumption about twice that of those who do not shiver and three times that occurring during anesthesia. Associated with the increased oxygen utilization are substantial increases in heart rate, cardiac index, and myocardial work.[32] The ideal physiologic balance of oxygen supply and demand is threatened when these patients emerge from anesthesia.

Nonshivering Thermogenesis

Neonates and small infants are also vulnerable to serious postoperative problems as a result of hypothermia. Because of their greater surface-to-volume ratio and higher metabolic rate, they tend to lose more heat to the environment. On emergence from anesthesia, they do not shiver; instead, they

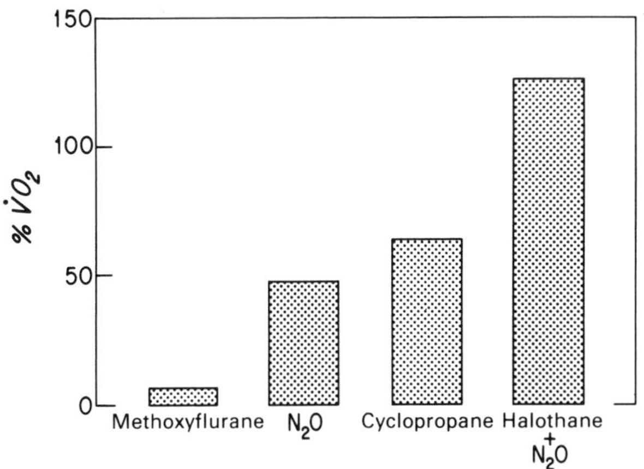

FIGURE 10-5. The effect of different anesthetics on postoperative oxygen consumption in the presence of hypothermia. V^{O^2}, oxygen consumption. (Roe CF, Goldberg MI, Blair CS, et al: The influence of body temperature on early postoperative oxygen consumption. Surgery 60:85, 1966.)

attempt thermal homeostasis by metabolizing brown fat (nonshivering thermogenesis), a process mediated through increased norepinephrine secretion.[33-35] The resultant increased rate of metabolism is accompanied by an increase in the proportion of the cardiac output (as much as 25%) diverted through the brown fat. Increased norepinephrine also produces pulmonary and peripheral vasoconstriction, predisposing to hypoxemia because of right-to-left shunting through the foramen ovale and ductus arteriosus in these infants.

TREATMENT OF POSTOPERATIVE HYPOTHERMIA

Treatment is largely symptomatic (Fig. 10-6). Warm blankets should be applied, although conductive heat transfer is very inefficient, in part because the cold patient emerging from anesthesia responds with peripheral vasoconstriction. If a passive approach is used, it does not matter whether the blanket is plastic or cotton; rather, it is the amount of skin surfaced covered.[36] Radiant heat or forced hot-air heaters are considerably more efficient in heat transfer and are especially effective in infants. Meperidine given to control shivering has been found effective after general anesthesia,[37-39] obstetric epidural anesthesia,[40] and cardiopulmonary bypass.[41] The effect is dose-related, with most adults requiring 25 to 50 mg intravenously. The mechanism is unknown. Of interest, morphine and fentanyl are ineffective in this application.[42]

PREVENTION OF INTRAOPERATIVE HYPOTHERMIA

Preventing hypothermia during anesthesia and surgery requires a multifaceted approach, especially in young children (Table 10-3). The mechanisms of heat loss are illustrated in Figure 10-2.

Maintenance of Operating Room Temperature

Morris and Wilkey have defined 21°C as a critical ambient operating room temperature at or above which body temperature is maintained.[42] All patients studied had an initial temperature decrease in the first 15 minutes, irrespective of room temperature. This decrease was attributed to undraping, cool skin-cleansing solutions, and lack of motion of the anesthetized patient. Heat loss occurs by radiation, convection, conduction, and evaporation.

In neonates, radiant heat loss is particularly important because of their relatively large ratio of body surface area to mass.[43] Even in a warmed isolette, an infant can become hypothermic if uncovered when the walls of the isolette are cool because of low ambient temperature. In this regard, the operating room can be considered a large isolette; to maintain the patient's temperature, a warm environment is necessary to minimize radiant heat loss (see Fig. 10-2).

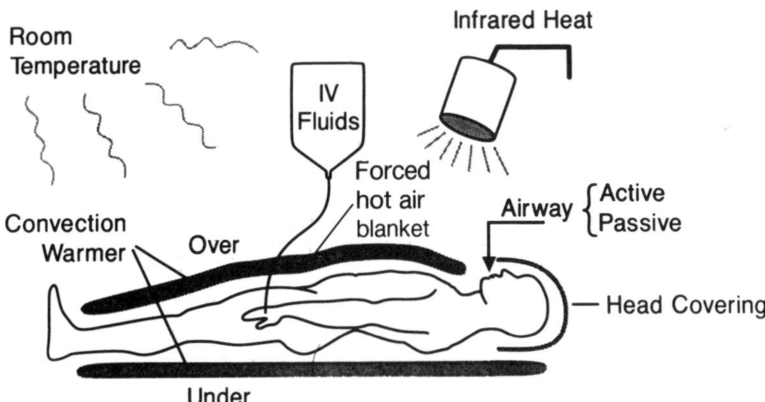

FIGURE 10-6. A number of options are available to control or maintain patient temperature during anesthesia. (Modified from Cork RC: Temperature monitoring. In Kirby RR, Gravenstein N (eds): Clinical anesthesia practice. Philadelphia; WB Saunders, 1994;436.)

TABLE 10-3
Prevention of Hypothermia

- Monitor body temperature
- Keep room warm
  - *Newborns and neonates:* >26.6°C
  - *Infants:* >25.5°C
  - *Adults:* >21.1°C
- Cover the patient
- Warm any blood transufsions
- Apply these techniques, *especially to infants*
  - Use a heating blanket
  - Apply drapes and wrap extremities
  - Use a radiant heat source
  - Heat fluids *(especially for irrigation)*
  - Use heated, humidified anesthetic gases

Protection From High Air Flow

In modern air-conditioned operating rooms, air flow velocity is sufficiently high to cool patients, especially infants and small children whose surface area is large relative to their weight. The orthopedic patient, cared for in the laminar-flow sterile chamber used in some institutions for total joint replacement, can cool markedly because of the wind chill factor from high air flow and convective heat loss. Similarly, the elderly patient awaiting vascular surgery in a cold operating room can become hypothermic during induction of anesthesia and surgical preparation.[44]

Conductive, Convective, Radiant, and Evaporative Heat Loss

Convective and radiant heat loss can be reduced by covering the patient with plastic sheeting.[45] Conductive loss to cool sheets and drapes occurs. Prevention of heat loss by a heating blanket is not of value in adults or children with a surface area greater than 0.5 m^2 (normally those older than 15 months of age or greater than 10 kg in weight) and adds the problem of protecting the patient from burns that may be caused by pooled cleansing solution or a faulty thermostat.[46] Evaporative heat loss may occur in the operating room at temperatures above 23°C, but more commonly, sweating is related to problems in anesthetic management.

Heated Humidification

Provision of heated, humidified inspired gas is a useful method to maintain or restore temperature and decrease the length of postoperative recovery.[47] Various methods have been advocated, such as heating the carbon dioxide absorber[48] and passing inspiratory gases through it; using a heated humidifier in the circle system[49–52]; using an artificial nose[53]; and using an ultrasonic nebulizer.[54,55] A limitation of the last method is the potential administration of a significant fluid load.

With the first two methods, measurement of the temperature of the heated gases before their administration is a reasonable precaution to prevent overheating. A system that warms and humidifies anesthetic gases prevents caloric expenditure for these functions. Also, cooling of aortic blood does not occur from the cool dry gases flowing into the trachea. In long cases, this prevention of insensible fluid loss also decreases fluid requirements. A potential for cross-infection occurs, unless reliable gas sterilization of individual units is maintained or disposable units are used.

Radiant Heat

Radiant heat lamps are effective to prevent heat loss in premature infants, neonates, and burned patients.[56,57] The lamp should be kept at least 70 cm from the patient's skin, and skin temperature should be monitored by a covered probe to prevent overheating (Fig. 10-7); a decrease of 25 cm in the distance from the heat source to the patient increases skin temperature to 38°C.

Radiant heat loss has been reduced in infants by a silver swaddle.[58] Similar in principle to the plastic sheeting mentioned previously,[45] this body wrap consists of an inner layer of polyethylene and an outer layer of aluminum foil. Areas are peeled open to insert monitors and intravenous catheters. Although this is an effective deterrent to heat loss, care must be taken to prevent pooling of cleansing solutions inside the wrap.

Forced Hot-Air Systems

Forced hot-air systems, which can be used to cover the patient's shoulders, chest, and outstretched arms intraoperatively, eliminate convective and radiant heat loss by blowing warm air over and around the covered areas. Typically, they lend themselves best to postoperative warming because the patient's entire body can be covered.[59]

Warming of Transfused Blood and Fluids

Warming of blood during transfusion has long been advocated, particularly when massive volumes are infused.[60] To bring

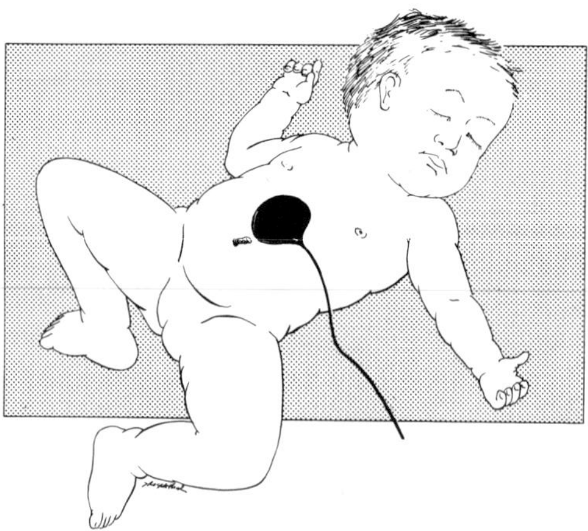

FIGURE 10-7. The skin thermometer monitors the heat from a radiant heat source. The thick adhesive cover that holds the thermistor in place also shields it from direct heating by the lamp. This ensures that the temperature recorded is that of the skin surface.

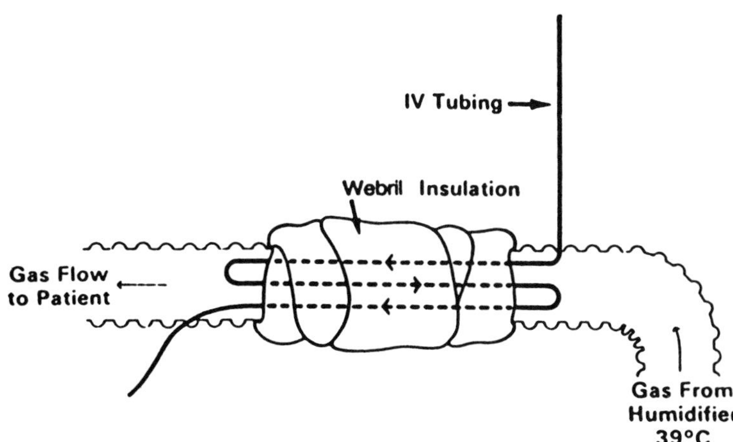

FIGURE 10-8. Set-up for warming in fluid. *IV*, intravenous. (Legend modified from Rosen KR, Rosen DA, Broadman L: A simple method for warming intravenous fluid in infants (letter). Anesthesiology 64:133, 1986.

500 mL of bank blood (4°C) to body temperature requires 32 kcal per hour, approximately 50% of basal metabolic heating output by a 70-kg person. Warming of cleansing solutions, intravenous fluids, and irrigation or cystoscopy fluids in children are important adjuncts to maintaining body temperature. One liter of intravenous fluid at 20°C decreases the temperature of a 70-kg person by approximately 0.2°C. Intravenous fluids may be partially warmed and can contribute to pediatric thermal homeostasis by having the intravenous tubing wrapped around the warm anesthesia circuit and by having it traverse under the heating blanket (Fig. 10-8).

TEMPERATURE MONITORS

What is the best method of monitoring temperature? Basic approaches include determination of central temperature and monitoring of noncentral, peripheral temperature.

Central Temperature

The recorded "central temperature" reflects the temperature of the blood flowing by the temperature-sensitive center of the hypothalamus (Aronsohn-Sachs center[26]). Temperature sensors placed on the tympanic membrane,[62] in the lower third of the esophagus,[63] or in the nasopharynx measure central temperature during anesthesia; a close relation exists among these parameters.[64]

The blood coursing adjacent to the tympanic membrane is similar in temperature to blood flowing in the branches of the internal carotid artery to the hypothalamus. A sensor placed in the lower third of the esophagus measures the temperature of aortic blood, but if it is in the proximal or middle third of the esophagus, it is influenced by either cool or heated anesthetic gases in the endotracheal tube.[65,66] The nasotracheal sensor is warmed by branches of the internal carotid artery. If the sensor is moved into the pharynx, cool air lowers the reading, an effect illustrating the importance of proper placement.

Peripheral Temperature

Rectal

Noncentral monitors measure local changes in temperature that depend on regional blood flow and other factors. They may not determine core temperature but are useful and convenient monitors of relative changes in body temperature. For example, a rapidly decreasing rectal temperature not explained by peritoneal lavage, prolonged cystoscopy, or replacement of cold bowel into the abdomen reflects decreased temperature in the tissues perfused by the inferior hemorrhoidal artery.

Axillary

Axillary temperature monitoring also is simple to perform. If the arm can be adducted to prevent air cooling of the probe, and if cold intravenous fluids given into a vein of that arm do not distort the response of the probe, this method is a useful guide to changes in temperature. However, axillary and extremity skin may not correlate well with core temperature.[64]

Forehead

Devices that use temperature-sensitive liquid crystals calibrated to yield digital images at the appropriate temperatures are available. The adhesive-backed disposable strip can be placed on the forehead, a location that is advantageous from a physiologic and anatomic standpoint. Vasoconstriction is delayed in this area, despite hypothermia. Twenty-three percent of heat loss, down to 15.5°C ambient temperature, occurs from the head. Below 15.5°C, this value increases to 40%. The skin in this area remains relatively well perfused even under thermal stress; thus these strips should track core temperature. Skin and core temperature can diverge widely, however, and therefore these devices have limited application (Table 10-4). Of note, in an effort to accommodate the offset between skin and core temperature, most of these devices incorporate a built-in 2°C to 6°C offset to give a "better"

TABLE 10-4
Offset Between Displayed and Actual Temperatures Measured by Liquid Crystal Temperature Indicators

LIQUID CRYSTAL TEMPERATURE INDICATOR	TEMPERATURE (°F) Claimed Accuracy	Offset MEAN	Offset RANGE
Stat Temp II*	±0.42	5.3	3.0–8.7
Stat Temp II WR*	±0.42	6.2	3.4–9.0
RediTemp, oval†	±0.04	4.5	3.2–5.2
RediTemp, strip†	±0.04	3.1	2.6–4.0
TriTemp‡	±0.5	3.5	3.0–4.2
Temp-a-Strip‡	—	0.6	0.2–1.0
Protect‡	±0.5	3.2	2.8–4.0
Crystalline‡	±0.5	4.9	4.5–5.0
EZ Temp§	—	1.7	0–2.5
Omni Combo‖	±0.5	3.5	2.7–3.6
Omni II‖	±0.5	5.0	3.8–5.8
Omni OR‖	±0.5	5.3	4.4–6.6
Omni Wide Range‖	±0.5	4.7	2.0–6.6
Anesthesia Monitor#	—	2.3	0.0–5.4

Mean offset was based on eight readings; displayed temperature was always greater than actual temperature.

* Trademark Medical, Fenton, MD.

† Medical Products of America, Highland, IL.

‡ Sharn, Tampa, FL.

§ Seven Cs, St. Louis, MO.

‖ Omnitherm, Florrisant, MO.

\# Clinitemp, Indianapolis, IN.

Shomaker TS, Bjoraker DG: Measurement offset with liquid crystal temperature indicators. Anesthesiology 73:A425, 1990.

indication of core temperature.[64] These devices should be used only to establish temperature trends and not to measure absolute temperature.

Summary

The most important factors in the choice of a temperature sensor are the location of the surgical incision and the experience of the anesthesiologist with a particular probe. All temperature sensors can injure the body orifice into which they are introduced; obvious care must be taken to prevent perforation of the eardrum, esophagus, or rectum.

THE IMPORTANCE OF TEMPERATURE MONITORING

Our knowledge of thermoregulatory responses should make us wary of even mild hypothermia. Until evidence is presented that complete abolition of compensatory increased heat production is the response to a decrease in core temperature, we should assume that thermoregulatory responses are functioning during general anesthesia.

Avoidance of Cold Stress

Avoidance of "cold stress" is vital in the newborn and in the sick premature neonate. Increased mortality, marked metabolic acidosis, and postoperative apnea compel the anesthesiologist to pay stringent attention to maintaining normothermia. Relatively simple methods, such as control of ambient operating room temperature and humidification of inspired gases, are effective. Roe and colleagues' findings of increased postoperative oxygen consumption after mild intraoperative hypothermia also indicate the necessity to monitor and maintain temperature at or near 37°C.[31] In addition, it has been suggested that hypothermia during anesthesia is followed by rebound hyperthermia.[59]

Detection of Malignant Hyperthermia

Finally, the possibility of malignant hyperthermia has made temperature monitoring particularly important. The early detection of a temperature increase of 0.5°C or more during surgery is important in controlling the febrile responses in septic patients. Recognition of possible iatrogenic pyrogenic responses during anesthesia is equally important: seven of the last eight cases in which we have observed increases in temperature to above 42°C were not attributable to malignant hyperthermia. Confirmation of the diagnosis of malignant hyperthermia early (eg, an increased end-tidal carbon dioxide value with a temperature elevation from 35°C to 37°C) aids in the diagnosis of unexplained tachycardia.

REFERENCES

1. Holdcroft A: Control of body temperature. In Holdcroft A (ed): Body temperature control in anaesthesia, surgery, and intensive care. London: Bailliere-Tindall, 1980: 12
2. Bligh J: Temperature Regulation in Mammals and Other Vertebrates. New York: American Elsevier, 1973
3. Himms-Hagen J: Nonshivering thermogenesis. Brain Res Bull 12:151, 1984
4. Hensel H, Zotterman Y: The response of the cold receptors to constant cooling. Acta Physiol Scand 22:96, 1951
5. Boulant JA, Hardy JD: The effect of spinal and skin temperatures on the firing rate and the thermosensitivity of preoptic neurones. J Physiol (Lond) 240:639, 1974
6. Boulant JA: The effect of firing rate on preoptical neuronal thermosensitivity. J Physiol (Lond) 240:661, 1974
7. Nicholls DG, Locke RM: Thermogenic mechanisms in brown fat. Physiol Rev 61:1, 1984
8. Benzinger TH, Pratt AW, Kitzinger C: The thermostatic control of human metabolic heat production. Proc Natl Acad Sci U S A 47:730, 1961
9. Cranston WI, Duff GW, Hellman RF, et al: Thermoregulation in rabbits during fever. J Physiol (Lond) 257:767, 1976
10. Myers RD, Yaksh TL: Thermoregulation around a new 'set-point' established in the monkey by altering the ratio of sodium to calcium ions within the hypothalamus. J Physiol (Lond) 218:609, 1971
11. Jell RM: Responses of rostral hypothalamic neurones to peripheral temperatures and to amines. J Physiol (Lond) 240:295, 1974
12. Cooper KE, Preston E, Veale WL: Effects of atropine, injected into a lateral cerebral ventricle of the rabbit, on fevers due to i.v. leucocyte pyrogen and hypothalamic and intraventricular injection of PGE_1. J Physiol (Lond) 254:729, 1976
13. Myers RD, Yaksh TL: Thermoregulation around a new 'set-point' established in the monkey by altering the ratio of sodium to calcium ions within the hypothalamus. J Physiol 218:609, 1971
14. Kubo K, Tsuzuki K, Sasaki T: What is the main physiological role of opioid peptides in thermoregulation? In Hales JRS (ed): Thermal physiology. New York: Raven Press, 1984
15. Donnerer J, Lembeck F: Heat loss reaction to capsaicin through a peripheral site of action. Br J Pharmacol 79:719, 1983

16. Clark WG, Cumby HR: Antagonism by antipyretics of the hyperthermic effect of a prostaglandin precursor, sodium arachidonate, in the cat. J Physiol (Lond) 257:581, 1976
17. Lin, MT, Chai CY: Effect of sodium acetylsalicylate on body temperature of monkeys during heat exposure. J Pharmacol Exp Ther 194:165, 1975
18. Benzinger TH: Heat regulation: homeostasis of central temperature in man. Physiol Rev 49:671, 1969
19. Stolwijk JAJ, Hardy JD: Partitional calorimetric studies of responses of man to thermal transients. J Appl Physiol 21:967, 1966
20. Wyndham CH, Williams CG, Loots H: Reactions to cold. J Appl Physiol 24:282, 1968
21. Wyndham CH, Ward JS, Strydom NB, et al: Physiologic reactions of caucasian and Bantu males on acute cold exposure. J Appl Physiol 19:583, 1964
22. Downey JA, Chiodi HP, Darling RC: Central temperature regulation in the spinal cord injured man. J Appl Physiol 22:91, 1967
23. Szyfelbein SK, Ryan JF: Thermoregulatory responses in burned children. Buenos Aires: International Congress on Burn Injuries, 1974
24. Benzinger TH: The diminution of thermoregulatory sweating during cold-reception at the skin. Proc Natl Acad Sci U S A 47: 1683, 1961
25. Hickey PR, Anderson ND: Deep hypothermia circulatory arrest: a review of pathophysiology and clinical experience as a basis for anesthetic management. J Cardiothorac Anesth 1:137, 1987
26. Sessler DI, Rubenstein EH, Moayeri AM: Physiologic response to mild perianesthetic hypothermia in humans. Anesthesiology 75:594, 1991
27. Dawkins MJR, Scopes JW: Non-shivering thermogenesis and brown adipose tissue in the human newborn infant. Nature 206: 201, 1965
28. Sessler DI, Olofsson CI, Rubinstein EH, et al: The thermoregulatory threshold in humans during halothane anesthesia. Anesthesiology 68:836, 1988
29. Sessler DI, Moayeri A, Stoen R, et al: Thermoregulatory vasoconstriction decreases heat loss. Anesthesiology 75:656, 1990
30. Sessler DI, Israel D, Pozos RS, et al: Spontaneous post-anesthetic tremor does not resemble thermoregulatory shivering. Anesthesiology 68:843, 1988
31. Roe CF, Goldberg MJ, Blair CS, et al: The influence of body temperature on early postoperative oxygen consumption. Surgery 60:85, 1966
32. Ralley FE, Wynands JE, Ramsay JG, et al: The effects of shivering on oxygen consumption and carbon dioxide production in patients rewarming from hypothermic cardiopulmonary bypass. Can J Anaesth 35:332, 1988
33. Silverman WA, Sinclair JC: Temperature regulation in the newborn. N Engl J Med 274:92, 1966
34. Sinclair JF: Heat production and thermoregulation in the small infant. Pediatr Clin North Am 17:147, 1970
35. Ryan JF, Vacanti FX: Temperature regulation. In Ryan JF, Todres ID, Cote CJ, et al (eds): A practice of anesthesia for infants and children. Orlando: Grune & Stratton, 1986: 19
36. Sessler DI, McGuire BS, Sessler AM: Perioperative thermal insulation. Anesthesiology 74:875, 1991
37. Holdcroft A, Hall GM, Cooper GM: Redistribution of body heat during anaesthesia. Anaesthesia 34:758, 1979
38. Claybon LE, Hirsh RA: Meperidine arrests postanesthesia shivering. Anesthesiology 53:S180, 1980
39. Pauca AL, Savage RT, Simpson S, et al: Effect of pethidine, fentanyl and morphine on post-operative shivering in man. Acta Anaesth Scand 28:138, 1982
40. Casey WF, Smith CE, Katz JM, et al: Intravenous meperidine for control of shivering during Caesarean section under epidural anaesthesia. Can J Anaesth 35:128, 1988
41. Guffin A, Girard D, Kaplan JA: Shivering following cardiac surgery: hemodynamic changes and reversal. J Cardiothorac Anesth 1:24, 1987
42. Morris RH, Wilkey BR: The effects of ambient temperature on patient temperature during surgery not involving body cavities. Anesthesiology 32:102, 1970
43. Rackow H, Salanitre E: Modern concepts in pediatric anesthesiology. Anesthesiology 30:208, 1969
44. Roizen MF, Sohn YJ, L'Hommedieu CS, et al: Operating room temperature prior to surgical draping: effect on patient temperature in recovery room. Anesthesiology 59:852, 1980
45. Telfer Brunton JLA, Thoms GMM, Blair I: Reduction of heat loss in neurosurgical patients using metallized plastic sheeting. Br J Anaesth 54:1201, 1982
46. Goudsouzian NG, Morris RH, Ryan JF: The effects of a warming blanket on the maintenance of body temperature in anesthetized infants and children. Anesthesiology 39:351, 1973
47. Conahan TJ, Williams CD, Apfelbaum JL: Airway heating reduces recovery room time (cost) in outpatients. Anesthesiology 67:128, 1987
48. Berry FA, Hughes-Davies DI: Method of increasing the humidity and temperature of the inspired gases in the infant circle system. Anesthesiology 37:456, 1972
49. Tovell RM, Lion KS, Lovell BS: Recent advances in inhalation therapy utilizing high humidity. Anesth Analg 40:105, 1961
50. Pflug AG, Aasheim GM, Foster C, et al: Prevention of postanaesthesia shivering. Can Anaesth Soc J 25:43, 1978
51. Morton GH, Flewellen EH II: Prevention of intraoperative hypothermia in geriatric patients. Anesth Analg 68:S204, 1989
52. Bissonnette B, Sessler DI, LaFlamme P: Inspired gas humidification prevents intraoperative hypothermia in infants and children. Anesth Analg 68:S28, 1989
53. Lin CY, Bodenstab PC, Yoon SM, et al: Reappraisal of heat-moisture exchanger. Anesth Analg 68(suppl):S166, 1989
54. Avery ME, Galina M, Nachman R: Mist therapy. Pediatrics 39: 160, 1967
55. Sara C, Currie T: Humidification by nebulization. Med J Aust 1:174, 1965
56. Smith RM: Temperature monitoring and regulation. Pediatr Clin North Am 16:643, 1969
57. Friedman F, Adams FH, Emmanouilides G: Regulation of body temperature of premature infants with low energy radiant heat. J Pediatr 70:270, 1967
58. Dick W, Kreuscher H, Luhker D: Prevention of heat loss during anesthesia and operation in the newborn baby and small infant. Acta Anaesthesiol Scand 37(suppl):134, 1970
59. Lennon RL, Hosking MP, Conover MA, et al: Evaluation of forced hot heat systems for rewarming hypothermic patients. Anesth Analg 70:424, 1990
60. Boyan CP: Cold or warm blood for massive transfusions? Ann Surg 160:282, 1964
61. Aronsohn E, Sach J: Die Beziehungen des Gehirns zur Korperwarme and zum Fieber. Arch Ges Physiol 37:232, 1885
62. Benzinger M: Tympanic thermometry in surgery and anesthesia. JAMA 209:1207, 1969
63. Whitby JD, Dunkin LJ: Cerebral, oesophageal and nasopharyngeal temperatures. Br J Anaesth 43: 673, 1971
64. Bissonnette B, Sessler DI, LaLamme P: Temperature monitoring sites in infants and children. Anesth Analg 68:S29, 1989
65. Kaufman RD: Relationship between esophageal temperature gradient and heart and lung sounds heard by esophageal stethoscope. Anesth Analg 66:1046, 1987
66. Siegel MN, Gravenstein N: Passive warming of airway gases (artificial nose) improves accuracy of esophageal temperature monitoring. J Clin Monit 6:89, 1990

FURTHER READING

Cork RC: Temperature monitoring. In Kirby RR, Gravenstein N (eds): Clinical anesthesia practice. Philadelphia: WB Saunders, 1994: 429

Kaplan RF: Hypothermia/hyperthermia . In Gravenstein N (ed): Manual of complications during anesthesia. Philadelphia: JB Lippincott, 1991: 11, 121

Lilly RB Jr: Temperature fluctuations. In Kirby RR, Gravenstein N (eds): Clinical anesthesia practice. Philadelphia: WB Saunders, 1994: 817

Ryan JF, Vacanti FX: Temperature regulation. In Ryan JF, Todres ID, Cote CJ, et al (eds): A practice of anesthesia for infants and children. Orlando: Grune & Stratton, 1986: 19

Complications in Anesthesiology, second edition,
edited by Nikolaus Gravenstein and Robert R. Kirby.
Lippincott-Raven Publishers, Philadelphia © 1996.

CHAPTER 11

Physiologic Disturbances Associated With Induced Hypothermia

Fredrick K. Orkin

Induced hypothermia is by no means a new technique in anesthesia. Indeed, the use of hypothermia during surgery predates anesthesia, at least as we know it, by thousands of years. Hippocrates was among the first to note the analgesic property of cold, and refrigeration anesthesia, as it came to be called, was commonly used before the modern era of anesthesia, the most celebrated instances being the painless amputations performed by Napoleon's surgeon general, Baron Larrey.[1]

Much more in keeping with our current use of hypothermia to decrease metabolism, however, are the early attempts by the 18th-century English physiologist Hunter to freeze fish in a state of suspended animation.[1] More than 50 years ago, Smith and Fay reported limited success in slowing the growth of cancer when cold was applied locally.[2] Induced hypothermia has enjoyed sporadic use in carotid artery and intracranial surgery to decrease cerebral metabolism during periods of hypoperfusion.[3,4] Our principal current use of induced hypothermia in cardiac surgery results largely from the demonstration by Bigelow and colleagues that hypothermia permits complete occlusion of blood flow to the heart and thus performance of intracardiac surgery in a bloodless field.[5,6]

This chapter surveys the problems associated with *induced* hypothermia and places special emphasis on alterations in physiologic function. The culprit, as will become apparent, is not the cold itself but rather the resultant physiologic alterations when they are inadequately monitored and controlled.

CLINICAL PRESENTATIONS

The Three Zones of Hypothermia

Hypothermia is the clinical state of subnormal body temperature. In clinical practice, "core" (rectal, esophageal, or tympanic) temperature is measured, and in general hypothermia is regarded as a temperature less than 35°C. Values down to about 32°C describe mild hypothermia, or a safe zone in which heat-conservation and heat-production mechanisms, such as peripheral vasoconstriction and shivering, are usually present. Between about 32°C and 24°C is a transitional zone, characterized by progressive depression of tissue metabolism, development of maximal vasoconstriction, and cessation of shivering. Below 24°C is the danger zone in which the human behaves as a poikilothermic organism, assuming the temperature of his or her surroundings.[7]

Accidental Hypothermia

Causes

Used without qualification, the term "hypothermia" conjures images of the elderly person brought to the emergency room severely hypothermic after prolonged exposure to cold. Although particularly common among the elderly, accidental hypothermia also is seen in neonates, immobile and unconscious persons, and others who become physically exhausted in a cold environment. Not unexpectedly, associated conditions include endocrine deficiency states (eg, myxedema, hypoglycemia, Addison's disease, and pituitary insufficiency), malnutrition, uremia, severe infection, cerebrovascular or other intracranial disease, myocardial infarction, cirrhosis, pancreatitis, and drug and ethanol ingestion.

Recognition

Accidental hypothermia frequently is not recognized, in part because most clinical thermometers do not record temperatures low enough and because the affected person may appear clinically dead. Unchecked, hypothermia often leads to fatal multiple-system failure that can include pneumonia, intractable ventricular dysrhythmias, congestive heart failure, pancreatitis, and cerebrovascular accidents.[8,9]

Survival requires that accidental hypothermia be recognized as a medical emergency and managed with prompt institution of aggressive therapy to raise body temperature, establish and maintain an airway, ensure oxygenation and blood volume expansion, and monitor for and treat dysrhythmias and acid–base and electrolyte disorders (eg, hypokalemia and acidosis).[8–11]

Unintentional Hypothermia

Causes and Effects

A far less catastrophic but much more common form of hypothermia is the unintentional hypothermia that results during anesthesia in a cold operating room (see Chap 10). Preanesthetic administration of sedative agents, anesthetics, and anesthetic adjuvants predisposes the patient to hypothermia by depressing the thermoregulatory center and voluntary muscular activity, increasing cutaneous vasodilatation, reducing peripheral thermal receptor sensitivity, and preventing shivering.

In addition, hypothermia alters aspects of the pharmacologic characteristics of inhalation anesthetics and adjuvant drugs. For example, muscle sensitivity to nondepolarizing neuromuscular blocking agents diminishes as body temperature decreases. Upon rewarming, the clinical effect of the residual relaxant is increased ("recurarization"), making the patient vulnerable to muscle weakness when it is least expected.

Shivering

Of greater concern, however, is the shivering that occurs upon emergence from anesthesia as the thermoregulatory system regains its integrity and attempts to return the body temperature to normal. The resultant greatly augmented utilization of oxygen stresses the respiratory and circulatory systems at a time when they may not be able to meet the demand fully. Hypoxemia and secondary problems, such as cardiac dysrhythmias, can appear with little warning. Particularly at risk for unintentional hypothermia and postoperative shivering are infants and small children, who lose heat more readily because of their greater ratio of body-surface area to volume.

Induced Hypothermia

In contrast to other presentations of hypothermia, induced hypothermia is a controlled and remarkably safe physiologic state. Uneventful recovery generally follows hypothermia induced to levels at which survival of accidental hypothermia is uncommon. This observation suggests that cold is not innately harmful and also that what determines morbidity is the manner in which hypothermia is managed.[10] Although hypothermia has been induced in a variety of ways,[12,13] today it is usually produced as an adjunct to extracorporeal circulation in cardiac surgery. To avoid complications, however, hypothermia once induced must be managed with keen awareness of the resultant alterations in physiologic functions.

ALTERATIONS IN CLINICAL PHYSIOLOGIC FUNCTION

Hypothermia produces physiologic disturbances in most tissues and organ systems (Table 11-1). Unfortunately, how a given patient will respond to induced hypothermia is often difficult to predict, for a variety of reasons. First, thermoregulation is probably subject to greater individual variation than are other body functions. Moreover, observations in humans have been modified necessarily by the concomitant administration of general anesthetics and other drugs as well as the patient's state of health. Still other observations were made in the uncontrolled setting of accidental hypothermia. Finally, too, observations made in other species are not directly applicable to humans.

Nonetheless, some generalizations can be made. Although the more salient disturbances are discussed here primarily by body system to facilitate discussion, the disturbances usually are interrelated. In addition, by themselves, the disturbances resulting from well-conducted induced hypothermia are generally remarkably benign and limited to the period of hypothermia.

Metabolism

Underlying the usefulness of induced hypothermia is the accompanying generalized depression of metabolism. Metabolic rate is quantitated most easily by measuring oxygen consumption. Whole-body oxygen consumption bears a direct linear relation to core temperature, decreasing approximately 50% for each 10°C change (Fig. 11-1). However, large temperature gradients develop between superficial and deep tissues; more importantly, tissues also vary innately in their oxygen requirements. In the most metabolically active tissues a threefold decrease in oxygen consumption occurs for each 10°C drop in temperature; these tissues are said to have a temperature coefficient (Q_{10}) of 3. In contrast, most physical processes, such as the diffusion of metabolic substrate, have a temperature coefficient close to 1.[10] Thus, as temperature decreases, a disproportionately greater decrease in the use of metabolic substrate results. Herein lies the metabolic benefit of hypothermia.

The beneficial effect of hypothermia may be offset, however, or, more likely, negated by shivering, which occurs involuntarily as a centrally mediated, nonautonomic response to decreased core temperature. The intense muscular activity that occurs during shivering increases heat production and thereby tends to restore euthermia. Initially an increase in muscle tone occurs that, in turn, increases basal heat production by 50% to 100%. This period is followed by the visible and more familiar vigorous muscular activity that results in a 50% to 500% increase in whole-body oxygen consumption.[14–16]

Nervous System Function

Central

Cerebral blood flow decreases in direct proportion to the decrease in body temperature, at a rate of 6.7% for each degree

Celsius.[17] Hence, at 30°C, cerebral blood flow is about half normal, and at 25°C about one fifth of its normothermic value. Concomitantly, mean systemic blood pressure decreases by only about 5% for each degree Celsius of temperature decrease, indicating that cerebrovascular resistance increases.[18,19] In the absence of shivering,[20] however, cerebral oxygen consumption falls at the same rate as does cerebral blood flow.[17-19] As a result, arteriovenous oxygen difference is unchanged, and, if cerebral perfusion is uninterrupted, cerebral hypoxia does not occur. Associated with decreases in cerebral metabolism and blood flow are decreases in brain volume, cerebral venous pressure, and cerebrospinal fluid volume.[21]

Coincident with the depression of cerebral metabolism is depression of all aspects of central nervous system function.[10] Subtle changes in consciousness accompany mild hypothermia, although the electroencephalogram appears normal, perhaps with slightly decreased wave frequency or amplitude. Consciousness is lost when body temperature drops below 28°C, at which point progressive electric slowing occurs, with the appearance of τ and then δ wave activity, before the electroencephalogram becomes isoelectric in the temperature range of 15°C to 20°C.[22]

Although the electroencephalographic changes occurring during hypothermia qualitatively resemble those caused by acute hypoxia, power spectrum analysis suggests that changes in electroencephalographic frequency (but not amplitude) may be useful in distinguishing thermal effects from those associated with hypoxia.[23] The autonomic nervous system and the respiratory and cardiovascular centers also exhibit pro-

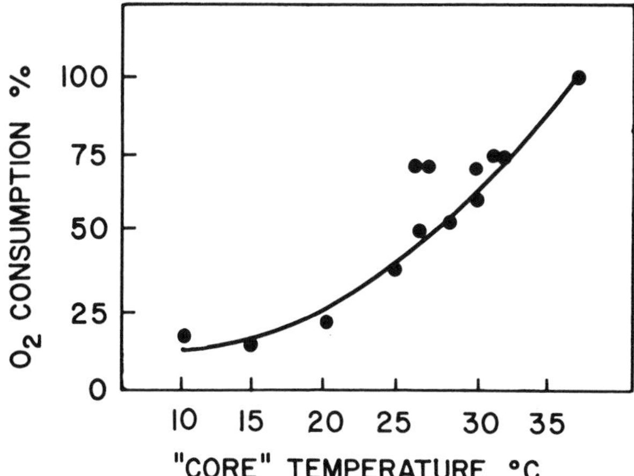

FIGURE 11-1. The relation between core temperature and whole-body oxygen consumption (compared with control values at 37°C), based on values taken from various studies. (Data from Dills DB, Forbes WH: Respiratory and metabolic effects of hypothermia. Am J Physiol 132:685, 1941; Spurr GB, Hutt BK, Horwath SM: Responses of dogs to hypothermia. Am J Physiol 179:139, 1954; Lougheed WH, Sweet WH, White JC, et al: Use of hypothermia in surgical treatment of cerebral vascular lesions: preliminary report. J Neurosurg 12:240, 1955; Severinghaus JW, Stupfel M, Bradley AF: Alveolar dead space and arterial to end-tidal carbon dioxide differences during hypothermia in dog and man. J Appl Physiol 10:349, 1957; Rosomoff HL: Pathophysiology of the central nervous system during hypothermia. Acta Neurochir Suppl 13:11, 1964; Blair E: Physiologic and metabolic effects of hypothermia in man. In Muschia XJ, Saunders JF (eds): Depressed metabolism. Proceedings of the First International Conference on Depressed Metabolism, Washington, DC, August 22–23, 1968. New York: American Elsevier, 1969.)

TABLE 11-1
Physiologic Effects of Hypothermia

CARDIOVASCULAR
↓ CO (↑ CO if shivering), ↑ SVR, central redistribution of blood → CHF, bradycardia → ventricular arrhythmias
METABOLIC
↓ Metabolic rate (↑ if shivering), ↓ tissue perfusion → metabolic acidosis, lipolysis → ↑ FFA, ↓ glucose utilization → hyperglycemia
PULMONARY
↑ PVR, ↓ hypoxic pulmonary vasoconstriction, ↑ anatomic dead space, ↓ ventilation (apnea in newborns)
HEMATOLOGIC
↑ Blood viscosity, shift of oxygen dissociation curve to left (↓ oxygen availability)
NEUROLOGIC
↑ CVR, ↓ CBF, EEG slowing → coma, ↓ MAC, ↓ CMR_{O_2}
DRUG DISPOSITION
↓ Hepatic blood flow, ↓ hepatic metabolism, ↓ renal blood flow, ↓ excretion, ↑ solubility of anesthetics, ↑ duration of muscle relaxant effect
SHIVERING (Usually in recovery room)
↑ Oxygen consumption to 500%, ↑ carbon dioxide production

CBF, cerebral blood flow; *CHF*, congestive heart failure; CMR_{O_2}, cerebral metabolic rate for oxygen; *CO*, cardiac output; *CVR*, cerebral vascular resistance; *EEG*, electroencephalogram; *FFA*, free fatty acids; *MAC*, minimum alveolar concentration; *PVR*, pulmonary vascular resistance; *SVR*, systemic vascular resistance.

Modified from Kaplan RF: Hypothermia/hyperthermia. In Gravenstein N (ed): Manual of complications during anesthesia. Philadelphia: JB Lippincott, 1991: 127.

gressive depression with hypothermia. However, reflexes (eg, gag, pupillary light, and deep tendon reflexes) usually remain intact until the temperature decreases below 25°C. Typically monosynaptic responses, such as muscle stretch, become polysynaptic or less pure during hypothermia, activating neighboring pathways.

Peripheral

Not unexpectedly, hypothermia is associated with generalized depression of conduction of the nerve impulse, the magnitude of which is directly related to the decrease in temperature. Thus, excitability and the rate of conduction are decreased in peripheral nerves and spinal pathways, and neuromuscular transmission is impaired. The larger, myelinated fibers are blocked first, whereas the small, unmyelinated sympathetic fibers are affected only during deep hypothermia.

Hypothermia-induced decreased conduction velocity and impaired transmitter release in peripheral nerves are reflected by temperature-related prolongation of the latency of cortical responses to somatosensory evoked potentials.[24] Also, as body temperature decreases, muscle tone becomes more prominent, with rigidity apparent at about 26°C. Spontaneous myoclonus, facial spasms, and other examples of muscle excitability may be noted at temperatures below 30°C.

Cardiovascular Function

The Heart

RATE. Heart rate increases transiently in response to the early sympathetic stimulation that accompanies hypothermia, especially if shivering is present.[25] Below 32°C to 34°C, cooling results in a proportional decrease in heart rate[26,27] that ends in ventricular fibrillation at about 25°C or in asystole at profound depths of hypothermia (eg, 10°C to 15°C). Probably caused by the direct effect of cold on the sinoatrial tissue, this bradycardia is not affected by atropine or vagotomy.

STROKE VOLUME AND CARDIAC OUTPUT. In the absence of anesthetic-induced cardiac depression, stroke volume is preserved down through the transitional zone of hypothermia[28] and then usually increases.[29] Given the relatively stable stroke volume, cardiac output necessarily mirrors the heart rate, rising initially and then falling proportionally with body temperature and, thus, tissue metabolism. Coronary blood flow is markedly diminished.[30]

MYOCARDIAL CONDUCTION AND IRRITABILITY. The most important cardiovascular effects of hypothermia are those affecting myocardial conduction and irritability. During mild hypothermia, an inapparent skeletal-muscle tremor caused by thermal muscle tone may completely obscure the P wave in the electrocardiogram. In addition to bradycardia, prolongation of the PR interval, QRS complex, and QT interval results from retarded depolarization and repolarization.[31]

The most characteristic electrocardiographic change below 31°C, consistently present below 25°C, is the J wave (the Osborn wave[32] or camel-hump sign), a slow deflection that is apparent in all leads and that arises during the terminal deflection of and in the same direction as the QRS complex (Fig. 11-2). Initially thought to represent a "current of injury," the J wave is no longer regarded as a presage of ventricular fibrillation.[33] Neither is the J wave pathognomonic of hypothermia, for it has been noted in other circumstances, such as cerebral injuries.[34] During deep hypothermia, the ST segment often is elevated or depressed and the T wave biphasic and then deeply inverted,[25] as if to suggest myocardial ischemia.[35]

PACEMAKER ACTIVITY. As cooling progresses, sinoatrial tissue tends to be inhibited, and lower areas assume pacemaker activity. When blood temperature has decreased to 27°C to 30°C, ECG evidence of myocardial irritability appears, though in a highly variable fashion. Irritability may appear first as an atrial ectopic focus or wandering atrial pacemaker but then insidiously changes to atrial fibrillation, usually with a slow ventricular response; sometimes an abrupt increase in heart rate occurs that interrupts the typical bradycardia of hypothermia.

A first-degree heart block may be present; a higher degree of block usually is observed only in patients with organic heart disease. As body temperature drops, other ectopic rhythms, such as atrial flutter, atrioventricular junctional rhythm, premature ventricular contractions, and ventricular fibrillation, also may appear. Ventricular fibrillation can develop without any forewarning in this part of the transitional zone of hypothermia.

Peripheral Circulation

RESISTANCE. The initial peripheral circulatory response to hypothermia is increased peripheral resistance caused by cutaneous vasoconstriction.[36] The latter condition results from the direct effect of cold on arterial walls[37] and reflex sympathetic stimulation initiated by cold receptors in the skin. Below 34°C, cutaneous vessels dilate as a direct effect of the cold,[38] but deeper vessels progressively constrict down to about 25°C, at which point generalized vasodilatation begins.

BLOOD VOLUME SHIFTS. Consequent to vasoconstriction, blood volume shifts to the deep capacitance vessels, particularly those in the liver and lungs, stimulating volume receptors and thereby probably contributing to "cold diuresis."[7] In addition, water moves extravascularly to the tissues,[39] and the hematocrit rises secondarily.[40] Hemoconcentration raises

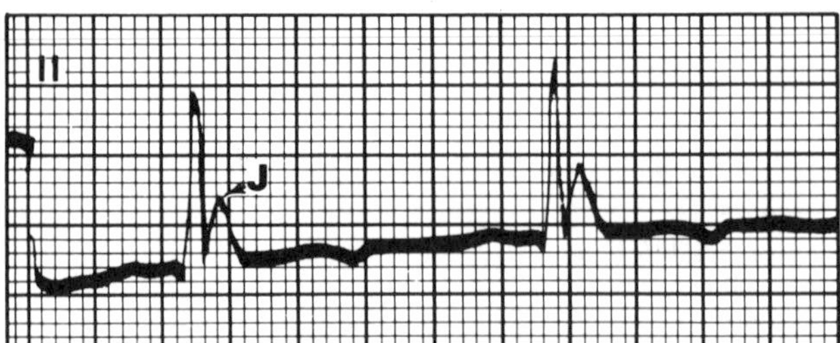

FIGURE 11-2. The characteristic J or Osborn wave of hypothermia appears during the terminal deflection of the QRS complex and may be mistaken for a T wave with a narrow QT interval.

blood viscosity and thereby increases peripheral resistance further.

BLOOD PRESSURE. Blood pressure rises initially during the transient period of peripheral vasoconstriction and then falls as body temperature decreases and cardiac depression develops. Clinically important hypotension, however, generally appears only below about 25°C.[41]

Adverse Effects

Hypothermia is detrimental when it is continued for more than 24 hours, a period that may be considered during treatment of cerebral resuscitation after cardiac arrest, head trauma, or near-drowning.[42,43] With time, the favorable reductions in both cardiac output and whole-body oxygen consumption are themselves diminished to less than 10% and 30% of control values, respectively; both remain depressed upon rewarming. Diffuse nonperfusion of capillary beds probably occurs during prolonged hypothermia, with resultant trapping of acid metabolites in the unperfused or underperfused tissues. Upon rewarming, vascular beds open and the accumulated metabolites enter the circulation and depress the cardiovascular system. Humans and animals usually die of shock and severe metabolic acidosis after prolonged hypothermia.[2,42,43]

Respiratory Function

The Lungs

As with cardiac function, the initial respiratory response to hypothermia is stimulation,[7,44] which is followed by depression in proportion to the decrements in body temperature and rate of metabolism.[45] In general, the respiratory rate, minute ventilation, and arterial carbon dioxide partial pressure decrease in parallel with one another. More important, however, is the decreased ventilatory responsiveness to increased carbon dioxide[45,46] and decreased oxygen inhalation,[46] even when anesthetic depth is constant relative to body temperature. If controlled ventilation is not instituted, spontaneous respiration ceases when body temperature reaches about 24°C. In addition to disturbances in respiratory control are changes in respiratory mechanics, albeit much less important in the clinical setting. These include increases in anatomic and physiologic dead space, apparently the result of bronchodilatation.[47]

The Blood

OXYHEMOGLOBIN DISSOCIATION. Respiratory function is also influenced by the complex ways in which gas transport is affected by temperature. The oxyhemoglobin dissociation curve shifts to the left in hypothermia. Thus, the partial pressure of oxygen in the tissues must fall to a lower-than-normal value before the hemoglobin gives up its oxygen. Although tissues can manage with remarkably little oxygen, oxygen-starved tissues could resort, theoretically, to anaerobic metabolism. That condition would result in acidosis that in turn would shift the curve toward the right again.

A more realistic mechanism for offsetting the shift in the dissociation curve is the increased solubility of oxygen in blood and other body fluids during hypothermia. For example, compared with its solubility at normal body temperature, dissolved oxygen is 19% greater at 30°C and 33% greater at 25°C. As large as these increases are, dissolved oxygen alone is insufficient to meet tissue oxygen requirements until the body temperature decreases to about 16°C.[48] Hypoxia does not occur during hypothermia, however, provided that tissue perfusion remains adequate.

CARBON DIOXIDE AND BICARBONATE. Carbon dioxide also is more soluble in blood and other body fluids during hypothermia; in fact, the increase in carbon dioxide dissolved in plasma is the same as that for oxygen. However, because dissolved carbon dioxide constitutes only about 5% of the total carbon dioxide carried in blood under normal circumstances, the increased solubility has only a limited effect on carbon dioxide transport during hypothermia.

Quantitatively more important is an increase in the plasma concentration of the bicarbonate ion that under normal circumstances accounts for 95% of carbon dioxide transport. Plasma bicarbonate concentration increases because the ionization of carbonic acid (formed when carbon dioxide hydrates in body fluids) to bicarbonate is favored even more as body temperature decreases and the activity of blood buffers increases, allowing them to accept more hydrogen ions.

These changes in carbon dioxide carriage, coupled with the decreased production of carbon dioxide during depressed metabolism, result in an arterial carbon dioxide partial pressure that is lower for any given pulmonary minute ventilation than it is at normal temperature. Respiratory alkalosis, in turn, is associated with a leftward shift of the oxyhemoglobin dissociation curve.

Renal Function

Renal function also is depressed reversibly during hypothermia, both because of decreased systemic blood pressure (secondary to the cardiovascular depression) and because of the direct cold effect. Typically, as renal blood flow progressively falls, renal vascular resistance rises, causing renal blood flow and glomerular filtration to decrease further.[49] However, because tubular reabsorption of water also is depressed, urine flow is only mildly decreased, if at all.[50]

In general, serum sodium and potassium levels remain normal, but the impairment of sodium and water reabsorption is great enough for relatively large volumes of dilute urine to be excreted ("cold diuresis") down to at least 20°C. With deep hypothermia, sufficiently large shifts of fluid may occur to result in hypovolemia during cooling and oliguria during rewarming.

Renal excretion of acid also is impaired, but acid–base disturbances are uncommon during induced hypothermia down to 27°C. In the absence of severe hypotension or myxedema or very uncommon disorders such as cryoglobulinemia or cold agglutinin disease that result in acute renal failure in a cold environment,[51] these changes are transient. Recovery of renal blood flow and filtration rate is about three-fourths complete within 2 hours of rewarming and is normal by the following day.[50]

Alimentary Function

The Gut

Hypothermia causes a reversible depression of smooth-muscle motility throughout the alimentary tract.[10] Thus, peristalsis is reduced in the esophagus, stomach, and intestines. Common manifestations include acute gastric dilatation (often with abdominal distension), paralytic ileus, and colonic dilatation. Gastric secretion and free-acid production are markedly depressed, as is the absorption of drugs from the intestine.

The Liver

GLUCOSE UTILIZATION. Splanchnic blood flow decreases directly in proportion to the decrease in temperature.[52,53] Although the liver continues to utilize oxygen and to avoid cellular hypoxia down to 25°C, it is less able to use the available glucose. This alteration is due in large part to the inhibition of insulin release from the pancreas and of the peripheral uptake of glucose.[54] As a result, blood glucose rises and remains elevated but without the development of ketoacidosis.

DRUG METABOLISM. A particularly important aspect of the liver's altered functioning is the generalized depression of drug metabolism. During induced hypothermia and general anesthesia, the liver's ability to conjugate steroids, excrete sodium sulfobromophthalein (Bromsulphalein), and detoxify and excrete drugs is impaired.[10]

Depression of drug metabolism has particular relevance when sodium nitroprusside is administered during hypothermic cardiopulmonary bypass. The initial step in the metabolism of this drug occurs nonenzymatically with hemoglobin within the red blood cell; the resultant free cyanide ions are converted to thiocyanate by the enzyme rhodanase in the liver and kidneys. Whereas clinical hypothermia does not affect the rate of the first step, theoretically it can retard detoxification of the cyanide ions that are released from the red blood cells and thereby increase the likelihood of cyanide toxicity when large doses of the drug are used.[55]

Coagulation

Although clinical experience suggests that hypothermia is associated with a bleeding tendency, substantive studies of coagulation are scant and controversial. Because clotting is enzymatically mediated, it stands to reason that hypothermia reduces the activity of humoral clotting factors. Some investigators have noted evidence of impaired coagulation only when the temperature is below 26°C,[56] when the cooling technique is improper, or when a surgical procedure is performed in addition to hypothermia.[57] Others have reported that clotting time increases as body temperature decreases.[58,59]

A short-lived, heparin-like substance that specifically inhibits factor Xa has been identified during deep hypothermia in dogs; however, the clinical relevance of this finding in humans is unknown.[60] The longer the period of hypothermia, the greater the prolongation of the clotting time, possibly because of the reversible, progressive thrombocytopenia associated with sequestration of platelets in the liver.[61,62] Wound cooling also has been shown to depress platelet function.[63]

Other clotting defects, such as fibrinolysis,[64] have been observed sporadically and probably are related to the surgical procedure rather than to the hypothermia. Similarly, disseminated intravascular coagulation has not been described in induced hypothermia, although occasionally it occurs during rewarming in cases of accidental hypothermia.

MANAGEMENT OF DISTURBANCES ASSOCIATED WITH INDUCED HYPOTHERMIA

General Considerations

Despite the many published reports on alterations in physiologic functioning associated with hypothermia, little has been written, particularly during the last 30 years, on the clinical management of the disturbances associated with induced hypothermia. In large part, this deficit reflects the use of induced hypothermia almost exclusively as an adjunct to cardiopulmonary bypass; during bypass procedures, cardiopulmonary support effectively treats many of the most serious disturbances associated with hypothermia, and complications from the bypass generally overshadow those from hypothermia. Nonetheless, some recommendations can be made.

Temperature Monitoring

As noted in the discussion of metabolism, large temperature gradients develop among the tissues as hypothermia progresses. These gradients are accentuated during rapid cooling and warming (Fig. 11-3).[65] However, even in the absence of rapid changes in body temperature, the gradients produced are sufficiently large to result in a continued decrease in body temperature after cooling has been discontinued. This unintentional, usually unpredictable downward drift in body temperature is termed "after-drop." Monitoring of several representative body temperatures allows a more adequate assessment of the progress of hypothermia (and of warming) and in particular of the magnitude of the temperature gradients. If these gradients are eliminated—that is, if the temperature is allowed to equilibrate before termination of cooling—after-drop should occur less frequently, and the resultant physiologic disturbances should be less severe.

Sites

Among the sites most commonly monitored are the rectum, esophagus, tympanic membrane, and nasopharynx. The highest temperature during normothermia is usually recorded in the rectum, which in general is regarded as representing core temperature. About 0.5°C lower than rectal, esophageal temperature reflects the temperature of the central blood volume, unless the probe is located in the proximal two thirds of the esophagus, where it is retrotracheal and influenced by room temperature or heated anesthetic gases passing through the trachea.[66,67] This effect can be overcome by inserting the esophageal probe 12 to 14 cm beyond the location where heart

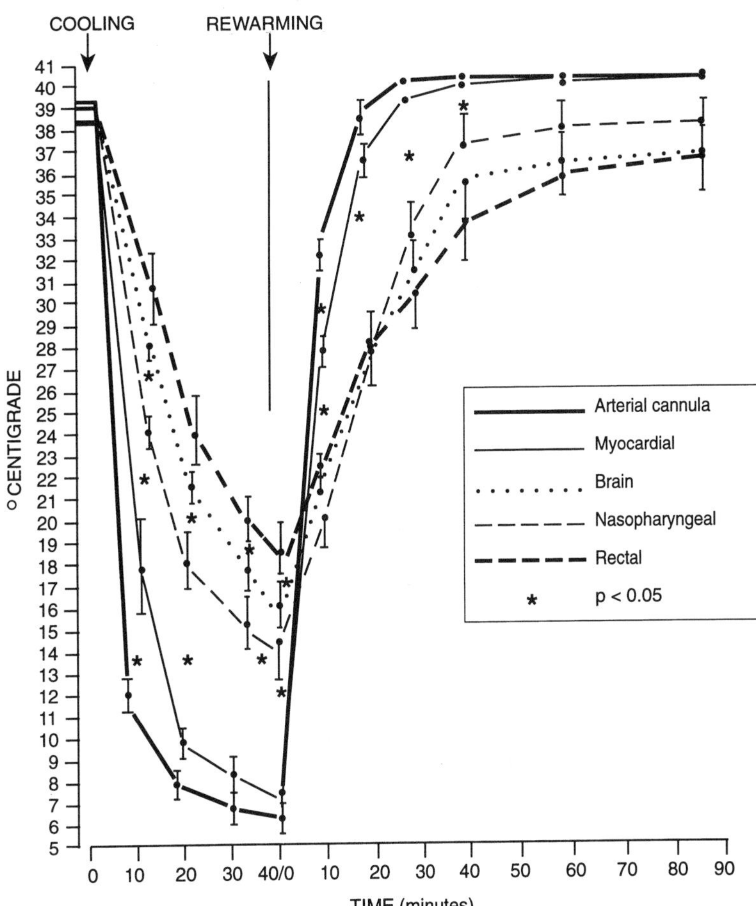

FIGURE 11-3. The figure dramatically shows the relationships of temperatures measured at various sites over time during cooling and rewarming from cardiopulmonary bypass. (Stefaniszyn HJ, Novicki RJ, Keith FM, et al: Is the brain adequately cooled during deep hypothermic cardiopulmonary bypass? Curr Surg 1983;40:296.)

and breath sounds are best heard[67] or by using a passive warming device (eg, an artificial nose).[68]

Close to esophageal temperature, tympanic membrane temperature reflects that of the nearby internal carotid artery, which supplies the thermoregulatory centers in the hypothalamus.[69] Although tympanic thermometry is simple, convenient, and provides reliable information, the probe can damage the membrane as well as cause aural bleeding.

Nasopharyngeal temperature reflects that of the brain, but only if the probe makes contact with the mucosa. Urinary bladder temperature has been shown to lag sufficiently behind nasopharyngeal temperature such that it reflects total body temperature more accurately during rewarming after cardiopulmonary bypass.[70] Because of changes in cutaneous blood flow, skin temperature varies so much that monitoring it has limited usefulness during induced hypothermia.

Arterial Blood Gas Analysis

Acidosis

Frequent assessment of arterial blood gas partial pressures and pH is essential to diagnose, treat, and prevent cardiorespiratory problems that are particularly likely during hypothermia. In addition to customary uses such as assessment of the adequacy of oxygenation, blood gas changes have been used to aid in early detection of and to guide therapy of developing acidosis in an attempt to minimize episodes of ventricular fibrillation. In current practice, however, provided that tissue perfusion remains adequate, acidosis in uncommon because ventilation is controlled.

Respiratory Alkalosis

A much more likely problem is respiratory alkalosis. This problem develops if ventilation is not decreased proportionately as metabolism slows and carbon dioxide becomes more soluble in body tissues and fluids. Respiratory alkalosis is especially undesirable because the concomitant physiologic changes counter the beneficial effects of hypothermia: these changes include cerebral hypoperfusion; increased ventricular irritability with ventricular dysrhythmias; and a leftward shift of the oxyhemoglobin dissociation curve with generalized reduction in tissue oxygen delivery. Serial blood gas analysis enables early detection and treatment of these acid–base disturbances as they are developing.

Assessment

The assessment of acid–base disturbances during hypothermia is complicated by the temperature dependence of the blood gas values. Although normal blood gas values in humans are well known for a body temperature of 37°C, "normal" values have not been established for the hypothermic state. Analysis is performed in an electrode system at 37°C, and nomograms are often used to correct the measured values to the patient's lower temperature.[71,72]

The question then arises: what are the ideal values, particularly of pH and arterial carbon dioxide partial pressure (Pa_{CO_2}), when reported values are "temperature corrected" (pH-stat) to the patient's actual body temperature or are "uncorrected" (α-stat) at the measuring electrode's temperature? At 37°C the more familiar arterial pH of 7.40 and P_{CO_2} of 40 mm Hg are "normal" regardless of patient temperature. The prevailing view, although not unanimously held, is that blood gas values should be reported at 37°C—in other words, that the α-stat method should be used.[73] Uncorrected values are not only simpler to use; they also offer ease of interpretation when serial measurements are made at different body temperatures.[74]

Intravenous Fluid Management

As during normothermic conditions, intravenous-fluid management must relate to the patient's state of hydration, electrolyte balance, and ongoing fluid losses. Hypothermia poses two additional considerations. Because of the depression of liver metabolism, glucose-containing infusions and excessive amounts of acid-citrate-dextrose blood should be avoided, if possible, during the period of hypothermia, to avoid the risk of hyperglycemia; however, mild hyperglycemia or citrate toxicity should not be treated because hypoglycemia is likely upon rewarming when the liver resumes normal metabolic function.

Fluid input and estimates of overall fluid loss should be monitored particularly closely if the period of hypothermia is more than a few hours because of the possibility of cold diuresis and posthypothermia oliguria. During prolonged hypothermia, serial measurements of urine and serum electrolytes also are needed to plan optimal fluid management. Potassium supplementation often is required during the diuretic phase.

MANAGEMENT OF SPECIFIC PROBLEMS

Shivering

Adverse Effects

As noted in the discussions of the metabolic and cerebral effects of hypothermia, shivering during induced hypothermia is not only counterproductive but also potentially threatening to the patient's well-being. The increased oxygen requirement imposed by shivering places undue and probably excessive demands on the cardiorespiratory systems.[14-16] Should respiratory obstruction occur during emergence from hypothermia, the small oxygen reserves available can be depleted rapidly and hypoxemia can develop. Patients with compromised cardiorespiratory reserve or neuromuscular disease are likely to have difficulty compensating for the increased demands imposed by shivering.

Treatment

The best treatment for shivering, as for most other complications, begins with prevention. Most anesthetic techniques used in association with hypothermia involve combinations of inhalation anesthetics, narcotics, and, especially, neuromuscular blocking agents to minimize, if not avoid, shivering. Postanesthetic shivering can be treated with radiant or conductive heat,[75] ventilation with warm, humidified oxygen,[76] narcotics such as meperidine,[77,78] and vasodilators such as nitroprusside.[79] Once shivering has occurred, the two quickest options until body temperature is normalized are probably intravenous meperidine, 25 to 50 mg, or muscle paralysis and sedation if the patient's lungs are being mechanically ventilated.

Cardiac Dysrhythmias

General Measures

Cardiac dysrhythmias are common when the body temperature falls below 30°C; they occur invariably below 28°C. The occurrence of the dysrhythmia during hypothermia should not prevent the clinician from considering and if necessary treating its many other potential causes: inadequate depth of anesthesia with secondary endogenous catecholamine release; exogenous administration of a catecholamine; electrolyte imbalance (eg, hypokalemia); hypotension with inadequate coronary perfusion; hypercapnia; and hypoxemia. If the more common causes can be excluded, conventional treatment for the specific dysrhythmia should be attempted if the disturbance has a deleterious effect on blood pressure. Propranolol in doses of 0.5 mg to a total dose of 1 to 2 mg has been advocated in anecdotal case reports,[80,81] but whether it is more effective than other therapies remains to be demonstrated.

Clinical experience suggests that during hypothermia most rhythm disturbances are recalcitrant to therapy, but this obstacle usually does not pose a problem because blood pressure and tissue perfusion are well maintained during short periods of well-monitored induced hypothermia. Ventricular fibrillation, the most serious complication of hypothermia, however, necessitates treatment, but below about 27°C, defibrillation is invariably ineffective. Therapy for fibrillation occurring in the absence of cardiopulmonary bypass (which would maintain tissue perfusion) should be directed at raising the body temperature to 28°C to 30°C, at which defibrillation is usually effective.

Drug Effects

The narcosis accompanying hypothermia results, not unexpectedly, in diminished anesthetic requirement. Minimal alveolar concentration (MAC) is reduced linearly as temperature falls, although the magnitude of this effect varies among anesthetics.[82-85] For example, a 10°C decrease in body temperature is associated with a 53% decrease in the MAC for halothane.[84] Similarly, depression of liver function results in slower metabolism of drugs such as sodium nitroprusside[56] and morphine.[86] In addition, because anesthetic gases are more soluble as temperature falls and because both blood flow and ventilation are reduced by hypothermia, emergence from anesthesia is likely to be prolonged.

The metabolism and elimination of nondepolarizing neuromuscular blocking agents also are depressed during hypothermia, but (with the exception of pancuronium[87]) there is an associated antagonism of their relaxant effect, and the net result is a prolongation of neuromuscular blockage at moderate levels of hypothermia.[88] Although no prolongation is observed at lesser degrees of hypothermia, upon rewarming the possibility exists that residual relaxant can have a clinically important effect. Unless the reduced requirement for anesthetics is considered and depth of anesthesia is monitored more carefully, overdose is likely.

REFERENCES

1. Armstrong Davison MH: Evolution of anaesthesia. Br J Anaesth 31:134, 1959
2. Smith LW, Fay T: Observations on human beings with cancer maintained at reduced temperature of 75-90 Fahrenheit. Am J Clin Pathol 10:1, 1940
3. Sedzimir CB, Dundee JW: Hypothermia in the treatment of cerebral tumors. J Neurosurg 15:199, 1958
4. Baker KZ, Young WL, Stone JG: Deliberate mild intraoperative hypothermia for craniotomy. Anesthesiology 8:361, 1994
5. Bigelow WG, Callaghan JC, Hopps JA: General hypothermia for experimental intracardiac surgery: use of electrophrenic respirations, artificial pacemaker for cardiac standstill, and radiofrequency rewarming in general hypothermia. Ann Surg 132: 531, 1950
6. Bigelow WG, Lindsay WK, Greenwood WF: Hypothermia: possible role in cardiac surgery—investigation of factors governing survival in dogs at low body temperature. Ann Surg 132:948, 1950
7. Hervey GR: Hypothermia. Proc R Soc Med 66:1053, 1973
8. Reuler JB: Hypothermia: pathophysiology, clinical settings, and management. Ann Intern Med 89:519, 1978
9. Coniam SW: Accidental hypothermia. Anaesthesia 34:250, 1979
10. Maclean D, Emslie-Smith D: Accidental hypothermia. Oxford: Blackwell Scientific Publications, 1977
11. Welton DE, Mattox KL, Miller RR, et al: Treatment of profound hypothermia. JAMA 240:2291, 1978
12. Little DM Jr: Hypothermia. Anesthesiology 20:842, 1959
13. Collins VJ: Hypothermia: total body (refrigeration anesthesia). In Anesthesiology. 2nd ed. Philadelphia: Lea & Febiger, 1976: 748
14. Wolff RC, Penrod KE: Factors affecting the rate of cooling in immersion hypothermia in dogs. Am J Physiol 163:580, 1950
15. Hegnauer AH, D'Amoto HE: Oxygen consumption and cardiac output in the hypothermic dog. Am J Physiol 178:138, 1954
16. Bay J, Nunn JF, Prys-Roberts C: Factors influencing arterial PaO_2 during recovery from anaesthesia. Br J Anaesth 40:398, 1968
17. Rosomoff, HL: Effects of hypothermia on physiology of the nervous system. Surgery 40:328, 1958
18. Michenfelder JD, Theye RA: Hypothermia: effect on canine brain and whole-body metabolism. Anesthesiology 29:1107, 1968
19. Lafferty JJ, Keyhah MM, Shapiro HM, et al: Cerebral hypometabolism obtained with deep pentobarbital anesthesia and hypothermia (30°C). Anesthesiology 49:159, 1978
20. Stone HH, Donnelly C, Frobese AS: Effect of lowered body temperature on cerebral hemodynamics and metabolism of man. Surg Gynecol Obstet 103:313, 1956
21. Rosomoff HL, Gilbert R: Brain volume and cerebrospinal fluid pressure during hypothermia. Am J Physiol 183:19, 1955
22. Scott JW: The EEG during hypothermia. Electroencephalogr Clin Neurophysiol 7:466, 1955
23. Levy WJ: Quantitative analysis of EEG changes during hypothermia. Anesthesiology 60:291, 1984
24. van Rheineck Leyssius, Kalkman CJ, Bovill JG: Influence of moderate hypothermia on posterior tibial nerve somatosensory evoked potentials. Anesth Analg 65:475, 1986
25. Hegnauer AH, Shriber WJ, Haterius HO: Cardiovascular response of the dog to immersion hypothermia. Am J Physiol 161: 455, 1950
26. Hook WE, Stormont RT: Effect of lowered body temperature on heart rate, blood pressure and electrocardiogram. Am J Physiol 133:334, 1941
27. Badeer H: Influence of temperature on S-A rate of dog's heart in denervated heart-lung preparation. Am J Physiol 167:76, 1951
28. Bullard RW: Cardiac output of the hypothermic rat. Am J Physiol 196:415, 1959
29. Popovic V, Kent KM: Cardiovascular responses in prolonged hypothermia. Am J Physiol 209:1069, 1965
30. Wells R: Microcirculation and the coronary blood flow. Am J Cardiol 29:847, 1972
31. Johansson B, Biorck G, Heager K, et al: Electrocardiographic observations on patients operated upon in hypothermia. Acta Med Scand 155:257, 1956
32. Osborn JJ: Experimental hypothermia: respiratory and blood *p*H changes in relation to cardiac function. Am J Physiol 175: 389, 1953
33. Emslie-Smith D, Sladden GE, Stirling GR: The significance of changes in the electrocardiogram in hypothermia. Br Heart J 21:343, 1959
34. Abbott JA, Chietlin MD: The nonspecific camel-hump sign. JAMA 235:413, 1976
35. Falk RB Jr, Denlinger JK, O'Neill MJ: Changes in the electrocardiogram associated with intraoperative epicardial hypothermia. Anesthesiology 46:302, 1977
36. Blair M, Austin R, Blount SG, et al: A study of the cardiovascular changes during cooling and rewarming in human subjects undergoing total circulatory occlusion. J Thorac Surg 33:707, 1957
37. Lynch JF, Adolph EF: Blood flow in small vessels during deep hypothermia. J Appl Physiol 11:192, 1957
38. Keatinge WR: Mechanism of adrenergic stimulation of mammalian arteries and its failure at low temperatures. J Physiol 174:184, 1964
39. D'Amato HE: Thiocyanate space and distribution of water in musculature of hypothermic dog. Am J Physiol 178:143, 1954
40. D'Amato HE, Hegnauer AH: Blood volume in hypothermic dog. Am J Physiol 173:100, 1953
41. Rose JC, McDermott TF, Lilienfield LS, et al: Cardiovascular function in hypothermic anesthetized man. Circulation 15:512, 1957
42. Steen PA, Michenfelder JD: Detrimental effects of prolonged hypothermia in cats and monkeys with and without regional cerebral ischemia. Stroke 10:522, 1979
43. Steen PA, Michenfelder JD: The detrimental effects of prolonged hypothermia and rewarming in the dog. Anesthesiology 52:224, 1980
44. Bigelow WG, Lindsay WK, Harrison RC, et al: Oxygen transport and utilization in dogs at low temperatures. Am J Physiol 160: 125, 1950
45. Sodipo JO, Lee DC: Comparison of ventilation responses to hypercapnia at normothermia and hypothermia during halothane anaesthesia. Can Anaesth Soc J 18:426, 1971
46. Regan MJ, Eger EI II: Ventilatory responses to hypercapnia and hypoxia at normothermia and moderate hypothermia during constant-depth halothane anesthesia. Anesthesiology 27:624, 1966
47. Severinghaus JW, Stupfel M: Respiratory dead space increases following atropine in man, and atropine, vagal or ganglionic blockade and hypothermia in dogs. J Appl Physiol 8:81, 1955
48. Nisbet HIA: Acid-base disturbance in hypothermia. Int Anesthesiol Clin 2:829, 1964
49. Page LB: Effects of hypothermia on renal function. Am J Physiol 181:171, 1955
50. Moyer JH, Morris GC Jr, DeBakey ME: Hypothermia: I. effect on renal hemodynamics and on excretion of water and electrolytes in dog and man. Ann Surg 145:26, 1957
51. Carloss HW, Tavassoli M: Acute renal failure from precipitation of cryoglobulins in a cool operating room. JAMA 244:1472, 1980
52. Hallet EB: Effect of decreased body temperature on liver function and splanchnic blood flow in dogs. Surgical Forum 5:362, 1955
53. Brauer RW, Holloway RJ, Krebs JS, et al: The liver in hypothermia. Ann N Y Acad Sci 80:395, 1959
54. Curry DL, Curry KP: Hypothermia and insulin secretion. Endocrinology 87:750, 1970

55. Blair E: Clinical hypothermia. New York: McGraw-Hill, 1964: 49
56. Moore RA, Geller EA, Gallagher JD, et al: Effect of hypothermic cardiopulmonary bypass on nitroprusside metabolism. Clin Pharmacol Ther 37:680, 1985
57. Bunker JP, Goldstein R: Coagulation during hypothermia in man. Proc Soc Exp Biol Med 97:199, 1958
58. Halinen MO, Suhonen RE, Sarajas HS: Characteristics of blood clotting in hypothermia. Scand J Clin Lab Invest Suppl 21 (suppl 101):65, 1968
59. Kopriva CJ, Sreenivasan N, Stefansson S, et al: Hypothermia can cause errors in activated coagulation time. Anesthesiology 53:585, 1980
60. Paul J, Cornillon B, Baguet J, et al: In vivo release of a heparin-like factor in dogs during profound hypothermia. J Thorac Cardiovasc Surg 82:45, 1981
61. Hessell EA II, Schemr G, Dillard DH: Platelet kinetics during deep hypothermia. J Surg Res 28:23, 1980
62. Thomas R, Hessel EA, Harker LA, et al: Platelet function during and after deep surface hypothermia. J Surg Res 31:314, 1981
63. Valeri R, Casidy G, Shabri K, et al: Hypothermia-induced platelet dysfunction. Ann Surg 205:175, 1987
64. Von Kaulla KN, Swan H: Clotting deviations in man associated with open-heart surgery during hypothermia. J Thorac Surg 36: 857, 1958
65. Cooper KE, Kenyon RF: A comparison of temperatures measured in the rectum, oesophagus and on the surface of the aorta during hypothermia in man. Br J Surg 44:616, 1957
66. Whitby JD, Dunkin LJ: Temperature difference in the oesophagus: the effects of intubation and ventilation. Br J Anaesth 41: 615, 1969
67. Kaufman RD: Relationship between esophageal temperature gradient and heart and lung sounds heard by esophageal stethoscope. Anesth Analg 66:751, 1987
68. Siegel MN, Gravenstein N: Passive warming of airway gases (artificial nose) improves accuracy of esophageal temperature monitoring. J Clin Monit 6:89, 1990
69. Benzinger M: Tympanic thermometry in surgery and anesthesia. JAMA 209:1207, 1969
70. Ramsay JG, Ralley FE, Whalley DG, et al: Site of temperature monitoring and prediction of afterdrop after open heart surgery. Can Anaesth Soc J 32:607, 1985
71. Severinghaus JW: Blood gas calculator. J Appl Physiol 21:1108, 1966
72. Kelman GR, Nunn JF: Nomograms for correction of blood PO_2, PCO_2, *p*H, and base excess for time and temperature. J Appl Physiol 21:1484, 1966
73. Ream AK, Reitz BA, Silverberg G: Temperature correction of P_{CO_2} and *p*H in estimating acid–base status: an example of the emperor's new clothes? Anesthesiology 56:41, 1982
74. Hansen JE, Sue DY: Should blood gas measurements be corrected for the patient's temperature? N Engl J Med 303:341, 1980
75. Sessler DI, Moayeri A: Skin surface warming, heat flux, and control of temperature. Anesthesiology 73:218, 1990
76. Pflug ARE, Aasheim GM, Foster C, et al: Prevention of post-anaesthesia shivering. Can Anaesth Soc J 25:43, 1978
77. Pauca AL, Savage RT, Simpson S, et al: Effect of pethidine, morphine, and fentanyl on post-operative shivering in man. Acta Anaesthesiol Scand 28:138, 1984
78. Lisman SR, Hatton WF, Bigatello LM: Intraoperative meperidine prevents postanesthetic shivering. Anesthesiol Rev 4:29, 1991
79. Noback CR, Tinker JH: Hypothermia after cardiopulmonary bypass in man: amelioration by nitroprusside-induced vasodilation during rewarming. Anesthesiology 53:277, 1980
80. Cole AFD, Jacobs JA: Propranolol in the management of cardiac arrhythmias during hypothermia. Can Anaesth Soc J 14:44, 1967
81. Finley WEI, Dykes WS: Cardiac arrhythmias during hypothermia controlled by propranolol. Anaesthesia 23:631, 1968
82. Cherkin A, Catchpoll JF: Temperature dependence of anesthesia in goldfish. Science 144:1460, 1964
83. Eger EI II, Saidman LJ, Brandstater B: Temperature dependence of halothane and cyclopropane anesthesia in dogs: correlation with some theories of anesthetic action. Anesthesiology 26:764, 1965
84. Regan MJ, Eger EI II: The effect of hypothermia in dogs on anesthetizing and apneic doses of inhalation agents. Anesthesiology 28:689, 1967
85. Munson ES: Effect of hypothermia on anesthetic requirement in rats. Lab Anim Sci 20:1109, 1970
86. Rink RA, Gray I, Rueckert RR, et al: Effect of hypothermia on morphine metabolism in isolated perfused liver. Anesthesiology 17:377, 1956
87. Horrow JC, Bartkowski RR: Pancuronium, unlike other non-depolarizing relaxants retains potency at hypothermia. Anesthesiology 58:357, 1983
88. Ham J, Miller RD, Benet LZ, et al: Pharmacokinetics and pharmacodynamics of *d*-tubocurarine during hypothermia in the cat. Anesthesiology 49:324, 1978

FURTHER READING

Davies LK: Hypothermia: Physiology and clinical use. In: Gravlee GP, Davis RF, Utley JR (eds): Cardiopulmonary bypass: principles and Practice. Baltimore: Williams & Wilkins, 1993: 140

Farmer JC: Temperature-related injuries. In Civetta JM, Taylor RW, Kirby RR (eds): Critical care. 2nd ed. Philadelphia: JB Lippincott, 1992: 899

Lilly RB: Temperature fluctuations. In Kirby RR, Gravenstein N (eds): Clinical anesthesia practice. Philadelphia: WB Saunders, 1994: 429

Sessler DI: Temperature monitoring. In Miller RD (ed): Anesthesia. 4th ed. New York: Churchill Livingstone, 1994: 1363

Complications in Anesthesiology, second edition,
edited by Nikolaus Gravenstein and Robert R. Kirby.
Lippincott-Raven Publishers, Philadelphia © 1996.

CHAPTER 12

Malignant Hyperthermia

The term malignant hyperthermia (MH) refers to the clinical syndrome classically occurring under general anesthesia and consisting of a rapidly rising temperature associated with a high mortality rate. The syndrome is a result of increased skeletal muscle metabolism that can proceed to severe rhabdomyolysis and biochemical changes and may lead to irreversible shock and death. Early mortality reached 70%. Earlier diagnosis and symptomatic treatment decreased this rate to 28%, and the introduction of dantrolene as a treatment modality in 1979 lowered it further to less than 10%.[1,2]

Numerous reviews and several symposia[3–12] have addressed all aspects of the syndrome since Wilson's group first used the term "malignant hyperthermia" in 1966,[13] several months before Gordon independently referred to malignant hyperpyrexia.[14] A lay organization, the Malignant Hyperthermia Association of the United States (32 South Main, P.O. Box 1069, Sherburne, NY 13460) has been established for public education and communication among affected families. A 24-hour, 7-day telephone service has been created for emergency consultation (MH Hotline, 209-634-4917, ask for index zero, MH consultant). The North American Malignant Hyperthermia Registry collates findings from biopsy centers in Canada and the United States and provides access to specific patient data, either via the hotline or by direct contact with Dr. Marilyn Larach, Department of Anesthesiology, Pennsylvania State University, Hershey, Pennsylvania, 17033-0850 (telephone 717-531-6936).

HISTORY

Clinical Observations

In the earliest reference to the syndrome, in 1929, Ombredanne described postoperative pallor and hyperthermia associated with high mortality in children who had received general anesthesia. He did not, however, detect a familial relation.[15] In 1960, Denborough and Lovell[16] described a 21-year-old Australian man with an open leg fracture who was more anxious about anesthesia than surgery. His anxiety was appropriate, as 10 members of his family had died during or after ether anesthesia.

Further evaluations of affected families came from Locher in Wausau, Wisconsin, in association with Britt and coworkers in Toronto.[17] Direct skeletal muscle involvement soon superseded loss of central temperature control as the favored etiologic theory. This observation was based on recognition of increased muscle metabolism or muscle rigidity early in the syndrome, reports of low threshold contracture responses by Kalow and coworkers,[18] and elevated values for the muscle enzyme creatine kinase (CK) in the blood of affected persons.

Animal Studies

An excellent animal model was discovered in several strains of inbred swine (eg, the Landrace, Pietrain, and Poland China). Early reports in the veterinary literature described pork unsuitable for consumption.[19–21] Stresses of the slaughter house resulted in increased muscle metabolism causing pale, soft, exudative pork.[20] Breeding patterns designed to produce a rapid growth rate and superior musculature increased the incidence of swine with pale, soft, exudative musculature and led to the definition and use of the term, porcine stress syndrome.[21] Any stress, such as separation, shipping, weaning, fighting, coitus, and slaughter, could lead to increased metabolism, acidosis, rigidity, fever, and death in the affected swine.

In 1966, Hall and colleagues[22] reported MH triggered by halothane and succinylcholine in stress-susceptible swine. When clinical and laboratory observations during anesthesia-induced MH were compared, the porcine and human forms were virtually identical. Harrison[23] described the efficacy of dantrolene in preventing and treating porcine MH in 1975. A multihospital evaluation of dantrolene for treatment of unanticipated human episodes during anesthesia confirmed its effectiveness in 1982.[1]

Paradoxical Findings

A review of the MH literature reveals several paradoxes. In 1979, Halsall and coworkers[24] noted that many patients known

TABLE 12-1
Signs of Malignant Hyperthermia

EARLY	LATE	AFTER CRISIS
Muscle rigidity	Hyperpyrexia (may be >43°C)	Muscle pain, edema
Tachycardia	Cyanosis	Central nervous system damage
Hypertension	Electrolyte abnormalities, lactic acidosis	Renal failure
Increased end-tidal carbon dioxide tension	Increased CK rhabdomyolysis	Continued electrolyte imbalance
Lactic acidosis	Myoglobinuria	Disseminated intravascular coagulation, cardiac failure

Modified from Layon AJ: Anesthesia: physiology and postanesthesia problems. In: Civetta JM, Kirby RR, Taylor RW, (eds): Critical care, 2nd ed. Philadelphia: JB Lippincott, 1992: 581.

to have MH had previous uneventful experiences with anesthetics later identified as MH triggers. This observation may have been partially explained by a delay in response caused by attendant use of depressants or nondepolarizing muscle relaxants.[25] Conversely, nontriggering anesthetics have been associated with apparent MH episodes, even in humans partially protected by dantrolene.[26,27] Furthermore, reports of awake triggering in stressed humans further complicate our understanding of the clinical syndrome.

The best indicator of susceptibility is still survival of an unequivocal episode. Second best is an in vitro muscle contracture test that is perhaps 95% reliable.[28,29] Although variations in laboratory techniques and interpretation still may exist, the North American Malignant Hyperthermia Registry, formed in 1987, has worked toward standardization of the test.

CLINICAL PRESENTATION

The onset of MH can be acute and dramatic, particularly during induction of general anesthesia with a potent volatile agent or the administration of succinylcholine. Frequently, however, the onset is delayed for hours and may not become overt until late in the case or during the recovery period.[30]

When clinical signs, such as muscle rigidity, tachycardia, or fever suggest MH, the association is not strong (Table 12-1) unless more than one abnormal sign is noted. A single suggestive adverse sign usually is not associated with MH. Only patients with two or more adverse anesthetic signs or laboratory tests were noted to be MH-susceptible in a series of children presenting for MH muscle biopsy studied by Larach and colleagues[30] (Table 12-2).

TABLE 12-2
Clinical Data Recorded During Initial Anesthetic and Relation to Biopsy Outcome

	BIOPSY RESULT			
	MH+	*MH−*		*Total*
ADVERSE REACTION	NO. (%)	NO. (%)	*Equivocal No.*	NO. (%)
Generalized muscle rigidity*	13 (76)	3 (12)	0	16 (38)
Masseter rigidity	10 (59)	11 (46)	0	21 (50)
Myoglobinuria	7 (41)	6 (25)	0	13 (31)
CK (U/L)				
>100	17 (100)	15 (62)	1	33 (79)
100–20,000	11 (65)	12 (50)	1	24 (57)
>20,000	6 (35)	2 (8)	0	8 (19)
Acidosis	5 (29)	4 (17)	0	9 (21)
Hypercapnia	4 (24)	0 (17)	0	4 (10)
Hypoxemia	1 (6)	1 (4)	0	2 (5)
Temperature elevation	4 (24)	9 (38)	1	14 (33)
Tachycardia	5 (29)	8 (33)	0	13 (31)
Arrhythmia	5 (29)	5 (21)	0	10 (24)
Total patients with adverse reactions	17 (100)	24 (100)	1	42 (100)

* MH+ group vs. MH− group, $P < 0.0001$.

Green Larach M, Rosenberg H, Larach DR, et al: Clinical report: prediction of malignant hyperthermia susceptibility by clinical signs. Anesthesiology 66:549, 1987.

The clinical signs and symptoms reflect a state of highly increased metabolism, both aerobic and anaerobic, resulting in intense production of heat, carbon dioxide, and lactic acid with associated metabolic and respiratory acidosis. The high proportion of skeletal muscle to body weight (40% to 50%) accounts for the markedly altered acid–base status and temperature increase. Rigidity occurs in all susceptible pigs and in about 75% of humans. The temperature may exceed 43°C (109.4°F); arterial carbon dioxide partial pressure (Pa_{CO_2}) may exceed 100 mm Hg; and pHa may be less than 7.00.

Laboratory Findings

Associated increases in muscle permeability cause elevated serum potassium, ionized calcium, CK, myoglobin, and sodium. Later serum potassium and calcium levels may decrease markedly, indicating renal excretion as well as fluid and electrolyte shifts.

Organ Dysfunction

Sympathetic hyperactivity including tachycardia, dysrhythmias, sweating, and hypertension, is often an early sign of MH. Early muscle edema is followed by generalized and cerebral edema, as increased cellular permeability accompanies metabolic exhaustion. In the late stages of MH, disseminated intravascular coagulation, and cardiac and renal failure can develop and often contribute to death.

Temperature Elevation

Although increasing temperature classically is associated with the syndrome, MH is a disorder of increased metabolism and need not exhibit temperature elevation. If heat loss exceeds production or cardiac output drops early, the temperature may rise late or not at all. Some believe that MH may involve a generalized membrane disorder affecting permeability of calcium in virtually all tissues, though direct support for this theory is still lacking.

Masseter Muscle Rigidity

Masseter muscle rigidity or trismus after succinylcholine administration is associated with a subsequent diagnosis of MH about 50% to 70% of the time,[31–35] but rarely signals the onset of an MH episode. It is defined as jaw muscle rigidity in association with limb muscle flaccidity after administration of succinylcholine. Its causes include MH, myotonia, and possibly other myopathic conditions.

Relation to Malignant Hyperthermia

There appear to be three patterns of masseter muscle response to succinylcholine (Fig. 12-1).[34] Subclinical masseter stiffening is a normal response to succinylcholine.[35] Because it is subclinical, it obviously does not interfere with mouth opening. A second and much less common response on the order of a 1% incidence is "jaw tightness interfering with intubation."[33] The most severe response is masseter muscle rigidity such that the mouth cannot be opened.[36] Of these masseter muscle responses to succinylcholine, the second group includes probably 1 in 100 children, of whom a small number will be MH susceptible. The third group, on the other hand, is much less common but has a 50% incidence of MH susceptibility.

Two retrospective American studies document a 1% incidence in children given succinylcholine after an inhalation induction with halothane.[32,33] This rather high incidence contradicts the 0.01% incidence reported in Denmark,[34] but it nonetheless forces a reexamination of trismus. Compelling evidence suggests that trismus occurs as a unique property of jaw muscle in some normal people. Several findings support this thesis: masseter muscles have unusual fiber types that respond with slow tonic contractures.[37] In vitro, halothane predisposes normal skeletal muscle to development of a contracture upon exposure to succinylcholine.[38] In vivo, normal children under deep anesthesia with halothane or enflurane have tighter jaw muscles after succinylcholine is given.[35,39]

Thus, trismus may be a benign response on many occasions. In such circumstance, Gronert believes that anesthesia may be continued safely.[40] Conversely, Rosenberg has argued that anesthesia should always be halted if possible, the patient observed for signs of MH, and treatment initiated if these develop.[41] If anesthesia must be continued, Rosenberg suggests use of nontriggering agents. An intermediate approach that has also been proposed is that in the presence of isolated muscle spasm, anesthesia can be continued safely using the same anesthetic so long as MH monitoring is in place.[42] These proponents support their view by citing the efficacy of dantrolene therapy and the lack of increase in long-term morbidity or mortality after isolated masseter spasm compared with outcome data for the entire pediatric population at their institution.[43]

Anesthesiologists must remember that MH will occur in a few patients who manifest trismus. Thus, the usual careful monitoring to detect signs of MH (end-tidal carbon dioxide tension, pulse, temperature, muscle tone elsewhere in the body, heat loss, venous or arterial blood gas partial pressures, and examination of urine for myoglobin) must be performed. Furthermore, patients in whom trismus develops should be considered for testing of MH susceptibility. Collection of such

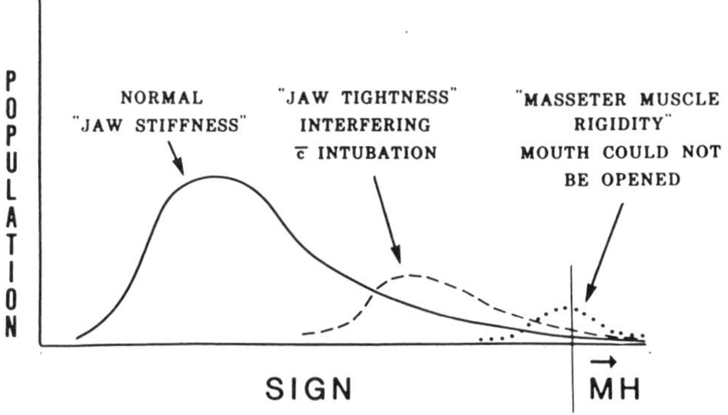

FIGURE 12-1. The spectrum of masseter muscle response to succinylcholine and the relationship to malignant hyperthermia (*MH*). (Kaplan RF: Hypothermia/hyperthermia. In Gravenstein N (ed): Manual of complications during anesthesia. Philadelphia: JB Lippincott, 1991: 138.)

data will help further our understanding of MH and provide the means whereby we can better determine the relation of masseter spasm to MH.

PATHOPHYSIOLOGY

Theory

The mechanism underlying the clinical picture of MH is best described as decreased control of intracellular calcium. Normally, the wave of depolarization from endplate to transverse tubule is somehow transferred to the sarcoplasmic reticulum (SR), resulting in release of calcium. The free, ionized, unbound, intracellular calcium concentration within the muscle cell increases from the relaxed level of 10^{-7} M to about 5×10^{-5} M. This increase in calcium removes troponin inhibition of the contractile elements, resulting in muscle contraction. The intracellular calcium pumps rapidly transfer calcium ion back into the SR, and relaxation occurs when the concentration is less than the mechanical threshold.

Contraction and relaxation require adenosine triphosphate (ATP); that is, both are energy-related processes that consume ATP provided by increased aerobic and anaerobic metabolism. Dantrolene reverses these effects by blocking SR calcium release without altering calcium reuptake.[44] Data obtained from humans and from swine support this theory.[45,46]

Abnormalities of Skeletal Muscle

Skeletal muscle is the only human tissue in which abnormalities associated with MH can be conclusively demonstrated. Although affected human muscle frequently has no histologic defect, a variety of nonspecific pathologic findings have been described. These include central cores, internal nuclei, target fibers, supercontracted fibrils, and marked variation in fiber diameter.[47]

Functional Changes

Functionally, affected muscle has exaggerated responses to various stimuli when compared with normal muscle, in both pigs and humans. During an MH episode, oxygen consumption ($\dot{V}O_2$) and glycolytic metabolism increase dramatically. A roughly three-fold increase in $\dot{V}O_2$ accompanies a 15- to 20-fold increase in blood lactate with attendant acid base abnormalities. Early changes are seen in the venous effluent, with decreases in pH and venous oxygen partial pressure and increases in carbon dioxide partial pressure, lactate, potassium, and temperature. The increases in lactate occur before any drop in venous oxygen partial pressure, indicating tissue hypoxia. Thus, the increased lactate probably indicates increased energy demands, reflecting a decrease in ATP that alters the balance between nicotinamide adenine dinucleotide and reduced nicotinamide adenine dinucleotide, forcing increased lactate production.

The earlier metabolic changes occur before alterations in heart rate, temperature, or circulating catecholamines. An increasing expired carbon dioxide (assuming constant ventilation) is the most sensitive early sign under general anesthesia.[48] Other signs of increased carbon dioxide production include increased mixed venous carbon dioxide partial pressure and hyperventilation in the spontaneously breathing patient. Muscle enzyme systems that have been studied for evidence of abnormalities include adenylate kinase, adenylate cyclase, and glutathione peroxidase. Such studies have proven inconclusive at best.

Heat Production

Heat production during acute MH derives from aerobic metabolism, glycolysis, neutralization of hydrogen ions, and hydrolysis of high-energy phosphate compounds involved in ion transport and contraction–relaxation. Initial heat production is due to increased aerobic metabolism, whereas lactate formation is responsible for later heat production. Precise calculations of the total energy expenditure are difficult due to unsteady metabolic and circulatory states, variable and uncontrolled heat loss, and production of heat by neutralization of acid.

Muscle Contracture

Muscle contractures that occur during MH can be differentiated from normal muscle contraction. Normal muscle contracts due to a propagated wave of depolarization that is brief and reversible. The nonpropagated, prolonged contracture of MH is similar to a muscle cramp and causes the rigidity that is seen clinically and that may be irreversible. These contractures are pharmacologically induced and observed in tissue baths for the in vitro study of MH.

Ideally, an intact muscle fiber from tendon to tendon would be preferable. Although such a fiber can be obtained from human intercostal muscle, for practical reasons, most contracture studies use cut muscle, usually from the quadriceps. These biopsy samples function adequately, but deteriorate quickly due to injury currents from the cut ends.[49,50]

The skinned fiber test is a further modification in which the sarcolemma and transverse tubules are mechanically or chemically[51] stripped away, leaving a preparation of SR and fibrils that can be manipulated in the laboratory. This technique requires more skill and preparation time than does fresh muscle contracture testing. It offers the advantages of requiring smaller amounts of muscle that can be frozen until preparation for chemically skinned fiber testing.[51] Mechanically skinned fiber testing can only be performed on fresh muscle.

Calcium Control Mechanisms

Several studies support the theory that MH is a disorder of calcium control. The SR is the intracellular organelle primarily responsible for control of intracellular calcium transients, and mitochondria serve a secondary reserve function in binding calcium. When intracellular calcium levels increase beyond the capabilities of the SR, the mitochondria begin to bind calcium. Thus, during acute MH, porcine muscle mitochondria begin to store calcium, and this process is reversed after treatment with dantrolene.[52]

Intrafibrillar ionized calcium in unstimulated MH-susceptible human intercostal muscle is elevated, as measured with a calcium selective microelectrode.[53] However, to have an increase in resting intracellular ionized calcium (observed by the same authors in porcine studies[54]) is paradoxical, as such increases of intracellular calcium should be associated with increased resting metabolism. This observation has not been made in susceptible humans or pigs. Perhaps the trauma of cellular microelectrode puncture evokes a stress response resulting in the increases in intracellular ionized calcium levels, as normal levels were observed when the intracellular calcium-selective dye Fura-2 was used to measure calcium.[55]

Intracellular calcium levels increase with initiation of porcine MH and are reversed by treatment with dantrolene.[52,55,56]

Transverse Tubules and the Sarcoplasmic Reticulum

The key to explaining MH is the link between the transverse tubules of skeletal muscle and the SR. Muscle physiologists have not yet explained this critical area of excitation–contraction coupling; it appears to be of likely concern in identifying the mechanisms underlying MH. However, initial investigations of the structure of this link and the involved receptors have been made. Recent studies identify the ryanodine receptor of skeletal muscle as a factor in the transfer of depolarization from the transverse tubule to SR to produce an intracellular release of calcium.[57] Furthermore, in susceptible swine, the ryanodine receptor has an altered calcium dependence with a markedly lower threshold for ryanodine inhibition of contractile activity.[57]

This finding may bear directly upon the mechanism of MH at a cellular level. Examination of the effects of volatile anesthetics upon skeletal muscle indicate that halothane does not act on the action potential of susceptible muscle via specific effects on sodium channels.[58] The volatile anesthetics alter calcium release from the SR at concentrations below their clinical effectiveness; at least in the rabbit, this alteration occurs at concentrations below those that alter calcium uptake.[59]

Studies of the intracellular organelles have focused on the SR and the mitochondria. The SR releases and reaccumulates calcium so rapidly that these processes are difficult to measure accurately. Accumulation of calcium by the SR is more efficient than by the mitochondria, suggesting a reserve function in the latter. Calcium binding by isolated SR can be estimated by the rate and capacity of calcium accumulation in the absence of oxalate. However, this measurement may not correspond to the mechanism or character of calcium uptake by the SR in vivo. Accurate measurements of SR calcium release remain technically problematic because of the difficulties in loading SR vesicles with sufficient amounts of labeled calcium.

Sarcoplasmic Reticulum Function

Studies of SR function have reported variable results,[60] partly because unphysiologic calcium concentrations were used in most. Although transport of calcium in the SR appears diminished in susceptible pigs and humans, differences from normal are not pronounced. Calcium binding and reuptake are decreased by about one third in susceptible pigs. Halothane in concentrations of 0.5% to 1% stimulates calcium binding to isolated SR from both normal and MH subjects. Higher concentrations of halothane progressively depress binding in both groups. Therefore, release of calcium by normal and MH SR is marked at high halothane concentrations, but is minimal at concentrations encountered during anesthesia.[60]

Cheah and associates' data suggest that abnormal mitochondrial release of fatty acids may adversely affect SR function in MH.[61,62] Other data suggest that a triglyceride lipase may be more important in heat and energy metabolism than phospholipase A_2 in the abnormalities of SR.[63] The calcium content of muscle from affected swine and humans is usually, but not always, less than normal.[64]

DANTROLENE. Dantrolene inhibits calcium release from the SR without affecting reuptake. This action specifically inhibits the hypermetabolism of MH and indirectly aids in evaluating SR action during MH. Because reuptake is not affected, abnormal SR function involves calcium release via factors acting beyond the end plate up to and including the SR. Until the precise mechanism of excitation–contraction coupling between the transverse tubules and the SR is determined in normal muscle, the specific defect involved probably will remain a mystery. A calcium-induced release of calcium has been noted to be abnormal in MH.[65] The usual normal transfer of depolarization from the transverse tubule to the SR is believed to occur by a depolarization-induced release of calcium.

Calcium-induced release of calcium may represent an abnormal pathway that is activated once MH is triggered. As mentioned previously, ryanodine receptors may participate in this action. Studies at room temperature suggested that dantrolene would not block a calcium-induced release of calcium, but this apparent lack of correlation with the physiologic state of MH is explained by the observation that dantrolene blocks this response at 37°C but not at 22°C.[66–68]

Mitochondrial Abnormalities

The mitochondria primarily provide ATP via aerobic metabolism, but also bind and store calcium. Isolated mitochondria from MH muscles have been shown to have diminished function when compared with normal muscles. However, this change is insufficient, by itself, to cause MH. Little evidence supports intracellular calcium release from the mitochondria by MH triggers. Evidence of increased calcium binding in the mitochondria is noted during MH,[52,69] perhaps due to decreased SR function. This change may, of itself, limit ATP production. Increased phospholipase or triglyceride lipase activity may alter SR function because of its effect in releasing long chain fatty acids that uncouple mitochondrial respiration and cause SR calcium release, but mitochondrial uncoupling as a proposed theoretical cause of MH has been discounted.[69]

Mitochondrial deficiencies alone do not explain the diminished aerobic responses in MH. The 3-fold increase in $\dot{V}O_2$ in MH contrasts poorly with the 10-fold increase seen in strenuous exercise. In view of the severe acid–base imbalances associated with depletion of muscle energy stores, the increase in $\dot{V}O_2$ seems paradoxically low. A limitation on mitochondrial energy production may be caused by several factors, including mitochondrial calcium binding, acid base disturbances and electrolyte imbalances.

Implications of Findings in Skeletal Muscle

Normal muscle can withstand the stresses of MH triggers that affect the membranes and disturb calcium homeostasis. In susceptible muscle, however, the membrane perturbation induced by halothane or the depolarization induced by succinylcholine may cause an earlier calcium release that strikingly stimulates greater calcium release.[66–68] This early calcium release, coupled with the lower mechanical threshold, may cause an MH response. Thus, MH muscle appears to exhibit abnormal excitation–contraction coupling, a conclusion supported by studies in pigs.[70] Although abnormal muscle may compensate temporarily, an increase in metabolism, temperature, and acidosis could cause a cascading loss of control. Even normal muscle may respond to extreme stress abnormally, as is seen in the "overstraining disease" or "capture myopathy" of wild animals after prolonged chase.[71]

Other Abnormalities

Central Nervous System

Central nervous system involvement is secondary to the increased temperature, acidosis, hyperkalemia, and hypoxia seen in fulminant MH. The late clinical picture of coma, areflexia, and fixed dilated pupils is related to acute cerebral edema with attendant intracranial hypertension. Recovery is variable and dependent on the duration and severity of the episode. Although high temperatures, to 42.5°C, can result in a flat electroencephalogram and coma, recovery may still be possible.[72] Early primary brain involvement is unlikely in MH. Studies in swine show normal cerebral $\dot{V}O_2$ and lactate production during MH episodes.

Peripheral Nervous System

Involvement of the peripheral nervous system is controversial. Histologic abnormalities of intramuscular axons, fiber type grouping, and target fibers seen in muscle are suggested as evidence. However, no good evidence shows that the muscle defect in MH is related to central or peripheral nervous system abnormalities.

Observations of porcine and human MH during regional anesthesia have led to contradictory data. Kerr, Wingard, and Gatz suggested a neural component when they noted that muscle rigidity with halothane was prevented in swine limbs anesthetized with epidural local anesthetic.[73] This phenomenon was also reported in an apparent episode of MH in a human undergoing epidural anesthesia.[74] Other porcine data, however, indicate that conduction anesthesia, while masking rigidity, does not prevent the hypermetabolic changes of MH.[75]

Sympathetic Nervous System

Whether activation of the sympathetic nervous system is a primary or secondary response in MH is unclear. Stress with its attendant sympathetic outflow can trigger MH in swine without exposure to anesthetic agents. Evidence of sympathetic hyperactivity with elevated levels of epinephrine and norepinephrine is found in both human and porcine MH. Many of the changes that occur during MH can be ascribed to sympathetic hyperactivity. However, increased levels of circulating catecholamines follow the changes in muscle metabolism and acid base balance that have already heralded an episode of MH. Furthermore, complete sympathetic denervation produced by total spinal anesthesia did not block development of halothane-induced MH in swine, though rises in circulating catecholamines were completely blocked.[75]

Many reports exploring the role of the sympathetic nervous system in MH have been published.[76–78] Swine studies demonstrating apparent triggering of MH by phenylephrine, an α-agonist, show an increase in muscle temperature preceding the rise in lactate levels. This finding contradicts previous studies showing that in succinylcholine-induced MH, lactate production increased before the onset of hyperthermia. A possible explanation of this apparent contradiction is that phenylephrine, by causing muscle vasoconstriction, results in tissue ischemia and increased heat production. This secondary effect then triggers the MH response.

Although hypoxia and hyperthermia are demonstrated triggers of MH, increased metabolism does not directly result from α- or β-agonists in susceptible porcine muscle.[79] Sympathetic antagonists may protect against or attenuate MH episodes by lowering body temperature and modifying acid base imbalances. But, although β-agonists have a beneficial effect on metabolism and fever in MH, their use does not alter survival.[78]

Blood

Abnormalities in blood components have been observed more consistently in swine than in humans. These include variations in ionic permeability, fragility, cholesterol content, and leukocyte antigens. Plasma pseudocholinesterase deficiency (fluoride-resistant gene) has been inconsistently associated with MH.[80] Platelet ATP stores and depletion by halothane have been used to predict susceptibility to MH, but evidence from several laboratories strongly suggests that this is not a reliable test. Disseminated intravascular coagulation can occur during MH, usually late. It may be related to release of tissue thromboplastin during fever, acidosis, hypoxia, hypoperfusion, and alterations of membrane permeability.

Cardiovascular System

Initial tachycardia and dysrhythmias during an MH episode are followed by hypotension, decreased cardiac output, and finally, cardiac arrest. Controversy continues over whether the heart is primarily involved, with intrinsic abnormalities, or secondarily affected by the hyperthermia, membrane permeability abnormalities, hyperkalemia, and acidosis associated with MH.

Porcine data support a secondary involvement. The increased myocardial $\dot{V}O_2$ in swine during MH is related to sympathetic stimulation without the localized increased lactate production or potassium efflux that would be expected of a primary MH response.[81] Porcine myocardium does not respond abnormally to even high doses of various sympathetic and inotropic stimulants, including various β- and α-adrenergic agonists, adenosine, carbachol, carbon dioxide, calcium, digoxin, and potassium. Cardiac symptoms in MH cannot be explained by altered function of α and β receptors, adenosine receptors, or cholinoceptors.[82]

Human patients susceptible to MH have been shown to have a higher incidence of sudden death,[83] nonspecific cardiomyopathies, and abnormal cardiac thallium scans[84] than the normal population. Examination of right ventricular biopsy specimens demonstrated only artifactual changes,[85] perhaps because of the difficulty of locating and identifying a structural abnormality in a disorder exhibiting abnormal function. Overall, evidence for myocardial involvement remains indirect. Higher mortality has been associated with certain drugs, such as cardiac glycosides,[5] but this relation may reflect a tendency to utilize these drugs in the more fulminant MH episodes with subsequent poor outcome. Cardiac muscle in susceptible swine is not triggered by calcium, digoxin, or potassium.[83]

GENETIC FACTORS

Incidence

The incidence of MH in children, adolescents, and young adults is about 1 in 15,000 anesthetics.[33] It drops to 1 in 50,000 or less in middle-aged and older patients.[86] MH is rare in infants and in adults older than 50 years. Approximately one half of susceptible patients will have received a previous general anesthetic without the development of MH.[24]

Inheritance

Denborough and colleagues, in their case descriptions of an affected family in 1960[16] and 1962,[87] noted an apparent autosomal dominant pattern of inheritance. This observation was supported by other early investigators. More recent investigations, however, suggest that two or more genes may be involved. Ellis and colleagues[88] described inheritance of two separate traits, myopathy and halothane contractures, in MH-affected families. These traits showed variable expressivity without evidence of reduced penetrance. That is, although both traits might not be found in every affected person, generation skipping did not occur. They concluded that MH was a polygenetic, multifactorial autosomal dominant trait. A family pedigree is shown in Figure 12-2.

Gender Linkage

Although gender linkage does not occur, a gender influence is seen, with men more commonly affected than women. This difference is marked between the ages of 16 and 30 years, perhaps accounting for the rarely reported cases of MH during pregnancy. After the age of 29 years, the incidence of episodes of MH decreases in both genders.

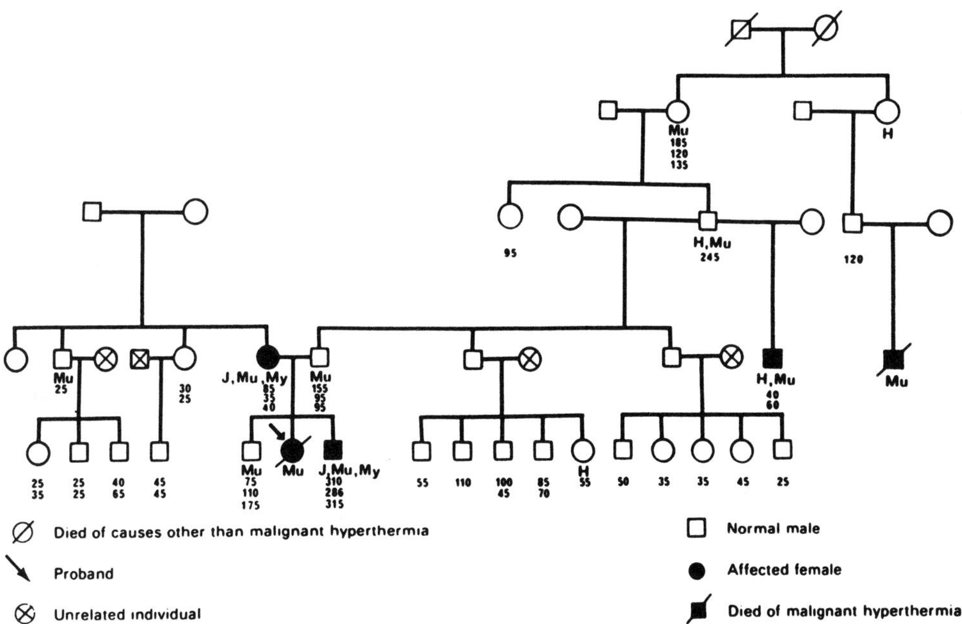

FIGURE 12-2. Pedigree of a family with malignant hyperthermia exhibiting atypical inheritance. The proband died during a rigid malignant hyperthermic reaction. The mother survived a similar rigid reaction. A second cousin of the proband's father died during a rigid crisis. In the mother, the proband's brother, and paternal stepuncle, muscle biopsy specimens tested positive for malignant hyperthermia. The mother exhibited a moderate elevation of the serum creatine kinase level on one occasion. Both brothers, the father, the grandfather, and the great-grandmother of the proband displayed significant elevations in serum creatine kinase. *H*, congenital inguinal hernia; *J*, joint hypermobility; *Mu*, excessive muscularity; *My*, muscle biopsy specimen positive for malignant hyperthermia; *numerals*, creatine kinase in international units. (Henschel EO (ed): Malignant hyperthermia: current concepts. New York: Appleton-Century-Crofts, 1977.)

Racial Characteristics

The racial distribution of MH is worldwide. The majority of reported cases have involved Caucasians, but Asians and Blacks are also affected. The incidence varies geographically, due to areas of genetic inbreeding and isolation.

TRIGGERING

Clinical and laboratory data in affected swine and humans indicate a decreased control of intracellular calcium, resulting in a release of free unbound ionized calcium from the storage sites that normally keep muscle relaxed. Subsequently, aerobic and anaerobic metabolism must increase to provide more ATP to drive the calcium pumps that maintain homeostasis across the sarcolemma into extracellular fluid and into the SR and mitochondria. Rigidity occurs when unbound myofibrillar calcium approaches the contractile threshold; rigid and nonrigid MH are unlikely to be different entities.

An acute MH episode might result from a series of minor defects in several areas leading to minimal increases in metabolism, heat production, and acid loads. These could then lead to a cyclic cascade and loss of control of enzyme systems and energy production as cellular temperature and acidosis increase. This process is accelerated by the lowered threshold for thermal inactivation of cellular function observed in susceptible muscle.[78] Widespread tissue and organ changes occur secondarily, leading to cell membrane breakdown with attendant increased permeability, edema, and further diminished perfusion.

Depolarization

The acute episode depends on three variables.[89] These are a genetic predisposition, the presence of a sufficiently potent anesthetic or nonanesthetic trigger, and the absence of inhibitory factors. Depolarization may be a significant factor in MH reactions whether these are anesthetic induced or "awake" (Table 12-3).[90–92]

Evidence against this theory of depolarization is the action of 4-aminopyridine, which increases acetylcholine release at the endplate but does not trigger hypermetabolism in susceptible swine.[93] Thus, extreme muscle activity or tension, either in the awake susceptible subject or in the susceptible person with increased muscle tension induced during anesthesia, results in exaggerated metabolism in susceptible subjects.[44]

TABLE 12-3
Evidence That Depolarization Is a Significant Factor in Malignant Hyperthermia

1. The mechanical threshold of susceptible muscle is lower than normal muscle, predisposing to easier development of contracture; halothane decreases muscle mechanical threshold
2. Succinylcholine and carbachol (equivalent of acetylcholine) depolarize normal and susceptible muscle; both trigger susceptible but not normal muscle
3. Electric stimulation triggers susceptible but not normal muscle
4. Nondepolarizing muscle relaxants delay MH episodes

Data from references 90–92.

Anesthetic Agents and Adjunctive Drugs

Anesthetic agents known to trigger MH include halothane, enflurane, isoflurane, sevoflurane, desflurane, methoxyflurane, cyclopropane, and ether as well as succinylcholine and decamethonium. The onset of MH can be delayed up to several hours by barbiturates, tranquilizers, or other depressants and by nondepolarizing muscle relaxants.[25,92,94,95]

Etomidate does not trigger MH, but is associated with a more rapid onset of the attack in swine when compared with pentothal.[96] Susceptible swine that received etomidate also demonstrated elevated lactate levels and temperatures without actually triggering. Halothane, used for identification of MH-susceptible swine, causes marked hind limb rigidity within 5 minutes. Prior exercise increases the severity and hastens the onset of these attacks in swine. A recent study showed that MH triggering in susceptible swine was delayed significantly with desflurane or isoflurane compared with halothane.[97] Times to MH onset were 20 ± 5, 48 ± 24, and 65 ± 28 minutes for halothane, isoflurane, and desflurane, respectively.

Susceptible humans respond much less predictably than swine to anesthetic triggers. Approximately half of affected humans previously have tolerated potent triggers without development of a recognized MH episode.[24] Factors that attenuate or mask an episode may include premedication, brief duration of anesthesia, and depressant induction agents. Reports of development of MH during nontriggering anesthetics and even after pretreatment with oral dantrolene[26,27,98] add to the diagnostic confusion. The prophylactic use of intravenous dantrolene, when indicated, should eliminate this phenomenon.[99]

Succinylcholine

Succinylcholine has several variant responses that can occur singly or in combination:

1. A muscle contracture, also noted in muscle that is myotonic or denervated
2. A change in muscle membrane permeability without contracture, resulting in the release of CK and myoglobin from muscle (even in normal patients, succinylcholine releases CK and myoglobin from muscle in small amounts). This response is exaggerated in the presence of halothane and attenuated by curare.[100]
3. An increase in metabolism, as in MH, usually associated with both muscle contracture and increased membrane permeability.

Although succinylcholine is a valuable and preferred relaxant in certain situations, its use presents a small but significant risk, partly as already detailed, and partly in the patient with occult muscle disease in whom an abrupt cardiac arrest may occur in association with hyperkalemia and rhabdomyolysis. Cases such as these occur rarely, but regularly, and occasionally present serious problems in resuscitation. In recognition of this complication, the manufacturers of succinylcholine modified their package inserts in 1993 to contraindicate the use of succinylcholine in children or adolescents except when used for emergency or rapid sequence type airway management. Significant controversy followed this action, with recommendations that the contraindication labeling be downscaled to a warning.

Nitrous Oxide

Nitrous oxide has been cited as a weak trigger of MH in humans, based on a single case report of elevated temperatures in an 11-year-old child undergoing dental care. However, the extensive use of this agent for susceptible swine and humans without adverse results makes it a very unlikely trigger. Susceptible swine given hyperbaric nitrous oxide did not trigger even with concentrations high enough to produce apnea.[102]

Nondepolarizing Muscle Relaxants

Nondepolarizing muscle relaxants attenuate or delay the triggering effects of volatile anesthetics and block the triggering effect of succinylcholine.[25,92,93] However, d-tubocurarine has been reported to be a triggering agent, based on elevated temperatures in two children from MH-affected families who received it as part of a nontriggering anesthetic.[103] Although d-tubocurarine has been associated with greater lactate production in environmentally stressed swine, it has not been shown to be a trigger in known susceptible swine. It is, therefore, unlikely that d-tubocurarine or pancuronium is a triggering agent; both have been used safely for susceptible patients. Vecuronium has been shown to be nontriggering in a study on MH-susceptible pigs,[104] and atracurium was safely used on a susceptible human.[105]

Antagonism of nondepolarizing muscle relaxants is more controversial. Although it has been performed without adverse effects in humans,[106] carbachol, and therefore acetylcholine, can provoke porcine MH.[87] Theoretically, reversal, including cholinergic drugs, could trigger MH. The agent 4-aminopyridine, which acts by releasing acetylcholine, does not trigger MH in swine.[78]

Local Anesthetics

Episodes of MH have been reported in the extremes of age and during regional as well as general anesthesia. The youngest reported case involved muscle rigidity in utero occurring just before birth.[107] The fetus presumably inherited the trait from the father and was triggered by anesthetic agents administered to the mother.

Suspicious events interpreted as MH triggering have been reported during epidural anesthesia with lidocaine[74] and spinal anesthesia with tetracaine.[108] Theoretical concerns have been expressed regarding the demonstrated calcium release from the SR by amides in laboratory animals; however, these studies involved local anesthetic concentrations far greater than those used clinically.[7] Furthermore, susceptible swine cannot be triggered into MH even when enormous doses of lidocaine are administered intravenously.[109]

Britt proposed possible triggering by lidocaine, but she and others also have commented on its use as a safe and perhaps effective treatment adjuvant in an acute episode of MH.[18,110] Another amide, bupivacaine, has been safely used for epidural analgesia during pregnancy in an affected patient without adverse effects,[111] nor does it trigger susceptible swine when given intravenously.[109] A report describing the safe use of mepivacaine in femoral nerve blocks combined with skin infiltration with lidocaine for muscle biopsies in possibly susceptible humans[112] should lay to rest the controversy and open the way to appropriate use of amide local anesthetics in affected persons.[113]

Timing

An MH episode may be delayed in onset for as long as 25 hours. One case report describes triggering after 26.5 hours of noncontinuous anesthesia for limb attachment that included enflurane, halothane, pancuronium, and two doses of succinylcholine.[114] This delayed response may be related to the attenuating effect of premedication or induction agents or to variable expressivity of the trait among susceptible persons.

The effects of prolonged stress on normal human muscle have not been fully studied, but observations of capture myopathy in wild animals raise some interesting questions. Further studies may demonstrate similar effects in stressed human muscle and help explain some of the reports of atypical or unusual events surrounding an apparent triggering episode.

Species Differences

Finally, species differences in MH triggering are known to occur; humans, pigs, dogs, cats, and horses have a more virulent form of MH than other studied species (eg, birds, rodents, and rabbits). This factor becomes important when animal studies are compared.

Awake Triggering

As previously described, susceptible swine can be easily triggered by a variety of environmental stresses. Exercise, heat, anoxia, apprehension, or excitement are specific factors. In the absence of triggering anesthetic agents, a possible mechanism for MH involves a hypermetabolic response to a neurotransmitter in association with unchanged responses to sympathetic stimulation. Muscle activity, which occurs in response to the cited factors, apparently results in uncontrolled, high levels of intracellular ionized calcium.

The reasons for this lack of intrinsic control are unclear, but they may be related to an abnormal and exaggerated response of susceptible muscle to stress. The elevated calcium results in greater than normal muscle $\dot{V}O_2$ and lactate production. Vasoconstriction that occurs secondary to sympathetic stimulation may raise lactate levels even further. These effects result in acidosis, hyperthermia, and further secondary sympathetic stress responses. Increasing temperature and ischemia result in an escalation into the vicious cycle of fulminant MH episode with further loss of control of calcium and eventual cardiovascular collapse.

Awake triggering in humans is less frequently observed than in swine and is rarely dramatic.[115] Episodes of MH triggered by anxiety in humans have been reported[116,117] and an increased incidence of unexplained sudden death,[83,118] sudden infant death syndrome,[119] and nonspecific cardiomyopathies[84,85] has been noted in susceptible families. Denborough and associates[120] also cite three cases of apparent MH episodes related to pneumonitis, combined exercise and alcohol, and treatment of schizophrenia with fluphenazine. All had positive muscle biopsies and responded to treatment with dantrolene (although response to this drug can be nonspecific and nondiagnostic).

Whether any of these reports truly represents awake human triggering is unclear. Furthermore, mechanisms explaining swine awake triggering may not be applicable in humans. Attempts to trigger MH in susceptible humans by severe exercise and fasting have been unsuccessful. No increased heat production occurred; however, in susceptible patients, higher insulin levels for given blood glucose levels did develop and no diet-induced thermogenesis occurred with exercise when these patients were compared with normal subjects.[121] More data need to be collected before the true nature and incidence of human awake triggering can be clarified.

ASSOCIATION WITH OTHER DISORDERS

Brownell has written a comprehensive review of MH and its relation to other diseases (Table 12-4).[122] In 1973, King and Denborough[123] first described a syndrome in four male children that was characterized by a slowly progressive myopathy, short stature, kyphoscoliosis, pectus carinatum, a distinctive facies, and susceptibility to MH.[124–126] Subsequently, several authors have described MH in other similarly affected males and at least one female.[124–126] MH has been reported with less consistency in several other disorders, including muscular dystrophy,[127–129] myotonia congenita,[130] central core disease,[131] sudden infant death syndrome,[119,132] and neuroleptic malignant syndrome (NMS).[133–142]

TABLE 12-4
Diseases Associated With Malignant Hypertermia

DISEASES ALMOST CERTAINLY RELATED
Central core disease

DISEASES POSSIBLY RELATED
- Duchenne muscular dystrophy
- King-Denborough syndrome
- Other myopathies
  - Schwartz-Jampel syndrome
  - Fukuyama congenital muscular dystrophy
  - Becker muscular dystrophy
  - Periodic paralysis
  - Myotonia congenita
  - Sarcoplasmic reticulum adenosine triphosphatase deficiency syndrome and mitochondrial myopathy

DISEASES OF COINCIDENTAL ASSOCIATION
- Sudden infant death syndrome
- Neuroleptic malignant syndrome
- Other diseases
  - Lymphomas
  - Osteogenesis imperfecta
  - Glycogen storage disease

Brownell AKW: Malignant hyperthermia: relationship to other diseases. Br J Anaesth 60:303, 1988.

Duchenne's Dystrophy

Patients with Duchenne's dystrophy, an X-linked recessive disorder, have a higher risk for MH susceptibility than does the normal population.[143] However, membrane fragility may lead to MH-like symptoms and/or rhabdomyolysis. The occasional occurrence of anesthetic disasters in this group, characterized by sudden cardiac collapse and poor response to resuscitation, may be hard to distinguish from an MH episode.

Occult Myopathies

These potentially and rapidly disastrous anesthetic events may occur in patients with occult myopathies of any type, and not necessarily related to MH or to the use of succinylcholine. Succinylcholine causes contractures in myotonic muscle, but this phenomenon is not usually related to MH. Myotonic goats do not proceed to full triggering of an episode even if halothane is added to the succinylcholine. A recent report suggests an association between myotonia and MH; it demonstrates that positive contracture responses may be observed in patients in whom rigidity developed after succinylcholine, or who have myotonia.[130] However, an association with clinical episodes of MH has not been demonstrated; in myotonia, rigidity appears in the absence of serious metabolic abnormalities.

Sudden Infant Death Syndrome

The relation to sudden infant death syndrome, or crib death, may be coincidental. It is based largely on studies of families of babies affected by the sudden infant death syndrome that reveal a higher than expected incidence of susceptibility to MH based on contracture studies.[119] Minimal correlative data exist and the area remains controversial.[132]

Neuroleptic Malignant Syndrome

Neuroleptic malignant syndrome (NMS) is related to central effects of psychoactive drugs including butyrophenones, phenothiazines, monoamine oxidase inhibitors and lithium.[134,139] The specific cause of NMS has been postulated as a spontaneous or iatrogenic derangement of the central nervous system's dopaminergic system. Neuroleptic agents often result in antagonism or depression of the actions of dopamine centrally. In addition, withdrawal of L-dopa may precipitate the syndrome. The reaction may not be specifically drug related, however, as a similar neuropsychiatric syndrome called lethal catatonia has also been described. Abrupt discontinuation of anti-parkinsonian agents and the use of dopamine depleting agents have also been reported to produce NMS.

Pathophysiology

Three key elements of the pathophysiologic processes involved in NMS are known. First, the patient usually has an impairment of motor function with generalized rigidity, akinesis, or extrapyramidal disturbances. Second, mental status deteriorates, with coma, stupor, or delirium. Third, hyperpyrexia develops, with deterioration and lability of other "vegetative functions," resulting in diaphoresis, blood pressure and heart rate fluctuations, and tachypnea. Onset is over days to weeks, in contrast to the acute onset of symptoms seen in true MH. It is apparently unrelated to duration of exposure to the neuroleptics, and subsequent rechallenge may not result in a recurrence.

Treatment

Treatment includes dantrolene, bromocriptine mesylate and amantadine hydrochloride (the latter two are dopamine agonists[140]), and general supportive measures. No controlled study evaluating the efficacy of the various treatment regimens exists. The rigidity associated with NMS can be relieved by nondepolarizing muscle relaxants if due to central drug effects, but dantrolene may be preferable as it will relax muscle tone while allowing spontaneous ventilation to persist. These patients can be extremely ill and require careful monitoring and support with special attention to control of acid base balance, muscle tone and hydration. The recovery period is prolonged due to the slow dissipation of the drug effects.

Susceptibility to Malignant Hyperthermia

MH-affected patients appear to be more susceptible to NMS,[141] but persons in whom NMS develops need not be MH susceptible.[142] Evidence obtained during general anesthesia suggests that NMS may not be associated with susceptibility to MH: patients with NMS have responded favorably to electroshock therapy and have tolerated succinylcholine without evidence of clinical MH.[137] This apparent lack of MH susceptibility may be attributable in part to the use of only a single trigger, succinylcholine, during a brief anesthetic. Nonetheless, careful metabolic monitoring disclosed no evidence of MH.

DIAGNOSIS

Diagnosis of an acute MH episode can be difficult, particularly when the onset is delayed,[30] and early signs are nonspecific (see Table 12-1). A fulminant episode associated with marked hypermetabolism and heat production must be treated promptly if permanent sequelae or death are to be prevented. In these cases, the diagnosis must be made early to ensure a good outcome. Ordinarily, MH would not be expected in cases where nontriggering anesthetics (ie, barbiturates, nondepolarizing relaxants, nitrous oxide, opiates, or benzodiazepines) are used, though rare exceptions have been reported.[26,27]

Clinical Findings

When potent volatile agents and depolarizing relaxants are used, MH should be considered if unexplained tachycardia, tachypnea, dysrhythmias, mottling of the skin, cyanosis, increased temperature, muscle rigidity, sweating or unstable hemodynamics occurs. If any of these signs is present, evidence of increased metabolism, hyperkalemia, or acidosis should be sought. Measurements of expired carbon dioxide during constant ventilation provides early, noninvasive evidence.[46,144] Other causes such as hyperthyroidism, pheochromocytoma, NMS, non-MH–related elevated temperature, and a circle system valve malfunction, causing increased inspired carbon dioxide must be ruled out. Some rare families manifest repeated hyperthermia during or after anesthesia, despite pretreatment with dantrolene and other various precautions.[145] These episodes did not feature clinical or laboratory evidence of MH. Thus, part of the differential diagnosis includes familial fever.

Blood Gas Analysis

Analysis of arterial blood gas partial pressures and pH demonstrate metabolic acidosis and may also show respiratory acidosis if the patient is unable to compensate for the metabolic increases. Central venous oxygen and carbon dioxide levels will show greater changes than those in arterial blood and are a more accurate measure of whole-body carbon dioxide stores. Peripheral venous blood gas analyses are also useful; carbon dioxide partial pressures greater than 55 mm Hg are abnormal, assuming adequate ventilation.

If arterial blood gas analysis demonstrates a $Paco_2$ greater than 60 mm Hg and a base deficit of −5 to −7 mEq/L or greater, the diagnosis can be made and treatment begun. Small children who have been fasting for long periods may have base deficits greater than −5 mEq/L because of smaller energy stores. Other disorders that may have acute onsets, such as hyperthyroidism and pheochromocytoma are included in the differential diagnosis and must be ruled out. The former can be differentiated by the lack of marked acid–base disturbances[146] and the latter by lack of a metabolic response.

Trismus and Rigidity

The diagnosis of MH after succinylcholine-induced trismus or rigidity can be difficult.[147–148] The association of succinylcholine-induced trismus or masseter spasm with MH is usually estimated to be 50% to 70%.[31,149–151] However, Schwartz and coworkers[32] in 1984 reported an incidence of 100% in 12 children in whom succinylcholine-induced masseter spasm occurred in the presence of halothane, as diagnosed by calcium uptake in thin sections of the muscle. They also noted an overall incidence of succinylcholine-induced masseter spasm of 1 of 800 anesthetics, and specifically in 1 of 100 halothane inductions followed by intravenous succinylcholine.

These results are controversial as the use of thin section calcium uptake for diagnosis of MH has not been confirmed.[152] Furthermore, a 1985 in vitro study by Fletcher and Rosenberg[38] showed that all muscle, normal and MH susceptible, that was preexposed to halothane, developed contractures with succinylcholine. They also demonstrated that muscle from patients with a clinical history of succinylcholine-induced masseter spasm and negative contracture studies developed abnormal contractures when exposed to halothane in the presence of succinylcholine. This sequence did not occur in nonsusceptible patients without a history of masseter spasm.

Further in vitro and in vivo studies need to be done to clarify this issue.

The proposed change in package labeling[101] and indications for succinylcholine use in children and adolescents, may eliminate this diagnostic dilemma by decreasing the number of patients exposed to succinylcholine. Good practice suggests that succinylcholine-induced trismus or rigidity should be treated conservatively, with cessation of the anesthetic, cancellation of the surgical procedure if possible, and careful monitoring for evidence of an MH episode. Even if a hypermetabolic response does not occur, CK and myoglobin should be monitored as massive rhabdomyolysis requiring appropriate hydration and diuresis can occur. Further evaluation including contracture testing to diagnose susceptibility to MH should be offered to the patient and family.

CONTRACTURE TESTING

Procedures

Contracture testing entails exposure of the muscle preparation to various contracture-producing drugs acting on the SR either directly or indirectly (Fig. 12-3). These drugs include caffeine, halothane or other potent volatile anesthetics, and potassium. Succinylcholine 1.1 mM can produce contractures in the tissue bath environment, but this effect is apparently due to the preservative rather than to succinylcholine itself.[153] Most laboratories report their results in terms of the amount of caffeine required to raise tension by one gram. Kalow and associates[154] proposed this concept and described the response as the caffeine or caffeine:halothane specific concentration.

Gronert takes into account the differences in tension due to varying cross-sectional area by expressing tension as the fraction of the peak observed tension.[48] Others, in Denborough's group, measure contracture responses to potassium and suxamethonium as well as halothane and caffeine.[155,156] Work by Fletcher and Rosenberg suggests that succinylcholine exposure combined with halothane produces contractures in muscle from patients with a history of masseter spasm in a situation in which succinylcholine or halothane alone were ineffective.[151]

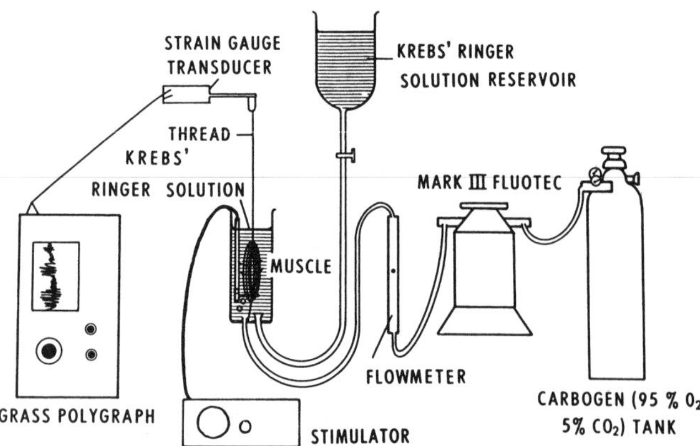

FIGURE 12-3. Experimental method for isolated isometric muscle contraction study. (Polygraph: Grass Instrument, Quincy, MA.)

European researchers have worked to standardize their technique to achieve consistent and comparable results.[157] North American laboratories are working toward the same goal. Whatever the method used, MH-susceptible muscle bundles produce low threshold responses, and interpretations of results from a given laboratory tend to be reproducible.

A major controversy concerning contracture testing concerns the use of halothane and caffeine in combination. Detractors believe that the broad range of responses indicates lack of specificity, whereas proponents hold that this broader range reveals a spectrum of susceptibility. Examination of intrafibrillar proteins has yielded inconsistent results.[158–160] Although differences in regard to nonhistone chromatin proteins have been detected, analysis by gel electrophoresis has yielded mixed results, and such tests are not predictive of MH susceptibility.

TREATMENT

Severity and Onset

When time permits, as in a slow onset or mild case of MH, the diagnosis should be confirmed by appropriate testing before instituting treatment. Discontinuation of the triggering anesthetic may be adequate treatment in these cases. However, if MH is fulminant ($Paco_2$ greater than 60 mm Hg and rising, base deficit less than −5 mEq/L and falling, and temperatures increasing 1.5°C every 15 minutes) treatment must be prompt and comprehensive (Table 12-5). Some patients may appear to have minimal metabolic and acid base changes in spite of a fulminant course. In these cases, an early drop in cardiac output with resultant poor tissue perfusion may mask the usual findings and can result in a rapid demise if not treated aggressively.

Dantrolene

Dantrolene specifically reverses the metabolic defect in MH but must be given while muscle perfusion is adequate. Symptomatic therapy also must be used to control body temperature, acid base balance, and renal function. Adjuvant drugs are rarely necessary if dantrolene is begun early enough. The discovery and application of this drug in treating MH has been the single most important factor in altering the morbidity and mortality figures in reported cases in humans[2] as well as in swine.[23] It rapidly slows metabolism, which results in a secondary return to normal levels of potassium and catecholamines. The body's homeostatic mechanisms can then rapidly restore arterial blood pressure, heart rate, and sympathetic activity back to normal.

Dose and Administration

For intravenous use, dantrolene is available in 20-mg bottles containing sodium hydroxide with pH value of 9 to 10 (to permit dissolution) and mannitol (to make the solution isotonic). It should be dissolved in sterile water to avoid a salting-out effect. When completely dissolved, the solution will be clear yellow to yellow-orange. Heating the solution under hot

TABLE 12-5

LOOK FOR • *tachycardia • muscle stiffness • hypercarbia • tachypnea • cardiac dysrhythmias • respiratory & metabolic acidosis • fever • unstable/rising blood pressure • cyanosis/mottling • myoglobinuria*

Emergency Therapy for

Malignant Hyperthermia

*** Revised 1993 ***

ACUTE PHASE TREATMENT

1. Immediately discontinue all volatile inhalation anesthetics and succinylcholine. Hyperventilate with 100% oxygen at high gas flows; at least 10 L/min. The circle system and CO_2 absorbent need not be changed.
2. Administer dantrolene sodium 2-3 mg/kg initial bolus rapidly with increments up to 10 mg/kg total. Continue to administer dantrolene until signs of MH (e.g. tachycardia, rigidity, increased end-tidal CO_2, and temperature elevation) are controlled. Occasionally, a total dose greater than 10 mg/kg may be needed. Each vial of dantrolene contains 20 mg of dantrolene and 3 grams mannitol. Each vial should be mixed with 60 mL of sterile water for injection USP without a bacteriostatic agent.
3. Administer bicarbonate to correct metabolic acidosis as guided by blood gas analysis. In the absence of blood gas analysis, 1-2 mEq/kg should be administered.
4. Simultaneous with the above, actively cool the hyperthermic patient. Use IV iced saline (not Ringer's lactate) 15 mL/kg q 15 min X 3.
   a. Lavage stomach, bladder, rectum and open cavities with iced saline as appropriate.
   b. Surface cool with ice and hypothermia blanket.
   c. Monitor closely since overvigorous treatment may lead to hypothermia.
5. Dysrhythmias will usually respond to treatment of acidosis and hyperkalemia. If they persist or are life threatening, standard anti-arrhythmic agents may be used, with the exception of calcium channel blockers (may cause hyperkalemia and CV collapse).
6. Determine and monitor end-tidal CO_2, arterial, central or femoral venous blood gases, serum potassium, calcium, clotting studies and urine output.
7. Hyperkalemia is common and should be treated with hyperventilation, bicarbonate, intravenous glucose and insulin (10 units regular insulin in 50 mL 50% glucose titrated to potassium level). Life threatening hyperkalemia may also be treated with calcium administration (e.g. 2-5 mg/kg of $CaCl_2$).
8. Ensure urine output of greater than 2 mL/kg/hr. Consider central venous or PA monitoring because of fluid shifts and hemodynamic instability that may occur.
9. Boys less than 9 years of age who experience sudden cardiac arrest after succinylcholine in the absence of hypoxemia should be treated for acute hyperkalemia first. In this situation calcium chloride should be administered along with other means to reduce serum potassium. They should be presumed to have subclinical muscular dystrophy.

POST ACUTE PHASE

A. Observe the patient in an ICU setting for at least 24 hours since recrudescence of MH may occur, particularly following a fulminant case resistant to treatment.
B. Administer dantrolene 1 mg/kg IV q 6 hours for 24-48 hours post episode. After that, oral dantrolene 1 mg/kg q 6 hours may be used for 24 hours as necessary.
C. Follow ABG, CK, potassium, calcium, urine and serum myoglobin, clotting studies and core body temperature until such time as they return to normal values (e.g. q 6 hours). Central temperature (e.g. rectal, esophageal) should be continuously monitored until stable.
D. Counsel the patient and family regarding MH and further precautions. Refer the patient to MHAUS. Fill out an Adverse Metabolic Reaction to Anesthesia (AMRA) report available through the North American Malignant Hyperthermia Registry (717) 531-6936.

CAUTION: This protocol may not apply to every patient and must of necessity be altered according to specific patient needs.

Names of on-call physicians available to consult in MH emergencies may be obtained 24 hours a day through:

MEDIC ALERT FOUNDATION INTERNATIONAL
(209) 634-4917
Ask for: INDEX ZERO

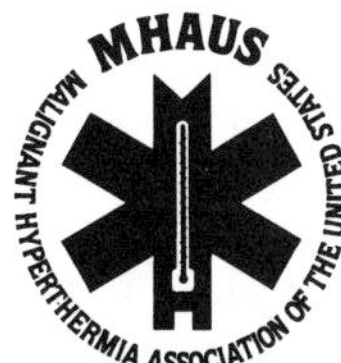

For Non-Emergency or Patient Referral Calls:
MHAUS
(203) 847-0407
P.O. Box 191
Westport, CT 06881-0191

3/93/12K

Malignant Hyperthermia Association of the United States. Westport, CT: 1993.

tap water or in an autoclave for a few minutes will help it to dissolve more rapidly. In a dire emergency, it may be mixed rapidly and administered through a standard blood filter to prevent infusion of undissolved crystals.

Seven to 12 bottles may be required to provide a therapeutic dose of 2.5 mg/kg in a large adult. Preparing dantrolene for such a patient will require the full-time efforts of three or four practitioners. Preoccupation with the symptomatic aspects of care, if it leads to a delay in the administration of dantrolene, may cause the patient's demise. Early dantrolene administration is the key to successful therapy.

Action

Dantrolene, as noted previously, acts by inhibiting SR calcium release without affecting reuptake. The specific site of action includes all components between the neuromuscular junction and the SR (ie, sarcolemma, transverse tubule, the "bridge" between the tubule and the SR, and the SR itself).[161] Dantrolene does not cause paralysis. At plateau effect twitch tension is inhibited more than response to a tetanic stimulus.[162,163] Usual clinical effects at maximum doses include moderate muscle weakness but adequate strength for deep breathing and coughing. The initial 2- to 2.5-mg/kg dose may be repeated every 5 minutes for a total of 10 mg/kg. Dantrolene has no serious side effects unless given for longer than 3 weeks. Oral preparations, used in the long-term treatment of spasticity, may result in cholestatic jaundice. Therapy for MH is summarized in Table 12-5.

Continuation of treatment and laboratory studies depends on the clinical course. Dantrolene should be repeated in a 1 mg/kg dose every 6 hours for 24 to 48 hours following the episode. If no sign of recurrence is present, it may then be discontinued.

Other Drugs

Historically, procaine was the drug treatment of choice,[9] and is still suggested as the treatment (in the form of procainamide) for dysrhythmias that do not respond to early adequate therapy for MH. Lidocaine once was abandoned for theoretical reasons, but the more recent literature[109,112,113] suggests that the amide local anesthetics are safe in human and porcine MH in the usual clinical dosages. Porcine data indicate that cardiac glycosides and calcium will not trigger MH episodes.[82] Their cautious use may be indicated in humans.

Suggested Therapeutic Adjuvants

Other suggested therapeutic adjuvants include the calcium channel blockers (ie, nimodipine, verapamil, nifedipine, and diltiazem)[164] and sympathetic antagonists such as propranolol. Calcium antagonists are associated with hyperkalemia and potentially increased mortality in vivo when used in conjunction with dantrolene,[165,166] and do not prevent or effectively treat MH in susceptible pigs.[167,168] Further, because of the risk of hyperkalemia with calcium antagonists and dantrolene, a MH episode may be triggered in susceptible skeletal muscle.[82]

The action of calcium antagonists is primarily on surface membranes of cardiac or smooth muscle, whereas dantrolene acts primarily on calcium release from the SR. β-Sympathetic agonists do not increase porcine MH survival. Propranolol may decrease myocardial $\dot{V}O_2$, but this effect can be disastrous in MH in which increased cardiac function is necessary for survival.

Hyperkalemia

Treatment of the accompanying hyperkalemia should be approached slowly. Serum potassium levels should be serially monitored (persistent elevations my prevent defibrillation). The most effective treatment of the associated hyperkalemia is reversal of MH by dantrolene. Frequently, depletional hypokalemia will follow the period of hyperkalemia and replacement of potassium may be necessary. The use of calcium to protect the heart during hyperkalemia is risky, and the administration of calcium is not effective in treating the hypocalcemia that occurs in MH. Calcium should be administered only for treatment of related dysrhythmias or for poor cardiac function associated with hypocalcemia.[169–171]

Neurologic Complications

Neurologic complications, including coma and paralysis, may occur in advanced cases in spite of satisfactory care during the MH episodes. Probable causes of neurologic dysfunction include inadequate cerebral oxygenation and perfusion for the increased metabolism as well as fever, acidosis, and potassium efflux. Intracranial pressure monitoring may be helpful in evaluating cerebral edema.

Disseminated Intravascular Coagulation

Disseminated Intravascular Coagulation or consumptive coagulopathy can also complicate a fulminant episode of MH. Suggested mechanisms include hemolysis, release of tissue thromboplastins due to increased membrane permeability or tissue damage, shock causing inadequate tissue perfusion or other unknown factors. The best therapy is early and adequate treatment of the underlying problem. Other care is symptomatic and may, in rare cases, include heparin.

Renal Dysfunction

Significant renal damage may occur secondary to poor perfusion and myoglobinuria. Dialysis may be required.

ANESTHESIA FOR SUSCEPTIBLE PATIENTS

Routine pretreatment with dantrolene has been reported to increase the risk of prolonged weakness or prolongation of the effects of nondepolarizing muscle relaxants.[163,172–175] For this reason, along with the relative rarity and minor nature of MH events during nontriggering anesthesia, many MH experts no longer recommend routine preoperative doses of dantrolene unless the patient has a history of awake stress-induced MH reaction, limited cardiac reserve, or renal insufficiency suggesting inability to tolerate stress or slight myoglobinuria.[176] The drug should be immediately available in the operating suite in either case.

Data from the maternal–fetal sheep model indicate a rapid equilibration, but that fetal levels were approximately 10% those of the mother.[177,178] In general, dantrolene is not recommended prepartum or to the small infant because it has an apparent sedative effect. At delivery, if dantrolene is needed for the mother, its administration should be withheld until after the cord is clamped. Intravenous pretreatment ensures adequate blood levels, which cannot be predicted after oral administration.[98,138]

General Anesthesia

General anesthetic agents may include nitrous oxide, barbiturates, etomidate, opiates, benzodiazepines, and nondepolarizing muscle relaxants including vecuronium and atracurium. To be avoided are all potent volatile agents and the depolarizing muscle relaxants, succinylcholine and decamethonium. Triggering episodes have been reported in humans in spite of these precautions.[26,27] Therefore, all patients must be monitored closely.

Regional Anesthesia

Regional anesthesia is safe and may be preferred for susceptible patients. Safe administration of both ester and amide local anesthetics has now been reported in susceptible humans,[112,179] so drug choice should be tailored to the individual case.

Apparatus

Precautions should be taken to avoid exposure to areas or machinery potentially contaminated by triggering agents. No longer is it necessary to provide a noncontaminated anesthetic machine by flushing with oxygen for a number of hours.[180] Removal or sealing of the vaporizers, replacement of the fresh gas outlet hose, and use of a disposable circle with a flush of 6 L per minute for 5 minutes suffice.[181] An equally satisfactory and economical method uses a nitrous oxide blender instead of an anesthetic machine.[182] Postoperatively, the patient should not recover near other patients who are expiring volatile gases. Isolated areas of the postanesthesia care unit or intensive care unit are safe alternatives for recovery from anesthesia.

Monitoring

Appropriate intraoperative monitoring for the susceptible patient will assist in early diagnosis, and should include the basic standards used in all safe anesthetics such as blood pressure, electrocardiogram, oxygen, and end-tidal carbon dioxide monitor. The latter is an excellent noninvasive indicator of metabolic hyperactivity if constant ventilation is maintained.[48] Noninvasive monitors of oxygenation such as pulse oximeters preclude vessel trauma. Central venous catheters and peripheral arterial cannulae are unnecessary for anesthetic management of an otherwise healthy susceptible patient, unless dictated by the procedure. Accurate core temperature measurements intra- and postoperatively are obviously also important.

Preanesthetic Assessment and Discussion

The anesthesiologist should spend adequate time with the susceptible patient preoperatively to discuss the anesthetic care and answer questions. Many of these patients will have undergone previous anesthetics without problem. However, some patients may have encountered physicians who refuse to anesthetize susceptible patients, thereby exaggerating their apprehensions and feelings of "abnormality." Careful explanation of preventive measures as well as assurance that appropriate treatment is readily available should an episode occur will minimize anxiety. With a confident approach by the physician, the patient will enter the therapeutic environment in a relaxed and comfortable state of mind.

Pregnancy

Care of the susceptible pregnant patient presents a few specialized problems. Monitoring and choice of anesthetic are based on the same guidelines used for nonpregnant patients. Regional anesthesia is well-accepted in obstetrics and often preferred by the patient. Both amide and ester agents have been used with safety in this population. Dantrolene pretreatment of the pregnant susceptible patient is controversial. Placental transfer does occur, although adverse reactions were not seen in fetuses after oral pretreatment of susceptible mothers.[177,178]

Muscle weakness associated with dantrolene may be more profound in the newborn, causing respiratory distress, especially if it is combined with other factors such as a cesarean delivery or maternal narcotic analgesia. This theoretical concern, as we have mentioned previously, can be eliminated by withholding the intravenous dantrolene until the umbilical cord is clamped. Of course, in a fulminant episode, it must be given. Further studies may clarify this clinical situation. Early diagnosis and adequate treatment are even more critical in the pregnant patient because cardiac and metabolic reserves are lower due to the demands and stresses of pregnancy and delivery.

Evaluation of Susceptibility

The subject of susceptibility has been comprehensively reviewed.[28] The suspect patient has a personal or family history of anesthetic problems, unexpected family deaths, or trismus. A detailed history and physical examination looking for evidence of subclinical abnormalities is the first step in evaluation for MH susceptibility. The history should include a genealogy of at least two generations to estimate exposure and response to triggering anesthetics.

Creatine Kinase

Measurement of serum CK provides a basic screening tool. These values should be determined in the resting patient without recent trauma or excessive exercise and with careful technique to avoid hemolysis. The CK is a reflection of muscle membrane stability and will be elevated in about 70% of affected humans and swine.

Many factors are known to be associated with elevated CK, including exercise, excessive tourniquet pressure, recent myocardial infarction, muscular dystrophy, hypothyroidism, intramuscular injections, muscle trauma, pregnancy, and alcoholism, to name a few. Falsely normal values can be obtained if the serum sample is exposed to light.

If the CK is elevated in a first-degree relative of a known susceptible person, this relative may also be considered susceptible without further invasive testing. However, a normal CK value in this situation is of no predictive value, and a muscle biopsy specimen is needed for contracture testing to make a reliable diagnosis.

Contracture Testing

Muscle contracture testing is done across the world using a variety of agents, including halothane, caffeine, halothane plus caffeine, succinylcholine, and potassium. Contraction thresholds are perhaps 95% reliable in evaluating susceptibility.[28,29] Porcine data suggest that cell injury may skew responses toward susceptible.[183] This aspect has not been directly studied in human biopsies. The pattern of mixed fiber types in human muscle precludes caffeine thresholds directly related to specific fiber types, such as has been seen at times in the pig. Contracture testing conceivably could be positive in patients with myopathies that have no clear relation with MH.[184] In these cases, a positive biopsy specimen may not indicate susceptibility.[138] Patients must not be given dantrolene before biopsy; to do so could mask the abnormal muscle response to triggering agents.[185]

SENSITIVITY AND SPECIFICITY. The predictive value of contracture testing in determining susceptibility in MH cannot be estimated. False positives due to cautious interpretations will be masked because these patients will never be exposed to triggering agents. Few false negative results have been reported.[186] The sensitivity of the tests used (frequency of positive results in true positives) is good in that positives correlate well with MH survivors and known susceptible swine.

Specificity (frequency of negative results in true negatives) will become known as patients with normal muscle biopsies are exposed to triggering anesthetics. These epidemiologic considerations are complicated by the variations in metabolic responses and consequent diagnostic dilemmas observed in MH-susceptible humans during anesthesia.

Contracture-testing results are based on the knowledge that susceptible persons have a lower threshold to contracture-producing drugs than do normal subjects. The muscle specimen must be viable (twitch response when stimulated electrically), as the contracture threshold may vary if the fiber is degenerating or acutely deteriorating.

HALOTHANE AND CAFFEINE. A major controversy exists regarding the combined use of halothane and caffeine. Experts agree that each drug alone accurately identifies susceptibility; however, combining the two agents yields a wide range of thresholds. This variability can be interpreted as the broad range inherent in a test lacking precision. It has also been interpreted as evidence for a wide spectrum of susceptibility within the affected population.[187] This controversy has not been settled by human or porcine data.

Standardization of contracture testing, organized by the Canadian MH Association, the Malignant Hyperthermia Association of the United States, and the North American Malignant Hyperthermia Registry should help to eliminate differences in protocols among the testing laboratories in North America, as well as to define more precisely the thresholds in normal people to caffeine alone, halothane alone, or to the combination of caffeine and halothane. These should then provide greater accuracy in diagnostic biopsies. In a recently published study of 350 muscle contracture studies, 49% tested normal.[186] Of these, the investigators believed that they identified 4 cases with false-negative results. The European protocol (exposure of muscle to incremental doses of halothane with a muscle contracture of ≥ 0.2 g considered abnormal) was used rather than the North American protocol (exposure to a single dose of 3% halothane with values for abnormal threshold responses determined by the individual laboratory director). Other differences of interpretation are present; hence the direct applicability of this study to MH detection in the United States and Canada is open to question. Nevertheless, the authors of that report[186] and an accompanying editorial[188] believe that contracture testing is generally reliable and should be continued while the diagnostic tests are developed and refined.

Other Tests

Other methods have been enthusiastically introduced and sometimes uncritically accepted, but these cannot be used as sole diagnostic tests in the absence of confirmatory data. What is needed in MH testing is an accurate, noninvasive or nondestructive measure of susceptibility.

MAGNETIC RESONANCE IMAGING. Magnetic resonance imaging probably has the greatest promise.[189] The difficulty is to standardize a stress, such as forearm ischemia, that will differentiate susceptible from normal tissue. In the absence of stress, susceptible persons or their tissues are not different from normal. As with so many tests, a major problem is to establish conditions whereby no overlap occurs between the ranges of normal and susceptible responses.

LYMPHOCYTE CALCIUM PRODUCTION. A nondestructive test introduced by Klipp and coworkers of Toronto involved the increase in ionized calcium produced by halothane in lymphocytes. Unfortunately, overlap occurred between results in pigs[190] and in humans[191] and the positive test results could not be confirmed by another laboratory.[192]

Other as-yet unconfirmed tests of susceptibility include halothane-induced disorders of red cell membranes,[193,194] and the use of a calcium iodophor that, in susceptible Pietrain pigs, elevated intracellular calcium concentrations in intercostal muscle.[195] In this particular situation, clear differentiation between normal and susceptible muscle was possible. We cannot at present predict the applicability of this test in humans or in muscle other than the intercostal.

ELECTROMYOGRAPHY. Noninvasive neuroelectrophysiologic tests have been studied looking for alternatives to invasive techniques of diagnosis. Electromyography shows an increased incidence of polyphasic action potentials of short duration in some susceptible patients but this is not diagnostic. Studies in swine vary, demonstrating longer motor unit potentials with greater amplitude, increased contraction and half-relaxation times, and prolonged time from stimulus to onset of contraction.

MOTOR UNIT COUNTING. Motor unit counting, though claimed to be more accurate in some studies, does not achieve the reproducibility of contracture testing. A porcine study clearly differentiates susceptible from nonsusceptible pigs by the use of multiple pulses and dantrolene.[196] Dantrolene alters normal responses more than susceptible ones in this situation. Further studies in this area are ongoing, but at present noninvasive testing alone cannot be relied upon to accurately diagnose MH susceptibility.

PHOSPHORYLASE RATIO. The phosphorylase ratio, the ratio of muscle phosphorylase A to total phosphorylase, has been noted to be higher in muscle from affected patients.[197] The same work repeated in patients receiving femoral nerve block rather than general anesthesia showed contradictory results, suggesting that apprehension in awake patients caused activation of phosphorylase.[198]

PLATELET ADENOSINE TRIPHOSPHATE DEPLETION. Halothane-induced platelet ATP depletion is claimed to be greater in platelets from affected patients[199]; however, other laboratories have been unable to confirm the accuracy of this technique.

MISCELLANEOUS TESTS. Calcium uptake data from muscle strips has not been confirmed and false positive results may be unacceptably high. Muscle ATP deletion was precise in affected swine, but has been disappointingly imprecise in human studies. Glutathione peroxidase assay, technically difficult, has not been confirmed as a predictive test. Electrophoresis of muscle from affected patients showed large amounts of low–molecular-weight proteins, but further testing in this area has not confirmed the validity of this type of analysis.[202]

New research is investigating the ryanodine receptor protein. The ryanodine receptor protein is made by the ryanodine gene, which probably lies very near the gene, causing MH susceptibility. Nelson has shown a defect in the ryanodine-sensitive calcium release channel from muscles of MH-susceptible patients.[201] If work in this area continues to support this relation, a serum test for MH susceptibility is conceivable.

For now, fresh muscle contracture testing remains the "gold standard" for diagnosis of susceptibility.[202] Several years ago the protocol for contracture testing was standardized among the laboratories in England, Scandinavia, and continental Europe. This protocol results in more precise definition of control values and what appears to be more accurate diagnosis of susceptibility. Efforts in the United States and Canada should develop an analogous standardized approach with similar results.

COUNSELING SUSCEPTIBLE PATIENTS

Once a diagnosis of MH susceptibility is made, either on the basis of an unequivocal episode or by muscle contracture testing, attention must be turned toward appropriate counseling of the patient and family. All family members should be counseled to include their relation to MH-affected persons when giving any medical history. Patients with known susceptibility should wear a Medic Alert bracelet identifying them as MH susceptible and listing major triggering anesthetics to be avoided. First degree relatives may also wish to wear these bracelets. Reassurance is important throughout the counseling period, as families will be naturally apprehensive about future anesthetics. Complete and detailed information will help allay anxieties. Ongoing information and communication with other affected families can be obtained by joining the Malignant Hyperthermia Association of the United States (the address is given at the beginning of this chapter).

CONCLUSION

MH is an inherited disorder in which, under triggering conditions usually related to anesthesia, skeletal muscle acutely increases $\dot{V}O_2$ and lactate production that results in a runaway cycle of heat production, acidosis, rigidity, sympathetic stimulation and increased cellular permeability.

The best accepted theory is that MH is caused by an inability to control calcium concentrations with the muscle fiber; it may involve a generalized alteration in cellular or subcellular membrane permeability. Episodes are triggered by potent volatile agents and succinylcholine in humans and swine; however, swine differ from humans in that they can be predictably triggered by excitement or stress while awake as well.

Inheritance appears to be controlled by more than one gene. Diagnosis is made by observation of tachycardia, rigidity, high temperatures and acid base alterations. Specific treatment by dantrolene should be initiated promptly. Symptomatic treatment of associated acid–base abnormalities and attendant complications should be added as needed.

General or regional anesthesia is safe for patients susceptible to MH, provided that if a general technique is chosen, care is taken to specially prepare the anesthesia machine and to avoid all anesthetic trigger agents.

Evaluation of susceptible patients includes a history, physical examination, and serum CK determinations before muscle biopsy for contracture testing. Efforts to find a noninvasive reliable test for evaluation of susceptibility continue. Challenges for the future include identification of the gene or genes responsible for MH, and elucidation of the mechanism that links exposure to the subsequent loss of calcium control.

REFERENCES

1. Kolb ME, Horne ML, Martz R: Dantrolene in human malignant hyperthermia: a multicenter study. Anesthesiology 56:254, 1982
2. Ranklev E, Fletcher R: Investigation of malignant hyperthermia in Sweden. Acta Anaesthesiol Scand 30:693, 1986
3. Britt BA: Etiology and pathophysiology of malignant hyperthermia. Fed Proc 38:44, 1979
4. Mitchell G, Heffron JJA: Porcine stress syndromes. Adv Food Res 28:167, 1982
5. Britt BA: Malignant hyperthermia. In Orkin FK, Cooperman LH (eds): Complications in anesthesiology. Philadelphia: JB Lippincott, 1982: 291
6. Gallant EM, Ahern CP: Malignant hyperthermia: responses of skeletal muscles to general anesthetics. Mayo Clin Proc 58: 758, 1983
7. Gronert GA: Malignant hyperthermia. Anesthesiology 53:395, 1980
8. Hall GM, Lucke JN, Lister D: Malignant hyperthermia: pearls out of swine? Br J Anaesth 52:165, 1980
9. Denborough MA: Malignant hyperpyrexia. Clinics in Anaesthesiology 2:669, 1984
10. Nelson TE, Flewellen EH: The malignant hyperthermia syndrome. New Engl J Med 309:416, 1983
11. Gordon RA, Britt BA, Kalow W (eds): International symposium on malignant hyperthermia. Springfield, IL: Charles C Thomas, 1973
12. Aldrete JA, Britt BA (eds): Second international symposium on malignant hyperthermia. New York: Grune and Stratton, 1978
13. Wilson RD, Nichols RJ Jr, Dent TE, et al: Disturbances of the oxidative-phosphorylation mechanism as a possible etiological factor in sudden unexplained hyperthermia occurring during anesthesia. Anesthesiology 27:231, 1966
14. Gordon RA: Malignant hyperpyrexia during general anesthesia. Can Anaesth Soc J 13:415, 1966
15. Ombredanne L: De l'influence de l'anesthesique-employé dans la genese des accidents post-operatoires de paleur-hyperthermie observes chez les nourrissons. Revue Medicale Francaise 10:617, 1929
16. Denborough MA, Lovell RRH: Anaesthetic deaths in a family. Lancet 2:45, 1960
17. Britt BA, Locher WG, Kalow W: Hereditary aspects of malignant hyperthermia. Can Anaesth Soc J 16:89, 1969
18. Kalow W, Britt BA, Terreau ME, et al: Metabolic error of muscle metabolism after recovery from malignant hyperthermia. Lancet 2:89, 1970
19. Herter M, Wilsdorf G: Die Bedeutung des Schweines fur die Fleischversorgung. Berlin: Arbeiten der Deutscher Landwirtschaft-Gesellschaft, 1914: 270
20. Briskey EJ: Etiological status and associated studies of pale, soft, exudative porcine musculature. Adv Food Res 13:89, 1964
21. Topel DG, Bicknell EJ, Preston KS, et al: Porcine stress syndrome. Modern Veterinary Practice 49:40, 1968
22. Hall LW, Woolf N, Bradley JWP, et al: Unusual reaction to suxamethonium chloride. Br Med J 2:1305, 1966
23. Harrison GG: Control of the malignant hyperpyrexic syndrome in MHS swine by dantrolene sodium. Br J Anaesth 47:62, 1975
24. Halsall PJ, Cain PA, Ellis FR: Retrospective analysis of anaesthetics received by patients before susceptibility to malignant hyperpyrexia was recognized. Br J Anaesth 51:949, 1979
25. Gronert GA, Milde JH: Variations in onset of porcine malignant hyperthermia. Anesth Analg 60:499, 1981
26. Fitzgibbons DC: Malignant hyperthermia following preoperative oral administration of dantrolene. Anesthesiology 54:73, 1981
27. Ruhland G, Hinkle AJ: Malignant hyperthermia after oral and intravenous pretreatment with dantrolene in a patient susceptible to malignant hyperthermia. Anesthesiology 60:159, 1984
28. Ording H: Diagnosis of susceptibility to malignant hyperthermia in man. Br J Anesth 60:287, 1988
29. Larach MG, Landis JR, Shirk SJ, Diaz M: The North American Malignant Hyperthermia Registry: Prediction of malignant hyperthermia susceptibility in humans: Improving sensitivity of the caffeine halothane contracture test (abstract). Anesthesiology 77:A1052, 1992
30. Larach MG, Rosenberg H, Larach DR, Broennle AM: Prediction of malignant hyperthermia susceptibility by clinical signs. Anesthesiology 66:547, 1987
31. Ellis Fr, Halsall PJ: Suxamethonium spasm: a differential diagnostic conundrum. Br J Anaesth 56:381, 1984
32. Schwartz L, Rockoff MA, Koka BV: Masseter spasm with anesthesia: incidence and implications. Anesthesiology 61:772, 1984
33. Carroll JB: Increased incidence of masseter spasm in children with strabismus anesthetized with halothane and succinylcholine. Anesthesiology 67:559, 1987
34. Ording H: Incidence of malignant hyperthermia in Denmark. Anesth Analg 64:700, 1985
35. Van der Spek AFL, Fang WB, Ashton-Miller JA, et al: The effects of succinylcholine on mouth opening. Anesthesiology 67:459, 1987
36. Flewellen EH, Nelson TE: Masseter spasm induced by succinylcholine in children: contracture testing for malignant hyperthermia—report of six cases. Can Anaesth Soc J 29:42, 1982
37. Butler-Browne GS, Eriksson PO, Laurent C, et al: Adult human masseter muscle fibers express myosin isozymes characteristic of development. Muscle Nerve 11:610, 1988
38. Fletcher JE, Rosenberg H: In vitro interaction between halothane and succinylcholine in human skeletal muscle: implications for malignant hyperthermia and masseter muscle rigidity. Anesthesiology 63:190, 1985
39. van der Spek AFL, Fang WB, Ashton-Miller JA, et al: Increased masticatory muscle stiffness during limb muscle flaccidity associated with succinylcholine administration. Anesthesiology 69:11, 1988
40. Gronert GA, Rosenberg H: Management of patients in whom trismus occurs following succinylcholine. Anesthesiology 68: 653, 1988
41. Rosenberg H: Trismus is not trivial. Anesthesiology 67:453, 1987
42. Littleford JA, Patil LR, Bose D, et al: Masseter muscle spasm in children: implications of continuing the triggering agents. Anesth Analg 72:151, 1991
43. Cohen M, Cameron BB, Duncan PG: Pediatric anesthesia morbidity and mortality in the perioperative period. Anesth Analg 70:160, 1990
44. Gronert GA, Mott J, Lee J: Aetiology of malignant hyperthermia. Br J Anaesth 60:253, 1988
45. Lopez JR, Alamo L, Caputo C, Wikinski J, Ledezma D: Intracellular ionized calcium concentration in muscles from humans with malignant hyperthermia. Muscle Nerve 8:355, 1985
46. Verburg MP, Oerlemans FTJ, van Bennekom CA, et al: In vivo induced malignant hyperthermia in pigs: I. physiological and biochemical chemical changes and the influence of dantrolene sodium. Acta Anaesthesiol Scand 28:1, 1984
47. Harriman DGF: Malignant hyperthermia myopathy: a critical review. Br J Anaesth 60:309, 1988
48. Baumgarten RK, Reynolds WJ: Early detection of malignant hyperthermia. Anesthesiology 63:123, 1985
49. Gronert GA: Contracture responses and energy stores in quadriceps muscle from humans age 7-82 years. Hum Biol 52:43, 1980
50. Rosenberg H, Reed S: In vitro contracture tests for susceptibility to malignant hyperthermia. Anesth Analg 62:415, 1983
51. Britt BA, Frodis W, Scott E, et al: Comparison of the caffeine skinned fibre tension (CSFT) test with the caffeine-halothane contracture (CHC) test in the diagnosis of malignant hyperthermia. Can Anaesth Soc J 29:550, 1982

52. Stadhouders AM, Viering WAL, Verburg MP, et al: In vivo induced malignant hyperthermia in pigs: III. Localization of calcium in skeletal muscle mitochondria by means of electron microscopy and microprobe analysis. Acta Anaesthesiol Scand 28:14, 1984
53. Lopez JR, Medina P, Alamo L: Dantrolene sodium is able to reduce the resting ionic [Ca^{2+}] in muscle from humans with malignant hyperthermia. Muscle Nerve 10:77, 1987
54. Lopez JR, Allen P, Alamo L, Ryan JF, Jones DE, Sreter F: Dantrolene prevents the malignant hyperthermic syndrome by reducing free intracellular calcium concentration in skeletal muscle of susceptible swine. Cell Calcium 8:385, 1987
55. Iaizzo PA, Klein W, Lehmann-Horn F: Fura-2 detected myoplasmic calcium and its correlation with contracture force in skeletal muscle from normal and malignant hyperthermia susceptible pigs. Pflugers Arch 411:648, 1988
56. Lopez JR, Allen PD, Alamo L, Jones D, Sreter FA: Myoplasmic free [Ca^{2+}] during malignant hyperthermia episode in swine. Muscle Nerve 11:82, 1988
57. Mickelson JR, Gallant EM, Litterer LA, Johnson KM, Rempel WE, Louis CF: Abnormal sarcoplasmic reticulum ryanodine receptor in malignant hyperthermia. J Biol Chem 263:9310, 1988
58. Ruppersberg JP, Rudel R: Differential effects of halothane on adult and juvenile sodium channels in human muscle. Pflugers Arch 412:17, 1988
59. Nelson TE, Sweo BA: Ca^{2+} uptake and Ca^{2+} release by skeletal muscle sarcoplasmic reticulum: differing sensitivity to inhalational anesthetics. Anesthesiology 69:571, 1988
60. Gronert GA, Heffron JJA, Taylor SR: Skeletal muscle sarcoplasmic reticulum in porcine malignant hyperthermia. Eur J Pharmacol 58:179, 1979
61. Cheah KS, Cheah AM: Skeletal muscle mitochondrial phospholipase A2 and the interaction of mitochondria and sarcoplasmic reticulum in porcine malignant hyperthermia. Biochem Biophys Acta 638:40, 1981
62. Cheah KS, Cheah AM, Waring JC: Phospholipase A2 activity, calmodulin, Ca2+ and meat quality in young and adult halothane-sensitive and halothane-insensitive British Landrace pigs. Meat Science 17:37, 1986
63. Fletcher JE, Rosenberg H, Michaux K, Tripolitis L, Lizzo FH: Triglyceride lipase, not phospholipase A2, activity is elevated in skeletal muscle from malignant hyperthermia susceptibles. Anesthesiology 69:A413, 1988
64. Britt BA, Endrenyi L, Barclay RL, Cadman DL: Total calcium content of skeletal muscle isolated from humans and pigs susceptible to malignant hyperthermia. Br J Anaesth 47:647, 1975
65. Endo M, Yagi S, Ishizuka T, et al: Changes in the Ca-induced Ca release mechanism in the sarcoplasmic reticulum of the muscle from a patient with malignant hyperthermia. Biomed Res 4:83, 1983
66. Ohta T, Endo M: Inhibition of calcium-induced calcium release by dantrolene at mammalian body temperature. Proceedings of the Japanese Academy 62:329, 1986
67. Mickelson JR, Ross JA, Reed BK, Louis CF: Enhanced Ca2+-induced calcium release by isolated sarcoplasmic reticulum vesicles from malignant hyperthermia susceptible pig muscle. Biochim Biophys Acta 862:318, 1986
68. Ohnishi ST, Waring AJ, Fang S-R G, Horiuchi K, Flick JL, Sadanaga KK, Ohnishi T: Abnormal membrane properties of the sarcoplasmic reticulum of pigs susceptible to malignant hyperthermia: modes of action of halothane, caffeine, dantrolene, and two other drugs. Arch Biochem Biophys 247:294, 1986
69. Ruitenbeek W, Verburg MP, Janssen AJM, et al: In vivo induced malignant hyperthermia in pigs: II. metabolism of skeletal muscle mitochondria. Acta Anaesthesiol Scand 28:9, 1984
70. Nelson TE, Flewellen EH, Arnett DW: Prolonged electromechanical coupling time intervals in skeletal muscle of pigs susceptible to malignant hyperthermia. Muscle Nerve 6:263, 1983
71. Harthoorn AM, van der Walt K, Young E: Possible therapy for capture myopathy in captured wild animals. Nature 247:577, 1974
72. Cabral R, Prior PF, Scott DF, Brierley JB: Reversible profound depression of cerebral electrical activity in hyperthermia. Electroencephalogr Clin Neurophysiol 42:697, 1977
73. Kerr DD, Wingard DW, Gatz EE: Prevention of porcine malignant hyperthermia by epidural block. Anesthesiology 42: 307, 1975
74. Klimanek J, Majewski W, Walencik K: A case of malignant hyperthermia during epidural analgesia. Anaesthesia, Resuscitation and Intensive Therapy 4:143, 1976
75. Gronert GA, Milde JH, Theye RA: Role of sympathetic activity in porcine malignant hyperthermia. Anesthesiology 47:411, 1977
76. Hall GM, Lucke JN, Lister D: Porcine malignant hyperthermia: V: fatal hyperthermia in the Pietrain pig, associated with the infusion of α-adrenergic agonists. Br J Anaesth 49:855, 1977
77. Lister D, Hall GM, Lucke JN: Porcine malignant hyperthermia: III. adrenergic blockade. Br J Anaesth 48:831, 1976
78. Gronert GA, Milde JH, Taylor SR: Porcine muscle responses to carbachol, α and β adrenoceptor agonists, halothane or hyperthermia. J Physiol (Lond) 307:319, 1980
79. Gronert GA, White DA: Failure of norepinephrine to initiate porcine malignant hyperthermia. Pflugers Arch 411:226, 1988
80. Gronert GA, Theye RA, Milde JH, et al: Catecholamine stimulation of myocardial oxygen consumption in porcine malignant hyperthermia. Anesthesiology 49:330, 1978
81. Bohm M, Roewer N, Schmnitz W, Scholz H, am Esch JS: Effects of β- and α-adrenergic agonists, adenosine, and carbachol in heart muscle isolated from malignant hyperthermia susceptible swine. Anesthesiology 68:38, 1988
82. Gronert GA, Ahern CP, Milde JH, White RD: Effect of CO_2, calcium, digoxin, and potassium on cardiac and skeletal muscle metabolism in malignant hyperthermia–susceptible swine. Anesthesiology 64:24, 1986
83. Wingard DW: Malignant hyperthermia: acute stress syndrome of man? In Henschel EO (ed): Malignant hyperthermia: current concepts. New York: Appleton-Century-Crofts, 1977: 79
84. Huckell VF, Staniloff HM, Britt BA, et al: Cardiac manifestations of malignant hyperthermia susceptibility. Circulation 58: 916, 1978
85. Mambo NC, Silver MD, McLaughlin PR, Huckell VF, et al: Malignant hyperthermia susceptibility: a light and electron microscopic study of endomyocardial biopsy specimens from nine patients. Hum Pathol 11:381, 1980
86. Gordon RA, Britt BA, Kalow W (eds): International symposium on malignant hyperthermia. Springfield, IL: Charles C Thomas, 1973
87. Denborough MA, Forster JFA, Lovell RRH, et al: Anaesthetic deaths in a family. Br J Anaesth 34:395, 1962
88. Ellis FR, Cain PA, Harriman DGF: Multifactorial inheritance of malignant hyperthermia susceptibility. In Aldrete JA, Britt BA (eds): Second international symposium on malignant hyperthermia. New York: Grune & Stratton, 1978: 329
89. Kalow W, Britt BA, Chan F-Y: Epidemiology and inheritance of malignant hyperthermia. Int Anaesthesiol Clin 17:119, 1979
90. Gallant EM, Gronert GA, Taylor SR: Cellular membrane potential and contractile threshold in mammalian skeletal muscle susceptible to malignant hyperthermia. Neurosci Lett 29:181, 1982
91. Ahern CP, Milde JH, Gronert GA: Electrical stimulation triggers porcine malignant hyperthermia. Research in Veterinary Science 39:257, 1985
92. Hall GM, Lucke JN, Lister D: Porcine malignant hyperthermia: IV. neuromuscular blockade. Br J Anaesth 48:1135, 1976
93. Hall GM, Cooper GM, Lucke JN, Lister D: 4-Aminopyridine fails to induce porcine malignant hyperthermia. Br J Anaesth 52:707, 1980
94. Flewellen EH, Nelson TE: In vivo and in vitro responses to magnesium sulfate in porcine malignant hyperthermia. Can Anaesth Soc J 27:363, 1980
95. McGrath CJ, Rempel WE, Addis PB, et al: Acepromazine and droperidol inhibition of halothane-induced malignant hyperthermia (porcine stress syndrome) in swine. American Journal of Veterinary Research 42:195, 1981

96. Suresh MS, Nelson TE: Malignant hyperthermia: is etomidate safe? Anesth Analg 64:420, 1985
97. Wedel DJ, Bammel SA, Milde JH, et al.: Delayed onset of malignant hyperthermia induced by isoflurane and desflurane compared with halothane in susceptible swine. Anesthesiology 78:1138, 1993
98. Flewellen EH, Nelson TE: Prophylactic and therapeutic doses of dantrolene for malignant hyperthermia. Anesthesiology 61: 477, 1984
99. Flewellen EH, Nelson TE, Jones WP, et al: Dantrolene dose response in awake man: implications for management of malignant hyperthermia. Anesthesiology 59:275, 1983
100. Tammisto T, Leikkonen P, Airaksinen M: The inhibitory effect of d-tubocurarine on the increase of serum-creatine-kinase activity produced by intermittent suxamethonium administration during halothane anesthesia. Acta Anaesthesiol Scand 11:333, 1967
101. Morell RC: FDA group urges sux label wording reduced to warning. Anesthesia Patient Safety Foundation Newsletter 9: 25, 1994
102. Gronert GA: Hyperbaric nitrous oxide and malignant hyperpyrexia. Br J Anaesth 53:1238, 1981
103. Britt BA, Webb GE, LeDuc D: Malignant hyperthermia induced by curare. Can Anaesth Soc J 21:371, 1974
104. Buzello W, Williams CH, Chandra P, Watkins ML: Preliminary studies on the response of malignant hyperthermia susceptible pigs to vecuronium. Anesth Analg 63:193, 1984
105. Michel PA, Fronefield HP: Use of atracurium in a patient susceptible to malignant hyperthermia. Anesthesiology 62:213, 1984
106. Ording H, Nielsen VG: Atracurium and its antagonism by neostigmine (plus glycopyrrolate) in patients susceptible to malignant hyperthermia. Br J Anaesth 58:1001, 1986
107. Sewall K, Flowerdew RMM, Bromberger P: Severe muscular rigidity at birth: malignant hyperthermia syndrome? Can Anaesth Soc J 27:279, 1980
108. Katz JD, Krich LB: Acute febrile reaction complicating spinal anaesthesia in a survivor of malignant hyperthermia. Can Anaesth Soc J 23:285, 1976
109. Harrison GG, Morrell DF: Response of MHS swine to IV infusion of lignocaine and bupivacaine. Br J Anaesth 52:385, 1980
110. Katz D: Recurrent malignant hyperpyrexia during anesthesia. Anesth Analg 49:225, 1970
111. Willatts SM: Malignant hyperthermia susceptibility. Anaesthesia 34:41, 1979
112. Berkowitz A, Rosenberg H: Femoral block with mepivacaine for muscle biopsy in malignant hyperthermia patients. Anesthesiology 62:651, 1985
113. Adragna MG: Medical protocol by habit: the avoidance of amide local anesthetics in malignant hyperthermia susceptible patients. Anesthesiology 62:99, 1985
114. Murphy AL, Conlay L, Ryan JF, Roberts JT: Malignant hyperthermia during a prolonged anesthetic for reattachment of a limb. Anesthesiology 60:149, 1984
115. Gronert GA, Thompson RL, Onofrio BM: Human malignant hyperthermia: awake episodes and correction by dantrolene. Anesth Analg 59:377, 1980
116. Sporn P, Steinbereithner K, Sluga E, et al: Tödliche maligne Hyperthermie-Krise In Der Prämedikationsphase. Anaesthesist 29:85, 1980
117. Fletcher R, Ranclev E, Olsson AK, et al: Malignant hyperthermia syndrome in an anxious patient. Br J Anaesth 53:993, 1981
118. Ranklev E, Fletcher R, Krantz P: Malignant hyperpyrexia and sudden death. Am J Forensic Med Pathol 6:149, 1985
119. Denborough MA, Galloway GJ, Hopkinson JC: Malignant hyperpyrexia and sudden infant death. Lancet 2:1068, 1982
120. Denborough MA, Collins SP, Hopkinson KC: Rhabdomyolysis and malignant hyperpyrexia. Br Med J 288:1878, 1984
121. Green JH, Ellis FR, Halsall PJ, Campbell IT, Currie S, Caddy J: Thermoregulation, plasma catecholamine and metabolite levels during submaximal work in individuals susceptible to malignant hyperthermia. Acta Anaesthesiol Scand 31:122, 1987
122. Brownell AKW: Malignant hyperthermia: relationship to other diseases. Br J Anaesth 60:303, 1988
123. King JO, Denborough MA: Anesthetic-induced malignant hyperpyrexia in children. J Pediatr 83:37, 1973
124. McPherson EW, Taylor CA Jr: The King syndrome: malignant hyperthermia, myopathy, and multiple anomalies. Am J Med Genet 8:159, 1981
125. Kaplan AM, Bergeson PS, Gregg SA, Curless RG: Malignant hyperthermia associated with myopathy and normal muscle enzymes. J Pediatr 91:431, 1977
126. Steenson AJ, Torkelson RD: King's syndrome with malignant hyperthermia potential outpatient risks. Am J Dis Child 141: 271, 1987
127. Sethna NF, Rockoff MA, Worthen HM, Rosnow JM: Anesthesia-related complications in children with Duchenne muscular dystrophy. Anesthesiology 68:462, 1988
128. Wang JM, Stanley TH: Duchenne muscular dystrophy and malignant hyperthermia: two case reports. Can Anaesth Soc J 33: 492, 1986
129. Sethna NF, Rockoff MA: Cardiac arrest following inhalation induction of anaesthesia in a child with Duchenne's muscular dystrophy. Can Anaesth Soc J 33:799, 1986
130. Heiman-Patterson T, Martino C, Rosenberg H, Fletcher J, Tahmoush A: Malignant hyperthermia in myotonia congenita. Neurology 38:810, 1988
131. Frank JP, Harati Y, Butler IJ, Nelson TE, Scott CI: Central core disease and malignant hyperthermia syndrome. Ann Neurol 7:11, 1980
132. Ellis FR, Halsall PJ, Harriman DGF: Malignant hyperpyrexia and sudden infant death syndrome. Br J Anaesth 60:28, 1988
133. Weinberg S, Twersky RS: Neuroleptic malignant syndrome. Anesth Analg 62:848, 1983
134. Caroff Sn, Rosenberg H, Fletcher JE, Heiman-Patterson TD, Mann SC: Malignant hyperthermia susceptibility in neuroleptic malignant syndrome. Anesthesiology 67:20, 1977
135. Krivosic-Horber R, Adnet P, Guevart E, Theunynck D, Lestavel P: Neuroleptic malignant syndrome and malignant hyperthermia: in vitro comparison with halothane and caffeine contracture tests. Br J Anaesth 59:1554, 1987
136. Araki M, Takagi A, Higuchi I, Sugita H: Neuroleptic malignant syndrome: caffeine contracture of single muscle fibers and muscle pathology. Neurology 38:297, 1988
137. Geiduschek J, Cohen SA, Khan A, Cullen BF: Repeated anesthesia for a patient with neuroleptic malignant syndrome. Anesthesiology 68:134, 1988
138. Gronert GA: Controversies in malignant hyperthermia. Anesthesiology 59:273, 1983
139. Guze BH, Baxter LR: Neuroleptic malignant syndrome. N Engl J Med 313:163, 1985
140. Granato JE, Stern BJ, Ringel A, et al: Neuroleptic malignant syndrome: successful treatment with dantrolene and bromocriptine. Ann Neurol 14:89, 1983
141. Caroff S, Rosenberg H, Gerber JC: Neuroleptic malignant syndrome and malignant hyperthermia. Lancet 1:244, 1983
142. Tollefson G: A case of neuroleptic malignant syndrome: in vitro muscle comparisons with malignant hyperthermia. J Clin Psychopharmacol 2:266, 1982
143. Rosenberg H, Heiman-Patterson T: Duchenne's muscular dystrophy and malignant hyperthermia: another warning. Anesthesiology 59:362, 1983
144. Liebenschutz F, Mai C, Pickerodt VMA: Increased carbon dioxide production in two patients with malignant hyperpyrexia and its control by dantrolene. Br J Anaesth 51:899, 1979
145. Lee DS, Adams JP, Zimmerman JE: Malignant hyperthermia: a possible new variant. Can Anaesth Soc J 32:268, 1985
146. Stevens JJ: A case of thyrotoxic crisis that mimicked malignant hyperthermia. Anesthesiology 59:263, 1983
147. Donlon JV, Newfield P, Sreter F, Ryan JF: Implications of masseter spasm after succinylcholine. Anesthesiology 49:298, 1978
148. Badgwell JM, Heavner JE: Masseter spasm heralds malignant

hyperthermia: current dilemma or merely academia gone mad? Anesthesiology 61:230, 1984
149. Christian AS, Ellis FR, Halsall J: Is there a relationship between masseteric muscle spasm and malignant hyperthermia? Br J Anaesth 56:1267, 1989
150. Flewellen EH, Nelson TE: Halothane-succinylcholine induced masseter spasm: indicative of malignant hyperthermia susceptibility? Anesth Analg 63:693, 1984
151. Rosenberg H, Fletcher JE: Masseter muscle rigidity and malignant hyperthermia susceptibility. Anesth Analg 65:161, 1986
152. Nagarajan K, Fishbein WN, Muldoon SM, Pezeshkpour G: Calcium uptake in frozen muscle biopsy sections compared with other predictors of malignant hyperthermia susceptibility. Anesthesiology 66:680, 1987
153. Galloway GJ, Denborough MA: Suxamethonium chloride and malignant hyperpyrexia. Br J Anaesth 58:447, 1986
154. Kalow W, Britt BA, Richter A: The caffeine test of isolated human muscle in relation to malignant hyperthermia. Can Anaesth Soc J 24:678, 1977
155. Sullivan JS, Denborough MA: Temperature dependence of muscle function in malignant hyperpyrexia-susceptible swine. Br J Anaesth 53:1217, 1981
156. Nelson TE, Austin KL, Denborough MA: Screening for malignant hyperpyrexia. Br J Anaesth 49:169, 1977
157. The European Malignant Hyperpyrexia Group: A protocol for the investigation of malignant hyperpyrexia (MH) susceptibility. Br J Anaesth 56:1267, 1984
158. Nelson TE, Schochet SS Jr: Malignant hyperthermia: a disease of specific myofiber type? Can Anesth Soc J 29:163, 1982
159. Gallant EM: Histochemical observations on muscle from normal and malignant hyperthermia-susceptible swine. American Journal of Veterinary Research 41:1069, 1980
160. Niebroj-Dobosz I, Mayzner-Zawadzka E: Experimental porcine malignant hyperthermia: the activity of certain transporting enzymes and myofibrillar calcium-binding protein content in the muscle fiber. Br J Anaesth 54:885, 1982
161. Morgan KG, Bryant SH: The mechanism of action of dantrolene sodium. J Pharmacol Exp Ther 201:138, 1977
162. Krarup C: The effect of dantrolene on the enhancement and diminution of tension evoked by staircase and by tetanus in rat muscle. J Physiol 311:389, 1981
163. Harrison GG: Dantrolene: dynamics and kinetics. Br J Anaesth 60:279, 1988
164. Ilias WK, Williams CH, Fulfer RT, Dozier SE: Diltiazem inhibits halothane-induced contractions in malignant hyperthermia-susceptible muscles in vitro. Br J Anaesth 57:994, 1985
165. Rubis AS, Zablocki AD: Hyperkalemia, verapamil, and dantrolene. Anesthesiology 66:246, 1987
166. Saltzman LS, Kates RA, Corke BC, et al: Hyperkalemia and cardiovascular collapse after verapamil and dantrolene administration in swine. Anesth Analg 63:272, 1984
167. Harrison GG, Wright IG, Morrell DF: The effects of calcium channel blocking drugs on halothane initiation of malignant hyperthermia in MHS swine and on the established syndrome. Anaesth Intensive Care 16:187, 1988
168. Gallant EM, Foldes FF, Rempel WE, Gronert GA: Verapamil is not a therapeutic adjunct to dantrolene in porcine malignant hyperthermia. Anesth Analg 64:601, 1985
169. Knochel JP: Serum calcium derangements in rhabdomyolysis. New Engl J Med 305:161, 1981
170. Murakawa M, Hatano Y, Magaribuchi T, Mori K: Should calcium administration be avoided in treatment of hyperkalemia in malignant hyperthermia? Anesth Analg 67:604, 1988
171. Harrison GG, Morrell DF, Jaros GG: Acute calcium homeostasis in MHS swine. Can Anaesth Soc J 34:377, 1987
172. Oikkonen M, Rosenberg PH, Bjorkenheim JM, Paetau A, Huopanieme T: Spinal block, after dantrolene pretreatment, for resection of a thigh muscle herniation in a young malignant hyperthermia susceptible man. Acta Anaesthesiol Scand 31: 309, 1987
173. Watson CB, Reierson N, Norfleet EA: Clinically significant muscle weakness induced by oral dantrolene sodium prophylaxis for malignant hyperthermia. Anesthesiology 65:312, 1986
174. Driessen JJ, Wuis EW, Gielen MJM: Prolonged vecuronium neuromuscular blockade in a patient receiving orally administered dantrolene. Anesthesiology 62:523, 1985
175. Allen GC, Cattran CB, Peterson RG, Lalande M: Plasma levels of dantrolene following oral administration in malignant hyperthermia–susceptible patients. Anesthesiology 69: 900, 1988
176. Kaplan RF: Malignant hyperthermia. In: Barash PG (ed): ASA Refresher Courses in Anesthesiology, Vol. 22. Philadelphia: JB Lippincott, 1994:169
177. Craft JB, Goldberg NH, Lim M, Landsberg E, Mazel P, Abramson FP, Stolte AL, Braswell ME Jr, Farina JP: Cardiovascular effects and placental passage of dantrolene in the maternal–fetal sheep model. Anesthesiology 68:68, 1988
178. Morison DH: Placental transfer of dantrolene. Anesthesiology 59:265, 1983
179. Khalil SN, Williams JP, Bourke DL: Management of a malignant hyperthermia susceptible patient in labor with 2-chloroprocaine epidural anesthesia. Anesth Analg 62:119, 1983
180. Ritchie PA, Cheshire MA, Pearce NH: Decontamination of halothane from anaesthetic machines achieved by continuous flushing with oxygen. Br J Anaesth 60:859, 1988
181. Beebe JJ, Sessler DI: Preparation of anesthesia machines for patients susceptible to malignant hyperthermia. Anesthesiology 69:395, 1988
182. Donahue JP, Schulz J: An alternative to purging an anesthetic machine for patients in whom malignant hyperthermia is a possibility. Anesthesiology 69:1023, 1988
183. Gallant EM, Fletcher TF, Goettl VM, Rempel WE: Porcine malignant hyperthermia: cell injury enhances halothane sensitivity of biopsies. Muscle Nerve 9:174, 1986
184. Heiman-Patterson TD, Rosenberg H, Fletcher JE, Tahmoush AJ: Halothane-caffeine contracture testing in neuromuscular diseases. Muscle Nerve 11:453, 1988
185. Lambert W: Dantrolene and caffeine contracture test. Can Anaesth Soc J 27:304, 1980
186. Isaacs H, Badenhorst M: False-negative results with muscle caffeine halothane contracture testing for malignant hyperthermia. Anesthesiology 79:5, 1993
187. Nelson TE, Flewellen EH, Gloyna DF: Spectrum of susceptibility to malignant hyperthermia: diagnostic dilemma. Anesth Analg 62:545, 1983
188. Larach MG: Should we use muscle biopsy to diagnose malignant hyperthermia susceptibility? Anesthesiology 79:1, 1993
189. Olgin J, Argov Z, Rosenberg H, Tuchler M, Chance B: Noninvasive evaluation of malignant hyperthermia susceptibility with phosphorus nuclear magnetic resonance spectroscopy. Anesthesiology 68:507, 1988
190. Klip A, Ramlal T, Walker D, Britt BA, Elliott ME: Selective increase in cytoplasmic calcium by anesthetic in lymphocytes from malignant hyperthermia-susceptible pigs. Anesth Analg 66:381, 1987
191. Klip A, Britt BA, Elliott ME, Pegg W, Frodis W, Scott E: Anaesthetic-induced increase in ionized calcium in blood mononuclear cells from malignant hyperthermia patients. Lancet 1:463, 1987
192. Smiley R, Greenberg S, Silverstein SC: Anesthetics increase cytosolic calcium in mononuclear cells from normal and MH-susceptible patients. Anesthesiology 69:A418, 1988
193. Ohnishi ST, Katagi H, Ohnishi T, Brownell AKW: Detection of malignant hyperthermia susceptibility using a spin label technique on red blood cells. Br J Anaesth 61:565, 1988
194. Thatte HS, Addis PB, Thomas DD, Bigelow DJ, Mickelson JR, Louis CF: Temperature-dependent abnormalities of the erythrocyte membrane in porcine malignant hyperthermia. Biochem Med Metab Biol 38:266, 1987
195. Reiss G, Monin G, Lauer C: Comparative effects of the ionophore A23187 on the mechanical responses of muscle in normal Pietrain pigs and pigs with malignant hyperthermia. Can J Physiol Pharm 64:248, 1986
196. Quinlan JG, Iaizzo PA, Gronert GA. Taylor SR: Use of dantrolene plus multiple pulses to detect stress-susceptible porcine muscles. J Appl Physiol 60:1313, 1986

197. Willner JH, Wood DS, Cerri C, et al: Increased myophosphorylase a in malignant hyperthermia. New Engl J Med 303:138, 1980
198. Traynor CA, Van Dyke RA, Gronert GA: Phosphorylase ratio and susceptibility to malignant hyperthermia. Anesth Analg 62:324, 1983
199. Solomons CC, Masson N: Malignant hyperthermia: platelet bioassay. Anesthesiology 60:265, 1984
200. Walsh MP, Brownell AK, Littman V, Paasuke RT: Electrophoresis of muscle proteins is not a method for diagnosis of malignant hyperthermia susceptibility. Anesthesiology 64:473, 1986
201. Nelson TE: Halothane effects on human malignant hyperthermia skeletal muscle single calcium-release channels in plasma lipid bilayers. Anesthesiology 76:588, 1992
202. Allen GC, Rosenberg H, Fletcher JC: Safety of general anesthesia for malignant hyperthermia susceptibility. Anesthesiology 72:619, 1990

FURTHER READING

Black JW, Muldoon SM: Clinical perspectives on malignant hyperthermia. Problems in Anesthesia 8:137, 1994

Britt BA: Malignant hyperthermia. Boston: Martinus Nijhoff, 1987

Ellis FR, Smith G: Symposium on malignant hyperthermia. Br J Anaesth 60:1988

Gronert GA, Antognini JF: Malignant hyperthermia. In Miller RD (ed): Anesthesia. 4th ed. New York: Churchill Livingstone, 1994: 1075

Complications in Anesthesiology, second edition,
edited by Nikolaus Gravenstein and Robert R. Kirby.
Lippincott-Raven Publishers, Philadelphia © 1996.

CHAPTER 13

Dental and Salivary Gland Complications

Andrew Herlich
Jeffrey G. Garber
Fredrick K. Orkin

Much of clinical anesthesia involves working in and about the oral cavity. Despite this working relationship with the mouth, most anesthesiologists have little knowledge of its hard and soft structures. Yet understanding and recognizing significant oral pathologic changes and differences in prosthetic restorations may help the clinician to avoid dental complications when providing anesthetic care.

The patient's expectations of competent anesthetic care include reasonable protection from dental injury, as evidenced by a growing body of case law. Protection from dental injury can be ensured only when precautionary measures based on a rational understanding of potential hazards are undertaken. Because recognition is the first step toward prevention, and because most dental complications during anesthetic care are a direct result of potential problems that have gone unrecognized, a major aim of this chapter is to promote basic awareness of normal and abnormal oral structure.

DENTITION

At birth, the oral cavity is usually devoid of teeth. The gum pads are relatively firm in comparison with other oral tissue but must be protected from trauma during airway manipulation. The oral structure of most significance to airway management is the tongue.

Primary

By the age of about 6 months, the primary (deciduous) dentition begins to erupt and by 2 years is usually complete (Table 13-1). When complete, the primary dentition consists of 20 teeth (10 maxillary and 10 mandibular). The morphologic features of primary teeth differ from those of permanent (adult, or succedaneous) teeth in several important ways. The primary teeth are smaller than their permanent analogues. The roots of primary teeth tend to be long and slender after initial development and are resorbed as eruption of the underlying adult teeth progresses. When the roots of these primary teeth have resorbed nearly completely, they are held in place by only ligamentous and soft-tissue attachments. Hence, excessive mobility results from the loss of alveolar support.[1]

Permanent

In general, the eruption of the permanent dentition begins at the age of 6 years and is complete by the age of 13 or 14 years, with the exception of the third molar teeth ("wisdom teeth") (see Table 13-1). The third molars have an extremely variable sequence of eruption, if they erupt at all.[2–4] A mixed dentition consisting of primary and permanent teeth is present during this period of exfoliation and eruption (see Table 13-1). When complete, the adult dentition consists of 16 maxillary teeth and 16 mandibular teeth.

OVERVIEW OF DENTAL COMPLICATIONS

Incidence

With the completion of several surveys of anesthesia departments and the review of malpractice liability claims, the spectrum and relative importance of dental complications has become known.[5] In one study, a questionnaire inquiring about dental complications was sent to the then-162 approved anesthesiology residency programs in the United States; 133 institutions responded.[5] During the 12-month study period,

TABLE 13-1
Development of Human Dentition

TOOTH	ERUPTION (age in yr)	ROOT COMPLETED (age in yr)	EXFOLIATION (age in yr)
PRIMARY DENTITION			
Maxillary			
Central incisor	7.5 mo	1.5	7
Lateral incisor	9 mo	2	8
Cuspid	18 mo	3.25	11
First molar	14 mo	2.5	9
Second molar	24 mo	3	11
Mandibular			
Central incisor	6 mo	1.5	6
Lateral incisor	7 mo	1.5	7
Cuspid	16 mo	3.25	10
First molar	12 mo	2.25	9
Second molar	20 mo	3	10
PERMANENT DENTITION			
Maxillary			
Central incisor	7–8	10	
Lateral incisor	8–9	11	
Cuspid	11–12	13–15	
First bicuspid	10–11	12–13	
Second biscuspid	10–12	12–14	
First molar	6–7	9–10	
Second molar	12–13	14–16	
Mandibular	6–7	9	
Central incisor			
Lateral incisor	7–8	10	
Cuspid	9–10	12–14	
First bicuspid	10–12	12–13	
Second biscuspid	11–12	13–14	
First molar	6–7	9–10	
Second molar	11–13	14–15	

Modified from Logan WHG, Kronfeld R: Development of the human jaws and surrounding structures from birth to the age of 15 years. J Am Dent Assoc 20:379, 1933, and Schour I, Massler M: The development of human dentition. J Am Dent Assoc 28:1153, 1941

1,135,212 tracheal intubations were performed, and 1223 dental injuries occurred, representing an incidence of about 1 dental injury per 1000 intubations. Because some injuries very likely escaped reporting, the true incidence of dental injury is undoubtedly higher.

Types of Injuries

The same study[5] found that almost half of the injuries involved dislodgment of loose teeth; 39% involved chipping or fracturing of natural teeth; and 12% related to damage to a dental prosthesis (permanent crown or partial denture) (Fig. 13-1). Forty percent of respondents used some method of tooth protection when treating patients with loose teeth or crowns: prefabricated rubber or plastic tooth guards (36.8%); taping of teeth (23.0%); skill and a gentle technique (20.7%); custom-made tooth guards (6.9%); and careful dental examination before anesthesia (6.9%).

Only 62.4% of respondents indicated that a hospital or departmental policy existed for the treatment or reimbursement of patients with anesthesia-related dental damage; 46% of responding departments paid for the necessary dental care.

Thirty-two dental injuries occurred during the period 1978 through 1982,[5] constituting an incidence of 1 dental injury per 1364 patients undergoing tracheal intubation. Dislodgment of one or more loose teeth occurred in 28% of these patients; chipping or fracturing of natural teeth in 44%; and damage to a dental prosthesis in the remaining 28%. The

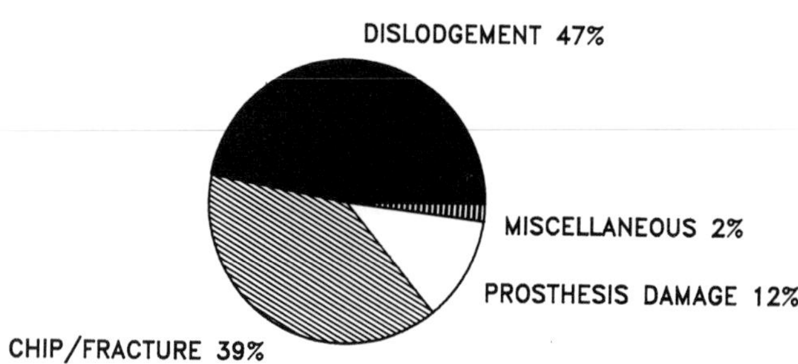

FIGURE 13-1. Distribution of 1223 dental injuries identified among 133 anesthesiology training programs in which 1,135,212 endotracheal intubations were performed during a 12-month period. (Modified from Lockhart PB, Feldbau EV, Gabel RA, et al: Dental complications during and after tracheal intubation. J Am Dent Assoc 112:480, 1986.)

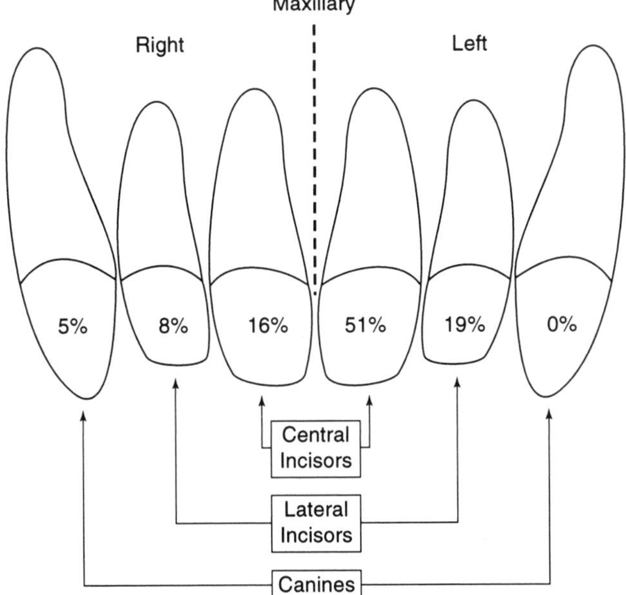

FIGURE 13-2. Location of 32 dental injuries to the anterior maxillary teeth occurring during anesthetic care in one large teaching hospital. (Modified from Lockhart PB, Feldbau EV, Gabel RA, et al: Dental complications during and after tracheal intubation. J Am Dent Assoc 112:480, 1986.)

locations of these injuries are shown in Figure 13-2. Three fourths of the injuries occurred during tracheal intubation in the operating room, whereas the others occurred at the time of extubation (9%), in the recovery room (9%), or at an unknown time (6%).

Informed Consent

Slightly over half of these injuries occurred during difficult or emergency intubations.[5] Of note, in each case the patient had a readily identifiable, preexisting oral condition that predisposed him or her to dental trauma. However, no documentation was found in the patient's chart to suggest that the patient had been informed about the risk of dental injury or that measures had been taken to prevent the injury. Twenty-four patients required dental treatment, the total cost of which (for all 24 patients) was $2800, in addition to an average of 2 hours administrative and legal time in each case.

Malpractice Liability

Perhaps not unexpectedly, dental injury is a common cause of a malpractice liability action. In a review of claims related to the administration of general anesthesia during the period from 1976 to 1983, the Risk Management Foundation found that the most frequent claims involved dental injury (Fig. 13-3).[5] Similarly, in a review of 541 claims closed during the period 1978 through 1980, the National Association of Insurance Commissioners reported that cases involving dental injury were as frequent as those involving cardiac arrest with brain damage (Fig. 13-4).[5]

PEDIATRIC COMPLICATIONS

During infancy, laryngoscopy may cause damage to the gum pads and soft oral mucosal linings. Trauma to the gum pads during laryngoscopy or with compression caused by the presence of an orotracheal tube may lead to infection and injury of the unerupted tooth buds and result in maleruption or abnormal development.[6,7] Traumatic injury to the oral mucosa of neonates and infants is particularly likely because of the relatively large tongue, which limits the working space available to the anesthesiologist. Macroglossia frequently contributes to the difficulty of maintaining the airway. When airway support is necessary, the use of lubricant facilitates the placement of an oropharyngeal airway and may prevent needless trauma.[6]

Young Children

Eruption of the primary dentition proceeds from about 6 months to 2 years of age. When children of this age undergo

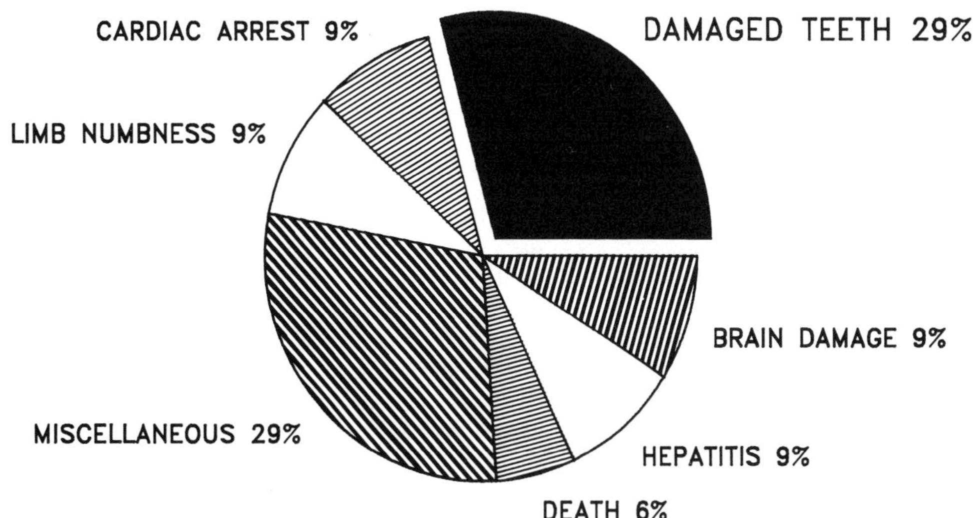

FIGURE 13-3. Distribution of the most frequent anesthesia-related malpractice liability claims relating to general anesthesia during the period 1976 to 1983 (Risk Management Foundation data). (Modified from Lockhart PB, Feldbau EV, Gabel RA, et al: Dental complications during and after tracheal intubation. J Am Dent Assoc 112:480, 1986.)

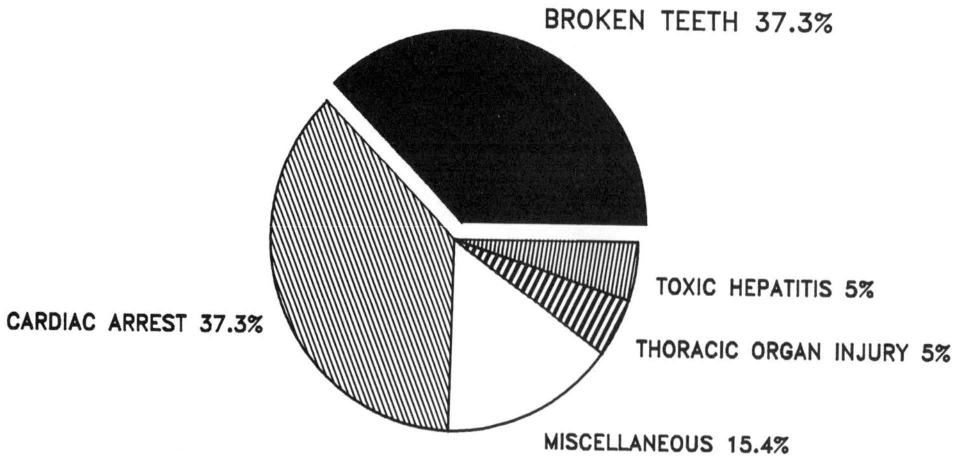

FIGURE 13-4. Distribution of complications from general anesthesia among 541 closed malpractice liability claims during a 36-month period from 1978 to 1980. The cases of cardiac arrest include brain damage, and those of thoracic organ injury exclude the heart and lungs (National Association of Insurance Commissioners' data.) (Modified from Lockhart PB, Feldbau EV, Gabel RA, et al: Dental complications during and after tracheal intubation. J Am Dent Assoc 112:480, 1986.)

surgery, anesthesiologists must be prepared to care for these teeth. Premature loss may lead to malocclusion and abnormal development of the permanent teeth. When developmentally complete, the slender roots of the primary teeth are prone to fracture during laryngoscopy if undue pressure is placed on them.

Oropharyngeal Airways

Oropharyngeal airways, frequently used as bite blocks during general anesthesia, contact the teeth in the incisor region and exert inappropriate forces (Fig. 13-5A). If additional force is exerted when the patient bites down on the airway, the likelihood of fracture or displacement of these incisor teeth is increased greatly. In one study, patients biting on oropharyngeal airways accounted for 55% of reported malpractice claims.[8] If a bite block is needed to prevent endotracheal tube compression, a suitable mouth prop, placed in the posterior portion of the mouth and supported by the molar teeth, is preferred (Fig. 13-5B). The molar teeth are positioned in a manner that evenly distributes the forces along their long axis and makes fracture less likely. Similarly, if a mouth gag is required for the surgical procedure (eg, tonsillectomy), a broad-bladed gag that distributes pressure over a wide area should be chosen.

Tooth Avulsion

Once development of the primary dentition is complete, a period follows in which these teeth are resorbed as the underlying permanent successors erupt. This process continues until the last primary molar is exfoliated at about the age of 11 years. As the primary roots are resorbed, the teeth lose their alveolar support and loosen. This process makes avulsion of these teeth considerably more likely during routine clinical manipulation in the mouth.

Preoperative visual examination alone is not sufficient to assess tooth mobility; the appearance of loose teeth is the same as that of other, nonmobile teeth. Children should be asked which teeth are loose, and examination should follow to determine the extent of mobility. When teeth can be moved easily by fingertip pressure, elective preoperative removal is indicated. If removal of a loose primary tooth during a general anesthetic is necessary, it can be accomplished easily by grasping the tooth with a gauze pad and applying a quick twisting and snapping motion. Caution must be taken, however, and a gauze pack must placed in the back of the mouth to prevent the tooth from being swallowed or aspirated. Should a tooth be avulsed and lost, it must be located and recovered. In almost all cases, the recovered primary tooth consists of only a crown, because normally the roots have been resorbed.

Oral Appliances

Because of the many advances in pediatric dentistry and the early recognition and treatment of orthodontic problems, anesthesiologists encounter a wide variety of oral appliances in daily practice. When premature loss of primary teeth has occurred, these appliances function to maintain spaces to correct malocclusions and to break existing oral habits, such as thumb-sucking and tongue-thrusting.

Oral appliances may have been fixed permanently in place, or they may be removable. Some may interfere with the space available for manipulations within the oral cavity and make placement of airway adjuncts difficult or impossible. In particular, appliances used to prevent thumb-sucking and tongue-thrusting often hang down from the hard palate and interfere with the free space above the tongue.

Removable space maintainers, such as orthodontic retainers, if not recognized, may loosen during airway manipulation and become obstructive hazards (Fig. 13-6). Particular care must be taken to avoid damaging permanent appliances; often they are quite costly. When necessary, dental consultation to ascertain the best methods for protection is indicated.

ADULT COMPLICATIONS

An adult's dentition, like a child's, presents potential hazards to unwary anesthesiologists.

Tooth Structure and Function

Teeth consist of enamel, a hard, heavily calcified outer layer; dentin, a softer, partially calcified organic matrix that underlies the enamel; and in the innermost region, pulpal tissue,

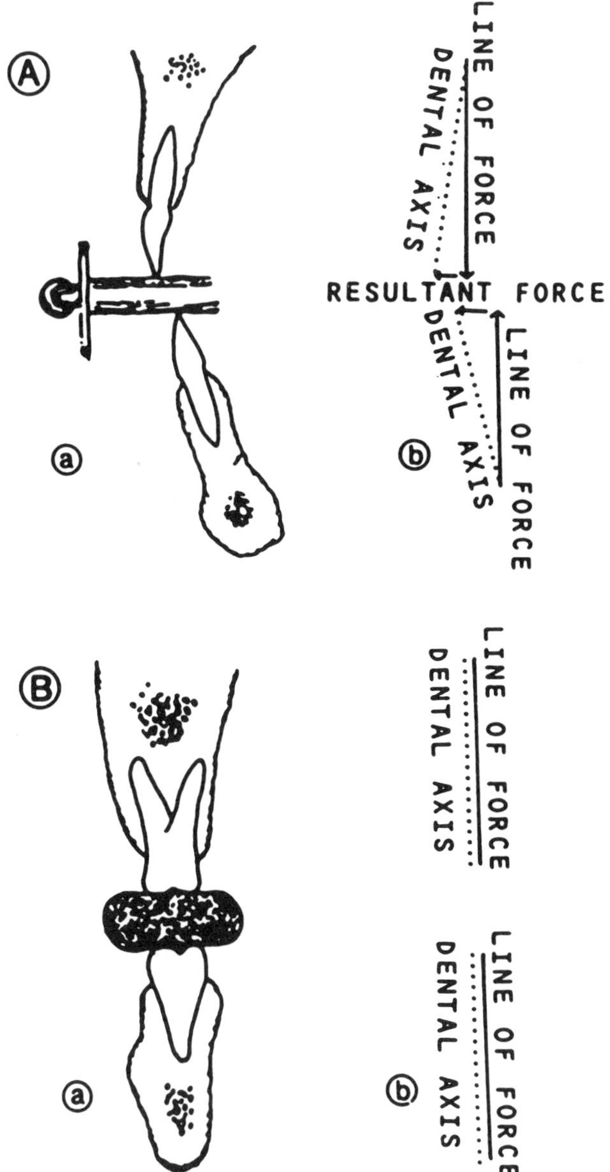

FIGURE 13-5. Lines of force and bite block. (**A**) Alignment of the incisor teeth (*a*) and associated lines of force (*b*). (**B**) Alignment of the premolar and molar teeth (*a*) and associated lines of force (*b*). (Dornette WHL, Hughes BH: Care of the teeth during anesthesia. Anesth Analg 38:211, 1959.)

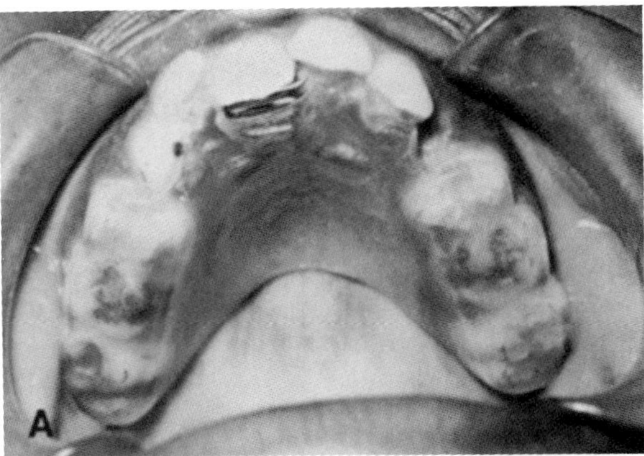

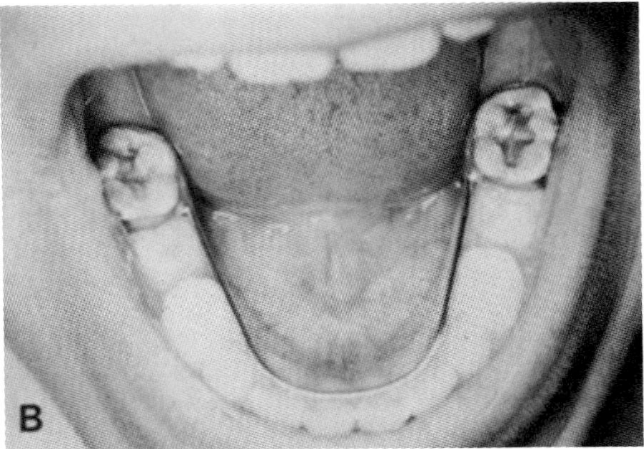

FIGURE 13-6. Orthodontic retainers that may dislodge during airway manipulations and result in airway obstruction. (Courtesy of John Hunter, D.D.S.)

composed of vascular and neural elements.[2,3,9] Normal teeth have an exposed crown, supported by roots housed within the alveolus of the maxilla and mandible.

Functionally, the anterior teeth, consisting of incisors and canines, have single roots and have crowns that slice food. The maxillary and mandibular antagonists overlap slightly in normal occlusion and have a slightly forward inclination, which subjects them to the risk of being used as a fulcrum during laryngoscopy. The posterior teeth, the premolars and molars, are multirooted and function to grind food and support occlusion. The multiple roots of the molar impart a significant lateral and vertical stability to the tooth in the arch.

Bite Block

Because of the stability of the posterior dentition, it is preferable to place a bite block in this area of the mouth as opposed to the more usual, anterior resting place (see Fig. 13-5). The bite block acts as a wedge between the vertex of the angle formed by the maxilla and the mandible and provides maximum separation between the anterior teeth. However, a bite block placed between the incisors permits only minimal mouth opening and subjects these teeth to a greater chance of fracture or displacement. The oropharyngeal airway should be used just as that and not as a bite block.[6] If an oropharyngeal airway is needed, a flexible plastic type is preferred.

Tooth Damage

Although the incisor teeth, positionally and structurally, are the most likely to fracture, few anesthesiologists use commercially produced rubber or plastic tooth guards during laryngoscopy. Applebaum and Bruce reported that only 2% of surveyed anesthesiologists used a tooth guard during intubation.[10] However, tooth guards probably are not necessary on a routine basis if the laryngoscopy is performed correctly. In addition, the tooth guard may give anesthesiologists a false sense of security, and fracture of the anterior teeth still can occur if excessive force is applied.[10] A guide to the classification and care of anterior tooth fractures is provided in Figure 13-7 and Table 13-2.

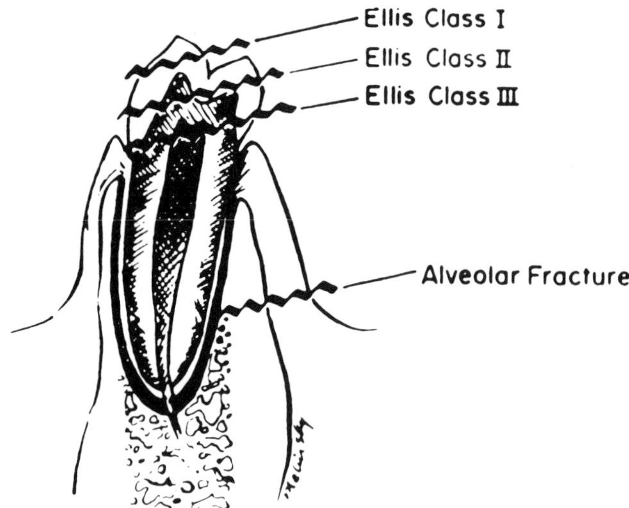

FIGURE 13-7. Classifications for fractured anterior teeth. Amsterdam JT, Hendler BH, Rose LF: Dental emergencies. In Schwartz GR, Safar P, Stone JH, et al (eds): Principles and practice of emergency medicine, 2nd ed. Philadelphia: WB Saunders, 1986:1564.)

Root Fractures

Rarely, a skilled anesthesiologist causes fracture, displacement, or avulsion of a permanent tooth. When one of these complications occurs, proper steps should be taken to minimize the possible sequelae. Fractures of the teeth may involve the crown or root, may be displaced or nondisplaced, and may not require treatment. Root fractures may easily go unnoticed until oral radiographs reveal them. They may be discovered when the patient complains of pain or excessive mobility. Little danger accrues to the patient during the intraoperative period, unless the root fracture is associated with avulsion.

Coronal Fractures

Coronal fractures may involve the outer enamel layer only (Ellis class I) or the underlying dentinal layer or vital pulp tissue (Ellis class II or III, respectively) as well. If a portion of the crown is displaced, location of the missing piece is imperative. Postoperatively, restorative dentistry can return fractured teeth to a satisfactory aesthetic appearance and normal function. Fractures within the dentinal layer may cause pain and thermal sensitivity. Symptomatic relief of this discomfort may be required until the tooth is restored. When the tooth is damaged to the point of exposure of the vital pulp tissue, postoperative pain usually is present, and prompt endodontic or oral surgical treatment is indicated.[11]

Partial or Total Avulsion

Partial or total avulsion of teeth, with the rarest of exceptions, can be avoided if the laryngoscopic procedure and airway placement are performed with care. Partially avulsed teeth usually can be pushed back into position immediately. Postoperatively, the tooth should be splinted to allow healing of the disrupted ligamentous attachment. The need for future endodontic treatment is likely. When total avulsion occurs, immediate retrieval of the tooth is necessary. Frequently the avulsed tooth is found in the mouth or nearby drapes. If the tooth cannot be located, complete radiographs of the head, neck, chest, and abdomen may be required. A posterior-anterior radiograph often does not allow distinction between airway or esophageal location, and therefore a lateral view may be necessary. The unconscious anesthetized patient can easily aspirate not only the avulsed tooth but also restorative portions of the tooth: the crown, inlay, silver filling, or composite filling.

If an avulsed tooth is found, reimplantation into its socket should be considered.[11,12] To preserve the delicate periodontal ligament attached to the tooth, it should be rinsed gently in cold isotonic saline or milk before reimplantation.[13] The reimplanted tooth should be shielded from further trauma and splinted as soon as possible.

Dental Disease That Predisposes to Injury

Rampant Caries

This condition involves decay of gross proportions, affecting almost all of the existing teeth. Young adults and children are those most likely to have this advanced disease. Particularly characteristic is the circumferential location of much of the decay in the cervical area of the crown, that is, at the gumline. Such decay undermines crown support and makes fracture more likely when forces are directed against it. Factors contributing to this aggressive carious process include irregularities in salivary composition, diet, oral hygiene, and composition of oral flora. Xerostomia resulting from head and neck radiation, Mikulicz's syndrome, and Sjögren's syndrome make

TABLE 13-2
Guide to Tooth Fracture Care

ELLIS CLASS	DEPTH	THERAPY
I	Enamel	Filing and filling
II	Enamel and dentin	Dressing, analgesics, and dental referral
III	Enamel, dentin, and pulp	Dressing, analgesics, and immediate dental referral
Alveolar fracture	Alveolar bone	Stabilization of teeth and referral to oral surgeon

Amsterdam JT, Hendler BH, Rose LF: Dental emergencies. In Schwartz GR, Safar P, Stone JH, et al (eds): Principles and practice of emergency medicine, 2nd ed. Philadelphia: WB Saunders, 1986, 1565.

the finding of cervical caries more likely.[13,14] Prolonged systemic steroid administration also increases the likelihood of cervical caries.[15] When this condition is noted by an anesthesiologist, additional care must be taken to prevent tooth fracture during laryngoscopy and airway insertion.

Periodontal Disease

Sometimes called "pyorrhea," periodontal disease probably is the most widespread chronic disease in the world. It primarily affects adults older than 25 years, and significant changes that would affect anesthetic care occur after the age of 40 years. It is best defined as a multifactorial disease resulting in inflammatory destruction of the bony and ligamentous support of the teeth.[16] The overlying gingival tissues also undergo characteristic inflammatory changes. The resulting tooth mobility from loss of supporting structures may be minimal, or, in advanced states, may cause spontaneous exfoliation or avulsion when the tooth is traumatized even slightly. For this reason, anesthesiologists must be aware of loose teeth preoperatively.

Periodontosis

An idiopathic degenerative destruction of alveolar bone, periodontosis is thought to be a very early and aggressive form of periodontal disease; therefore it also is of interest to anesthesiologists. It tends to affect persons between puberty and age 30 years and is more common in black than in white persons. During this age span, one normally would not expect to find advanced tooth mobility, as occurs in this condition. The most severely affected teeth are the incisors and first molars. The teeth appear extruded and loosened, with significant gingival changes.[15]

Dentinogenesis Imperfecta

Dentinogenesis imperfecta, also known as "hereditary opalescent dentin," is a rare, dominantly inherited disturbance that affects both primary and permanent dentition. The teeth have an opalescent brown color and, because they are structurally weak, are fractured or abraded easily. Associated with this condition, some patients have osteogenesis imperfecta, characterized by unusually brittle bones and, in many cases, blue sclerae. Any airway manipulation may damage the weak teeth.[4,14] Frequently, they are fitted with full coverage crowns soon after eruption.

Problems Related to Dental Prostheses

Prosthetic correction of dental disease involves the splinting, replacement, or repair of mobile, missing, or broken teeth. These appliances may be fixed or removable, and they may involve individual teeth, groups of teeth, or complete arches. The restorations may improve aesthetics, function, or both. They are particularly prone to breakage and are likely to cause airway interference or obstruction.

Individual Crowns and Bridges

Individual crowns or bridges (a series of crowns joined together) are subject to the greatest risk of fracture and avulsion. Crowns and bridges may be made from porcelain, from porcelain fused to metal (gold or nonprecious metal), from pure metal, from acrylic fused to metal, or from pure acrylic.[19] Usually the porcelain and acrylic portions are liable to fracture under pressure from undue forces. Porcelain crowns are particularly delicate and usually are found in the front of the mouth. Any tooth prepared for a crown is weakened structurally and is therefore at greater risk of fracture (Fig. 13-8).[8]

All fixed restorations such as crowns and bridges require cement. Difficult or improper laryngoscopy may result in dislodgment of the prosthesis as a result of breakage of the cement bond. If dislodgment of a crown or bridge occurs, retrieval of the dislodged piece and protection of the remaining tooth structure with an oil-soluble lubricant, such as petroleum jelly, are sufficient initial therapy.

Removable Dentures

Removable prosthetic appliances likely to be encountered by anesthesiologists include partial and full dentures. A partial denture in most instances consists of a metal framework of chromium-cobalt overlaid by acrylic in which porcelain or plastic teeth are embedded. The partial denture is held in place by metal arms or clasps that partially surround selected teeth.

PARTIAL DENTURES. Partial dentures tend to exert excessive force on the teeth to which they are clasped, potentially

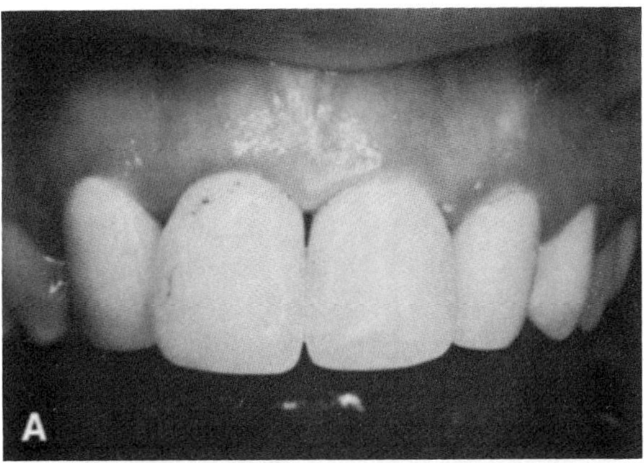

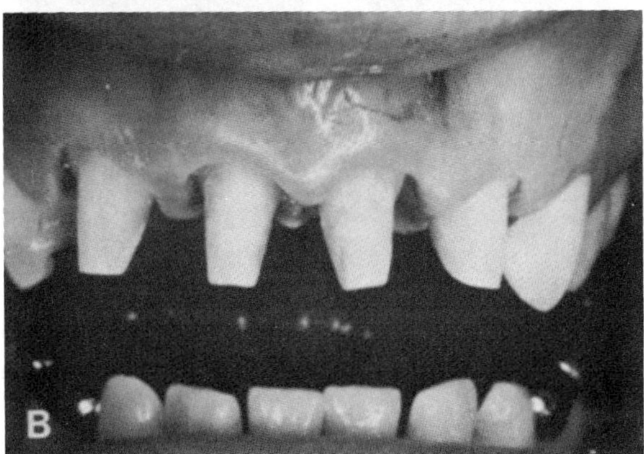

FIGURE 13-8. (**A**) Aesthetically pleasing crowns; (**B**) underneath, structurally weak teeth. (Courtesy of John Hunter, DDS)

leading to advanced loss of bony support with resultant tooth mobility and risk of avulsion. Anesthesiologists should ask these patients to remove the partial denture during the preoperative visit so they can inspect the edentulous area and surrounding teeth for evidence of trauma, mobility, and loss of structural integrity (eg, broken teeth). Patients also should be instructed to remove a partial denture before surgery, because dislodgment may occur and lead to airway obstruction.[18,19] Prostheses too may be swallowed and require surgical removal[4] (Fig. 13-9).

FULL DENTURES. As the name implies, full dentures replace a complete arch of teeth. For the most part, they are made from processed acrylic bases with either porcelain or plastic teeth.[20] Full dentures, like other prosthetic devices, are prone to fracture and may become an obstructive hazard because they are not permanently secured in the mouth. As with partial dentures, anesthesiologists should inspect the oral mucosa under the dentures for areas of trauma and describe any that are found in the preoperative note. In most cases, patients are instructed to remove their dentures before surgery. However, sometimes tight-fitting dentures worn during surgery aid the fitting of a mask and airway management by supporting the facial skin and musculature. When laryngoscopy is attempted, the dentures should be removed and stored in water for return to the patient after surgery.[6,8]

Because dental prostheses are costly and frequently affect the patient's psyche, it behooves the anesthesiologist during the preoperative visit to ask the simple question, "Do you have any caps, crowns, or bridges?" Knowing the answer to this question permits the anesthesiologist to plan appropriately and may prevent much intra- and postoperative difficulty.

Problems Related to Skeletal Abnormalities

Complications involving the teeth and their prosthetic replacements are more likely to occur in patients in whom laryngoscopy and placement of artificial airways are technically more difficult. Certainly patients with known orofacial skeletal abnormalities must be assessed particularly carefully to minimize dental trauma, because difficult airway management and manipulation are likely to be encountered. Other skeletal changes that involve the occlusive function of the temporomandibular joint may greatly increase the difficulty of airway management and thereby increase the likelihood of dental complications.

Mandible and Maxilla

Skeletal malposition of the mandible frequently increases the difficulty of orotracheal intubation. Problems during intubation may occur especially if the patient has excessively protruding (prognathic) or retruding (retrognathic) mandibles that had not been examined preoperatively. Arch shape and position should alert the clinician to possible difficulties. The narrow, arched maxilla and mandible usually cause a technically more difficult laryngoscopy.

Temporomandibular Joint

Although they are rare, occasional hyperplastic or hypertrophic anomalies of the coronoid process cause significant limitation of mandibular movement.[21,22] More commonly, temporomandibular joint abnormalities or dysfunction may decrease mandibular movement sufficiently to make airway

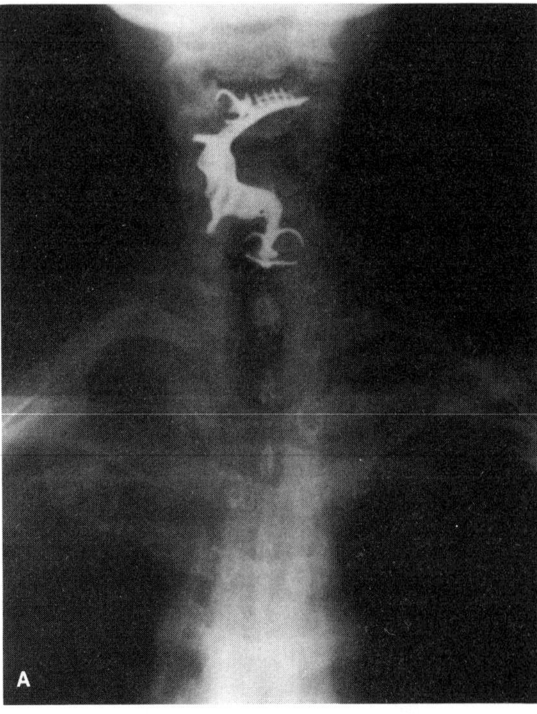

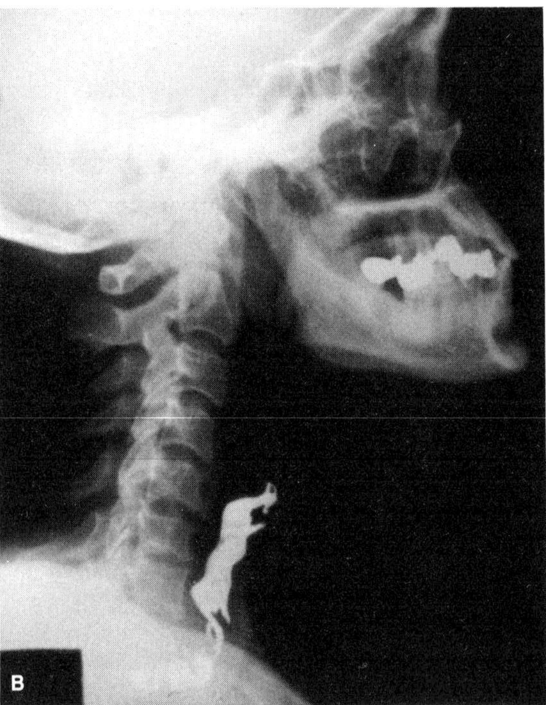

FIGURE 13-9. AP and lateral neck radiographs of a patient in whom a partial denture was accidentally dislodged during airway manipulation.

maintenance difficult. One unusual type of temporomandibular joint derangement is that of unilateral closed lock, in which case the mouth can be opened only with a forward jaw thrust with lateral displacement of the mandible toward the affected side.[23] The patient, having accommodated to it, may be completely unaware that he or she has this condition. Arthritic and traumatic changes of the temporomandibular joint are the most likely causes; others include acute reversible traumatic arthritis and condylar head and neck fractures.[3,24,25]

Soft-tissue Injury

Oral soft-tissue injury may occur during anesthetic care.[10,26,27] Difficult laryngoscopy, especially with extended periods of cricoid pressure, can result in transient lingual nerve injury. Typically, numbness appears and taste is lost on the 1st postoperative day, but these complications disappear within 1 to 4 weeks.[26,27] Laceration or abrasion of the lips, palate, and cheeks, with possible ulceration and infections, may occur as the result of placement of the laryngoscope blade.

RECOMMENDATIONS

Anesthesiologists must maintain constant awareness of the problems that may be encountered in the mouth. The special importance of teeth in our society and the ease with which they may be damaged during the administration of anesthesia prompt several general suggestions.[5,28]

As part of the preoperative visit, the anesthesiologist should note which of the patient's teeth are loose, decayed, or heavily restored; whether other oral disease that weakens support of the teeth is present; where prosthetic devices are located; and whether direct laryngoscopy and tracheal intubation are likely to be difficult as a result of a skeletal abnormality. In children the location of recently erupted teeth should be noted as well, because both primary and permanent teeth have only partially formed roots when they erupt. Abnormal findings should be mentioned briefly in the preanesthetic note.

When the risk of dental complications seems high, the anesthesiologist should inform the patient of the risk and should consider ways to minimize it. Steps taken to minimize risk may include greater care in direct laryngoscopy and orotracheal intubation, the use of a nasopharyngeal rather than an oropharyngeal airway or nasotracheal rather than orotracheal intubation, general anesthesia without intubation, and regional anesthesia instead of general anesthesia. However, regardless of the anesthetic technique used, unavoidable dental complications may occur as a result of actions necessary in an emergency and constitute a risk that the patient must accept should he or she agree to surgery.

Should a dental complication occur, the anesthesiologist should seek dental consultation in addition to describing the injury in the patient's chart. Displaced teeth should be placed in chilled isotonic saline for later reimplantation. If lost teeth and prostheses cannot be found, appropriate radiographs must be obtained. Finally, the anesthesiologist should tell the patient and family members of any dental complication that may have occurred and be prepared to furnish dental consultation and necessary care.[5,28–30]

SALIVARY GLAND ENLARGEMENT

Salivary gland enlargement in association with general anesthesia is an unusual complication first described in 1968.[31] Since then, several additional reports have appeared, so a fuller description of the syndrome can be given.[32–37]

In general, the condition occurs as a benign, painless, though often puzzling and alarming enlargement of the salivary glands (Fig. 13-10). Onset is variable, sometimes beginning shortly

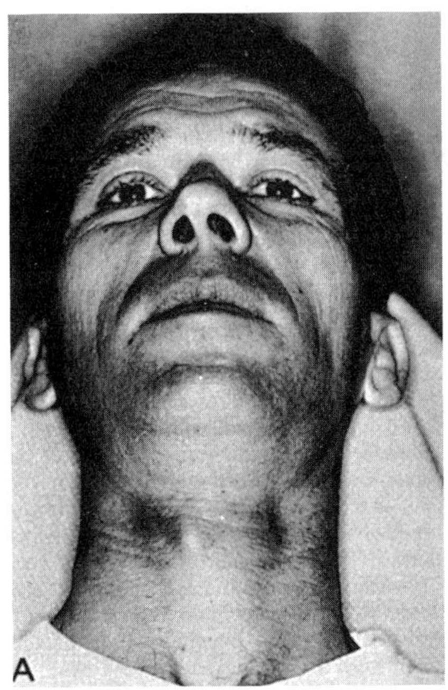

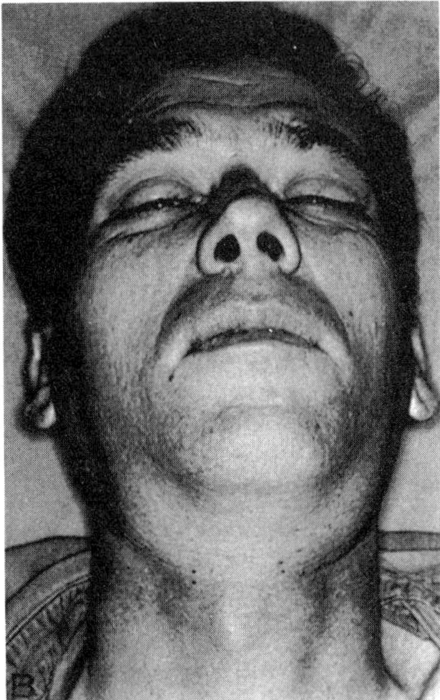

FIGURE 13-10. (**A**) Before and (**B**) immediately after peroral endoscopy, showing bilateral submaxillary swellings. (Slaughter RL, Boyce HW Jr: Submaxillary salivary gland swelling developing during peroral endoscopy. Gastroenterology 57:85, 1969.)

after induction of anesthesia (within 15 minutes), sometimes just before the termination of anesthesia, or, rarely, several hours later. Usually, all three glands are involved bilaterally. The severity of the disorder ranges from a barely noticeable swelling to a massive enlargement that actually impairs the airway.

Typically, the symptoms include fever, dry mouth, and pain and tenderness of the involved glands. Salivary gland enlargement is usually transient, lasting several hours at most, although in occasional cases patients have sialadenopathy for several days. Long-term sequelae have not been reported. Case reports suggest that enlargement occurs in about 0.16% to 0.20% of patients undergoing general anesthesia.

Causes

Several well-known causes of salivary gland enlargement include mumps, suppurative parotitis,[38] lymphoma, leukemia, sarcoidosis, Sjögren's syndrome, and salivary duct stones. Acute parotitis with hyperamylasemia has been described in patients undergoing whole-brain radiation therapy.[39] None of these conditions, however, accounts for the salivary gland enlargement associated with general anesthesia. In fact, its exact cause is not known, but several factors probably are involved.

Enlargement often follows a period of coughing and straining that results in increased venous pressure and engorgement of the glands. Reflexes initiated by manipulation in the mouth (eg, airway insertion, laryngoscopy, or tracheal intubation with straining on the endotracheal tube[37]) may stimulate parasympathetic hyperactivity and glandular hyperemia. Drugs, especially atropine and succinylcholine, may be inciting agents. Anticholinergic agents given to susceptible patients may cause inspissation of secretions, whereas succinylcholine stimulates autonomic ganglia and thereby acutely increases salivary gland secretion. Manual pressure or laryngoscopy can obstruct a salivary duct when secretion is stimulated. The exact mechanism is, at best, a matter of speculation.

Salivary gland enlargement also has been observed in patients undergoing endoscopy by the oral route, as reported in the gastroenterologic literature.[40,41] Because patients undergoing endoscopy do not receive general anesthesia, intraoral and pharyngeal stimulation are probably the most important etiologic factors. Of note is that the salivary gland enlargement may not resolve until the endotracheal tube is removed.[32]

Management

No special treatment is required; the adenopathy disappears in minutes, hours, or (rarely) days. In one reported case, salivary gland enlargement was associated with malignant hyperthermia[42]; in this situation, of course, prompt treatment for the metabolic derangement of hyperthermia is mandatory.

REFERENCES

1. McDonald RE, Avery DR: Development and morphology of the primary teeth in dentistry for the adolescent and child. 6th ed. St. Louis: Mosby-Year Book, 1994: 53
2. Ash MM Jr: Wheeler's dental anatomy, physiology and occlusion. 7th ed. Philadelphia: WB Saunders, 1994: 24
3. DuBrul EL: Sicher's oral anatomy. 7th ed. St. Louis: CV Mosby, 1980: 210
4. Zegarelli EV, Kutsler AW: Diagnosis of diseases of the mouth and jaws. 2nd ed. Philadelphia: Lea and Febiger, 1978: 503
5. Lockhart PB, Feldbau EV, Gabel RA, et al: Dental complications during and after tracheal intubation. J Am Dent Assoc 112:480, 1986
6. Dornette WHL, Hughes BH: Care of the teeth during anesthesia. Anesth Analg 38:206, 1959
7. Boice JB, Krous HF, Foley JM: Gingival and dental complications of orotracheal intubation. JAMA 236:957, 1976
8. Solazzi RW, Ward RJ: The spectrum of medical liability cases. Int Anesthesiol Clin 22:43, 1984
9. Seltzer S: Endodontology: biologic considerations in endodontic procedures. 2nd ed. Philadelphia: Lea & Febiger, 1988: 1
10. Applebaum EL, Bruce DL: Tracheal intubation. Philadelphia: WB Saunders, 1976: 81
11. Hale ML: Traumatic injuries of the teeth and alveolar processes. In Kruger GO (ed): The textbook of oral surgery. 6th ed. St. Louis: CV Mosby, 1984: 357
12. Boyne PJ: Tissue transplantation. In Kruger GO (ed): The textbook of oral surgery. 6th ed. St. Louis: CV Mosby, 1984: 296
13. Courts FJ, Mueller WA, Tabeling HJ: Milk as an interim storage medium for avulsed teeth. Pediatric Dentistry 5:183, 1983
14. Bhaskar SN: Synopsis of oral pathology. 7th ed. St Louis: CV Mosby, 1986: 635
15. Herlich A: Dental complications of anesthesia. Progress in Anesthesiology 4:250, 1990
16. Spolsky V: The epidemiology of gingival and periodontal disease. In Carranza FA Jr (ed): Glickman's periodontology. 7th ed. Philadelphia: WB Saunders, 1990: 302
17. Craig RG: Restorative dental materials. 8th ed. St Louis: CV Mosby, 1989: 113, 397, 481, 499
18. Mehta RM, Pathak PN: A foreign body in the larynx. Br J Anaesth 45:755, 1973
19. Nash PJ: A foreign body in the larynx. Br J Anaesth 48:371, 1976
20. Hearthwell CM Jr, Rahn AO: Syllabus of complete dentures. 4th ed. Philadelphia: Lea & Febiger, 1986: 309
21. Patane PS, Ragno JR, Mahla ME: Temporomandibular joint disease and difficult intubation. Anesth Analg 67:483, 1988
22. Shurman J: Bilateral hypertrophy of the coronoid processes. Anesthesiology 42:491, 1975
23. Allison ML, Wallance WR, Von Wyl H: Coronoid abnormalities causing limitation of mandibular movement. Journal of Oral Surgery 27:229, 1969
24. Shira RB, Alling CC: Traumatic injuries involving the temporomandibular joint articulation. In Schwartz L, Chayes CM (eds): Facial pain and mandibular dysfunction. Philadelphia: WB Saunders, 1968: 129
25. Guralnick W, Kaban LB, Merrill RG: Temporomandibular joint afflictions. N Engl J Med 299:123, 1978
26. Jones BC: Lingual nerve injury: a complication of intubation. Br J Anaesth 43:730, 1971
27. Teichner RL: Lingual nerve injury: a complication of orotracheal anaesthesia. Br J Anaesth 43:413, 1971
28. Wright RB, Manfield FFV: Damage to teeth during the administration of general anesthesia. Reprinted from notices of the Medical Protection Society of Great Britain. Anesthesia and Analgesia: Current Research 53:405, 1974
29. Guarnieri DM, Prevoznik SJ: Preoperative evaluation. In Longnecker DE, Murphy FL (eds): Introduction to anesthesia. 8th ed. Philadelphia: WB Saunders, 1992: 19
30. Jackson C, Jackson CL: Bronchoesophagology. Philadelphia: WB Saunders, 1950: 13
31. Attas M, Sabawala PB, Keats AS: Acute transient sialadenopathy during induction of anesthesia. Anesthesiology 29:1050, 1968
32. Bonchek LI: Salivary gland enlargement during induction of anesthesia. JAMA 209:1716, 1969
33. Reilly DJ: Benign transient swelling of the parotid glands following general anesthesia: 'anesthesia mumps.' Anesth Analg 49:560, 1970
34. Smith GL, Mainous EG, Crowell NT: Unilateral submandibular gland swelling after induction of general anesthesia: report of case. Journal of Oral Surgery 30:911, 1972

35. Couper JL: Benign transient enlargement of the parotid glands associated with anesthesia. S Afr Med J 47:316, 1973
36. Matsuki A, Wakayama S, Oyama T: Acute transient swelling of the salivary glands during and following endotracheal anaesthesia. Anaethesist 28:125, 1975
37. Rubin MM, Cozzi G, Meadow E: Acute transient sialadenopathy associated with anesthesia. Oral Surg Oral Med Oral Pathol 61: 227, 1986
38. Perry RS: Recognition and management of acute suppurative parotitis. Clin Pharmacol 4:566, 1985
39. Cairncross JG, Salmon J, Kim JH, et al: Acute parotitis and hyperamylasemia following whole-brain radiation therapy. Ann Neurol 7:385, 1980
40. Gordon MJ: Transient submandibular swelling following esophagogastroduodenoscopy. Dig Dis 21:507, 1976
41. Shields HM, Soloway RD, Long WB, et al: Bilateral recurrent parotid gland swelling after endoscopy. Gastroenterology 73: 164, 1977
42. Katz DF: Recurrent malignant hyperpyrexia during anesthesia. Anesth Analg 49:225, 1970

FURTHER READING

Bhaskar SN: Synopsis of oral pathology. 7th ed. St Louis: CV Mosby, 1986: 635

Clokie C, Metcalf I, Holland A: Dental trauma in anesthesia. Can J Anaesth 36:675, 1989

Dornette WHL: Care of the teeth during endoscopy and anesthesia. Clin Anesth 8:213, 1972

Lockhart PB, Feldbau EV, Gabel RA, et al: Dental complications during and after tracheal intubation. J Am Dent Assoc 112:480, 1986

McDonald RE, Avery DR (eds): Dentistry for the adolescent and child. St Louis: Mosby-Year Book, 1994: 53

Roberts JT: Fundamentals of tracheal intubation. New York: Grune & Stratton, 1983

Complications in Anesthesiology, second edition,
edited by Nikolaus Gravenstein and Robert R. Kirby.
Lippincott-Raven Publishers, Philadelphia © 1996.

CHAPTER 14

Pulmonary Aspiration of Gastric Contents

Christopher F. James

HISTORY

In 1848, Simpson proposed that the first reported anesthetic death had been caused by pulmonary aspiration and asphyxia, rather than the anesthetic itself. A young girl had been given brandy during chloroform anesthesia for the extraction of a toe nail. During the anesthetic, "her lips, which had been previously of good colour, became suddenly blanched, and she sputtered slightly at the mouth, as one in epilepsy." She was given water and brandy, "a little of which she swallowed with difficulty." Her physician gave more brandy, and "she rattled in her throat" and then died. Although early reports implicated the new anesthetic, chloroform, Simpson argued that she might have been saved

> by simply removing the chloroform napkin from her face . . . but with the best of motives and intentions water and brandy were poured into the girl's mouth. They were, of course, allowed to rest in and fill up the pharynx. . . The girl died, then as I conceive, from the *nimia cura medicine*—choked or asphyxiated by the very means intended to give her life.[1]

Nearly a century later, reports during the late 1930s and early 1940s documented pathologic effects on the lung of pulmonary aspiration of stomach contents.[2-4] However, it was not until 1946 that Mendelson reported the pulmonary aspiration syndrome so completely that it is commonly termed "Mendelson syndrome."[5] In Mendelson's study, 66 cases of aspiration occurred among 44,016 cases of obstetric patients undergoing general anesthesia for vaginal delivery. He described the symptoms of aspiration of liquid gastric contents, which included wheezing, dysrhythmia, cyanosis, and tachycardia. He also described the effects of acidic versus nonacidic aspirate on the lungs of rabbits. With this foundation, subsequent studies during the subsequent 50 years have reported on various types and amounts of aspirates, their consequences, and modes of prevention and treatment.

INCIDENCE AND OUTCOME

Regurgitation Versus Aspiration

Although the true incidence of aspiration during anesthesia is unknown, it continues to be a major contributing factor in anesthetic-related morbidity and mortality. In some mortality studies, aspiration accounts for as many as 20% of all anesthetic-related deaths and is purported to be the cause of death in 1 per 5000 anesthetized patients.[6-8] Whereas aspiration after vomiting may be obvious, regurgitation during anesthesia frequently is clinically silent and therefore difficult to diagnose.

Numerous studies of regurgitation and aspiration during general anesthesia have been reported since the early 1950s; the incidence of regurgitation has ranged from 4% to 26%, with the incidence of resultant aspiration as great as 76% but typically 10% to 20%.[9-12] Later studies using more contemporary anesthetic techniques revealed an overall incidence of regurgitation during anesthesia as high as 15%, with an incidence as great as 30% during upper abdominal procedures.[13-16] In turn, pulmonary aspiration resulting from regurgitation occurred in as many as 9% of the patients in these more recent studies. Among surgical outpatients, a group that may be at greater risk for pulmonary aspiration, this complication has been remarkably rare: in a survey of 181 institutions performing ambulatory surgery, possible or definite aspiration occurred in only 0.017% of patients treated in 1985.[17]

Morbidity and Mortality

Because of the diverse types of aspirates, morbidity may range from mild pneumonitis to severe respiratory distress syndrome with associated cardiac decompensation and renal failure. Mortality after pulmonary aspiration of gastric contents has ranged from 3% to as great as 70%.[5,18-20] One of the most comprehensive studies noted the mortality after aspiration to be 5%.[16]

PHYSIOLOGY

Fundamental Concepts

Pulmonary aspiration of gastric contents results from passive regurgitation or active vomiting and associated depression of protective laryngeal reflexes. Regurgitation and vomiting cannot be understood fully without consideration of the physiologic functions of the esophagogastric junction and stomach.

The Lower Esophageal Sphincter

The lower esophageal sphincter lies 2 to 5 cm superior to the esophagogastric junction. Although no anatomic difference is discernible between the sphincter and the rest of the esophagus, physiologically it remains tonically constricted to prevent reflux of stomach contents into the upper esophagus. Moreover, a small portion of the esophagus lies inferior to the diaphragm and is moved into the stomach lumen by the compression of the diaphragmatic crura, creating a flutter valve that closes the sphincter during markedly increased intra-abdominal pressure.[21]

The Stomach

The stomach serves three main functions: to store large quantities of food in the fundus and corpus (typically as much as 2 L), to mix food with gastric secretions, and to empty gastric contents into the duodenum.

GASTRIC SECRETIONS. Gastric secretions include a hypertonic hydrochloric acid solution (pH 0.87) from the parietal cells and the nonacid component of pepsinogen and mucus.[22] The volume of gastric secretions averages 80 mL per hour or 2 L per day, contributing substantially to the gastric contents. Marked variation in gastric secretion rate ranges from less than 10 mL per hour between digestive periods to as great as 500 mL per hour during the cephalic phase associated with hunger.[21]

EMPTYING. Gastric emptying is promoted by peristaltic waves in the antrum and is opposed by resistance from the pylorus. Neurogenic and hormonal factors in the stomach and duodenum regulate gastric emptying. Stretching of the stomach by the presence of food elicits vagal and local myenteric reflexes that promote emptying. Moreover, certain types of food induce gastrin release from the antrum, which not only causes gastric acid secretion but also promotes gastric emptying and constricts the esophagogastric sphincter. Typically, solids pass more slowly than liquids, and high-calorie solids more slowly than low-calorie ones; fatty foods delay emptying most, whereas protein is intermediate, and carbohydrates delay emptying the least. Feedback mechanisms from the duodenum slow the rate of gastric emptying when a larger volume of food is in the duodenum and when the gastric contents are hyperosmolar or hypo-osmolar, are extremely acidic, or contain a large portion of protein or fat.

ALTERATIONS IN MOTILITY. A diverse group of disorders—diabetes mellitus, myxedema, peptic ulcer disease, and electrolyte disorders—reduce gastric motility. Whereas alcohol, narcotic analgesics, and atropine-like drugs also decrease gastric emptying, metoclopramide, domperidone, and propranolol hasten it.[23] A myriad of intrinsic and extrinsic factors make prediction of the time required for gastric emptying in a given clinical situation difficult at best. Liquids may pass into the duodenum in minutes to 1 hour, whereas solids may take more than 4 hours. Gastric emptying in the preoperative period may be delayed (>24 hours) by pain, anxiety, trauma, obstetric labor, gastrointestinal obstruction, increased intra-abdominal pressure (resulting from, for example, ascites, gravid uterus, or obesity), and administration of narcotic analgesics.

Regurgitation

Regurgitation is the passive, retrograde flow of gastric contents from the stomach, through the lower esophageal sphincter, and into the esophagus. Gastric contents can then enter the pharynx. With alteration in laryngeal reflexes or with laryngeal incompetence, pulmonary aspiration can occur.

Predisposing Factors

Despite the previously described anatomic and physiologic barriers at the esophagogastric junction, reflux of gastric contents into the esophagus can occur at pressures as low as 23 cmH_2O and at even lower pressures if the fundoesophageal angle decreases.[24,25]

INCOMPETENCY OF THE LOWER ESOPHAGEAL SPHINCTER. Other anatomic causes of lower esophageal sphincter incompetence include abdominal tumors and masses (eg, gravid uterus), collagen vascular disease (eg, scleroderma), and the presence of a nasogastric tube. In addition, common physiologic occurrences such as coughing, straining, and obstructive breathing efforts markedly increase intragastric pressure and thus promote reflux. Hiatal hernia without evidence of regurgitation may have no effect on esophagogastric sphincter competence. In a cat model, the minimum gastric volume required to produce regurgitation under general anesthesia was 8.0 mL/kg.[26]

DRUG EFFECTS. Many drugs commonly used in anesthesia also affect the lower esophageal sphincter. These include morphine, meperidine, diazepam, promethazine, droperidol, general anesthetics, and nondepolarizing neuromuscular blocking agents. Anticholinergic agents, such as atropine, scopolamine, and glycopyrrolate, decrease esophagogastric sphincter tone[27–30] (Table 14-1). A wide variety of other factors, including ethanol, cigarette smoking, caffeine, theophylline, and a fatty meal, cause similar reduction in tone. In contrast, metoclopramide and domperidone increase sphincter tone.[30,31] The effect of succinylcholine on the gastroesophageal sphincter tone is complex; succinylcholine has been shown to increase intragastric pressure and to increase lower esophageal sphincter pressure, thereby preserving the trans-sphincteric pressure gradient.[32]

TABLE 14-1
Effect of Drugs Used in Anesthesia on Lower Esophageal Sphincter Tone

INCREASE	DECREASE	NO CHANGE
Metoclopramide	Atropine	Propranolol
Domperidone	Glycopyrrolate	Oxprenolol
Prochlorperazine	Dopamine	Cimetidine
Cyclizine	Sodium nitroprusside	Ranitidine
Endrophonium	Ganglion blockers	Atracurium
Neostigmine	Thiopentone	? Nitrous oxide
Histamine	Tricyclic antidepressants	
Suxamethonium	β-Adrenergic stimulants	
Pancuronium	Halothane	
Metoprolol	Enflurane	
α-Adrenergic stimulants	Opiates	
Antacids	? Nitrous oxide	

Cotton BR, Smith G: The lower oesophageal sphincter and anaesthesia. Br J Anaesth 56:38, 1984.

LARYNGEAL COMPETENCE. Laryngeal incompetence can lead to pulmonary aspiration. Normally, the lungs are protected from regurgitated stomach contents by reflex closure of the glottis in response to a wide variety of noxious stimuli. However, this protective airway reflex diminishes with age,[33] explaining occasional aspiration in the conscious person.[34] Depression of this reflex also occurs after the administration of ketamine,[35] methohexital,[36] neuroleptanalgesia,[37] and translaryngeal local anesthetic block.[38] Even the inhalation of 50% nitrous oxide from a loosely fitting nasal mask for dental analgesia may be associated with aspiration.[39] Anesthetic-related depression of the glottic reflex lasts at least 2 h and sometimes as long as 8 h after tracheal extubation, even in patients who appear alert.[40] This depression of laryngeal competence is attributable in part to the mechanical effect of tracheal intubation, as distinct from residual anesthesia.[41]

Vomiting

Stimuli

Unlike regurgitation, which can occur without any clinical signs or symptoms, vomiting is a very active process with multiple afferent and efferent neural limbs. Distention or irritation of the stomach and duodenum are among the strongest stimuli. Other factors exciting afferent stimuli include increased intracranial pressure and renal pelvic, bladder or uterine distension. Also, positive-pressure ventilation via face mask in the perioperative period may be a strong stimulus for vomiting.

Impulses are transmitted to the vomiting center of the medulla by vagal and sympathetic afferent fibers. Other than the irritating stimuli in the gastrointestinal tract, certain drugs, such as narcotics, directly stimulate the chemoreceptor trigger zone of the area postrema in the floor of the fourth ventricle, which, in turn, stimulates the vomiting center. Efferent impulses from the vomiting center stimulate the upper gastrointestinal tract via cranial nerves and the diaphragm and abdominal musculature via the spinal nerves.

Motor Action

The motor actions of vomiting include an initial deep inspiration with no further respiration during vomiting and relaxation of the cricopharyngeus produced by raising of the hyoid bone in the larynx. The glottis is closed as are the posterior nares when the soft palate is lifted. Downward contraction of the diaphragm, contraction of the abdominal muscles, and relaxation of the lower esophageal sphincter allow expulsion of gastric contents into the esophagus.[21,42]

PATHOLOGY

Types of Aspirates

After Mendelson described the signs and symptoms of aspiration of gastric contents in pregnant patients at term, he produced similar pathologic effects in rabbits by injecting highly acidic liquid into their tracheas.[5] In 1952, Teabeaut showed that a liquid aspirate with a pH below 2.5 would produce pneumonitis in rabbits.[43] Subsequent animal studies demonstrated that larger volumes of acidic aspirates produced greater morbidity and mortality (Fig. 14-1).[44–46] Although some variation occurs among species regarding the level of pH that produces pulmonary damage, liquid aspirate with a pH below 2.5 is considered sufficiently acidic; solutions with pH above 2.5 are considered nonacidic or neutral in regard to causing pulmonary parenchymal injury.

Acid Liquid Aspirate

ANATOMIC CHANGES. Acidic liquid aspirate has been widely studied in animal models. In dogs, gastric juice containing methylene blue is evident on the surface of isolated and ventilated lungs 12 to 18 seconds after tracheal instillation of very acidic liquid aspirate (pH 1.0).[45] This acidic aspirate produces areas of macroscopic necrosis on the surface of the lungs and extensive atelectasis within 3 minutes of aspiration.

Light microscopic findings 1 hour after aspiration include epithelial degeneration of the bronchi, pulmonary edema, and

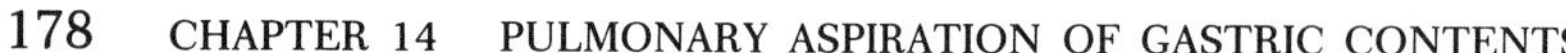

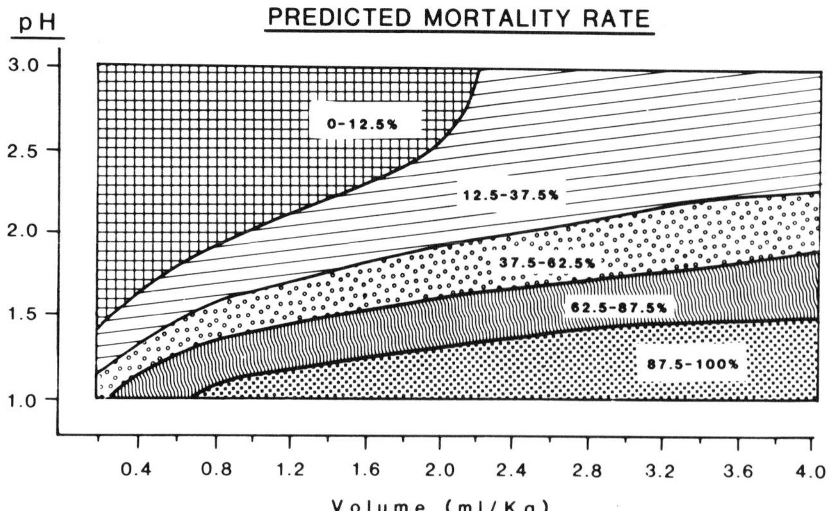

FIGURE 14-1. Predicted mortality rates (percentages) after aspiration. *Shaded areas,* the mortality rate intervals predicted for specific pH values and volumes of solution aspirated. (James CF, Modell JH, Gibbs GP, et al: Pulmonary aspiration: effects of volume and pH in the rat. Anesth Analg 63:667, 1984.)

hemorrhage. In a rat model, a biphasic injury pattern occurs with a marked increase in capillary leakage and no applicable inflammatory response at 1 hour, followed by a significant neutrophil response and further increase in capillary leakage in 4 hours.[47]

Ultrastructural examination reveals necrosis of type I alveolar cells and laminated inclusion bodies in the pulmonary transudate. By 24 hours, extensive alveolar consolidation is present, caused by the acute inflammatory cell infiltrate and abundant fibrin deposition in the alveolar spaces. Separation of the vascular endothelium from the alveolar basement membrane occurs.[48] Hyaline membranes form by 48 hours, and by 72 hours, bronchial epithelium begins to regenerate, fibroblasts proliferate, and the acute inflammatory response decreases.[49] Two weeks to 2 months after acid aspiration, parenchymal scarring with pleural retractions is extensive.

CARDIOPULMONARY RESPONSES. Pulmonary aspiration of liquid leads to airway closure with decreased lung compliance, most likely as a result of a reflex parasympathetic response.[50] Moreover, with the alveolar cell capillary damage of acid aspiration, fluid and protein move into the alveoli and interstitium and decrease surfactant activity. These anatomic responses, in turn, increase airway resistance, decrease pulmonary compliance and functional residual capacity, and substantially increase intrapulmonary physiologic shunt. Thus, liquid acid aspiration results in marked hypoxia. Severe hypotension can occur as a result of significant loss in intravascular volume via transudation into the pulmonary interstitium and alveoli. Pulmonary artery pressure and pulmonary vascular resistance initially increase after acid aspiration; however, subsequent pulmonary artery pressures may be normal or lower than normal in association with a decreased cardiac output caused by decreased intravascular volume.[18,50,51]

BLOOD GAS AND ACID–BASE CHANGES. Arterial oxygen partial pressure (Pa_{O_2}) decreases acutely, whereas changes in pH and arterial carbon dioxide partial pressure (Pa_{CO_2}) vary. Hypocapnia may occur initially as a result of tachypnea in response to the pulmonary insult. However, hypercapnia may ensue after frank respiratory failure. A respiratory alkalosis is common initially and may be followed by metabolic acidosis caused by inadequate oxygen delivery to the tissues.

Nonacidic or Neutral Liquid Aspirate

Liquid with a pH greater than 2.5 produces less severe lesions than an acid aspirate. As opposed to the acidic aspirate, little alveolar cell necrosis is seen. However, the early responses to a nonacidic liquid aspirate also include pulmonary edema, separation of the vascular endothelium from the basement membrane, and peribronchial polymorphonuclear cell infiltrate.[48,52]

CARDIOPULMONARY CHANGES. Early physiologic responses to the aspiration of nonacidic liquid may be indistinguishable from those of acid aspiration because of the nonspecific pulmonary responses to the aspiration of any fluid—that is, reflex airway closure, interstitial pulmonary edema, and decreased pulmonary compliance contributing to an immediate and significant decrease in arterial oxygen tension.[50,53] An increase in intrapulmonary physiologic shunt, which is more easily reversible because the tissue necrosis associated with nonacidic aspirates is minimal, is also evident. However, the aspiration of a large volume of nonacidic liquid can severely impair ventilation–perfusion ratios, markedly compromise pulmonary function, and cause death by mechanisms similar to drowning.[54]

Particulate Aspirate

Aspirate containing large particles accounted for 7.5% of the cases of aspiration in Mendelson's series.[5] Two of the five patients who aspirated solid material died of suffocation. Perioperatively, most gastric aspirates do not contain large particulate matter, but instead small, nonobstructive food particles. The severity of the pulmonary reaction to aspiration of particulate matter varies according to the size and chemical composition of the particles and the associated fluid.[43,55]

HISTOLOGIC FINDINGS. The initial histologic changes of particulate aspiration (acidic or nonacidic) are similar to those from liquid acid aspiration; however, by the 2nd or 3rd day, the dominant cellular infiltrate consists of a mononuclear and granulomatous response and small food particles may be present.[43,53,55] By week 3, light microscopic findings include minimal fibrosis and focal granulomas, but no evidence of hyaline membranes.

CARDIOPULMONARY CHANGES. Hypoxemia occurs early and may be more severe than with liquid acid aspiration. These changes also are attributable to increased airway resistance, decreased pulmonary compliance and functional residual capacity, and increased pulmonary venous admixture. However, the fluid shift from the intravascular compartment to the pulmonary tissue is less extensive than with liquid acid aspiration. In contrast to the effects of liquid aspiration, Pa_{CO_2} increases and pH_a decreases after particulate aspiration. If the particulate matter is very acidic, marked tissue damage with hemorrhagic pulmonary edema and alveolar wall necrosis may be present and more extensive than with acid liquid aspiration. Likewise, hypoxemia, hypercarbia, and acidosis are more severe with this type of aspiration.[53]

Miscellaneous Aspirates

Common aspirates other than gastric contents include blood, saliva, alcohol in intoxicated patients, and meconium in newborn infants. Similar to any liquid aspiration, these substances also produce acute hypoxemia, increase venous admixture, and decrease lung compliance.[56,57]

Of these substances, blood results in the most self-limiting insult (unless large quantities are aspirated) with no metabolic acidosis or increase in pulmonary artery pressure.[12,58] Similarly, aspiration of saliva (pH 6 to 7) only increases pulmonary artery pressure slightly. Alcohol has physiologic effects similar to those of saliva.[58] However, in animal studies, ethanol aspiration results in a marked inflammatory response and bronchiolitis obliterans.[59]

Meconium aspiration (pH 5.5 to 7) can cause mechanical obstruction, depending on the amount and consistency of the meconium, and often results in hypercapnia, acidosis, pneumothorax, and pneumomediastinum. Meconium aspiration also produces chemical pneumonitis.[57]

PREDISPOSING FACTORS

General Considerations

From the preceding discussion, it is clear that many factors predispose to pulmonary aspiration of gastric contents. These factors may affect gastric pH, gastric volume or pressure, gastroesophageal sphincter tone, and laryngeal competence (Table 14-2).[5,19,20,60–63]

In a retrospective study of patients known to have aspirated gastric contents, sedative drug overdose accounted for 36% of the disorders leading to aspiration, and general anesthesia accounted for another 26%.[56] Ninety-two percent of the cases of aspiration occurring during general anesthesia involved emergency surgical and obstetric cases.[56] Patients undergoing emergency surgical procedures are particularly at risk from aspiration of gastric contents because of decreased intestinal motility resulting from pain, trauma, and analgesic drug administration.[16] Similarly, outpatients tend to have increased gastric fluid, presumably because of anxiety.[64]

Equally noteworthy is the presence of antecedent airway problems (eg, laryngospasm, difficult intubation, bronchospasm, or other ventilatory problems) in the majority of cases of pulmonary aspiration during anesthesia.[16]

TABLE 14-2
Risk Factors in Gastric Aspiration

PERIOPERATIVE
- Parturition
- Emergency
- Obesity
- Outpatient status
- Gastrointestinal dysfunction
- Hiatal hernia
- Scleroderma
- Intestinal obstruction
- Esophageal diverticulae
- Gastroesophageal reflux

DEPRESSED CONSCIOUSNESS
- Head injury
- Drug overdose
- Metabolic coma
- Infection of central nervous system
- Seizure
- Hypothermia
- Sepsis

LARYNGEAL INCOMPETENCE
- Central nervous system disease causing bulbar dysfunction
- Guillain-Barré syndrome
- Multiple sclerosis
- Brain stem cerebrovascular accident
- Posterior fossa tumor
- Muscular dystrophy
- Myasthenia gravis
- Amyotrophic lateral sclerosis
- Traumatic vocal cord paralysis
- Extensive surgery of pharynx and hypopharynx

NASOGASTRIC FEEDING

ARTIFICIAL AIRWAYS
- Tracheotomy tube
- Endotracheal tube

GASTROINTESTINAL HEMORRHAGE

Goodwin S: Aspiration syndromes. In Civetta JM, Taylor RW, Kirby RR (eds): Critical care, 2nd ed. Philadelphia: JB Lippincott, 1992: 1262.

Specific Risk Factors

Pregnancy

The pregnant patient is particularly at risk for aspiration of gastric contents for a variety of reasons, including mechanical, hormonal, and iatrogenic factors. The gravid uterus increases intra-abdominal and intragastric pressures, which may increase even more during delivery (Fig. 14-2). Although the distortion of the esophagogastric junction and the stomach by the gravid uterus may promote esophageal reflux, gastric emptying time is prolonged.[65]

Hormonal factors peculiar to pregnancy include increased levels of gastrin, which increases gastric acidity and volume; progesterone, which can decrease gastroesophageal sphincter tone; and decreased levels of motilin, which decreases gastrointestinal sphincter tone and delays gastric emptying.[66–68]

Iatrogenic factors include sedative and narcotic administration during labor, which prolongs gastric emptying and also may depress protective airway reflexes. Moreover, the lithotomy position commonly used for examinations during labor and for delivery increases intragastric pressure.[25]

Although these mechanical and iatrogenic factors are not active until the latter part of pregnancy, the hormonal factors act in the first trimester and may continue into the early postpartum period. Gastric emptying has been shown to be delayed at 12 to 14 weeks gestation.[69] Moreover, the lithotomy position during the first trimester of pregnancy is associated with a significant reduction in lower esophageal sphincter pressure.[70] Thus, the pregnant patient is predisposed to a greater risk of aspiration from early gestation until the early postpartum period. There is no conclusive safe delivery-to-surgery interval; therefore, preventive measures should be used at least until 48 hours, with decreasing concern approaching 6 weeks postpartum, which is considered the baseline state.

Impaired Consciousness and Airway Reflexes

Patients with impaired consciousness and depressed airway reflexes should be protected from aspiration by careful positioning. A head-up or sitting position, if possible, aids in preventing regurgitation and the risk of pulmonary aspiration. However, in obtunded patients who may already have regurgitated, a head-down tilt or lateral position enables secretions and regurgitated gastric contents to drain from the pharynx (Fig. 14-3).

The geriatric population also is subject to this risk because of the progressive impairment of protective airway reflexes with age,[33] which may be compounded by preoperative sedative drug administration, as mentioned earlier. Moreover, pharyngeal weakness and abnormal cricopharyngeal relaxation have been documented in the elderly, with a 7% incidence of aspiration in asymptomatic subjects over the age of 65 years undergoing a barium-swallow study.[71]

Motor Dysfunction

Motor dysfunction of the pharynx and cricopharyngeus muscle or upper esophageal sphincter can result from a number of disorders, including collagen-vascular disease, muscular dystrophies, myasthenia gravis, cerebrovascular accident, multiple sclerosis, Parkinsonism, and transient pharyngeal weakness in newborns and infants.[72] As noted earlier, laryngeal incompetence or failure of glottic closure in response to noxious stimuli can occur in any patient during the perioperative administration of ketamine, methohexital, neuroleptanalgesia, nitrous oxide, potent inhalational anesthetics, laryngeal nerve blocks, or unconscious sedation.[35–39] Moreover, laryngeal incompetence, as an effect of general anesthetic agents or tracheal intubation, can persist during the postoperative period.[40,41]

Trauma

In addition to the possibility of impaired consciousness resulting from head injury, acute gastric dilatation after trauma is a common finding. The incidence in children is as high as 44% versus 25% for adults. Serious complications associated with gastric dilatation have included pulmonary aspiration.[73]

Cardiopulmonary resuscitation also poses a high risk for pulmonary aspiration. In one study, 46% of patients had full stomachs at autopsy, and the incidence of pulmonary aspiration during unsuccessful cardiopulmonary resuscitation was 29%.[74] Similar to patients at risk during anesthetic induction, cricoid pressure should be considered during cardiopulmonary resuscitation, if feasible.

PREVENTION

Several methods may be employed to decrease the risk of aspiration (Table 14-3).

Avoidance of Oral Intake

Avoiding oral intake before general anesthesia was advocated from the time of the first demonstrations of clinical anesthesia almost 150 years ago. For example, in 1858, in his early trea-

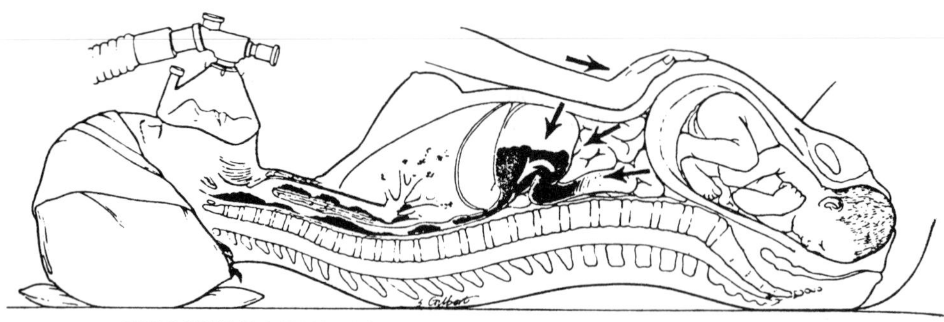

FIGURE 14-2. Pulmonary aspiration of gastric contents during delivery after regurgitation caused by marked increase in intra-abdominal and intragastric pressures. (Bonica JJ: Principles of obstetric analgesia and anesthesia. Philadelphia: FA Davis, 1967.)

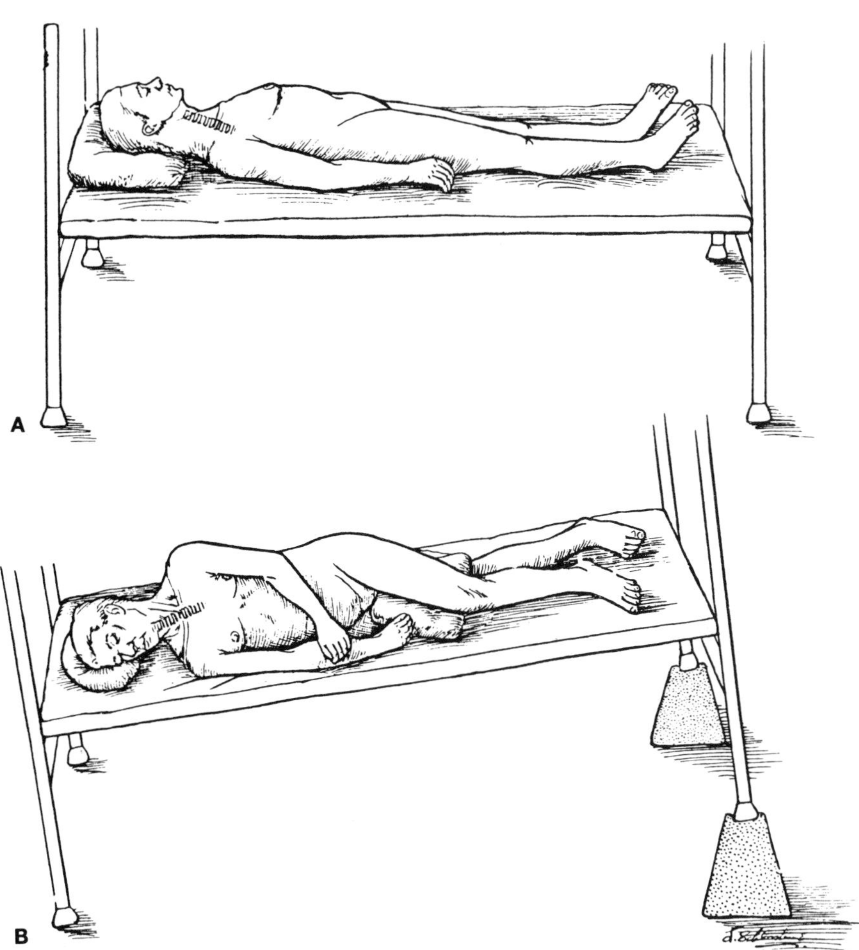

FIGURE 14-3. The position of the trachea with changes in position of the unconscious patient. (**A**) In the supine position, in the absence of protective airway reflexes, pooling of secretions occurs, and aspiration of regurgitated or vomited gastric contents is encouraged. (**B**) In the lateral position with head-down tilt, tracheal pooling and aspiration are less likely. (Cameron JL, Zuidema GD: Aspiration pneumonia: magnitude and frequency of the problem. JAMA 219:1194, 1972.)

tise on chloroform anesthesia, Snow noted that "chloroform is very apt to cause vomiting, if inhaled whilst there is a quantity of food in the stomach."[75] Although early anesthesiologists knew that vomitus could cause tracheal obstruction, the threat of regurgitation of stomach contents was not widely recognized for about 100 years. Current practice requires that the adult patient be maintained in nil per os status for at least 6 hours before anesthesia for elective surgery, with shorter fasts for young children and infants.

Shorter Nil Per Os Periods

British and Canadian and, more recently, American practitioners have questioned the ritualistic fast over the past decade, given that fasting threatens dehydration, increases patient anxiety, and results in unpleasant hunger and thirst. Moreover, gastric secretions may be increased by hunger and emotional stimuli. In one study, patients received a light breakfast consisting of a slice of buttered toast and a cup of tea or coffee with milk 2 to 3 hours before surgery; the volumes and acidity of gastric contents were similar to those of other patients undergoing a conventional overnight fast.[76] Others also noted unchanged gastric contents after the ingestion of 100 mL of water, coffee, or orange juice 2 to 3 hours before anesthesia.[77–79]

Pediatric Patients

There is particular interest in reevaluating the preoperative fast for children. One study found gastric volume and pH unchanged in children aged 5 to 10 years who had received 6 or 10 mL/kg of apple juice 2.5 hours before anesthesia; however, they were less thirsty and less irritable.[80] This practice recently has been extended to pediatric cardiac surgical patients with no increase in gastric volume or lower pH in children who ingested clear liquids 2 to 3 hours before anesthesia induction.[81]

Critical Minimum Fasting Period

Although oral intake of clear fluids several hours before anesthesia for elective surgery may be reasonable, the critical minimum period of fasting is unknown. Moreover, the preoperative fast should not be liberalized to include food other than clear liquids, because the aspiration of particulate material is severe, regardless of its acidity.[53] Neither should the fast be liberalized in the case of obstetric patients and those awaiting emergency procedures. In a study of obstetric patients given tea and toast less than 4 hours before cesarean section, the patients who were fed had significantly higher gastric vol-

TABLE 14-3
Methods to Reduce the Risk of Pulmonary Aspiration Syndrome

REGURGITATION

- Decrease gastric volume
  - Stop intake (nil per os)
  - Facilitate emptying (metoclopramide)
- Sellick's maneuver (cricoid pressure)
- Head-up position
- Surgery
  - Nissen fundoplication
  - Gastric division

ASPIRATION

- Maintain consciousness
- Lateral and head-down position
- Endotracheal tube
- Surgery
  - Tracheostomy
  - Laryngotracheal closure
  - Laryngeal diversion
  - Laryngeal stent
  - Total laryngectomy
  - Epiglottoaryeglottopexy

GASTRIC ACIDITY

- Antacids
  - Particulate
  - Clear
- Histamine H_2-receptor antagonists
  - Cimetidine
  - Ranitidine

Goodwin S: Aspiration syndromes. In Civetta JM, Taylor RW, Kirby RR (eds): Critical care, 2nd ed. Philadelphia, JB Lippincott, 1992: 1267.

umes (73 versus 33 mL) than the patients who were maintained in nil per os status overnight.[82]

Delay of Surgery

When possible, consider delaying surgery if recent oral intake of liquid or solid material has occurred.

Reduction of Gastric Acidity or Volume

Consider reducing gastric acidity (sodium citrate) or volume (metoclopramide) by pharmacologic agents in clinical circumstances posing especially great risk for aspiration pneumonitis.

Regional or Local Anesthesia

Consider regional or local anesthesia in patients at particular risk for aspiration, whenever possible, to reduce the risk. However, the risk of pulmonary aspiration is still present during regional anesthesia with sedation,[35–39] toxic reactions to local anesthetic agents, or an accidental high level of spinal or epidural analgesia.

Awake Intubation

Consider awake intubation, either nasally or orally, before inducing general anesthesia in neonates, in patients considered to have difficult airways, or in patients with other hazardous conditions such as active oropharyngeal or gastrointestinal bleeding or facial trauma. A fiberoptic bronchoscope may be especially useful in these circumstances.[83]

Rapid-Sequence Induction

Rapid-sequence induction with intravenous agents and simultaneous application of cricoid pressure, followed immediately by tracheal intubation, should be undertaken when regional anesthesia or awake intubation is not possible in patients thought to be at risk for aspiration. Although aspiration can occur anytime during a general anesthetic, the most dangerous periods are induction and emergence.

During induction, every attempt should be make to minimize the time during which the airway is unprotected and to insert a cuffed endotracheal tube promptly that remains in place until the patient regains protective airway reflexes.

Variations

Many variations have been proposed to the standard rapid-sequence induction technique. Intravenous induction agents may include precurarization with d-tubocurarine or pancuronium. An induction dose of thiopental (3 to 4 mg/kg) or ketamine (1 to 2 mg/kg) is given and is immediately followed by succinylcholine (1 to 2 mg/kg), higher dosage being required when a defasciculating dose of nondepolarizing muscle relaxant has been used.

Pancuronium (0.15 mg/kg) can be substituted for succinylcholine when the latter is inadvisable or contraindicated; such a substitution also obviates the use of a desfasciculating agent.[84] Because of the prolonged action of pancuronium with higher dosages, some investigators have recommended the intermediate-duration, nondepolarizing muscle relaxants, atracurium or vecuronium, using either a large intubating dose or a priming dose followed by a smaller intubating dose.[85–88] However, the onset time still is not as rapid as with succinylcholine; moreover, priming doses may lead to weakness, which also places the patient in jeopardy. The newest nondepolarizing agent, rocuronium, produces relaxation in approximately 90 seconds.

Use of Cricoid Pressure

Sellick's maneuver, applied simultaneously during induction of general anesthesia, was described in 1961 (Fig. 14-4).[89] Using this technique, Sellick demonstrated that the esophageal lumen is completely collapsed at pressure as high as 100 cmH_2O.[89] In contrast, intragastric pressure generated from fasciculations after succinylcholine administration is well below 50 cmH_2O.[32] Cricoid pressure should be maintained until the endotracheal tube cuff has been inflated, breath sounds are noted to be equal bilaterally, and end-tidal carbon dioxide is detected. In special situations such as increased intracranial

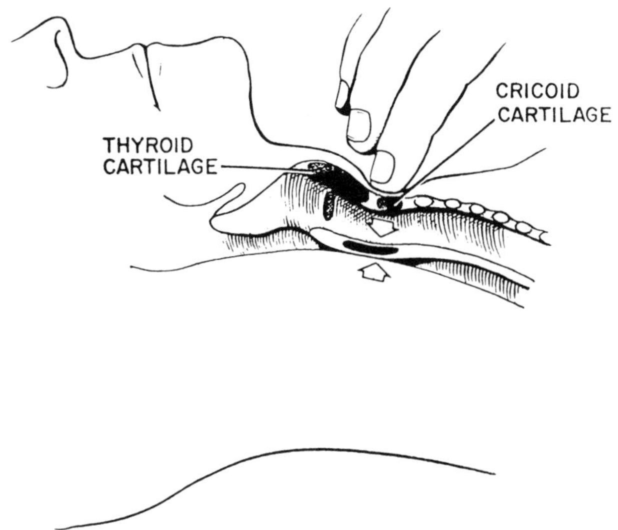

FIGURE 14-4. Posterior pressure on the cricoid cartilage (Sellick's maneuver) occludes the esophagus and thereby prevents regurgitation. (Hamelberg W, Bosomworth PP: Aspiration pneumonitis. Springfield: Charles C Thomas, 1968:26.)

pressure, alone or combined with cardiac ischemia or instability, the rapid-sequence induction can be modified to include manual ventilation. Cricoid pressure should still be used because it is effective and essentially without risk, despite concerns of esophageal rupture during vomiting.[90–92]

Use of Tubes With High-Volume, Low-Pressure Cuffs

Although the incidence of aspiration is less with high-volume, low-pressure endotracheal tube cuffs than with older low-volume, high-pressure cuffs or uncuffed tubes, silent aspiration can still occur intraoperatively or in the intensive care setting.[93–95] The cuff pressure, wall thickness, and other design aspects of the endotracheal tube can also influence the incidence of silent aspiration.[96,97] Aspiration with cuffed tubes can also occur after extubation. If fluid (gastric contents, blood or saliva) is in the area between the cuff and vocal cords, distal movement can occur when the cuff is deflated and the endotracheal tube is removed.[98,99] A recent study demonstrated a 16% incidence of gastroesophageal reflux, the majority of cases occurring during emergence and in the recovery room associated with bucking and coughing.[100]

Nasogastric Suction

Consider passing a naso- or orogastric tube during the operative procedure, once the airway has been secured, to remove as much of the gastric contents as possible. This maneuver should decrease the risk of aspiration during extubation and emergence from anesthesia, although gastric contents cannot be totally removed.[101] Patients especially predisposed to pulmonary aspiration should be awake (eg, able to respond appropriately to commands) before extubation. Despite their conscious state, they must be watched carefully in the recovery room and intensive care unit because laryngeal incompetence may persist for several hours after extubation.[40,41]

New Airway Devices

Recently, new airway devices, such as the laryngeal mask and the combitube, have been introduced as options for the clinician when securing the airway via tracheal intubation is difficult or unattainable. One of these devices, the laryngeal mask airway, has been available in England since the late 1980s and often is used in routine cases as an alternative to tracheal intubation. Despite the potential advantages of the laryngeal mask airway in maintaining a patent airway under spontaneous or controlled ventilation, several cases of pulmonary aspiration have occurred because the laryngeal mask does not protect the airway from regurgitated material.[102] The incidence of regurgitation with the laryngeal mask airway is reported as high as 25%.[103] An additional consideration is that cricoid pressure may prevent the airway's insertion.[104]

REDUCING THE RISK OF PNEUMONITIS

Should pulmonary aspiration occur, the nature and extent of lung injury depends on the type and quantity of the aspirate, as noted earlier.

General Considerations

Definition of the risk for pneumonitis is controversial. The accepted criteria for aspiration pneumonitis are a critical combination of gastric contents with a pH below 2.5 and a volume greater than 25 mL.[105] Although substantial evidence supports the pH value, the value of 25 mL (or 0.4 mL/kg) for gastric volume is less well established.[43,106] This volume is based on limited data obtained from *Rhesus* monkeys that had received an intratracheal dose of highly acidic liquid (pH 1.2) and suffered pneumonitis from volumes of 0.8 mL/kg.[107] Rats that aspirate liquid solutions with extremely low pH (1.0), even at low volumes (0.3 mL/kg), incur a high mortality. In contrast, mortality is much lower with solutions with higher pH (>1.8) and much higher volumes (>1 mL/kg).[46] This observation strongly suggests that no single volume is critical, but the pH of the aspirate is.

In another report, the pH of the aspirated solution was the critical determinant of the amount of lung injury.[47] Maximal nonlethal lung injury occurred at pH 1.5 with a linear relationship between injury and volume of aspirate of less than 1.2 mL/kg; volumes of 71.2 mL/h did not increase lung injury.[47] To further elucidate the role of volume in lung aspiration, a recent study in primates also revealed that a higher critical volume of 0.8 mL/kg at pH 1 caused severe pneumonitis versus no mortality at volumes of 0.4 mL/kg and 0.6 mL/kg.[108]

If one accepts the current criteria for the risk of pneumonitis should aspiration occur, emergency, pregnant, postpartum, pediatric, obese patients and outpatients are at risk.[105,109–122] A postpartum study revealed that 60% of inpatients undergoing elective surgical procedures are also at risk. Moreover, 40% of all postpartum patients and 26% of inpatients had gastric contents with pH below 1.4, which may suggest an even greater risk for pneumonia should aspiration occur.[11]

Pharmacologic Agents

In the perioperative period, pharmacologic measures have focused mainly on neutralizing gastric acidity and reducing gastric volume. Given the infrequent occurrence of pulmonary aspiration and, undoubtedly, the great difficulty in conducting a controlled clinical trial, no documentation exists that the administration of pharmacologic agents affects the incidence of pulmonary aspiration.

Antacids

Antacids have been recommended as a prophylactic measure to neutralize gastric acidity since Mendelson's original report.[106,107] Although particulate antacids have been shown to decrease gastric acidity effectively, the pulmonary aspiration of particulate antacids in dogs produces a marked bronchopneumonia with a persistent inflammatory reaction.[123] A nonparticulate antacid, sodium citrate, is safer than particulate antacids after food aspiration in the dog.[124] Moreover, 30 mL of 0.3 M sodium citrate (pH 8.4) decreases gastric acidity effectively in humans.[125–128]

Commercially available buffering solutions, Bicitra (pH 4.2) and Alka-Seltzer Effervescent, taken as two tablets dissolved in 30 mL of distilled water (pH 6.8), do not produce severe pulmonary pathologic effects when aspirated in the dog and also decrease gastric acidity effectively in humans.[117,129,130] For optimal reduction of gastric acidity, these nonparticulate antacids should be administered within 60 minutes of anesthetic induction and may need to be repeated intraoperatively for longer procedures because their duration of action is short.[128]

Major concerns about antacid administration include increasing gastric volume, inadequate mixing with gastric contents, and possible promotion of nausea and vomiting.[119,120,131] Moreover, the rate of gastric emptying determines the efficacy of antacids.[132] Nonobstetric patients with a strong history and symptoms of esophageal reflux, and patients receiving narcotics preoperatively, probably should not be given anything orally, including antacids, because increased stomach volume may further increase the probability of regurgitation and vomiting.

Histamine H_2-Receptor Blocking Agents

CIMETIDINE. In clinical studies cimetidine effectively decreases gastric acidity perioperatively in adults, children, and obstetric patients.[133–137] However, data on the effect of cimetidine on gastric volume are conflicting.[134,137,138] Because cimetidine acts on subsequent gastric secretions rather than preexisting contents, it should be given, by any route, at least 60 to 90 minutes before anesthetic induction for maximal effect. Therefore, its use is precluded for many emergency procedures.[135,139] In these circumstances, a clear antacid should be administered instead of cimetidine.

Many side effects have been reported with cimetidine, notably acute toxic reactions that are rare and life threatening and may not be solely attributable to cimetidine. Dysrhythmias, bradycardia, hypotension, and cardiac arrest have occurred during rapid intravenous administration of cimetidine.[140–143] Likewise, hematologic abnormalities including bone marrow suppression have been reported.[144]

Other side effects include somnolence, mental confusion, nausea, vomiting and diarrhea, gynecomastia, dry mouth, and muscular pain.[145] Cimetidine also prolongs the action of various drugs such as propranolol, lidocaine, benzodiazepines, morphine sulphate, theophylline, barbiturates, phenytoin, carbamazepine, and warfarin by inhibiting microsomal drug metabolism in the liver and reducing hepatic blood flow.[145–155] The concomitant administration of oral antacids, metoclopramide, or both may reduce the absorption of oral cimetidine and, thereby, decrease its effectiveness.[152]

RANITIDINE. Another H_2-receptor antagonist, ranitidine, also has been shown to decrease gastric acidity effectively.[153] Ranitidine has a longer duration of action than cimetidine and, thus, offers more protection during emergence from anesthesia.

Studies of ranitidine are more limited, and only minor side effects have been reported: headache, mental confusion, dizziness, nausea, skin rash, constipation, and transient increases in serum aminotransferase levels.[154] Except for bradycardia after intravenous use,[155] no major cardiovascular effects have been noted.

Like cimetidine, reports on hematologic abnormalities are inconclusive except for a transient case of neutropenia.[156] Ranitidine may decrease hepatic blood flow but has minimal to no effect on the microsomal enzyme system in the liver, and thus has not been shown to prolong the hepatic clearance of various drugs.[157] Coadministration of oral antacids reduces the bioavailability of ranitidine.[158]

FAMOTIDINE. A newer histamine H_2-receptor antagonist, Famotidine, has been shown to be as effective as cimetidine and ranitidine in decreasing gastric acidity.[159] Potential advantages of famotidine include its longer duration of action, with suppression of gastric secretions for over 12 hours, and negligible effects on hepatic blood flow and drug enzyme induction.[160]

ANTICHOLINERGIC DRUGS. Atropine and glycopyrrolate, also have been used to decrease gastric acidity. They have a variable effect on pH and volume and are definitely inferior to histamine H_2-receptor antagonists and antacids.[119,161] One study noted that the preinduction addition of glycopyrrolate to cimetidine was no more effective than cimetidine.[151] Moreover, these anticholinergic agents also decrease esophagogastric sphincter tone and, thus, may increase the risk of regurgitation and pulmonary aspiration of gastric contents (see Table 14-1).[28,29]

METOCLOPRAMIDE AND DOMPERIDONE. These agents decrease gastric volume without affecting gastric acidity.[53] They have upper gastrointestinal stimulatory properties and also increase esophagogastric sphincter tone.[31,162,163]

However, the effectiveness of metoclopramide in reducing gastric volume when it is administered preoperatively is inconsistent,[116,162,164] as is the effectiveness of both agents to reduce vomiting during emergence and in the early postoperative period.[165-167]

Combinations of metoclopramide and cimetidine or ranitidine are very effective in decreasing gastric acidity and volume.[168-171] The potential problem with the coadministration of metoclopramide and cimetidine is reduction in the absorption of cimetidine as a result of the increased gastric-emptying properties of metoclopramide.[152] Moreover, the previous administration of anticholinergic drugs and narcotics may reduce the efficacy of metoclopramide.[172]

Adverse effects of metoclopramide include somnolence, nervousness, and extrapyramidal symptoms caused by dopamine antagonism in the central nervous system.[163,173] Other problems include stimulation of prolactin secretion, and occasional hypotensive episodes after intravenous administration.[163,174] The dopamine receptor-blocking agent properties of domperidone are thought to be limited to the peripheral nervous system; thus this drug does not have extrapyramidal side effects.[166]

OMEPRAZOLE. A substituted benzimidimazole, omeprazole decreases gastric fluid volume and acidity by producing rapid, prolonged inhibition of the parietal cell enzyme responsible for the final common pathway of gastric acid secretion. This antisecretagogue awaits comparison with the more familiar antacids and histamine H_2-receptor blocking agents.[175]

ONDANSETRON. Ondansetron is a new antiemetic, a selective S-hydroxytryptamine subtype 3 receptor antagonist. Although it has no known effect on gastric volume or pH, it has been shown to markedly decrease the incidence of nausea and vomiting in the postoperative period. The advantage of ondansetron includes its lack of cholinergic, dopaminergic, or histaminergic effects.[176,177] Ondansetron may be useful in the early postoperative period, especially in patients predisposed to pulmonary aspiration as laryngeal incompetence may persist for hours after extubation.

DIAGNOSIS

Despite all precautionary and preventive measures, pulmonary aspiration may still occur. If regurgitation or vomiting is not observed, diagnosis often is difficult, because clinical signs in mild cases can be quite subtle. Symptoms include tachypnea, tachycardia, refractory laryngospasm, bronchospasm, or any combination thereof. Râles and rhonchi may be heard on auscultation of the chest. A chest radiograph may not demonstrate the full extent of the subsequent pathologic changes,[161,178] and radiographic changes can be delayed for 6 to 24 hours following aspiration.

Although bronchoscopy usually is not advocated for diagnosis of pulmonary aspiration, erythematous lesions of the carina, main stem bronchi, and subsegmental bronchi have been demonstrated by fiberoptic bronchoscopy after suspected pulmonary aspiration.[179,180] Regardless of whether pulmonary aspiration is documented or only suggested, the patient's ventilatory and hemodynamic states should be assessed immediately. A blood gas analysis should also be obtained because a decrease in Pa_{O_2} occurs consistently with any type of aspiration.

TREATMENT

The success of treatment depends on prompt recognition of immediate institution of vigorous measures to relieve respiratory obstruction, thereby assuring adequate gas exchange and minimizing damage to the lungs.

Airway

Clear the airway as soon as possible after pulmonary aspiration is observed or suspected. If the patient is not awake and alert, the trachea should be intubated and suctioned, although suctioning often does not remove all aspirated material and most of the peripheral pulmonary injury already will have occurred.[45] Tracheal suctioning may stimulate coughing, bring up some aspirated material, and, thus, help confirm a presumptive diagnosis. Immediate bronchoscopy should be performed only when particulate matter obstructs the airway. An essential part of therapy is frequent suctioning of the airway. Periodic repositioning of the patient and chest physiotherapy helps to reduce further complications in dependent portions of the lungs.

Oxygenation

Improve oxygenation with supplemental oxygen and, depending on the patient's respiratory status and arterial blood gas values, institute mechanical ventilation. First, an initially high fraction of inspired oxygen should be administered and then decreased to lower the risk of oxygen toxicity and eventually to detect ventilation/perfusion mismatch and intrapulmonary shunt.

Positive Airway Pressure

If the patient is awake, alert, and cooperative, up to 15 and possibly even 20 cmH_2O of continuous positive airway pressure (CPAP) may be administered by mask; greater pressure promotes opening of the esophagogastric junction and, thus, may increase the risk of further regurgitation and aspiration. If higher levels of continuous positive airway pressure are required, or if the patient is not alert, tracheal intubation should be performed.

A variety of methods are used to determine the most beneficial level of continuous positive airway pressure (CPAP) or positive end-expiratory pressure (PEEP), each of which involves increasing pressure incrementally until some physiologic end-point is reached: "best PEEP," with the end-point being improved lung compliance; "optimum PEEP," with minimization of intrapulmonary venous admixture; "appropriate PEEP," with minimization of the arterial–end tidal carbon dioxide partial pressure gradient; and adjustment of PEEP or CPAP according to arterial oxygen partial pressure.[181-184]

Pulmonary Lavage

Pulmonary lavage is not warranted in the majority of cases of pulmonary aspiration. Damage to the lungs by acidic liquid occurs within 12 to 18 seconds[45]; moreover, no demonstrated improvement occurs with lavage. On the contrary, an increased risk of greater pulmonary damage is present from spread of aspirate. However, lavage under direct vision via bronchoscopy can be performed, with a small amount of saline, to loosen impacted particulate matter or secretions when they are thought to be obstructing the airway.

Corticosteroids

Corticosteroid administration for pulmonary aspiration of gastric contents first was advocated in the early 1960s.[185] The rationale for its use reflected the ability of steroids to decrease inflammation, stabilize lysosomal membranes, prevent leukocyte and platelet aggregation, and shift the oxyhemoglobin dissociation curve to the right (increasing oxygen release in the periphery).

Although several studies demonstrated improvement in the gross and microscopic appearance of lungs after acid aspiration,[185] deficiencies in experimental design rendered their conclusions tenuous at best.[186–189] Subsequent well-designed studies failed to show any improvement in morphologic changes or morbidity and mortality rates.[49,190–192] Moreover, corticosteroids may delay the inflammatory response and also facilitate secondary bacterial infection.[193]

Prophylactic Antibiotic Agents

Pulmonary infection after aspiration is difficult to assess. Any benefit for prophylactic antibiotic agents is outweighed by altering the normal flora of the respiratory tract, leading to infection with resistant organisms.[193] Initially, antibiotics should be reserved for patients who have aspirated grossly contaminated material (eg, feculent aspirate, carious teeth, or pus from pharyngeal abscess).[45,194] Otherwise, antibiotics should be withheld and the patient monitored for clinical evidence of infection.

Temperature elevation alone is not sufficient reason for therapy; leukocytosis, pulmonary infiltrates, thick sputum, and fever may be nonspecific responses to chemical pneumonitis.[190] Antibiotics should be administered according to the results of Gram-stained smears, as well as cultures from well-collected sputum specimens (*ie*, using a protected brush technique). Therapy should be adjusted appropriately when culture and sensitivity reports become available.

Hydration

Aggressive intravenous fluid replacement may be warranted to treat hypovolemia, which occurs with highly acidic and even neutral aspirates because of the shift of fluid from the vascular bed into the pulmonary interstitium and alveoli. In severe cases, a central venous or pulmonary artery catheter should be inserted to guide fluid management; to facilitate the determination of cardiac output and the sampling of mixed venous blood; or to permit continuous mixed venous saturation measurements, and calculation of intrapulmonary venous admixture. Alterations in oxygenation, acid–base status, hydration, and cardiac function all affect renal function: thus, a physiologic basis should be sought for renal impairment before therapy (eg, diuretic agents) is instituted prematurely.

POSTSCRIPT

When Mendelson first described the syndrome of aspiration pneumonitis,[5] the instance in obstetric patients was 15 per 10,000. Forty years later a computer-generated review from Sweden documented that the incidence of aspiration in cesarean section also was 15 per 10,000.[16] In the general surgical population it was only 5 per 10,000. Thus the obstetric patient remains a particular concern, not only because of her own risk but also because of that to the fetus.

REFERENCES

1. Simpson JY: Remarks on the alleged case of death from the action of chloroform. Lancet 1:175, 1848
2. Apfelbach CW, Christianson OO: Alterations in respiratory tract from aspirated vomitus. JAMA 108:503, 1937
3. Irons EE, Apfelbach CW: Aspiration bronchopneumonia. JAMA 115:584, 1940
4. Fetterman GH, Moran TJ: Food aspiration pneumonia. Pennsylvania Medical Journal 45:810, 1942
5. Mendelson CL: The aspiration of stomach contents into the lungs during obstetric anesthesia. Am J Obstet Gynecol 52: 191, 1946
6. Marx GF, Mateo CV, Orkin LR: Computer analysis of post-anesthetic deaths. Anesthesiology 39:54, 1973
7. Harrison GG: Anaesthetic-associated mortality. S Afr Med J 48:550, 1974
8. Bodlander FMS: Deaths associated with anaesthesia. Br J Anaesth 47:36, 1975
9. Weiss WA: Regurgitation and aspiration of gastric contents during inhalation anesthesia. Anesthesiology 11:102, 1950
10. Berson W, Adriani J: 'Silent' regurgitation and aspiration during anesthesia. Anesthesiology 15:644, 1954
11. Culver GA, Makel HP, Beecher HK: Frequency of aspiration of gastric contents by the lungs during general anesthesia and surgery. Ann Surg 133:289, 1951
12. Marshall BM, Gordon RA: Vomiting, regurgitation and aspiration in anesthesia: I. Can Anaesth Soc J 5:274, 1958
13. Blitt CD, Gutman HL, Cohen DD, et al: 'Silent' regurgitation and aspiration during general anesthesia. Anesth Analg 49: 707, 1970
14. Turndorf H, Rodis ID, Clark TS: 'Silent' regurgitation during general anesthesia. Anesth Analg 53:700, 1974
15. Carlsson C, Islander G: Silent gastropharyngeal regurgitation during anesthesia. Anesth Analg 60:655, 1981
16. Olsson GL, Hallen B, Hambraeus-Jonzon K: Aspiration during anaesthesia: a computer-aided study of 185,358 anaesthetics. Acta Anaesthesiol Scand 30:84, 1986
17. Kallar SK: Aspiration pneumonitis: fact or fiction? Problems in Anesthesia 2:29, 1988
18. Awe WC, Fletcher WS, Jacob SW: The pathophysiology of aspiration pneumonitis. Surgery 60:232, 1966
19. Arms RA, Dines DE, Tintsman TC: Aspiration pneumonia. Chest 65:136, 1974
20. Cameron JL, Mitchel WH, Zuidema GD: Aspiration pneumonia: clinical outcome following documented aspiration. Arch Surg 106:49, 1973
21. Guyton AC: Textbook of medical physiology. 7th ed. Philadelphia: WB Saunders, 1986: 754
22. Hollander F: The composition and mechanism of formation of gastric acid secretion. Science 110:57, 1949

23. Nimmo WS: Drugs, diseases and altered gastric emptying. Clin Pharmacokin 1:189, 1976
24. Clark CG, Riddoch ME: Observations on the human cardia at operation. Br J Anaesth 34:875, 1962
25. Spence AA, Moir DD, Finlay WEI: Observations of intragastric pressure. Anaesthesia 22:249, 1967
26. Plourde G, Hardy JF: Aspiration pneumonia: assessing the risk of regurgitation in the cat. Can Anaesth Soc J 33:345, 1986
27. Hall AW, Moossa AR, Clark J, et al: The effects of premedication drugs on the lower oesophageal high pressure zone and reflux status of *Rhesus* monkeys and man. Gut 16:347, 1975
28. Brock-Utne JG, Rubin J, McAravey R, et al: The effect of hyoscine and atropine on the lower oesophageal sphincter. Anaesth Intensive Care 5:223, 1977
29. Brock-Utne JG, Rubin J, Welman S, et al: The effect of glycopyrrolate (Robinul) on the lower oesophageal sphincter. Can Anaesth Soc J 25:144, 1978
30. Brock-Utne JG, Rubin J, Welman S, et al: The action of commonly used antiemetics on the lower oesophageal sphincter. Br J Anaesth 50:295, 1978
31. Brock-Utne JG, Downing JW, Dimopoulos GE, et al: The effect of domperidone on lower esophageal sphincter tone in late pregnancy. Anesthesiology 52:321, 1980
32. Smith G, Dalling R, Williams TIR: Gastroesophageal pressure gradient changes produced by induction of anaesthesia and suxamethonium. Br J Anaesth 50:1137, 1978
33. Pontoppidan H, Beecher HK: Progressive loss of protective reflexes in the airway with the advance of age. JAMA 174: 2209, 1960
34. Clark MM: Aspiration of stomach contents in a conscious patient: a case report. Br J Anaesth 35:133, 1963
35. Taylor PA, Towey RM: Depression of laryngeal reflexes during ketamine anesthesia. Br Med J 2:688, 1971
36. Wise CC, Robinson JS, Heath MJ, et al: Physiological response to intermittent methohexitone for conservation dentistry. Br Med J 2:540, 1969
37. Brock-Utne JC, Winning TJ, Rubin J, et al: Laryngeal incompetence during neuroleptanalgesia in combination with diazepam. Br J Anaesth 48:699, 1976
38. Claeys DW, Lockhart CH, Hinkle JE: The effects of transtracheal block and Innovar on glottic competence. Anesthesiology 38:485, 1973
39. Rubin J, Brock-Utne JG, Greenberg M, et al: Laryngeal incompetence during experimental 'relative analgesia' using 50% nitrous oxide in oxygen. Br J Anaesth 49:1005, 1977
40. Tomlin PJ, Howarth FH, Robinson JS: Postoperative atelectasis and laryngeal incompetence. Lancet 1:1402, 1968
41. Burgess GE III, Cooper JR Jr, Marino RJ, et al: Laryngeal competence after tracheal extubation. Anesthesiology 45:73, 1979
42. Brown HG: The applied anatomy of vomiting. Br J Anaesth 35:136, 1963
43. Teabeaut JR II: Aspiration of gastric contents: an experimental study. Am J Pathol 24:51, 1952
44. Exarhos ND, Logan WD, Abbott OA, et al: The importance of pH and volume in tracheobronchial aspiration. Dis Chest 47: 167, 1965
45. Hamelberg W, Bosomworth PP: Aspiration pneumonitis: experimental studies and clinical observations. Anesth Analg 43: 669, 1964
46. James CF, Modell JH, Gibbs CP, et al: Pulmonary aspiration: effects of volume and pH in the rat. Anesth Analg 63:667, 1984
47. Kennedy TP, Johnson KJ, Kunkel RG, et al: Acute acid aspiration lung injury in the rat: biphasic pathogenesis. Anesth Analg 69:87, 1989
48. Alexander IGS: The ultrastructure of the pulmonary alveolar vessels in Mendelson's (acid pulmonary aspiration) syndrome. Br J Anaesth 40:408, 1968
49. Downs JB, Chapman RL Jr, Modell JH, et al: An evaluation of steroid therapy in aspiration pneumonitis. Anesthesiology 40: 129, 1974
50. Colebatch HJH, Halmgyi DFJ: Reflex airway reaction to fluid aspiration. J Appl Physiol 17:787, 1962
51. Cameron JL, Caldini P, Toung JK, et al: Aspiration pneumonia: physiologic data following experimental aspiration. Surgery 72:238, 1972
52. Harboro RP, Honi J: Microscopic changes in living lung after fluid aspiration. Anesth Analg 49:835, 1970
53. Schwartz DJ, Wynne JW, Gibbs CP, et al: The pulmonary consequences of aspirations of gastric contents at pH values greater than 2.5. Am Rev Respir Dis 121:119, 1980
54. Modell JH, Graves SA, Ketover A: Clinical course of 91 consecutive near-drowning victims. Chest 70:231, 1976
55. Moran TJ: Experimental food-aspiration pneumonia. Arch Pathol 52:350, 1951
56. Halmagyi DFJ, Colebatch HJG, Starzecki B: Inhalation of blood, saliva, and alcohol: consequences, mechanisms, and treatment. Thorax 17:244, 1962
57. Vidyasagar D, Yeh TF, Harris V, et al: Assisted ventilation in infants with meconium aspiration syndrome. Pediatrics 56: 208, 1975
58. Perel A, Downs JB, Crawford CA, et al: Continuous positive airway pressure improves oxygenation in dogs after the aspiration of blood. Crit Care Med 11:868, 1983
59. Moran TJ, Hellstrom HR: Experimental aspiration pneumonia: V. acute pulmonary edema, pneumonia and bronchiolitis obliterans produced by injection of ethyl alcohol. Am J Clin Pathol 27:300, 1957
60. Bynum LJ, Pierce AK: Pulmonary aspiration of gastric contents. Am Rev Respir Dis 114:1129, 1976
61. Landay MJ, Christensen EE, Bynum LJ: Pulmonary manifestations of acute aspiration of gastric contents. Am J Roentgenol 131:587, 1978
62. Cameron JL, Reynolds J, Zuidema GD: Aspiration in patients with tracheostomies. Surg Gynecol Obstet 136:68, 1973
63. Hoyt J: Aspiration pneumonitis: patient risk factors, prevention, and management. Intensive Care Med 5:S2, 1990
64. Ong BY, Palahniuk RJ, Cumming M: Gastric volume and pH in out-patients. Can Anaesth Soc J 25:36, 1978
65. Davison JS, Davison MC, Hay DM: Gastric emptying time in late pregnancy and labour. J Obstet Gynecol Br Commonwealth 77:37, 1970
66. Attia RR, Ebeid AM, Fischer JE, et al: Maternal, fetal and placental gastrin concentrations. Anaesthesia 37:18, 1982
67. Van Thiel DH, Gavaler JS, Joshi SN, et al: Heartburn of pregnancy. Gastroenterology 72:666, 1977
68. Christofides ND, Ghatei MA, Bloom SR, et al: Decreased motilin concentrations in pregnancy. Br Med J 285:1453, 1982
69. Simpson KH, Stakes AF, Miller M: Pregnancy delays paracetamol absorption and gastric emptying in patients undergoing surgery. Br J Anaesth 60:24, 1988
70. Jones MJ, Mitchell RWD, Hindocha N, et al: The lower oesophageal sphincter in the first trimester of pregnancy: comparison of supine with lithotomy positions. Br J Anaesth 61: 475, 1988
71. Piaget F, Fouillet J: Le pharynx et l'oesophage seniles étude clinique radiologique et radiocinematographique. J Med Lyon 40:951, 1959
72. Kilman WJ, Goyal RK: Disorders of pharyngeal and upper esophageal sphincter motor function. Arch Intern Med 136: 592, 1976
73. Cogbill TH, Bintz M, Johnson JA, et al: Acute gastric dilatation after trauma. J Trauma 27:1113, 1987
74. Lawes EG, Baskett PJF: Pulmonary aspiration. Intensive Care Med 13:379, 1982
75. Snow J: On chloroform and other anaesthetics: their action and administration. London: Churchill, 1858
76. Kallar SK, Everett LL: Potential risks and preventive measures for pulmonary aspiration: new concepts in preoperative fasting guidelines. Anesth Analg 77:171, 1993
77. Sutherland AD, Maltby JR, Sale JP, et al: The effect of preoperative oral fluid and ranitidine on gastric fluid volume and pH. Can J Anaesth 34:117, 1987
78. McGrady EM, Macdonald AG: Effect of the preoperative administration of water on gastric volume and pH. Br J Anaesth 60:803, 1988

79. Hutchinson A, Maltyb JR, Reid CRG: Gastric fluid volume pH in elective inpatients: I. coffee or orange juice versus overnight fast. Can J Anaesth 35:12, 1988
80. Splinter WM, Stewart JA, Muir JG: Large volumes of apple juice preoperatively do not affect gastric pH and volume in children. Can J Anaesth 37:36, 1990
81. Nicolson SC, Dorsey AT, Schreiner MS: Shortened preanesthetic fasting interval in pediatric cardiac surgical patients. Anesth Analg 74:694, 1992
82. Lewis M, Crawford JS: Can one risk fasting the obstetric patient for less than 4 hours? Br J Anaesth 59:312, 1987
83. Ovassapian A, Krejcie TC, Telich SJ, et al: Awake fiberoptic intubation in the patient at high risk of aspiration. Br J Anaesth 62:13, 1989
84. Brown EM, Krishnaprasad D, Smiler BG: Pancuronium for rapid induction technique for tracheal intubation. Can Anaesth Soc J 26:489, 1979
85. Waldburger JJ, Neilsen CH, Mulroy MF: Evaluation of atracurium for rapid-sequence endotracheal intubation. Anesthesiology 61:A290, 1984
86. Schwarz S, Ilias W, Lackner F, et al: Rapid tracheal intubation with vecuronium: the priming principle. Anesthesiology 62: 388, 1985
87. Nagashima H, Nguyen HD, Lee S, et al: Facilitation of rapid endotracheal intubation with atracurium. Anesthesiology 61: A289, 1984
88. Foldes F: Rapid tracheal intubation with non-depolarizing neuromuscular blocking drugs: the priming principle. Br J Anaesth 56:663, 1984
89. Sellick BA: Cricoid pressure to control regurgitation of stomach contents during induction of anaesthesia. Lancet 2:404, 1961
90. Fanning GL: The efficacy of cricoid pressure in preventing regurgitation of gastric contents. Anesthesiology 32:553, 1970
91. Notcutt WG: Rupture of the oesophagus following cricoid pressure? Anaesthesia 36:911, 1981
92. Sellick BA: Rupture of the oesophagus following cricoid pressure? Anaesthesia 37:213, 1982
93. Spray SB, Zuidema GD, Cameron JL: Aspiration pneumonia: incidence of aspiration with endotracheal tubes. Am J Surg 131:701, 1976
94. Pavlin EG, Van Nimwegan D, Hornbein TF: Failure of a high-compliance low-pressure cuff to prevent aspiration. Anesthesiology 42:216, 1975
95. Browning DH, Graves SA: Incidence of aspiration with endotracheal tubes in children. J Pediatr 102:582, 1983
96. Bernhard WN, Cottrell JE, Sivakumaran C, et al: Adjustment of intracuff pressure to prevent aspiration. Anesthesiology 50: 363, 1979
97. Petring OU, Adelhoj B, Jensen BN, et al: Prevention of silent aspiration due to leaks around cuffs of endotracheal tubes. Anesth Analg 65:777, 1986
98. Mehta S: The risk of aspiration in presence of cuffed endotracheal tubes. Br J Anaesth 44:601, 1972
99. Whiffler K, Andrew WK, Glyn Thomas RG: The hazardous cuffed endotracheal tube: aspiration on extubation. S Afr Med J 61:240, 1982
100. Illing L, Duncan PG, Yip R: Gastroesophageal reflux during anaesthesia. Can J Anaesth 39:446, 1992
101. Holdsworth JD, Furness RMB, Roulston RG: A comparison of apomorphine and stomach tubes for emptying the stomach before general anesthesia in obstetrics. Br J Anaesth 46:526, 1974
102. Nanji GM, Maltby JR: Vomiting and aspiration pneumonitis with the laryngeal mask airway. Can J Anaesth 39:69, 1992
103. Barker P, Langton JA, Murphy PJ, et al: Regurgitation of gastric contents during general anaesthetic using the laryngeal mask airway. Br J Anaesth 69:514, 1992
104. Ansermino JM, Blogg CE: Cricoid pressure may prevent insertion of the laryngeal mask airway. Br J Anaesth 69:465, 1992
105. Roberts RB, Shirley MA: Reducing the risk of acid aspiration during cesarean section. Anesth Analg 53:859, 1974
106. Taylor G, Pryse-Davies J: The prophylactic use of antacids in the prevention of the acid-pulmonary-aspiration syndrome (Mendelson's syndrome). Lancet 1:288, 1966
107. Roberts RB: Aspiration and its prevention in obstetrical patients. Int Anesthesiol Clin 15:49, 1977
108. Raidoo DM, Rocke DA, Brocke-Utne JG, et al: Critical volume for pulmonary acid aspiration reappraisal in a primate model. Br J Anaesth 65:248, 1990
109. James CF: Maternal mortality. Sem Anesthesia 11:76, 1992
110. Blouw R, Scatciff J, Craig DB, et al: Gastric volume and pH in postpartum patients. Anesthesiology 45:456, 1976
111. James CF, Gibbs CP, Banner T: Postpartum perioperative risk of aspiration pneumonia. Anesthesiology 61:756, 1984
112. Salem MR, Wong AY, Mani M, et al: Premedicant drugs and gastric juice pH and volume in pediatric patients. Anesthesiology 44:216, 1976
113. Coté CJ, Goudsouzian NG, Liu LMP, et al: Assessment of risk factors related to the acid aspiration syndrome in pediatric patients: gastric pH and residual volume. Anesthesiology 56: 70, 1982
114. Vaughan RW, Bauer S, Wise L: Volume and pH of gastric juice in obese patients. Anesthesiology 43:686, 1975
115. Wheatley RG, Kallus FT, Reynolds RC, et al: Milk of magnesia is an effective preinduction antacid in obstetric anesthesia. Anesthesiology 50:514, 1979
116. Wyner J, Cohen SE: Gastric volume in early pregnancy: effect of metoclopramide. Anesthesiology 57:209, 1982
117. Chen CT, Toung TJK, Haupt HM, et al: Evaluation of the efficacy of Alka-Seltzer Effervescent in gastric acid neutralization. Anesth Analg 63:325, 1984
118. Manchikanti L, Roush JR: Effect of preanesthetic glycopyrrolate in cimetidine on gastric fluid pH and volume in outpatients. Anesth Analg 63:40, 1984
119. Stoelting RK: Responses to atropine, glycopyrrolate, and Riopan of gastric fluid pH and volume in adult patients. Anesthesiology 48:367, 1978
120. Foulkes E, Jenkins LC: A comparative evaluation of cimetidine and sodium citrate to decrease gastric acidity: effectiveness at the time of induction of anaesthesia. Can Anaesth Soc J 28: 29, 1981
121. Coombs DW, Hooper D, Colton T: Pre-anesthetic cimetidine alteration of gastric fluid volume and pH. Anesth Analg 58: 183, 1979
122. Capan LM, Rosenberg AD, Carni A, et al: Effect of cimetidine–metoclopramide combination on gastric fluid volume and acidity. Anesthesiology 59:A402, 1983
123. Gibbs CP, Schwartz DJ, Wynne JW, et al: Antacid pulmonary aspiration in the dog. Anesthesiology 51:380, 1979
124. Gibbs CP, Kuck EJ, Hood IC, et al: Antacid plus foodstuff aspiration in the dog. Anesthesiology 53:S307, 1980
125. Lahiri SK, Thomas TA, Hodgson RMH: Single-dose antacid therapy for the prevention of Mendelson's Syndrome. Br J Anaesth 45:1143, 1973
126. Gibbs CP, Spohr L, Schmidt D: The effectiveness of sodium citrate as an antacid. Anesthesiology 57:44, 1982
127. Frank M, Evans M, Flynn P, et al: Comparison of the prophylactic use of magnesium trisilicate mixture B.P.C., sodium citrate mixture or cimetidine in obstetrics. Br J Anaesth 56:355, 1984
128. Dewan DM, Floyd HM, Thistlewood JM, et al: Sodium citrate pretreatment in elective cesarean section patients. Anesth Analg 64:34, 1985
129. Eyler SW, Cullen BG, Murphy ME, et al: Antacid aspiration in rabbits: a comparison of Mylanta and Bicitra. Anesth Analg 61: 288, 1982
130. Gibbs CP, Banner TC: Effectiveness of Bicitra as a preoperative antacid. Anesthesiology 61:97, 1984
131. Holdsworth JD, Johnson K, Mascall G, et al: Mixing of antacids with stomach contents: another approach to the prevention of acid aspiration (Mendelson's) syndrome. Anaesthesia 35:641, 1980
132. O'Sullivan GM, Bullingham RE: Noninvasive assessment by radiotelemetry of antacid effect during labor. Anesth Analg 64: 95, 1985

133. Weber L, Hirshman CA: Cimetidine for prophylaxis of aspiration pneumonitis: comparison of intramuscular and oral dosage schedules. Anesth Analg 58:426, 1979
134. Toung T, Cameron JL: Cimetidine as a preoperative medication to reduce the complications of aspiration of gastric contents. Surgery 87:205, 1980
135. Goudsouzian N, Cote CJ, Liu LMP, et al: The dose-response effects of oral cimetidine on gastric pH and volume in children. Anesthesiology 55:533, 1981
136. Johnston JR, McCaughey W, Moore J, et al: Cimetidine as an oral antacid before elective caesarean section. Anaesthesia 37: 26, 1982
137. Hodgkinson R, Classenberg R, Joyce TH, et al: Comparison of cimetidine (Tagamet) with antacid for safety and effectiveness in reducing gastric acidity before elective cesarean section. Anesthesiology 59:86, 1983
138. Pickering BG, Palahniuk RJ, Cumming M: Cimetidine premedication in elective caesarean section. Can Anaesth Soc J 27:33, 1980
139. Stoelting RK: Gastric fluid Ph in patients receiving cimetidine. Anesth Analg 57:675, 1978
140. Cohen J, Weetman AP, Dargie HJ, et al: Life-threatening arrhythmias and intravenous cimetidine. Br Med J 2:768, 1979
141. Jeffreys DB, Vale JA: Cimetidine and bradycardia. Lancet 1: 828, 1978
142. Mahon WA, Kolton M: Hypotension after intravenous cimetidine. Lancet 1:828, 1978
143. Shaw RG, Mashford ML, Desmond PV: Cardiac arrest after intravenous injection of cimetidine. Med J Aust 2:629, 1980
144. Chang HK, Morrison SL: Bone-marrow suppression associated with cimetidine. Ann Intern Med 91:580, 1979
145. Freston JW: Cimetidine: II. adverse reactions and patterns of use. Ann Intern Med 97:728, 1982
146. Puurunen J, Pelonen O: Cimetidine inhibits microsomal drug metabolism in the rat. Eur J Pharmacol 55:335, 1979
147. Feely J, Wilkinson GR, Wood AJJ: Reduction of liver blood flow and propranolol metabolism by cimetidine. N Engl J Med 304:692, 1981
148. Feely J, Wilkinson GR, McAllister CB, et al: Increased toxicity and reduced clearance of lidocaine by cimetidine. Ann Intern Med 96:592, 1982
149. Klotz U, Reimanns I: Delayed clearance of diazepam due to cimetidine. N Engl J Med 302:1012, 1980
150. Lam AM, Clement JL: Effect of cimetidine premedication on morphine-induced ventilatory depression. Can Anaesth Soc J 31:36, 1984
151. Jackson JE, Powell JR, Wandaell M, et al: Cimetidine decreases theophylline clearance. Am Rev Respir Dis 123:619, 1981
152. Gugler R, Brand M, Somogyi A: Impaired cimetidine absorption due to antacids and metoclopramide. Eur J Clin Pharmacol 20:225, 1981
153. Andrews AD, Brock-Utne JG, Downing JW: Protection against pulmonary acid aspiration with ranitidine. Anaesthesia 37:22, 1982
154. Zeldis JB, Friedman LS, Isselbacher KJ: Ranitidine: a new H_2-receptor antagonist. N Engl J Med 309:1368, 1983
155. Camarri G, Chirone E, Fanteira G, et al: Ranitidine-induced bradycardia. Lancet 2:160, 1982
156. Herrera A, Sabal-Celigny P, Dresch C, et al: Ranitidine. N Engl J Med 310:1604, 1984
157. Knodell RG, Holtzman JL, Crankshaw DL, et al: Drug metabolism by rat and human hepatic microsomes in response to interaction with H_2-receptor antagonists. Gastroenterology 82: 84, 1982
158. Mihaly GW, Marino AT, Webster LK, et al: High dose of antacid (Mylanta II) reduces bioavailability of ranitidine. Br Med J 285: 998, 1982
159. Dubin SA, Silverstein PI, Wakefield ML, et al: Comparison of the effects of oral famotidine and ranitidine on gastric volume and pH. Anesth Analg 69:680, 1989
160. Langtry HD, Grant SM, Goa KL: Famotidine. An updated review of the pharmacodynamic and pharmacokinetic properties, and therapeutic use in peptic ulcer disease and other allied diseases. Drugs 38:551, 1989
161. Baraka A, Saab M, Salem MR, et al: Control of gastric acidity by glycopyrrolate premedication in the parturient. Anesth Analg 56:642, 1977
162. Howard FA, Sharp DS: Effect of metoclopramide on gastric emptying during labour. Br Med J 1:446, 1973
163. Schulze-Delrieu K: Metoclopramide. N Engl J Med 305:28, 1981
164. Cohen SE, Jasson J, Talafre M-L, et al: Does metoclopramide decrease the volume of gastric contents in patients undergoing cesarean section? Anesthesiology 61:604, 1984
165. Diamond MJ, Keeri-Szanto M: Reduction of postoperative vomiting by preoperative administration of oral metoclopramide. Can Anaesth Soc J 27:36, 1980
166. Fragen RJ, Caldwell N: A new benzimidazole antiemetic, domperidone, for the treatment of postoperative nausea and vomiting. Anesthesiology 49:289, 1978
167. Cohen SE, Woods WA, Wyner J: Antiemetic efficacy of droperidol and metoclopramide. Anesthesiology 60:67, 1984
168. Solanki DR, Suresh M, Ethridge HC: The effects of intravenous cimetidine and metoclopramide on gastric volume and pH. Anesth Analg 63:599, 1984
169. Rao TLK, Madhavareddy S, Chinthagada M, et al: Metoclopramide and cimetidine to reduce gastric fluid pH and volume. Anesth Analg 63:1014, 1984
170. Manchikanti L, Marrero TC, Roush JR: Preanesthetic cimetidine and metoclopramide for acid aspiration prophylaxis in elective surgery. Anesthesiology 61:48, 1984
171. Manchikanti L, Colliver JA, Marrero TC, et al: Ranitidine and metoclopramide for prophylaxis of aspiration pneumonitis in elective surgery. Anesth Analg 64:903, 1984
172. Nimmo WS, Wilson J, Prescott LF: Narcotic analgesics and delayed gastric emptying during labour. Lancet 1:890, 1975
173. Grimes JD, Hassan MN, Preston DN: Adverse neurologic effects of metoclopramide. Can Med Assoc J 126:23, 1982
174. Park GR: Hypotension following the intravenous injection of metoclopramide. Anaesthesia 36:75, 1981
175. Cruickshank RH, Morrison DA, Bamber PA, et al: Effect of I.V. omeprazole on the pH and volume of gastric contents before surgery. Br J Anaesth 63:536, 1989
176. Scuderi P, Wetchler B, Sung YF: Treatment of postoperative nausea and vomiting after outpatient surgery with the 5-HT_3 antagonist ondansetron. Anesthesiology 78:15, 1993
177. McKenzie R, Kovac A, O'Connor T, et al: Comparison of ondansetron versus placebo to prevent postoperative nausea and vomiting in women undergoing ambulatory gynecologic surgery. Anesthesiology 78:21, 1993
178. LeFrock JL, Clark TS, Davies B, et al: Aspiration pneumonia: a ten-year review. Am Surg 45:305, 1979
179. Campinos L, Duval G, Couturier M, et al: The value of early fiberoptic bronchoscopy after aspiration of gastric contents. Br J Anaesth 55:1103, 1983
180. Wolfe JE, Bone RC, Ruth WE: Diagnosis of gastric aspiration by fiberoptic bronchoscopy. Chest 70:458, 1976
181. Suter PM, Fairley HB, Isenberg MD: Optimum end-expiratory airway pressure in patients with acute pulmonary failure. N Engl J Med 292:284, 1975
182. Downs JB, Modell JH: Patterns of respiratory support aimed at pathophysiologic conditions. ASA Refresher Courses in Anesthesiology 5:71, 1977
183. Murray IP, Modell JH, Gallagher TJ, et al: Titration of PEEP by the arterial minus end-tidal carbon dioxide gradient. Chest 85:100, 1984
184. Downs JB, Klein EF Jr, Modell JH: The effect of incremental PEEP on PaO_2 in patients with respiratory failure. Anesth Analg 52:210, 1973
185. Bannister WK, Sattilaro AJ, Otis RD: Therapeutic aspects of aspiration pneumonitis in experimental animals. Anesthesiology 22:440, 1961
186. Lewinski A: Evaluation of methods employed in the treatment of the chemical pneumonitis of aspiration. Anesthesiology 26: 37, 1965

187. Bosomworth PP, Hamelberg W: Etiologic and therapeutic aspects of aspiration pneumonitis: experimental study. Surg Forum 13:158, 1962
188. Lawson DW, Defalco AJ, Phelphs JA, et al: Corticosteroids as treatment for aspiration of gastric contents: an experimental study. Surgery 59:845, 1966
189. Dudley WR, Marshall BE: Steroid treatment for acid-aspiration pneumonitis. Anesthesiology 40:136, 1974
190. Wynne JW, Modell JH: Respiratory aspiration of stomach contents. Ann Intern Med 87:466, 1977
191. Chapman RL Jr, Downs JB, Modell JH, et al: The ineffectiveness of steroid therapy in treating aspiration of hydrochloric acid. Arch Surg 108:858, 1974
192. Chapman RL Jr, Modell JH, Ruiz BC, et al: Effect of continuous positive-pressure ventilation and steroid on aspiration of hydrochloric acid (pH 1.8) in dogs. Anesth Analg 53:556, 1974
193. Wynne JW, Reynolds JC, Hood CI, et al: Steroid therapy for pneumonitis induced in rabbits by aspiration of foodstuff. Anesthesiology 51:11, 1979
194. Vilinskas J, Schweizer RT, Foster JH: Experimental studies on aspiration of contents of obstructed intestine. Surg Gynecol Obstet 135:568, 1972

Complications in Anesthesiology, second edition,
edited by Nikolaus Gravenstein and Robert R. Kirby.
Lippincott-Raven Publishers, Philadelphia © 1996.

CHAPTER 15

Negative-Pressure Pulmonary Edema

Cheri Sulek

Negative-pressure pulmonary edema is a complication of acute and chronic upper-airway obstruction that is likely underrecognized and misdiagnosed by anesthesiologists. The predominant pathophysiologic mechanism is the development of a markedly negative (subambient) intrapleural pressure during inspiration against a closed glottis, ultimately producing increased pulmonary microvascular pressure. The risk factors for and causes of upper-airway obstruction are numerous, but in general the clinical course of postobstructive pulmonary edema is self-limited with supportive treatment only. The diagnosis often is confused with pulmonary aspiration of gastric contents because the two entities may initially be indistinguishable in presentation and precipitating factors.

HISTORICAL PERSPECTIVE

Early Studies

The association between upper-airway obstruction and the development of pulmonary edema was first described in 1927,[1] but the first case was not reported until 1973.[2]

Negative Pleural Pressure

In 1919, Davies and associates studied the ventilatory response to increased inspiratory and expiratory resistance in humans and noted an elevated respiratory rate and hypoxemia.[3] In 1921, Graham observed the production of pleural fluid during inspiration and expiration in an isolated edematous lung model.[4] He proposed that negative intrapleural pressure developed during inspiration, contributing to the formation of pleural fluid.

Upper-Airway Obstruction

In 1927, Moore and Binger[1] expanded the previous work by Davies and associates and were the first to recognize the association between upper-airway obstruction and the development of pulmonary edema in animals. The effect of an increase in inspiratory resistance, simulating partial upper-airway obstruction, was determined in spontaneously breathing, anesthetized animals. Some animals remained hypoxic after relief of the obstruction, and the lungs at autopsy were described as congested with frothy fluid in the trachea. It is of interest that the intratracheal pressure ranged only from -11 to -20 cm H_2O.

Inspiratory Loading

In 1942, Warren and coworkers described the effects of subambient pressure in the chest.[5] The right lymphatic duct was cannulated in anesthetized, spontaneously breathing animals, and lymph production was recorded during inspiratory loading. When animals inspired against resistance, creating a markedly subambient intrapleural pressure (to as low as -56 cm H_2O), transudation of fluid and red blood cells from the pulmonary capillaries into the interstitial space was observed. In further experiments by Warren and coworkers, lung lymph flow was increased during periods of hypoxia in animals not subjected to inspiratory resistance, leading to speculation that hypoxia may alter pulmonary capillary permeability.[5] The clinical significance of these observations was not recognized until years later.

The association between asphyxial deaths and pulmonary edema at autopsy was recognized by Swann in 1964.[6] In further studies, he noted that pulmonary congestion was prominent in asphyxial deaths in animals after strangulation, brain injury, drowning, and barbiturate overdose.

Smith-Eriksen and Bo demonstrated that interstitial edema in an isolated rabbit lung model increased eightfold when the intrapleural pressure was decreased by less than 5 cm H_2O in the presence of a closed airway.[7] Of considerable clinical relevance is that the intrapleural pressure created in this model was within the normal range seen with inspiration. In 1986 Lloyd and colleagues simulated upper-airway obstruction in awake sheep by inspiratory loading with 20 cm H_2O and recorded lung lymph flow and hemodynamic parameters.[8] Lung lymph flow increased without a documented change in mean pulmonary artery pressure; however, it was hypothesized that pulmonary microvascular hydrostatic pressure increased. This study provided a better understanding of the pathogenesis of negative-pressure pulmonary edema.

Human Case Studies

The first recognized pediatric case of negative-pressure pulmonary edema was reported in 1973[2] and the first adult case in 1977.[9] From 1977 to 1990, only 77 cases of upper-airway obstruction associated with pulmonary edema were reported.[10] The true incidence is unknown; however, it is likely much higher than reported, considering the frequency of upper-airway obstruction in the perianesthetic period and the probability that many cases may be misdiagnosed as aspiration syndromes.

EPIDEMIOLOGIC CHARACTERISTICS

Negative-pressure pulmonary edema may be misdiagnosed or go clinically unrecognized in mild cases. It usually becomes clinically evident after relief of upper-airway obstruction but can be delayed in presentation. The causes of upper-airway obstruction are numerous and can be acute or chronic (Table 15-1). Laryngospasm and upper-airway tumors account for 50% of adult cases of postobstructive pulmonary edema. Laryngospasm is the most common inciting event.[10,11] The time to onset of pulmonary edema after obstruction ranges from 3 to 150 minutes.

TABLE 15-1
Causes of Upper-Airway Obstruction

ACUTE
Laryngospasm
Foreign-body aspiration
Bronchospasm
Airway trauma
Interrupted hanging
Obstruction of endotracheal tube
Malpositioned laryngeal mask airway
Supraglottitis
Tumor
Croup
Strangulation
Excessive sedation
Retropharyngeal or peritonsillar abscess
Laryngotracheobronchitis
CHRONIC
Tonsillar or adenoidal hypertrophy
Goiter
Acromegaly
Obstructive sleep apnea with obesity
Nasopharyngeal mass

Acute Airway Obstruction

Despite the frequency of laryngospasm in children, postobstructive pulmonary edema is rare. It is not clear why negative-pressure pulmonary edema is not common after laryngospasm, because children have extremely compliant chest walls and can generate large negative intrapleural pressures. In the past, before the institution of pulse oximetry as a standard of care in anesthesia, mild cases may have been unrecognized. Croup, supraglottitis, and laryngotracheobronchitis account for more than 50% of these pulmonary edema cases in children less than 10 years of age.[12] Other causes of acute upper-airway obstruction include aspiration, strangulation, interrupted hanging, retropharyngeal or peritonsillar abscess, Ludwig's angina, angioedema, bronchospasm, excessive sedation, biting on an endotracheal tube, and malposition of a laryngeal mask airway.[12–14]

Chronic Airway Obstruction

Chronic upper-airway obstruction may occur as a result of obstructive sleep apnea, adenoidal or tonsillar hypertrophy, nasopharyngeal mass, goiter, or acromegaly.[12,15] In adults who have obstructive sleep apnea, chronic hypoventilation and hypoxemia may result in cor pulmonale and intermittent pulmonary edema due to intermittent upper-airway obstruction.

Risk Factors

Perianesthetic risk factors identified by Lorch and Sahn in a review of cases include obesity with obstructive sleep apnea; anatomically difficult intubations; and nasal, oral or pharyngeal surgery or pathologic lesions.[16] Patients with these risk factors probably should be fully awake at the time of extubation and must be observed closely in the postanesthesia care unit. However, the period of observation is controversial and should be individualized.

Young male athletes also appear to be at an increased risk because they can generate markedly negative intrapleural pressures ($\leqslant -100$ cm H_2O).[17] In these cases, negative-pressure pulmonary edema has also been termed "athlete's pulmonary edema," or the "APE syndrome." In human volunteers, obstructive periods of as little as 10 to 30 seconds have precipitated pulmonary edema and profound hypoxemia.[18]

PATHOGENESIS AND PATHOPHYSIOLOGIC FEATURES

Starling Forces

The pathogenesis of negative-pressure pulmonary edema is multifactorial (Table 15-2). The predominant mechanism, as noted, is the generation of a markedly subambient intrapleural pressure during inspiration against a closed glottis. An understanding of the Starling forces that control fluid exchange along the pulmonary capillaries is important, because only 0.5 μm of tissue separates the pulmonary capillaries from the alveoli.[19] The forces associated with transcapillary fluid flux ($\dot{Q}f=+$) are represented by the Starling equation:

TABLE 15-2
Balance of Forces in Negative-Pressure Pulmonary Edema

FAVORING EDEMA: INSPIRATION
Müller maneuver
Increased venous return
Increased microvascular pressures
Increased pulmonary capillary permeability
Negative intrapleural pressure
Increased pulmonary blood flow
Increased left ventricular afterload
Hypoxia and hyperadrenergic state
OPPOSING EDEMA: EXPIRATION
Valsalva's maneuver
Decreased venous return
Decreased microvascular pressure
Positive pleural pressure
Decreased pulmonary blood volume
DECOMPENSATED STATE
Relief of obstruction
Increased venous return
Interstitial or alveolar pulmonary edema
Decreased airway pressure
Increased microvascular pressure

$$\dot{Q}f = Kf([Pc - Pi]) - \delta[\pi c - \pi i]),$$

where Kf = the filtration coefficient; Pc = pulmonary capillary hydrostatic pressure; Pi = interstitial hydrostatic pressure; δ = the reflection coefficient; πc = capillary colloid oncotic pressure; and πi = interstitial colloid oncotic pressure. δ represents the effectiveness of the endothelium in preventing the movement of solutes (primarily albumin) across the membrane. A δ value of 0 represents free permeability (no barrier function), and 1 represents total impermeability to proteins.

Normally, a small net flux of fluid passes out of the capillaries and into the interstitium of the peribronchial and perivascular spaces.[7,8] The lymphatic vessels in the peribronchial and perivascular spaces usually are able to clear this lymphatic fluid effectively. Large, rapid effluxes may overcome the lymphatic drainage capacity. In such cases, fluid ultimately crosses into the alveoli in later stages.

Müller Maneuver

During attempted inspiration against a closed glottis, known as a Müller maneuver, a markedly subambient intrapleural pressure develops and is transmitted to the perivascular and interstitial spaces (see Table 16-2).[18] Before inspiration is initiated, the normal intrapleural pressure is −5 cm H_2O.[19] It decreases to −7 to −8 cm H_2O during normal active inspiration. The intrapleural pressures may decrease to −50 to −100 cm H_2O when inspiration is attempted against a closed glottis.[12] The threshold level of subambient pressure necessary to produce edema is not known and may vary considerably among individuals (as may be demonstrated by the Starling equation).

Ventricular Preload and Afterload

This pleural pressure decrement is transmitted ultimately to the pulmonary interstitium and increases venous return to the right heart. Elevated hydrostatic pressure in the pulmonary capillaries increases the transcapillary hydrostatic pressure gradient and thus predisposes the patient to pulmonary edema.[20] In addition, subambient intrapleural pressure during systole increases left ventricular afterload, resulting in elevated left ventricular end-diastolic volume and pressure, decreased left ventricular stroke volume and ejection fraction, and increased pulmonary microvascular pressure.[20,21]

Ventricular Interdependence

As the right ventricle distends with increasing venous return, the interventricular septum shifts leftward, and left ventricular volume and compliance decrease (ventricular interdependence), resulting in further elevation of left ventricular end-diastolic pressure. Negative intrapleural pressure also increases the transmural pressure across the aorta and left ventricle, thereby augmenting afterload.[21]

Pulmonary Capillary Permeability

Pulmonary capillary permeability is thought to increase with negative intrapleural pressure.[10] In general, when pulmonary vascular compliance is low, increased blood volume to the pulmonary circulation alters membrane permeability, predisposing membrane integrity to physical disruption and ultimately resulting in transudation of fluid and red blood cells. This disruption has been observed experimentally and clinically.

Hypoxia and the Hyperadrenergic State

Hypoxia and the hyperadrenergic state that accompany upper-airway obstruction probably also contribute to the development of pulmonary edema.[22] The hyperadrenergic state can be induced by upper-airway obstruction alone and is augmented by hypoxia. Hypoxia and metabolic acidosis increase vasoconstriction at the precapillary level,[23] elevate pulmonary microvascular pressure, alter pulmonary capillary membrane permeability, and are myocardial depressants.[10] Increased sympathetic nervous system activity causes centralization of the circulating blood volume with translocation of blood from the systemic to the pulmonary circulation, thereby further elevating pulmonary microvascular pressure.

The hyperadrenergic state also may contribute to the alteration of pulmonary capillary membrane integrity. Neurogenic pulmonary edema sustained after a variety of central nervous system insults supports the role of the autonomic nervous system in edema development.[24] Permeability defects in the pulmonary capillaries and an elevated pulmonary microvascular pressure caused by intense catecholamine release have been suggested as the major pathogenic mechanisms.

Valsalva's Maneuver

Expiration against a closed glottis (Valsalva's maneuver) creates an auto–positive end-expiratory pressure (PEEP) effect that favors distention of the alveoli and prevents pulmonary edema until the obstruction is relieved (see Table 15-2).[11] During expiration against a closed glottis, the trapping of air results in sustained inflation and PEEP. Even with a Valsalva's maneuver, mean intratracheal pressure during obstruction is subambient.[10]

Positive intrapleural pressure decreases venous return, pulmonary microvasculature pressure, and left ventricular afterload.[25] In the clinical situation, after the obstruction is relieved, the auto-PEEP effect dissipates, promoting pulmonary edema formation (see Table 15-2). A balance of subambient inspiratory and positive expiratory pressures during a fixed upper-airway obstruction prevents the development of pulmonary edema until the obstruction is relieved. With a variable upper-airway obstruction, however, the Müller maneuver predominates, manifesting as clinically evident pulmonary edema before relief of the upper-airway obstruction.[11]

PRESENTATION

Symptoms

Recognition of patients with predisposing factors for upper-airway obstruction is important. Clinical signs of upper-airway obstruction include stridor, respiratory distress, paradoxical chest movement, and use of accessory respiratory musculature. Pulmonary edema acutely manifests as dyspnea, tachypnea, cyanosis, wheezing, and the production of abundant pink, frothy secretions. Hypoxia, hypercapnia, and metabolic acidosis ensue.

Time Course

Eighty percent of cases of negative-pressure pulmonary edema occur within minutes after relief of upper-airway obstruction.[10] Delayed onset is rare, but has been reported after 4 to 6 hours in some cases (particularly in strangulation).[9,25] Because the spectrum of presentation ranges from mild to severe, some cases go unrecognized. Severity probably is related to the duration of obstruction and degree of pulmonary capillary injury.

Some investigators advocate prolonged observation after extubation in patients in whom upper-airway obstruction develops or in patients who have predisposing risk factors even when pulmonary edema is not clinically evident.[16,22,26] The use of pulse oximetry in the operating room and postanesthesia care unit probably identifies any risk in most patients. Signs and symptoms of negative-pressure pulmonary edema often are subtle, manifesting only as a modest decrease in oxygen saturation on pulse oximetry, a sign that may be evident only when the patient is breathing room air. Pulmonary edema usually is self-limited and may be evident only on radiographic examination of the chest (Fig. 15-1).

Resolution

Radiographically confirmed alveolar or interstitial edema[10,22] usually resolves within 12 to 24 hours. However, in some cases resolution takes longer; the time required presumably is related to the degree of injury or physical disruption of the pulmonary microvasculature.

Hemodynamic Alterations

Hemodynamic monitoring reveals normal values for central venous, pulmonary artery, and pulmonary capillary wedge pressures.[10] Pulmonary capillary pressure, as distinguished from pulmonary artery occlusion pressure, is likely elevated; however, direct measurement in humans is not possible.[23] The visual-inspection method of determining pulmonary capillary pressure uses the occlusion pressure tracing but often is not feasible or is inaccurate. An increased pulmonary capillary pressure cannot be predicted by pulmonary artery pressure or pulmonary artery occlusion pressure: these parameters are normal in a variety of clinical situations in which pulmonary capillary pressure is increased.[23]

DIFFERENTIAL DIAGNOSIS

The differential diagnosis of perianesthetic pulmonary edema varies and should be pursued because the treatment depends on the cause (Table 15-3).

Aspiration of Gastric Contents

If negative-pressure pulmonary edema is ruled out, the primary alternative diagnosis is the aspiration of gastric contents and development of pneumonia. Aspiration pneumonia also may be self-limited and require only supportive treatment, depending on the quantity and quality (ie, pH and particulate nature) of the aspirate. Direct laryngoscopy or fiberoptic bronchoscopy may be helpful in the identification of particulate aspiration. Chest radiographs frequently are not helpful in distinguishing between the two entities. Massive aspiration can appear identical to negative-pressure pulmonary edema, and unilateral negative-pressure pulmonary edema can occur.

Acute Respiratory Distress Syndrome

The acute respiratory distress syndrome must be excluded, based on patient risk factors; however, rapid clinical improvement in postobstructive negative-pressure pulmonary edema will assist in confirmation of the diagnosis.

Intravascular Volume Excess

Iatrogenic volume overload also should be considered and can be determined by measurement of central venous or pulmonary capillary wedge pressure. Treatment of this problem involves fluid restriction, vasodilation, and administration of diuretic agents that are not advocated in negative-pressure pulmonary edema.

Cardiac Abnormalities

Cardiogenic factors must be excluded, especially in patients with a preexisting history of cardiac disease or identifiable cardiac risk factors. Ischemic events, dysrhythmias, or de-

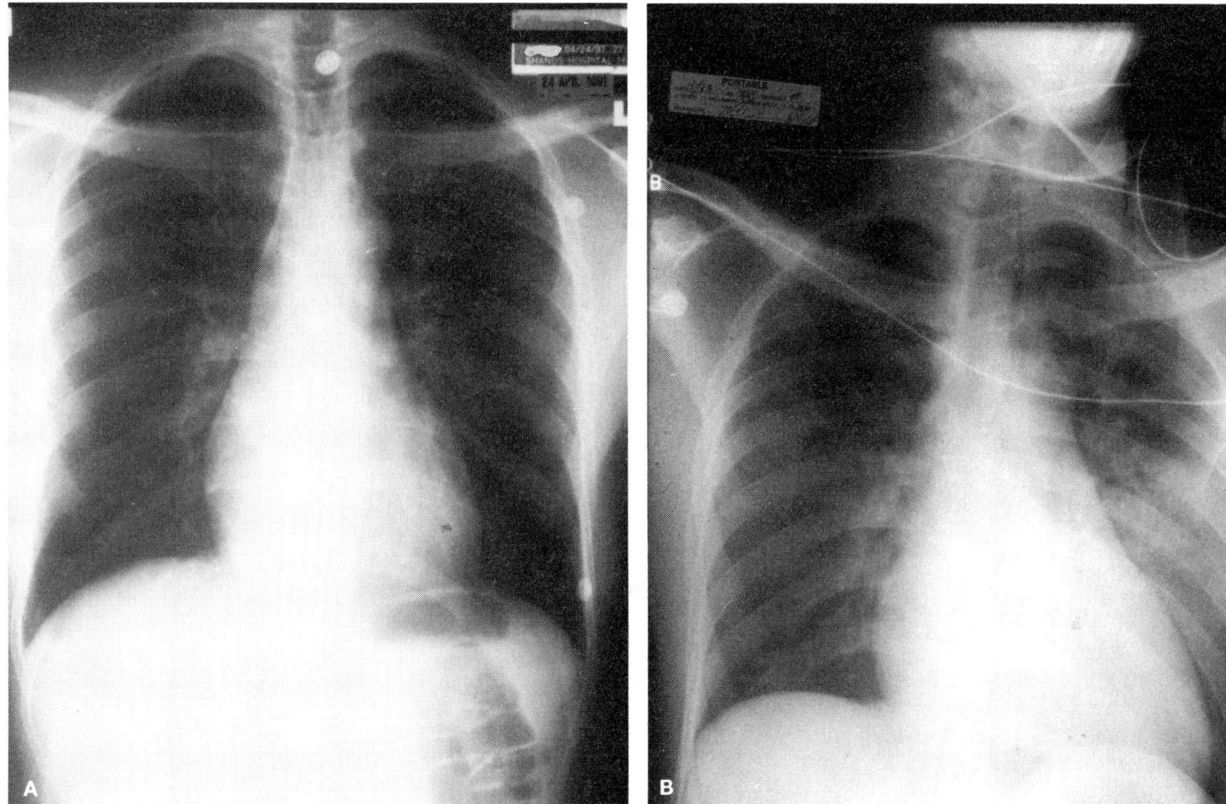

FIGURE 15-1. (A) Normal preoperative chest radiograph of a male patient scheduled for elective surgery. (B) Postextubation chest radiograph of the same patient, who experienced transient pulse oximetric hemoglobin oxygen desaturation (Spo_2 = 86%) immediately after tracheal extubation. Bilateral interstitial edema is present. The anesthesiologist described a brief period of "laryngospasm" (20 to 30 seconds), which, in association with the decrease in Spo_2, prompted radiographic examination. Continuous positive airway pressure by face mask was applied for 4 hours and resulted in total resolution of the pulmonary edema.

compensation resulting from valvular disease should be ruled out. Ischemic changes and rhythm disturbances sometimes are detected by a standard electrocardiogram, and a transthoracic or transesophageal echocardiogram may assist in detecting wall motion abnormalities, quantitating ejection fraction, and assessing valvular function.

Miscellaneous Causes

Pulmonary embolus should be excluded in patients with predisposing factors or with surgical procedures that may precipitate such an event (ie, orthopedic or cardiac procedures). Anaphylaxis also must be considered; a review of recently administered medications is essential.

TABLE 15-3
Differential Diagnosis of Perianesthetic Pulmonary Edema

- Negative-pressure pulmonary edema
- Aspiration of gastric contents
- Acute respiratory distress syndrome (ARDS)
- Congestive heart failure
- Volume overload
- Anaphylaxis

Modified from Sulek CA: Negative pressure pulmonary edema. Current Reviews in Clinical Anesthesia 13:9, 1992.

TREATMENT

Ventilatory Support

Treatment of negative-pressure pulmonary edema is primarily supportive and includes maintenance of a patent airway and administration of supplemental oxygen (Table 15-4).[11] Aggressive intervention usually is not required when the diagnosis is suggested; however, patients should be monitored in an intensive care setting until the condition resolves. Ensuring a patent airway may require placement of an endotracheal tube and possibly mechanical ventilation. In case reports compiled by Lang and coworkers, 85% of adults and children required intubation; 50% required mechanical ventilation; and 50% required application of continuous positive airway pressure or PEEP.[10]

Maintenance of the airway and oxygenation initially may be attempted without intubation; some patients may need only supplemental oxygen, continuous positive airway pressure administered by mask, or both. In general, in patients with

TABLE 15-4
Treatment of Negative-Pressure Pulmonary Edema

- Supportive measures
- Maintenance of patent airway
- Oxygen
- Continuous positive airway pressure
- Mechanical ventilation
- Careful monitoring (seldom aggressive or invasive)

Sulek CA: Negative pressure pulmonary edema. Current Reviews in Clincal Anesthesia 13:9, 1992.

severe pulmonary edema the trachea will be reintubated in the operating room or postanesthesia care unit. In most patients requiring mechanical ventilation the trachea can be extubated within 24 hours as the edema resolves. For those who require mechanical ventilation, PEEP almost always improves oxygenation and limits the amount of oxygen used.

Fluid Management

Fluid restriction and diuretic agents are not advocated for patients in whom the diagnosis of negative-pressure pulmonary edema is clear. These patients may be hypovolemic as a result of massive fluid transfer to the lungs, and this therapy will only make their condition worse.

Miscellaneous

Aggressive hemodynamic monitoring usually is unnecessary but occasionally can be helpful in the differential diagnosis. In the past, treatment with steroids was used, but currently it is not advocated. Patients who have upper-airway obstruction or who have predisposing risk factors but do not immediately manifest pulmonary edema need close monitoring in the postanesthesia care unit. The duration of observation, as noted previously, is controversial. Negative-pressure pulmonary edema usually is benign and self-limited and produces no long-term sequelae. Occasionally, however, cases can be fulminant and even life-threatening. Even in these instances the condition usually resolves rapidly once the diagnosis is recognized and treatment is instituted.

Prevention

Aggressive treatment of upper-airway obstruction may prevent the development of negative-pressure pulmonary edema. Patients with signs of upper-airway obstruction should be treated early. The anesthesiologist should not struggle for long periods to overcome the obstruction with a mask; a small dose, 5 to 20 mg, of succinylcholine usually is all that is needed. Attention should be paid to the possibility that the endotracheal tube is kinked, and the patient should be prevented from biting the tube. Some investigators advocate the immediate use of a mask for continuous positive airway pressure in children after relief of epiglottitis and croup to reduce the risk of postobstructive pulmonary edema; however, this approach is anecdotal and has not proven clinically efficacious[22,25,27] and probably does not work well in adults.

CONCLUSIONS

Negative-pressure pulmonary edema is probably more common than most anesthesiologists realize, considering the relative frequency of upper-airway obstruction in the perianesthetic period. In subtle cases the diagnosis may be missed, and in severe cases it may be confused with aspiration, which many anesthesiologists are quick to diagnose because it is potentially lethal. The events preceding negative-pressure pulmonary edema may resemble those leading to aspiration (ie, a patient's struggling, or difficulty or failure in intubating the airway), and the clinical presentation may be identical. In the past, mild cases of postobstructive pulmonary edema may have been unrecognized, but pulse oximetry now allows their detection.

REFERENCES

1. Moore RL, Binger CAL: The response to respiratory resistance: a comparison of the effects produced by partial obstruction in the inspiratory and expiratory phases of respiration. J Exp Med 45:1065, 1927
2. Capitanio MA, Kirkpatrick JA: Obstructions of the upper airway in children as reflected on the chest radiograph. Pediatr Radiol 107:159, 1973
3. Davies HWA, Haldane JS, Priestley JG: The response to respiratory resistance. J Physiol 53:60, 1919
4. Graham EA: Influence of respiratory movements on the formation of pleural exudates. JAMA 76:784, 1921
5. Warren MF, Peterson DK, Drinker CK: The effects of heightened negative pressure in the chest, together with further experiments upon anoxia in increasing the flow of lung lymph. Am J Physiol 137:641, 1942
6. Swann HE: The development of pulmonary edema during the agonal period of sudden asphyxial deaths. J Forensic Sci 9:360, 1964
7. Smith-Ericksen N, Bo G: Airway closure and fluid filtration in the lung. Br J Anaesth 51:475, 1979
8. Lloyd JE, Nolop KB, Parker RE, et al: Effects of inspiratory loading on lung fluid balance in awake sheep. J Appl Physiol 60:198, 1986
9. Oswalt CE, Gates GA, Holmstrom FMG: Pulmonary edema as a complication of acute airway obstruction. JAMA 238:1833, 1977
10. Lang SA, Duncan PG, Shephard DAE, et al: Pulmonary oedema associated with airway obstruction. Can J Anaesth 37:210, 1990
11. Herrick JA, Mahendran B, Penny FJ: Postobstructive pulmonary edema following anesthetics. J Clin Anesth 2:116, 1990
12. Timby J, Reed C, Zeilender S, et al: Mechanical cause of pulmonary edema. Chest 98:973, 1990
13. Warner LO, Beach ATP, Martino JD: Negative pressure pulmonary oedema secondary to airway obstruction in an intubated infant. Can J Anaesth 35:507, 1988
14. Ezri T, Priscu V, Szmuk P, et al: Laryngeal mask and pulmonary edema (letter). Anesthesiology 78:219, 1993
15. Goldhill DR, Dalgleish JG, Lake RHN: Respiratory problems and acromegaly. Anaesthesia 37:1200, 1982
16. Lorch DG, Sahn SA: Post-extubation pulmonary edema following anesthesia induced by upper airway obstruction: are certain patients at increased risk? Chest 90:802, 1986
17. Anderson AF, Alfrey D, Lipscomb AB Jr: Acute pulmonary edema, an unusual complication following arthroscopy: a report of three cases. Arthroscopy 6:235, 1990
18. Robotham J: Obstructive airways disease in infants and children. In Kirby RR, Taylor RW (eds): Respiratory failure. Chicago: Year Book Medical Publishers, 1986: 169

19. West JB: Respiratory physiology, 3rd ed. Baltimore: Williams & Wilkins, 1985: 31, 106
20. Kollef MH, Pluss J: Noncardiogenic pulmonary edema following upper airway obstruction. Medicine (Baltimore) 70:98, 1991
21. Buda AJ, Pinsky MR, Ingels NB, et al: Effect of intrathoracic pressure on left ventricular performance. N Engl J Med 301: 453, 1979
22. Willms D, Shure D: Pulmonary edema due to upper airway obstruction in adults. Chest 94:1090, 1988
23. Cope DK, Grimbert F, Downey JM, et al: Pulmonary capillary pressure: a review. Crit Care Med 20:1043, 1992
24. Colice GL, Matthay MA, Bass E, et al: Neurogenic pulmonary edema. Am Rev Respir Dis 130:941, 1984
25. Galvis AG, Stool SE, Bluestone CD: Pulmonary edema following relief of acute upper airway obstruction. Ann Otol 89:124, 1980
26. Glasser SA, Siler JN: Delayed onset of laryngospasm-induced pulmonary edema in an adult outpatient (letter). Anesthesiology 62:370, 1985
27. Kamal RS, Agha S: Acute pulmonary edema: a complication of upper airway obstruction. Anaesthesia 39:464, 1984

FURTHER READING

Cascade PN, Alexander GD, Mackie DS: Negative pressure pulmonary edema after endotracheal intubation. Radiology 186:671, 1993

Cozanitis DA, Pesonen E, Zaki HA: Acute pulmonary oedema due to laryngeal spasm. Anaesthesia 37:1198, 1982

Jackson FN, Rowland V, Corssen G: Laryngospasm-induced pulmonary edema. Chest 78:819, 1980

Lagler U, Russi E: Upper airway obstruction as a cause of pulmonary edema during late pregnancy. Am J Obstet Gynecol 156:643, 1987

Lee KWT, Downes JJ: Pulmonary edema secondary to laryngospasm in children. Anesthesiology 39:347, 1983

Olsen KS: Naloxone administration and laryngospasm followed by pulmonary edema. Intensive Care Med 16:340, 1990

Sulek CA: Negative pressure pulmonary edema. Current Reviews in Clinical Anesthesia 13:9, 1992

Szucs RA, Floyd HL: Laryngospasm-induced pulmonary edema. Radiology 170:446, 1980

Weissman C, Damask MC, Yang J: Noncardiogenic pulmonary edema following laryngeal obstruction. Anesthesiology 60:163, 1984

Complications in Anesthesiology, second edition,
edited by Nikolaus Gravenstein and Robert R. Kirby.
Lippincott-Raven Publishers, Philadelphia © 1996.

CHAPTER 16

Bronchospasm

Thomas J. Gal

Patients with obstructive airway diseases such as asthma and chronic bronchitis exhibit exaggerated bronchoconstriction when exposed to a variety of physical, chemical, and pharmacologic stimuli. During the course of anesthesia severe bronchospasm may develop in these patients and other select groups as a result of airway manipulation, irritation of the tracheobronchial tree, or a host of other factors that provoke histamine release. This chapter reviews some of the factors that modify normal and abnormal airway reactivity. The goal is to provide a background for practical decisions regarding the diagnosis and management of perioperative bronchospasm and to minimize its occurrence and severity.

NORMAL BRONCHOMOTOR TONE

A slight degree of tonic constriction exists in all normal airways in humans. This bronchial smooth muscle tone is maintained largely by efferent vagal activity and can be readily abolished by the administration of an antimuscarinic drug such as atropine or glycopyrrolate.[1] The physiologic significance of this normal resting bronchoconstriction is unclear. Widdincombe and Nadel suggested that the resultant airway caliber provides an ideal balance between the conflicting forces of anatomic dead space and airway resistance.[2] Thus, conditions exist for optimal efficiency of gas exchange and the work of breathing. This normal tone also has been ascribed the role of rendering large cartilaginous airways less compressible in the condition of high pleural pleural pressures associated with forced exhalation and coughing.[3] The same muscle tone possibly confers stability on the smaller bronchioles, thereby minimizing their tendency to close at low lung volumes during normal breathing.

AIR-FLOW RESISTANCE AND MECHANISMS OF BRONCHIAL HYPERACTIVITY

The heightened bronchial reactivity so characteristic of patients with obstructive airway disease has been attributed to a variety of factors, among them reduced airway caliber, hypertrophy of airway smooth muscle, and increased accessibility of the stimuli to target cells. Baseline airway caliber can influence the bronchoconstrictive response significantly. Changes in air-flow resistance are inversely related to the fourth power of the airway radius during laminar flow and to the fifth power in turbulent flow. Thus, any decrease in the radius of an already narrow airway produces a greater degree of airway obstruction than the same absolute decrease in the radius of a larger or dilated airway.[4]

Airway Hypertrophy and Hyperplasia

Hypertrophy and hyperplasia of airway smooth muscle also are observed in patients with chronic bronchitis and asthma[5] and may play a role in increasing airway reactivity. The increased muscle mass is capable of producing greater wall tension and presumably a greater degree of airway narrowing. This mechanism is likely to be important in severe disease but does not account for the hyperreactivity that occurs in milder disease and in normal subjects after viral infections[6] and exposure to pollutants.[7] In the latter cases, damage to airway epithelium has been suggested to be the major factor producing airway hyperactivity. This damage may be associated with an increase in receptor sensitivity caused by removal of the barrier to the irritant stimuli, which thereby have greater access to the subepithelial receptors.[8]

ARCHITECTURE OF THE TRACHEOBRONCHIAL TREE

The airways originate in a single tube, the trachea, which penetrates each lung as a mainstem bronchus. More distally the airways continue to branch in an irregular, dichotomous pattern (Fig. 16-1). Although each branch has a reduced diameter compared with that of its parent, the total cross-sectional area of the airways progressively increases. The airways are conveniently divided into three zones, each with specific structural and functional characteristics.[9]

Conductive Zone

The first of these, the conductive zone, consists of the trachea, the cartilaginous bronchi, and the nonalveolated bronchioles,

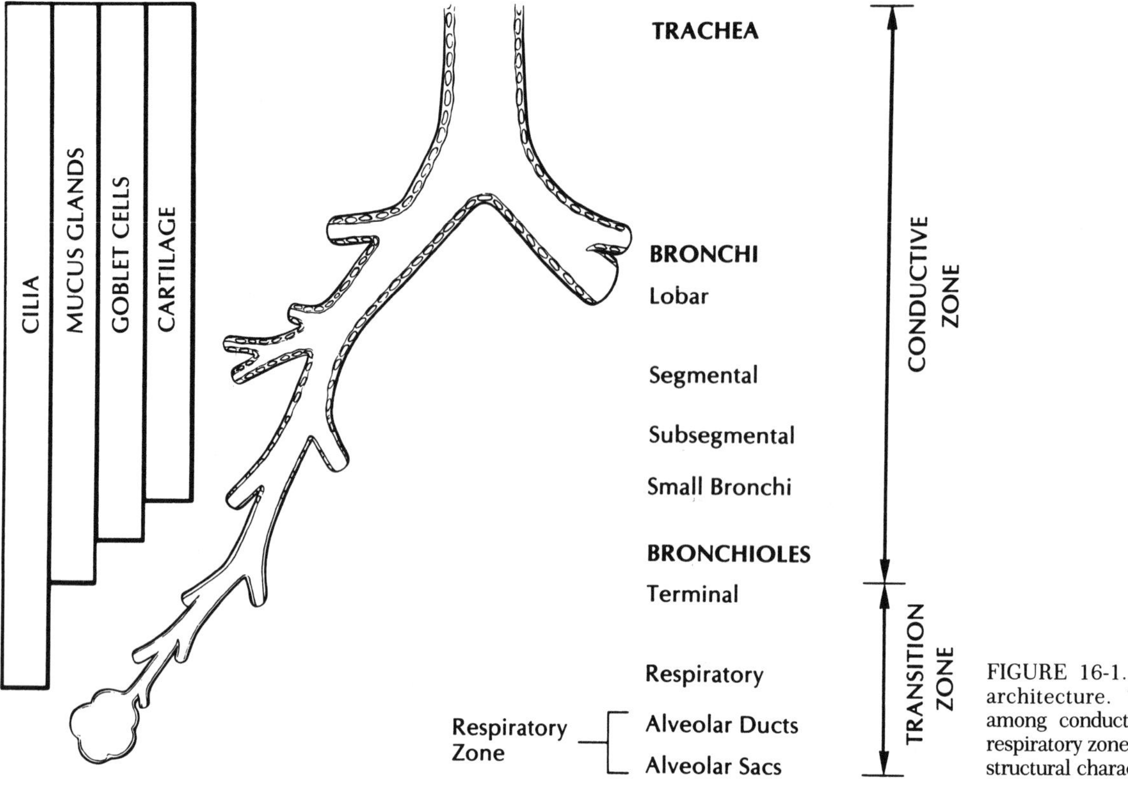

FIGURE 16-1. Branching airway architecture. The relationships among conductive, transition, and respiratory zones and the changes in structural characteristics are shown.

which include the terminal bronchioles. This area comprises the greater part of the length but a smaller part of the volume of the respiratory tract and functions primarily to distribute air to peripheral lung regions.

Transition Zone

A second area, the transition zone, has the dual functions of distributing air and facilitating gas exchange. This zone includes the respiratory bronchioles, alveolar ducts, and alveolar sacs, all of which constitute the greatest part of the total volume of the respiratory tract.

Respiratory Zone

The final, respiratory zone consists entirely of alveoli, whose sole function is the exchange of gas between air and the bloodstream. A unit of lung that is recognizable both anatomically and functionally is the acinus. It consists of lung components distal to the terminal bronchiole and includes portions of both transition zone and respiratory zone structures.

Surface Characteristics

Epithelium

Along the respiratory tract, the surface characteristics and the structure of the airways change. Only the epithelial covering extends throughout (see Fig. 16-1). The cilia appear on the epithelium in the respiratory bronchioles, at which point the "ciliary escalator" begins its mouthward journey. Goblet cells are found only above the terminal bronchioles, whereas mucus glands extend down into the terminal bronchioles.

Cartilage

The units of cartilage that provide structural integrity in the trachea and mainstem bronchi are horseshoe shaped. In lobar and segmental bronchi the cartilage is arranged in irregular plates that form much of the walls. Cartilage becomes increasingly sparse as the small (1- to 2-mm) bronchioles are approached. In contrast, the proportion of muscle increases in the bronchial wall as the lumen size decreases in the peripheral airways.[10]

BRONCHIAL SMOOTH MUSCLE TONE

Airway tone responds to autonomic, nonadrenergic, noncholinergic,[10] and sensory receptor influences. The autonomic and sensory receptors alter bronchial smooth muscle tone principally via parasympathetic pathways. In patients with bronchospastic disease the decreased threshold of these receptors to noxious stimuli results in exaggerated reflex bronchoconstriction.

Slowly Adapting Stretch Receptors

The slowly adapting pulmonary stretch receptors are abundant deep within the smooth muscle of the posterior tracheal wall but are also found in the walls of the bronchi and small airways. These receptors appear to be involved in regulating the rate and depth of breathing and are responsible for the classic Hering-Breuer inflation reflex.[11] They respond slowly to inflation, deflation, and bronchodilation.

Rapidly Adapting Irritant Receptors

Another group, the rapidly adapting irritant receptors, are found throughout the mucosa of all the cartilaginous airways but are most prominent in the trachea and especially at the carina. They respond to mechanical irritation, thermal stimuli, and irritants such as inhaled particles or gases. Airway edema and histamine release also elicit their activity, which results in reflex cough, bronchoconstriction, and mucus secretion.

Juxtapulmonary Receptors

A final group of receptors, the juxtapulmonary receptors, lie adjacent to pulmonary capillaries between alveoli in the interstitium. They appear to respond to pulmonary congestion, edema, inflammation, and exercise and play a prominent role in producing the unpleasant sensation of dyspnea that accompanies states such as pulmonary congestion.

SITES OF AIRWAY OBSTRUCTION

The large central airways account for approximately 80% of the measurable resistance to air flow.[12] Bronchoconstriction in these areas results in readily measurable marked airway obstruction. The smaller, more peripheral bronchioles account for the remaining 20% of airway resistance. Dramatic decreases in the caliber of these small airways may occur without appreciably affecting total airway resistance. Because these airways are the site of early obstructive lung disease, they often are termed the "silent zone."

Ventilatory obstruction may result from a variety of airway defects, some of which do not involve active bronchospasm but can mimic it clinically (Table 16-1). The possibility of these lesions must be considered in the examination of any patient with airway obstruction and possible bronchospasm.

TABLE 16-1
Causes of Ventilatory Obstruction

UPPER-AIRWAY DISEASE
Tumors of the larynx or pharynx
Laryngeal edema or infection
Foreign body
Tracheomalacia
Tracheal stenosis
PERIPHERAL-AIRWAY DISEASE
Bronchitis
Bronchiectasis
Asthma
PULMONARY PARENCHYMAL DISEASE
Emphysema (loss of airway support)

TABLE 16-2
Factors Contributing to Bronchospasm

IRRITANT RECEPTOR RESPONSE (PARASYMPATHETIC)
Inhaled stimulant
Mechanical stimulant (tracheal intubation)
MEDIATOR RELEASE (ALLERGIC)
Histamine
Slow-reacting substance of anaphylaxis (a mixture of leukotrienes)
VIRAL INFECTIONS
PHARMACOLOGIC FACTORS
β-Adrenergic blockade
Prostaglandin inhibition (eg, aspirin or indomethacin)
Anticholinesterases
Alcohol
EXERCISE

PATHOPHYSIOLOGIC FEATURES OF BRONCHOSPASM

Diverse factors contribute to bronchospasm in patients with obstructive airway disease (Table 16-2). In children with asthma, bronchospasm usually develops during exposure to allergen or from the edema and inflammation associated with viral infections. Treatment regimens, therefore, consist primarily of mediator inhibitors and anti-inflammatory drugs.

In adults with airway obstruction, allergy is far less important than irritant reflex mechanisms. Irritant-induced bronchoconstriction constitutes the most significant problem in the anesthetic management of these patients. Tracheal intubation, for example, is a strong irritating stimulus, especially if some bronchocarinal stimulation occurs.[13] Therefore, an understanding of the pathways involved in this parasympathetic reflex arc (Fig. 16-2) is important, as is knowledge of the multiple sites at which the reflex can be interrupted pharmacologically. Antimuscarinics are nonselective and inhibit pre- and postjunctional receptors equally. Lidocaine blocks the airway reflex response to irritation. Volatile anesthetics appear to block airway reflexes as well as exert a direct relaxing effect on airway smooth muscle. In most cases, the compounds that interrupt the reflex are more effective in preventing acute onset rather than preexisting bronchospasm.

AIRWAY SMOOTH MUSCLE: PHARMACOLOGIC APPROACHES

The airway smooth muscle, which extends from the trachea to the alveolar ducts, operates under the influence of the autonomic nervous system. Parasympathetic innervation by the vagus nerves extends down to the terminal bronchioles and has been demonstrated histologically (see Fig. 16-2). Little evidence exists for direct innervation of bronchial smooth muscle by the sympathetic nervous system; the sympathetic influence is instead exerted primarily by circulating β_2 active catecholamines.

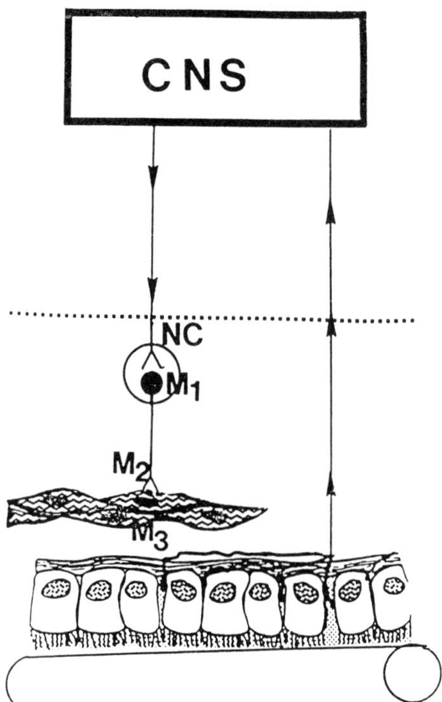

FIGURE 16-2. Diagrammatic representation of the parasympathetic efferent neural pathways that affect airway caliber. The afferent fibers arise from the epithelial layer of the airway lumen, which is depicted as a simple tube. *CNS*, central nervous system; *NC*, nicotinic cholinergic; M_1, muscarinic receptors in ganglia within the airway wall (below dotted line); M_2, prejunctional muscarinic receptors; M_3, postjunctional muscarinic receptors on airway smooth muscle.

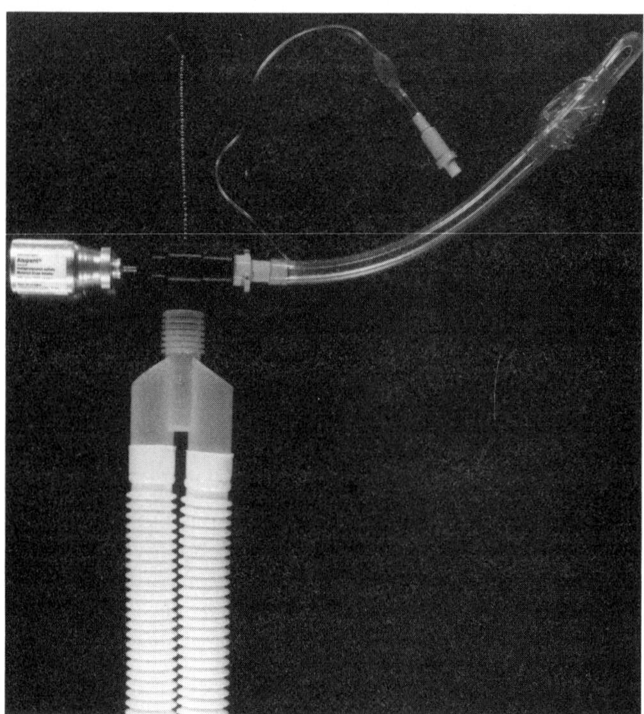

FIGURE 16-3. A fluorocarbon aerosol generator in place in the anesthetic circuit with the aid of an elbow adapter. (Metered dose manifold, Boehringer Laboratories, Ridgefield, CT.)

Routes of Drug Administration

Drugs that alter airway caliber can be administered orally or parenterally or by inhalation of aerosol. Oral medications play a prominent role in maintenance therapy of bronchospasm. In perioperative management, intravenous and aerosol routes of administration assume greater utility. With aerosol therapy, high concentrations of bronchodilators can be administered directly to the airways. The onset of action is comparable to direct intravenous administration, but therapeutic effects are not usually associated with the same high systemic blood levels.

With hand-held fluorocarbon propellant canisters (metered-dose inhalers), medication can be administered preoperatively in cooperative patients. Because many patients do not use these devices properly, demonstration and supervision is essential. For anesthetized patients, adaptors can be obtained commercially or can readily be constructed for drug administration directly into the anesthetic circuit at the endotracheal tube (Figs. 16-3 and 16-4). The medication should be administered as close to the patient's airway as possible. Pressure on the canister during the initial phase of inspiration administers the puff of aerosol, which emerges from the endotracheal tube and is deposited in the airway. The deposition of aerosol is enhanced by a slow, deep inspiration followed by a pause before exhalation. This technique can be accomplished readily by manual squeezing of the reservoir bag or in conjunction with normal ventilator cycling. It is not uncommon to require five to ten metered doses to achieve a clinical effect because of the significant drug loss that occurs via deposition along the inner wall of the endotracheal tube. Drug delivery is enhanced by use of a reservoir or spacer device placed in the inspiratory limb of the anesthetic circuit adjacent to the Y-piece.[15]

Specific Bronchodilator Drugs

A variety of bronchodilator drugs can be administered by metered-dose inhalers (Table 16-3).

β-Adrenergic Agents

EPINEPHRINE AND ISOPROTERENOL. Epinephrine, a natural catecholamine, has been used for decades and is the prototype for all sympathomimetic agents. It is still regarded by many clinicians as the initial therapy, in 0.1- to 0.5-mL subcutaneous doses of 0.1% solution, for young asthmatic patients. Isoproterenol, another potent β-agonist drug, is usually administered as an aerosol. Responses to both compounds are mediated via β_1 and β_2 receptors (Table 16-4). Thus, the desirable β_2 effect of bronchodilation is often accompanied by adverse β_1 effects of cardiac stimulation, resulting in tachydysrhythmia and ventricular ectopy.

β_2-SELECTIVE DRUGS. Substituted catecholamines provide more β_2 selectivity and a longer duration of action. The most notable of these compounds are albuterol, terbutaline, and bitolterol. Bitolterol may prove to be the longest-acting compound of the group: its duration of action is greater than 8 hours with aerosol therapy and outlasts that of albuterol.[16] Terbutaline is currently available only in oral and parenteral

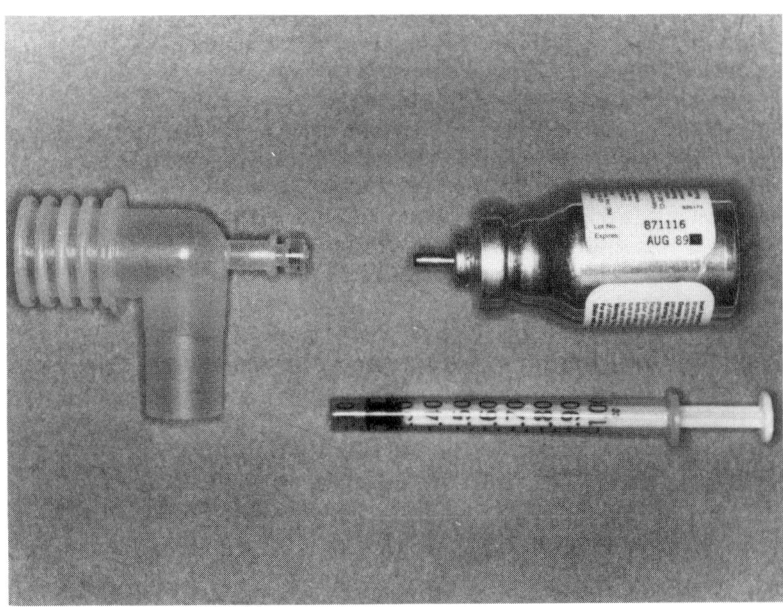

FIGURE 16-4. An elbow adapter with a cut-off tuberculin syringe tip inserted to allow administration by metered dose inhaler. (Koska AJ, Bjoraker DG: An anesthetic adapter for all metered dose inhalers that is readily available to all (letter). Anesth Analg 69: 266, 1989)

forms, both of which are associated with tachycardia and unpleasant muscle tremors.

Currently the most popular relatively β_2-selective drug is albuterol, which is available in a metered-dose inhaler producing about 100 μg per puff; the usual dose is two puffs. The onset of action with albuterol aerosol is relatively slow compared with that of isoproterenol, which reaches its peak effect 5 to 6 minutes after inhalation. Albuterol also is effective in 5 to 6 minutes but may take as long as 30 to 60 minutes to reach maximal effect. An intravenous preparation of albuterol

TABLE 16-3
Metered-dose Inhaler Bronchodilators

Drug	Company	Concentration (μg per puff)
Terbutaline		
Brethaire	Geigy	200
Albuterol		
Proventil	Schering	90
Ventolin	Glaxo	
Metaproterenol		
Alupent	Boehringer Ingelheim	650
Metaprel	Dorsey	
Isoetharine		
Bronkometer	Winthrop-Breon	340
Bitolterol		
Tornalate	Winthrop-Breon	370
Isoproterenol		
Isuprel Mistometer	Winthrop-Breon	130
Medihaler-Iso	Riker	75
Isoproterenol and phenylephrine		
Duo-Medihaler	Riker	160 isoproterenol, 240 phenylephrine
Epinephrine*		
Asthmahler	Norcliff Thayer	160
Bronitin Mist	Whitehall	160
Bronitin Mist	Winthrop-Breon	160
Medihaler-Epi	Riker	160
Primatene Mist	Whitehall	160
Ipratropium		
Atrovent	Boehringer Ingelheim	18

* Other concedntrations available: 200 and 270 μg per puff.

Gold MI, Marcial E: An anesthetic adaptor for all metered dose inhalers (letter) Anesthesiology 68:965, 1988.

TABLE 16-4
Effects of β-Adrenergic Agents in Humans

β_1-ADRENERGIC EFFECTS
Cardiac stimulation
Chronotropic
Inotropic
Lipolysis (increase in free fatty acids)
β_2-ADRENERGIC EFFECTS
Vasodilation
Bronchodilation
Inhibition of histamine release
Uterine relaxation
Muscle tremor
Lactic acidemia

currently is not available, and its therapeutic usefulness would be doubtful. Spiro and colleagues[19] have shown that if the drug is given by intravenous injection, the initial plasma concentrations can be great enough to abolish β_2 selectivity, such that bronchodilation and tachycardia occur to the same degree. Therein lies the advantage of aerosol therapy, which can produce bronchodilation without high systemic levels of drug.

Use of β antagonists risks increasing bronchoconstriction; however, parenteral labetalol to treat hypertension and/or esmolol to achieve β blockade appears to be tolerated without adverse increase in airway reactivity.[17,18]

Methylxanthines

THEOPHYLLINE. Theophylline derivatives have been used to treat bronchospasm for more than 50 years and are regarded as the drugs of choice by many physicians.[20] For years the bronchodilator effect of theophylline was thought to result in part from inhibition of the phosphodiesterase that reduces degradation of cyclic adenosine monophosphate. This mechanism has been questioned by evidence that the theophylline concentrations required to increase cellular concentrations of cyclic adenosine monophosphate are many times those that produce smooth muscle relaxation and bronchodilation. Therefore, theophylline's action is speculated to result from adenosine antagonism. Additional data in subjects with normal airways support the hypothesis that bronchodilation with theophyllines also may occur as a result of catecholamine release.[21]

AMINOPHYLLINE. Aminophylline, the ethylene diamine salt of theophylline, is considered the standard maintenance therapy for patients with bronchospasm, despite its rather narrow therapeutic range. The role of aminophylline in the treatment or prevention of bronchospasm likely to be associated with anesthesia or surgery is controversial. Its potential for generating dysrhythmias during general anesthesia and the lack of objective data concerning its efficacy have led to questions about its overall perioperative role.[22]

Meta-analysis does not support the use of aminophylline for treatment of acute bronchospasm in the emergency room.[23] Nelson has even suggested that its usefulness in treating acute bronchospasm in the emergency department has been overemphasized and leads to underuse of adrenergic drugs.[24] This view is supported by the data of Rousing and coworkers, who noted that sympathomimetic agents administered by the subcutaneous or aerosol route were superior to intravenous aminophylline in the treatment of acute bronchospasm.[25]

Corticosteroids

Although their mechanism of action remains unclear, steroids are commonly used to manage chronic bronchospasm. Their efficacy is enhanced by aerosol therapy. Lower doses minimize the adrenal cortical suppression accompanying prolonged oral administration. Inhaled steroids are not effective for treatment of acute bronchospasm, however.

In the preoperative preparation of patients with reactive airway disease and in the treatment of intraoperative bronchospasm, parenteral steroids are important. Doses equivalent to 1 to 2 mg/kg of hydrocortisone (eg, 0.2 to 0.4 mg/kg of prednisone) are recommended to obtain a good clinical response. In steroid-treated patients the doses usually are doubled, because lower plasma corticoid concentrations result from similar doses compared with untreated patients.[26] Preoperative steroid administration 1 to 2 hours before induction is particularly important because the beneficial effects of steroids may not be fully manifest for several hours. Steroids also enhance and prolong the response to β-adrenergic agents.[27]

Anticholinergic Agents

ATROPINE. The anticholinergic drugs, or, more precisely, antimuscarinic compounds, have been used for centuries to treat asthma. They largely have been neglected in modern treatment because of the troublesome systemic side effects associated with atropine administration. However, quaternary ammonium cogeners of atropine are poorly absorbed across biologic membranes. When administered as aerosols, they produce significant prolonged bronchodilation that is relatively free of side effects.[28,29] Such agents offer an alternative or complementary approach to treating airway obstruction, particularly in conditions of chronic bronchitis. This approach is especially useful in patients who experience tremor and tachycardia with β-adrenergic drugs and those whose bronchodilator response is incomplete despite optimum therapy with sympathomimetic agents, theophyllines, and steroids. Ipratropium bromide is available as an aerosol (see Table 16-3).

GLYCOPYRROLATE. Glycopyrrolate, a compound familiar to anesthesiologists, produces bronchodilation of significantly longer duration when injected intravenously in doses of 1.0 mg than that produced by atropine.[30] Such large doses are required to prevent or reverse reflex bronchospasm. The smaller doses used in routine premedication produce significant bronchodilation but do not appear to be effective in blocking the efferent limb of the irritant reflex. The latter is important during general anesthesia, in which airway instrumentation may initiate such reflexes.

The bronchodilating action of the anticholinergic agents is relatively slow in onset (20–30 min) compared with that of the sympathomimetic agents (4–6 min), whether by inhalation or parenteral administration. They therefore appear to be more effective when used as prophylaxis than as treatment for active bronchospasm. This effect can be readily accomplished by intravenous administration before induction of anesthesia.

IPRATROPIUM. Ipratropium is as effective as atropine but has fewer side effects. It has a slow onset and prolonged duration of action. Fifty percent of its effect occurs at 3 minutes, 80% at 30 minutes, and 100% at 90 to 120 minutes.[31] The dose by nebulizer is 125 to 500 μg and by metered-dose inhaler is 8 μg.

EFFECTS ON AIRWAY SECRETIONS. One long-standing concern with the use of anticholinergic agents is that they reduce the volume of secretions. Clinicians have feared that this therapy would render respiratory secretions more viscid and apt to occlude airways. Evidence for this effect is scant and subjective. Bronchospasm is usually accompanied by increased output of bronchial mucus. A narrowed airway lumen is occluded by the mucus more easily than one dilated by anticholinergic therapy. Furthermore, concerns about altering the viscosity of secretions and causing inspissation are not supported by existing data that indicate that these drugs alter the volume of secretions but not their chemical composition.[32]

THE AIRWAY AND ANESTHETIC DRUGS

Intravenous Induction Agents

Thiopental / Propofol

The usual clinical induction doses of thiopental leave airway reflexes largely intact and may be associated with bronchospasm if instrumentation of the airway occurs before adequate anesthesia is established. The observations of Schnider and Papper[33] indicate that thiopental per se is not the cause of bronchospasm and is therefore not contraindicated for induction of anesthesia in patients with airway disease.[34] Propofol appears to decrease airway resistance in COPD and possibly also in asthma patients.[35,36]

Ketamine

EFFECT ON AIRWAY SECRETIONS. Ketamine has been suggested as the induction agent of choice for patients with bronchospastic disease, especially if rapid induction is necessary. Salivary and tracheobronchial mucous gland secretions are increased by ketamine. This effect necessitates prophylactic administration of an antisialagogue such as glycopyrrolate. An increase in the dose of glycopyrrolate (0.5 to 1.0 mg intravenously) further protects against irritant reflex bronchospasm.[37]

BRONCHIAL SMOOTH MUSCLE EFFECTS. Ketamine has been shown to cause bronchial smooth muscle relaxation in vitro and to be as effective as enflurane or halothane in preventing mediator-induced bronchospasm in dogs.[38] The latter effect appears to be related to ketamine's sympathomimetic properties, because the protective effect is abolished by β-adrenergic blockade.

Clinical data identifying bronchodilating actions of ketamine in humans are scant and are confined largely to subjective observations. One study provided measurements of total respiratory resistance, but the results were confounded by the administration (after control measurements) of muscle relaxants to patients in whom the trachea had been intubated.[39] Muscle relaxation, by reducing chest wall and abdominal muscle tone, could have accounted for a large portion of the decrease in respiratory resistance. However, because none of the patients experienced a worsening of bronchospasm, ketamine may well be a useful agent in treatment of the bronchospastic patient, especially in emergency situations that require rapid tracheal intubation.

Narcotic Analgesics

Narcotic analgesia in patients with chronic airway obstruction is controversial because of its well-known inhibition of the respiratory responses to hypoxia and hypercapnia. Opioids alter the activity of various other neural pathways, including the human cough reflex.[40] Morphine inhibits vagally mediated bronchoconstriction in patients with mild asthma.[41]

Although no objective data are available, large doses of narcotics probably block airway reflexes in a fashion similar to their suppression of cardiovascular reflexes. Because such large doses of morphine are associated with increases in plasma histamine,[42] use of fentanyl or sufentanil seems prudent for general anesthesia supplementation. It should be remembered, however, that balanced anesthesia with nitrous oxide and narcotics is relatively "light" and therefore may not be the anesthetic of choice for patients with reactive airway disease.

Inhalation Anesthetics

Inhalation of anesthetic concentrations of halothane produces bronchodilation. Although this action was originally believed to result from augmentation of β-adrenergic responses, more recent evidence indicates that depression of airway reflexes and direct relaxation of airway smooth muscle are also important mechanisms.[43]

Halothane has been considered the agent of choice for the patient with bronchospastic disease; however, its myocardial depressant action and dysrhythmic effects in the presence of circulating catecholamines prevent it from being ideal. Enflurane and isoflurane are equally effective in preventing and reversing bronchoconstriction when significant levels of anesthesia (1.5 × minimum alveolar concentration) are achieved.[44] This depth of anesthesia may be difficult to establish before tracheal intubation in patients with airway disease because of major ventilation–perfusion mismatching that impedes the uptake of anesthetic agents. At lower doses of inhaled anesthetic, halothane is the most effective at reversing bronchoconstriction, at least in the canine model.[45]

Lidocaine

Lidocaine has been reported to be effective in the treatment of intraoperative bronchospasm.[46] Intravenous lidocaine administered to produce clinically useful blood concentrations (1 to 2 μg/mL) prevents reflex bronchoconstriction, presumably by blockade of vagal afferent fibers.[47] Aerosols of lidocaine offer no advantage over intravenous administration and may provoke bronchospasm in susceptible persons because of direct irritation.

Lidocaine given intravenously (1 to 2 mg/kg) immediately before airway instrumentation appears useful to prevent troublesome reflex bronchoconstriction. In debilitated, elderly patients with chronic airway obstruction, infusions of lidocaine (2 to 3 mg/min) also may be useful to minimize airway reactivity. In these patients, suppression of airway reflexes with inhalation anesthetics may not be possible without profound cardiovascular depression.

Neuromuscular Blocking Agents

Long-acting Relaxants

The administration of d-tubocurarine is associated with histamine release. Because of the potential bronchoconstrictive actions of histamine, curare usually is not used in the treatment of patients with asthma. Crago and coworkers[48] noted no changes in respiratory resistance in normal subjects receiving curare but marked increases in patients with preexistent airway obstruction. They concluded that the latter group is highly susceptible to the effects of substances such as histamine that provoke bronchospasm. Their recommendations that curare be avoided in the treatment of patients with significant airway obstruction and that pancuronium, which produced no changes in flow resistance, be used instead seem entirely prudent. Doxacurium is not associated with histamine release.

Intermediate-acting Relaxants

It is perhaps best to avoid the use of atracurium and mivacurium, which in larger doses or after rapid administration can be associated with histamine release. Vecuronium, which does not provoke histamine flux, may be used satisfactorily. Because of its limited duration of action, it is best suited for relatively short cases, tracheal intubation, or both.

Reversal

A factor of equal importance concerns the need to reverse the actions of nondepolarizing blocking agents. In patients with airway obstruction, the muscarinic actions of cholinesterase inhibitors such as neostigmine may increase airway secretions and precipitate bronchospasm. Larger-than-customary doses of glycopyrrolate (>0.5 mg) or atropine (>1.0 mg) should be used to minimize this possibility. Antagonism of neuromuscular blockade in asthmatic patients who are not actively wheezing at the time of antagonism does not seem to be a clinical problem.

PREOPERATIVE IDENTIFICATION OF REACTIVE AIRWAY DISEASE

Careful preoperative identification of a risk for development of intraoperative or postoperative bronchospasm is important in planning a rational technique for anesthesia and postoperative care. The many important areas that should be considered in eliciting the history of at-risk patients are summarized in Table 16-5.

Upper-Airway Infection

One of the most important factors associated with an increase in bronchial hyperreactivity is a history of a recent upper respiratory tract infection. The clinical state of asthmatic and bronchitic patients often deteriorates markedly when they have viral respiratory tract infections.[49] In normal subjects, viral upper respiratory tract infections cause striking bronchial reactivity.[6] This response persists for 3 to 4 weeks after infection.[50] Because the bronchoconstriction occurs via vagal reflexes, full blocking doses of atropine (2 mg) or glycopyrrolate (1 mg) should be considered before induction if general anesthesia is required.

Smoking

Also at increased risk for airway reactivity are patients with a prominent smoking history, particularly a history of cough and sputum production. In many of these patients, chronic bronchitis has not yet been diagnosed, and findings on routine pulmonary function tests may be only minimally abnormal. In some cases an anesthetic history is very helpful to anticipate a likelihood of increased airway reactivity.

Wheezing and Bronchospasm

Many patients provide an actual history of wheezing attacks. This history of wheezing does not always reliably predict reactive airway disease.[51] In many cases bronchial provocation testing or the demonstration of reversible airway obstruction by spirometry may be required to establish the diagnosis. However, if patients require no medications, and the history, physical examination, and spirometric test indicate insignificant respiratory dysfunction, selection of anesthetic techniques least apt to incite bronchospasm is all that is likely to be necessary.

TABLE 16-5
Reactive Airway Disease: Important Factors in Preoperative History

- Recent upper respiratory tract infection
- Prominent smoking history
- Cough or sputum production
- Previous anesthetics
- History of wheezing attacks
- Hospitalization
- Medications

Any medications being taken by patients who experience recurrent attacks of bronchospasm should be identified; the clinician then can to decide whether that therapy should be continued and formulate a rational plan for treating bronchospasm during and after surgery. Medications other than bronchodilators may have a significant influence on airway function. One example is therapy with nonselective β-adrenergic blocking agents, such as propranolol: in patients with asthma and bronchitis, significant persistent bronchoconstriction may develop after propranolol therapy. This increased airway tone appears to result from unopposed parasympathetic activity because it can be readily antagonized by anticholinergic therapy.[52] Esmolol appears useful when β-adrenergic blockade is necessary in the treatment of patients with obstructive lung disease.[18] Because significant tachycardia is less apt to occur with glycopyrrolate,[30] the latter agent appears to be preferable to atropine.

ANESTHETIC APPROACH TO PREVENTION OF BRONCHOSPASM

Regional Anesthesia

Regional anesthesia (when effective) obviates instrumentation of the airway and hence minimizes airway reflexes. Regional techniques are not feasible, however, in upper abdominal surgery because of the high levels of sensory and motor block that are necessary. This sensory deprivation may produce anxiety in the patient with asthma and thereby incite bronchospasm. More important, the loss of expiratory muscle power may compromise the condition of patients who have airway obstruction and who rely on active exhalation for adequate gas exchange.[53] These patients may experience additional respiratory difficulties because of surgical positioning and the likely need for sedatives and analgesics.

General Anesthesia

During general anesthesia for a patient with hyperactive airways, the primary aim of the anesthesiologist is to prevent airway constriction, and, if it does occur, to minimize its severity so that it is readily reversible. Inhalation anesthetics can accomplish these goals by enhancing sympathetic responses, relaxing airway smooth muscle, and blocking irritant reflexes, but only after a significant depth of surgical anesthesia has been established.

Tracheal Intubation

Tracheal intubation ideally should not be attempted before an adequate depth of anesthesia has been achieved. However, the significant ventilation–perfusion mismatching in most patients with airway obstruction often delays the achievement of this state. In this case, intravenous local anesthetics such as lidocaine (1 to 2 mg/kg) and cholinergic antagonists such as glycopyrrolate (0.5 to 1.0 mg) are helpful adjunctive pretreatments to prevent airway constriction. β-Adrenergic aerosols such as albuterol administered 1 to 2 hours in advance may also be helpful before induction of general anesthesia. If rapid induction and tracheal intubation are essential, intravenous ketamine (1 to 2 mg/kg) and possibly propofol (2–3 mg/kg) are logical alternatives to thiopental as an induction agent.

Tracheal Extubation

Of equal concern in patients with airway disease is the appropriate time to extubate. Removal of the endotracheal tube during "deep" anesthesia to minimize reactive bronchospasm is often unsafe. The residual effects of anesthetics, which include ventilation–perfusion mismatching, persist for several hours. Many of these patients require ventilatory support in the postanesthesia care unit. Additional intravenous lidocaine, anticholinergic agents, inhaled sympathomimetic agents, and even small doses of opioids may be required to permit toleration of tracheal intubation without severe reflex bronchospasm.

DIFFERENTIAL DIAGNOSIS OF INTRAOPERATIVE BRONCHOSPASM

Episodes of wheezing during anesthesia are not uncommon and may result from many phenomena other than simple reactive bronchospasm. The spectrum of causes for intraoperative wheezing (Table 16-6) must be considered before definitive treatment of bronchospasm is initiated.

Tube Malposition

Bronchial intubation may result in dramatic increases in airway pressure during mechanical ventilation because gas delivery is confined to one lung. The presence of the tube at the

TABLE 16-6
Causes of Intraoperative Wheezing

BRONCHOSPASTIC DISEASE
- Asthma
- Chronic obstructive airway disease

INDUCED BRONCHOSPASM DURING ANESTHESIA
- Tracheal intubation
- Aspiration of gastric contents
- Allergic reactions (to blood or drugs)
- Light anesthesia or surgical stimulation
- Pulmonary embolization
- Negative airway pressure
- Irritation of carina by endotracheal tube

CONDITIONS MIMICKING BRONCHOSPASM
- Airway obstruction
  - Kinked tube
  - Overinflated occlusive cuff
  - Secretions or airway edema

Kirby RR: Respiratory system. In Gravenstein N (ed): Manual of complications during anesthesia. Philadelphia: JB Lippincott, 1991:326.

carina also may stimulate the very abundant and sensitive irritant receptors in this area and actually produce reflex bronchospasm. More commonly, this irritation is manifested by persistent coughing and straining and a need for high inflation pressures. Administration of muscle relaxants to differentiate this condition from actual bronchoconstriction is emphasized.[54]

Tube Obstruction

Excessive lung-inflation pressures also may result from mechanical obstruction of the endotracheal tube, whether from kinking, inspissated secretions, or overinflation of the cuff. Usually this obstruction is associated with audible noises throughout the inspiratory and expiratory phases of respiration. Diagnosis may be inferred by failure in the attempt to pass a suction catheter but may be verified only by fiberoptic bronchoscopy.

Rapid Bellows Descent

Older mechanical ventilators available for anesthetic applications incorporate a bellows that ascends during inspiration and descends during expiration. The rapid descent of the bellows produces subambient pressures within the anesthetic circuit and accelerates expiratory flow in a manner comparable to that during mild expiratory effort. The result is a wheezing sound during the final portion of expiration. The sounds occur not because of active airway constriction but rather because the airways undergo dynamic collapse as they reach their expiratory flow limits.

Pulmonary Edema

Early in the development of pulmonary edema, interstitial fluid accumulates around bronchioles in a cufflike fashion. This phenomenon is believed to be responsible for the increased airway resistance associated with pulmonary congestion and results in wheezing most prominent near the end of exhalation. Cooperman and Price noted that this wheezing was a prominent early sign in surgical patients who had pulmonary edema.[55] Obviously, effective treatment must be directed at correcting cardiac failure, noncardiogenic causative factors, or both, rather than at producing bronchodilation.

Tension Pneumothorax

Another condition that may manifest clinical signs similar to those of actual bronchospasm is tension pneumothorax. Recognition of pneumothorax is often delayed because of the similarity of the signs and also because many of the patients in whom pneumothoraces occur have chronic obstructive airway disease.[56] Wheezing results presumably from bronchiolar compression associated with the reduced volume of the affected lung. Hypotension and tachycardia are early signs of pneumothorax and may help in differentiation from true bronchospasm, but definitive diagnosis and treatment may be confirmed only by a chest radiograph or demonstration of gas escape through a large-bore needle inserted anteriorly into the second intercostal space.

Aspiration of Gastric Contents

Aspiration of gastric contents into the tracheobronchial tree also must be considered as a cause of bronchospasm, although it is less likely to occur in patients whose tracheas are intubated. The aspirate stimulates irritant receptors and results in constriction of the major airways. In most cases airway constriction is self-limited, and efforts should be devoted to correcting gas-exchange abnormalities.

Pulmonary Embolization

Correction of gas exchange also is appropriate for cases of pulmonary embolism. Wheezing in this situation is believed to be related to the release of bronchoconstrictive amines into peripheral airways. The importance of wheezing as a major finding in pulmonary embolism is disputed.

THERAPEUTIC APPROACH TO INTRAOPERATIVE BRONCHOSPASM

Increased Depth of Anesthesia

When the diagnosis of bronchospasm is established during a general anesthetic, initial therapy may consist simply of increasing anesthetic depth. However, profound levels of inhalation anesthesia may not be totally effective in cases of severe bronchospasm and may produce severe hypotension and arrhythmias.[57] Despite these cardiovascular limitations, anecdotal reports continue to tout deep inhalation anesthesia to treat status asthmaticus.[58]

Neuromuscular Paralysis

In anesthetized patients who are not already paralyzed, skeletal muscle relaxation is essential because vigorous expiratory efforts may worsen airway obstruction. Paralysis also helps in the determination of whether the increased airway pressures and the difficulty in ventilation are due to bronchospasm or merely to straining and coughing in response to the endotracheal tube. If ventilation improves with paralysis, the cause of the ventilatory disturbance is not likely to be bronchoconstriction.

Oxygen

The decreased airway caliber associated with bronchoconstriction profoundly affects distribution of gases within the lung, the major effect of which is inadequate ventilation of many lung units. The net result of this maldistribution relative to perfusion is arterial hypoxemia. The pulmonary vasodilating properties of many bronchodilating agents further worsen these effects. Thus, increase in the inspired oxygen concentration to as high a level as needed to achieve a normal oxygen saturation is required.

Pharmacologic Support

Therapy with intravenous lidocaine (2 mg/kg) and atropine (1 to 2 mg) or glycopyrrolate (1 mg) may be helpful in reversing some of the bronchoconstriction, but these agents are far more valuable for prophylaxis. Corticosteroids (hydrocortisone 4 mg/kg) also are more appropriate for prophylaxis because of delays in their onset of action.

The cornerstone of the treatment of intraoperative bronchospasm is inhalation of sympathomimetic agents such as albuterol via metered-dose inhaler. These agents can be administered conveniently (Figs. 16-3 and 16-4) and produce bronchodilation more rapidly and effectively than does intravenous aminophylline.[25] It must be reiterated that as many as five to ten puffs may be required, because less than 10% of the metered dose actually passes through the endotracheal tube and into the airway.[59] This loss of drug to condensation on the inner surface of the endotracheal tube is even more pronounced with smaller tubes. Another approach is to attach an ultrasonic nebulizer in the anesthetic circuit, although a similar phenomenon may occur. In both approaches, the end point is the response to therapy or undesired side effects, rather than administration of an arbitrary dose. Additional measures to treat refractory wheezing include intravenous lidocaine (1 to 2 mg/kg) and an anticholinergic agent.

Recommended therapy for intraoperative bronchospasm also includes intravenous aminophylline (5 mg/kg administered over a 10- to 20-minute period followed by an infusion of 0.9 mg/kg/h) if no previous therapy with theophyllines has been used. In patients already receiving theophyllines with a known serum concentration, this level can be increased by 2 μg/mL for every milligram per kilogram given. Thus, if the level is subtherapeutic (eg, 5 μg/ml) or marginally therapeutic (eg 10 μg/ml), it can be raised to 15 to 20 μg/ml. Acute administration intraoperatively in patients in whom the preoperative level is not known may result in blood concentrations that approach the toxic range. Interaction with halothane is apt to produce cardiac dysrhythmias. In addition, the potential interaction of aminophylline with the sympathomimetic agents commonly used to treat bronchospasm must be considered. Aminophylline use in the anesthetized patient remains controversial, not only because of cardiotoxicity and dysrhythmias, but also because of questions concerning its efficacy. It should therefore be considered a second- or third-line drug after inhalation of sympathomimetics, intravenous lidocaine, and anticholinergic therapy.[24]

REFERENCES

1. Detroyer A, Yernault JC, Rodenstein D: Effects of vagal blockade on lung mechanics in normal man. J Appl Physiol 46:217, 1979
2. Widdincombe JG, Nadel JA: Airway volume, airway resistance and work and force of breathing: theory. J Appl Physiol 18:863, 1963
3. Olsen CR, Stevens AE, McIlroy MB: Rigidity of trachea and bronchi during muscular constriction. J Appl Physiol 23:27, 1967
4. Benson MK: Bronchial hyperreactivity. Br J Dis Chest 69:227, 1975
5. Takizawa T, Thurlbeck WM: Muscle and mucus gland size in the major bronchi of patients with chronic bronchitis, asthma, and asthmatic bronchitis. Am Rev Respir Dis 104:331, 1971
6. Empey DW, Laitinen LA, Jacobs L, Gold WM, Nadel JA: Mechanism of bronchial hyperreactivity in normal subjects after upper respiratory tract infection. Am Rev Respir Dis 113:131, 1976
7. Golden JA, Nadel JA, Boushey HA: Bronchial hyperirritability in healthy subjects after exposure to ozone. Am Rev Respir Dis 118:287, 1978
8. Nadel JA: Autonomic control of airway smooth muscle and airway secretions. Am Rev Respir Dis 115(suppl 2):117, 1977
9. Fraser RG, Pare JAP: Structure and function of the lung. In Organ physiology, 2nd ed. Philadelphia: WB Saunders, 1977
10. Barnes PJ, Baraniwk JN, Belvisi MG: Neuropeptides in the respiratory tract. Am Rev Respir Dis 144:1187, 1991
11. Hammouda M, Wilson WH: Reflex slowing of respiration accompanying the changes in intrapulmonary pressure. J Physiol (Lond) 88:284, 1937
12. Macklem PT, Mead J: Resistance of the central and peripheral airways measured by a retrograde catheter. J Appl Physiol 22: 395, 1967
13. Dohi S, Gold MK: Pulmonary mechanics during general anesthesia: the influence of mechanical irritation of the airway. Br J Anaesth 51:205, 1979
14. Brichart JF, Gunst SJ, Warner DO, et al: Halothane, enflurane and isoflurane depress the peripheral vagal motor pathway in isolated canine tracheal smooth muscle. Anesthesiology 74:325, 1991
15. Rav JI, Harwood RJ, Groff JL: Evaluation of reservoir device for metered-dose bronchodilator delivery to intubated adults. An in vitro study. Chest 102:924, 1993
16. Orgel HA, Kemp JP, Tinkleman DG, et al: Bitolterol and albuterol metered-dose aerosols: comparison of two long acting $beta_2$ adrenergic bronchodilators for treatment of asthma. J Allergy Clin Immunol 75:55, 1985
17. Wallen JD: Beta-adrenergic blockers in the hypertensive asthmatic patient. Chest 88:801, 1985
18. Gold MR, William G, Cocca-Spofford D, et al: Esmolol and ventilatory function in cardiac patients with COPD. Chest 100:1215, 1991
19. Spiro SG, Johnson AJ, May CS, Paterson JW: Effect of intravenous injection of salbuta molsin asthma. Br J Clin Pharmacol 2:495, 1975
20. McFadden ER: Methylxanthines in the treatment of asthma: the rise, the fill and the possible rise again. Ann Intern Med 115:323, 1991
21. Mackay AD, Baldwin CJ, Tattersfield AE: Action of intravenously administered aminophylline on normal airways. Am Rev Respir Dis 127:609, 1983
22. Stirt JA, Sullivan SF: Aminophylline. Anesth Analg 60:587, 1981
23. Littenberg B: Aminophylline treatment in severe acute asthma. A meta-analysis. JAMA 259:1678, 1988
24. Nelson HS: Beta adrenergic agonist. Chest 82(suppl):33, 1982
25. Rousing TH, Fanta CH, Goldstein DH, Snapper JR, McFadden ER: Emergency therapy of asthma: comparison of the acute effects of parenteral and inhaled sympathomimetics and infused aminophylline. Am Rev Respir Dis 122:365, 1980
26. Dwyer J, Lazarus L, Hickie JB: A study of cortisol metabolism in patients with chronic asthma. Aust Ann Med 16:297, 1967
27. Morris HG: Mechanism of action and therapeutic role of corticosteroids in asthma. J Allergy Clin Immunol 75:1, 1985
28. Gal TJ, Suratt PM, Lu Y: Glycopyrrolate and atropine inhalation: comparative effects on normal airway function. Am Rev Respir Dis 129:871, 1984
29. Gros NJ, Skorodin MS: Anticholinergic, antimuscarinic bronchodilators. Am Rev Respir Dis 129:856, 1984
30. Gal TJ, Surratt PM: Atropine and glycopyrrolate effects on lung mechanics in normal man. Anesth Analg 60:85, 1980
31. Ziment I: Anticholinergic agents. Clin Chest Med 7:355, 1986
32. Keal EE: Physiological and pharmacological control of airway secretions. In Proctor DF, Reid LM (eds): Respiratory defense mechanisms. New York: Dekker, 1977: 357
33. Schnider SM, Papper EM: Anesthesia for the asthmatic patient. Anesthesiology 22:886, 1961
34. Kingston HGG, Hirshman CA: Perioperative management of the patient with asthma. Anesth Analg 63:844, 1984
35. Conti G, Dellutri D, Vilardi V: Propofol induces bronchodilation in mechanically ventilated chronic obstructive pulmonary disease (COPD) patients. Acta Anaesthesiol Scand 37:105, 1993
36. Brown RH, Pizov R, Mennes M, et al: The incidence and relative risk of wheezing during induction of anesthesia in asthmatics. Anesthesiology 77:A1209, 1992

37. Gal TJ: Perioperative approach to patients with chronic obstructive pulmonary disease. Current Reviews in Clinical Anesthesia 5:163, 1985
38. Hirshman CA, Downes H, Farbood A, Bergman NA: Ketamine block of bronchospasm in experimental canine asthma. Br J Anaesth 51:713, 1979
39. Huber FC, Reves JG, Gutierrez J, Corssen G: Ketamine: its effect on airway resistance in man. South Med J 65:1176, 1972
40. Chakravarty NK, Matellana A, Jensen R, Borison HL: Central effects of antitussive drugs on cough and respiration. J Pharmacol Exp Ther 117:127, 1956
41. Eschenbacher WL, Bethel RA, Boushey HA, Sheppard D: Morphine sulfate inhibits bronchoconstriction in subjects with mild asthma whose responses are inhibited by atropine. Am Rev Respir Dis 130:363, 1984
42. Rosow CE, Moss J, Philbin DM, Savarese JJ: Histamine release during morphine and fentanyl anesthesia. Anesthesiology 56: 93, 1982
43. Hirschman CA, Edelstein G, Peetz S, Wayne R, Downes H: Mechanism of action of inhalational anesthesia on airways. Anesthesiology 56:107, 1982
44. Hirschman CA, Bergman NA: Factors influencing intrapulmonary airway calibre during anaesthesia. Br J Anaesth 65:30, 1990
45. Brown RH, Zerhani EA, Hirschman CA: Comparison of low concentrations of halothane and isoflurane as bronchodilators. Anesthesiology 78:1097, 1993
46. Brandus V, Joffe S, Benoit CV, Wolff WI: Bronchial spasm during general anesthesia. Can Anaesth Soc J 17:269, 1970
47. Downes H, Gerber N, Hirshman CA: I.V. lignocaine in reflex and allergic bronchoconstriction. Br J Anaesth 52:873, 1980
48. Crago RR, Bryan AC, Laws AK, et al: Respiratory flow resistance after curare and pancuyronium measured by forced oscillation. Can Anaesth Soc J 19:607, 1972
49. Lambert HP, Stern H: Infective factors in exacerbations of bronchitis and asthma. Br Med J 3:323, 1972
50. Little JW, Hall WJ, Douglass RG, Mudhockar GS, Speers DM, Patel K: Airway hyperreactivity and peripheral airway dysfunction in influenza infection. Am Rev Respir Dis 118:295, 1978
51. Pratter MR, Hingston DM, Irwin RS: Diagnosis of bronchial asthma by clinical evaluation: an unreliable method. Chest 84: 42, 1983
52. MacDonald AG, Ingram CG, McNeill RS: The effect of propranolol on airway resistance. Br J Anaesth 39:919, 1967
53. Paskin S, Rodman T, Smith TC: The effect of spinal anesthesia on the pulmonary function of patients with chronic obstructive pulmonary disease. Ann Surg 169:35, 1969
54. Gold MI: Anesthesia for the asthmatic patient. Anesth Analg 49: 881, 1970
55. Cooperman LH, Price H: Pulmonary edema in the operative and postoperative period: a review of 40 cases. Ann Surg 172: 883, 1970
56. Gold MI, Joseph SI: Bilateral tension pneumothorax following induction of anesthesia in two patients with chronic obstructive airway disease. Anesthesiology 38:93, 1973
57. Gold MI, Helrich M: Pulmonary mechanics during general anesthesia: V. status asthmaticus. Anesthesiology 32:422, 1970
58. Schwartz SH: Treatment of status asthmaticus with halothane. JAMA 251:2688, 1984
59. Crogan SJ, Bishop MJ: Delivery efficiency of metered dose aerosols given via endotracheal tubes. Anesthesiology 70:1008, 1989

FURTHER READING

Gal TJ: Bronchial hyperresponsiveness and anesthesia: physiologic and therapeutic perspectives. Anesth Analg 78:559, 1994

Kirby RR: Respiratory system. In Gravenstein N (ed): Manual of complications during anesthesia. Philadelphia: JB Lippincott, 1991: 303

McFadden ER: Asthma: general lectures, pathogenesis, and pathophysiology. In Fishman AP (ed): Pulmonary diseases and disorders, 2nd ed, vol 2. New York: McGraw-Hill, 1988: 1295

Complications in Anesthesiology, second edition,
edited by Nikolaus Gravenstein and Robert R. Kirby.
Lippincott-Raven Publishers, Philadelphia © 1996.

CHAPTER 17

Airway Obstruction and Tracheal Intubation

Henry Rosenberg
Henrietta Kotlus Rosenberg

Patency of the airway is a *sine qua non* of safe anesthesia. Airway obstruction can occur at any time during administration of a general anesthetic, particularly in patients with predisposing structural abnormalities. Ideally, the anesthesiologist and anesthetist should be able to identify any potential airway disorder before induction of anesthesia and should be ready to use special techniques to ensure easy access to the airway and adequate respiratory exchange. These techniques may include adjustment of head position, awake intubation, fiberoptic bronchoscopy, percutaneous or surgical cricothyroidotomy, tracheotomy, and on rare occasions even institution of cardiopulmonary bypass. Hence, a plan to diagnose the causes of airway obstruction and to establish airway patency must be available before induction of anesthesia.

CAUSES OF AIRWAY OBSTRUCTION

General Considerations

Partial or complete airway obstruction may occur at any time in the perioperative period. Obstruction that occurs on induction of anesthesia is a frightening experience and requires rapid diagnosis and treatment. However, even when such obstruction cannot be predicted, knowledge of the patient's condition helps to diagnose the cause and locate the site of obstruction and allows proper treatment to be selected. Abnormalities that may cause difficult intubation are listed in Table 17-1.[1–26]

Preventive Measures

Preventive measures are of even greater value. For example, anesthesia for a patient with a mass lesion of the pharynx can be induced more safely with a mask than with an intravenous technique using a muscle relaxant because airway obstruction may occur on relaxation of the soft tissues, and the anesthesiologist's view of the trachea can be obstructed by the mass. In a patient with a substernal thyroid, intubation with an endotracheal tube that is smaller than the predicted size is often advisable, because the tracheal lumen may be narrowed by the mass. Awake intubation frequently is preferable before induction of general anesthesia. A variety of techniques may be used.[27]

Syndromes Associated With Obstructive Phenomena

Compromise of the airway can occur as a result of changes in the mouth, pharynx, trachea, or bronchi. Table 17-1 presents in detail some of the unusual syndromes that can be associated with airway obstruction. Although difficult intubation does not always ensue, the anesthesiologist should be aware of its possibility with each of these syndromes, regardless of any past history of airway compromise.

Disorders of the Neck and Mandible

Mobility of the neck and opening of the mouth are important for the alignment of the tracheo-oral axes and visualization of the glottis (Fig. 17-1). Often, functional impairment relating to these structures is apparent (as in cases of fractures and trauma); sometimes the disability must be sought. Patients with various forms of arthritis (rheumatoid[18,20] or juvenile[21]) and congenital anomalies (Klippel-Feil syndrome,[28] diabetic stiff-joint syndrome,[6] or coronoid process hyperplasia[4]) require careful testing of neck mobility and mouth opening.

Oral, Nasal, and Pharyngeal Lesions

Congenital Abnormalities and Infantile Tumors

Many congenital abnormalities have in common macroglossia, hypoplasia of the mandible, or both, which can make

(text continues on page 214)

TABLE 17-1
Abnormalities That Affect Intubation of the Airway

SITE OF ABNORMALITY	CONGENITAL/ METABOLIC	TRAUMATIC	INFECTIOUS	INFLAMMATORY	NEOPLASTIC	NEUROLOGIC	OTHER
Head, neck, and jaws	Inability to extend the head (Klippel-Feil syndrome,[1] achondroplasia,[2] large encephalocele[3]) Inability to achieve optimal head position (craniosynostoses, encephalocele) Inability to open mouth widely (coronoid hyperplasia,[4] Hurler's syndrome,[5] diabetic stiff joint syndrome[6])	Maxillary or mandibular fracture, cervical fracture, burns	Trismus resulting from infection, fracture, or osteomyelitis		Tumors of tongue and palate with bony extension and trismus		Immobility of neck, ankylosing spondylitis,[18] scleroderma,[19] wired jaw, rheumatoid arthritis of temporomandibular joint,[20] effects of radiation, juvenile chronic polyarthritis (Still's disease)[21]
Oral cavity	Microstomia, macroglossia (lymphangioma, muscular hypertrophy, Down syndrome), micrognathia (hypoplasia of mandible[5]) Treacher Collins syndrome,[7] Pierre Robin syndrome[5]), first arch syndrome, trisomy 18	Burns, caustic ingestion, macroglossia[10] (resulting from decreased venous return or trauma), lesions after posterior pharyngeal flap repair (surgery for cleft palate repair[11])	Ludwig's angina,[12] Vincent's angina		Tumors of tongue, palate, floor of mouth; thyroglossal duct cyst; aberrant thyroid		Angioneurotic edema, radiation changes, epidermolysis bullosa,[22] pemphigus, hemorrhagic diathesis or surgery with dissection of blood to base of tongue

Nose	Choanal atresia, agenesis of the nose	Broken nose	Adenoid hyperplasia		Polyps, hemangiomas, cysts, solid tumors, encephalocele		Foreign bodies
Pharynx	Cystic hygroma,[5] lymphoid hyperplasia (Hurler's syndrome,[5] Niemann-Pick disease, Gaucher's disease)	Burns, caustic ingestion	Retropharyngeal abscess, hypertrophied tonsils with or without abscess (infectious mononucleosis,[13] bacterial infection)		Carcinoma and sarcoma, fibroma (Gardner's syndrome[15]), other benign growths, hemangioma	Paralysis of pharyngeal muscles (myasthenia gravis, Guillain-Barré syndrome, cerebrovascular accident, syringomyelia)	Retropharyngeal intubation,[23] foreign body,[23,24] angioneurotic edema, epidermolysis bullosa, submucosal hemorrhage (hemophilia)
Larynx and glottis	Laryngeal stenosis, cysts, laryngomalacia, laryngocele[8]	Burns, external injury, posttraumatic stenosis		Epiglottitis,[14] laryngitis, arthritis and ankylosis of small joints of the larynx	Polyps and papillomas,[16] epiglottic cysts, carcinoma, hemangioma		Foreign body (cafe coronary syndrome); bilateral midline abductor paralysis; paralysis of recurrent laryngeal nerves (birth trauma, surgery);[25] laryngeal stenosis caused by acromegaly;[26] laryngeal spasm during anesthesia; glottic edema from allergic reactions
Trachea and bronchus	Stenosis, tracheomalacia, vascular rings[9] (double aortic arch, right aortic arch); may occur at any point through main bronchi			Laryngotracheobronchitis, retropharyngeal abscess	Papillomas, benign tumors, granuloma, hemangioma, mediastinal mass,[17] thyroid and esophageal tumors		Foreign body; hemorrhage resulting from trauma or carcinoma

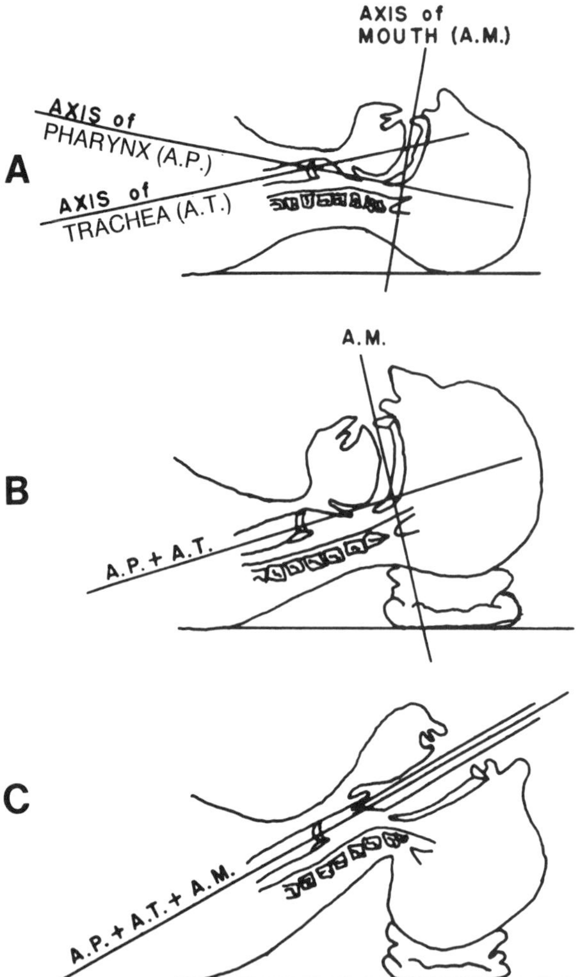

FIGURE 17-1. Proper position for laryngoscopy and tracheal intubation. (A) Axes of the mouth, pharynx, and trachea are shown, with the head in the customary, neutral position. (B) Axes of the pharynx and trachea are superimposed, with the head resting on a firm pad or folded sheets. (C) All three axes are aligned by flexion of the cervical spine and extension at the atlanto-occipital joint.

airway maintenance and tracheal intubation difficult (Fig. 17-2).[28-30] Even after surgical repair of these lesions, the airway still may remain narrowed, and the patient may be subject to airway obstruction.

Infants may have large tumor masses protruding from the oral cavity that fill the mouth and impede intubation.[5] Conventional radiologic evaluation and computed tomographic scans often are necessary to assess the degree of airway compromise.[31] Because neonates are obligate nose-breathers, obstruction of nasal passages resulting from choanal atresia or birth trauma can be life-threatening, unless measures are taken to keep the mouth open or establish a nasal airway.[28]

Oropharyngeal Infection

Inflammation of the submandibular space, as in Ludwig's angina,[12] is rather uncommon today. Submandibular infection or hemorrhage causes obstruction by pushing up the tongue and dissecting through tissue planes into the pharynx.[12,32] Spontaneous retropharyngeal hematoma also has been reported.[33] Foreign body perforation and extension of tonsillar infection to form a retropharyngeal abscess (Fig. 17-3) are more common causes of tracheal deviation and narrowing. If special precautions are not taken in patients with oral and pharyngeal infection, bleeding and rupture of abscesses can occur, with the resulting risk of airway obstruction and aspiration.[13]

Previous Surgery and Radiation Therapy

Airway maintenance and tracheal intubation often are difficult during general anesthesia in patients who have undergone extensive intraoral cancer surgery. The tissues are distorted by changes caused by radiation and surgery. They may be friable, depending on the stage of healing. Furthermore, radiation can cause induration of tissues, resulting in loss of the normal elasticity of the oral and pharyngeal structures.

Miscellaneous Lesions

The pharynx is the site of partial respiratory obstruction for a variety of reasons. Cystic hygromas may be large and require

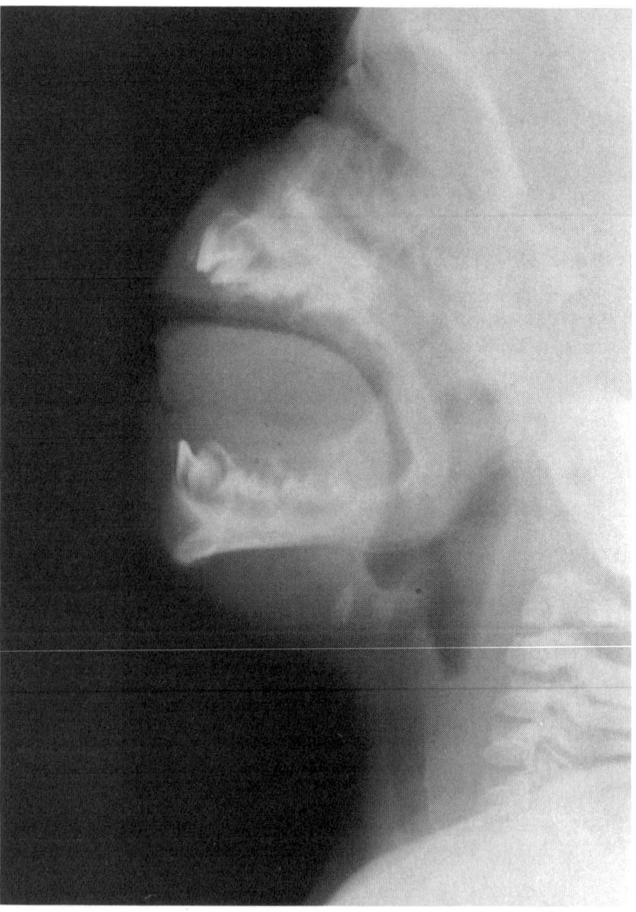

FIGURE 17-2. Lateral neck radiograph of a 24-month-old child with Down syndrome. Orotracheal intubation would be extremely difficult in this child because of macroglossia; the nasopharynx and upper airway are otherwise normal.

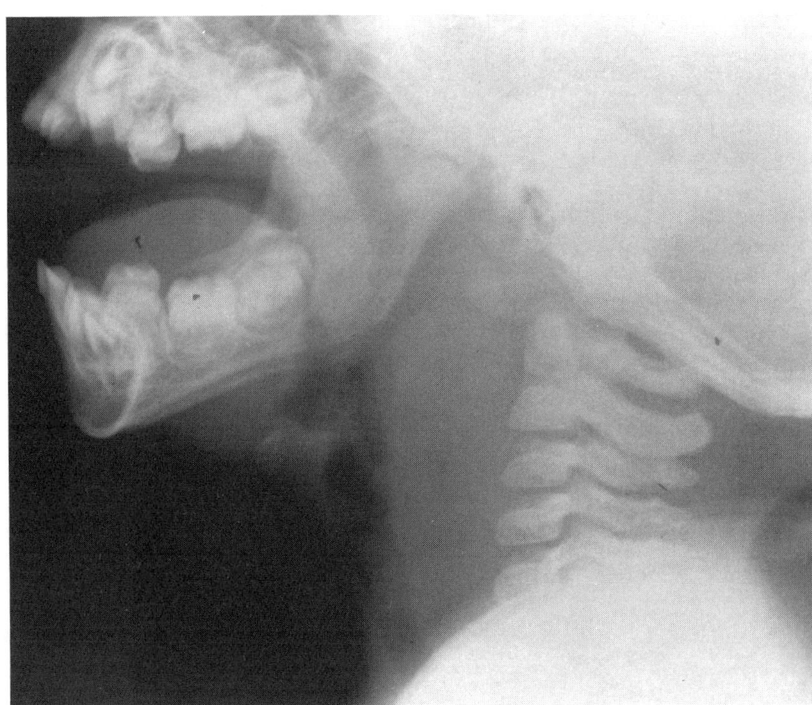

FIGURE 17-3. Lateral neck radiograph of an 18-month-old infant with a large retropharyngeal abscess. Marked thickening of the retropharyngeal and retrotracheal soft tissues makes tracheal intubation difficult because of the resultant displacement of the glottis.

several surgical procedures for complete removal. Each procedure carries an attendant threat of airway compromise.[5] Mucopolysaccharidoses and lipid storage diseases may cause obstruction because of lymphoid hyperplasia.[5,34]

With mass lesions of the pharynx, complete airway obstruction can occur after muscle relaxation from general anesthesia or muscle relaxants. A pharyngeal mass makes visualization of the glottis difficult or may cause airway obstruction that necessitates emergency tracheotomy (Fig. 17-4). In other cases, although the airway may be maintained, intubation of the trachea may require special techniques such as fiberoptic laryngoscopy or bronchoscopy.[27]

Lesions of the Glottis and Trachea

General Considerations

The airway is narrowest at the larynx, which therefore is a potentially hazardous site for respiratory obstruction, especially in infants. Mucosal edema of 1 mm in the infantile larynx reduces the glottic cross-sectional area from 14 to 6 mm^2.[35]

Narrowing of the trachea from intrinsic or extrinsic lesions may be asymptomatic. Causes of a narrowed trachea or bronchus include substernal thyroid,[36] subglottic hemangioma,[37] and mediastinal masses (Fig. 17-5).[17,38,39] Vascular rings and infectious processes of the pharynx frequently result in narrowing of the trachea or its branches.[8] Acromegalic patients may show decreased internal diameter of the cricoid and thickened soft tissues as well.[26,40]

Tracheomalacia

Chronic compression of the trachea resulting from a tumor or a vascular structure (Fig. 17-6) may cause tracheomalacia. The presence of the tumor and fibrotic tissue may stent the trachea. However, after reduction of the compression and any support it provided, the trachea may collapse. Tracheotomy or passage of a tube past the narrowed area is then needed.

Glottic Obstruction

Patients with lesions that partially obstruct the glottis often refuse to lie down because airway obstruction can occur when they are supine. The characteristic sitting position facilitates more efficient use of accessory muscles of respiration. Therefore, anesthesia should be induced in the sitting position, and provisions made for immediate cricothyrotomy or tracheotomy in the event the airway becomes completely obstructed.

Muscle Relaxation

Muscle relaxants frequently are associated with airway problems in patients who have tracheal and glottic narrowing or throat trauma. Normal muscle tone is important to stent the trachea and provide a clear air passage. In particular, a patient with a lacerated trachea should not be paralyzed, because the free ends of the trachea may separate further after muscle relaxation.[41,42]

Supraglottitis

Supraglottitis (epiglottitis) occurs in children from ages 2 to 7 years. It is a life-threatening condition, because swelling may narrow the glottis or lead to total obstruction. Once treated routinely by tracheotomy, supraglottitis today is managed by tracheal intubation with general anesthesia induced by mask in the operating room. Equipment for bronchoscopy, tracheotomy, or both must be immediately available. Intu-

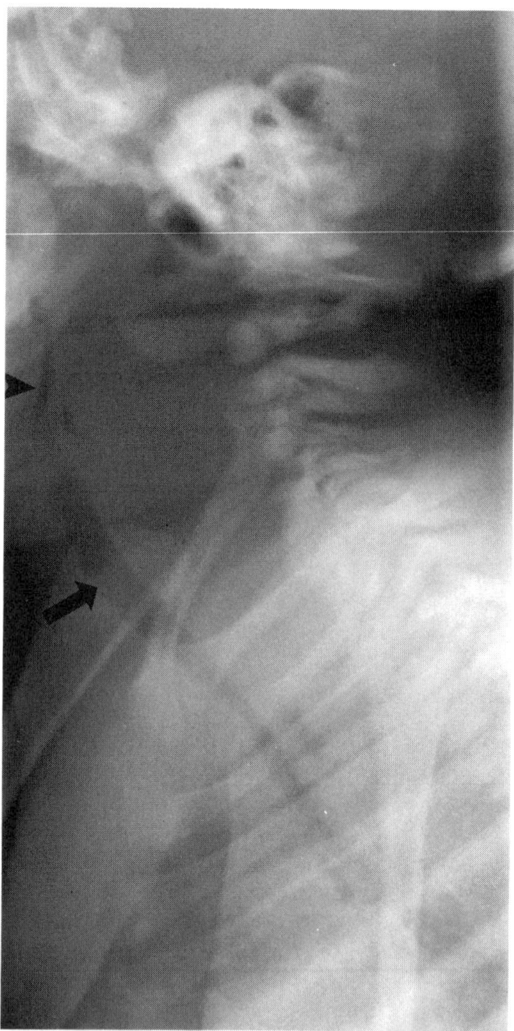

FIGURE 17-4. Lateral neck radiograph of a newborn infant with marked anterior bowing and narrowing of hypopharyngeal airway (*arrowhead*) and anterior displacement of cervical trachea (*arrow*) caused by large esophageal duplication.

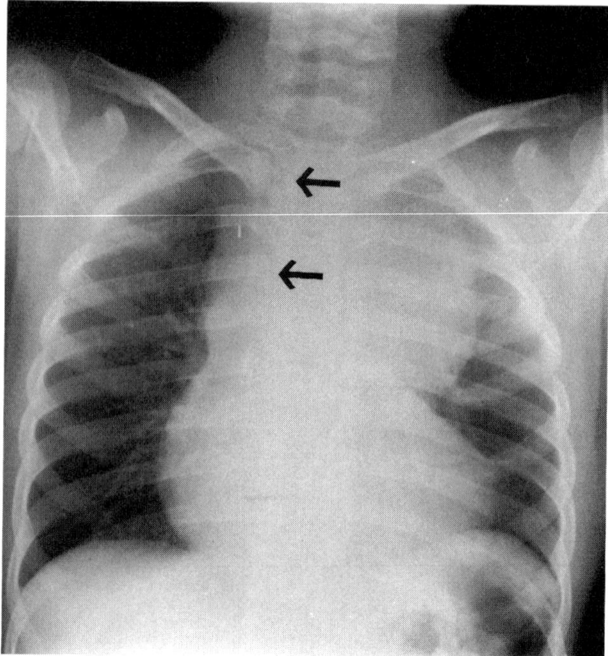

FIGURE 17-5. Plain-film radiograph of an 8-year-old girl with a large anterior mediastinal, non-Hodgkin's lymphomatous mass just superior to the heart. This mass causes right lateral bowing and displacement of the trachea (*arrows*) in the PA view.

bation is maintained for 24 to 48 hours. Before extubation, laryngoscopy is performed again to ensure that the swelling has subsided. Supraglottitis occurs only occasionally in adults, who more often than children have epiglottic abscess. Early tracheal intubation is recommended for both adults and children.[43]

Juvenile Papillomatosis of the Larynx

Another condition that merits special attention is papillomatosis of the larynx (Fig. 17-7).[16] Infants and children with papillomatosis require repeated surgery for removal of the polyps. They, too, are best treated with general anesthesia and without muscle relaxants, because the glottic opening may not be visible in the presence of the multiple polyps. Bear in mind, however, that bag-and-mask ventilation is not always effective. Another hazard is the seeding of affected tissue into the trachea and bronchi, which may cause polyps to develop in these structures.[44]

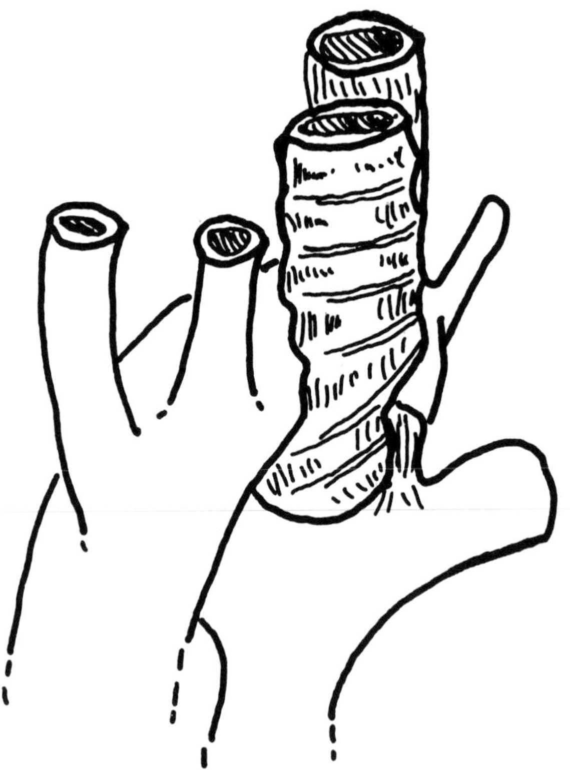

FIGURE 17-6. Tracheal compression caused by a tight ligamentum arteriosum.

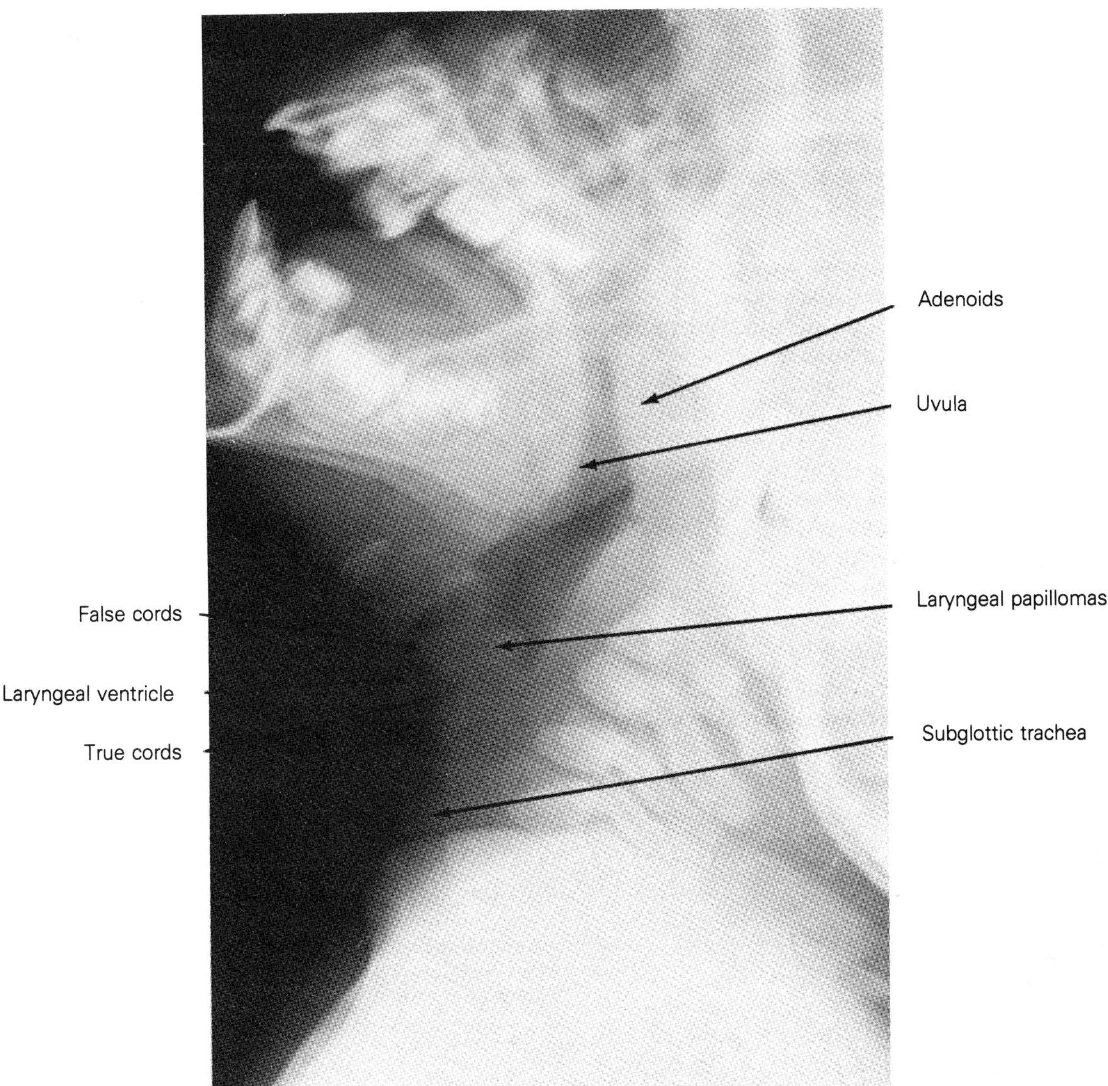

FIGURE 17-7. Glottic narrowing resulting from multiple laryngeal papillomas.

MANAGEMENT

Fundamental Considerations

Tracheal intubation is not always necessary to maintain airway patency, even in emergency situations. Oropharyngeal and nasopharyngeal airways usually relieve the most common type of airway compromise—soft-tissue obstruction—and may help in other situations as well.

Although nasal airways are easier to insert, they may cause epistaxis, mucosal damage, and bacteremia. Improper placement of an oral airway may push the tongue posteriorly and aggravate soft-tissue obstruction. Neither airway protects against pulmonary aspiration.

Positioning of the Head and Neck

Proper positioning of the patient's head and neck simplifies access to the glottis and trachea.[45,46] Often, a difficult intubation is made easy merely by placing one or two folded sheets or firm pads under the occiput. The main problem in visualization of the glottic opening is the proper alignment of the axes of the trachea, the mouth, and the pharynx (see Fig. 17-1). Alignment is achieved by flexing the neck, thereby straightening the cervical spine, and extending the head at the atlanto-occipital joint. The purpose of the laryngoscope blade is to lift the tongue and epiglottis up and away from the airway to provide a view of the vocal cords once the axes are in proper alignment.

Special Problems in Infants and Young Children

In infants and young children, because the head is large relative to the trunk, only slight neck flexion is necessary. Flattening of the shoulders often is needed to prevent displacement of the glottis beneath the mandible. Straight rather than curved blades are preferred for pediatric intubation because the epiglottis is usually long and floppy and protrudes posteriorly at 45° to the anterior pharyngeal wall. In infants the glottis is opposite the C2 to C4 vertebral bodies, whereas in adults it is opposite C5 and C6; it also is more superior in children than in adults.[36] Pulling of the tongue with a forceps is a simple maneuver that can aid in the intubation of a child with Treacher Collins syndrome.[46]

Ancillary Measures

Other routine aids to laryngoscopy are adequate jaw and soft-tissue relaxation, airway anesthesia, or both. Patient "cooperation" during airway instrumentation usually is provided by adequate general anesthesia and muscle paralysis or topical anesthesia and psychological preparation. Occasionally, however, anesthesia and paralysis make laryngoscopy difficult when the larynx moves more anteriorly after relaxation of oral and pharyngeal muscles.[47] At least two laryngoscopy blades of different sizes should be readily available before intubation, in both adults and children.

Difficult Intubation

Visualization of the Glottic Opening

Even with optimal position of the head and neck in patients without obvious difficult airway features, the glottis is sometimes impossible to visualize. Cass and colleagues,[48] White and Kander,[49] and Benumof[27] analyzed the anatomic factors that predispose patients to difficult intubation. In patients who are unable to extend their heads, flex their necks, or open their mouths widely, intubation is more difficult, as might be expected. Factors that predispose patients to difficult intubations include[49] a short muscular neck and a full set of teeth; a receding lower jaw with obtuse mandibular angles; protrusion of the upper incisors and reduced space between the angles of the mandible, with a high arched palate; and increased distance from the upper incisors to the posterior border of the ramus of the mandible.

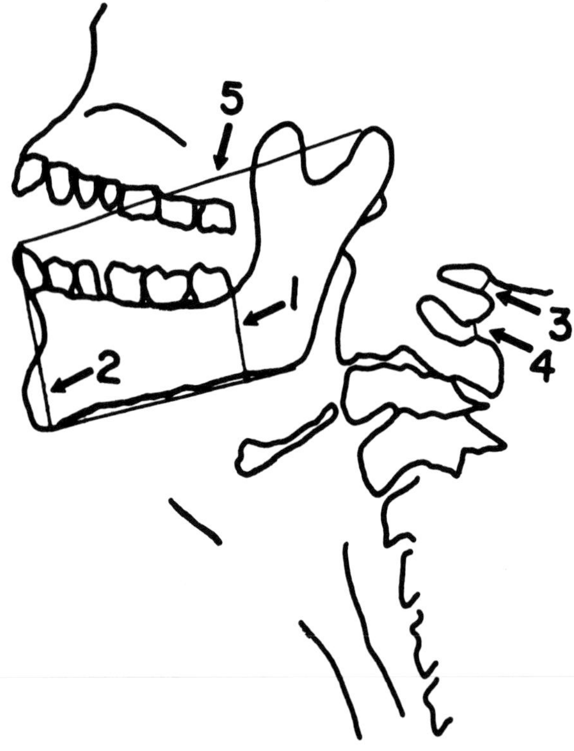

FIGURE 17-8. Measurements relevant in assessing the difficulty of laryngoscopy in adult: increased posterior depth of the mandible (*1*); increased anterior depth of the mandible (2); reduction in the distances between the occiput and the spinous process of C1 (3) and the occiput and the C1–C2 interspinous gap (*4*); and effective mandibular length less than 3.6 times the posterior depth of the mandible (5). Effective mandibular length by itself however, is no different in those in whom laryngoscopy is difficult. (White A, Kander PL: Anatomical factors in difficult direct laryngoscopy. Br J Anaesth 47:468, 1975)

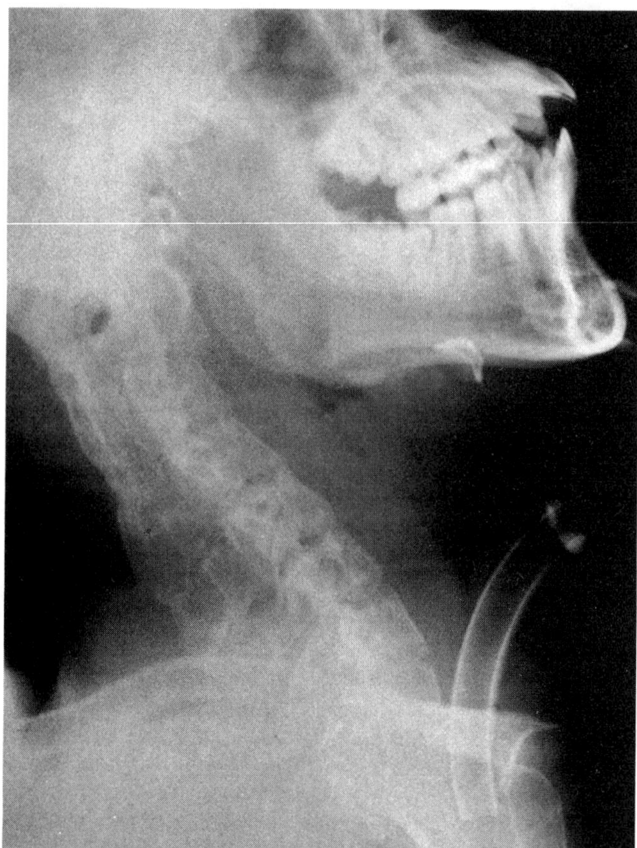

FIGURE 17-9. Lateral neck radiograph of a 19-year-old achondroplastic dwarf whose neck could not be hyperextended because of a cervical spine fusion for C2–C3 subluxation. Endotracheal intubation proved impossible, and emergency tracheostomy was performed after respiratory arrest during a viral illness.

Radiographic Findings

White and Kander analyzed the position of teeth on radiographs.[49] They concluded that protruding upper incisors do not make intubation difficult and that the size of the bodies of the cervical spinous processes do not differ significantly in patients in whom direct laryngoscopy is easy to perform and in those in whom it is difficult. They found, however, that the following factors were important in making direct laryngoscopy difficult (Figs. 17-8 and 17-9): increased posterior depth

TABLE 17-2
Miscellaneous Causes of Difficult Intubation

ENLARGED TONSILS AND ADENOIDS CAUSED BY INFLAMMATION OR TUMORS (Lymphoma)
RETROPHARYNGEAL ABSCESS
CYSTIC HYGROMA
RETROPHARYNGEAL TUMORS
Teratoma
Neurofibroma
Neuroblastoma
NASOPHARYNGEAL MENINGOENCEPHALOCELE
MYXEDEMATOUS THICKENING OF RETROPHARYNGEAL SOFT TISSUES
PHARYNGEAL TUMORS
Benign polyps
Dermoids
Teratomas
Thyroglossal duct cysts
Neuroblastoma
Neurofibromas
Hemangiomas
LARYNGEAL AND UPPER-TRACHEAL TUMORS
Papillomas
Subglottic hemangioma
ENLARGED THYROID
MIDDLE- AND LOWER-TRACHEAL COMPRESSION
Enlarged thyroid
Mediastinal masses
Teratoma
Lymphoma
Ecotopic thyroid

of the mandible (possibly by hindering displacement of the soft tissues by laryngoscopy); increased anterior depth of the mandible; reduced distance between the occiput and the spinous process of C1 and to a lesser extent the C1-to-C2 interspinous gap, thus narrowing limits of head extension; and reduced mobility of the mandible because of temporomandibular joint dysfunction.[49]

Physical Assessment

A common clinical observation is that a chin-to-thyroid cartilage distance of less than 3 to 4 cm (two fingerbreadths) hampers visualization of the glottis. In the absence of jaw measurements, an inability to visualize the faucial pillars (palatoglossal and palatopharyngeal arches) and uvula when the seated, awake patient protrudes his or her tongue, can help predict the degree of difficulty likely with direct laryngoscopy.[50,51]

Miscellaneous causes of difficult intubation are listed in Table 17-2. Patients in whom for any reason intubation is difficult should be apprised of the problem so that they may advise anesthesiologists in the future. Patients should wear identification bracelets noting this difficulty.

Mechanical Problems Associated With Endotracheal Tubes

Insertion of an endotracheal tube does not always guarantee that the airway is patent. In addition to malposition, several problems have been associated with endotracheal tubes (Table 17-3).[52–58]

TABLE 17-3
Causes of Endotracheal Tube Obstruction

CUFFS
Protrusion of the cuff past the end of the tube
Overinflation of the cuff, with part of the cuff covering the end of the tube
Overinflation of the cuff, leading to compression of the tube
Asymmetric expansion of the cuff, leading to bevel compression against the tracheal wall
TUBES
Blistering of the luminal wall
Foreign body in the tube
Mucus, blood or local anesthetic jelly plugs
Kinking
ARMORED TUBES
Kinking below the connector and above the spiral winding
Separation of the inner wall of the tube
MISCELLANEOUS
Obstruction in the connector to the tube (eg, a manufacturer's defect or foreign body)
Sheared plastic coating of stylet
Displacement of tube due to change in position of the head

Cuff Herniation and Slippage

Herniation and slippage of the inflatable cuff past the end of the tube are rare with modern plastic tubes and glued-on cuffs. However, compression of the tube lumen by overexpansion of the balloon can occur,[56] and a foreign body in the tube lumen can pose a problem.[57] Extraluminal causes of endotracheal tube obstruction include anatomic abnormalities such as aortic knuckle[59] and double aortic arch that indent the trachea[60] as well as intrinsic weakness of the tracheal cartilage, as seen in Marfan syndrome.[61]

Armored Tubes

Armored tubes present special problems.[52] Because they consist of two coatings of latex that enclose spiral metal windings, the inner layer may peel away and cause obstruction of the lumen. Air has been reported to dissect from the cuff under the latex coating and to cause separation and obstruction during the course of an anesthetic procedure.[52] An armored tube may kink between the connector and the spiral winding or may kink if the patient bites on the tube.

Assessment

When airway obstruction occurs after intubation, mechanical problems with the tube should always be considered. Removal of air from the balloon, passage of a suction catheter through the tube, and, finally, removal of the tube itself are steps that should be taken.

PATIENT EXAMINATION

Preoperative assessment of all patients should include a history of airway problems. Of particular importance are previous surgery or injury or radiation to the airway or adjacent structures; a history of difficult intubation; hoarseness or awakening from sleep short of breath; dyspnea on exertion in the absence of heart disease; congenital heart disease; and recent infection of the mouth, pharynx, or teeth.

Lesions occurring below the glottis usually do not affect the quality of the voice, whereas laryngeal lesions are associated with hoarseness and occasionally with stridor or aphonia. Wheezing may indicate narrowing of the airway. Infants may have a history of difficulties during feedings; occasional cyanosis or dysphonia; use of accessory muscles of respiration; or relief of respiratory difficulties when the head is extended.[9,28,36]

Special Concerns

Oropharyngeal Lesions

Lesions in the mouth or pharynx sometimes lead to difficulties in articulation, especially when the pharyngeal musculature is dysfunctional. In some cases, the patient's voice sounds nasal. Croupy cough is characteristic of lesions about the glottis. Preoperative examination should include inspection of the mouth and pharynx; assessment of the patient's ability to open the jaw, extend the head, and flex the neck; determination of tracheal deviation; and examination of a chest radiograph for tracheal deformity and mediastinal masses.

Stridor

Stridor is an important sign. Inspiratory stridor usually indicates obstruction at or above the vocal cords, whereas expiratory stridor and wheezing may be associated with bronchial obstruction. Extreme narrowing of the airway below the vocal cords may be associated with both inspiratory and expiratory stridor. A history of frequent respiratory infections, croup, or pain on swallowing are other clues to the diagnosis of airway lesions.

Temporomandibular Joint Movement

Limitation of movement at the temporomandibular joint may be indicated by the inability of the patient to move his or her lower incisors anterior to the upper incisors.

Radiographic Findings

When a diagnosis is questionable, lateral neck and chest radiographs, xeroradiograms, and computed tomographic scans are valuable.[31,62–64] Although xeroradiograms are useful (Fig. 17-10), the computed tomographic scan is now the diagnostic choice for delineating the airway and mediastinal detail when the results of plain-film radiography are questionable (Figs. 17-11 to 17-13).

DIFFICULT INTUBATION

When difficulty is anticipated,[2] alternatives to routine techniques of intubation are inhalation induction; awake intubation with sedation and topical anesthesia; nasotracheal intubation; fiberoptic laryngoscopy or bronchoscopy[65,66]; passage of a guide retrograde or anterograde[67–69]; tracheotomy, cricothyroidotomy, and transtracheal ventilation[27]; tactile orotracheal intubation[70]; blind transillumination of the trachea,[71] and the Bullard laryngoscope.[72,73] A possible alternative to intubation is the laryngeal mask airway[74,75] or the esophageal tracheal Combitube (Sheridan Catheter Corp, Argyle, NY).[76–78]

Fiberoptic Laryngoscopy and Bronchoscopy

The fiberoptic bronchoscope is an important aid to achieve control of the airway before induction of anesthesia when tracheal intubation is expected or found to be difficult. It is likely the single most commonly used ancillary technique. During the more than 25 years since a fiberoptic choledoscope was first reported to facilitate nasotracheal intubation,[79] many sizes and styles of fiberoptic laryngoscopes and bronchoscopes have been designed specifically for various applications in anesthesia.[27]

Preintubation Preparation

Optimal results require a well-planned and coordinated technique, which begins with discussing the procedure with patient

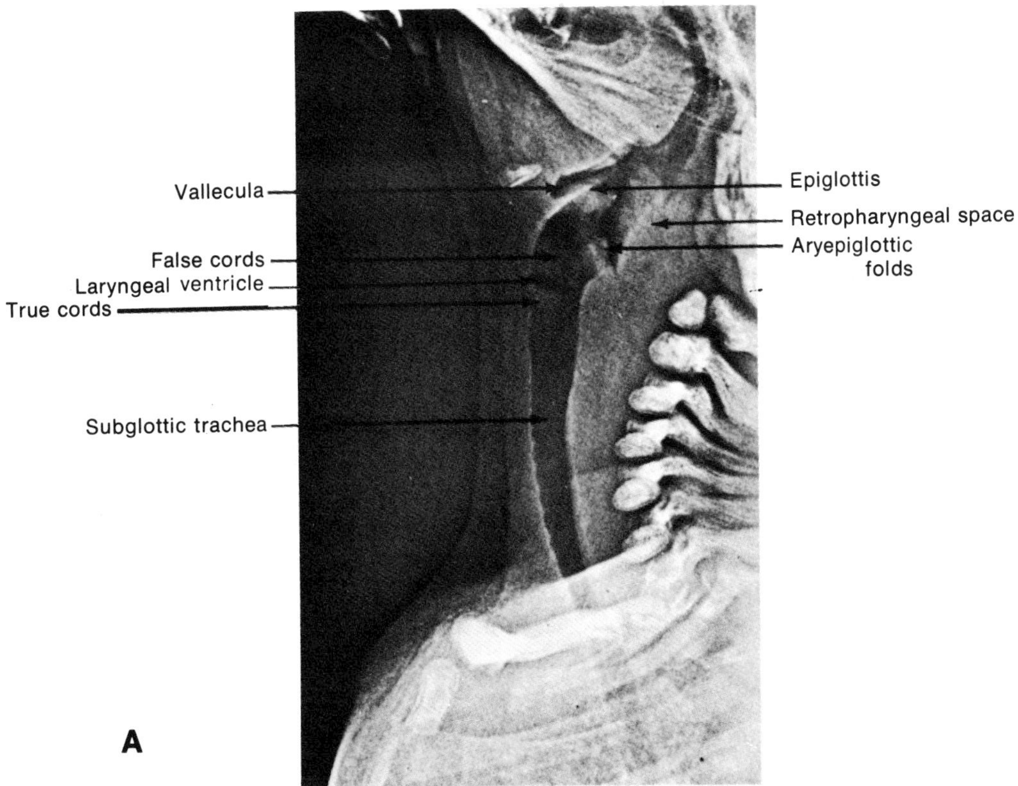

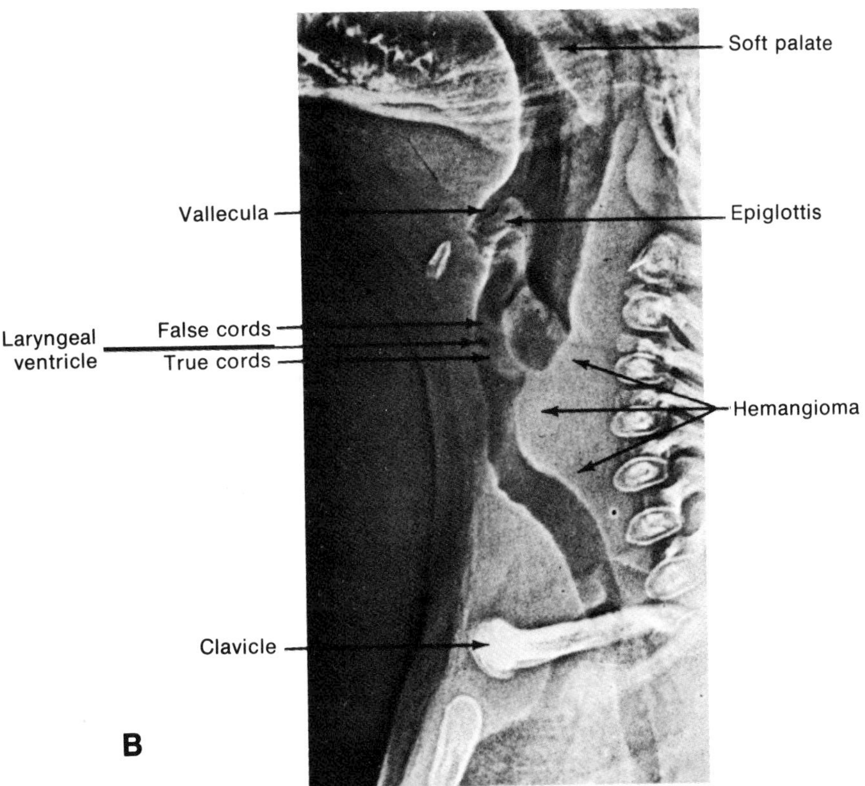

FIGURE 17-10. Xeroradiograms may be helpful in evaluating the airway. (A) Normal appearance on examination. (B) Subglottic hemangioma in a child. (Courtesy of John Scott, M.D., Department of Radiology, Albany Medical School).

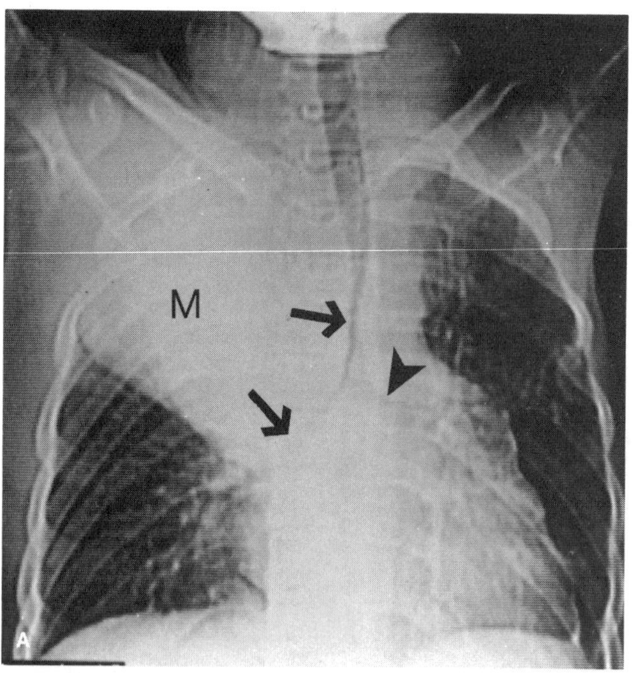

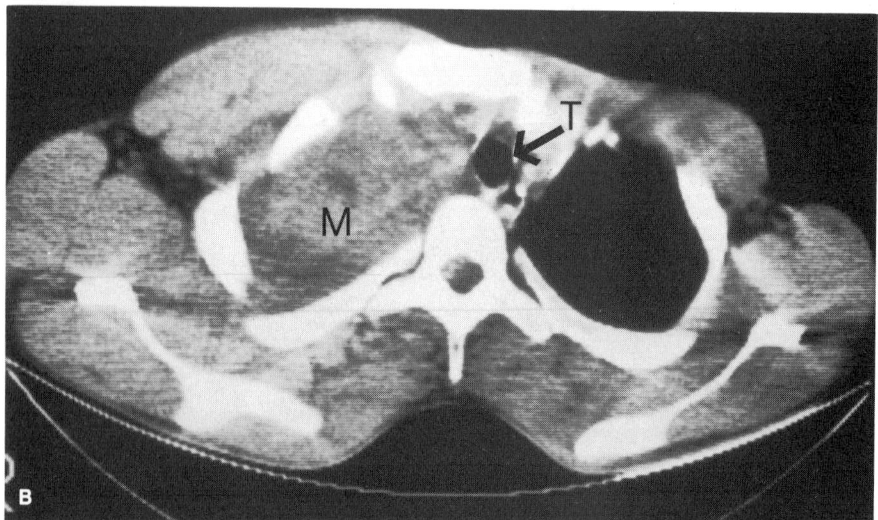

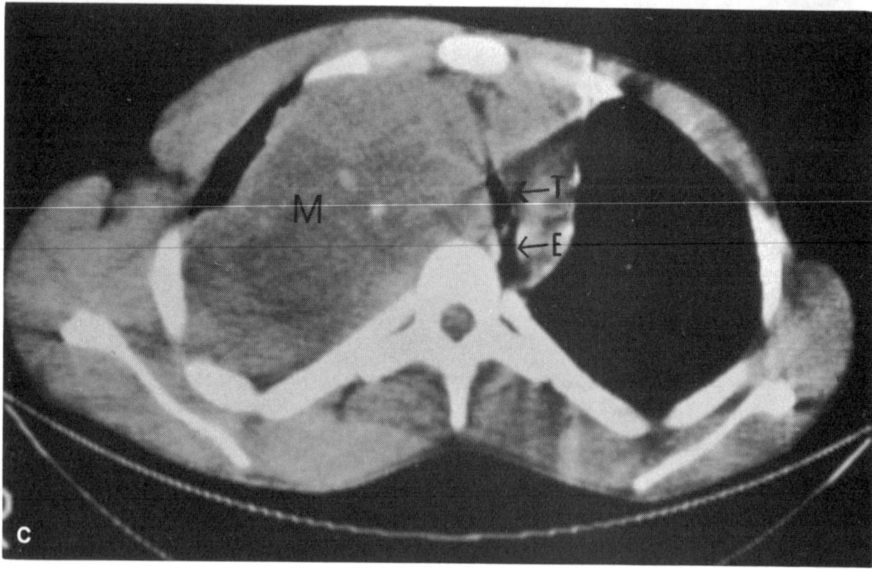

FIGURE 17-11. Radiologic studies in a 16-year-old with a large, metastatic soft tissue tumor. (A) A plain PA radiograph. The mass (*M*) is causing narrowing of the trachea and right mainstem bronchus (*arrows*); the large left mainstem bronchus is normal (*arrowhead*). (B) A CT scan through the superior thorax shows the right-sided mass (*M*) and slight left lateral deviation of the minimally compressed trachea (*T*). (C) A CT scan at the level of the distal trachea reveals the mass (*M*), which contains hypodense areas and calcifications. The trachea (*T*) is markedly compressed and displaced laterally. *E*, esophagus.

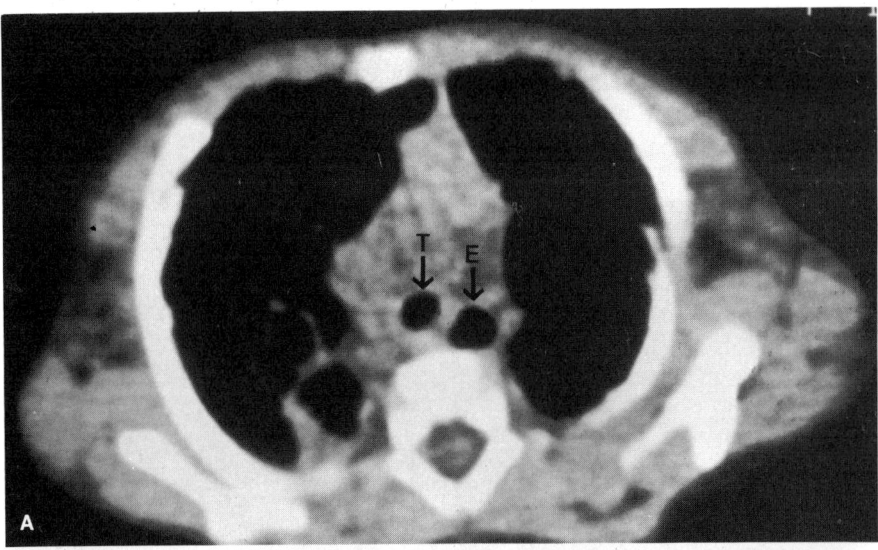

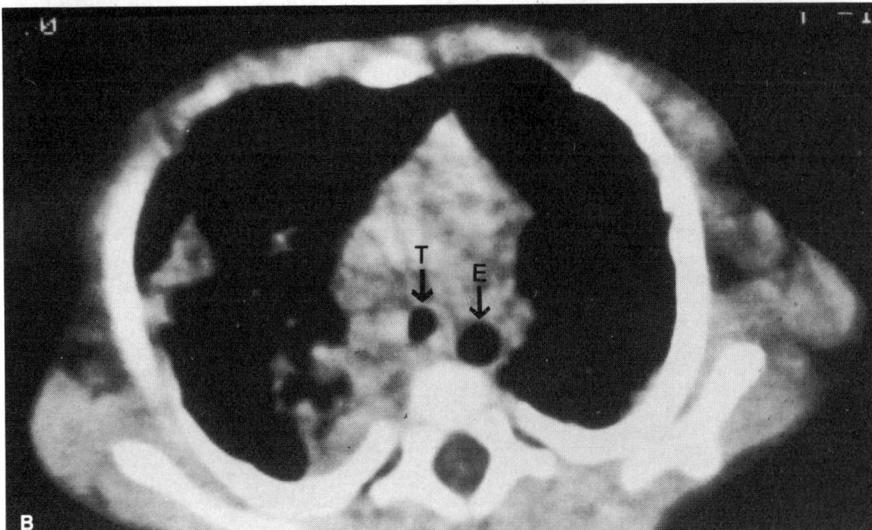

FIGURE 17-12. Computed tomographic scans of the upper thorax of an 8-month-old with tracheal stenosis. (A) This view demonstrates the normally rounded trachea (*T*) as well as scarring, fibrosis, and atelectasis in the right lung. The esophagus (*E*) is distended with air. (B) At a slightly lower level there is narrowing and deformity of the trachea (*T*) above the carina. *E*, esophagus.

during the preoperative visit. Light sedation, oral or intravenous, with a benzodiazepine before arrival in the operating room suite allays anxiety. Addition of an anticholinergic drug is important to lessen secretions that might otherwise impair visualization and impede absorption of topical anesthesia.

In the operating room, appropriate monitoring is established, and additional sedatives and short-acting narcotics are given, as needed. Topical anesthesia, consisting of cocaine or a mixture of lidocaine and phenylephrine or other vasoconstrictor, is applied to the nasal mucosa and pharyngeal and laryngeal structures.

When difficult intubation is expected and fiberoptic nasotracheal intubation is anticipated, it should be tried initially rather than after several attempts at more conventional approaches. Fiberoptic intubation is much more difficult after bleeding, edema, and secretions have obstructed the view of expected landmarks and structures.

Technique

Although the technical details of fiberoptic nasotracheal intubation (the more common application) differ among users, the fiber bundle over which the endotracheal tube is passed must be lubricated sufficiently so that the tube slides smoothly. Care must be taken to keep the lubricant away from the lens; immersion of the tip in warm saline or an antifog spray applied to the lens is helpful. An endotracheal tube of appropriate length and diameter is positioned over the proximal end; the flexible bundle tip then is inserted into a preselected naris and advanced into the hypopharynx. As structures are identified, the instrument is advanced and flexed anteriorly to visualize the larynx. It then is inserted through the vocal cords, at which point flexion is released. It is then advanced until the carina is visualized, at which time the endotracheal tube is passed over the instrument. After removal of the broncho-

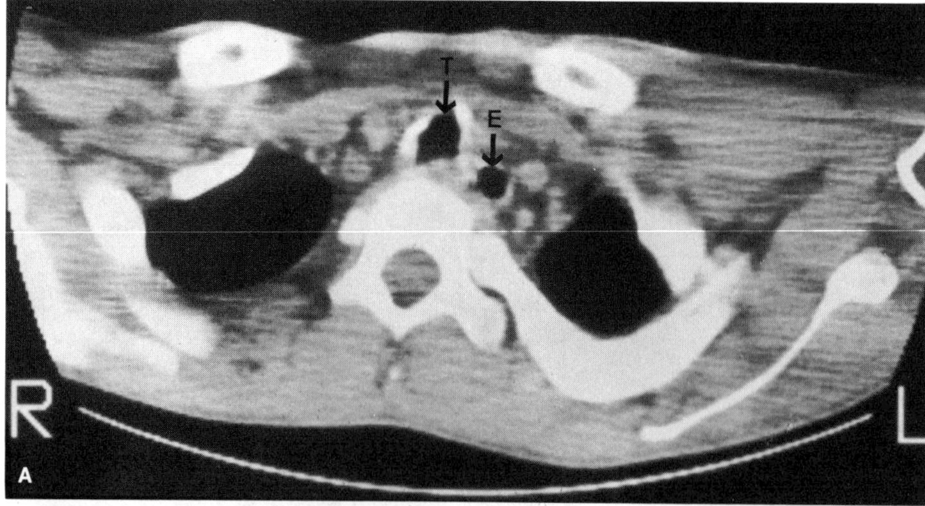

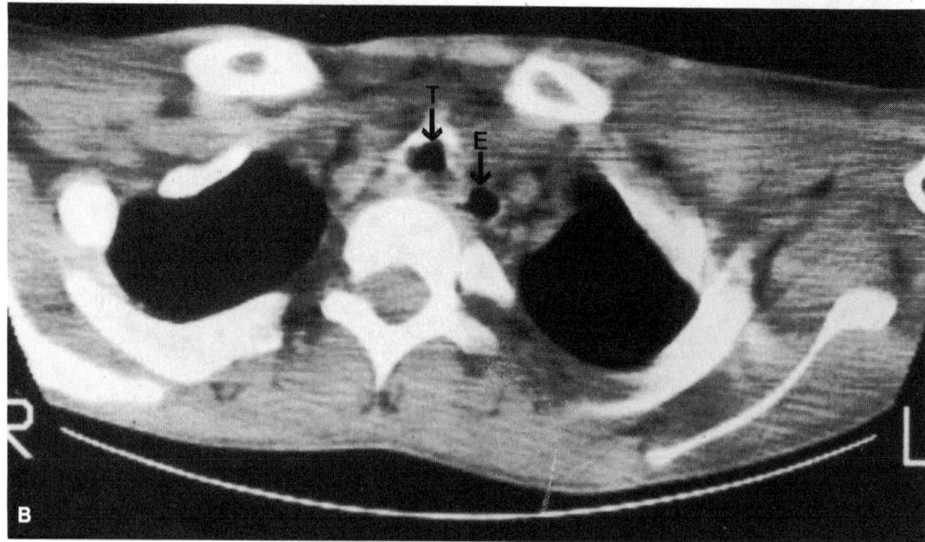

FIGURE 17-13. Computed tomographic scans of the upper thorax of a 20-year-old patient after tracheal reconstruction. (A) The trachea (*T*) has bright walls because of the presence of synthetic material; there is almost triangular deformity of the trachea. *E*, esophagus. (B) At a slightly lower level, the reconstructed trachea (*T*) becomes more narrow and deformed at a level just above the carina. *E*, esophagus.

scope, the endotracheal tube is positioned and secured, and breath sounds are verified.

Failure to Intubate

Despite the best of plans, fiberoptic intubation sometimes is unsuccessful.[27,80] Although the most common reason is inexperience on the part of the endoscopist, other reasons include secretions, blood, tissue edema, fogging of the lens, insufficient light or improper focus, inability to pass the tube over the fiberscope, distortion of anatomic structures, soft-tissue traction, a large floppy epiglottis, and severe cervical flexion deformity.

Potential Complications

Potential complications include laryngospasm; bronchospasm; bleeding; trauma; and pulmonary aspiration of gastric contents, blood, or oral secretions. Measures to prevent aspiration, especially in the patient with a full stomach, must be exercised.

ANESTHETIC INDUCTION AND PERIOPERATIVE MANAGEMENT

No routine method of induction of maintenance of anesthesia can be applied to all patients with airway compromise. Each case must be evaluated in light of individual conditions and possible causes as well as the anesthetist's skills and resources. Algorithms for management of the difficult airway have been published by Benumof[27] and by the American Society of Anesthesiologists (Fig. 17-14).

Muscle relaxation from general anesthesia may contribute to soft-tissue obstruction. In addition, mucus or blood on the larynx during light anesthesia can cause laryngospasm. Distortion resulting from surgery and secretions make reintubation extremely difficult in many instances. Patients with obstructive lesions in any area of the respiratory tract should be examined carefully before extubation, particularly after surgical procedures, as well as before intubation. Uvular edema[81] and macroglossia[82] are among the more obvious causes of postoperative airway obstruction. A less obvious cause is intraoperative nerve injury, especially that involving the glossopharyngeal and hypoglossal nerves.[83,84]

DIFFICULT AIRWAY ALGORITHM

1. Assess the likelihood and clinical impact of basic management problems:

   A. Difficult Intubation
   B. Difficult Ventilation
   C. Difficulty with Patient Cooperation or Consent

2. Consider the relative merits and feasibility of basic management choices:

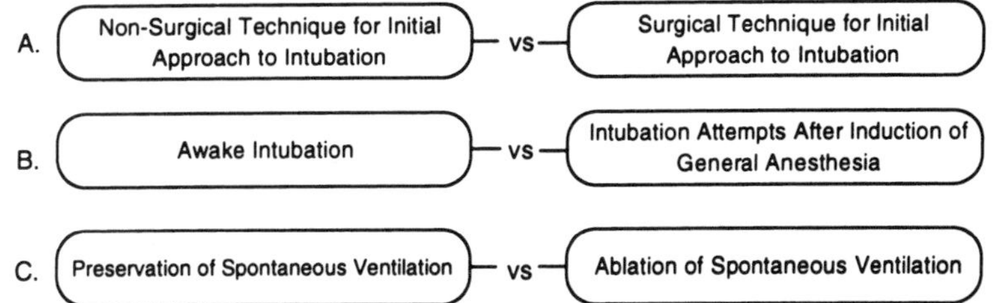

3. Develop primary and alternative strategies:

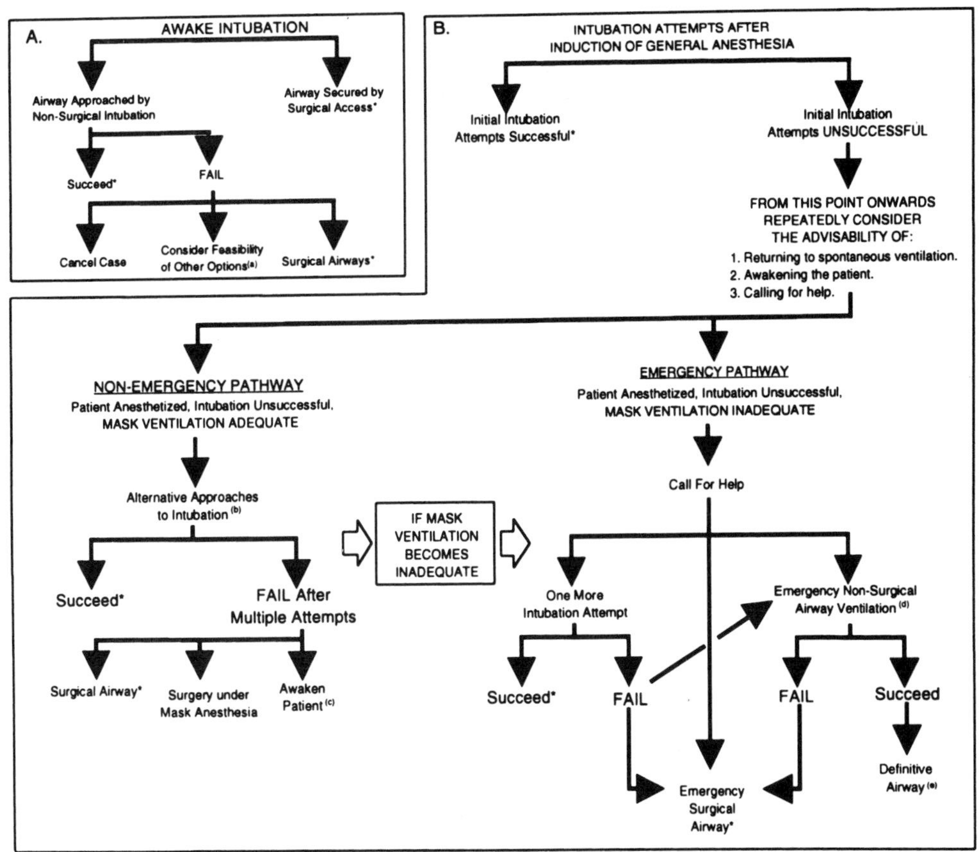

* CONFIRM INTUBATION WITH EXHALED CO_2

(a) Other options include (but are not limited to): surgery under mask anesthesia, surgery under local anesthesia infiltration or regional nerve blockade, or intubation attempts after induction of general anesthesia.

(b) Alternative approaches to difficult intubation include (but are not limited to): use of different laryngoscope blades, awake intubation, or tube changer, light wand, retrograde intubation, and surgical airway access.

(c) See awake intubation

(d) Options for emergency non-surgical airway ventilation include (but are not limited to): transtracheal jet ventilation, laryngeal mask ventilation, or esophageal-tracheal combitube ventilation.

(e) Options for establishing a definitive airway include (but are not limited to): returning to awake state with spontaneous ventilation, tracheotomy, or endotracheal intubation.

FIGURE 17-14. Management algorithm for the difficult airway. (The American Society of Anesthesiologists: Practice guidelines for management of the difficult airway: a report by the American Society of Anesthesiologists Task Force on management of the difficult airway. Anesthesiology 78:597, 1993.)

In general, when special techniques are required to ensure a patent airway, the trachea should be extubated after the patient's reflexes have returned completely and he or she is able to open the eyes and respond to commands. Often there is concern about trauma or edema to the airway; one approach to rule out this sequela is to deflate the tube cuff after suctioning the patient's mouth and then briefly obstruct the endotracheal tube to determine if the patient is able to move any air around it. Another useful approach to consider is to extubate the trachea after placing a tube exchange stylet through the endotracheal tube and taping it in place. If the patient maintains adequate respiration around this partial obstruction, it is unlikely that sufficient edema is present to worsen the respiratory status after complete extubation. Conversely, if the patient shows evidence of respiratory distress, reintubation is a relatively simple matter of sliding an endotracheal tube over the tube changer, following which the tube changer is removed.

ACKNOWLEDGMENT

The authors would like to give special thanks to Dr. Jason Brajer and Dr. Pietro Colonna-Romano for help with manuscript review.

REFERENCES

1. Jones ACP, Pelton DA: An index of syndromes and their anaesthetic implications. Can Anaesth Soc J 23:207, 1976
2. Berkowitz ID, Raja SN, Bender KS, et al: Dwarfs: pathophysiology and anesthetic implications. Anesthesiology 73:739, 1990
3. Cordon RA: Anesthetic management of patients with airway problems. Int Anesthesiol Clin 10:37, 1972
4. Shurman J: Bilateral hypertrophy of the coronoid processes. Anesthesiology 42:491, 1975
5. Bougas TP, Smith RM: Pathologic airway obstruction in children. Anesth Analg 37:137, 1958
6. Salzarullo HH, Taylor LA: Diabetic 'stiff joint syndrome' as a cause of difficult endotracheal intubation. Anesthesiology 64: 366, 1986
7. Ross EDT: Treacher-Collins syndrome: an anaesthetic hazard. Anaesthesia 18:350, 1963
8. Ferguson CF: Treatment of airway problems in the newborn. Ann Otol Rhinol Laryngol 76:762, 1967
9. Fearon B: Respiratory distress in the newborn. Otolaryngol Clin North Am 1:147, 1968
10. McAllister RG: Macroglossia: a positional complication. Anesthesiology 40:199, 1974
11. Jackson P, Whitaker LA, Randall P: Airway hazards associated with pharyngeal flaps in patients who have the Pierre-Robin syndrome. Plast Reconstr Surg 58:184, 1976
12. Bennett JH: Anesthetic management for drainage of abscess of the submandibular space (Ludwig's angina). Anesthesiology 4: 25, 1943
13. Meyers EF, Chapin B: Anesthetic management of emergency tonsillectomy and adenoidectomy in infectious mononucleosis. Anesthesiology 42:490, 1975
14. Blanc VF, Weber ML, Levuc C, et al: Acute epiglottitis in children: management of 27 consecutive cases with nasotracheal intubation with emphasis on anaesthetic considerations. Can Anaesth Soc J 24:1, 1977
15. Pappas MT, Katz J, Finestone SC: Problems in anesthetic and airway management with Gardner's syndrome: report of a case. Anesth Analg 50:340, 1971
16. Stein AA, Volk BM: Papillomatosis of trachea and lung. Arch Pathol 68:468, 1959
17. Amaranth L, Frankmann DB, Andersen NB: An unusual airway obstruction secondary to congenital malformation of the thoracic inlet. Anesthesiology 43:106, 1975
18. Sinclar JR, Mason RA: Ankylosing spondylitis: the case for awake intubation. Anaesthesia 39:3, 1984
19. Birkham J, Heifetz M, Harm S: Diffuse cutaneous scleroderma: an anaesthetic problem. Anaesthesia 27:89, 1972
20. Gardner DL, Holmes F: Anaesthetic and postoperative hazards in rheumatoid arthritis. Br J Anaesth 33:258, 1961
21. D'Arcy EJ, Fell RH, Ansell BM, et al: Ketamine and juvenile chronic polyarthritis (Still's disease). Anesthesia 31:624, 1976
22. Reddy ARR, Wong PHW: Epidermolysis bullosa: a review of the anaesthetic problems and case reports. Can Anaesth Soc J 19: 536, 1972
23. Barnard J: An unusual accident during intubation. Anaesthesia 3:126, 1948
24. Nash PJ: A foreign body in the larynx. Br J Anaesth 48:371, 1976
25. Butsch JL, Butsch WL, DaRosa JFT: Bilateral vocal cord paralysis. Arch Surg 111:828, 1976
26. Hassan SZ, Matz GJ, Lawrence AM, et al: Laryngeal stenosis in acromegaly: a possible cause of airway difficulties associated with anesthesia. Anesth Analg 55:57, 1976
27. Benumof JL: Management of the difficult airway: with special emphasis on awake tracheal intubation. Anesthesiology 75:1087, 1991
28. Pelton DA, Whalen JS: Airway obstruction in infants and children. Int Anesthesiol Clin 10:123, 1972
29. Salem MR, Mathrubhutham M, Bennett EJ: Difficult intubation. N Engl J Med 295:879, 1976
30. Sklar GS, King BD: Endotracheal intubation and Treacher-Collins syndrome. Anesthesiology 44:247, 1976
31. Isdale JM: The role of radiology in the assessment of the acutely ill neonate. Int Anesthesiol Clin 13:49, 1975
32. O'Leary AM: Acute upper airway obstruction due to arterial puncture during percutaneous central venous cannulation of the subclavian vein. Anesthesiology 73:780, 1990
33. Mackenzie JW, Jellicoe JA: Acute upper airway obstruction. Anaesthesia 41:57, 1986
34. Woolley MM, Morgan S, Hays BR: Heritable disorders of connective tissue in surgical anesthetic problems. J Pediatr Surg 2: 325, 1967
35. Holinger PH, Johnston KC: Factors responsible for laryngeal obstruction in infants. JAMA 143:1229, 1950
36. Shambaugh GE, Seed R, Kurn A: Airway obstruction in substernal goiter: clinical and therapeutic implications. Journal of Chronic Diseases 26:737, 1973
37. Lee MH, Ramanathan S, Chalon J, et al: Subglottic hemangioma. Anesthesiology 45:459, 1976
38. Barash PG, Tsai B, Kitahata LM: Acute tracheal collapse following mediastinoscopy. Anesthesiology 44:67, 1976
39. Hall KD, Friedman M: Extracorporeal oxygenation for induction of anesthesia in a patient with an intrathoracic tumor. Anesthesiology 42:493, 1975
40. Kitahata LM: Airway difficulties associated with anaesthesia in acromegaly. Br J Anaesth 43:1187, 1971
41. Donchin Y, Vered IY: Blunt trauma to the trachea. Br J Anaesth 48:1113, 1976
42. Ellis FR: Management of the cut throat. Anaesthesia 21:253, 1966
43. Bishop MJ: Epiglottitis in the adult. Anesthesiology 55:701, 1981
44. Hitz HB, Oesterlin E: A case of multiple papillomata of the larynx with aerial metastases to the lungs. Am J Pathol 8:333, 1932
45. Bannister FB, MacBeth RG: Direct laryngoscopy and tracheal intubation. Lancet 2:651, 1944
46. Miyabe M, Dohi S, Homa E: Tracheal intubation in an infant with Treacher-Collins syndrome: pulling out the tongue by a forceps. Anesthesiology 62:213, 1985
47. Sivarajan M, Fink RB: The position and state of the larynx during general anesthesia and muscle paralysis. Anesthesiology 72:439, 1990
48. Cass NM, James NR, Lines V: Intubation under direct laryngoscopy. Br Med J 2:488, 1956

49. White A, Kander PL: Anatomical factors in difficult direct laryngoscopy. Br J Anaesth 47:468, 1975
50. Mallampati SR, Gatt SP, Gugino LD, et al: A clinical sign to predict difficult tracheal intubation: a prospective study. Can Anaesth Soc J 32:429, 1985
51. Tham ES, Gatt SP, Gugino LD, et al: Effects of posture, phonation, and observer on Mallampati classification. Br J Anaesth 68:32, 1992
52. Bachaud R, Fortin G: Airway obstruction with cuffed flexometallic tracheal tubes. Can Anaesth Soc J 23:330, 1976
53. Blitt CD, Wright WA: An unusual complication of percutaneous internal jugular vein cannulation: puncture of an endotracheal tube cuff. Anesthesiology 40:306, 1974
54. Chiu TM, Meyers EF: Defective disposable endotracheal tube. Anesth Analg 55:437, 1976
55. Dorsch JA, Dorsch SE: Understanding anesthesia equipment, 2nd ed. Baltimore: Williams & Wilkins, 1984: 377
56. Ketover AK, Feingold A: Collapse of a disposable endotracheal tube by its high-pressure cuff. Anesthesiology 45:108, 1975
57. Kloss J, Petty C: Obstruction of endotracheal intubation by a mobile pedunculated polyp. Anesthesiology 43:380, 1975
58. Stark DCC: Endotracheal tube obstruction. Anesthesiology 45: 467, 1976
59. Martin J, Hutchinson B: Tracheal tube obstruction by a prominent aortic knuckle. Anaesthesia 41:86, 1985
60. Moorthy SS, Haselby KA, Stein KD: Airway obstruction with esophageal monitors in a patient with double aortic arch. Anesthesiology 63:465, 1985
61. Mesrobian RB, Epps JE: Midtracheal obstruction after Harrington rod placement in a patient with Marfan's syndrome. Anesth Analg 65:411, 1986
62. Moorthy SS, Lo Sasso AM, King H, et al: Evaluation of larynx and trachea by xeroradiography. Anesth Analg 55:598, 1976
63. Griscom NT: Computed tomographic determination of tracheal dimensions in children and adolescents. Radiology 145:361, 1982
64. Northrip DR, Bohman B, Tsueda K: Total occlusion and superior vena cava syndrome in a child with an anterior mediastinal tumor. Anesth Analg 65:1079, 1986
65. Dellinger RP: Fiberoptic bronchoscopy in adult airway management. Crit Care Med 18:882, 1990
66. Heffner JE: The technique of fiberoptic bronchoscopy for difficult intubations. J Crit Illness 25:83, 1988
67. Audenaert SM, Montgomery CL, Stone B, et al: Retrograde-assisted fiberoptic tracheal intubation in children with difficult airways. Anesth Analg 73:660, 1991
68. Powell WF, Ozdil T: A translaryngeal guide for tracheal intubation. Anesth Analg 46:231, 1967
69. Carlson CC, Perkins HM, Veltkamp S: Solving a difficult intubation. Anesthesiology 64:537, 1986
70. Stewart R: Tactile orotracheal intubation. Ann Emerg Med 13: 175, 1984
71. Williams RT: Lighted stylet and endotracheal intubation. Anesthesiology 66:851, 1987
72. Gorback MS: Management of the challenging airway with the Bullard laryngoscope. J Clin Anaesth 3:473, 1991
73. Borland LM, Casselbrant M: The Bullard laryngoscope: a new indirect oral laryngoscope (pediatric version). Anesth Analg 70: 105, 1990
74. Benumof JL: Laryngeal mask airway: indications and contraindications. Anesthesiology 77:843, 1992
75. Maltby JR, Loken RG, Watson NC: The laryngeal mask airway: clinical appraisal in 150 patients. Can J Anaesth 37:509, 1990
76. Frass M, Johnson JC, Atherton GL, et al: Esophageal tracheal combitube (ETC) for emergency intubation: anatomical evaluation of ETC placement by radiography. Resuscitation 18:95, 1989
77. Frass M, Frenzer R, Zahler J, et al: Ventilation via the esophageal tracheal combitube in a case of difficult intubation. J Cardiothorac Anesth 1:565, 1987
78. Bigenzahn W, Pesau B, Frass M: Emergency ventilation using the combitube in cases of difficult intubation. Eur Arch Otorhinolaryngol 248:129, 1991
79. Murphy P: A fibre-optic endoscope for nasal intubation. Anaesthesia 22:489, 1967
80. Katsnelson T, Frost EA, Farcon E, et al: When the endotracheal tube will not pass over flexible fiberoptic bronchoscope. Anesthesiology 76:151, 1992
81. Haselby KA, McNeice WL: Respiratory obstruction from uvular edema in a pediatric patient. Anesth Analg 62:1127, 1983
82. Mayhew JF, Miner M, Katz J: Macroglossia in a 16-month-old child after craniotomy. Anesthesiology 62:683, 1985
83. Gorski DW, Rao TK, Scarff TB: Airway obstruction following surgical manipulation of the posterior cranial fossa, an unusual complication. Anesthesiology 54:80, 1981
84. Levelle JP, Martinez OA: Airway obstruction after bilateral carotid endarterectomy. Anesthesiology 63:220, 1985

FURTHER READING

American Society of Anesthesiologists: Practice guidelines for management of the difficult airway: a report by the American Society of Anesthesiologists task force on management of the difficult airway. Anesthesiology 78:597, 1993

Florete O: Airway management. In Civetta JM, Taylor RW, Kirby RR (eds): Critical care, 2nd ed. Philadelphia, JB Lippincott Co, 1992: 1419

King TA, Adams AP: Failed tracheal intubation. Brit J Anaesth 65: 400, 1990

Patton C: The critical airway: classic problems. Current Reviews in Clinical Anesthesia 11:81, 1991

Rigor BM: Management of difficult airway and failed intubation. Current Reviews in Clinical Anesthesia 10:16, 1990

Walker RWM, Darowski M, Morris P, et al: Anesthesia and mucopolysaccharidoses—A review of airway problems in children. Anaesthesia 49:1078, 1994

Complications in Anesthesiology, second edition,
edited by Nikolaus Gravenstein and Robert R. Kirby.
Lippincott-Raven Publishers, Philadelphia © 1996.

CHAPTER 18

Hazards of Tracheal Intubation

David C. Flemming
Fredrick K. Orkin
Robert R. Kirby

Intubation of the trachea for surgical procedures began in 1878, when MacEwen of Glasgow performed an orotracheal intubation in an awake patient before administration of chloroform for a mandibular resection.[1] His reasoning included two of the tenets of tracheal intubation[2]: intubation allows easier access to the surgical field during head and neck surgery, and intubation "guarantees" the integrity of the airway.

Methods for intubation did not become established clinically until the 1920s, when troops returned for repair of their war-torn faces. Rowbotham and Magill[3,4] described equipment and techniques that enabled Sir Harold Gilles to perform his remarkable facial reconstructions. These techniques, and those popularized by Waters, Guedel, and Rovenstine[5,6] in America, developed into an essential part of modern anesthetic practice over the subsequent 75 years.

Originally, intubation was practiced only when it was essential to conduct surgery. Hazards were recognized but were confined to dangers inherent in the intubation process; however, Langton-Hewer suggested in 1924 that intubation made anesthesia easier and safer and should be used far more extensively, noting in particular the ease with which general anesthesia could be maintained during cholecystectomy in the "bucolic drayman."[7]

In the 1950s it became clear that life could be maintained past its common termination in respiratory failure by tracheal intubation and mechanical ventilation. The proliferation of intensive care units that began in the 1960s demonstrated that long-term intubation with crude equipment and techniques was associated with new problems. Despite the current effort to improve intubation techniques and equipment, we still are unable to guarantee that tracheal intubation will be benign. Before intubation is undertaken, assessment of the benefits relative to the attendant risks is always necessary.

INCIDENCE OF COMPLICATIONS AND PREDISPOSING FACTORS

Problems of Study

Knowledge of hazards and their incidence comes from experience, conferences on morbidity, and published reports. Despite numerous studies, the incidence of each complication is difficult to state. The field is changing rapidly, with technological improvements being introduced continually. For example, the incorporation of high-volume, low-pressure cuffs for endotracheal tubes in the early 1970s was thought to have resulted in a reduction of tracheal injury after long-term intubation, but this widely accepted "fact" has not been substantiated.[8–11] Numerous factors predisposing to injury vary from population to population. Thus, the incidence of each complication is variable, and estimates made only a few years ago may not be valid now.

Patient Factors

Complications are in part dependent on the patient.[12] Infants, children, and adult women, all of whom have a relatively small larynx and trachea, are more susceptible to airway narrowing from mucosal edema. This observation follows from the Hagen-Poiseuille law, which states that resistance to flow in tubes varies inversely as the fourth power of the radius of that tube for laminar flow and as the fifth power of the radius for turbulent flow.

The patient whose trachea is difficult to intubate is likely to sustain more injury. Similarly, patients with chronic or debilitating diseases are less able to tolerate the tissue trauma encountered during long-term tracheal intubation. An increased risk for complications related to tracheal intubation should be identified and the patient cautioned, whenever possible, and appropriate documentation should be made in the medical record. Written cautions improve communication of the potential problem to an anesthesiologist administering a future anesthetic. There is growing opinion that the patient with a truly "difficult airway" should wear a bracelet or necklace engraved with a suitable warning in case incapacitation prevents him or her from alerting the anesthesiologist.

Equipment and Preparation

Complications are influenced by the intubation process and the equipment used. A hurried intubation in a poorly prepared patient (inadequate muscle relaxation or anesthesia; incorrect head position; or poor visualization) often is injurious.[8] Care must be taken to avoid these mistakes.

Endotracheal Tubes

SIZE OF THE TUBE AND DURATION OF INTUBATION. Some determinants of injury are associated directly with the endotracheal tube. The longer a tube is in place and the larger its diameter, the greater is the possibility for complications.[12–15] However, the work of spontaneous breathing is significantly increased by a small-diameter tube, as is the risk of cuff-induced injury.[9,16,17]

TUBE MATERIALS AND STERILIZATION. Although early studies suggested that plastic was superior to rubber as a material for endotracheal tubes, subsequent work showed that various ingredients in the plastic—for example, catalysts, antioxidants, and plasticizers—are tissue irritants.[18,19] When tubes are reused, residual cleaning agent may remain in and on the plastic and result in tissue irritation and injury. This problem was a potent stimulus for the almost universal adoption of disposable tubes in the United States. If they are inadequately aerated, gas-sterilized tubes may contain ethylene oxide that is released and that injures airway mucosa; water and ethylene oxide form an irritant, ethylene glycol.

TUBE-INDUCED DAMAGE. The standard endotracheal tube, because of its shape, exerts significant pressure on the arytenoid cartilages, the posterior half of the vocal cords, and the posterior tracheal wall (Fig. 18-1). Minimization of tube-induced mucosal injury has been thought to necessitate the use of tubes with the smallest diameter and for the shortest time possible, as well as tubes with a pronounced pharyngeal curve (eg, Oxford or Lindholm tubes), the contour of which conforms better to that of the upper airway.[19–21] The tradeoff is the need for increased cuff volume to effect a seal and a high possibility of cuff-induced damage.[9–11]

Movement of the tube in the airway with each breath is another source of injury. This problem occurs because the tube is fixed externally; however, the tracheobronchial tree moves with ventilation, especially with positive-pressure ventilation, coughing, swallowing, and head movement, all of which contribute to mechanical stresses within the airway.[13,19,22]

EARLY TRACHEOTOMY. Because airway injury may be unavoidable during long-term intubation, some have argued that tracheotomy should be performed earlier in patients requiring prolonged ventilatory support.[20] Others dispute that recommendation, stating that tracheotomy induces new, different, and more severe complications than those resulting from intubation for at least 3 weeks with conventional endotracheal tubes.[8]

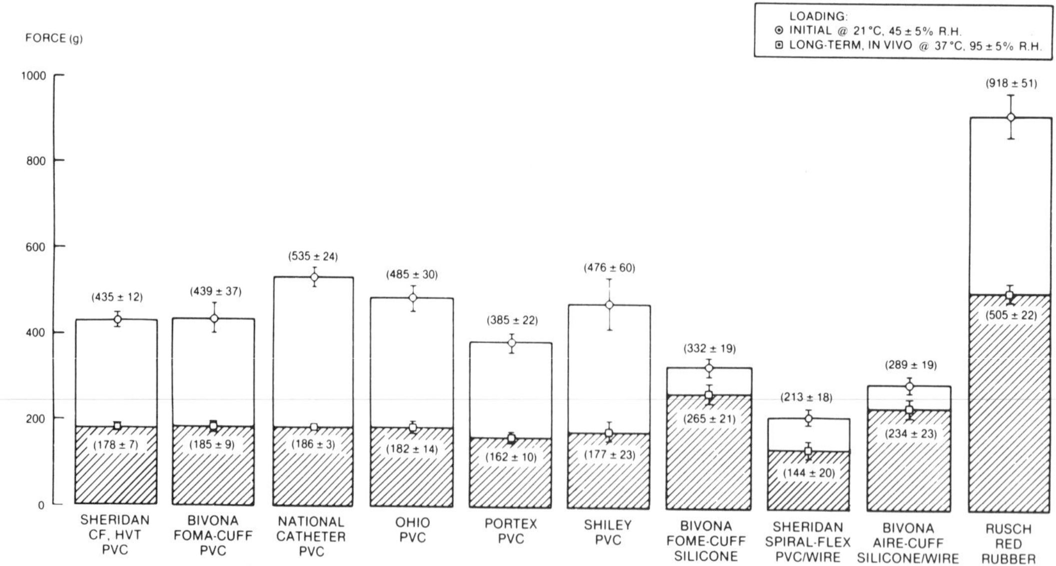

FIGURE 18-1. Bending forces (mean ± standard deviation) required to bring various models of tracheal tubes to anatomic conformity. *RH*, relative humidity. *PVC*, polyvinylchloride. (Steen JA: Impact of tube design and materials on complications of tracheal intubation. Problems in Anesthesia 2:221, 1988.)

CUFF DAMAGE. Much of the tracheal injury is associated with the pressure exerted by the endotracheal tube cuff, which in turn is influenced by cuff design.[9-11,19,20,23,24] Until about 1970, cuffs were high-pressure, low-volume types that often inflated eccentrically, thereby exerting extreme and uneven pressure against the tracheal wall. Since the early 1970s, cuff design has incorporated high volumes with low pressure that is distributed more evenly over a large surface area and theoretically results in less mucosal and submucosal injury. These large, floppy cuffs, however, offer less protection from pulmonary aspiration than did the high-pressure types they supplanted.[25] Also, in patients with severely reduced lung compliance who require high peak inflation pressures, the cuffs must be overinflated. Hence, their low-pressure characteristics are lost, and severe damage often results from prolonged use.[9-11]

HAZARDS REQUIRING IMMEDIATE RECOGNITION AND MANAGEMENT

A description of the hazards of intubation may be based on grades of therapeutic urgency, of which three primary categories are apparent (Table 18-1).

TABLE 18-1
Complications of Tracheal Intubation According to Graded Therapeutic Urgency

HAZARDS REQUIRING IMMEDIATE RECOGNITION AND MANAGEMENT
Spinal cord and vertebral column injury
Airway perforation
Barotrauma
Inadvertent bronchial intubation
Airway obstruction
Circuit leaks
Difficult extubation
Airway fires
Nasopharyngeal trauma associated with nasotracheal intubation
Esophageal intubation
Aspiration of foreign materials
Disconnection and dislodgment
Laryngeal and airway edema
ACUTE TRAUMA OF LESSER SIGNIFICANCE
Sore throat
Lip and tooth injury
Corneal abrasion
Epistaxis
CHRONIC EFFECTS OF EROSION AND HEALING
Trachea: granuloma formation
Synechiae
Webs
Chondritis
Stenosis, fibrosis
Nerve injury
Vocal cord paralysis

Spinal Cord and Vertebral Column Injury

Ordinarily the neck is extended and the head brought anteriorly into the sniffing position to facilitate visualization for laryngoscopy. This position may be difficult to obtain because of jaw or neck stiffness accompanying trismus, arthritis, ankylosing spondylitis, radiation therapy, or burns; an anterior larynx accompanying a narrow receding mandible, heavy musculature, or a short neck; or distortion of the upper airway by tumor or trauma. Cervical spine malformation, instability, tumor, osteoporosis, or fracture predispose to spine or cord damage with forceful hyperextension of the neck.

Laryngoscopy

When a patient has one or more of these predisposing factors, laryngoscopy must be gentle and careful. The head should be maintained in neutral position, with the help of an assistant if necessary. Alternative methods that do not involve neck manipulation or direct laryngoscopy, such as blind nasal, transillumination, or fiberoptic techniques, should be considered.[12] Because these techniques take time to perform, they entail additional risk when pulmonary ventilation has been interrupted long enough for arterial oxyhemoglobin desaturation to begin.

In the zeal to accomplish tracheal intubation, the anesthesiologist must not forget that the patient needs oxygen and not necessarily a endotracheal tube. Oxygen should be administered by mask between attempted intubations. In difficult circumstances, immediate cricothyrotomy or, much less frequently, tracheotomy may be preferable.[26] Equipment for and training of personnel in these techniques is increasingly a standard of care in the operating room.

Autonomic Reflexes

Direct laryngoscopy and tracheal intubation are intense stimuli, causing brisk autonomic responses.[27] Hypertension, tachycardia, cardiac dysrhythmias, bronchospasm, and bronchorrhea are common; bradycardia and hypotension also may occur. These problems emerged as a by-product of medical progress, when the advent of muscle relaxants enabled tracheal intubation without the need for deep planes of anesthesia.

All patients undergoing laryngoscopy under light planes of anesthesia experience these responses to some extent. Patients with preexisting hypertensive cardiovascular disease are doubly at risk, having both brisker pressor reflexes and generalized vascular disease with the attendant risks of pulmonary edema, myocardial ischemia and infarction, and cerebrovascular accident (Fig. 18-2).[28,29] Though brief, the circulatory responses are severe enough to upset the delicate balance between myocardial oxygen supply and demand in patients with coronary artery disease.

Given the inability of these patients to meet the resultant increased myocardial oxygen demand, an attempt should be made to abort these circulatory responses. Increasing the depth of anesthesia, treating the sympathetic response more directly (eg, with labetalol for hypertension, or with propran-

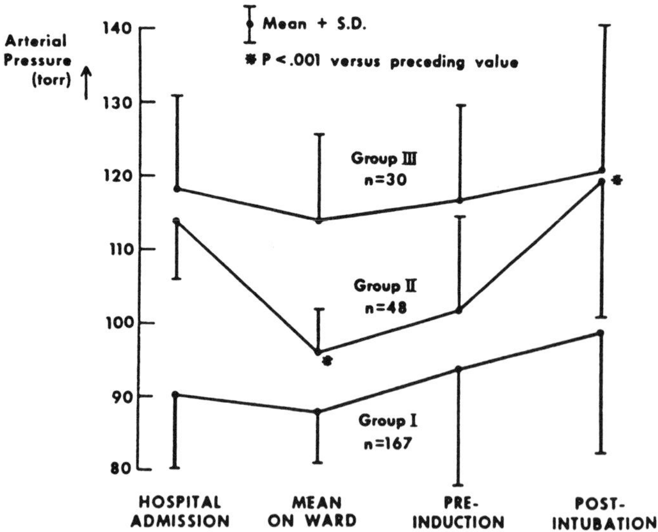

FIGURE 18-2. Mean arterial blood pressure in response to hospital admission and endotracheal intubation in three groups of patients. A significant increase in blood pressure occurred following intubation only in the group of patients who were hypertensive (>140/90 mm Hg) at the time of admission but who were otherwise normotensive during hospitalization. *SD,* standard deviation. (Bedford RF, Feinstein B: Hospital admission blood pressure: a predictor for hypertension following endotracheal intubation. Anesth Analg 59:368, 1980.)

olol, esmolol, or both for tachycardia) may be indicated. These responses may provoke additional complications such as hypotension and bronchospasm.

Prevention

As with many anesthetic problems, prevention is preferable to treatment, and many options are available for the control or attenuation of the circulatory responses (Table 18-2).

PAIN CONTROL. One approach to pain control involves blocking the patient's perception of pain by using deeper levels of inhalation anesthesia as well as supplemental doses of rapidly acting potent narcotics, lidocaine, or both. The depth of inhalation anesthesia needed to prevent these responses is unknown. However, the required dose must be substantial, because that needed to prevent coughing during tracheal intubation is about 30% greater than the 1.5 to 1.6 × minimum alveolar concentration needed to block circulatory responses to skin incision.[30–32] Thus, supplemental doses of rapidly acting narcotics that offer dose-related protection against circulatory responses are used commonly (see Table 18-2).[33–35] Intravenous lidocaine also may be used.[36,37]

BLOCKING AGENTS. A second approach to prevention involves administration of drugs that block specific circulatory responses: nitroprusside,[38] hydralazine,[39] or nitroglycerin[40] for hypertension; intravenous labetalol[41] 0.25 mg/kg and esmolol[42] 500 μg/kg/min for 4 minutes and then 300 μg/kg/min through induction for tachycardia; and atropine for bradycardia. Administration of an appropriate dose as pretreatment in this dynamic situation is empirical (ie, based on patient response).

LOCAL ANESTHETICS. Block of laryngeal sensory nerves by topical administration of lidocaine and block of laryngeal or glossopharyngeal nerves may be effective. Implementation of these techniques can be stressful and may not anesthetize all tissues affected by laryngoscopy. Application of topical anesthesia to the trachea (eg, lidocaine 3.0 mg/kg as an aerosol[43]) after the induction of general anesthesia requires direct laryngoscopy, which often has cardiovascular effects apart from those associated with tracheal intubation. Inhalation of lidocaine mist before induction of anesthesia may be a rapid and effective method for achieving topical anesthesia before laryngoscopy and intubation; however, documentation of efficacy has not yet been published.

LARYNGEAL MASK. The laryngeal mask may be substituted for a conventional endotracheal tube in some cases. Most of the advantages of tracheal intubation can be obtained with the laryngeal mask, the blind insertion of which does not involve the use of a laryngoscope.[26,44,45] Resultant circulatory responses attributable to laryngoscopy are thereby eliminated.

Airway Fires

Formerly associated with flammable anesthetics, the use of which ended in the mid-1970s, fires and explosions now occur occasionally in association with newer surgical techniques, such as radiofrequency electrocautery and a variety of laser applications.

Laser Surgery

Laser technology, in particular, has simplified the ablation of both benign and neoplastic tissue in the airway; however, laryngeal application of laser surgery usually requires tracheal

TABLE 18-2
Prevention of Circulatory Responses to Laryngoscopy and Intubation

INCREASING DEPTH OF INHALATIONAL AGENTS
NARCOTICS
Fentanyl
2 μg/kg intravenously: partially effective
6 μg/kg intravenously: usually effective[33]
11 to 15 μg/kg intravenously: almost completely protective
Alfentanil
10 μg/kg or more: protective[35]
VASOACTIVE AGENTS
Sodium nitroprusside[38]
Hydralazine[39]
Nitroglycerin[40]
Labetalol[41]
Esmolol[42]
Atropine
LOCAL ANESTHETICS
Topical lidocaine[43]
Intravenous lidocaine[37]
Block of sensory nerves

intubation. Among the most catastrophic intraoperative events is an airway fire caused by ignition of the endotracheal tube by the laser[46–48] or by electrocautery.[49] Oxygen-rich inspired gas mixtures fuel brisk conflagration, creating the potential for sudden, severe, airway damage by heat and fumes from the burning endotracheal tube. Treatment involves immediate removal of the endotracheal tube; institution of ventilation by face mask; endoscopy and bronchoscopy to evaluate the extent of trauma; and supportive respiratory care appropriate to the degree of impairment. Clinically, the respiratory impairment resembles that caused by airway damage in a house fire.

ENERGY AND IGNITION. Avoiding or at least reducing the risk of airway fires requires an appreciation of the physical principles underlying laser energy and ignition as well as knowledge of airway management for the surgical procedures.[50–52] One option is the avoidance of the endotracheal tube, when possible, and the use instead of jet (Venturi) ventilation through a bronchoscope or metal injector[53]; insufflation; or ventilation through a tracheotomy caudal to the site of laser application. Although the ignitable endotracheal tube is avoided, these ventilatory techniques pose other problems, such as hypoventilation and barotrauma, and the inspired gases still may support combustion.

TUBE TYPES. Approaches to the prevention of airway fires also involves protection of the endotracheal tube or use of special, noncombustible tubes. Originally, tubes were protected by wrapping them with an aluminum foil tape to at least 1 cm below the vocal cords. This reflective metallic covering was intended to shield the endotracheal tube and dissipate heat. However, the wrapping also reflects the laser beam, perhaps onto other structures; may be traumatic to adjacent laryngeal tissue; and may slip off, resulting in airway obstruction[54] or tube ignition. Tube ignition also may occur at the unwrapped cuff[47] or because of differences among tapes in the degree of protection offered.[48,55]

Alternatively, flexible stainless steel tubes are used,[56] but they are more traumatic to adjacent tissues than are conventional plastic or rubber tubes. Similarly, plastic tubes coated with metallic particles afford some protection by withstanding several applications of a laser beam. Cuff ignition is avoided by filling the cuff with saline instead of air and placing a moist pledget over it.

NITROUS OXIDE, HELIUM, NITROGEN, AND PEEP. Regardless of the type of endotracheal tube protection adopted, nitrous oxide should not be used because it supports combustion.[57] Inert gases such as helium[58] or nitrogen, instead of nitrous oxide, and lower concentrations of oxygen (eg, <40%)[57,58] have been recommended, based on laboratory simulations. Flushing the pharynx with nitrogen by catheter also has been suggested. The endotracheal tube should be affixed loosely so that it can be removed rapidly should ignition occur. Because fires always begin near end expiration and because PEEP (5 cm) with an FIO_2 of .4 prevents ignition, routine use of PEEP during laser operations on the airway in which tubes with PVC components (cuff or body) are used is recommended.[59]

Airway Perforation

Mechanical trauma during tracheal intubation can result in airway perforation, which may be regarded as one end of the broad spectrum of injury, the other extreme of which includes mild abrasion. Injury may result from the tube, laryngoscope, stylet, or other related equipment. Predisposing factors include anatomic difficulties (eg, difficult intubation), blind intubation, poor positioning, hurried intubation, poor visualization, inadequate muscle relaxation, and inexperience on the part of the clinician. The site of injury can be almost anywhere between the point of insertion and the alveoli, and clinical signs vary.

Nasal Intubation

Nasal intubation frequently causes laceration of the nasal mucosa and hemorrhage but also may result in turbinate fractures. Nasotracheal and nasogastric tubes may dissect posteriorly and descend behind the posterior pharyngeal wall; the more flexible nasogastric tubes may even pierce the cribriform plate and coil up within the cranium. Predisposing to these complications is obstruction of the nasal passage by the convoluted turbinates.

Even in the absence of gross trauma, nasotracheal intubation causes sufficient mechanical damage to superficial epithelial layers to produce mucociliary slowing in about 65%[60] and bacteremia in about 5.5% of patients.[61] Typically, the bloodborne microbes include the nasopharyngeal commensal organisms (eg, *Streptococcus viridans*) implicated in both endocarditis and systemic infection. Paranasal sinusitis may also occur, especially with prolonged nasotracheal intubation.[62]

Barotrauma

Airway rupture at levels lower than the nasal passages causes leakage of air into subcutaneous and peribronchial tissues, lung interstices, and, with progression, pleural and pericardial cavities. Though not always well circumscribed, these sites of air collection result in clinical features that help to define the site of rupture and to guide therapy. The collection of pulmonary interstitial air results in progressive loss of pulmonary compliance, and the larger volumes associated with pericardial and pulmonary tamponade may produce circulatory collapse. Abrupt circulatory collapse is often the initial sign of the large pleural collections occurring in tension pneumothorax.

Esophageal Intubation

When visualization of the larynx is difficult, the endotracheal tube occasionally is mistakenly inserted into the esophagus. Recognition of this error must be prompt to avoid the devastating effects of prolonged hypoxia. Paradoxically, the almost universally accepted practice of preoxygenation before induction of general anesthesia not only enables a longer apneic period for tracheal intubation (which is often helpful in difficult intubations) but also delays the onset of the hypoxemia for as long as 11 minutes. Thus, the secondary signs of hypoxemia, cyanosis, tachycardia, and dysrhythmias, followed by bradycardia, hypotension, and cardiac arrest, can occur after surgery has begun, confounding detection of the underlying problem.

The American Society of Anesthesiologists' ongoing study of closed claims emphasizes the significance of esophageal intubation cases, which constitute 18% of respiratory-related claims (Table 18-3).[63]

Signs

Esophageal intubation is characterized typically by absence of breath sounds over the chest, a gurgling sound in the epigastrium, and progressive abdominal distention, and, later, secondary signs of hypoxemia. Although esophageal intubation usually is detected by clinical signs, sometimes even careful, experienced practitioners are misled by observations that suggest that tracheal placement has been achieved. In 48% of cases of esophageal intubation in the closed-claims study,[63] breath sounds allegedly were auscultated. Fortunately, capnography and other technology to detect carbon dioxide in expired respiratory gas, direct visualization, and fiberoptic bronchoscopy allow esophageal intubation to be detected promptly.

Allowing the misplaced tube to remain in situ while the trachea is correctly intubated may prevent regurgitated gastric contents from entering the trachea. After correct endotracheal tube placement, the stomach should be decompressed because a distended stomach can lead to regurgitation, vomiting, or perforation.

Bronchial Intubation

Because of acute branching of the left bronchus at the carina, an endotracheal tube, when passed beyond this point, usually enters the right mainstem bronchus. Asymmetric chest expansion, unilateral absence of breath sounds, and, with time, arterial blood gas abnormalities are diagnostic features. Clinical diagnosis is rarely difficult; occasionally a chest radiograph is required to confirm the diagnosis in the operating room. This examination is mandatory in the intensive care unit, where the margin for error is less than in the operating room.

When inadvertent bronchial intubation is discovered, the tube should be withdrawn several centimeters and the lungs hyperinflated sufficiently to expand atelectatic segments. For longstanding atelectasis, bronchoscopy may be required to remove mucus plugs. The incidence of this complication can be minimized by measuring the endotracheal tube along the length of the airway before its insertion. In general, insertion to a depth of 21 cm from the teeth is appropriate for adult women and 23 cm for adult men.[64] Adherence to this recommendation prevents mainstem intubation in men and women of average height (168 to 174 cm and 158 to 174 cm, respectively). If a cuffed tube is used, the cuff location can be readily ballotted by partial compression of the pilot balloon and then ballottement along the length of the trachea with the other hand until pulsations are felt in the pilot balloon. If the cuff is identified higher in the neck, then the tube is simply advanced until the cuff is ballotted in the suprasternal notch. Conversely, if the cuff cannot be ballotted, it is carefully withdrawn until it is identified in the suprasternal notch. It should be remembered, however, that head flexion can force an appropriately placed tube into a mainstem bronchus (Fig. 18-3).

Pulmonary Aspiration

During induction of anesthesia, laryngoscopy, and intubation, a variety of materials can be aspirated into the trachea. These include teeth, blood, parts of the laryngoscope, adenoidal tissue, and, most commonly, regurgitated or vomited stomach contents.

Airway Obstruction

After the endotracheal tube has been inserted, patency of the airway still may be lost. Gradual kinking of the tube as it warms or drying of accumulated secretions can give rise to an obstruction of slow onset that may appear as a decrease in

TABLE 18-3
Distribution of Claims for Adverse Respiratory Events

EVENT	CASES (no.)	RESPIRATORY CLAIMS (% of 522)	TOTAL CLAIMS (% of 1541)
Inadequate ventilation	196	38	13
Esophageal intubation	94	18	6
Difficult tracheal intubation	87	17	6
Airway obstruction	34	7	2
Bronchospasm	32	6	2
Aspiration	26	5	2
Premature tracheal extubation	21	4	1
Unintentional tracheal extubation	14	3	1
Inadequate fraction of inspired oxygen	11	2	1
Endobronchial intubation	7	1	<1
Total	522	100	34

Caplan RA: Adverse respiratory events in anesthesia: a closed-claims analysis. Anesthesiology 72:829, 1990.

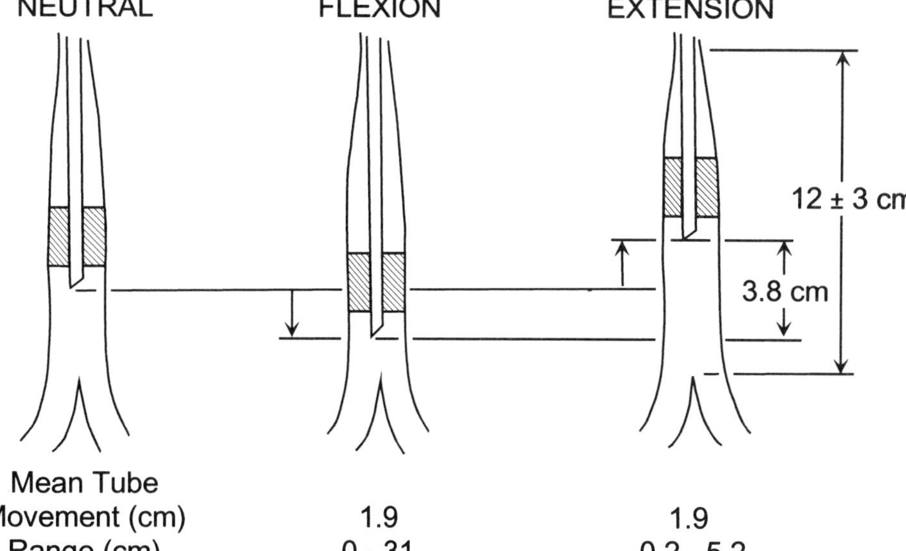

FIGURE 18-3. Mean endotracheal tube movement with flexion and extension of the neck from a neutral position. Mean tube movement between flexion and extension is about one-third to one-fourth the length of an adult trachea (12 ± 3 cm). (Conrardy PA, Goodman LR, Lainge F, et al: Alteration of endotracheal tube position: flexion and extension of the neck. Crit Care Med 4:9, 1976.)

compliance coupled with wheezing breath sounds resembling bronchospasm; in this situation bronchodilators often are given, in error. Acute, complete obstruction is much less ambiguous in its presentation. A problem that permits inhalation but prevents exhalation may present as circulatory collapse in the same manner as does tension pneumothorax or as rupture of the lungs with pneumothorax and subcutaneous emphysema.

Mechanical Problems

Mechanical problems that must be excluded[12,13] include separation of the interior latex coat of an armored tube; herniation of the endotracheal cuff; kinking, especially with the neck flexed; gradual accumulation of dried blood and secretions in the tube lumen; slow collapse of the tube by the cuff; occlusion of the endotracheal tube bevel against the tracheal wall; and blockage of the hoses leading to the patient by foreign bodies, external pressure, or incorrectly applied one-way valves in the circle absorber system.

Lack of Adequate Humidification

Prolonged ventilation with dry gases causes dehydration of tracheal mucus or blood, and the crusts that form may completely obstruct the endotracheal tube. This sequence of events is particularly likely with the use of nasal tubes that are longer and of smaller diameter than oral tubes and during pediatric anesthesia or intensive care. Humidification of the inspired gas helps to prevent the airway obstruction and mucosal damage that could result.

Negative-pressure Pulmonary Edema

If a patient is allowed to breathe spontaneously through a partially or totally obstructed airway, the marked inspiratory decrease in pleural pressure can result in sudden, often massive, acute pulmonary edema.[65] The condition may be mistaken for aspiration, anaphylaxis, or heart failure.

Remedial Steps

If time allows, evaluation of an obstruction problem should include passage of a suction catheter through the endotracheal tube to confirm its patency and then deflation and reinflation of the cuff. Should these measures not be successful or if little time is available, extubation and ventilation with a mask or a new endotracheal tube should be performed.

Disconnection and Dislodgment

One of the more serious and common mechanical complications of tracheal intubation is disconnection of the tube from the rest of the breathing circuit. This problem was the most frequent "critical incident" recalled in a study of human error and equipment failure.[66] Ordinarily this type of disconnection is readily discovered by the anesthesiologist. However, when the patient's head is not accessible or when the mechanical ventilator that is used (eg, the hanging bellows, in which the bellow descends during expiration) continues to cycle despite the leak, the physician may be deluded into believing that the patient is being adequately ventilated. Alarms to alert personnel of an airway disconnection are recommended, as are anti-disconnection devices.

Securement techniques appropriate to the nature of the surgery or accessibility of the tube are needed to prevent accidental dislodgment. Adhesive tape, adhesive solutions, and stainless steel wire to secure the tube to the teeth are tools that may be considered, but more important is the development of plans to cope with dislodgment should this problem occur.

Circuit Leaks

Circuit leaks cause hypoventilation and dilution of the inspired mixture by entry of air into the system. With spontaneous or manual ventilation and with mechanical ventilation when the bellows descends during inspiration (in newer models), collapse of the ventilator bellows provides visual indication that the leak exceeds the fresh gas inflow. However, older ventilators with hanging bellows may give no visual warning; the greater the leak, the more easily the bellows falls to its original position and in doing so entrains more air.

Continuous monitoring with a thoracic stethoscope and monitoring of inspired oxygen concentration, which will be reduced by dilution with air, and of end-tidal carbon dioxide partial pressure, which may increase, can reveal a developing leak. Cyanosis, a decrease in pulse oximeter oxygen saturation, or the hypertension and tachycardia of hypercapnia have been the presenting sign.

Evaporative Cooling

Evaporative water loss in children who are breathing dry gases causes heat loss in the vaporization of water. Humidification of inspired gas offers some thermal conservation, particularly when infants and smaller children are anesthetized. Humidification may also be useful in diminishing the incidence of sore throat and irritation of the tracheal mucosa.

Difficult Extubation

On occasion, endotracheal tubes are difficult to remove. Usually this problem results from use of oversized tubes or cuffs that are not or cannot be deflated.[67] A sore throat, attributable to local trauma, is more common after extubation is achieved; these patients, especially children, should be monitored carefully for the onset of postintubation croup. In rare instances, a endotracheal tube may be sutured mistakenly to the trachea or bronchial stump during surgery.

Laryngeal and Tracheal Edema

Any irritant stimulus, such as pressure from an oversized endotracheal tube, dryness of inhaled gas, allergy to laryngeal sprays, or chemical irritation from rubber or ethylene oxide–sterilized tubes can initiate an inflammatory response, producing mucosal edema in the larynx or trachea. The edema encroaches on the lumen and thereby increases airway resistance. This problem is especially acute in young children, in whom a disproportionate increase in resistance with a decrease in lumen radius results in croup. The peak incidence of this problem occurs at 1 to 3 years of age, affecting almost 4% of children in whom the trachea is intubated.[68,69]

Presentation

Croup may occur within hours of extubation and produce a barking, brassy cough and varying degrees of respiratory obstruction. Dyspnea, stridor, tachypnea, tachycardia, and suprasternal retraction are common. Should resolution be followed by scar formation, subglottic stenosis may then become evident but only several weeks or months after the initial insult.

Prevention

Prevention of this complication begins with avoiding irritant stimuli, particularly an oversized endotracheal tube, and avoiding intubation in the presence of upper respiratory tract infection. A leak around the endotracheal tube in pediatric cases should always be present, and use of a face mask during anesthesia should be encouraged where possible.

Treatment

Should postintubation croup occur, the beneficial roles of humidification of the inspired gases, application of cool mist, administration of oxygen, and administration of racemic epinephrine by aerosol are well established.[68] Steroids may be effective, but this therapy is not proven definitely to help. Helium–oxygen mixtures are suggested as a means of improving oxygen flow through edematous airways.[70]

TISSUE EROSION AND HEALING

Pathogenesis

The presence of an endotracheal tube may lead to edema, desquamation, inflammation, and ulceration of the airway.[9] The first three conditions usually are self-limited, whereas ulceration is more serious. Typically it occurs over the posterior half of the vocal cords, the medial arytenoid and posterior cricoid surfaces, and the anterior portion of the trachea. Severity may be related to the duration of intubation, but this association is not established.[8]

Although tracheotomy protects the larynx from further injury, trauma still may occur at sites of the inflated cuff and to a lesser degree at the tip of the tube. Healing occurs by epithelial regeneration, although granuloma and polyps may develop in an ulcerated area.[9] The damage to the tissues may be unrecognized, and the sequelae may appear only after prolonged intubation or months after extubation, when scarring diminishes tracheal diameter markedly.

Prevention

To prevent these injuries, endotracheal tube cuffs have been redesigned to produce the lowest possible lateral tracheal wall pressure. The principal change, as discussed previously, has been the substitution of a large-volume, low-pressure cuff for the small-volume, high-pressure types of the past. Other initiatives historically included stretching the cuff before use,[71] periodically deflating or inflating only during inspiration,[11] and using a fluted cuff, a foam-filled cuff, or pressure-regulating devices. Nonetheless, trauma still occurs[8,72–74] and frequently is serious.[9–11]

Tracheal Erosion

Erosion of the trachea into peritracheal tissue has been observed frequently, with the symptoms depending on the eroded tissue. For example, erosion into the esophagus gives rise to a tracheoesophageal fistula with subsequent pulmonary aspiration. Erosion into the brachiocephalic artery results in aspiration of blood and potential exsanguination. Dysphonia, hoarseness, and laryngeal incompetence may result from erosion into paratracheal nerves. Tracheomalacia, with possible tracheal collapse, results from erosion confined to the tracheal cartilages.

Tracheotomy is associated with tracheal erosion, particularly into the esophagus or brachiocephalic artery, more often than is laryngotracheal intubation. Tracheotomy tubes generally sit lower in the trachea and have a built-in, fixed curve. They are more rigid and do not necessarily conform to the shape or morphologic features of the trachea, potentially causing pressure on tissues at the tube tip. Furthermore, hoses connected to the short tracheotomy tube are capable of exerting great leverage against the tracheal wall unless they are very carefully supported.

Erosion of Other Tissues

Tube pressure also damages skin at the site of insertion. Securement devices as well as adhesive tapes and solution can erode the skin of the face, ears, and scalp. Salivary gland erosion can lead to suppurative parotitis. Meticulous care in tube placement may help to reduce the incidence of chronic pressure sequelae; however, the difficulty of continuous observation of all potential sites of injury makes it likely that these injuries will continue to occur.

Healing and Granuloma Formation

Eroded tissues are ultimately replaced by scar tissue that retracts, leading to stenosis of the trachea, larynx, or nares. Granuloma occurs in 1 in 800[75] to 1 in 20,000[76] tracheal intubations, more commonly in women than men and only rarely in children. The posterior laryngeal wall is the common site of erosion and is the site of abundant overgrowth of granulation tissue. Granuloma causes cough, hoarseness, and throat discomfort. It can be prevented by minimizing the trauma associated with laryngoscopy and intubation. When it occurs, however, surgical excision usually is required.

Synechiae

Eroded vocal cords and processes may adhere together, especially when air flow through the cords is diminished by tracheostomy.[77] Surgical correction is required.

Membranes and Webs

Membranes and webs may form over sites of laryngeal and tracheal ulceration. Typically they are thick and gray. If they tear away from their site of attachment, respiratory obstruction may ensue.

Chondritis

After several days the inflammatory response to laryngeal ulceration extends to involve the laryngeal cartilages. Eventually a chondritis or chondromalacia may occur.

Stenosis and Fibrosis

This serious complication occurs several months after tracheal intubation. It is the end result in a continuum beginning with erosion of the tracheal wall, weakening of the cartilages, and healing with fibrosis.[9] Commonly associated with prolonged intubation, stenosis occurs more often in adults than in children. Stenosis usually occurs at the site of cuff inflation or, less commonly, at the tip of the tube. The symptoms include a dry cough, dyspnea, and signs of respiratory obstruction. Treatment includes dilatation in the early stages and resection of the stenotic segment should the lumen size be reduced to 4 to 5 mm.[78,79]

Vocal Cord Paralysis

Vocal cord paralysis can be unilateral or bilateral. Symptoms of respiratory obstruction occur with bilateral paralysis, whereas hoarseness occurs after unilateral paralysis. It may originate from pressure exerted by the distended cuff on branches of the recurrent laryngeal nerve; hence the paralysis usually is transient.

Nerve Injury

Transient weakness, numbness, and paralysis of the tongue occurs occasionally after laryngoscopy, presumably from pressure on the laryngeal or hypoglossal nerves. The complication is short-lasting.[80]

COMPLICATIONS OF LESSER CLINICAL SIGNIFICANCE

Although it is the most common complication, sore throat is also one of the most benign and transient. The pain on swallowing lasts no more than 24 to 48 hours and can be alleviated to some extent by having the patient inspire humidified air. Topical anesthesia applied to the endotracheal tube may lessen the severity of this complication.

Other minor complications include corneal abrasion, lip and tooth injury, and epistaxis after nasal intubation. The latter can be minimized by previous application of a nasal decongestant (eg, phenylephrine 0.25%) or cocaine, which shrinks the nasal mucosa.

REFERENCES

1. MacEwen W: Clinical observations on the introduction of tracheal tubes by the mouth instead of performing tracheotomy or laryngotomy. Br Med J 2:122 and 163, 1880
2. Atkinson RG, Rushman GB, Lee JA: A synopsis of anaesthesia, 8th ed. Bristol: John Wright and Sons, 1977: 237
3. Rowbotham ES: Intratracheal anaesthesia by the nasal route for operations on the mouth and lips. Br Med J 2:590, 1920
4. Rowbotham ES, Magill IW: Anaesthetics in plastic surgery of the face and jaws. Proc R Soc Med 14:17, 1921
5. Waters RM, Guedel AE: Endotracheal anesthesia: a new technique. Ann Otol Rhinol Laryngol 40:1139, 1931
6. Waters RM, Rovenstine EA, Guedel AE: Endotracheal anesthesia and its historical development. Anesth Analg 12:196, 1933
7. Langton-Hewer C: The endotracheal administration of nitrous oxide-ethanesol as the routine anaesthetic of choice for major surgery. Br J Anaesth 1:113, 1924

8. Stauffer JL, Olson DE, Petty TL: Complications and consequences of endotracheal intubation and tracheotomy. Am J Med 70:65, 1981
9. Guyton DC: Endotracheal and tracheotomy tube cuff design: Influences on tracheal damage. Critical Care Update 1:1, 1990
10. Guyton DC, Banner MJ, Kirby RR: High-volume, low-pressure cuffs: are they always low pressure? Chest 100:1076, 1991
11. Jaeger JM, Wells NC, Kirby RR, et al: Mechanical ventilation of a patient with decreased lung compliance and tracheal dilatation. J Clin Anesth 4:147, 1992
12. Applebaum EL, Bruce DL: Tracheal intubation. Philadelphia: WB Saunders Company, 1976: 77
13. Blanc VF, Tremblay NAG: The complications of tracheal intubation: a new classification with a review of the literature. Anesth Analg 53:202, 1974
14. Bunegin L, Albin MS, Ruiz M, et al: Prolonged intubation affects tracheal blood flow during normotension and induced hypotension (abstract). Anesthesiology 63:A5, 1985
15. Stout DM, Bishop MJ, Dwersteg JF, et al: Correlation of endotracheal tube size with sore throat and hoarseness following general anesthesia. Anesthesiology 67:419, 1987
16. McGinnis Ge, Shively KG, Patterson RL, et al: An engineering analysis of intratracheal tube cuffs. Anesth Analg 50:557, 1971
17. Banner MJ, Kirby RR, Blanch PB, et al: Decreasing imposed work of breathing apparatus to zero using pressure support ventilation. Crit Care Med 21:1333, 1993
18. Stetson JB, Guess WL: Causes of damage to tissues by polymers and elastomers used in the fabrication of tracheal devices. Anesthesiology 33:635, 1970
19. Steen JA: Impact of tube design and material on complications of tracheal intubation. Problems in Anesthesia 2:211, 1988
20. Lindholm CE: Prolonged endotracheal intubation: a clinical investigation with specific reference to its consequences for the larynx and the trachea and to its place as an alternative to intubation through a tracheostomy. Acta Anaesthesiol Scand Suppl 33, 1969
21. Bishop MJ, Fink BR, Hibbard AW, et al: Quantification of intralaryngeal pressure exerted by endotracheal tubes. Ann Otol Rhinol Laryngol 92:444, 1983
22. Baron SH, Kahlmoos HW: Laryngeal sequelae of endotracheal anesthesia. Ann Otol Rhinol Laryngol 60:767, 1951
23. Hilding AC: Laryngotracheal damage during intratracheal anesthesia: demonstration by staining the unfixed specimen with methylene blue. Ann Otol Rhinol Laryngol 80:565, 1971
24. Cooper JD, Grillo HC: Analysis of problems related to cuffs on intratracheal tubes. Chest 62:21(Suppl), 1972
25. Pavlin EG, Van Nimwegan D, Hornbein TF: Failure of high-compliance low-pressure cuff to prevent aspiration. Anesthesiology 42:216, 1975
26. Benumof JL: Management of the difficult and adult airway: With special emphasis on awake tracheal intubation. Anesthesiology 75:1087, 1991
27. Bedford RF: Circulatory responses to tracheal intubation. Problems in Anesthesia 2:201, 1988
28. Prys-Roberts C, Greene LT, Meloche R, et al: Studies of anaesthesia in relation to hypertension: II. haemodynamic consequences of induction and endotracheal intubation. Br J Anaesth 43:531, 1971
29. Bedford RF, Feinstein B: Hospital admission blood pressure: a predictor for hypertension following endotracheal intubation. Anesth Analg 59:367, 1980
30. Yakaitis RW, Blitt CD, Angiulo JP: End-tidal halothane concentration for endotracheal intubation. Anesthesiology 47:386, 1977
31. Yakaitis RW, Blitt CD, Angiulo JP: End-tidal enflurane concentration for endotracheal intubation. Anesthesiology 50:59, 1979
32. Roizen MF, Horrigan RW, Frazer BM: Anesthetic doses that block adrenergic (stress) and cardiovascular responses to incision: MAC-BAR. Anesthesiology 54:390, 1981
33. Kautto HM: Attenuation of the circulatory responses to laryngoscopy and intubation by fentanyl. Acta Anaesthesiol Scand 26:217, 1982
34. Chen CT, Toung TJK, Donham RT, et al: Fentanyl dosage for suppression of circulatory response to laryngoscopy and endotracheal intubation. Anesthesiology Review 13:37, 1986
35. Crawford DC, Fell D, Achola KJ, et al: Effects of alfentanil on the pressor and catecholamine responses to tracheal intubation. Br J Anaesth 59:707, 1987
36. Abou-Madi MN, Keszler H, Yacoub JM: Cardiovascular reactions to laryngoscopy and tracheal intubation following small and large intravenous doses of lidocaine. Can Anaesth Soc J 24:12, 1977
37. Tam S, Chung F, Campbell M: Intravenous lidocaine: optimal time of injection before tracheal intubation. Anesth Analg 66: 1036, 1987
38. Stoelting RK: Attenuation of blood pressure response to laryngoscopy and tracheal intubation with sodium nitroprusside. Anesth Analg 58:116, 1979
39. Davies MJ, Cronin KD, Cowie RW: The prevention of hypertension at intubation: a controlled study of intravenous hydralazine on patients undergoing intracranial surgery. Anaesthesia 36:147, 1981
40. Gallagher JD, Moore RA, Jose AB, et al: Prophylactic nitroglycerin infusions during coronary artery bypass surgery. Anesthesiology 64:785, 1986
41. Van Aken H, Puchstein C, Hidding J: The prevention of hypertension at intubation. Anaesthesia 37:82, 1982
42. Gold MI, Brown M, Coverman S, et al: Heart rate and blood pressure effects of esmolol after ketamine induction and intubation. Anesthesiology 64:718, 1986
43. Denlinger JK, Ellison N, Ominsky AJ: Effects of intratracheal lidocaine on circulatory responses to tracheal intubation. Anesthesiology 41:409, 1974
44. Brain AIJ: The laryngeal mask: a new concept in airway management. Br J Anaesth 55:801, 1983
45. Brain AIJ, McGhee TD, McAteer EJ, et al: The laryngeal mask airway: development and preliminary trials of a new type of airway. Anaesthesia 40:356, 1985
46. Snow JC, Norton ML, Saluja TS, et al: Fire hazard during CO_2 laser microsurgery on the larynx and trachea. Anesth Analg 55: 146, 1976
47. Ossoff ARG: Laser safety in otolaryngology: head and neck surgery—anesthetic and educational considerations for laryngeal surgery. Laryngoscope 99(suppl 48):1, 1989
48. Hirshman CA, Smith J: Indirect ignition of the endotracheal tube during carbon dioxide laser surgery. Arch Otolaryngol 106: 639, 1980
49. Simpson JL, Wolf GL: Endotracheal tube fire ignited by pharyngeal electrocautery. Anesthesiology 65:76, 1986
50. Hermens JM, Bennet MJ, Hirshman CA: Anesthesia for laser surgery: a review. Anesth Analg 62:218, 1983
51. Van Der Spek AFL, Spargo PM, Norton ML: The physics of lasers and implications for their use during airway surgery. Br J Anaesth 60:709, 1988
52. Paes ML: General anaesthesia for carbon dioxide laser surgery within the larynx. Br J Anaesth 59:1610, 1987
53. Oliveri RM, Ruder CB, Abramson AL: Jet ventilation for laryngeal microsurgery. Br J Anaesth 53:1010, 1981
54. Kaeder CS, Hirshman CA: Acute airway obstruction: a complication of aluminum tape wrapping of tracheal tubes in laser surgery. Can Anaesth Soc J 26:138, 1979
55. Sosis MB: Evaluation of five metallic tapes for protection of endotracheal tubes during CO_2 laser surgery. Anesth Analg 68: 392, 1989
56. Hirshman CA, Leon D, Porch D, et al: Improved metal endotracheal tube for laser surgery of the airway. Anesth Analg 59: 789, 1980
57. Wolf GL, Simpson JI: Flammability of endotracheal tubes in oxygen- and nitrous oxide–enriched atmosphere. Anesthesiology 67:236, 1987
58. Pashayan AG, Gravenstein JS, Cassisi NJ, et al: The helium protocol for laryngotracheal operations with CO_2 laser: a retrospective review of 523 cases. Anesthesiology 68:801, 1988
59. Pashayan AG, San Giovanni C, Davis LE: Positive end-expiratory pressure lowers the risk of laser-induced polyvinylchloride tracheal tube fires. Anesthesiology 79:83, 1993
60. Elwany S, Mekhamer A: Effect of nasotracheal intubation on nasal mucociliary clearance. Br J Anaesth 59:755, 1987
61. Dinner M, Tjeuw M, Artusio JF: Bacteremia as a complication of nasotracheal intubation. Anesth Analg 66:460, 1987

62. Willatts SW, Cochrane DF: Paranasal sinusitis: a complication of nasotracheal intubation. Br J Anaesth 57:1026, 1985
63. Caplan RA, Posner KL, Ward RJ, et al: Adverse respiratory events in anesthesia: a closed claim analysis. Anesthesiology 72:828, 1990
64. Owen RL, Cheney FW: Endobronchial intubation: a preventable complication. Anesthesiology 67:255, 1987
65. Sulek CA: Negative pressure pulmonary edema. Current Reviews in Clinical Anesthesia 13:9, 1992
66. Cooper JB, Newbower RS, Kitts RJ: An analysis of major errors and equipment failures in anesthesia management: consideration for prevention and detection. Anesthesiology 60:34, 1984
67. Hartley M, Vaughan RS: Problems associated with tracheal extubation. Br J Anaesth 71:561, 1993
68. Jordon WS, Graves CL, Elwyn RA: New therapy for postintubation laryngeal edema and tracheitis in children. JAMA 212: 585, 1970
69. Pender JW: Endotracheal anesthesia in children: advantages and disadvantages. Anesthesiology 15:495, 1954
70. Duncan PG: Efficacy of helium-oxygen mixtures in the management of severe viral and post-intubation croup. Can Anaesth Soc J 26:206, 1979
71. Geffin B, Pontoppidan H: Reduction of tracheal damage by the prestretching of inflatable cuffs. Anesthesiology 31:462, 1969
72. Klainer AS, Turndorf H, Wu W, et al: Surface alterations due to endotracheal intubation. Am J Med 58:674, 1975
73. Loeser EA, Hodges M, Gliedman J, et al: Tracheal pathology following short-term intubation with low- and high-pressure endotracheal tube cuffs. Anesth Analg 57:577, 1978
74. Mackenzie CF, Shin B, McAslan TC, et al: Severe stridor after prolonged endotracheal intubation using high-volume cuffs. Anesthesiology 50:235, 1979
75. Howland WS, Lewis JS: Post-intubation granulomas of the larynx. Cancer 9:1244, 1965
76. Snow JC, Harano M, Balough K: Postintubation granuloma of the larynx. Anesth Analg 45:425, 1966
77. Kirchner JA, Sasaki CT: Fusion of the vocal cords following intubation and tracheostomy. Transactions of the American Academy of Ophthalmology and Otolaryngology 77:88, 1973
78. Geffin B, Bland J, Grillo HC: Anesthetic management of tracheal resection and reconstruction. Anesth Analg 48:884, 1969
79. Webb WR, Ozdemir IA, Ikins PM, et al: Surgical management of tracheal stenosis. Ann Surg 179:819, 1974
80. Teichner RL: Lingual nerve injury: a complication of orotracheal intubation. Br J Anaesth 43:413, 1971

FURTHER READING

Applebaum EL, Bruce DL: Tracheal intubation. Philadelphia: WB Saunders Company, 1976

Bishop MJ (ed): Physiology and consequences of tracheal intubation. Problems in Anesthesia 2:1, 1988

Latto IP, Rosen M: Difficulties in tracheal intubation. London: Ballière-Tindall, 1985

Miller KA, Harkin CP, Bailey PL: Postoperative tracheal extubation (review article). Anesth Analg 80:149, 1995

Sykes WS: Essays on the first hundred years of anaesthesia, vol 2. Edinburgh: E & S Livingstone, 1960: 95

Complications in Anesthesiology, second edition, edited by Nikolaus Gravenstein and Robert R. Kirby. Lippincott-Raven Publishers, Philadelphia © 1996.

CHAPTER 19

Pneumothorax

J. Kenneth Denlinger

Pneumothorax was recognized as a potential hazard of mechanical ventilation shortly after the introduction of tracheal intubation, in the 19th century.[1] As early as 1828, excessive pressure applied to the trachea by a bellows was known to produce lung rupture. As a result, it was suggested that the handles of the bellows be equipped with a safety "stop-catch" to prevent overdistention of the lungs.[1] In 1912, several cases of pulmonary overdistention resulting in death were reported.[2]

Although pneumothorax does not occur as frequently as originally was feared by investigators who introduced positive-pressure ventilation, case reports of intraoperative pneumothorax continue to appear. The incidence of iatrogenic pneumothorax has increased markedly in the past two to three decades as a result of more frequent use of subclavian and internal jugular venipuncture, pulmonary artery catheterization,[3] prolonged mechanical ventilation[4–9], and external cardiac massage.[10] Increased application of new and old diagnostic and therapeutic procedures—laparoscopy, thoracentesis, amniocentesis, fiberoptic bronchoscopy,[11] jet ventilation (with or without laser surgery of the airway),[12–16] and acupuncture—has resulted in a variety of other causes of pneumothorax.

Because tension pneumothorax may be manifested by unexplained hypotension or wheezing during anesthesia, prompt diagnosis of the complication is often difficult. Rapid cardiorespiratory failure can occur with positive-pressure ventilation, and enlargement of the enclosed gas-filled space is accelerated by inward diffusion of nitrous oxide. Although pneumothorax can be treated easily and successfully, it has been associated with significant mortality during mechanical ventilation.

An understanding of the pathophysiologic features and clinical presentation of pneumothorax will permit this potentially fatal anesthetic complication to be recognized early and treated aggressively.

PATHOPHYSIOLOGIC FEATURES

Pneumothorax can occur by way of three mechanisms: (1) intrapulmonary alveolar rupture, with retrograde perivascular dissection of air, which produces mediastinal emphysema; (2) injury to the visceral pleura, with escape of air into the pleural space; or (3) interruption of the parietal pleura, with entry of air from adjoining structures (peritoneal cavity, mediastinum, or thoracic wall). Although simple lung collapse occurring by way of any of these mechanisms may be relatively innocuous, tension pneumothorax is a life-threatening emergency.

Intrapulmonary Alveolar Rupture

Mechanism

The mechanism by which intrapulmonary alveolar rupture (Table 19-1) leads to pneumothorax is diagrammed in Figure 19-1. Macklin and Macklin distinguished partitional alveoli, surrounded by other alveoli, from marginal alveoli, which adjoin blood vessels and bronchi.[17] Distention of partitional alveoli by excessive airway pressure is limited by distention of surrounding alveoli; therefore, rupture is unlikely. Distention of marginal alveoli is more likely to result in alveolar wall rupture at the interface with adjoining vascular and bronchial structures. In this situation, perivascular gas then escapes from the site of alveolar rupture and dissects toward the hilum of the lung and mediastinum; gas then ruptures through the mediastinal pleura. The perivascular spread of gas can be distributed as tiny bubbles throughout the lung, in some cases producing pulmonary interstitial emphysema. This interstitial emphysema can cause pulmonary ventilation–perfusion abnormalities, which may persist after reexpansion of the collapsed lung.

Pressure Gradients

Normal intrapleural pressure during quiet, spontaneous ventilation is slightly subatmospheric (−3 to −6 mm Hg). However, intrapleural pressures exceeding ±100 mm Hg may be observed during coughing, laryngospasm, and initial expansion of the lungs at birth. These pressures are physiologic extremes, required at times for maintenance of the lung's structural integrity. Instantaneous airway or pleural pressures of this magnitude may be relatively unimportant among the causes of alveolar rupture. Rather, alveolar rupture is related to disten-

TABLE 19-1
Causes of Alveolar Rupture

- Positive-pressure ventilation
  - Positive end-expiratory pressure?
  - Continuous positive airway pressure?
- Chronic obstructive lung disease
  - Bullae
  - Blebs
- Hypovolemia
- Cough
- Necrotizing pneumonia
- Blast injury

tion that occurs when a pressure gradient is maintained across the alveolar wall for some time.[18]

The safe limits of time and pressure in humans have not been determined. A sustained intrabronchial pressure of 24 mm Hg regularly produces interstitial emphysema in dogs.[19] In humans, phasic pressures of less than 25 mm Hg are reported to be relatively safe; pressures from 30 to 80 mm Hg are potentially dangerous; and pressures greater than 80 mm Hg are definitely hazardous.[20]

Expiratory Obstruction

Expiratory obstruction that produces excessive positive airway pressure and tension pneumothorax has resulted from malfunction of expiratory valve mechanisms in anesthesia breathing systems.[21,22] In one case, a valve disk was misplaced during reassembly of an anesthesia circle-absorber system and resulted in lung rupture by way of this mechanism.[23] Lung inflation by delivery of oxygen at a pressure of 50 pounds per square inch from the flush valve of an anesthesia machine to an Ayres T-piece system also has been reported to cause pneumothorax.[24]

Simple inattention and failure to observe the distended breathing bag during controlled manual ventilation also predisposes to alveolar rupture. Other mechanical causes of excessively high inflation pressure produced by interference with exhalation include overinflation of a tracheal cuff, with cuff herniation over the tip of the endotracheal tube; asymmetric inflation of a tracheal cuff, causing the beveled tube orifice to rest against the tracheal wall; and tube compression by an overinflated cuff further distended by nitrous oxide.

Excessive Stretching of Normal Alveoli

Excessive stretching of normal alveoli is another mechanism by which pneumothorax may occur in some lung diseases characterized by a patchy distribution of atelectasis.[25,26] Aspiration of meconium in the neonate and segmental airway obstruction by any cause limit the expansion of some pulmonary segments and increase that of others, predisposing the latter to alveolar rupture. The increased risk of pneumothorax in neonates with respiratory distress syndrome or diaphragmatic hernia may be due to pulmonary dysplasia in addition to segmental lung overdistention.

Weakening of Alveolar Septa

Intrapulmonary rupture also may be related to weakening of the alveolar septa, such as that accompanying pulmonary infection. The increased incidence of pneumothorax in necrotizing pneumonia, chronic lung disease, cystic fibrosis, some collagen diseases, and hypovolemic shock may be related to alveolar structural abnormalities and airway obstruction.

Injury to Visceral Pleura

Mechanisms

Air also can enter the pleural space through a rent in the visceral pleura (Fig. 19-2 and Table 19-2). The increased in-

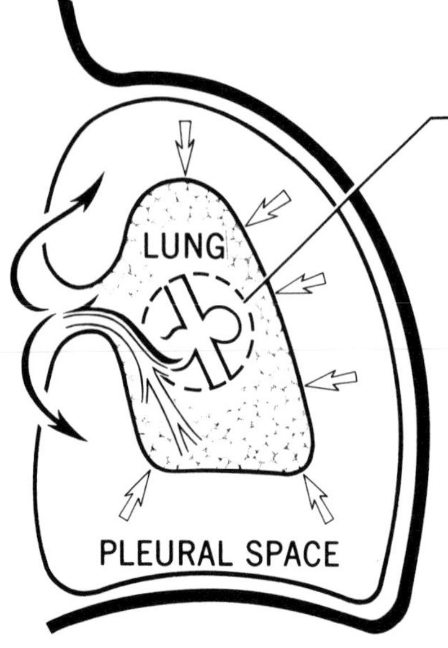

Alveolar rupture (magnified schematically) may be due to:

A. Increased airway pressure
   1. Expiratory valve dysfunction
   2. Overstretch of normal alveoli in segmental lung disease
   3. Cough, Valsalva
B. Weakened alveolar septum
   1. Infection (e.g. necrotizing pneumonia)
   2. Chronic lung disease (e.g. emphysema)
   3. Hypovolemic Shock

FIGURE 19-1. A pneumothorax that results from intrapulmonary rupture, perivascular dissection of air to the hilum, and rupture of the mediastinal pleura.

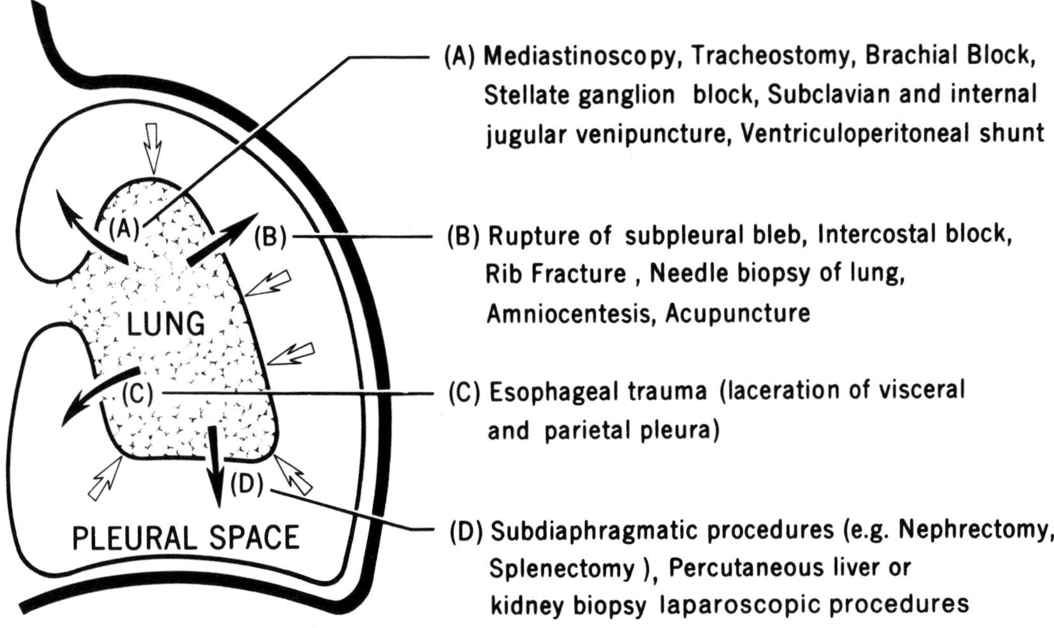

FIGURE 19-2. A pneumothorax that results from a break in the visceral pleura.

cidence of pneumothorax in parturient patients may result from "bearing down" and rupture of a subpleural bleb during labor. Pneumothorax after laryngospasm, bronchospasm, or cough presumably also results from rupture of an emphysematous bleb. A direct connection is then established between the terminal bronchus and the pleural space (forming a bronchopleural fistula). In these cases, the ruptured emphysematous bleb can function as a valve that permits flow of gas unidirectionally from the bronchus to the pleural space. A pressure gradient from the terminal bronchus to the pleural space results in progressive accumulation of pleural gas and can eventuate in tension pneumothorax.

The causes of pleural injury that may lead to pneumothorax are many and varied. The most common are thoracic trauma with fracture of the ribs and iatrogenic disorders resulting from needle puncture of incision of the pleura. Laparoscopic procedures represent an increasingly common cause as well.

TABLE 19-2
Causes of Visceral Pleural Rupture

- Nerve blocks
  - Intercostal
  - Interscalene
  - Supraclavicular
  - Infraclavicular
- Vascular cannulation
  - Internal jugular
  - Subclavian
- Tracheostomy
- Liver biopsy
- Lung biopsy
- Kidney biopsy

Needle Puncture

Pleural laceration during internal jugular and especially subclavian venipuncture is fairly common. Pneumothorax is a known complication of intercostal, thoracic, paravertebral, brachial plexus (especially supraclavicular and interscalene approaches), phrenic, and stellate ganglion nerve blocks. Although air can enter the thorax through the needle at the time of administration of the nerve block, typically this type of pneumothorax develops 6 to 12 hours after the block, suggesting that air passes slowly and progressively through a pleural rent.[27]

Tracheotomy and Other Operative Procedures

Pleural trauma may occur during tracheotomy (especially in children), other neck procedures, mediastinoscopy, thoracotomy, and subdiaphragmatic procedures (eg, nephrectomy).[28-31] Pneumothorax resulting from pleural trauma has occurred after percutaneous liver biopsy, renal biopsy, nephrectomy, splenectomy, adrenalectomy, and ventriculoperitoneal shunt insertion.[18-32] It also has been reported after acupuncture.[33] Pleural laceration in utero, during amniocentesis, is known to cause neonatal pneumothorax.[34] When visceral pleural discontinuity by any cause occurs, airway pressures that ordinarily would be safe can produce tension pneumothorax.

Injury to Parietal Pleura

Air also can enter the pleural space through a break in the parietal pleura, as may occur with open chest trauma (Fig. 19-3 and Table 19-3). Artificial air conduits, including open chest tubes or cardiac pacemaker wire sheaths,[35] also have

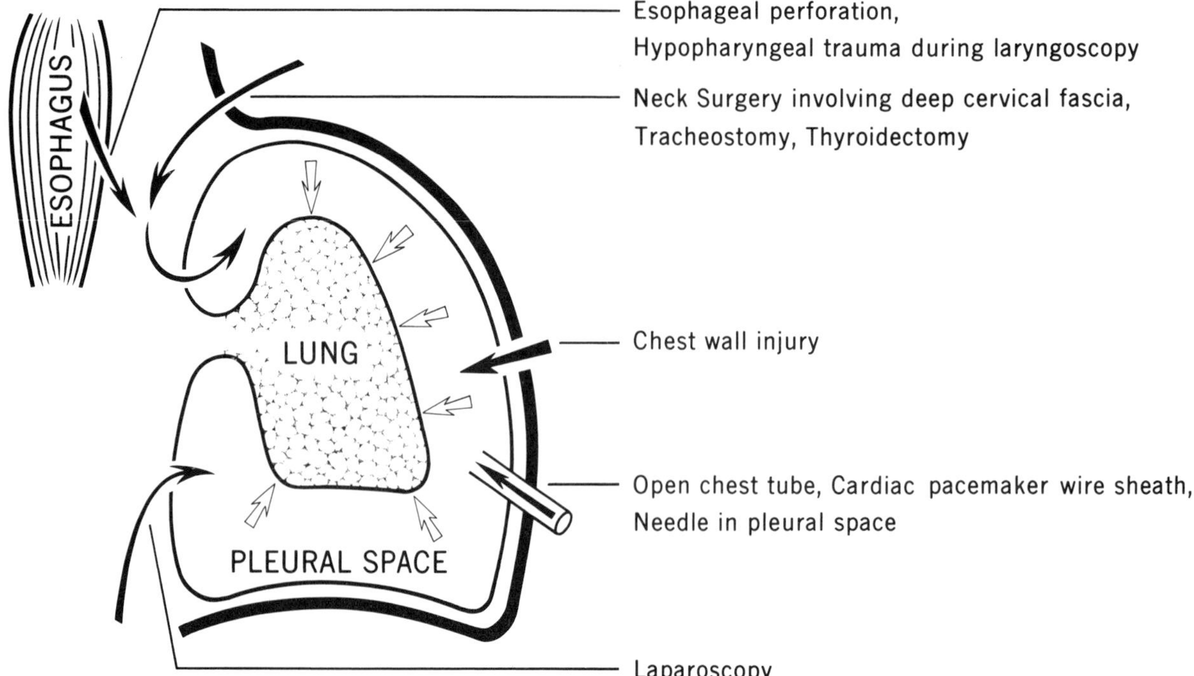

FIGURE 19-3. A pneumothorax that results from a break in the parietal pleura.

caused pneumothorax by this mechanism. Pneumoperitoneum induced to facilitate laparoscopy or the procedure itself may result in retroperitoneal, para-aortic air dissection, with mediastinal pleural rupture and pneumothorax.[36–38] Alternatively, diaphragmatic defects provide a pathway by which peritoneal gas enters the chest. Finally, pneumothorax sometimes complicates thyroidectomy, tracheotomy, stellate ganglionectomy, or radical neck dissection, in which exposure of the deep cervical fascia provides a portal by which air enters the mediastinum.

The pretracheal layer of the deep cervical fascia invests the trachea and extends directly into the mediastinum. Simple exposure of the cervical fascia to the atmosphere probably is not sufficient to produce pneumothorax. Dissection of air along the cervical fascia usually is associated with excessive negative airway pressures developed during obstructed or labored respiration.

TABLE 19-3
Causes of Parietal Pleural Rupture

- Penetrating trauma
  - Bullet
  - Knife
- Perforation
  - Tracheal
  - Mediastinal
  - Esophageal
- Operative procedures
  - Tracheotomy
  - Nephrectomy
  - Rib resection
  - Laparoscopy
  - Spinal fusion

Paratracheal air dissection results in pneumomediastinum followed by pneumothorax as the mediastinal parietal pleura ruptures. Air also may enter the mediastinum by way of esophageal or hypopharyngeal perforation.[39] Positive-pressure ventilation by face mask during induction of anesthesia in a patient with hypopharyngeal or esophageal perforation has been reported as a cause of tension pneumothorax.[40]

TENSION PNEUMOTHORAX

Hemodynamic Effects

Tension pneumothorax can produce hypotension, increased pulmonary artery pressures, and circulatory collapse by several mechanisms.

Hypoxia and Acidosis

Hypoventilation produces hypoxia and hypercapnia, leading to circulatory depression. Studies in goats subjected to progressive pneumothorax by pleural air injection indicated that severe hypoxia, respiratory acidosis, tachycardia, and a decrease in stroke volume occurred before the obstruction to venous return was significant enough to interfere with cardiac output.[41] These investigators concluded that severe hypoxia is a more likely explanation for the hemodynamic sequelae of pneumothorax than is mechanical venous obstruction, as traditionally was thought.

Obstruction to Venous Return

Mechanical obstruction to systemic venous return occurs as the mediastinal structures are displaced toward the contralateral hemithorax. A decrease in cardiac filling is associated with decreased stroke volume and arterial hypotension. Initially, this effect is masked by an increased heart rate, which serves to maintain cardiac output under conditions of decreased stroke volume. Both the compressive effect of the pneumothorax on the pulmonary vasculature as well as hypoxic pulmonary vasoconstriction probably contribute to the increase in pulmonary artery pressures seen during tension pneumothorax.[42]

Coronary Air Embolization

Cardiovascular depression is not always reversible, even when the chest is promptly decompressed by thoracostomy. It has been hypothesized that in these rare instances, pulmonary interstitial air gains entry to the pulmonary circulation and that embolization to the coronary arteries ensues.[42] Air has been observed in the coronary circulation of patients who have died after tension pneumothorax and cardiac arrest. Experimental lung rupture in dogs has produced coronary air embolization and reversal of pulmonary artery flow, with retrograde air entry into the right ventricle.[42] Although these data perhaps are not directly applicable to humans, they may explain the observed association of coronary air embolism and pulmonary overdistention.

The Hazard of Nitrous Oxide

Anesthetic-induced expansion of an enclosed gas-filled space, such as a pneumothorax, can contribute to rapid development of tension pneumothorax. The solubility of nitrous oxide in blood is 34 times greater than that of nitrogen. Therefore, blood exposed to an air-filled pneumothorax discharges nitrous oxide into the space much more rapidly than nitrogen is absorbed into the blood, provided that the partial pressure gradients of the two gases are similar.

Eger and Saidman quantitated the rate of increase of intrapleural gas volume in dogs breathing 68% to 78% nitrous oxide (Fig. 19-4).[43] The initial 300 mL of air placed in the pleural space doubled in 10 minutes, tripled in 45 minutes, and, in one dog, quadrupled in 2 hours. Thus, administration of high concentrations of nitrous oxide is contraindicated in patients with pneumothorax or in patients who have intrapulmonary cysts or nonventilated bullae. Of note, the presence of a chest tube does not guarantee that a pneumothorax is completely evacuated; the pneumothorax may be loculated, or the chest tube may be obstructed. It is therefore prudent to avoid nitrous oxide, even if a chest tube is in place.

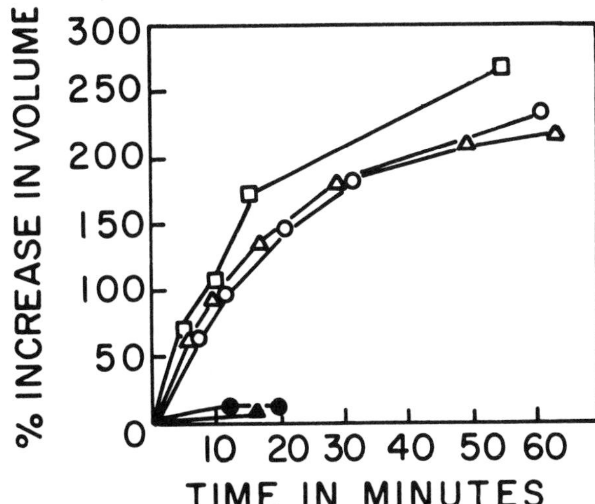

FIGURE 19-4. An increase in intrapleural gas volume occurs on administration of nitrous oxide (*open squares, open circles,* and *open triangles*), as opposed to a change in volume on administration of oxygen plus halothane (*solid* triangles and *solid circles*). (Eger EI, Saidman LJ: Hazards of nitrous oxide anesthesia in bowel obstruction and pneumothorax. Anesthesiology 26:64, 1965.)

CLINICAL PRESENTATION

The clinical presentation of pneumothorax depends on the patient's level of consciousness, associated cardiopulmonary disease, and age, and on whether the pneumothorax is simple or under tension.

Awake Adults

In the awake adult, pneumothorax is first evidenced by tachycardia, cough, and chest pain that often is referred to the shoulder area and is accentuated by deep breathing or a change in posture. Progressive expansion of the pneumothorax leads to tachypnea, dyspnea, and cyanosis. Severe hypoxia eventually produces loss of consciousness and cardiovascular collapse.

Physical examination reveals breath sounds that are decreased over the involved hemithorax; frequently, expiratory wheezing is heard, and hyperresonance and decreased vocal fremitus may be elicited. Air in the mediastinum may be evidenced by a mediastinal "crunch" heard on auscultation (Hamman's sign). The trachea may be deviated contralaterally if the pneumothorax is under tension, and subcutaneous emphysema may be observed.

Electrocardiographic changes mimicking acute myocardial infarction have been reported.[44] Left-sided tension pneumothorax typically produces low voltage in the precordial leads. However, before the aforementioned symptoms appear, the presence of pulmonary interstitial gas as subpleural air cysts may be detected on the chest radiograph as the first sign of barotrauma.[45] With continued exposure to high transpulmonary pressure, these small air collections portend tension pneumothorax.

Anesthetized Patients

Detection of pneumothorax in the anesthetized patient presents a more difficult diagnostic challenge. Frequently, the first signs are tachycardia and hypotension. These nonspecific findings usually direct the clinician to consider more common problems, such as anesthetic overdose or hypovolemia. As the pneumothorax expands, reduction in pulmonary compliance becomes evident. Increased airway pressure is required to maintain ventilation, and subcutaneous emphysema may appear.

As in the awake patient, examination of the chest reveals

decreased breath sounds, wheezing, and hyperresonance on the affected side. Central venous pressure may be elevated, and the trachea may be deviated away from the affected side. Progressive hypoxia and hypercapnia lead to obvious cyanosis, cardiac dysrhythmias, and finally circulatory arrest. The diagnosis of unilateral tension pneumothorax often can be aided by comparison of physical signs elicited over each hemithorax. However, tension pneumothorax may occur bilaterally, with decreased air entry, wheezing, and hyperresonance over the entire thorax.

The Postoperative Period

In the postoperative period, pneumothorax must be considered in the differential diagnosis of either respiratory or circulatory distress. Intraoperative pleural trauma can result in a pneumothorax that develops slowly and that first appears as postoperative restlessness in the patient. In a large series of patients requiring mechanical ventilation, the most reliable signs of tension pneumothorax were subcutaneous emphysema, tachycardia, decreased breath sounds, hyperresonance, and hypotension.[4] These signs invariably were associated with increasing arterial carbon dioxide partial pressure and decreasing arterial oxygen partial pressure.

The Neonate

Pneumothorax in the neonate is evidenced by tachypnea, increased irritability, grunting, retractions, and cyanosis. The chest may bulge on one side, and the apical cardiac impulse may be shifted. A sudden appearance of cyanosis and bradycardia in any neonate with pulmonary disease necessitating respiratory care should alert the physician to the immediate possibility of tension pneumothorax.

INCIDENCE

Pneumothorax complicating anesthesia is sufficiently uncommon that precise data describing its incidence are not available, except in relation to specific high-risk procedures. Moore and Bridenbaugh found a 1% incidence of pneumothorax after supraclavicular brachial plexus block.[27] Percutaneous needle biopsy of the lung is associated with pneumothorax in approximately 30% of cases.[46] Etiologic classification of 544 cases of pneumothorax by Steier and colleagues revealed that 209 were attributable to complications of hospital care, such as subclavian venipuncture and external cardiac massage.[4] Of the remaining instances, 179 were related to various types of chest trauma; 150 developed "spontaneously"; and 6 were thought to be related to pulmonary infection.

Mechanical Ventilation

The incidence of pneumothorax in patients requiring mechanical ventilation ranges from 0.5% to 39%.[6,7] Initially, the use of positive end-expiratory pressure (PEEP) in the treatment of patients with respiratory failure was believed to increase pneumothorax and pneumomediastinum greatly. Yet subsequent studies found that adult patients treated with PEEP plus mechanical ventilation showed no greater incidence of pneumothorax than did those treated with mechanical ventilation alone.[9,47] In only 14% of patients treated with high levels of PEEP (18 mm Hg or greater) did pneumothorax develop.[48]

Neonatal Respiratory Distress Syndrome

The incidence of pneumothorax in neonates with respiratory distress syndrome increases with the severity of the disease and with the aggressiveness of the therapy used to treat it.[25,49,50] In one study of infants with respiratory distress syndrome, pneumothorax occurred in 2 (3.5%) of 58 infants who did not receive assisted ventilation and in 14 (11%) of 124 infants who received treatment with continuous positive airway pressure.[48] Pneumothorax occurred in 12 (24%) of 49 infants who were initially treated with continuous positive airway pressure but later required mechanical ventilation with PEEP. Of 64 infants with severe respiratory distress syndrome who were initially treated with mechanical ventilation plus PEEP, pneumothorax occurred in 21 (33%). Although most infants with pneumothorax receive some form of positive-pressure ventilation, the complication probably results from the underlying severe pulmonary lesions that necessitate ventilatory assistance rather than from the inflation pressures per se.[50]

The incidence of spontaneous pneumothorax is higher in neonates than in any other age group. Routine radiographic screening revealed pneumothorax in 1% to 2% of neonates shortly after birth. However, the incidence of symptomatic pneumothorax requiring treatment is only 0.05% to 0.07%.[51]

DIFFERENTIAL DIAGNOSIS

Bronchospasm

The clinical presentation of pneumothorax can mimic that of bronchospasm during anesthesia. Pneumothorax and bronchospasm are more likely to occur in patients with chronic lung disease, and both are associated with wheezing, increased airway pressure, diminished breath sounds, cyanosis, and hypotension.[52] Anesthetic-induced bronchospasm may occur after tracheal intubation in patients with bronchial asthma, especially when the tracheobronchial tree is instrumented during light planes of anesthesia.

Pulmonary embolism and anaphylaxis are other causes of bronchospasm during anesthesia. The differential diagnosis must also include mechanical problems resulting from overinflation of the tracheal cuff, aspiration of a foreign body, or bronchial intubation. Deflation of the tracheal cuff and repositioning of the endotracheal tube often results in improved ventilation and cessation of wheezing in these cases. These mechanical airway difficulties are more common than true bronchospasm during modern anesthesia practice and therefore should be excluded immediately.

Because the signs of pneumothorax are so similar to those of true bronchospasm, recognition of pneumothorax during anesthesia is sometimes delayed while bronchodilator therapy is begun. Administration of aminophylline and/or beta agonists to the hypoxic, hypercapnic patient for a condition misdiagnosed as bronchospasm is dangerous and may result in fatal cardiac dysrhythmias.

Because the urgency of this situation does not usually permit definitive diagnosis by chest radiograph, pneumothorax must be distinguished on the basis of physical signs: hyperresonance, tracheal deviation, shifted cardiac impulse, and subcutaneous emphysema. The "scratch sign," elicited by scratching the skin over each hemithorax while listening through a stethoscope placed over the sternum, has been described as a valuable aid in the detection of unilateral tension pneumothorax.[53] A loud and harsh sound elicited over the hemithorax constitutes a sign positive for pneumothorax. When pneumothorax is strongly suggested, the diagnosis is confirmed by demonstration of gas escape through a large-bore needle inserted in the midclavicular sagittal plane into the second intercostal space and by resolution of other signs, such as hypoxemia, hypotension, and difficult ventilation.

Congestive Heart Failure or Myocardial Depression

Because tachycardia and hypotension are early signs of pneumothorax during anesthesia, congestive heart failure or anesthetic-induced cardiac depression must be included in the differential diagnosis. Pulmonary edema due to left ventricular failure also causes decreased pulmonary compliance, wheezing, and increased venous pressure, as in pneumothorax. Ischemic electrocardiographic changes may occur both in pulmonary edema and in pneumothorax. However, frank pulmonary edema is associated with pink, frothy fluid during tracheal aspiration, and pneumothorax is suggested by the finding of hyperresonance, tracheal deviation, and subcutaneous emphysema.

In at least one case report, tension pneumothorax was recognized only after thoracotomy was performed for direct cardiac massage, as a resuscitative measure after circulatory collapse.[54] In this case, thoracotomy might have been avoided by simple aspiration of air from the pleural space, had the diagnosis of pneumothorax been considered.

Pleural or Mediastinal Fluid

Rapid accumulation of pleural or mediastinal fluid from an infiltrated or improperly positioned central venous catheter, as well as hemothorax complicating central venipuncture, may produce cardiorespiratory signs simulating pneumothorax in the anesthetized patient. Pleural fluid is distinguished by dullness to percussion and is confirmed by chest radiograph or by thoracentesis.

Restlessness and Delirium

Pneumothorax must be considered in the differential diagnosis of postoperative restlessness and emergence delirium. In the presence of postoperative restlessness and tachypnea, administration of narcotics without careful evaluation of oxygenation, ventilation, and physical examination of the chest is never justified. In the awake patient, chest pain associated with tachycardia, tachypnea, and cough resulting from pneumothorax must be differentiated from that resulting from pulmonary embolism or myocardial infarction.

TREATMENT

Oxygen

As soon as pneumothorax is suggested, the patient should receive supplemental oxygen. Oxygen administration not only treats hypoxemia but also helps to reduce the gas pocket volume: oxygen washes out nitrogen or, during general anesthesia, nitrous oxide from the expanding gas space and is then better reabsorbed than either nitrogen or nitrous oxide. In addition, a high inspired oxygen fraction reduces the partial pressure of nitrogen (or nitrous oxide) in tissue, an effect that in turn facilitates absorption of gas from closed body spaces. In fact, oxygen therapy has been used successfully to treat pneumothorax in patients refusing conventional tube thoracostomy drainage.[55]

Needle Aspiration or Tube Thoracostomy

In general, a pneumothorax large enough to produce symptoms should be treated by needle aspiration or tube thoracostomy. In many cases, a small (<20%), asymptomatic pneumothorax after nerve block or minor pleural trauma resolves spontaneously and requires only observation. Many cases of neonatal pneumothorax develop slowly after birth and resolve spontaneously. However, neonatal pneumothorax that shows a rapid onset and is symptomatic should be treated. Repeated needle aspiration may be inadvisable because of the possibility of repeated trauma. Cardiac laceration and death have been reported after repeated needle aspiration of a pneumothorax in the neonate.[56]

Immediate treatment of tension pneumothorax usually is accomplished by insertion of a large-bore needle anteriorly through the second intercostal space in the midclavicular line. Several methods have been described for continued drainage of the pleural space. The Clagett-S needle is a blunt-tipped, S-shaped needle that has multiple drainage openings and that may be inserted intrapleurally to maintain lung expansion.[46] Insertion of 3-French silicone Silastic tube over a rigid stylet also has been advocated for the treatment of pneumothorax complicating radiologic procedures.[46] However, the most reliable method for obtaining proper pleural drainage and maintaining lung expansion is the insertion of a standard chest tube. A small plastic intravenous catheter threaded over or through a needle is not recommended for anything beyond the acute treatment phase because of subsequent problems with catheter kinking, obstruction, and displacement.[57]

Reexpansion Pulmonary Edema

Intercostal air drainage for reexpansion of pneumothorax is occasionally associated with pulmonary edema.[58] Although the mechanism is uncertain, the complication is associated with pneumothoraxes that are especially large, are evacuated rapidly, or have been present for more than a few days.

PREVENTION

Consideration of Predisposing Factors

Because the incidence of iatrogenic pneumothorax seems to be increasing, careful consideration of the risk–benefit ratio should precede certain procedures, such as subclavian venipuncture. The mortality and morbidity related to pneumothorax, however, need not be great if adequate observation of the patient is maintained. A pneumothorax should be considered a possibility whenever a central venous catheter is inserted by way of the subclavian[4] or internal jugular vein,[59] especially just before or after induction of anesthesia. Any otherwise unexplained hemodynamic deterioration in a patient with a recently placed (<3 days previously) central venous catheter should provoke an evaluation for pneumothorax as part of the differential diagnosis. Positive airway pressure and the use of high concentrations of nitrous oxide may convert a small, previously asymptomatic pneumothorax into a rapidly expanding tension pneumothorax.

Practitioners who perform intercostal, subclavian, perivascular, or interscalene nerve blocks; acupuncture; laparoscopy; bronchoscopy; percutaneous liver biopsy; or other procedures associated with pneumothorax should be prepared to treat this potential complication without delay.

Avoidance of High Inflation Pressures

Although high inflation pressures sometimes are required to reexpand atelectatic pulmonary segments, care should be exercised to avoid excessive airway pressure during anesthetic administration. Proper functioning of each anesthesia breathing system must be checked before use, and new or reassembled equipment should be inspected carefully. Poorly compliant breathing bags should not be used because of the higher peak pressures produced during unrecognized distention of the bag.[60]

Awareness of the Risk Factors

Avoidance of airway obstruction or of excessive negative airway pressure during neck surgery prevents most cases of pneumothorax that are due to air dissection along the deep cervical fascia into the mediastinum. Cases involving blunt chest trauma or fractured ribs should be managed with regional anesthesia, when possible, to prevent pneumothorax. Neonates requiring mechanical ventilation have a lower incidence of pneumothorax when pancuronium is used[61]; this therapy also hastens recovery of their underlying lung disease.[62] When positive-pressure ventilation is required in the management of chest trauma, tension pneumothorax should be strongly considered and treated at its earliest indication—at any sign of otherwise unexplained clinical deterioration.

Some of the mechanical factors predisposing to pulmonary barotrauma are listed in Table 19-4. A few are amenable to alternatives in therapy such as reduction of airway pressure by adjustment of ventilator inspiratory waveforms or rates; control of infection; and prevention of hypovolemia.[63,64]

TABLE 19-4
Mechanical Factors Responsible for Barotrauma

- High airway pressure
- Rapid respiratory rate
- Infection
  - Pulmonary
  - Systemic
- Diffuse alveolar injury
- Hypovolemia

REFERENCES

1. Gillespie NA: The history of endotracheal anesthesia. In Bamforth BJ, Siebecker KL (eds): Endotracheal anesthesia. Madison: University of Wisconsin Press, 1963: 6
2. Woolsey WC: Intratracheal insufflation anesthesia. New York State Journal of Medicine 12:167, 1912
3. Damen J, Bolton D: A prospective analysis of 1,400 pulmonary artery catheterizations in patients undergoing cardiac surgery. Acta Anaesthesiol Scand 30:386, 1986
4. Steier M, Ching N, Roberts EB, et al: Pneumothorax complicating continuous ventilatory support. J Thorac Cardiovasc Surg 67:17, 1974
5. Downs JB, Chapman RL: Treatment of bronchopleural fistula during continuous positive pressure ventilatory support. Chest 72:141, 1977
6. Cullen DJ, Caldera DL: The incidence of ventilator-induced pulmonary barotrauma in critically ill patients. Anesthesiology 50:185, 1979
7. Petersen GW, Baier H: Incidence of pulmonary barotrauma in a medical ICU. Crit Care Med 11:67, 1983
8. Mathru M, Rao TL, Venus B: Ventilator-induced barotrauma in controlled mechanical ventilation vs. intermittent mandatory ventilation. Crit Care Med 11:359, 1983
9. Pepe PE, Hudson LD, Carrico CJ: Early application of positive end-expiratory pressure in patients at risk for the adult respiratory-distress syndrome. N Engl J Med 311:281, 1984
10. Hillman K, Albin M: Pulmonary barotrauma during cardiopulmonary resuscitation. Crit Care Med 14:606, 1986
11. Simpson FG, Arnold AG, Purvis A, et al: Postal survey of bronchoscopic practice by physicians in the United Kingdom. Thorax 41:311, 1986
12. Vincken W, Cosio MG: Clinical applications of high-frequency jet ventilation. Intens Care Med 10:275, 1984
13. Wetmore SJ, Key JM, Suen JY: Complications of laser surgery for laryngeal papillomatosis. Laryngoscope 95:798, 1985
14. Shapshay SM, Beamis JF Jr: Safety precautions for bronchoscopic Nd-YAG laser surgery. Otolaryngol Head Neck Surg 94:175, 1986
15. Ferrari HA, Renner GJ, Luebrecht SM, et al: High-frequency jet ventilation: applications for endoscopy and surgery of the airway. South Med J 79:941, 1986
16. Rontal E, Rontal M, Wenokur ME: Jet insufflation anesthesia for endolaryngeal laser surgery: a review of 318 consecutive cases. Laryngoscope 95:990, 1985
17. Macklin MT, Macklin CC: Malignant interstitial emphysema of the lungs and mediastinum as an important occult complication in many respiratory diseases and other conditions. Medicine (Baltimore) 23:281, 1944
18. Hamilton WK: Atelectasis, pneumothorax, and aspiration as postoperative complications. Anesthesiology 22:708, 1961
19. Marcotte RJ, Phillips FJ, Adams WE, et al: Differential intrabronchial pressures and mediastinal emphysema. J Thorac Surg 9:346, 1940
20. Nennhaus HP, Javid H, Julian O: Alveolar and pleural rupture. Arch Surg 94:136, 1967
21. Martin JT, Patrick RT: Pneumothorax: its significance to the anesthesiologist. Anesth Analg 39:420, 1960
22. Aragon SB, Dolwick MF, Buckley S: Pneumomediastinum and

subcutaneous emphysema during third molar extraction under general anesthesia. J Oral Maxillofac Surg 44:141, 1986
23. Dean HN, Parsons DE, Raphaely RC: Case report: bilateral tension pneumothorax from mechanical failure of anesthesia machine due to misplaced expiratory valve. Anesth Analg 50:195, 1971
24. Arens JF: A hazard in the use of an Ayres T-piece. Anesth Analg 50:943, 1971
25. Berg TJ, Pagtakhan RD, Reed MH, et al: Bronchopulmonary dysplasia and lung rupture in hyaline membrane disease: influence of continuous distending pressure. Pediatrics 55:51, 1975
26. Siegel JH, Stoklosa JC, Borg U, et al: Quantification of asymmetric lung pathophysiology as a guide to the use of simultaneous independent lung ventilation in posttraumatic and septic adult respiratory distress syndrome. Ann Surg 202:425, 1985
27. Moore DC, Bridenbaugh LD: Pneumothorax: its incidence following brachial plexus block analgesia. Anesthesiology 15:475, 1954
28. Furgang FA, Saidman LJ: Bilateral tension pneumothorax associated with mediastinoscopy. J Thorac Cardiovasc Surg 63: 329, 1972
29. Meade JW: Tracheotomy: its complications and their management. N Engl J Med 265:529, 1961
30. Stromberg BV: Complications in plastic surgical anesthesia. Clin Plast Surg 12:91, 1985
31. Daugirdas JT, Leehey DJ, Popli S, et al: Subxiphoid pericardiotomy for hemodialysis-associated pericardial effusion. Arch Intern Med 146:1113, 1986
32. Portnoy HD, Croissant PD: Two unusual complications of a ventriculoperitoneal shunt. J Neurosurg 39:775, 1973
33. Goldberg I: Pneumothorax associated with acupuncture. Med J Aust 1:941, 1973
34. Hyman CJ, Depp R, Pakravan P, et al: Pneumothorax complicating amniocentesis. Obstet Gynecol 41:43, 1973
35. Linde LM, Mulder DG: Pneumothorax after externalization of cardiac pacemaker wires. N Engl J Med 272:682, 1965
36. McConnell MS, Finn JC, Feeley TW: Tension hydrothorax during laparoscopy in a patient with ascites. Anesthesiology 80: 1390, 1994
37. Chui PT, Gin T, Chung SCS: Subcutaneous emphysema, pneumomediastinum, and pneumothorax complicating laparoscopic vagotomy: report of two cases. Anaesthesia 48:978, 1993
38. Mangar D, Kirchhoff GT, Leal JJ, et al: Pneumothorax during laparoscopic Nissen fundoplication. Can J Anaesth 41:854, 1994
39. Hawkins DB, House JW: Postoperative pneumothorax secondary to hypopharyngeal perforation during anesthetic intubation. Ann Otol Rhinol Laryngol 83:556, 1974
40. Dundee JW: Tension pneumothorax during the induction of anaesthesia. Anaesthesia 10:74, 1955
41. Rutherford RB, Hurt HH Jr, Brickman RD, et al: The pathophysiology of progressive tension pneumothorax. J Trauma 8: 212, 1968
42. Lenaghan R, Silva YJ, Walt AJ: Hemodynamic alterations associated with expansion rupture of the lung. Arch Surg 99:339, 1969
43. Eger EI, Saidman LJ: Hazards of nitrous oxide anesthesia in bowel obstruction and pneumothorax. Anesthesiology 26:61, 1965
44. Summers RS: The electrocardiogram as a diagnostic aid in pneumothorax. Chest 63:127, 1973
45. Albelda SM, Gefter WB, Kelley MA, et al: Ventilator-induced subpleural air cysts: clinical, radiographic, and pathologic significance. Am Rev Respir Dis 127:360, 1983
46. Sargent EN, Turner AF: Emergency treatment of pneumothorax: a simple catheter technique for use in the radiology department. Am J Roentgenol Radium Ther Nucl Med 109:531, 1970
47. Kumar A, Pontoppidan J, Falke KJ, et al: Pulmonary barotrauma during mechanical ventilation. Crit Care Med 1:181, 1973
48. Kirby RR, Downs JB, Civetta JM, et al: High level positive end-expiratory pressure (PEEP) in acute respiratory insufficiency. Chest 67:156, 1975
49. Ogata ES, Gregory GA, Kitterman JA, et al: Pneumothorax in the respiratory distress syndrome: incidence and effect on vital signs, blood gases and pH. Pediatrics 58:177, 1976
50. Jones RM, Rutter N, Cooper AC, et al: Pneumothorax in the neonatal period. Anaesthesia 38:948, 1983
51. Chernick V, Reed MH: Pneumothorax and chylothorax in the neonatal period. J Pediatr 76:624, 1970
52. Gold MI, Joseph SI: Bilateral tension pneumothorax following induction of anesthesia in two patients with chronic obstructive airway disease. Anesthesiology 38:93, 1973
53. Lawson JD: The scratch sign: a valuable aid in the diagnosis of pneumothorax. N Engl J Med 264:88, 1961
54. Fitzgerald TB, Johnstone MW: Diaphragmatic defects and laparoscopy. Br Med J 2:604, 1970
55. Butler DA, Orlowski JP: Nitrogen washout therapy for pneumothorax. Cleve Clin Q 50:311, 1983
56. Shim WKI, Philip AGS: Danger of needle aspiration in pneumothorax in the newborn. JAMA 223:691, 1973
57. Withers JN, Fishback ME, Kiehl PV, et al: Spontaneous pneumothorax: suggested etiology and comparison of treatment methods. Am J Surg 108:772, 1964
58. Waqaruddin M, Bernstein A: Reexpansion pulmonary edema. Thorax 30:54, 1975
59. Arnold S, Feathers RS, Gibbs E: Bilateral pneumothoraces and subcutaneous emphysema: a complication of internal jugular venipuncture. Br Med J 1:211, 1973
60. Johnstone RE, Smith TC: Rebreathing bags as pressure-limiting devices. Anesthesiology 38:193, 1973
61. Greenough A, Wood S, Morley CJ, et al: Pancuronium prevents pneumothoraces in ventilated premature babies who actively expire against positive pressure inflation. Lancet 1:1, 1984
62. Pollitzer MJ, Reynolds EOR, Shaw DG, et al: Pancuronium during mechanical ventilation speeds recovery of lungs of infants with hyaline membrane disease. Lancet 1:346, 1984
63. Lenaghan R, Silva YJ, Walt AJ: Hemodynamic alteration associated expansion rupture of the lung. Arch Surg 99:339, 1969
64. Räsänen J, Downs JB: Modes of ventilatory support. In Kirby RR, Banner MJ, Downs JB (eds): Clinical applications of ventilatory support. New York: Churchill Livingstone, 1990: 173

FURTHER READING

Brown DL, Kirby RR: Pulmonary barotrauma. In Civetta JM, Taylor RW, Kirby RR (eds): Critical care, 2nd ed. Philadelphia: JB Lippincott, 1992: 1437

Hillman K: Pulmonary barotrauma. Clinics in Anaesthesiology 3:877, 1985

Powner DJ: Pulmonary barotrauma in the intensive care unit. J Intensive Care Med 3:224, 1988

Complications in Anesthesiology, second edition,
edited by Nikolaus Gravenstein and Robert R. Kirby.
Lippincott-Raven Publishers, Philadelphia © 1996.

CHAPTER 20

Hypoxemia and Hypercapnia During and After Anesthesia

Hillary F. Don

Hypoxemia is defined as a lower than normal partial pressure of oxygen in arterial blood (Pa_{O_2}). It does not include abnormalities of amount or type of hemoglobin. The interpretation of a normal value of Pa_{O_2} must consider the inspired oxygen fraction (FI_{O_2}), barometric pressure, the arterial carbon dioxide partial pressure (Pa_{CO_2}), and the posture and age of the subject. At sea level in the supine subject, the relation of Pa_{O_2} to age can be approximated as follows[1]:

$$Pa_{O_2} = 100 - 0.5 \times \text{age (in years) mm Hg}$$

This relation presumes normal alveolar carbon dioxide partial pressure (PA_{CO_2}) and Pa_{CO_2}. If the PA_{CO_2} and Pa_{CO_2} are reduced, alveolar oxygen partial pressure (PA_{O_2}) will increase, as exemplified by a simplified form of the alveolar gas equation:

$$PA_{O_2} = PI_{O_2} - \frac{PA_{CO_2}}{R} \text{ mm Hg}$$

where PI_{O_2} = the partial pressure of oxygen in dry inspired gas, and R = the respiratory quotient. Hypocapnia may, therefore, disguise a defect in oxygen exchange.

Hypercapnia exists when the Pa_{CO_2} is higher than the predicted normal level for the subject. Unlike Pa_{O_2}, Pa_{CO_2} remains remarkably constant with advancing age. With hypercapnia, the minute production of carbon dioxide ($\dot{V}_{CO_2}$) may or may not be excreted from the body. Elevation of Pa_{CO_2} and, therefore, of the alveolar carbon dioxide fraction, increases the removal of carbon dioxide with a given minute ventilation of expired alveolar gas. As the Pa_{CO_2} rises, carbon dioxide excretion initially will be less than its production. However, as a steady state develops at a higher Pa_{CO_2} level, excretion must become equal to production, or the Pa_{CO_2} will continue to rise.

HYPOXEMIA

General Considerations

Hypoxemia may be divided into two categories based on the PA_{O_2}.

1. Reduced PA_{O_2}: The Pa_{O_2} will parallel a reduction in PA_{O_2}. A decrease in PA_{O_2} is caused by either a reduced FI_{O_2} or a reduction in alveolar minute ventilation.
2. Normal or increased PA_{O_2}: An increase in the normally small difference between PA_{O_2} and Pa_{O_2} may occur. This alteration is sometimes called "venous admixture," because, conceptually, the Pa_{O_2}, which "should" be the same as that of the alveolus, is reduced, as if admixture with venous blood had occurred.

Three causes of venous admixture are described: diffusion defect; abnormal distribution of ventilation–perfusion ($\dot{V}_A/\dot{Q}$) ratios, with areas of the lungs in which alveolar minute ventilation, although reduced relative to perfusion, is greater than zero; and complete failure of ventilation of perfused parts of the lung ($\dot{V}_A/\dot{Q} = 0$), sometimes called a "shunt." Recognition of the latter category is important, because hypoxemia resulting from complete failure of ventilation is resistant to correction by increasing the FI_{O_2}.

Significance

Body tissues have a critical dependence on oxygen supply. Two factors must be considered: the content of oxygen in the arterial blood (Ca_{O_2}) and the actual level of Pa_{O_2}, which creates a driving pressure for movement of oxygen from the plasma to the tissues.

Arterial Blood Oxygen Content

The Ca_{O_2} is the sum of dissolved oxygen and that combined with hemoglobin (Hb_{O_2}). Dissolved oxygen ($Pa_{O_2} \times 0.003$ mL/dL of blood or plasma) is only a small fraction of Hb_{O_2} ([1.37 × hemoglobin] at 100% saturation). The shape of the oxygen–hemoglobin dissociation curve (Fig. 20-1) is such that even at a Pa_{O_2} of 40 mm Hg, hemoglobin is still approximately 75% saturated with oxygen. Below this partial pressure, a rapid reduction in Ca_{O_2} occurs.

Although a Pa_{O_2} below 40 mm Hg may be clinically unacceptable in terms of Ca_{O_2}, oxygen transport, which is the product of Ca_{O_2} and cardiac output, is the important consideration in terms of oxygen delivery to the capillary beds. Hence, an increase in hemoglobin, cardiac output, or both can restore oxygen transport toward normal levels in the face of a low Pa_{O_2}.

Capillary–Tissue Oxygen Partial Pressure Gradient

The second significant aspect in determining a satisfactory level of Pa_{O_2} is the pressure gradient that drives oxygen from the capillary bed to the tissue. If the gradient is low, the defect will not be corrected by changes in hemoglobin or cardiac output. It can be partially compensated by a shift of the Hb_{O_2} dissociation curve to the right, aiding the release of oxygen to the tissues. Such a shift is found with increases in hydrogen ion concentration, Pa_{CO_2}, temperature, and 2,3-diphosphoglycerate (see Fig. 20-1).[1] In states of chronic hypoxemia, increased levels of 2,3-diphosphoglycerate are present.

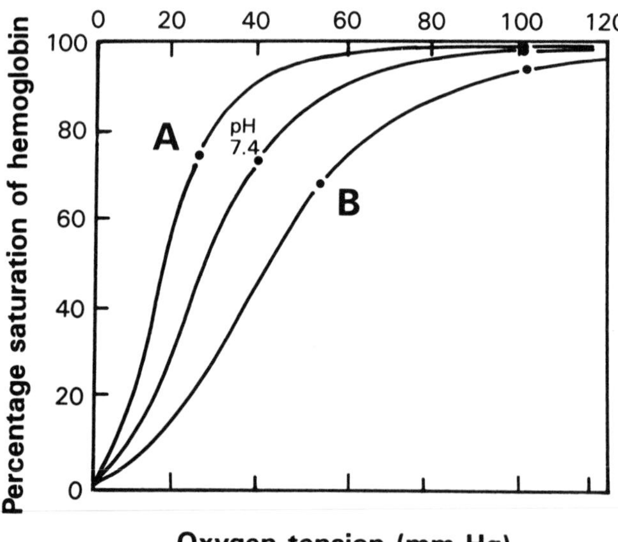

FIGURE 20-1. The shift in the Hb_{O_2} curve associated with changes in pH, P_{CO_2}, temperature, and 2,3-diphosphoglycerate concentration. The center curve is the normal curve under standard conditions; the other two curves show the leftward displacement (*curve A*) caused by a decrease and the rightward shift (*curve B*) caused by an increase in hydrogen ion concentration, temperature, P_{CO_2}, and 2,3-diphosphoglycerate concentration. (Cane RD, Rasanen J: Hypoxemia. In Kirby RR, Gravenstein N (eds): Clinical anesthesia practice. Philadelphia: WB Saunders, 1994:783.)

Critical Arterial Oxygen Partial Pressure

Determining the Pa_{O_2} that interferes with tissue oxygen delivery at the tissues is difficult. In a study by Cullen and Eger, hypoxemia (Pa_{O_2} = 38 mm Hg) reduced the minimum alveolar concentration (MAC) of halothane in dogs.[2] The investigators suggested that at this level of Pa_{O_2} cerebral oxygen uptake is impaired. That this phenomenon was not due merely to a reduction in Ca_{O_2} was supported by subsequent experiments, in which an equivalent reduction was produced by a decrease in hemoglobin.[3] In this situation, MAC was not reduced, suggesting that it was the "driving force" of Pa_{O_2} that was important. Therefore, a Pa_{O_2} below 40 mm Hg is unacceptable clinically, but not principally because of a failure of oxygen transport; rather, lowering of the oxygen-driving pressure is the significant factor.

Safety Margin

In determining an unsatisfactory level of Pa_{O_2} the available safety margin must be considered. When a patient is unstable, changes in cardiac output or a further increase in the impairment of gas exchange may drastically reduce Ca_{O_2} if the Pa_{O_2} approximates a value that is near the descending slope of the oxygen dissociation curve (see Fig. 20-1). Unless the avoidance of a high level of Pa_{O_2} is mandatory for some other reason (eg, chronic lung disease), the Pa_{O_2} should be maintained greater than or equal to 60 mm Hg, which represents a Hb_{O_2} saturation of greater than or equal to 90%.

Pulmonary Vascular Resistance

Apart from its effect on oxygen availability to tissues, hypoxemia is also potentially harmful to pulmonary vascular resistance. In spontaneously breathing dogs anesthetized with pentobarbital, the 1st minute of hypoxemia (Pa_{O_2} = 28 mm Hg) produces a 42% increase in pulmonary vascular resistance, which then falls to control levels. This return to normal in the presence of continued hypoxemia is caused by the accompanying hyperventilation and hypocapnia. The increase in pulmonary vascular resistance is not prevented by α- and β-adrenergic blockade.[4] Although the mechanism that mediates hypoxic pulmonary vasoconstriction is unknown, evidence suggests that local rather than nervous or humoral mechanisms are involved. Clinically, this effect of hypoxemia is significant, particularly in patients with chronic lung and cardiac disease.

Associated Disease States

Patients with certain disease states are peculiarly susceptible to hypoxemia. In sickle cell anemia, sickle cell hemoglobin C, and sickle cell β-thalassemia, hypoxemia is a well recognized trigger of sickle cell crisis.

Diagnosis

Hypoxemia can be diagnosed with certainty only by measurement of Pa_{O_2} or measurement of arterial oxygen saturation. With the routine availability and reliability of pulse oximeters, this is the most efficient way to rapidly diagnose and assess the degree of hypoxemia. It is useful to note that once the saturation is less than or equal to 90%, the corresponding Pa_{O_2} can be approximated by subtracting 30 from the saturation value. Cyanosis represents the presence of more than 5 g of desaturated hemoglobin per deciliter of blood. Changes in environmental lighting, the color of drapes and other surroundings, the amount of hemoglobin (especially severe anemia), and observer variation make the clinical diagnosis of cyanosis notoriously unreliable.[5] In addition, cyanosis may occasionally be apparent without hypoxemia, such as with either methemoglobinemia and sulfhemoglobinemia.[6] Similarly, hypoxemia can be present with no evident cyanosis (eg, in the patient with anemia).

Ventilatory Alterations

During anesthesia with spontaneous ventilation, the pathophysiologic changes induced by hypoxemia usually are qualitatively preserved. In experiments on dogs, Cullen and Eger[7] and Gray and colleagues[8] reported that hypoxemia (Pa_{O_2} = 26 to 31 mm Hg) produced by lowering FI_{O_2} during anesthesia with halothane or methoxyflurane is associated with the changes listed in Table 20-1.

In dogs, first awake and then anesthetized with halothane (1.1% end-tidal), Weiskopf and colleagues showed that the ventilatory response to hypoxemia is reduced during anesthesia.[9] In the awake dog, the minute ventilation of expired gas increases markedly as Pa_{O_2} is lowered to about 40 mm Hg. Halothane anesthesia depresses the hypoxic response by about 50% when animals are normocapnic, and by about 60% when they are hypercapnic. When end-tidal halothane is increased to 1.7%, severe hypotension results, and the ventilatory response to hypoxemia is almost completely extinguished.

Hypoxemia in the conscious state normally potentiates the effect of hypercapnia on ventilation. During anesthesia with halothane in the same experiments, hypoxemia has the reverse effect; as Pa_{O_2} was lowered, the slope of the ventilatory response to hypercapnia is reduced. Thiopental, pentobarbital, and, to a lesser extent, ketamine, all have been shown to depress the hypoxemic ventilatory drive when compared with the awake state.[10] In volunteers, subanesthetic levels of halothane severely impair the normal ventilatory responses to hypoxemia and to a low dose of doxapram. The mechanism of this impairment is postulated to be depression of the peripheral chemoreceptor pathway at the carotid bodies.[11]

TABLE 20-1
Changes in Respiratory Function After Reduction of Inspired Oxygen Fraction in Anesthetized Subjects[7,8]

- Increased frequency of respiration, with little change in V_T
- An increase in minute expired volume and alveolar minute ventilation
- An increase in the fraction of dead space ventilation (ratio of dead space to V_T)*
- A decrease in Pa_{CO_2} and an increase in pH

* The mechanism of this increase is unclear because cardiac output increased and V_T changed insignificantly.

Circulatory Alterations

Cardiovascular function in response to hypoxemia also changes during anesthesia.[2,7,8] Cardiac output, heart rate, and mean arterial pressure increase; oxygen consumption ($\dot{V}_{O_2}$) remains unchanged; oxygen delivery and systemic vascular resistance fall. A metabolic acidosis develops as the period of hypoxemia is extended.

Changes in Arterial Carbon Dioxide Partial Pressure

Cullen and Eger compared their results with those of further experiments on dogs in which Pa_{O_2} was reduced to 30 mm Hg, but Pa_{CO_2} was maintained at control levels by increasing inspired carbon dioxide partial pressure.[2] The results were similar: Cardiac output and heart rate increased; systolic blood pressure also rose slightly. However, arterial pH fell, because the increasing metabolic acidosis was not compensated by hypocapnia. Calculated Ca_{O_2} decreased to a greater extent during hypoxemia with normocapnia compared with that in dogs in which Pa_{CO_2} was allowed to fall. This difference was thought due to the shift of the Hb_{O_2} dissociation curve to the right with decreased pH.

Anesthetic Effects

With increasing depth of anesthesia during spontaneous breathing, the cardiovascular and respiratory effects of hypoxemia are preserved. However, delivered oxygen falls at the deepest level of anesthesia.

Cullen and Eger studied spontaneously breathing dogs during halothane anesthesia.[7] With moderate hypoxemia (Pa_{O_2} = 40 to 42 mm Hg), the frequency of respiration, heart rate, and systolic blood pressure increase up to an alveolar concentration of 2% halothane. During severe hypoxemia (Pa_{O_2} = 30 to 32 mm Hg), the animals preserved the respiratory and cardiovascular response, with end-tidal halothane concentrations ranging from 0.76% to 1.25%, but sudden respiratory arrest occurred at deeper levels of anesthesia.

Mechanical Ventilation

Mechanical ventilation with intermittent positive pressure may alter the cardiovascular response to hypoxemia. In studies of dogs anesthetized with pentobarbital or chloralose and urethane, with decamethonium for muscle paralysis, hypoxemia (Pa_{O_2} = 34 mm Hg) was associated with a reversal of the normal signs: heart rate decreased; mean systolic arterial pressure and peripheral vascular resistance increased; and cardiac output was unaltered.[12] The investigators suggested that mechanisms resulting from increased ventilation contributed significantly to the circulatory responses to hypoxemia during spontaneous breathing. This effect of mechanical ventilation is obviously significant during clinical anesthesia if it alters the cardiovascular response to hypoxemia.

Hypothermia

Moderate hypothermia also may alter the response to hypoxemia. Regan and Eger found in a study with anesthetized dogs that surface cooling the animal to 28°C almost completely abolished the increase in minute ventilation seen at 37°C.[13] At 32°C, a slight increase in ventilation with hypoxemia occurred.

β-Adrenergic Blockade

β-Adrenergic blockade in dogs does not alter the cardiovascular response to normocapnic hypoxemia (Pa_{O_2} approximately 30 mm Hg) induced for 90 seconds during mechanical ventilation with halothane.[14] In this case, the predominant effect of hypoxemia was an increase in cardiac output, stroke volume, and myocardial contractility. The investigators concluded that a possible mechanism for the altered cardiac performance is that hypoxemia leads to an increase in coronary blood flow, which, in turn, decreases the carbon dioxide partial pressure and increases pH in coronary sinus blood. Similar changes in these parameters increase the contractility of isolated cardiac muscle.

Anesthetic-related Causes

Several mechanisms are potentially responsible (Table 20-2).

Reduced Fraction of Inspired Oxygen

The accidental administration of a low FI_{O_2} from improper settings, mechanical failure, or misconnection of the oxygen delivery system is a potential hazard during anesthesia. Inadequate FI_{O_2} may also result from an obstructed fresh gas flow hose or an inadequate fresh gas flow rate (ie, $\dot{V}_{O_2}$ consumption and/or oxygen leaks and/or gas sampling exceeds oxygen delivery. Oxygen cylinders occasionally have contained a gas other than oxygen. Attachment of an oxygen cylinder to the wrong yoke should be prevented by the pin-indexing safety system, but attachment to the incorrect yoke has occurred after insertion of multiple washers.

Bulk oxygen systems supplying piped oxygen have reduced some of the problems associated with oxygen delivery but have introduced others. The central oxygen supply may be filled with other gases (eg, nitrogen) or may become exhausted. Infrequently, the oxygen and nitrous oxide pipelines may be accidentally switched. Finally, the central oxygen supply may be improperly attached to the anesthesia machine.

FLOWMETER DEFECTS. A supply of the correct gas at the correct yoke on the anesthesia machine still does not guarantee its delivery to the patient. Incorrect setting of the flowmeter or use of the wrong flowmeter, when more than one oxygen flowmeter is available, may occur. An open or cracked flowmeter results in loss of oxygen. Because flowmeters are gas-specific and each tube and bobbin is specifically calibrated, any exchange of components can result in hypoxic gas mixtures. The accidental delivery of high flows of other gases, eg nitrous oxide, has also resulted in dilution of the expected FI_{O_2} on machines where proportioning or interlock devices are absent or malfunction.

CIRCUIT PROBLEMS. Once the correct gas mixture is obtained, faults in the use or assembly of the apparatus may result in failure to deliver the mixture to the patient. Within the anesthetic circuit, sticking or incorrectly assembled valves result in rebreathing and reduction of FI_{O_2}. Many safeguards have been introduced to prevent such accidents. "Fail-safe" systems that alarm or shut off gases other than oxygen usually are effective. Continuous in-line monitoring of oxygen concentration with an audible alarm is mandatory.[15] Visual and auditory alarms must be part of the monitoring system, in the event that oxygen concentration falls below a preset limit. Nevertheless, failure of the oxygen monitoring system remains a hazard during anesthesia.

TABLE 20-2
Possible Causes of Hypoxemia During Anesthesia

REDUCED PA_{O_2}
Reduced FI_{O_2}
Reduced alveolar minute ventilation
NORMAL PA_{O_2} (Venous Admixture)
Diffusion defect (rare)
$\dot{V}_A/\dot{Q}$ abnormality (flow >0)
$\dot{V}_A/\dot{Q}$ abnormality (flow = 0; shunt)

Reduced Alveolar Ventilation

During spontaneous ventilation, increasing the depth of general anesthesia with any currently used potent inhalational agent results in increase of PA_{CO_2}. Therefore, as predicted by the alveolar gas equation (given above), PA_{O_2} will fall, and a previously adequate FI_{O_2} may now be associated with hypoxemia. Similarly, with controlled ventilation, mechanical failure of the apparatus, breathing circuit, or carbon dioxide absorber may raise PA_{CO_2} and thereby lower PA_{O_2}.

Increased Venous Admixture

The induction and maintenance of general anesthesia are usually accompanied by an alteration of gas exchange in the lungs. Venous admixture increases, so that PA_{O_2} must be increased to maintain Pa_{O_2} at the preanesthesia level. The causes of this interference with oxygenation are multifactorial.

In 1955, total compliance (chest wall plus lung) was demonstrated to be reduced during general anesthesia.[16] Subsequent studies showed that this change probably resulted from a reduction in lung compliance.[17] Since that time, many studies have shown an increase in alveolar-to-arterial oxygen partial pressure gradient ($PA\text{-}a_{O_2}$) during anesthesia with low (21% to 40%) or high (100%) oxygen concentrations.

Reduced Functional Residual Capacity

An explanation for the alterations in gas exchange may relate to changes in functional residual capacity (FRC). During anesthesia, FRC is reduced with spontaneous[18,19] and controlled ventilation.[20,21] With controlled ventilation, FRC is reduced independently of the size of tidal volume (V_T).[22] The reduction of FRC is found to occur within minutes, and possibly even within 20 seconds of induction. The reduction in FRC does not increase with duration of anesthesia.

The magnitude of the decrease in FRC is independent of the FI_{O_2}, but a greater decrease in FRC during anesthesia is found with increasing age and height-weight ratio.[18,19,21] Factors that influence the decrease in FRC during anesthesia are similar to those that influence impairment of gas exchange. Increase in $PA\text{-}a_{O_2}$ and shunt is found as soon as a steady state can be established after induction (within 7 minutes)[23]; is not progressive with time[24] and, possibly, is greater with increased age.[21]

CLOSING CAPACITY. The alterations in FRC and gas exchange might be explained by the relation of end-expiratory lung volume to closing capacity (CC) (Fig. 20-2). CC is the absolute lung volume at which the airways start to close. If FRC is near or below CC, areas of the lung may stay closed during part or all of the V_T exchange. Failure of ventilation may lead to absorption atelectasis beyond these closed airways. The effect on gas exchange is to increase the lung regions where ventilation is low relative to perfusion (low $\dot{V}_A/\dot{Q}$), or zero (eg, a shunt). The decrease in FRC during anesthesia, in fact, can be correlated with increase in $PA\text{-}a_{O_2}$.[21,25]

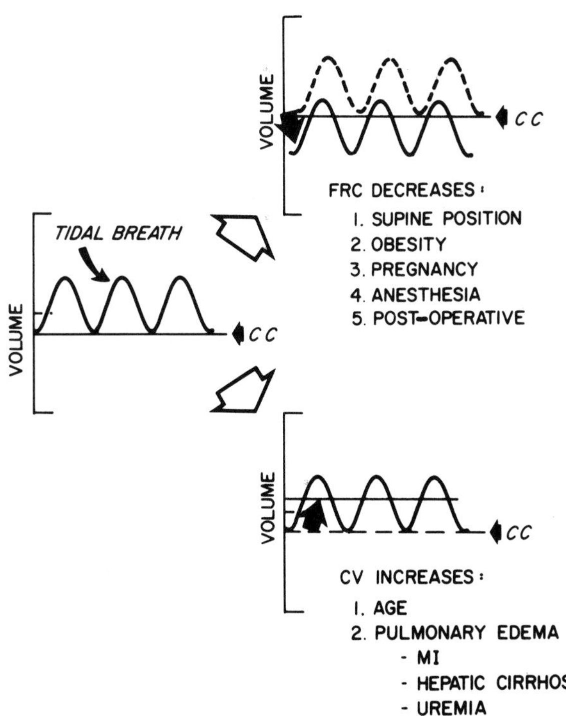

FIGURE 20-2. The relation between CC and FRC can be disturbed by decreasing FRC (*top*) or increasing CC (*bottom*). *MI*, myocardial infarction.

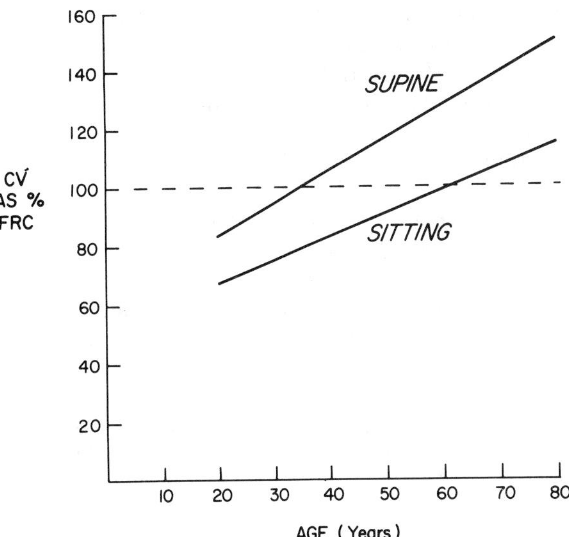

FIGURE 20-3. The variations in CV (or, more accurately, CC) as a percentage of FRC with age, in the sitting and supine positions. The difference is attributable primarily to a reduction in FRC on assumption of the supine position. (Adapted from Don HF, Craig DB, Wahba WM, et al: The measurement of gas trapped in the lungs at functional residual capacity and the effects of posture. Anesthesiology 35:582, 1971.)

Two studies measured CC during anesthesia; investigators found that it did not change with either spontaneous or controlled ventilation as a consequence of general anesthesia.[22,26] FRC falls, and the difference between FRC and CC correlates with $PA\text{-}a_{O_2}$; as CC exceeds FRC, $PA\text{-}a_{O_2}$ increases.[22] In one study, CC, FRC, and $PA\text{-}a_{O_2}$ were not altered by an increase in V_T from 5 to 10 mL/kg.[22] This finding is unexpected, because, if the defect is associated with airway closure, less closure would be expected with a high V_T. In conflict with some of this data, another study demonstrated a significant reduction in CC during anesthesia. This study measured CC by applying negative pressure at the airway, a technique that makes the results more difficult to interpret.[27]

GAS TRAPPING. The occurrence of airway closure during anesthesia has been demonstrated by measuring the volume of gas trapped in the lung.[28] This can be demonstrated by manual hyperinflation of the patient's lungs after equilibration with helium in a closed circuit. A decrease in helium concentration is interpreted as representing trapped gas. When anesthesia causes FRC to fall from a value above the CC, the volume of trapped gas increases from 0.12% of total lung capacity (TLC) to 3.36% of TLC. If gas trapping continues through a long case, FRC may begin to increase.

POSITION. Compared with sitting, the supine position is associated with a decrease in FRC (Fig. 20-3). Derangement of gas exchange is therefore more likely to occur in the supine position, as FRC approximates or falls below CC. One study during anesthesia with controlled ventilation in the sitting position did not demonstrate a decrease in FRC.[29] Anesthesia with nitrous oxide and spontaneous breathing in seated patients, on the other hand, was associated with a decrease in FRC within 20 seconds.[30]

MISCELLANEOUS FACTORS. The decrease in FRC accompanying induction of general anesthesia could be caused by an increase in the blood or water content within the thoracic cage, without necessarily any change in the contour or position of the chest wall or diaphragm. However, several studies show that the diaphragm shifts cephalad after induction of anesthesia; also, the cross-sectional area of the chest wall is reduced at that time, with a slight decrease in central blood volume and no change in extravascular lung water.[31] In addition, one study demonstrated the appearance of crescent-shaped densities in dependent parts of the lungs after induction of general anesthesia. These densities did not increase with continued anesthesia and were not affected by changes in $F_{I_{O_2}}$. The authors suggested that the densities represented atelectasis.[32]

Summary

The induction of general anesthesia is associated with an almost immediate decrease in FRC. This reduction is not progressive with time; is greater in older and more obese subjects; occurs in patients with spontaneous or controlled ventilation; is independent of the $F_{I_{O_2}}$; and may be minimized in the sitting position. General anesthesia is also associated with an increased $P_{A}\text{-}a_{O_2}$ gradient and shunt, which are influenced by factors similar to those affecting FRC. The increase in $P_{A}\text{-}a_{O_2}$ often is related to the decrease in FRC. Because of the relation of FRC to CC, gas trapping and areas of reduced (or zero) $\dot{V}_A/\dot{Q}$ may be produced in the lungs. Although this hypothesis is attractive, the changes in FRC and $P_{A}\text{-}a_{O_2}$ may not be causally related but, instead, have a common source.

Why the decrease of FRC occurs during anesthesia is incompletely understood. An intuitive explanation is that the increased tone in the abdominal muscles, observed in many patients breathing spontaneously under general anesthesia, is responsible. However, induction of total neuromuscular blockade with succinylcholine during halothane anesthesia does not alter the FRC in adults.[18] Cinefluoroscopic studies in three supine, adult subjects demonstrated that either general anesthesia or muscle paralysis with succinylcholine resulted in the same degree of cephalad movement of the diaphragm.[33] However, with spontaneous ventilation, the dependent diaphragm moved to a greater extent than did the nondependent portion, whereas with controlled ventilation these findings were reversed (Fig. 20-4). One might infer an overall difference in the resultant $\dot{V}_A/\dot{Q}$ changes. FRC generally falls after induction of general anesthesia accompanied by complete neuromuscular block and mechanical ventilation. The exception to this observation is a study suggesting that a considerable increase in FRC occurs after injection of succinylcholine during anesthesia with fentanyl and droperidol.[34] Alternative explanations for the decrease in FRC during anesthesia are an increase in central blood volume, alterations in lung elasticity, and a loss of inspiratory muscle tone.[19,35]

Therapeutic Implications

Techniques that increase lung volume should improve gas exchange during anesthesia. Results with positive end-expiratory pressure (PEEP) have been variable, and only small decreases in $P_{A}\text{-}a_{O_2}$ have been produced.[22,35] In one study a greater improvement of oxygenation with PEEP was found in patients anesthetized with Innovar,[36] which may have a greater effect on reducing FRC than other agents.[34] The mean lung volume will also be a function of the size of the tidal breath and the respiratory frequency. The significance of increased V_T and "sighs" has been disputed but apparently is of little or no value and may even be deleterious if decreased venous return and increased dead space result.

In the presence of existing abnormal venous admixture, a

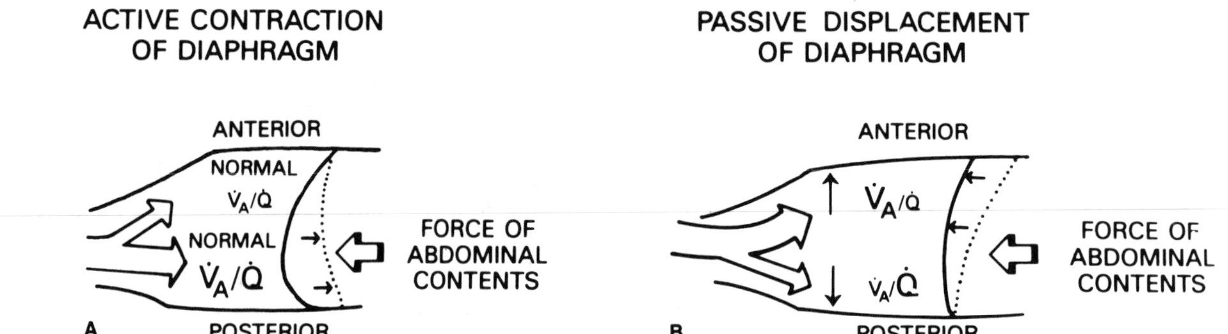

FIGURE 20-4. (**A**) Spontaneous breathing in the awake or anesthetized patient is associated with better $\dot{V}_A/\dot{V}_Q$ matching throughout the lungs. The shorter posterior radius of curvature leads to greater diaphragmatic force of contraction and lung excursion. (**B**) Paralysis renders the diaphragm flaccid. Manual or mechanical ventilation moves the anterior diaphragm most where it is unimpeded by abdominal contents, while perfusion is predominantly posterior. (Adapted from Rasanen J, Downs JB: Modes of mechanical ventilatory support. In Kirby RR, Banner MJ, Downs JB (eds): Clinical applications of ventilatory support. New York: Churchill Livingstone, 1990:173.)

decrease in cardiac output increases $P_{A}\text{-}a_{O_2}$ and causes a further decline in Pa_{O_2} due to a decrease in mixed venous oxygen content ($C\bar{v}_{O_2}$). Hence, maintenance or even increase of cardiac output is potentially desirable from this standpoint. Inhibition of hypoxic pulmonary vasoconstriction might also be important in producing decreased Pa_{O_2} with constant shunt. Regional $\dot{V}_A/\dot{Q}$ matching is controlled, in part, by local vasoconstriction in the presence of local alveolar hypoxia. General anesthetics have variable inhibitory effects on this response, but intravenous anesthetic agents do not seem to influence the response to hypoxia.

A shift to the left of the Hb_{O_2} dissociation curve may also increase $P_{A}\text{-}a_{O_2}$ in the presence of venous admixture by reducing $C\bar{v}_{O_2}$. General anesthetic agents shift the curve slightly but consistently to the right.[37] Lidocaine has no effect on the Hb_{O_2} relation.[38] "Therapeutic" manipulation of the curve is of no proven benefit.

Therefore, general anesthesia has an intrinsic effect of increasing $P_{A}\text{-}a_{O_2}$ in some patients. This change is augmented by changes in cardiac output or hemoglobin content. Whether hypoxemia is produced, however, depends on the $F_{I_{O_2}}$: A $F_{I_{O_2}}$ of at least 0.3 is recommended if hypoxemia is to be avoided. Epidural and spinal analgesia have no influence on $P_{A}\text{-}a_{O_2}$ or shunt.[39,40]

Factors Causing Hypoxemia

Apart from the expected increase in venous admixture associated with general anesthesia, hypoxemia can be caused by specific, abnormal, aggravating factors (Table 20-3).

Esophageal Intubation

Esophageal intubation leads to profound hypoxemia and is lethal if not detected and remedied almost immediately.

Intubation of One Mainstem Bronchus

Intubation of one mainstem bronchus, accidental or deliberate, usually produces an increase in $P_{A}\text{-}a_{O_2}$, as any shift of perfusion away from the under-ventilated lung is incomplete. Various maneuvers have been recommended to detect the presence of bronchial intubation, but none is completely reliable, except examination of the chest radiograph or fiberoptic bronchoscopic inspection.

TABLE 20-3
Factors Leading to Intraoperative Hypoxemia

- Esophageal intubation
- Mainstem bronchial intubation
- Tracheal suctioning
- Aspiration of foreign material
- Pulmonary edema
- Pulmonary embolism
- Bronchospasm
- Pneumothorax
- Atelectasis
- Airway obstruction

Deliberate ventilation of one lung during anesthesia for surgery inside the thorax invariably produces an increase in $P_{A}\text{-}a_{O_2}$ and, depending on the $F_{I_{O_2}}$, hypoxemia. In a series of 11 patients in whom one lung was mechanically ventilated and the other allowed to collapse, mean Pa_{O_2} ($F_{I_{O_2}} = 1.0$) was 160 mm Hg. In six of these patients, the Pa_{O_2} was less than 100 mm Hg. PEEP of 5 cmH_2O did not improve oxygenation.[41] However, insufflation of oxygen into the nonventilated lung to create positive airway pressure (10 cmH_2O) improves Pa_{O_2}.[42]

If the equivalent of one-lung ventilation is produced by surgical retraction, a similar increase in $P_{A}\text{-}a_{O_2}$ occurs.[43] In this study of 200 patients with a $F_{I_{O_2}}$ of 0.5, four had a Pa_{O_2} less than 60 mm Hg, and two had values under 50 mm Hg.

Tracheal Suctioning

Suction catheters inserted through the endotracheal tube in patients treated with mechanical ventilation will reduce Pa_{O_2} for a period of time (3 to 4 minutes) after reinstitution of ventilation. The length of time that suction is applied affects the increase of $P_{A}\text{-}a_{O_2}$. Hyperinflation after suctioning reduces the severity. Boutros showed that mean Pa_{O_2} fell from 81 to 70 mm Hg 60 seconds after tracheal suctioning when a $F_{I_{O_2}}$ of 0.25 was breathed.[44] Unfortunately, the individual values of Pa_{O_2} were not given. In assessing the apparent hazard of a procedure, the occurrence of a life-threatening Pa_{O_2} in even one patient is of greater significance than the mean Pa_{O_2}. A careful technique of conventional tracheal suctioning, with preoxygenation, a catheter of small diameter (approximately one-half the internal diameter of the endotracheal tube), and application of negative pressure only during withdrawal of the catheter followed by several manual hyperinflations will minimize this problem. Newer, closed systems do not require disconnection of the ventilator circuit; hence ventilation can be maintained during suctioning.

Aspiration of Foreign Material

Pulmonary edema or obstruction, with consequent hypoxemia, may result from aspiration of foreign material. Aspiration can occur even in the presence of an endotracheal tube with an inflated cuff.[45]

Pulmonary Edema

Pulmonary edema is rare during anesthesia, even with the large volumes of intravenous fluids commonly infused. It may be associated with hypersensitivity reactions to infused blood, to its components, or to drugs. However, its occurrence with forced spontaneous inspiration against a partially or totally obstructed airway (negative pressure pulmonary edema) is increasingly recognized.[46–48]

Pulmonary Embolism

Hypoxemia occurs probably because of abnormal anatomic shunts, bronchoconstriction, and atelectasis. Possible sources of emboli are blood clots, amniotic fluid, entrained or infused air, blood transfusion, fat, or foreign bodies. Irrigation of an anal fistula with hydrogen peroxide has been reported to cause near-fatal embolism with bubbles of oxygen.[49]

Bronchospasm

With or without an antecedent history of asthma, bronchospasm may develop during anesthesia. It has been reported after the use of many drugs, possibly because they release histamine or cause an anaphylactic or anaphylactoid reaction. Commonly used muscle relaxants (ie, atracurium, d-tubocurarine, pancuronium, and succinylcholine) have been implicated. Severe bronchospasm results in hypercapnia and hypoxemia, but milder forms may cause hypoxemia with normocapnia or hypocapnia.

Pneumothorax

Pneumothorax may occur with any percutaneous or surgical procedure around the thorax, neck, or diaphragm. Disruption of the lung is particularly likely to occur if high inflation pressures are used or are applied to limited areas of the lung (eg, by oxygen flow through a bronchoscope).

Pulmonary Collapse

Pulmonary collapse during anesthesia is rare. Etiologic factors include obstruction, hypoventilation, compression, and altered alveolar and airway surface tension. One-sided bronchial intubation, deliberate or otherwise, leads to collapse of the contralateral lung and sometimes of the right upper lobe if a right-sided tube is inserted and the right upper lobe ventilation slot is not properly positioned opposite the right upper lobe bronchus orifice.

Airway Obstruction

Many factors contribute, including soft tissue swelling, upper-airway obstruction due to the tongue, laryngospasm, foreign body, or endotracheal tube obstruction.

Postoperative Hypoxemia

A variety of conditions predispose to postoperative hypoxemia and are summarized in Table 20-4. In normal, conscious humans, hypoxemia stimulates the cardiovascular and respiratory systems. Increases in cardiac output, pulse rate, minute ventilation, and V_T occur. In contrast, experiments with controlled ventilation in conscious humans suggest the cardiovascular response is obtunded, and pulse rate does not necessarily increase with hypoxemia.[50] Symptoms of hypoxemia are nonspecific and include dyspnea and central nervous system changes, such as restlessness, confusion, and irritability. They may be found in patients who develop postoperative hypoxemia. Cyanosis can be present but is often not detectable.[5] Severe hypoxemia causes both cardiovascular and respiratory depression, with hypotension, bradycardia, and decrease in minute ventilation.

TABLE 20-4
Factors Influencing Postoperative Hypoxemia

- Hypoxemia can occur after any type of surgical procedure, even those of short duration. It occurs with greater severity and frequency after procedures near the diaphragm.
- The causes are unknown. A decrease in FRC of approximately 20% occurs after upper abdominal surgery. Whether this is a primary, causative phenomenon or is a result of other changes in the lung or chest wall has not been determined.
- No alteration in anesthetic technique influences the incidence, including regional analgesia, humidification, controlled ventilation, and continuous positive-pressure ventilation.
- Postoperative epidural analgesia and pulmonary physiotherapy do not prevent hypoxemia (but may reduce its severity).
- Prolonged surgery, obesity, advanced age, increased ratio of CC to FRC preoperatively, and preexisting lung disease predispose patients to hypoxemia.

Anesthesia and Surgery

Anesthesia and surgical procedures are commonly associated with postoperative hypoxemia, depending on the length of exposure and the site of operation. In a recent series of 500 consecutive patients presenting to the postanesthesia care unit (PACU), 37% required supplemental oxygen in the PACU and 12% on discharge to the ward to maintain an oxygen saturation greater than 94%, or their preoperative values if they were lower. Sixty-three percent of patients in the PACU in this series never required any supplemental oxygen.[51] The magnitude and duration of the decrease in Pa_{O_2} is directly related to the proximity of surgery to the diaphragm. When procedures performed under general anesthesia last less than 22 minutes and spontaneous ventilation occurs without thoracic, abdominal, or oral incisions, no postoperative decrease in mean Pa_{O_2} occurs.[52] However, even in this small series a 52-year-old woman had a postoperative Pa_{O_2} of 74 mm Hg, compared with a preanesthesia level of 92 mm Hg. This decrease in oxygen partial pressure was accompanied by a reduction of Pa_{CO_2} to 27 mm Hg; in other words, had the Pa_{CO_2} been equal to or greater than 40 mm Hg, the Pa_{O_2} would have been less than or equal to 60.

In similar procedures lasting longer (45 to 120 minutes), a decrease in Pa_{O_2} occurred up to 90 minutes after cessation of general anesthesia. Values at 3 hours had returned to preoperative levels.[52]

A more significant decline in Pa_{O_2} is found after abdominal surgery. After lower abdominal surgery, the mean Pa_{O_2} during room air breathing is reduced by 9.5 mm Hg at 24 hours.[53] After upper abdominal surgery, the decrease is greater[53] and may persist from 5 to 7 days.[54,55] The deficit in oxygen is greatest between the 1st and 3rd days.[54] Hypoxemia is found in patients with normal or low Pa_{CO_2} and without clinical or radiographic evidence of pulmonary disease. If a thoracic incision is involved, the decrease in Pa_{O_2} may persist at least 10 to 15 days.[54]

Increased Shunt and Ventilation–Perfusion Inequality

Hypoxemia that develops in patients with a normal PA_{O_2} is due either to an increase in $\dot{V}_A/\dot{Q}$ maldistribution or to an increased shunt. Evidence is conflicting. One study of 18 patients showed that 24 hours after upper abdominal surgery, shunt had increased from a mean of about 1% to 5% of the cardiac output.[56] The total venous admixture, however, increased from 5.2% to 23.4%. Hence, the predominant effect was thought to be due to uneven distribution of $\dot{V}_A/\dot{Q}$ ratios.

A later study also examined patients after upper abdominal surgery.[55] On the 1st, 3rd, and 6th days, $PA\text{-}a_{O_2}$ was significantly increased due to an increase in shunt, without $\dot{V}_A/\dot{Q}$ changes. In another study, it was demonstrated that both shunt and $\dot{V}_A/\dot{Q}$ inequality were increased 1 to 2 hours after surgery.[57] The overall conclusion is that venous admixture increases after anesthesia; whether this abnormality is due to shunt, to $\dot{V}_A/\dot{Q}$ mismatch, or to both cannot be stated with confidence.

Mechanisms that produce these changes are somewhat speculative. Changes in pulmonary function that have been documented after surgery and anesthesia are discussed in the following paragraphs.

REDUCTION IN FUNCTIONAL RESIDUAL CAPACITY. A 20% reduction from the preoperative value persists for approximately 12 days after abdominal surgery. This effect is greatest after upper abdominal surgery, is less after lower abdominal surgery, and is least after surgery outside the abdomen and thorax.[58]

DECREASE IN VITAL CAPACITY. A decrease in vital capacity persists for at least 12 days after abdominal surgery. Both expiratory reserve volume and inspiratory capacity are reduced. Vital capacity after upper abdominal surgery has been reported to be 45% of preoperative values. The corresponding figure for lower abdominal surgery is 60%.[59] Forced vital capacity and its component expired in 1 second are also reduced.

REDUCTION IN AVERAGE TIDAL VOLUME. A value of about 80% of preoperative levels occurs after upper abdominal surgery, but is unchanged after inguinal herniorrhaphy. Upper abdominal surgery also markedly decreases the rate at which larger than normal tidal breaths occur. In one study, sighs (defined as 200% of preoperative mean V_T) were found not to occur.[60] This effect was not seen after lower abdominal surgery.

INCREASE IN RESPIRATORY RATE. An increase of 50% is observed on the 2nd day after upper abdominal surgery, compared with a 10% increase after inguinal herniorrhaphy.[60]

Relation of Functional Residual Capacity to Closing Capacity

A popular explanation of the alteration in gas exchange after anesthesia and surgery involves the relation of FRC to CC. Because CC is the lung volume at which airways start to close, tidal breathing within CC will result in either total failure of ventilation to parts of the lung or reduced ventilation. Measurement of the difference indicates an inverse relation of FRC − CC with $PA\text{-}a_{O_2}$ after upper abdominal surgery as follows:

$$P(A\text{-}a)_{O_2} = 28.5 - 14.6(FRC - CC)\ \text{mm Hg}$$

where FRC and CC are measured in liters.[58] In that study, mean values for CC decreased slightly after the surgical procedures. Thus the reduction in FRC − CC is due solely to a decrease in FRC.

A study by Fibuch and colleagues demonstrated that the preoperative values of FRC/CC in patients undergoing upper or lower abdominal surgical procedures have an inverse relation to postoperative changes in $PA\text{-}a_{O_2}$ when the patients breathed 100% oxygen.[61]

Causes of Reduction in Functional Residual Capacity

ATELECTASIS. Lung volume may be reduced by atelectasis as a primary event. Immobility, depressed or absent cough reflex, altered ciliary activity, small V_T, and reduced inspired humidity are factors that predispose to collapse. However, radiographic evidence of atelectasis usually is not found. Failure of CC to decrease significantly after anesthesia also has been suggested as evidence against atelectasis. Pulmonary edema is unlikely to be a primary cause of the decrease in FRC, for it should cause an increase in CC due to the formation of edema fluid around small airways.

CHANGES IN LUNG AND CHEST WALL FUNCTION. Lung volume could be changed by alterations in the chest wall and abdomen. Wound dressings, abdominal binders, pneumoperitoneum, or distended bowel may increase cephalad displacement of the diaphragm. A common radiographic observation is that the left hemidiaphragm can be considerably elevated by air in the stomach. The supine position also exaggerates low lung volume.

INCREASED EXPIRATORY MUSCLE TONE. Increased abdominal muscle tone due to pain or reflex stimulation tends to reduce lung volume. However, abolishing pain after abdominal surgery by epidural analgesia did not increase FRC in one study.[62] Similarly, Pa_{O_2}, $PA\text{-}a_{O_2}$, and Pa_{CO_2} in patients breathing either air or 100% oxygen are not altered acutely by the relief of pain after abdominal surgery.[63] These studies suggest that pain-induced increase of expiratory muscle tone is not the mechanism of reduced FRC after abdominal surgery.

Diagnosis

Hypoxemia must be recognized as an ever-present postoperative threat, even if it is difficult to detect by physical examination. Routine pulse oximetry in the postoperative period leads to detection and, if coupled with intervention, may improve outcome.[64] In a significant step in this direction, the American Society of Anesthesiologists has included pulse oximetry monitoring as a standard of care in the PACU.[65]

Disorders

Factors involved in the development of hypoxemia in "routine" anesthetic practice were described in the foregoing sections. Specific disorders that are associated with hypoxemia, some of which have been described earlier, may also occur postoperatively.

Pulmonary Edema

Pulmonary edema is relatively uncommon.[66] The combination of high (>15 mm Hg) left atrial or pulmonary artery occlusion pressure (PAOP) with high or normal cardiac output may be seen with fluid overload or cardiac disease. A high PAOP in conjunction with a low cardiac output occurs in congestive heart failure. More commonly, pulmonary edema is associated with a low PAOP. Postoperatively, this occurrence may result from drugs; blood, white cell, or platelet transfusions; aspiration; sepsis; pulmonary embolism (air, fat, foreign body, amniotic fluid); airway obstruction; hypoproteinemia; or crystalloid fluid overload.

Myocardial Infarction

Myocardial infarction occurs in less than 0.1% of patients undergoing operations or diagnostic procedures. Although infarction is uncommon, its occurrence is usually associated with hypoxemia. The cause of hypoxemia is unexplained, but it may be associated with pulmonary edema and increased CC.

Pulmonary Thromboembolism

Hypoxemia results from unexplained mechanisms. Anatomic shunts, atelectasis, and bronchoconstriction probably occur. The incidence in surgical patients may seem surprisingly low unless sensitive diagnostic techniques are used. Diagnosed pulmonary embolism occurred in 0.4% of 54,183 adult patients in one survey, of whom 0.06% were postoperative surgical patients.[67] However, when photoscanning techniques were used on the 3rd or 4th day after surgery, slightly over half (56%) of 54 patients studied had evidence of thromboembolism. This incidence was reduced to 19% of 58 patients if prophylactic subcutaneous heparin was used.[68]

Of significance, between 0.1% and 1.0% of patients undergoing major surgery die of pulmonary embolism (4.7% of all surgical deaths in one study, as many as 15% in others). Over time, the mortality rate has decreased, presumably a reflection of increased appreciation, prophylactic anticoagulation, sequential calf and thigh compression stockings, earlier ambulation, and other preventive measures.[69]

Aspiration Pneumonia

Aspiration pneumonia can occur even in the presence of a cuffed endotracheal tube. Two syndromes have been described. In 44,016 pregnant patients between 1932 and 1945, aspiration of stomach contents occurred in 66 patients (0.16%) during delivery. In five cases, solid material was aspirated, and symptoms of obstruction occurred. Forty patients aspirated liquid material and showed delayed onset of expiratory rhonchi and, in some cases, pulmonary edema.[70] Differentiation of negative-pressure pulmonary edema is difficult to impossible in many cases.[48]

Hypoventilation

Common causes of reduced alveolar ventilation are airway obstruction, sedation, or partial paralysis of the respiratory muscles. An increase in $P_{A_{CO_2}}$ inevitably will cause a decrease in $P_{A_{O_2}}$ (as shown by the alveolar gas equation), and hence, hypoxemia, unless the inspired oxygen is increased.

Low Cardiac Output

In the presence of existing venous admixture, a reduced cardiac output causes a decrease in Pa_{O_2}.[71] The probable mechanism is that the decrease in $C\bar{v}_{O_2}$, which accompanies a low cardiac output, further dilutes the oxygen in pulmonary capillary blood, thereby reducing the Pa_{O_2}.

Increase in Oxygen Consumption

By a similar mechanism, increased $\dot{V}_{O_2}$ tends to lower $C\bar{v}_{O_2}$, producing hypoxemia, unless a compensatory increase in cardiac output occurs. Normally, this factor is not significant postoperatively; either little increase in $\dot{V}_{O_2}$ occurs, or a proportionately greater increase in cardiac output results, causing an increase in $C\bar{v}_{O_2}$.[72] However, $\dot{V}_{O_2}$ may be substantially increased during shivering, hyperactivity, fever, or after tissue trauma.

Decrease in Oxygen-carrying Capacity

A similar effect on decreasing $C\bar{v}_{O_2}$ occurs if a compensatory increase in cardiac output does not occur. Hence, anemia tends to cause hypoxemia in the presence of venous admixture.

Posthyperventilation Hypoxemia

After a period of hyperventilation, reduced body stores of carbon dioxide are replenished from the metabolic $\dot{V}_{CO_2}$. Hence, alveolar ventilation is reduced, causing a reduction in $P_{A_{O_2}}$ and Pa_{O_2}. A normal level of ventilation is usually achieved within 1 hour. In a group of 13 patients who had been hyperventilated for an average of 2.75 hours during anesthesia and surgery, the Pa_{O_2} fell to a mean low of 72 mm Hg when they breathed room air. Three patients experienced a Pa_{O_2} less than 60 mm Hg.[73]

Diffusion Hypoxemia

Diffusion hypoxemia also has been described. The elimination of anesthetic concentrations of nitrous oxide involves excretion of large volumes of this gas due to its high solubility in blood. This movement of nitrous oxide from blood to alveolus diminishes $P_{A_{O_2}}$, and consequently, Pa_{O_2}. In 20 patients when the gas mixture was changed from 80% nitrous oxide and 20% oxygen to air, the mean Pa_{O_2} decreased by 11%. This drop was maximal within 2 minutes and had returned to control values in 4 minutes in 75% of subjects. A Pa_{O_2} less than 60 mm Hg was found in four patients. Spontaneous rather than controlled ventilation during the study was associated with a greater drop (18 mm Hg) in Pa_{O_2} that took slightly longer to return to control levels.[74]

The additive effect of diffusion hypoxemia and posthyperventilation hypoxemia has been calculated; results suggest that PA_{O_2} will fall to a low of approximately 73 mm Hg within 5 minutes after 1 hour of controlled ventilation with 79% nitrous oxide.[1]

TREATMENT OF HYPOXEMIA

Hypoxemia usually can be corrected by enrichment of the FI_{O_2}. Whether hypoxemia will be present after a surgical procedure in an individual patient is impossible to reliably predict; hence the appeal and acceptance of the routine use of pulse oximetry in the PACU. The mean value for Pa_{O_2}, published for a group of subjects after a particular type of procedure can be a dangerous statistic if applied clinically. More important to examine in any published series is the range of values found. If a single patient in a group shows a Pa_{O_2} of 40 mm Hg, this life-threatening value is possible, even though the mean Pa_{O_2} value is 85 mm Hg for the group. Supplemental oxygen frequently is administered to every patient recovering from anesthesia and surgery. If this practice is not followed, each patient should be monitored with pulse oximetry to detect what otherwise might be unrecognized, developing hypoxemia.[51,75] Of note is that because the routine administration of supplemental oxygen also does not guarantee resolution of hypoxemia, it is impossible to argue convincingly against routine pulse oximetry in this setting.

Oxygen Therapy

A relatively low FI_{O_2} (<0.35) generally is felt to be adequate for reversal of hypoxemia after "routine" surgery. However, the greater decline in Pa_{O_2} in older subjects suggests that a higher FI_{O_2} is necessary.[76] After upper abdominal surgery, the Pa_{O_2} during air breathing can be calculated as follows:

$$Pa_{O_2} \simeq 81 - (0.28 \times \text{age [in years]})\ \text{mm Hg}$$

with a FI_{O_2} of 0.35 to 0.4:

$$Pa_{O_2} \simeq 166 - (1.12 \times \text{age [in years]})\ \text{mm Hg}$$

The difference between the actual fraction of oxygen delivered by a piece of equipment and the FI_{O_2} must be appreciated.[77] For example, a flow of 5 L/min through nasal prongs provided a FI_{O_2} of only 0.25 during normal breathing in two adult volunteers. A face mask with a flow of 10 L/min with an actual delivered oxygen fraction of 1.0 provided a FI_{O_2} of 0.52 in the trachea during normal breathing. With a flow of 15 L/min, the FI_{O_2} still only rose to 0.54.[77]

Positive End-Expiratory Pressure

In patients with severe lung disease, supplementation of the FI_{O_2} may not correct hypoxemia. Spontaneous ventilation with PEEP or continuous positive airway pressure is frequently used. Raised end-expiratory pressure delivered with a mask can avoid the need for tracheal intubation and mechanical ventilation.[78,79] However, we have found this method to be impractical. Tracheal intubation and mechanical ventilation are usually indicated. Although arguments have been raised that only hypoventilation requires mechanical ventilation, the greater V_T delivered mechanically usually will restore Pa_{O_2} to life-supporting levels. If this approach, in turn, is still associated with hypoxemia, the FRC can be elevated by PEEP.[80]

Hazards

It is common practice to augment inspired oxygen concentration after anesthesia and surgery. With the routine use of pulse oximetry, this practice may be due for reevaluation as a matter of economy and, in some cases, safety as well. Although no contraindication exists to oxygen administration for patients who are hypoxemic, recognition of the hazards of therapy dictates that its administration must always be undertaken with its potential complications in mind.

PHYSICAL PROBLEMS. The first category includes physical problems such as trauma from dry gas or equipment (mask or cannula). Equipment failure or errors in administration (eg, the delivery of nitrous oxide instead of oxygen) can ironically aggravate the very problem being treated.

FUNCTIONAL PROBLEMS. The second category is functional hazards: atelectasis or reduced alveolar ventilation. Atelectasis is thought to be produced by the absorption of oxygen beyond closed airways, although the data on its occurrence are conflicting.[18,81] Alveolar ventilation may be reduced if the administration of oxygen removes a hypoxemic drive to breath. Suppression of ventilation is more likely in the patient who has chronic lung disease, metabolic alkalosis, central nervous system disease, obesity, or chest wall abnormalities such as kyphoscoliosis. It also is more likely in patients who have received drugs that depress ventilation, such as narcotics. Depression of ventilation by the administration of oxygen is unusual unless chronic hypercapnia exists.

CYTOTOXIC HAZARDS. The third category comprises cytotoxic hazards, which are thought to result from an increased rate of generation of partially reduced oxygen products (free radicals) within the cell. Minor changes of pulmonary oxygen toxicity are seen as diminished vital capacity and substernal chest pain. More prolonged exposure may result in changes in the interstitium of the lung accompanied by reduced pulmonary compliance, severe hypoxemia, and a diffuse bilateral infiltrate on the chest radiograph—the adult respiratory distress syndrome.[82] In premature neonates, retinopathy of prematurity with permanent visual impairment may result from hyperoxia.

Pain and Analgesia

Epidural Local Anesthetics

Pain and its relief have been thought to modulate gas exchange. Epidural analgesia to a sensory level of the fourth thoracic dermatome has no influence on Pa_{O_2}, Pa_{CO_2}, or FRC.[39] Epidural analgesia after upper abdominal surgery also has been shown to produce no acute change in Pa_{O_2} or $PA\text{-}a_{O_2}$ in patients breathing air or oxygen.[63,65] FRC also is not altered by pain relief using epidural analgesia.[62] Whether the effect of prolonged pain relief by epidural analgesics is more beneficial to postoperative gas exchange is disputed. When compared with the use of morphine, epidural block with bupivacaine after upper abdominal or hip surgery, had no influence on Pa_{O_2}, $PA\text{-}a_{O_2}$, Pa_{CO_2}, vital capacity, or peak expiratory flow rate.[39,65] On the other hand, Holmdahl and Modig demonstrated a lowered $PA\text{-}a_{O_2}$ after upper abdominal surgery in patients in whom pain relief was provided by epidural analgesia.[72] The differences in these results are difficult to explain. One explanation is that the impaired gas exchange observed when parenteral morphine was used for pain relief was due to the comparatively large amounts of narcotic administered. In no study, however, has a significant increase in Pa_{CO_2} been shown, and most patients characteristically demonstrated mild hyperventilation. Narcotic analgesics in excess may be associated with hypercapnia, which will cause hypoxemia, depending on the FI_{O_2}. The use of narcotic antagonists is associated with reduction in Pa_{CO_2} and therefore improvement of Pa_{O_2}.

Even the addition of chest physiotherapy to a program of epidural analgesia does not alter the impaired gas exchange after surgery on the upper abdomen or hip. However, the overall hospital stay is shortened by epidural analgesia.[83,84]

Intravenous Narcotics

Continuous ventilatory monitoring after major surgery has shown that periods of oxygen desaturation, obstructive apnea, paradoxic breathing, and low ventilatory rate are common with a continuous intravenous infusion of morphine. These changes are exaggerated during sleep. In contrast, significant oxygen desaturation does not occur if analgesia is produced solely by local anesthetic agents administered either epidurally or intercostally.[83,85]

Epidural Narcotics

Since 1979, the epidural and intrathecal injection of narcotics has become popular. This technique produces satisfactory and prolonged (eg, 12 to 24 hours) pain relief after a wide variety of operations (eg, thoracotomy, abdominal procedures, orthopedic surgery), without the concomitant sympathetic blockade and hypotension that often accompany local anesthetic epidural techniques.[86] However, the so-called selective analgesia produced by narcotics poses the possibility of severe respiratory depression, occurring both early (eg, 1 to 2 hours) and late (eg, 6 to 24 hours) after injection. Less common after intrathecal use, the early respiratory depression is thought to be due to systemic levels of the narcotic and is more frequent with lipid soluble agents, such as meperidine and fentanyl. The late depression of breathing is believed to be due to rostral spread in the cerebrospinal fluid and is more frequent with agents that have low lipid solubility, eg morphine.

Factors that increase the incidence of respiratory depression are advanced age, high dosage, the supine and Trendelenburg positions, concomitant or recent use of parenteral narcotics or other respiratory depressants, lack of tolerance to narcotics, raised intraabdominal or intrathoracic pressure, preexisting pulmonary disease, and, in the case of the epidural technique, unintended dural puncture.[87] Respiratory depression can be prevented by a continuous intravenous infusion of naloxone, titrated so that it does not interfere with analgesia. Usually, 400 μg added to 500 to 1000 mL of the maintenance intravenous solution running at 75 to 150 mL per hour is sufficient.

Other Considerations

Activity and Positioning

Early mobilization and chest physiotherapy may be of value to increase lung volume and aid pulmonary secretion clearance. The upright position seems to be beneficial, because it is associated with an increase in FRC compared with the supine position. In a study of obese patients after intra-abdominal surgery, Pa_{O_2} was higher, and $PA\text{-}a_{O_2}$, lower in the semirecumbent position than in the supine position.[88]

Respiratory Care

Prevention of pulmonary complications and hypoxemia with incentive spirometry has been investigated.[89] Mean Pa_{O_2} increased in 10 patients breathing either air or oxygen after surgery; changes in Pa_{CO_2} and $PA\text{-}a_{O_2}$ were not reported, however. Treatment with intermittent positive-pressure breathing is controversial. Used discretely in patients with reduced vital capacities, intermittent positive-pressure breathing probably aids inflation of the lungs and clearance of retained secretions. Stock and coworkers reported that intermittent face-mask continuous positive airway pressure was superior to incentive spirometry and intermittent positive-pressure breathing.[90]

HYPERCAPNIA

Cardiovascular Responses

Awake Subjects

Carbon dioxide activates the central nervous system, producing sympathoadrenal responses, resulting in increased myocardial contractility, tachycardia, and hypertension. Acting directly, carbon dioxide dilates peripheral arterioles and depresses myocardial contractility. The net effect was studied by Cullen and Eger in 41 healthy young adult male volunteers.[91] During awake spontaneous breathing and with an elevation of Pa_{CO_2} from approximately 40 to 50 mm Hg, the investigators observed the following changes: Heart rate increases 26%; stroke volume rises 11%; cardiac output increases 32%; mean arterial pressure increases 10%; mean right atrial pressure is unchanged; total peripheral resistance falls 14%; and myocardial contractility increases.

Sechzer and coworkers showed in 12 healthy, awake, spontaneously breathing male volunteers that systolic and diastolic pressures increased progressively as Pa_{CO_2} was raised to values as high as 100 mm Hg.[92] Heart rate increased, but cardiac dysrhythmias were uncommon. The plasma levels of catecholamines (epinephrine and norepinephrine) also correlated with Pa_{CO_2}. Signs and symptoms produced by hypercapnia included headache, hiccups, nausea, vomiting, sweating, shivering, twitching, belligerence, restlessness, excitement and hallucinations. At acutely induced Pa_{CO_2} levels above 80 mm Hg, most subjects lose consciousness.

Anesthetized Subjects

General anesthesia modifies the cardiovascular responses to hypercapnia created by an elevation of inspired carbon dioxide. Deliberate studies of severe hypercapnia in patients are rare, for obvious reasons. However, moderate hypercapnia to a Pa_{CO_2} of 60 mm Hg has been studied. Cardiac output increases with increasing Pa_{CO_2} during anesthesia with nitrous oxide plus halothane, enflurane, and isoflurane. This increase in cardiac output is, however, less than that observed during hypercapnia in the awake state. The only exception occurs during anesthesia with 1.5% halothane in 70% nitrous oxide, when cardiac output decreases as Pa_{CO_2} rises.[93]

Heart rate rises during anesthesia in response to hypercapnia, but to a lesser extent than stroke volume. Hence, the increase in cardiac output during anesthesia is predominantly due to an increase in stroke volume.

Systemic blood pressure also rises when Pa_{CO_2} is increased from 40 to 50 mm Hg, except during anesthesia with halothane (1.5% end-tidal concentration) in oxygen or 70% nitrous oxide, when it remains unchanged, and with isoflurane (1.8% end-tidal concentration) when it decreases. With a wide range of anesthetic agents, the increase in mean systemic pressure ranges from one to eight mm Hg for an increase in Pa_{CO_2} of 40 to 50 mm Hg.

In summary, the cardiovascular parameters most easily measured during anesthesia, systemic blood pressure and pulse rate, increase during mild hypercapnia ($Pa_{CO_2} = 50$ mm Hg), but these increases are too small and nonspecific to be useful in detecting a 10 mm Hg increase in Pa_{CO_2}. They are independent of whether breathing is controlled or spontaneous.

Apneic Oxygenation

Higher levels of Pa_{CO_2} have been described during "apneic" oxygenation. Frumin studied eight patients made apneic with succinylcholine or d-tubocurarine during or after surgical procedures.[94] Anesthesia was maintained with intermittent intravenous injections of thiopental. Pa_{CO_2} rose at the rate of 3.0 mm Hg/min, with a range of 2.7 to 4.9 mm Hg/min. The mean value for the highest Pa_{CO_2} achieved was 166 mm Hg, with a range of 130 to 250 mm Hg. Mean systemic blood pressure rose by 26% of preapneic values. Systolic pressure increased by 45 mm Hg from a mean value of 115 mm Hg before apnea. In one subject in whom Pa_{CO_2} rose to 250 mm Hg, systolic blood pressure increased from 120 to 150 mm Hg. The increase in blood pressure seems to be independent of surgical stimulation, because in half of the subjects, the test apneic period was produced after the completion of surgery. Plasma epinephrine and norepinephrine values were elevated in three subjects.

Equipment Malfunction

Profound hypercapnia has been reported in cases in which an error in equipment assembly has led to an elevated Pa_{CO_2}. An 18-year-old patient, spontaneously breathing and anesthetized via a closed circuit, was noted to have a Pa_{CO_2} of 234 mm Hg due to the absence of one-way valves in the circuit.[95] At that time, systolic pressure was 120 mm Hg, with a regular pulse rate of 130 beats/min. Tachypnea, dilated pupils, perspiration, and flushing of the face were noted. Inspired anesthetic concentration was increased, as the signs were thought to represent a light level of anesthesia. After Pa_{CO_2} had been returned slowly to 40 mm Hg, systolic blood pressure was 130 mm Hg, with a pulse rate of 125 beats/min.

A second report involved a 60-year-old man who was mechanically ventilated during anesthesia using nitrous oxide, oxygen, and d-tubocurarine. A flow of carbon dioxide that was unrecognized at the time produced an inspired concentration of approximately 35%. During the initial 10 minutes of anesthetic administration, cyanosis was noted. This cyanosis disappeared, and the patient was said to be "damp." An arterial sample showed that the Pa_{CO_2} was 248 mm Hg. At that time, systolic blood pressure was 115 mm Hg, with a pulse rate of 100 beats/min. The inspired carbon dioxide flow was then stopped. Systolic blood pressure was approximately 90 mm Hg, and the pulse rate, 70 beats/min when Pa_{CO_2} was normal.[96]

Such extreme examples of hypercarbia and presence of carbon dioxide in the inspired gas are reliably prevented by the routine use of capnometry. Because modern anesthesia machines are not designed for carbon dioxide addition to the breathing circuit, and soda lime canisters no longer have a bypass valve, such causes have been eliminated by changes in equipment design. Table 20-5 offers a differential diagnosis for carbon dioxide in the inspired gas of a circle system, ie carbon dioxide rebreathing.

Chronic Lung Disease

In hypercapnia due to chronic lung disease, high Pa_{CO_2} can be present while the patient is awake, with little or no change in vital signs, even in the presence of considerable acidemia. We have observed one patient who experienced an increased Pa_{CO_2} from 60 to 105 mm Hg and decreased arterial pH to 7.0; no change in vital signs or mental state occurred.

Dysrhythmias

Cardiac dysrhythmias were once suggested as the most reliable circulatory indicator of hypercapnia.[97] However, they are by no means universally found. In a series of 18 patients anesthetized with thiopental and succinylcholine, no dysrhythmias were noted when Pa_{CO_2} was about 70 mm Hg.[98] Whether dysrhythmias occur seems to depend on the surgical stimulation, the age and physical fitness of the patient, and the type of

TABLE 20-5
Differential Diagnosis of Carbon Dioxide Rebreathing

FAULT	INSPIRATORY CARBON DIOXIDE	↓ PI_{CO_2} WITH ↑ FGF	CHANGE IN V_T*
Open rebreathing valve	+	+	0
Exhausted carbon dioxide absorbent (including channeling)	+	+	0
Incompetent expiratory valve	+	−	0
Incompetent inspiratory valve	±	−	↓

PI_{CO_2}, partial pressure of inspired carbon dioxide; FGF, fresh gas flow.
* V_T measured in expiratory limb.
Good ML, Paulus DA: Equipment. In Gravenstein N (ed): Manual of complications during anesthesia. Philadelphia: JB Lippincott, 1991:101.

anesthetic agent. Halothane in particular seems to predispose the patient to arrhythmias associated with hypercapnia.

Ventilatory Responses

The ventilatory response to inhaled carbon dioxide in conscious humans is increased minute ventilation. This response is blunted, but not usually eliminated, during anesthesia. For example, during halothane anesthesia, V_T and minute ventilation, though not respiratory rate, increase with a Pa_{CO_2} of as great as 70 mm Hg.

Hypoxemia

Hypercapnia can result in hypoxemia by two mechanisms. First, carbon dioxide displaces oxygen in the alveolar gas. Consider the alveolar gas equation, where it becomes clear that when patients breathe air, ie $FI_{O_2} = 0.21$, they cannot exceed a Pa_{CO_2} greater than 90 mm Hg because the displacement of alveolar oxygen produces a Pa_{O_2} of approximately 20 mm Hg, which is incompatible with survival. Even enriched inspired oxygen mixtures may not protect against low Pa_{O_2} if high levels of carbon dioxide are inspired.

The second mechanism is a rightward shift of the Hb_{O_2} dissociation curve. The significance of this factor can be judged by the calculations of Prys-Roberts and coworkers (see Fig. 21-1).[96] At a Pa_{O_2} of 104 mm Hg and a Pa_{CO_2} of 250 mm Hg, the arterial saturation would only be 90% as a consequence of the rightward shift of the curve, whereas at a normal Pa_{CO_2}, without the curve shifted the oxygen saturation would be very close to 100%.

The increase in cardiac output associated with hypercapnia, on the other hand, tends to improve arterial oxygenation. The $PA\text{-}a_{O_2}$ will decrease because of an increase in $C\bar{v}_{O_2}$. Pulmonary venous admixture is not altered by hypercapnia.

Anesthetic-related Causes

Increase in Carbon Dioxide Production

Measurement of $\dot{V}_{CO_2}$ during anesthesia is complicated by the size of the body stores of carbon dioxide, which affect the rate at which a new steady state will be achieved after an alteration in alveolar ventilation. Normally, $\dot{V}_{CO_2}$ is approximately 3 mL/kg/min. This is reduced to approximately 80% of the basal state during anesthesia. An increased $\dot{V}_{CO_2}$ is found with increased body temperature. This change is particularly marked in the syndrome of malignant hyperthermia. A modest increase in $\dot{V}_{CO_2}$ results when glucose is infused intravenously instead of normal saline. An artifactual increase in carbon dioxide "production" will be created when carbon dioxide is insufflated into a body cavity and then absorbed into the body (eg, during laparoscopy).

Intrinsic Lung Disease

Disturbance of the distribution of $\dot{V}_A/\dot{Q}$ ratios has been shown in lung models to impair carbon dioxide output as much as oxygen uptake.[99] Uncompensated, this disturbance will cause an elevation of Pa_{CO_2}. However, this increase in Pa_{CO_2} will usually provoke an increase in minute ventilation and a return toward a normal Pa_{CO_2}, with persisting hypoxemia. General anesthesia is associated with an increase in shunt, as was discussed earlier. Without compensatory hyperventilation, an increase in Pa_{CO_2} will occur. An increase in the alveolar dead space also occurs and has yet to be explained.

Pathologic Changes

Additional pathologic changes causing hypercapnia may occur. Atelectasis causes an increase in shunt and dead space and an increase in Pa_{CO_2} when patients are mechanically ventilated at a set minute volume. This increase usually is easily overcome by increasing the ventilation. Similarly, pulmonary embolism (eg, air, blood clot, fat, or tumor) causes an increase in alveolar dead space. Pulmonary edema, with its multitude of causes, may produce similar changes. Hypovolemia due to blood loss or extravasation of extracellular fluid into the so-called third space decreases systemic and pulmonary artery perfusion pressures and increases alveolar dead space.

Central Depression of Ventilation

The carbon dioxide level in blood and extracellular fluid usually is preserved at a constant level because of its involvement in acid-base regulation and cellular function. The potential effect on Pa_{CO_2} of increases in dead space due to lung disease will be offset by the respiratory centers, which tend to establish normocapnia. Failure to control ventilation appropriately results in hypercapnia. Whereas failure of oxygenation is usually a consequence of intrinsic lung disease, an increase in Pa_{CO_2} is most often the result of failure of ventilatory control. Although this statement bears the drawbacks of any generalization, it is made to emphasize this point. Obvious overlap occurs; for example, severe chronic lung disease causes increased Pa_{CO_2}.

Anesthetized Subjects

Inhalational Agents. In studies in anesthetized volunteers, the resting Pa_{CO_2} rises with increasing inspired concentrations of inhaled anesthetic agents. At the same level of MAC, halothane, methoxyflurane, cyclopropane, and fluroxene were associated with an increase in Pa_{CO_2} in decreasing order of intensity. At 2 MAC, for example, Pa_{CO_2} is approximately 70 mm Hg with halothane, and 42 mm Hg with fluroxene.[99] The predominant effect of these agents is to cause rapid, shallow breathing. Again at 2 MAC, halothane was associated with a decrease in V_T from a mean of approximately 400 mL to 150 mL. Respiratory frequency increased from approximately 15 to 30 breaths/min.

A V_T of 100 mL is common with halothane concentrations of 2.5 MAC. Although this V_T seems less than that of the anatomic dead space, physiologic dead space decreases with decreasing V_T, such that the ratio of dead space to V_T remains relatively constant throughout a wide range.

The exception among the inhalation agents is diethyl ether, which maintains Pa_{CO_2} from light to deep planes of anesthesia. The ventilatory response to increased inspired carbon dioxide is reduced with all agents, including ether. For example, with halothane (2 MAC) the response is only one-fifth that of the conscious state.

Except with diethyl ether, therefore, spontaneous breathing is usually associated with an increase in Pa_{CO_2} during inhalational anesthesia. This effect is modified by factors that increase ventilation (eg, surgical stimulation, metabolic acidosis). The information concerning the older agents is presented for historical interest and to form a basis for comparison with modern inhalational agents, because neither is used in the United States.

Narcotics. Narcotics depress ventilation and increase Pa_{CO_2} primarily by decreasing the rate of breathing, with less effect on V_T.[100]

Decrease in Work Capacity

An impairment of the ability of the respiratory pump may result in hypercapnia. For example, patients with neuromuscular disease, such as myasthenia gravis, or patients given muscle relaxants may develop an increase in Pa_{CO_2}. However, in awake volunteers given incremental intravenous doses of d-tubocurarine, the slope of the carbon dioxide response curve is not altered significantly.[101] Multiple fractured ribs or trauma to the diaphragm may result in a reduction in the effectiveness of the ventilatory pump, with consequent hypercapnia. Increases in airway resistance or a decrease in compliance also may result in hypercapnia.

Increase in Inhaled Carbon Dioxide

Expiratory or inspiratory valve incompetence and failure or exhaustion of the soda lime absorbing system also result in high inspired carbon dioxide concentrations. Carbon dioxide rebreathing also occurs when inadequate fresh gas flows are used with any of the Mapleson type circuits because they rely on a high fresh gas flow to purge the inspiratory gas reservoir of carbon dioxide.

Postoperative Hypercapnia

The characteristic disorders of gas exchange after anesthesia and surgery are an increase in shunt and mild to moderate hyperventilation. Two factors commonly thought to cause elevation of Pa_{CO_2} are abdominal distention and pain. However, neither has been demonstrated to do so. Elevated Pa_{CO_2} levels in the postoperative period cannot be attributed to "atelectasis" or "abdominal pain"; some other factor, usually not related to intrinsic lung disease, must be sought.

Central Depression of Ventilation

The clinical picture of the patient with elevated Pa_{CO_2} levels and no dyspnea or tachypnea is a clue to the presence of central depression of ventilation. This problem, however, may be complicated by concomitant intrinsic lung disease in which some degree of dyspnea and tachypnea may be found.

NARCOTICS. The effect of narcotics on the respiratory centers is probably the most common precipitating factor. They may have been used for the induction or maintenance of anesthesia and often have an exceptionally prolonged effect. We have seen patients with depressed mental status and elevated Pa_{CO_2} 10 days after intravenous morphine; these were reversed by intravenous naloxone. This prolonged effect seems particularly evident in patients with renal failure.[102] However, one patient with apparently normal renal and hepatic function developed a slow respiratory rate (reversed with naloxone) 10 days after the use of methadone (30 mg) for maintenance of anesthesia.[103] Drug synergism also occurs between narcotics and sedatives, and thus one may see an exaggerated respiratory depression when these drugs have been used in combination.[104]

Metabolic Alkalosis

Metabolic alkalosis commonly is related to removal of gastric contents and a resultant hypochloremic alkalosis. An elevated Pa_{CO_2} may result. Large volumes of homologous blood transfusion also produce alkalosis as citrate is metabolized. Failure to find compensatory changes in Pa_{CO_2} may be due to the duration and rate of onset of the alkalosis. The elevated Pa_{CO_2} does not require treatment, for it provides a more normal pH. The reduction in minute ventilation may predispose to atelectasis, and delay weaning from mechanical ventilation. It is best treated by slow correction of the metabolic alkalosis or administration of acetazolamide to promote renal excretion of bicarbonate through carbonic anhydrase inhibition. Two 500 mg boluses 4 hours apart usually suffice in combination with potassium chloride administration.

High Levels of Inspired Oxygen and Chronic Pulmonary Lung Disease

High levels of inspired oxygen administered to patients with chronic hypercapnia who therefore have a hypoxic respiratory drive may depress ventilation. This effect can be a prominent, though unusual, feature of chronic pulmonary disease. In 26 patients with emphysema, breathing of 100% oxygen caused a mean increase in Pa_{CO_2} from 49 to 62 mm Hg. In 9 of these patients with a normal Pa_{CO_2} (34 to 44 mm Hg) who breathed air, Pa_{CO_2} rose to a mean of 53 mm Hg.[105] High inspired oxygen sometimes is given to a patient in whom chronic lung disease is not recognized.

Patients with similar abnormalities of pulmonary function may have a normal or high Pa_{CO_2}. In those who develop hypercapnia, the work of breathing may be greater; or they may represent individuals who, in a normal distribution, would have a flattened carbon dioxide response, even without existing lung disease. Hence, some patients without lung disease may respond to high oxygen concentrations by developing an elevated Pa_{CO_2}. This should be suspected in patients who have an abnormal baseline oxygen saturation and can be verified by an arterial blood gas analysis that demonstrates an elevated Pa_{CO_2}.

Surgery in the Cervical Region

The term "Ondine's curse" was coined by Severinghaus and Mitchell to describe failure of automaticity of ventilation after cervical cordotomy for chronic pain.[106] This problem can occur after unilateral or bilateral cordotomy. It also has been described after anterior surgery at the third to fourth cervical interspace without cordotomy.[107] We have seen an elderly patient in whom methyl methacrylate cement was placed in the region of the third cervical vertebral body; this patient was discovered to be lethargic with a slow respiratory rate and a Pa_{CO_2} of 200 mm Hg 24 hours postoperatively. Her respiratory control returned to normal within 36 hours. No evidence for other causes of hypercapnia, such as narcotic effect was found.

Increased Work of Breathing

Upper-airway obstruction may cause hypercapnia. In obese, hypoventilating subjects, tracheotomy has been shown to restore normal Pa_{CO_2}.[108] Similarly, in children adenoidectomy has been associated with the relief of hypercapnia, hypoxemia, and pulmonary hypertension. In the postoperative period, upper-airway obstruction can lead to an elevated Pa_{CO_2}. Insertion of a nasopharyngeal airway may reverse the hypercapnia. Fatigue can result from abnormal respiratory muscle loading, deranged lung or chest wall mechanisms, and high ventilatory demand.[109] Increased work of breathing may also be a result of a small endotracheal tube, partial airway obstruction, or an inadequate ventilator–breathing circuit arrangement.[110]

Decreased Work Capacity

Failure to reverse the effect of neuromuscular blocking agents will result in partial paralysis. Patients so affected hypoventilate, even when vital capacity is greater than the V_T. The effect is as if the respiratory centers leave a small margin of reserve available in the ventilatory pump. Paralysis with pancuronium, d-tubocurarine, and metubine is prolonged in patients with renal disease. The effect of the nondepolarizing muscle relaxants may be potentiated by aminoglycoside antibiotics (eg, neomycin, streptomycin, and gentamicin).

Other Causes

Two or more factors may combine to produce hypercapnia. For example, an obese patient, with mild upper-airway obstruction, who is breathing high inspired oxygen and has developed a slight metabolic alkalosis from vomiting, can develop severe hypercapnia if given even a small dose of narcotic.

TREATMENT OF HYPERCAPNIA

During Anesthesia

The diagnosis of hypercapnia is made by the measurement of increased Pa_{CO_2}, end-tidal carbon dioxide partial pressure (PET_{CO_2}), or both. Measurement of the partial pressure of carbon dioxide in a peripheral venous sample during anesthesia gives an excellent indication of Pa_{CO_2} (Table 20-6).

With the advent of routine capnometry, airway PET_{CO_2} has become the most common method for diagnosing hypercapnia intraoperatively. However, use of capnometry to aid in this assessment must be made with an understanding of factors that are responsible for the differences between Pa_{CO_2} and PET_{CO_2}. In patients with healthy lungs, the Pa_{CO_2}-PET_{CO_2} difference is usually less than or equal to 6 mm Hg. However, patients with arteriolar chronic lung disease may manifest differences greater than 10 mm Hg.[111] Therefore, if it is clinically important to know the precise Pa_{CO_2}, capnometry does not replace arterial blood gas analysis.[110]

Once hypercapnia is diagnosed, when and how should it be treated? High levels of Pa_{CO_2} can be tolerated safely. In a study of 44 patients during anesthesia for thoracic and nonthoracic surgery, hypercapnia occurred in all patients. In the majority, maximal Pa_{CO_2} was 100 mm Hg, and in many cases a peak of 175 to 200 mm Hg was found.[112] In a series of 22 patients undergoing major abdominal surgery, with spontaneous ventilation, using a face mask and "closed-circuit" halothane, most values for Pa_{CO_2} were in the range of 50 to 90 mm Hg. In the latter half of each operation, some patients had Pa_{CO_2} levels as high as 160 mm Hg.[113]

In spite of these case reports, a Pa_{CO_2} above 50 mm Hg in a usually eucapnic patient probably should be avoided during anesthesia. The treatment, obviously, is assisted or controlled ventilation. Attention to equipment, flowmeters, valves, soda lime, and unnecessary dead space are essential to prevent the development of hypercapnia.

A number of reported hazards accrue to lowering an elevated Pa_{CO_2} too rapidly. Cardiac dysrhythmias often are thought to be precipitated. However, this phenomenon is not supported by all investigators.[94,95] Hypotension also has been reported, but does not occur consistently and is usually only found if Pa_{CO_2} is sufficiently elevated for a prolonged period.[97] Long-

TABLE 20-6
Differences in Peripheral Venous and Arterial Blood Gas Values During Anesthesia With Three Inhalation Anesthetics

	ISOFLURANE (n = 15)	ENFLURANE (n = 16)	HALOTHANE (n = 17)
P_{CO_2}	−1.2 ± 1.6	−1.5 ± 2.1	−1.6 ± 1.6
pH	0.01 ± 0.01	0.01 ± 0.01	0.02 ± 0.2
Base excess (mEq/L)	0.09 ± 0.56*	0.03 ± 0.75*	0.20 ± 0.33
P_{O_2}	49.5 ± 36.9	39.4 ± 29.1	56.9 ± 52.1
F_{IO_2}	0.65 ± 0.98	0.57 ± 0.44	0.69 ± 0.45

Values are means ± SD.
* With these exceptions, all arteriovenous values were significantly different at the 0.05 level.
Williamson DG, Munson ES. Correlation of peripheral venous and arterial blood gas values during general anesthesia. Anesth Analg 61:951, 1982.

standing hypercapnia usually produces increases in bicarbonate through renal compensation. Acute reduction to a normal Pa_{CO_2} will produce significant alkalosis of cerebral interstitial fluid.

After Surgery

After surgery, the same considerations apply to hypercapnia as in the intraoperative period: What is the danger, and what level of Pa_{CO_2} should be treated? In a patient who has received morphine, who is sleeping but arousable, and who has a Pa_{CO_2} of 50 mm Hg and pH of 7.32, reversal of the narcotic effect simply to improve these value seems unnecessary. Considerations for the treatment of hypercapnia are listed in Table 20-7.

Reversal of the Cause

NALOXONE. The initial treatment is reversal of the cause. Narcotic analgesic effects can be reversed with naloxone, which has the advantage of not causing respiratory depression and is relatively safe. However, it can cause transient nausea and vomiting and systemic hypertension, which may provoke congestive heart failure or rupture of a cerebral aneurysm. It can also cause pulmonary edema without systemic hypertension, producing a clinical picture similar to that of neurogenic pulmonary edema.[114] Its duration of action is short, so administration may have to be repeated at intervals. Obviously, it will also reverse the analgesic effects of the narcotic. Small, titrated, incremental doses, eg 20 to 40 μg, avoid these problems.

When the necessity for tracheal intubation is being considered in an obtunded patient with hypercapnia, we frequently give a trial of naloxone, particularly when the patient's drug history is not clear. If hypercapnia is associated with previous drug use other than narcotics, physostigmine may be beneficial. This anticholinesterase has been reported to reverse the central nervous system depressant effects of ketamine, phenothiazines, benzodiazepines, tricyclic antidepressants, and droperidol. Its reversal of the depressant effect of diazepam is disputed and outdated.[115] Flumazenil, a benzodiazepine receptor antagonist, can be used for reversal of benzodiazepine effect and reportedly is useful in the diagnosis and treatment of patients with coma of unknown etiology.[116]

ANCILLARY MEASURES. General stimulation and arousal are beneficial and are one of the benefits of postoperative intermittent positive-pressure breathing and chest physiotherapy. Metabolic alkalosis can be reversed slowly with acetazolamide, 0.1 N hydrochloric acid, or arginine hydrochloride. These agents are usually indicated in patients with a severe primary metabolic alkalosis (base excess greater than 15). Correction of upper-airway obstruction obviously is helpful. Simple insertion of a nasopharyngeal airway may be curative.

TABLE 20-7
Considerations in the Treatment of Hypercapnia

- Is the pH at a dangerous level (<7.25)?
- Is the condition likely to progress, or is it stable?
- Is it associated with any other harmful effect, such as arrhythmias or hypoxemia due to hypercapnia or atelectasis due to hypoventilation?
- What is the mental state of the patient?
- What are the comparative dangers of the treatments of hypercapnia?

Reduction in Arterial Oxygenation

Lowering the F_{IO_2} can reduce the Pa_{CO_2} if the etiology is interference with the patient's hypoxic respiratory drive. In such patients, care must be taken not to produce life-threatening hypoxemia in the treatment of relatively benign hypercapnia, particularly in the postoperative period, when oxygen demands may be greater and the patient's status is likely to undergo sudden fluctuations. This technique of controlled inspired oxygen requires expert nursing and medical attention and should be accompanied by pulse oximetry monitoring.

Treatment of any underlying lung disease is also important. Intermittent positive pressure breathing, incentive spirometry, spontaneous breathing with PEEP or continuous positive airway pressure, bronchodilators, chest physiotherapy, nasotracheal suctioning, mobilization, and humidification of the inspired gas all have a role when wisely and discretely used.

Tracheal Intubation and Mechanical Ventilation

In an intensive care environment, tracheal intubation and mechanical ventilation are relatively benign procedures. In a series of 88 adult cardiac patients, we could not detect a complication attributable to 24 hours of postoperative mechanical ventilation. However, in a series of 50 pediatric patients after cardiac surgery, an approximate 30% incidence of complications due to tracheal intubation and mechanical ventilation was noted. Airway obstruction, accidental extubation, postextubation airway obstruction, and accidental disconnection of the mechanical ventilator occurred. Therefore, examination of the environment in which the patient will be treated is important in determining the possible hazards.

Guidelines

Blood Gas Values. The patient's mental state should be monitored closely when mechanical ventilation is considered. An awake, alert patient is a less likely candidate. Not infrequently, we have decided against mechanical ventilation in patients with Pa_{CO_2} levels greater than 80 mm Hg on the basis of their clear mental status. The rate of change of Pa_{CO_2} is also an important factor. For example, two values of 55 mm Hg, found at a 1-hour interval, suggest the patient is stable. An increase in Pa_{CO_2} after 1 hour suggests continuing deterioration.

Physical Signs. If the patient is distressed, has tachypnea or dyspnea, or is working hard to breathe, with intercostal muscle retraction and a tracheal "tug," intubation and mechanical ventilation often are indicated. Hypoxemia (Pa_{O_2} <55 mm Hg) with a FI_{O_2} that is as high as can be justified by the combination of low Pa_{O_2} and high Pa_{CO_2} also indicate the need for intubation and mechanical ventilation. We have not found that measurement or calculation of $PA\text{-}a_{O_2}$, V_T, vital capacity, or dead space ventilation are valuable in making the decision. When hypercapnia is likely to be transient, intubation should be avoided if other techniques can be used. If personnel are available to determine the need for and to perform tracheal intubation on short notice, the decision to intubate also may be delayed. Sometimes, the decision to intubate is based on the clinical impression that the patient "looks bad" or "will go sour," and not on measurable quantities. In general, however, tracheal intubation and mechanical ventilation should be instituted if the patient's well-being is seriously in question.

REFERENCES

1. Marshall BE, Wyche MQ Jr: Hypoxemia during and after anesthesia. Anesthesiology 37:178, 1972
2. Cullen DJ, Eger EI II: The effects of hypoxia and isovolemic anemia on the halothane requirement (MAC) of dogs: I. the effect of hypoxia. Anesthesiology 32:28, 1970
3. Cullen DJ, Eger EI II: The effects of hypoxia and isovolemic anemia on the halothane requirement (MAC) of dogs: III. The effects of acute isovolemic anemia. Anesthesiology 32:46, 1970
4. Malik AB, Kidd BSL: Time course of pulmonary vascular response to hypoxia in dogs. Am J Physiol 224:1, 1973
5. Comroe JH, Botelho S: The unreliability of cyanosis in the recognition of arterial anoxemia. Am J Med Sci 214:1, 1947
6. Schmitter CR Jr: Sulfhemoglobinemia and methemoglobinemia: uncommon causes of cyanosis. Anesthesiology 43:586, 1975
7. Cullen DJ, Eger EI II: The effects of halothane on respiratory and cardiovascular responses to hypoxia in dogs: a dose–response study. Anesthesiology 33:487, 1970
8. Gray IG, Nisbet HIA, Olley PM, et al: Cardiovascular and respiratory responses to severe hypoxaemia under anaesthesia: II. spontaneous and controlled ventilation during methoxyflurane anaesthesia. Can Anaesth Soc J 20:637, 1973
9. Weiskopf RB, Raymond LW, Severinghaus JW: Effects of halothane on canine respiratory responses to hypoxia with and without hypercarbia. Anesthesiology 41:350, 1974
10. Hirshman CA, McCullough RE, Cohen PJ, et al: Hypoxic ventilatory drive in dogs during thiopental, ketamine, or pentobarbital anesthesia. Anesthesiology 43:628, 1975
11. Knill RL, Clement JL: Site of selective action of halothane on the peripheral chemoreceptor pathway in humans. Anesthesiology 61:121, 1984
12. Kontos HA, Mauck HP Jr, Richardson DW, et al: Mechanism of circulatory responses to systemic hypoxia in the anesthetized dog. Am J Physiol 209:397, 1965
13. Regan MJ, Eger EI II: Ventilatory responses to hypercapnia and hypoxia at normothermia and moderate hypothermia during constant-depth halothane anesthesia. Anesthesiology 27: 624, 1966
14. Roberts JG, Föex P, Clarke TNS, et al: Haemodynamic interactions of high-dose propranolol pretreatment and anaesthesia in the dog: II. the effects of acute arterial hypoxaemia at increasing depths of halothane anaesthesia. Br J Anaesth 48: 403, 1976
15. American Society of Anesthesiologists: Standards for basic intraoperative monitoring. In Directory of Members. Park Ridge, IL: American Society of Anesthesiologists, 1994:735
16. Nims RG, Conner EH, Comroe JH: The compliance of the human thorax in anesthetized patients. J Clin Invest 34:744, 1955
17. Howell JBL, Peckett BW: Studies of the elastic properties of the thorax of supine anaesthetized paralyzed human subjects. J Physiol 136:1, 1957
18. Don HF, Wahba M, Cuadrado L, et al: The effects of anesthesia and 100 per cent oxygen on the functional residual capacity of the lungs. Anesthesiology 32:521, 1970
19. Hewlett AM, Hulands GH, Nunn JF, et al: Functional residual capacity during anaesthesia: II. spontaneous respiration. Br J Anaesth 46:486, 1974
20. Laws AK: Effects of induction of anaesthesia and muscle paralysis on functional residual capacity of the lungs. Can Anaesth Soc J 15:325, 1968
21. Hewlett AM, Hulands GH, Nunn JF, et al: Functional residual capacity during anaesthesia: III. artificial ventilation. Br J Anaesth 46:495, 1974
22. Hedenstierna G, McCarthy G, Bergstrom M: Airway closure during mechanical ventilation. Anesthesiology 44:114, 1976
23. Nunn JF: Factors influencing the arterial oxygen tension during halothane anaesthesia with spontaneous respiration. Br J Anaesth 36:327, 1964
24. Panday J, Nunn JF: Failure to demonstrate progressive falls in arterial PO_2 during anaesthesia. Anaesthesia 23:38, 1968
25. Hickey RF, Visick WD, Fairley HB, et al: Effects of halothane anesthesia on functional residual capacity and alveolar–arterial oxygen tension difference. Anesthesiology 38:20, 1973
26. Gilmour I, Burnham M, Craig DB: Closing capacity measurement during general anesthesia. Anesthesiology 45:477, 1976
27. Juno P, Marsh HM, Knopp TJ, et al: Closing capacity in awake and anesthetized paralyzed man. J Appl Physiol 44:238, 1978
28. Don HF, Wahba WM, Craig DB: Airway closure, gas trapping, and the functional residual capacity during anesthesia. Anesthesiology 36:533, 1972

29. Rehder K, Sittipong R, Sessler AD: The effects of thiopental–meperidine anesthesia with succinylcholine paralysis on functional residual capacity and dynamic lung compliance in normal sitting man. Anesthesiology 37:395, 1972
30. Shah J, Jones JG, Galvin J, et al: Pulmonary gas exchange during induction of anaesthesia with nitrous oxide in seated subjects. Br J Anaesth 43:1013, 1971
31. Hedenstierna G, Strandberg A, Brismar B, et al: Functional residual capacity, thoracoabdominal dimensions, and central blood volume during general anesthesia with muscle paralysis and mechanical ventilation. Anesthesiology 62:247, 1985
32. Bismar B, Hedenstierna G, Lundquist H, et al: Pulmonary densities during anesthesia with muscular relaxation: a proposal of atelectasis. Anesthesiology 62:422, 1985
33. Froese AB, Bryan AC: Effects of anesthesia and paralysis on diaphragmatic mechanics in man. Anesthesiology 41:242, 1974
34. Kallos T, Wyche MQ, Garman JK: The effects of Innovar on functional residual capacity and total chest compliance in man. Anesthesiology 39:558, 1973
35. Bergman NA, Tien YK: Contribution of the closure of pulmonary units to impaired oxygenation during anesthesia. Anesthesiology 59:395, 1983
36. Patton CM Jr, Dannemiller FJ, Broennle AM: CPPB during surgical anesthesia: effect on oxygenation and blood pressure. Anesth Analg 53:309, 1974
37. Smith TC, Colton ET III, Behar MG: Does anesthesia alter hemoglobin dissociation? Anesthesiology 32:5, 1970
38. Carden WD, Petty WC: The lack of effect of lidocaine on oxyhemoglobin dissociation. Anesthesiology 38:177, 1973
39. Wahba WM, Craig DB, Don HF, et al: The cardio-respiratory effects of thoracic epidural anaesthesia. Can Anaesth Soc J 19: 8, 1972
40. Askrog VF, Smith TC, Eckenhoff JE: Changes in pulmonary ventilation during spinal anesthesia. Surg Gynecol Obstet 119: 563, 1964
41. Aalto-Setälä M, Heionen J, Salorinne Y: Cardiorespiratory function during thoracic anaesthesia: a comparison of two-lung ventilation and one-lung ventilation with and without $PEEP_5$. Acta Anaesthesiol Scand 19:287, 1975
42. Brown DL, Davis RF: A simple device for oxygen insufflation with continuous positive airway pressure during one-lung ventilation. Anesthesiology 61:481, 1984
43. Thomas DF, Campbell D: Changes in arterial oxygen tension during one-lung anaesthesia. Br J Anaesth 45:611, 1973
44. Boutros AR: Arterial blood oxygenation during and after endotracheal suctioning in the apneic patient. Anesthesiology 32: 114, 1970
45. Blitt CD, Gutman HL, Cohen DD, et al: 'Silent' regurgitation and aspiration with general anesthesia. Anesth Analg 49:707, 1970
46. Willms D, Shure D: Pulmonary edema due to upper airway obstruction in adults. Chest 94:1090, 1988
47. Kollef MH, Pluss J: Noncardiogenic pulmonary edema following upper airway obstruction. Medicine 70:91, 1991
48. Sulek CA: Negative pressure pulmonary edema. Current Reviews in Clinical Anesthesia 13:11, 1992
49. Tsai S, Lee T, Mok MS: Gas embolism produced by hydrogen peroxide irrigation of an anal fistula during anesthesia. Anesthesiology 63:316, 1985
50. Hanson EL, O'Connor NE, Drinker PA: Hemodynamic response to controlled ventilation during hypoxia in man and animals. Surgical Forum 23:207, 1972
51. Dibenedetto R, Graves SA, Gravenstein N: Pulse oximetry monitoring can change routine oxygen supplementation practices in the PACU. Anesth Analg 78:365, 1994
52. Marshall BE, Millar RA: Some factors influencing post-operative hypoxaemia. Anaesthesia 20:408, 1965
53. Diament ML, Palmer KNV: Postoperative changes in gas tensions of arterial blood and in ventilatory function. Lancet 2: 180, 1966
54. Knudsen J: Duration of hypoxaemia after uncomplicated upper abdominal and thoracoabdominal operations. Anaesthesia 25: 372, 1970
55. Siler JN, Rosenberg H, Mull TD, et al: Hypoxemia after upper abdominal surgery: comparisons of venous admixture and ventilation/perfusion inequality components, using a digital computer. Ann Surg 179:149, 1974
56. Georg J, Hornum I, Mellemgaard K: The mechanism of hypoxaemia after laparotomy. Thorax 22:382, 1967
57. Kitamura H, Sawa T, Ikezono E: Postoperative hypoxemia: the contribution of age to the maldistribution of ventilation. Anesthesiology 36:244, 1972
58. Alexander JI, Spence AA, Parikh RK, et al: The role of airway closure in postoperative hypoxaemia. Br J Anaesth 45:34, 1973
59. Beecher HK: The measured effect of laparotomy on respiration. J Clin Invest 12:639, 1933
60. Zikria BA, Spencer JL, Kinney JM, et al: Alterations in ventilatory function and breathing patterns following surgical trauma. Ann Surg 179:1, 1974
61. Fibuch EE, Rehder K, Sessler AD: Preoperative CC/FRC ratio and postoperative hypoxemia. Anesthesiology 43:481, 1975
62. Wahba WM, Don HF, Craig DB: Postoperative epidural analgesia: effects on lung volumes. Can Anaesth Soc J 22:519, 1975
63. Hollmen A, Saukkonen J: The effects of postoperative epidural analgesia versus centrally acting opiate on physiological shunt after upper abdominal operation. Acta Anaesthesiol Scand 16: 147, 1972
64. Grundy BL, Crampton CA, Hardcastle JF, et al: Postoperative hypoxia on a surgical ward: telemetered pulse oximetry, abstract. J Clin Monit 7:120, 1991
65. American Society of Anesthesiologists: Standards for postanesthesia care. Park Ridge, IL: American Society of Anesthesiologists, Oct 12, 1988; last amended Oct 19, 1994
66. Cooperman LH, Price HL: Pulmonary edema in the operative and postoperative period: a review of 40 cases. Ann Surg 172: 883, 1970
67. Levy RP, Laus VG, Miraldi FD: The frequency and detection of serious postoperative thromboembolic disease. Surg Gynecol Obstet 140:903, 1975
68. Lahnborg G, Bergstrom K, Friman L, et al: Effect of low dose heparin on incidence of postoperative pulmonary embolism detected by photoscanning. Lancet 1:329, 1974
69. Dismuke SE, Wagner EH: Pulmonary embolism as a cause of death: the changing mortality in hospitalized patients. JAMA 255:2039, 1986
70. Mendelson CL: The aspiration of stomach contents into the lungs during obstetric anesthesia. Am J Obstet Gynecol 52: 191, 1946
71. Philbin DM, Sullivan SF, Bowman FO, et al: Postoperative hypoxemia: contribution of the cardiac output. Anesthesiology 32:136, 1970
72. Holmdahl MH, Modig J: The role of regional block versus parenteral analgesics in patient management with special emphasis on the treatment of postoperative pain. Br J Anaesth 47:264, 1975
73. Salvatore AJ, Sullivan SF, Papper EM: Postoperative hypoventilation and hypoxemia in man after hyperventilation. N Engl J Med 280:467, 1969
74. Roesch R, Stoelting R: Duration of hypoxemia during nitrous oxide excretion. Anesth Analg 51:851, 1972
75. Cane RD, Rasanen J: Hypoxemia. In Kirby RR, Gravenstein N (eds): Clinical anesthesia practice. Philadelphia: WB Saunders, 1994: 782
76. Davis AG, Spence AA: Postoperative hypoxemia and age. Anesthesiology 37:663, 1972
77. Gibson RL, Comer PB, Beckham RW, et al: Actual tracheal oxygen concentration with commonly used oxygen equipment. Anesthesiology 44:71, 1976
78. Bersten AD, Holt AW, Vedig AE, et al: Treatment of severe pulmonary edema with continuous positive airway pressure delivered by face mask. N Engl J Med 325:1825, 1991
79. Smith RA, Kirby RR, Gooding JM: Continuous positive airway pressure (CPAP) by face mask. Crit Care Med 8:483, 1980
80. Kirby RR, Downs JB, Civetta JM, et al: High level positive end

expiratory pressure (PEEP) in acute respiratory insufficiency. Chest 67:156, 1975

81. Register SD, Downs JB, Stock MC, et al: Is 50% oxygen harmful? Crit Care Med 15:598, 1987
82. Jackson RM: Pulmonary oxygen toxicity. Chest 88:900, 1985
83. Dixon CL, Sefton W, Gravenstein N: Epidural analgesia after donor nephrectomy decreases duration of hospitalization (abstract). Regional Anesthesia 17:75, 1992
84. Pflug AE, Murphy TM, Butler SH, et al: The effects of postoperative peridural analgesia or pulmonary therapy and pulmonary complications. Anesthesiology 41:8, 1974
85. Catley DM, Thornton C, Jordan C, et al: Pronounced, episodic oxygen desaturation in the postoperative period: its association with ventilatory pattern and analgesic regimen. Anesthesiology 63:20, 1985
86. Brown DL, Flynn JF, Owens BD: Pain control. In Civetta JM, Taylor RW, Kirby RR (eds): Critical care. Philadelphia: JB Lippincott, 1992: 219
87. Cousins MJ, Mather LE: Intrathecal and epidural administration of opioids. Anesthesiology 61:276, 1984
88. Vaughan RW, Bauer S, Wise L: Effect of position (semirecumbent versus supine) on postoperative oxygenation in markedly obese subjects. Anesth Analg 55:37, 1976
89. Bartlett RJ, Brennan ML, Gazzaniga AB, et al: Studies on the pathogenesis and prevention of postoperative pulmonary complications. Surg Gynecol Obstet 137:925, 1973
90. Stock MC, Downs JB, Gauer PK, et al: Prevention of postoperative respiratory complications with CPAP, incentive spirometry, and conservative therapy. Chest 87:151, 1985
91. Cullen DJ, Eger EI II: Cardiovascular effects of carbon dioxide in man. Anesthesiology 41:345, 1974
92. Sechzer PH, Egbert LD, Linde HW, et al: Effect of CO_2 inhalation on arterial pressure, ECG and plasma catecholamines and 17-OH corticosteroids in normal man. J Appl Physiol 15: 454, 1960
93. Hornbein TF, Martin WE, Bonica JJ, et al: Nitrous oxide effects on the circulatory and ventilatory responses to halothane. Anesthesiology 31:250, 1969
94. Frumin JM, Epstein RM, Cohen G: Apneic oxygenation in man. Anesthesiology 20:789, 1959
95. Schultz EA, Buckley JJ, Oswald AJ, et al: Profound acidosis in an anesthetized human: report of a case. Anesthesiology 21: 285, 1960
96. Prys-Roberts C, Smith WDA, Nunn JF: Accidental severe hypercapnia during anaesthesia: a case report and review of some physiological effects. Br J Anaesth 39:257, 1967
97. Price HL: Effects of carbon dioxide on the cardiovascular system. Anesthesiology 21:652, 1960
98. Fraioli RL, Sheffer LA, Steffenson JL: Pulmonary and cardiovascular effects of apneic oxygenation in man. Anesthesiology 39:588, 1973
99. Larson CP Jr, Eger EI II, Maullem M, et al: The effects of diethyl ether and methoxyflurane on ventilation: II. a comparative study in man. Anesthesiology 30:174, 1969
100. Davie I, Scott DB, Stephen GW: Respiratory effects of pentazocine and pethidine in patients anaesthetized with halothane and oxygen. Br J Anaesth 42:113, 1970
101. Gal TJ, Smith TC: Partial paralysis with *d*-tubocurarine and the ventilatory response to CO_2: an example of respiratory sparing? Anesthesiology 45:22, 1976
102. Don HF, Dieppa RA, Taylor P: Narcotic analgesics in anuric patients. Anesthesiology 42:745, 1975
103. Norris JV, Don HF: Prolonged depression of respiratory rate following methadone analgesia. Anesthesiology 45:361, 1976
104. Ben Shlomo I, Abd-El-Khalim H, Ezry J, et al: Midazolam acts synergistically with fentanyl for the induction of anaesthesia. Br J Anaesth 64:45, 1990
105. Wilson RH, Hoseth W, Dempsey ME: Respiratory acidosis. I. Effects of decreasing respiratory minute volume in patients with severe chronic pulmonary emphysema, with specific reference to oxygen, morphine and barbiturates. Am J Med 10: 464, 1954
106. Severinghaus JW, Mitchell RA: Ondine's curse: failure of respiratory center automaticity while awake. Clin Res 10:122, 1962
107. Krieger AJ, Rosomoff HL: Sleep induced apnea: II. respiratory failure after anterior spinal surgery. J Neurosurg 39:181, 1974
108. Sackner MA, Landa J, Forrest T: Periodic sleep apnea: chronic sleep deprivation related to intermittent upper airway obstruction and central nervous system disturbance. Chest 67:164, 1975
109. Banner MJ, Blanch PB, Kirby RR: Imposed work of breathing and methods of triggering a demand-flow continuous positive airway pressure system. Crit Care Med 21:183, 1993
110. Roussos C: Respiratory muscle fatigue and ventilatory failure. Chest 97:895, 1990
111. Chopin C, Fesard P, Mangalaboy J, et al: Use of capnography in diagnosis of pulmonary embolism during acute respiratory failure of chronic obstructive pulmonary disease. Crit Care Med 18:353, 1990
112. Ellison RG, Ellison LT, Hamilton WF: Analysis of respiratory acidosis during anesthesia. Ann Surg 141:375, 1955
113. Birt C, Cole P: Some physiological effects of closed circuit halothane anaesthesia. Anaesthesia 20:258, 1965
114. Prough DS, Roy R, Bumgarner J, et al: Acute pulmonary edema in healthy teenagers following conservative doses of intravenous naloxone. Anesthesiology 60:485, 1984
115. Spaulding BC, Choi SD, Gross JB, et al: The effect of physostigmine on diazepam-induced ventilatory depression: a double-blind study. Anesthesiology 61:551, 1984
116. Winkler E, Almog S, Krieger D, et al: Use of flumazenil in the diagnosis and treatment of patients with coma of unknown etiology. Crit Care Med 21:538, 1993

FURTHER READING

Nunn, JF: Applied respiratory physiology, 4th ed. Oxford: Butterworth-Heinemann, 1993

Shapiro BW, Peruzzi WT: Clinical application of blood gases, 5th ed. St. Louis: Mosby-Year Book, 1994

Complications in Anesthesiology, second edition,
edited by Nikolaus Gravenstein and Robert R. Kirby.
Lippincott-Raven Publishers, Philadelphia © 1996.

CHAPTER 21

Air Embolism

Robert F. Bedford

Since the early 19th century, air embolism has been a potential complication of surgical and diagnostic procedures, particularly those performed with the patient in the sitting position.[1,2] A partial list of additional precipitating factors includes any procedure that requires externalization of the circulatory system (open heart surgery,[3] liver transplantation,[4] hemodialysis,[5] and pressurized intravascular infusions); any procedure that requires gas insufflation (Rubin's test,[6] laparoscopy,[7] therapeutic pneumothorax, gastrointestinal endoscopy,[8] pneumoencephalography,[9] pneumocystometry,[10] arthrography,[11] and epidural anesthesia administered by the technique of loss of resistance to air); any procedure that provides continuity between the atmosphere and the low-pressure venous circulation[12] (central venous catheterization[13,14] and catheter introducer sheath insertion[15]), especially those involving large areas of exposed tissue (scalp flap,[16] mastectomy,[17] spinal fusion,[18] and total hip arthroplasty[19]); thoracic trauma[20] (blast injury, thoracentesis, excessive positive airway pressure, and open chest wounds); and miscellaneous events (equipment failure during vacuum abortion[21] and cunnilingus[22]).

TYPES OF AIR EMBOLI

It is important to differentiate among embolization of air to the arterial circulation, embolization to the venous pulmonary circulation, and embolization to both circulations ("paradoxical air embolism").

Systemic Arterial Air Embolism

Systemic arterial embolization alone is most commonly a complication of extracorporeal bypass procedures or thoracic trauma. The primary threat of air in the systemic arterial system is the risk of embolization to the coronary or the cerebral circulation.

Coronary Arteries

Air embolized to the coronary arteries may be fatal because interruption of blood flow produces ischemia-induced terminal dysrhythmias or myocardial infarction or both.

Cerebral Vasculature

Embolization to the cerebral circulation can produce ischemic neurologic deficits that may range from transient impairment lasting several days to complete cerebral infarction.

Severity of Injury

The severity of injury resulting from systemic arterial air embolism depends on the volume of air entering the arterial tree and its subsequent distribution to end-arteries. Injected air bubbles are often seen during arteriographic studies without evidence of sequelae; however, some patients who have sustained arterial air embolism during cardiopulmonary bypass have had severe neurologic impairment postoperatively.[23]

Diagnosis and Treatment

Recognition of arterial air embolism may be facilitated by Doppler ultrasound monitoring in the cardiopulmonary bypass circuit or by transcranial Doppler monitoring during cardiopulmonary bypass, but the diagnosis is commonly made only in retrospect, when a patient awakens with neurologic complications. Specific therapy after arterial embolization is possible only with immediate pressurization in a hyperbaric chamber.[24]

Venous Pulmonary Air Embolism

Causes

By far the most common type of perioperative air embolism is limited to the venous pulmonary circulation. Embolization

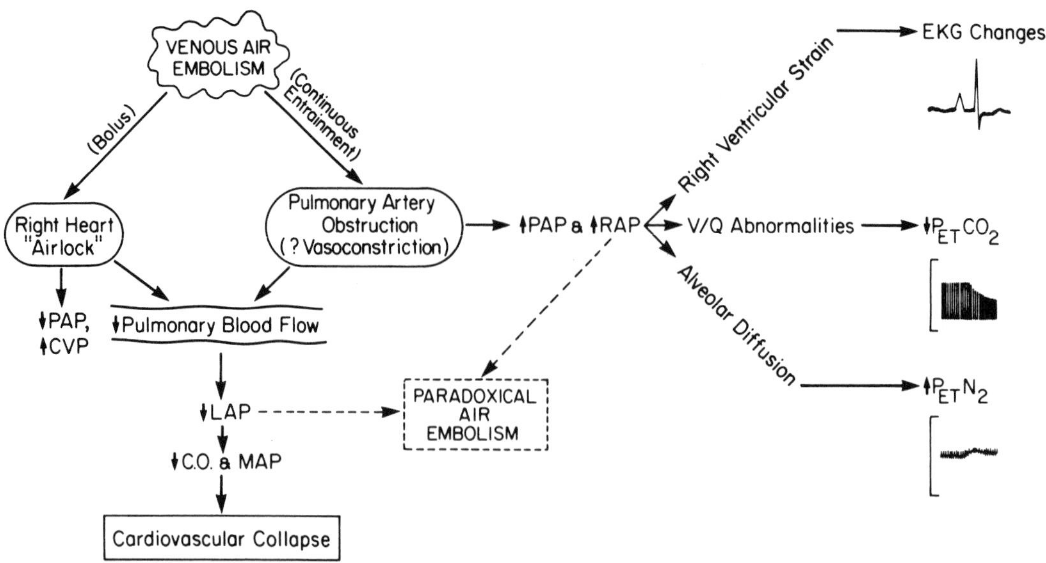

FIGURE 21-1. Pathophysiologic manifestation of venous air embolism. Venous air embolism leads to an air lock in the right heart after bolus infusion or progressive pulmonary artery obstruction after continuous entrainment. Either mechanism can lead to a significant decrease in pulmonary blood flow and subsequent cardiovascular collapse. *CO,* cardiac output; *CVP,* central venous pressure; *EKG,* electrocardiographic; *LAP,* left atrial pressure; *MAP,* mean arterial pressure; *PAP,* pulmonary arterial pressure; $P_{ET}CO_2$, end-tidal carbon dioxide tension; $P_{ET}N_2$, end-tidal nitrogen tension; *RAP,* right atrial pressure. (Lucas WJ: How to manage air embolism. Problems in Anesthesia 1:291, 1987.)

occurs when a vein is opened above heart level, where venous pressure is subatmospheric. If the vein is prevented from collapsing by connective tissue or bone, air can be entrained. Although this problem is not rare in hepatic, orthopedic, and major gynecologic operations, it occurs most frequently in neurosurgical operations performed with the patient in the sitting position, in which a large hydrostatic gradient is present between the operative site and the heart. Some investigators have reported an incidence of air embolism as high as 66% in patients undergoing suboccipital craniectomy.[25]

Pathophysiologic Features

Air bubbles in the venous circulation usually enter as a fine stream, passing with the blood flow through the right heart and out into the pulmonary circulation (Fig. 21-1). Pulmonary vascular resistance increases in proportion to the volume of air embolized[26] and results in impaired left atrial filling. Increases in pulmonary arterial and right ventricular pressures may result in increases in right atrial pressure if the volume of air embolized is sufficient (Fig. 21-2).[27] Decreased left ventricular filling may cause a decrease in systemic arterial pressure, whereas right ventricular strain often is accompanied by ectopic ventricular beats.

The classic studies by Durant and colleagues[28] in animals demonstrated that the embolus forms an "air lock" in the right heart. Passage of blood into the pulmonary circulation is thereby decreased or absent. They also demonstrated that placement of the animal in left lateral decubitus permitted cardiac output to be maintained. In patients in the sitting po-

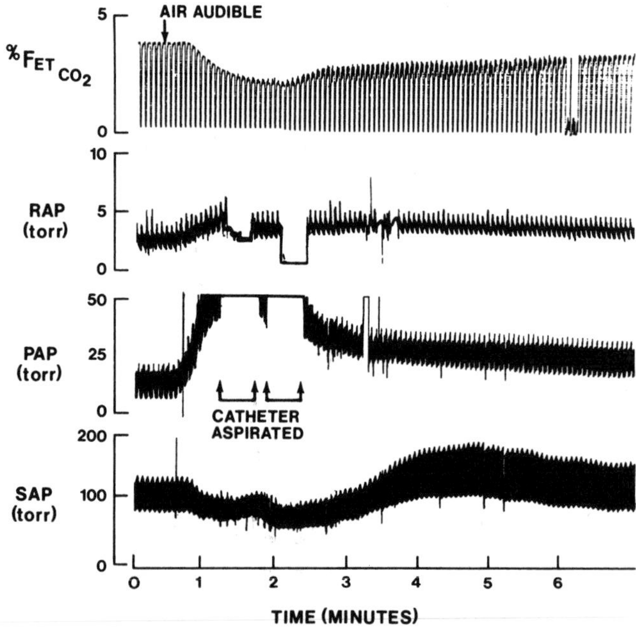

FIGURE 21-2. Strip-chart record of venous air embolism. Almost immediately after Doppler sounds indicate air embolism, there is a marked decrease in end-tidal carbon dioxide fraction (FET_{CO_2}) and a marked increase in pulmonary arterial pressure (*PAP*). During the decrease in systemic arterial pressure (*SAP*), negative deflections indicate beats dropped because of ventricular premature contractions. The breaks in the right atrial pressure (*RAP*) and PAP traces indicate attempts to aspirate air bubbles from the circulation. (Marshall WK, Bedford RF: Use of a pulmonary artery catheter for detection and treatment of venous air embolism: a prospective study in man. Anesthesiology 52:131, 1980.)

sition, they noted that the air lock developed in the main pulmonary arteries (Fig. 21-3). The principal route of egress for venous pulmonary air embolism appears to be exhalation of the air crossing the pulmonary alveolar capillary membrane, as long as cardiac output is maintained. This process has been verified by end-tidal nitrogen analysis.[29]

Paradoxical Air Embolism

Paradoxical air embolism (air bubbles that pass from the venous pulmonary circulation to the systemic arterial circulation) may occur in the presence of a patent foramen ovale[30] (present in 25% to 30% of the population[31]) or, on occasion, may develop in the absence of an intracardiac septal defect.[32,33] Cucchiara and associates[30] have demonstrated paradoxical air embolism graphically by using two-dimensional echocardiography to follow air bubbles passing from the right atrium to the left atrium and out the left ventricle during neurosurgical operations (Fig. 21-4).

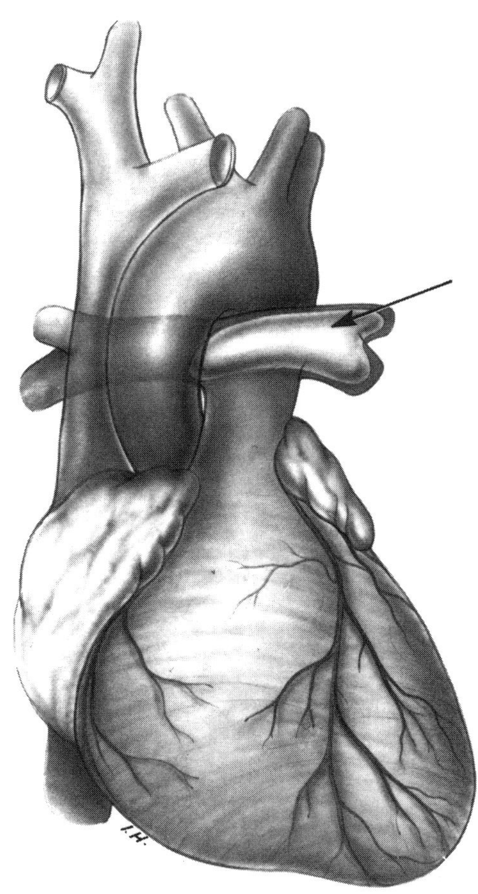

FIGURE 21-3. Angiographic findings during venous air embolism in a patient in the sitting position. Air lock has developed in the main pulmonary arteries (*arrow*). (Bedford RF: Venous air embolism: a historical perspective. Seminars in Anesthesia 2:169, 1983. Modified from Durant TM, et al: Body position in relation to venous air embolism: a roentgenologic study. Am J Med Sci 227:509, 1954.)

CLINICAL CORRELATES

Lethal "Dose"

The immediate consequences of venous air embolism are related to the volume of air embolized and the rate of entrainment or infusion. Morbidity and mortality studies in laboratory animals (usually dogs in the supine position) show that more than 6 to 10 mL/kg of air injected as a bolus will produce cardiovascular collapse and death if an air lock develops in the right heart.[28,34-36] Although a comparable dose in humans has not been investigated, I am aware of a 5-year-old patient who received a bolus injection of 2 mL/kg. Symptoms included profound systemic hypotension from which the child was successfully resuscitated only after closed-chest cardiac massage and administration of intravenous ephedrine. Presumably, a slightly larger volume would have proven to be fatal. Ordway has calculated that an average air infusion rate of 70 to 150 mL/s is fatal.[12]

Cardiopulmonary Effects

Continuous infusions of intravenous air result in predictable increases in pulmonary arterial and right ventricular pressures followed by impairment in arterial oxygenation and carbon dioxide elimination. Changes in heart rate, ventricular ectopic beats, and an increase in central venous pressure occur only with moderately large air emboli, whereas arterial hypotension and changes in heart tones (an augmented S_2, a systolic or continuous "mill-wheel" murmur) develop only with truly massive air embolism.[27,35,37,38] Pulmonary dysfunction may become apparent shortly after venous air embolism, with hypoxemia; hypercapnia; decreased compliance; and acute onset of bronchospasm, pulmonary edema, or both.[39-42] Although this syndrome has not been well defined, it is presumed to be related to disruption of the alveolar capillary membranes when air bubbles enter the pulmonary arterial circulation.

DIAGNOSIS

Even massive venous air embolism may be very difficult to ascertain during operations in which it is unexpected. Anesthesia personnel should remain aware of its possibility, especially in procedures in which the risk is greatest (eg, procedures in which incision is made above the heart level), to facilitate correct diagnosis. Usually in this situation, air embolism is suggested when an acute reduction in end tidal CO_2 or blood pressure, ventricular ectopy, and changes in heart tones occur. Gasping respirations may be noted if the patient is not paralyzed.

If a central venous catheter is in place, central venous pressure increases markedly. An attempt should be made to recover air by aspirating through the catheter with a syringe, an approach that has both therapeutic and diagnostic value.[43,44] Sudden intraoperative cardiovascular collapse often is blamed on the anesthesiologist; recovery of air clearly indicates that the problem is not attributable to anesthetic negligence.

Neurosurgical procedures performed in the sitting position

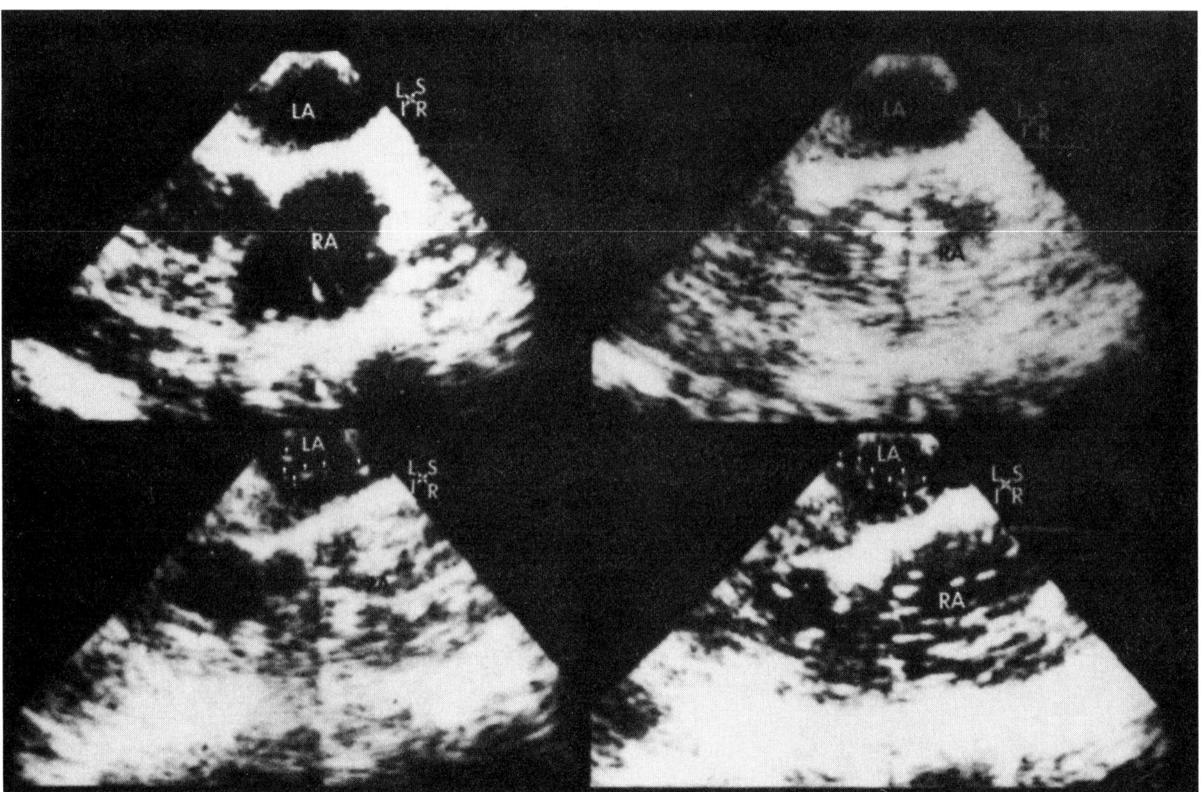

FIGURE 21-4. Two-dimensional echocardiographic findings during venous air embolism. Air bubbles (*white flecks*) appear first in the right atrium (*RA*) and then in the right ventricle. With progression of the embolism and an increase in right atrial pressure, air bubbles are driven across the interatrial septum into the left atrium (*LA*) and then pass into the left ventricle. (Cucchiara RF, Nugent M, Seward JB, et al: Air embolism in upright neurosurgical patients: detection and localization by two-dimensional transesophageal echocardiography. Anesthesiology 60:353, 1984.)

generally are thought to be associated with the highest incidence of intraoperative air embolism. Thus, multiple monitoring modalities are used during these operations to optimize both the diagnosis and the treatment of this complication. They are discussed here in the order of their sensitivities (Table 21-1) and relative invasiveness.[45]

Doppler Ultrasound

For more than two decades, the monitoring of reflected ultrasound from the right atrium with a Doppler flowmeter has been recognized as an extremely sensitive method for detecting the passage of air bubbles into the right heart.[46] En-

TABLE 21-1
Monitoring to Detect Venous Air Embolism

TECHNIQUE OR PARAMETER	SENSITIVITY ($mL \cdot kg^{-1} \cdot min^{-1}$ air entrainment)
Precordial Doppler ultrasound	0.1–0.25
Transesophageal Doppler ultrasound	0.1–0.25
Transesophageal echocardiography	<0.1–0.25
End-tidal carbon dioxide tension	0.25–0.5
End-tidal nitrogen tension	0.25–0.5
Central venous pressure (increase)	0.5
Pulmonary arterial pressure (increase)	0.5–0.75
Mean arterial pressure (decrease)	0.75–1.25
Electrocardiography (ventricular dysrhythmias)	1.25
Esophageal stethoscope (mill-wheel murmur)	1.5
Cardiovascular collapse	2.0

Modified from Pashayan AG: Monitoring the neurosurgical patient. Problems in Anesthesia 1:104, 1987.

trainment of air as slow as 0.1 mL/kg/min can be identified from a change in tone of the Doppler signal; frequently, therapeutic maneuvers can be initiated to stop air entrainment before symptoms of cardiovascular compromise develop.

Precordial Placement

The 2-Hz ultrasound transceiver is usually best positioned over the right parasternum at the level of the fourth to sixth intercostal space, where a typical triple-beat atrial signal is obtained. In some patients, a left parasternal position is needed. Placement of the ultrasound beam over the right atrium can be verified by rapidly injecting 5 to 10 mL of saline solution through a central or even a peripheral venous catheter. The normal atrial signal is disrupted by the saline injection, resulting in a "swishing" sound similar to the roar of a wave breaking on the shore.[47] A single, intense ejection signal is heard when the Doppler transceiver is placed over the left ventricle. This location is not useful for detecting incoming air bubbles, and no alteration occurs when saline is injected through a central venous catheter.

Transesophageal Placement

Because anatomic variation may make precordial placement of a Doppler probe difficult, a more recently developed approach is transesophageal probe placement.[45,48] The transesophageal probe not only is capable of detecting venous air emboli but also can be used to detect air bubbles in the left heart as might occur with an intracardiac defect, during cardiopulmonary bypass or surgery involving the pulmonary veins.

Although the precordial Doppler device is extremely sensitive, it repeatedly has been shown to be unable to detect air embolism in approximately 5% of cases.[49,50] These failures perhaps are related to malpositioning or slippage of the transceiver head during monitoring, or perhaps to the entrance of such a fine stream of air bubbles into the circulation that no noticeable alteration in audible Doppler signal occurs. Whatever the cause of the false-negative Doppler signal, in many instances large volumes of air have been recovered from central venous catheters, when only a Doppler, and no other air embolism detection monitor, was in use.[51,52] In contrast, when other monitors of venous air embolism were used clinically, only small volumes of air were recovered from the catheters, presumably because the diagnosis was made before massive air embolism occurred.[49]

Two-dimensional Echocardiography

Two-dimensional echocardiography, which provides graphic detail of cardiac structures (see Fig. 21-4), possesses sensitivity and specificity exceeding that of precordial Doppler monitoring (0.02 mL/kg).[37,45] Observation of the progress of air bubbles passing through the heart, detection of paradoxical air embolism,[30,53] and assessment of therapeutic maneuvers are possible with this technique. Transesophageal echocardiographic monitoring usually is atraumatic but has been associated with esophageal burns and reports of postoperative vocal cord paralysis when used for prolonged periods when the patient's neck is flexed.[54] The equipment is extremely expensive, currently more than $150,000 per unit.

Capnometry

Monitoring of end-expired carbon dioxide has proven to be a useful means of diagnosing air embolism. As air bubbles are ejected into the pulmonary circulation, alveolar capillary flow is temporarily obstructed. An abrupt reduction in the concentration of exhaled carbon dioxide follows, because wasted ventilation increases (see Fig. 21-2). The incidence of air embolism detected with capnometry has been shown to be about half that of Doppler detection,[25,45,49] an observation verified in animal studies.[27,35,37,45]

A potential problem with capnometry is confusion between changes induced by a reduction in cardiac output and those caused by air embolism (Fig. 21-5). Although failure of a Doppler signal to register is unlikely when an air embolus is detected by capnometry, in cases of doubt, the prudent course is to treat the patient as though air embolism has occurred.

Superior Vena Cava Catheter

As mentioned previously, a central venous catheter placed in the superior vena cava is useful both as a diagnostic and as a therapeutic tool. Aspiration of even a single air bubble confirms the diagnosis; in the event of a massive embolus, the ability to aspirate part of the intracardiac air contributes to overall management. In approximately 90% of adults, central venous catheters can be placed easily via an antecubital vein.[55] They have been used effectively in resuscitation from air embolism for more than 100 years.[56] Since its introduction into clinical practice in 1966,[43] central venous catheterization has been an accepted technique whenever a significant risk of air embolism is thought to exist.

Positioning

Studies by Bunegin and colleagues[57] with use of a mechanical model of the right heart have shown that placement of a single orifice catheter 3 cm above the junction of the superior vena cava and the right atrium or a multi-orifice catheter with its tip 2 cm below the superior vena cava–right atrium junction appears to be the most effective position for recovery of incoming air bubbles. This finding has been confirmed in upright dogs,[58] in which 40% of the volume of air emboli could be recovered from the superior vena cava, compared with only 15% from the right atrium. Apparently, a vortex is created in the superior vena cava by the mixing of bubbles and blood, rendering this site the optimal location for recovery of embolized air.

Placement of a catheter in the superior vena cava cannot be ensured either by an intraoperative chest radiograph or by advancement of the catheter tip until right ventricular pressures are recorded and subsequent withdrawal of the catheter. The tip of a single-orifice catheter can be positioned with electrocardiographic guidance by using the saline-filled central catheter as a V lead. A change from negative to biphasic P waves indicates passage past the sinoatrial node[59] and into the right atrium (Fig. 21-6). More recently, however, mul-

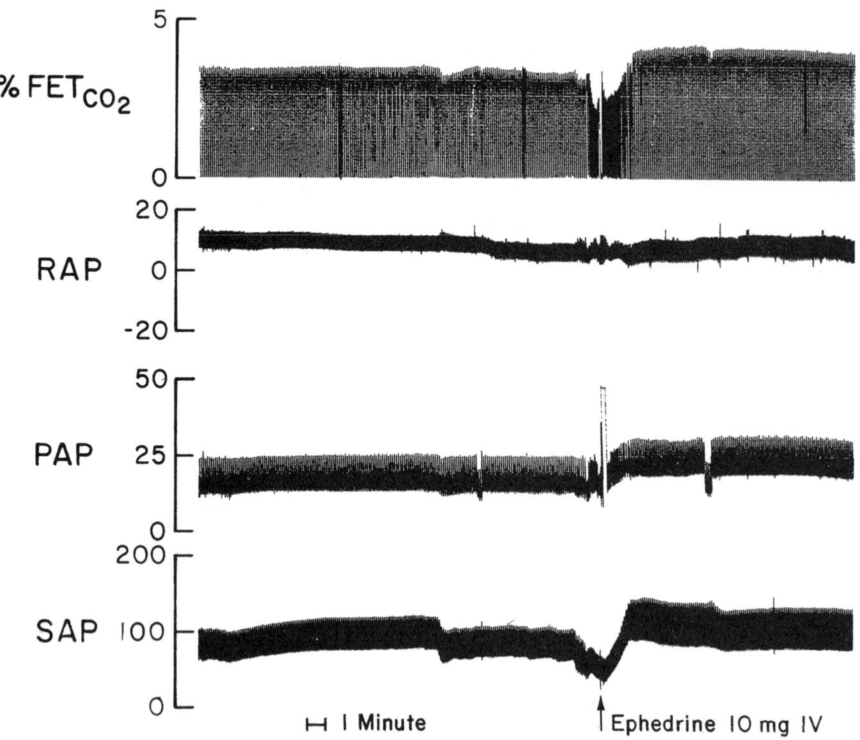

FIGURE 21-5. Abrupt reductions in systemic arterial pressure (*SAP*) and cardiac output resulting in acute decreases in end-tidal carbon dioxide fraction (FET_{CO_2}) that mimic the effect of air embolism, except that pulmonary arterial pressure (*PAP*) remains unchanged until vasopressor is given via the pulmonary artery. *IV*, intravenous; *RAP*, right atrial pressure. (Bedford RF, Marshall WK, Butler A, et al: Cardiac catheters for diagnosis and treatment of venous air embolism. J Neurosurg 55:610, 1981.)

tiorifice catheters have been advocated for recovery of air bubbles.[60] Ideally, the catheter should be left with the tip at the sinoatrial node and the multiple aspirating orifices in the superior vena cava. It should be borne in mind, however, that its location in this position increases the risk of cardiac perforation, particularly in long cases.

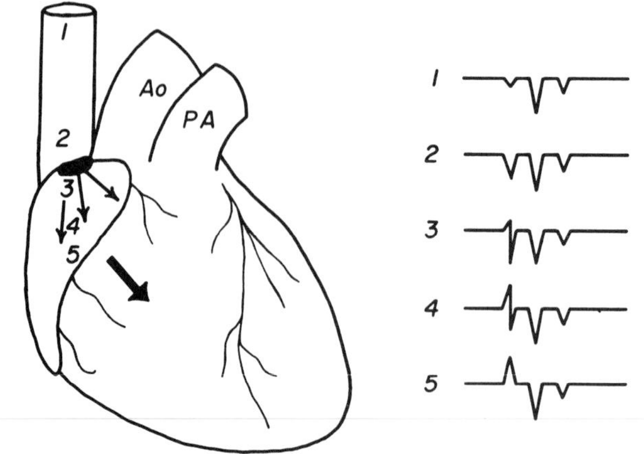

FIGURE 21-6. Changes in lead V of an electrocardiogram when the tip of the catheter enters the right heart. (*1, 2*) The P, QRS, and T vectors (*arrows*) point away from the catheter, and all waves are predominantly negative (with greater amplitude at 2). Just beyond the sinoatrial node (*3*), the initial deflection of the P wave is positive, because the first portion of the vector points toward the catheter tip. (*4*) The P wave is equally biphasic, and (*5*) the P wave is positive. *Ao*, aorta; *PA*, pulmonary artery. (Michenfelder JD, Martin JT, Altenburg BM, et al: Air embolism during neurosurgery: an evaluation of right-atrial catheters for diagnosis and treatment. JAMA 208:1353, 1969.)

Problems

The major problem with reliance on central venous catheters for recovery of embolized air is that inevitably some of the air will pass the catheter, either during the interval between an indication of air embolus by one of the monitors and the application of suctioning, or during the changing of aspirating syringes. Furthermore, changes in right atrial pressure are a relatively late indication of air embolism.[27,35,37] During posterior fossa surgery, reliance on aspiration of air results in a positive diagnosis only approximately 7% of the time,[44] compared with 55% of the time for Doppler monitoring.[25]

Pulmonary Artery Catheterization

Advantages

Some clinicians use pulmonary artery catheterization to monitor patients who are at high risk for venous air embolism.[41,49,61–63] Changes in pulmonary artery pressure reflect the severity of air embolism, indicate the effects of treatment, and are less subject to misinterpretation than Doppler or end-tidal carbon dioxide monitoring. Furthermore, during posterior fossa surgery, pulmonary arterial pressure monitoring facilitates the differentiation of cardiovascular changes caused by air embolism from those caused by cranial nerve or brain stem stimulation (see Fig. 21-5).

Although this technique theoretically affords access for recovery of air bubbles from both the pulmonary artery and the right atrium, no instance of massive withdrawal of air from a pulmonary artery catheter has been reported. The length and small bore of a pulmonary artery catheter lumen also make brisk aspiration difficult. Proponents of pulmonary artery catheterization believe that the device affords such early diagnosis that the source can be treated before massive air embolism occurs.[49]

INTERATRIAL PRESSURE GRADIENT DETERMINATION. Pulmonary artery catheterization also permits evaluation of right and left atrial pressures, thus indicating any possible risk for paradoxical air embolism.[64] The interatrial pressure gradient seems to reflect the propensity of the foramen ovale to open in seated patients who are simultaneously monitored with two-dimensional echocardiography. The interatrial pressure gradient tends to change unfavorably during prolonged operations with the patient in the sitting position because of a reduction in left atrial pressure. Thus, these patients are at risk for paradoxical air embolism even if only relatively small amounts of air enter the venous circulation.

Modalities that tend to keep left atrial pressure greater than right atrial pressure include augmentation of intravenous fluid replacement[65] and lowering of the head of the operating table to prevent peripheral pooling of blood.[25] When an unfavorable interatrial pressure gradient is noted immediately when the patient is placed in the sitting position, the surgeon should be notified and strongly advised to use a less hazardous position.

Although the incidence of venous air embolism is greater in the sitting position than in the supine position, a retrospective review of 579 posterior fossa craniotomies found that this higher incidence (45% versus 12% supine) was not associated with a different incidence of perioperative cardiopulmonary complications.[66] When an unfavorable interatrial pressure gradient develops during an operation, discontinuation of nitrous oxide is advisable, because 50% nitrous oxide will effectively double the size of the embolus, and 70% will triple it.[67]

Indications

Because pulmonary artery catheterization is a highly invasive procedure with definite hazards even when placed via an antecubital vein, most advocates suggest limiting its use to posterior fossa operations performed with the patient in the sitting position where both air embolism and neurogenic cardiovascular changes are anticipated.

TREATMENT

When air embolism is recognized, treatment must be directed toward several goals (Table 21-2).

Prevention of Further Air Entrainment

The first step, arresting air entrainment, requires notifying the surgeon that air embolism has been detected. If the Doppler monitor is functioning properly, the surgeon will hear the embolus as soon as the anesthesiologist does. The anesthesiologist must assess the severity of the situation and initiate nonsurgical treatment.

TABLE 21-2
Goals of Treatment

1. Cessation of further air entry into the venous system
2. Prevention of expansion of the air embolus with nitrous oxide
3. Evacuation of the embolized air from the heart or pulmonary artery
4. Maintenance of cardiac output to facilitate exhalation of the air via the pulmonary circulation
5. Meticulous respiratory care until the effects of possible pulmonary compromise have been evaluated

Occlusion and Flooding the Operative Field

Frequently the surgeon recognizes the venous structure that was just lacerated and can occlude it promptly. If, however, the site cannot be determined, the operative field must be flooded promptly with saline to allow time for the pulmonary vasculature to recover from the initial effects of the embolus.

Dependent Positioning

If practical, the operative site can be moved toward a more dependent position, thus raising venous pressure at the incision site above atmospheric pressure and causing venous bleeding, which facilitates identification of the involved vessels.

Bilateral Jugular Venous Compression

During operations with the patient in the sitting position, when changes in position are difficult to make, initial bilateral jugular venous compression to raise cerebral venous pressure acutely may be more practical than dependent positioning.[68] This maneuver should be used only with the knowledge and agreement of the neurosurgeon. It may be accompanied by bradycardia (carotid sinus stimulation) and may be hazardous in patients with carotid artery disease.

Increase of Venous Pressure

Acutely increasing venous pressure with positive end-expiratory pressure, military antishock trousers, Valsalva's maneuver, or acute fluid challenge may prevent further air entrainment. However, an increase in right atrial pressure may also open a probe-patent foramen ovale and cause paradoxical embolization of air already in the right atrium.[69,70]

Cessation of Nitrous Oxide

At the same time that the diagnosis of air embolism is made, nitrous oxide should be discontinued to prevent bubble expansion. High-flow 100% oxygen must be initiated in an attempt to remove as much nitrous oxide as possible from the breathing circuit and the patient. Although some investigators have suggested that the reintroduction of nitrous oxide may serve to test the reserve of the pulmonary vasculature after air entrainment has stopped,[61–63] this practice has been challenged on the grounds that neurologic damage might be aggravated if paradoxical embolization has occurred and intracerebral air bubbles are then expanded.[71]

Central Vascular Aspiration of Air

Recovery of air from the heart should be attempted by aspiration through a central venous or pulmonary artery catheter if one is in place. As much as 40% of embolized air can be recovered from the superior vena cava of upright dogs.[58] Dramatic reports have been published of patients being resuscitated by aspiration through a central venous catheter.[51,52,72–74] Hence, this maneuver appears to have as much therapeutic benefit today as it did when first used in dogs more than 100 years ago.[56]

Durant's Positioning

The remaining air will travel to the lungs, where it will be exhaled, assuming that cardiac output can be maintained. The left lateral decubitus (Durant's position), as noted above, is effective in resuscitating both dogs and humans from air embolism by preventing air lock in the right heart.[28,75] This maneuver is fairly drastic, however, in neurosurgical procedures performed with the patient in the sitting position.

Maintenance of Cardiac Output

If needed, inotropic vasopressors (ie, ephedrine, and in severe cases, epinephrine) should be given to treat hypotension and to promote passage of air out of the right heart. Closed-chest cardiac massage should be instituted promptly if the aforementioned maneuvers do not restore normal cardiovascular function.[76] Once air entrainment has been stopped, these patients usually respond promptly to resuscitative maneuvers.

Respiratory Care

Pulmonary dysfunction can be a significant problem after massive air embolism, with impairment of compliance and gas exchange persisting into the postoperative period.[41,42] Therefore, when air embolism is severe enough to cause hemodynamic changes, serial blood gas determinations should be performed. In these cases the patient should be treated for noncardiac pulmonary edema with appropriate levels of positive end-expiratory pressure if significant hypoxemia ensues. The patient's trachea should be left intubated and the patient's lungs mechanically ventilated postoperatively until an assessment of both pulmonary and neurologic status can be made.

PREVENTION

Air embolism will always be a possible complication during anesthesia, although abandonment of the sitting position for neurosurgery would help significantly to reduce its occurrence.[50,66] Death due to air embolism is relatively rare in procedures known to be associated with this complication; death now is reported primarily in unusual or unexpected circumstances when the patient is not monitored and the anesthetist is unprepared. Constant vigilance and inclusion of gas embolism in the differential diagnosis of cardiovascular collapse are the best preparation for this complication.

REFERENCES

1. Amussat JZ: Recherches sur l'introduction accidentale de l'air dans les veins. Paris: Germer Baillière, 1839: 255
2. Ericksen JE: On the proximate cause of death after spontaneous introduction of air into the veins, with some remarks on the treatment of the accident. Edinburgh Medical and Surgical Journal 61:1, 1844
3. Lawrence FG, McKay HA, Sherensky RT: Effective measures in the prevention of intraoperative aeroembolus. J Thorac Cardiovasc Surg 62:731, 1971
4. Khoury GF, Mann ME, Porot MJ, et al: Air embolism associated with veno-venous bypass during orthotopic liver transplantation. Anesthesiology 67:848, 1987
5. Manuel MA, Stewart WK, Tulley FM, et al: Air embolism monitor for use in hemodialysis. Lancet 2:1356, 1971
6. Rubin IC: Uterotubal insufflation. St. Louis: CV Mosby, 1947: 354
7. Rose DK, Cohen MM, Soutter DI: Laparoscopic cholecystectomy: the anaesthetist's point of view. Can J Anaesth 39:809, 1992
8. Lowdon JD, Tidmore TL Jr: Fatal air embolism after gastrointestinal endoscopy. Anesthesiology 69:622, 1988
9. Jacoby J, Jones JR, Ziegler J, et al: Pneumoencephalography and air embolism: simulated anesthetic death. Anesthesiology 20:336, 1959
10. Merrill DC: Air cystometry and embolism. Urology 4:495, 1974
11. Saha AK: Air embolism during anaesthesia for arthrography in a child. Anaesthesia 31:1231, 1976
12. Ordway CB: Air embolus via CVP catheter without positive pressure: presentation of case and review. Ann Surg 179:479, 1974
13. Conahan TJ: Air embolization during percutaneous Swan-Ganz catheter placement. Anesthesiology 50:360, 1979
14. Leicht CH, Waldman J: Pulmonary air embolism in the pediatric patient undergoing central catheter placement: a report of two cases. Anesthesiology 64:519, 1986
15. Cohen MB, Mark JB, Morris RW, et al: Introducer sheath malfunction producing insidious air embolism. Anesthesiology 67: 573, 1987
16. Roth AG, Dado DV: Venous air embolism during removal of tissue expander in a supine child. Anesthesiology 68:457, 1988
17. Alexander JI, Lewis AAM: Air embolism during mastectomy. Anaesthesia 24:618, 1969
18. Frankel AS, Holzman RS: Air embolism during posterior spinal fusion. Can J Anaesth 35:511, 1988
19. Spiess BD, Sloan MS, McCarthy RJ, et al: The incidence of venous air embolism during total hip arthroplasty. J Clin Anesth 1:25, 1988
20. Thomas AN, Stephens BG: Air embolism: a cause of morbidity and death after penetrating chest trauma. J Trauma 14:633, 1974
21. Munsick RA: Air embolism and maternal death from therapeutic abortion. Obstet Gynecol 39:688, 1972
22. Fatteh A, Leach WB, Wilkinson CA: Fatal air embolism in pregnancy resulting from orogenital sex play. Forensic Sci 2:247, 1973
23. Gallagher EG, Pearson DT: Ultrasonic identification of sources of gaseous microemboli during open heart surgery. Thorax 28: 247, 1973
24. Kindwall EP: Massive surgical air embolism treated with brief recompression to six atmospheres followed by hyperbaric oxygen. Aerospace Medicine 44:663, 1973

25. Bedford RF: Venous air embolism: a historical perspective. Seminars in Anesthesia 2:169, 1983
26. Josephson S: Pulmonary hemodynamics during experimental air embolism. Scand J Clin Lab Invest 26:6, 1970
27. English JB, Westenskow D, Hodges MR, et al: Comparison of venous air embolism monitoring methods in supine dogs. Anesthesiology 48:425, 1978
28. Durant TM, Long J, Oppenheimer MJ: Pulmonary (venous) air embolism. Am Heart J 33:269, 1947
29. Losee JM, Sherrill D, Virtue RW, et al: Quantitative detection of venous air embolism in the dog by mass spectrometry measurement of end-tidal nitrogen (abstract). Anesthesiology 57: A146, 1982
30. Cucchiara RF, Nugent M, Seward JB, et al: Air embolism in upright neurosurgical patients: detection and localization by two-dimensional transesophageal echocardiography. Anesthesiology 60:353, 1984
31. Hagen PT, Scholz DG, Edwards WD: Incidence and size of patent foramen ovale during the first 10 decades of life: an autopsy study of 965 normal hearts. Mayo Clin Proc 59:17, 1984
32. Marquez J, Sladen A, Gendell H, et al: Paradoxical cerebral air embolism without an intracardiac septal defect. J Neurosurg 55:997, 1981
33. Butler BD, Hills BA: The lung as a filter for microbubbles. J Appl Physiol 47:537, 1979
34. Wolffe JB, Robertson HF: Experimental air embolism. Ann Intern Med 9:162, 1935
35. Adornato DC, Gildenberg PL, Ferrario CM, et al: Pathophysiology of intravenous air embolism in dogs. Anesthesiology 49: 120, 1978
36. Hoff BH, Benedetto AR, Nusynowitz ML, et al: Rapid infusion air embolism: effects of IPPV and high frequency ventilation (HFV) (abstract). Anesthesiology 57:A85, 1982
37. Glenski JA, Cucchiara RF, Michenfelder JD: Comparison of venous air embolism monitoring methods in dogs: an evaluation of transesophageal echocardiography and transcutaneous O_2 and CO_2 monitoring (abstract). Anesthesiology 61:A160, 1984
38. Furuya H, Suzuki T, Okumura F, et al: Detection of air embolism by transesophageal echocardiography. Anesthesiology 58:124, 1983
39. Chandler WF, Dimsheff DG, Taren JA: Acute pulmonary edema following venous air embolism during a neurosurgical procedure. J Neurosurg 40:400, 1974
40. Still JA, Lederman DS, Renn WH: Pulmonary edema following air embolism. Anesthesiology 40:194, 1974
41. Perschau RA, Munson ES, Chapin JC: Pulmonary interstitial edema after multiple venous air emboli. Anesthesiology 45:364, 1976
42. Kizer K, Goodman PC: Radiologic manifestations of venous air embolism. Radiology 144:35, 1982
43. Michenfelder JD, Terry HR, Daw EF, et al: Air embolism during neurosurgery: a new method of treatment. Anesth Analg 45: 390, 1966
44. Michenfelder JD, Martin JT, Alternburg BM, et al: Air embolism catheters for diagnosis and treatment. JAMA 208:1353, 1969
45. Lucas WJ: How to manage air embolism. Problems in Anesthesia 1:288, 1987
46. Maroon JC, Goodman JM, Horner TG, et al: Detection of minute venous air emboli with ultrasound. Surg Gynecol Obstet 127: 1236, 1968
47. Tinker JH, Gronert GA, Messick JM Jr, et al: Detection of air embolism: a test for positioning of right atrial catheter and Doppler probe. Anesthesiology 43:104, 1975
48. Martin RW, Colley PS: Evaluation of transesophageal Doppler detection of air embolism in dogs. Anesthesiology 58:117, 1983
49. Bedford RF, Marshall WK, Butler A, et al: Cardiac catheters for diagnosis and treatment of venous air embolism. J Neurosurg 55:610, 1981
50. Albin MS: The paradox of paradoxical air embolism: PEEP, valsalva, and patent foramen ovale—should the sitting position be abandoned? Anesthesiology 61:222, 1984
51. Albin MS, Carroll RG, Maroon JC: Clinical considerations concerning detection of venous air embolism. Neurosurgery 3:380, 1978
52. Albin MS, Babinski M, Maroon JC, et al: Anesthetic management of posterior fossa surgery in the sitting position. Acta Anaesthesiol Scand 20:117, 1976
53. Furuya H, Okumura F: Detection of paradoxical air embolism by transesophageal echocardiography. Anesthesiology 60:374, 1984
54. Cucchiara RF, Nugent M, Seward JB, et al: Air embolism in upright patients: detection and localization by two-dimensional transesophageal echocardiography. Anesthesiology 60:353, 1984
55. Cucchiara RF, Messick JM, Gronert GA, et al: Time required and success rate of percutaneous right atrial catheterization: description of a technique. Can Anaesth Soc J 27:572, 1980
56. Senn N: An experimental and clinical study of air embolism. Ann Surg 3:197, 1885
57. Bunegin L, Albin MS, Helsel PE, et al: Positioning the right atrial catheter: a model for reappraisal. Anesthesiology 55:343, 1981
58. Motomatsu K, Adachi H, Uno T, et al: Evaluation of catheter placement for treatment of venous air embolism in the sitting position. Fukuoka Igaku Zasshi 70:66, 1979
59. Robertson JT, Schick RW, Morgan F, et al: Accurate placement of ventriculo-atrial shunt for hydrocephalus under electrocardiographic control. J Neurosurg 18:255, 1961
60. Colley PS, Artru AA: Bunegin-Albin catheter improves air retrieval and resuscitation from lethal air embolism in upright dogs. Anesth Analg 68:298, 1989
61. Munson ES, Paul WL, Perry JC, et al: Early detection of venous air embolism using a Swan-Ganz catheter. Anesthesiology 42: 223, 1975
62. Marshall WK, Bedford RF: Use of a pulmonary artery catheter for detection and treatment of venous air embolism. Anesthesiology 52:131, 1980
63. Shapiro HM, Yoachim J, Marshall LF: Nitrous oxide challenge for detection of residual pulmonary gas following venous air embolism. Anesth Analg 61:304, 1982
64. Perkins-Pearson NAK, Marshall WK, Bedford RF: Atrial pressures in the seated position: implications for paradoxical air embolism. Anesthesiology 57:493, 1982
65. Bedford RF, Perkins NAK, Colohan A: Intravenous fluid loading for prevention of paradoxical air embolism in the sitting position. J Neurosurg 62:839, 1985
66. Black S, Ockert DB, Oliver WC, et al: Outcome following posterior fossa craniectomy in patients in the sitting or horizontal positions. Anesthesiology 69:49, 1988
67. Munson ES, Merrick HC: Effect of nitrous oxide on venous air embolism. Anesthesiology 27:783, 1966
68. Bedford RF, Grady S, Park TS: Impact of head elevation, jugular compression, and PEEP on intracranial venous pressure in children (abstract). Anesthesiology 61:A386, 1984
69. Perkins NAK, Bedford RF: Hemodynamic consequences of PEEP in seated neurosurgical patients: implications for paradoxical air embolism. Anesth Analg 63:429, 1984
70. Gross CM, Wann S, Johnson G: Valsalva maneuver contrast echocardiography, a new technique for improved detection of right to left shunting in patients with systemic embolism. Am J Cardiol 49:955, 1982
71. Butler B: Pulmonary air embolism and nitrous oxide challenge (letter). Anesth Analg 61:956, 1982
72. Michenfelder JD: Central venous catheters in the management of air embolism: whether as well as where (editorial). Anesthesiology 55:399, 1981
73. Campkin TV: Air embolism: placement of central venous catheters. Anesthesiology 56:406, 1982
74. Merill DG, Samuels SI, Silberberg GD: Venous air embolism of uncertain etiology. Anesth Analg 61:65, 1982
75. Hamby WB, Terry RN: Air embolism in operations done in the sitting position: a report of 5 fatal cases and one of rescue by simple maneuver. Surgery 31:212, 1952
76. Ericsson JA, Gottlieb JD, Sweet RB: Closed chest cardiac mas-

sage in the treatment of venous air embolism. N Engl J Med 270:1353, 1964

FURTHER READING

Bedford RF: Perioperative air embolism. Seminars in Anesthesia 6: 163, 1987

Kirby RR: Respiratory system. In Gravenstein N (ed): Manual of complications during anesthesia. Philadelphia: JB Lippincott, 1991: 338

Orebaugh SL: Venous air embolism: clinical and experimental considerations. Critical Care Medicine 20:1169, 1992

Pashayan AG: Monitoring the neurosurgical patient. Problems in Anesthesia 1:104, 1987

Complications in Anesthesiology, second edition,
edited by Nikolaus Gravenstein and Robert R. Kirby.
Lippincott-Raven Publishers, Philadelphia © 1996.

CHAPTER 22

Cardiac Dysrhythmias

John L. Atlee III
Donn M. Dennis

Cardiac dysrhythmias are among the most common anesthetic complications and are frequently the result of other anesthetic misadventures. Indeed, the first recorded death during anesthesia, that of Hannah Greener in 1848,[1] was most likely due to a cardiac dysrhythmia, ventricular fibrillation, as the result of the "sensitizing" action of chloroform.

Although lethal cardiac dysrhythmias are rare in well-managed cases, all dysrhythmias are potentially dangerous. They can be deleterious when bradycardia is accompanied by atrioventricular (AV) dyssynchrony with a reduction in cardiac output; when they produce an imbalance between myocardial oxygen supply and demand; or if they are likely to progress to life-threatening dysrhythmias. Any tachydysrhythmia increases myocardial oxygen demand and, by shortening diastole, reduces oxygen supply as well. Finally, multiform or "R on T" premature ventricular preexcitation can provoke potentially lethal dysrhythmias.

Cardiac dysrhythmias should always be suspected as the cause of sudden hemodynamic imbalance. A common example during general anesthesia is a sudden reduction in blood pressure associated with little change in heart rate. A glance at the electrocardiogram (ECG) often shows AV junctional rhythm to be the cause (isorhythmic AV dissociation). Reducing the depth of inhalation anesthetic agent, or the substitution of another more balanced anesthetic technique, often is all that is required to terminate the dysrhythmia and resulting hypotension.

This chapter focuses on electrophysiologic mechanisms, causes, recognition, and current management of intraoperative dysrhythmias. In addition, newer concepts in the classification of antidysrhythmic drugs will be discussed. It is assumed that the reader has basic ECG knowledge. Detailed discussion of those aspects of ECG pertinent to anesthesiology can be found elsewhere.[2–6]

CARDIAC ELECTROPHYSIOLOGY

Cardiac Action Potential

The cardiac action potential has five distinct phases in *fast-response fibers* (atrial and ventricular muscle and Purkinje fibers) (Fig. 22-1*A* and Table 22-1). *Slow-response fibers*, those found in the sinoatrial (SA) and AV nodes, have little overshoot during phase 0, lack a distinct phase 1, and arise from a lower level (more positive voltage) of resting membrane potential (see Fig. 22-1*B*). The phases of the cardiac action potential are the result of passive ion fluxes down electrochemical gradients established by active ion pumps and exchange mechanisms.[6]

Resting Membrane Potential

The resting membrane potential (phase 4), recorded by a microelectrode during electric quiescence in diastole, represents the potential difference, in millivolts, between the inside and outside of the cell. Depending on the cell type and distribution of potassium, sodium, calcium, and chloride ions across the cell membrane, this difference ranges from −50 to −60 mV in SA node fibers to −90 to −95 mV in Purkinje fibers.

SODIUM, POTASSIUM, AND CHLORIDE. The distribution of potassium ions across the cell membrane is the principal determinant of the resting membrane potential, because during diastole the cell membrane is quite permeable to potassium but relatively impermeable to sodium and calcium. Intracellular potassium and sodium concentrations remain high and low, respectively, because of the *sodium pump*, which is fueled by sodium–potassium adenosine triphosphatase. The

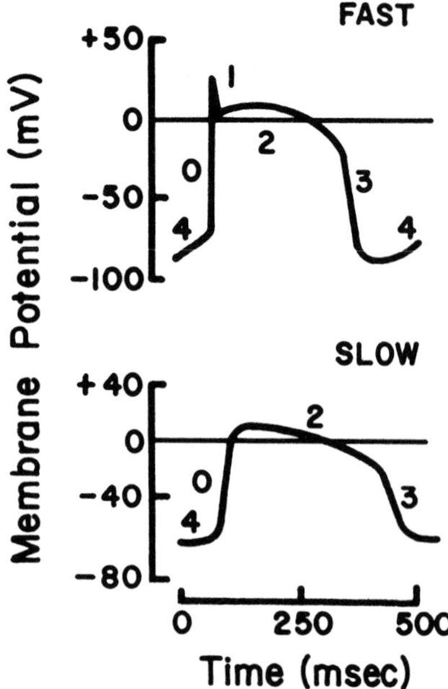

FIGURE 22-1. Cardiac action potential contours in fast-response fibers (*top*) and slow-response fibers (*bottom*).

sodium pump transports three sodium ions outward against its electrochemical gradient for two potassium ions inward against its chemical gradient.

Negative intracellular charges, presumably due to large polyvalent ions such as proteins, do not cross the cell membrane and also help to maintain intracellular negativity during phase 4. Chloride ions distribute passively in accordance with the resting membrane potential, and the chloride ion concentration inside the cell is low because the negative potential inside the cell drives chloride ions out.

CALCIUM. Calcium ions contribute little to the resting membrane potential. However, changes in the concentration of calcium ions inside cells can affect cellular membrane permeability to other ions. For example, an increase of intracellular calcium increases potassium conductance. The concentration of calcium ion inside the cell is affected by several mechanisms, especially uptake by the sarcoplasmic reticulum. In addition, a sodium-calcium exchange appears to occur across the cell membrane, which depends in part on maintenance of the sodium ion concentration gradient by the sodium pump.

Under normal conditions, one intracellular calcium ion is exchanged for two or three extracellular sodium ions. Under some pathologic conditions, or in the presence of digitalis, extracellular calcium ions may be exchanged for intracellular sodium. Cells that gain intracellular sodium tend also to gain intracellular calcium, which is thought to be important in the genesis of digitalis-induced dysrhythmias, as well as to dysrhythmias resulting from loss of the resting membrane potential.

Rapid Depolarization

FAST-RESPONSE FIBERS. After an appropriate stimulus to a fast-response fiber, the action potential is initiated by a sudden and marked increase in cell membrane permeability to sodium ions that lasts 1 to 2 ms. The maximal rate at which depolarization occurs during phase 0 (max, phase 0) is a measure of the rapidity of sodium ion entry (fast inward current) via its ion-specific channel, and a major determinant of *conduction velocity* for the propagated action potential.[7]

Any intervention that causes a subthreshold reduction (to less than the threshold potential of −70 to −60 mV for activation of the fast-inward current) partially inactivates the sodium ion channels and, consequently, causes a reduction in the magnitude (overshoot, phase 0) and rate of sodium ion influx (max, phase 0). Thus, a subthreshold reduction in resting membrane potential results in reduced *membrane responsiveness* and impaired conduction. Conversely, enhanced membrane responsiveness with greater negative levels of resting membrane potential leads to improved conduction.

SLOW-RESPONSE FIBERS. In contrast, action potentials of slow-response fibers have very slow upstrokes during phase 0 with a reduced level of overshoot and max, phase 0. Phase 0 of slow-response fibers is mediated by a slow inward, predominantly calcium ion current, termed the slow channel current ($I_{Ca\text{-}L}$). This current is blocked by verapamil and other calcium ion-entry blocking agents, and requires a longer time for activation (10 to 20 ms versus 1 to 2 ms) and inactivation (50 to 500 ms versus 1 to 2 ms) than the fast inward sodium ion current. Finally, the activation or threshold potential for the slow channel current is −40 to −30 mV, so that current flows through the fast and slow channels during the latter part of phase 0.

Early Rapid Repolarization

After phase 0 in fast-response fibers, the cell membrane repolarizes both rapidly and transiently. This sequence is partly owing to inactivation of the fast inward (sodium ion) current (I_{Na}) and to inactivation of a transient outward (potassium ion) current (I_{to}), and possibly to the inward movement of chloride ion through its own channel (I_{Cl}).[8] Phase 1 is well-defined and separated from phase 2 in Purkinje fibers and some atrial and ventricular muscle fibers.

Plateau

Membrane conductance falls to low values for all ions during phase 2. In spite of its large electrochemical gradient, conductance remains low for the outward potassium ion back-

TABLE 22-1
Phases of the Cardiac Action Potential in Fast-response Fibers

PHASE	
0	Rapid depolarization
1	Early rapid repolarization
2	Plateau
3	Final rapid repolarization
4	Resting membrane potential

ground current. The net result is that potassium ions can enter the cell more easily than they can exit. Sodium ion conductance is low owing to inactivation of the sodium ion channel. Minor ionic movements during phase 2 include adenosine triphosphate–dependent sodium–potassium exchange (sodium pump), calcium ion influx via the slow channel current (the slow channel current turns off slowly during phase 2), and possibly the inward movement of sodium ion via an ion-specific channel blocked by tetrodotoxin.[9]

Final Rapid Repolarization

Repolarization during phase 3 is primarily the result of an activated outward potassium current called the delayed rectifier current (I_K). Another potassium current, the inward rectifier (I_{K1}), is responsible for maintaining the resting membrane potential near the potassium equilibrium potential in atrial, AV nodal, His-Purkinje and ventricular cells. Repolarization is also the result of time-dependent inactivation of the slow channel current. As the net membrane current becomes more outward, the membrane potential shifts in a negative direction. As repolarization continues, potassium ion conductance increases, and repolarization self-perpetuates in a regenerative manner.

Normal Automaticity

Spontaneous phase 4 (diastolic) depolarization is a normal property of fibers found in the SA node, certain parts of the atria, the muscle of the mitral and tricuspid valves, the distal AV node, and Purkinje fibers. When this process leads to the initiation of action potentials, *normal automaticity* exists. Usually, the rate of diastolic depolarization in the SA node exceeds that in other potentially automatic sites, termed latent pacemakers. The SA node maintains dominance ("sinus dominance") by the mechanism of overdrive suppression. This control is mediated by enhanced activity of the sodium ion pump: when latent pacemakers are driven faster than their intrinsic rate, the enhanced outward current generated by this pump suppresses automaticity in these cells.[10]

Ionic Basis

The ionic basis for normal automaticity differs between Purkinje and SA node fibers. For diastolic depolarization to occur, a net gain of intracellular positive charges must occur during phase 4.

PURKINJE FIBERS. In Purkinje fibers, this gain is thought to result from a decrease in outward current carried by potassium ion while a relatively constant current carried by sodium ion moves inward. A slow inward (pacemaker) current, also carried by sodium ion, depolarizes the cell to threshold, whereupon the fast-inward (sodium ion) current is activated.[11]

SINOATRIAL NODE FIBERS. Diastolic depolarization in SA node fibers is the result of decreased outward flux of potassium ion (but not the same outward potassium ion current as in Purkinje fibers), activation of the pacemaker (sodium ion) current (I_f), and progressive activation of the slow-inward (calcium ion) current.[12,13] The resulting net increase in intracellular positive charges brings the cell membrane to threshold potential, at which time the slow-inward (calcium ion) current is fully activated giving rise to the upstroke of the action potential. The absence of I_{K1} in SA nodal cells is important in letting small currents (ie, I_f) regulate the pacemaker rate.

Passive Membrane Electric Properties

Passive membrane properties, as opposed to the active properties, include membrane resistance, capacitance, and cable properties.[14] With active properties, the response is greater than the applied stimulus, thereby adding energy to the system. With passive properties, the response is proportional to the applied stimulus and does not add energy to the system. The speed of conduction depends on both active (eg, membrane responsiveness) and passive membrane electric properties.

Resistance and Capacitance

In addition to resistance to current flow, the cardiac cell membrane can store charges (capacitance of opposite sign on its two sides). Resistive and capacitive charges cause the membrane to take a certain amount of time to respond to the applied stimulus, because the charges across the membrane must first be altered. A value referred to as the membrane time constant (capacitance × resistance) reflects this property; it is the time taken for membrane voltage to reach 63% of its final value after application of a steady current.

Cable Properties

When aligned end-to-end, cardiac cells behave like a long electric cable in which current flows more easily along cells than it does across the cell membrane. When current is introduced at a point, most of it flows along the cell, but some leaks out. Consequently, the voltage change of a cell distal to the site of current introduction is less than at the current injection site. A measure of this particular cable property is the space or length constant (λ), which is a distance along the cell membrane that the membrane potential is 37% of its value at the current injection site. For Purkinje fibers, this value is normally about 2 mm and for ventricular muscle fibers, 0.8 mm.

Current Flow

Because the current loop in an electric circuit must be closed, current must flow back to its point of origin. Local circuit currents pass across side-to-side (nexus) connections between cells and exit across the cell membrane to close the loop and complete the circuit. Through these local circuit currents, the transmembrane potential of each cell can influence that of its neighbor. As a result, a cell that is more negative inside in comparison with its neighbor will depolarize slightly (becomes more positive), whereas its neighbor polarizes (becomes more negative), and vice versa. This *electrotonic influence* of neighboring cells on one another is determined principally by the length constant for the fiber, and is due to the passive spread of current, or the cable properties of the membrane.

Loss of Membrane Potential

Many of the recognized causative and contributing factors to perioperative cardiac dysrhythmias, including myocardial ischemia, excess catecholamines, digitalis toxicity, and electrolyte imbalance can produce a loss (ie, more positive value) of resting membrane potential. Normal cardiac cells in an abnormal environment and vice versa, or abnormal cells in an abnormal environment, can singly or collectively reduce the resting membrane potential of adjacent cells.

Prolongation of Conduction Time and Heart Block

A loss of resting membrane potential prevents attainment of the large negative potentials required to reactivate all the fast (sodium ion) channels after excitation accompanying the previous cardiac cycle. At a resting membrane potential of −60 to −70 mV, half of the sodium ion channels are inactivated, whereas at −50 mV or less, all are inactivated. At a resting membrane potential of −50 mV, the slow-inward (predominately calcium ion) current is activated to generate phase 0 of the action potential. A smaller number of available sodium ion channels reduce the magnitude of the fast-inward current during phase 0. Hence, the upstroke velocity (max, phase 0) and amplitude of the action potential are reduced, both of which prolong conduction time, even to the point of conduction block.

Reentrant Dysrhythmias

Action potentials whose upstroke velocity and amplitude are dependent on the magnitude of current through partially inactivated sodium ion channels are termed *depressed fast responses*.[15] Depressed fast-response action potential contours often resemble those of slow-response fibers (see Fig. 22-1*B*). Also, they are likely to be heterogeneous because they occur in different cardiac fibers and in response to a variety of interventions,[16] or in the presence of nonuniform disease processes. As a result, varying degrees of depression of the fast response create areas that conduct with minimally reduced velocity, or, in more severely depressed zones, areas of complete block. Such uneven changes in conduction favor the development of reentrant dysrhythmias. In addition, depressed fast-response fibers may exhibit abnormal forms of automaticity or triggering.

Abnormal Automaticity

Pacemaker Mechanisms

Disorders of automaticity can result from an increase or decrease in the rate of diastolic depolarization associated with ionically normal pacemaker mechanisms in SA node and Purkinje fibers (normal automaticity), or they can result from diastolic depolarization due to ionically abnormal pacemaker mechanisms in atrial and ventricular muscle and Purkinje fibers (abnormal automaticity). Thus, the patient with persistent sinus tachycardia or inappropriate sinus bradycardia has an altered normal mechanism for automaticity. However, abnormal mechanisms for automaticity are more likely responsible for ventricular tachycardia in the setting of acute myocardial infarction. Whereas automaticity normally is not a property of working myocardial cells, myocardial ischemia may induce automaticity in such cells. Based on the rate response to catecholamines for pacemaker fibers exhibiting normal automaticity and on studies in vivo during stellate ganglion stimulation, it is unlikely that heart rates much greater than 200 beats/min are to be due to enhanced normal automaticity.[17–19]

Reduction of Resting Membrane Potential

When the resting membrane potential of working atrial and ventricular fibers is reduced to less than about −60 mV by disease or experimental methods, spontaneous diastolic depolarization may occur and cause repetitive impulse formation (Fig. 22-2).[17,20–22] Purkinje fibers that exhibit normal automaticity at normal levels of resting membrane potential (−70 to −90 mV) also show abnormal forms of automaticity when their resting membrane potential is the range of −40 to −60 mV. However, if a low level of resting membrane potential were the only criterion for abnormal automaticity, then (normal) SA node automaticity would have to be considered abnormal. Consequently, an important distinction between the

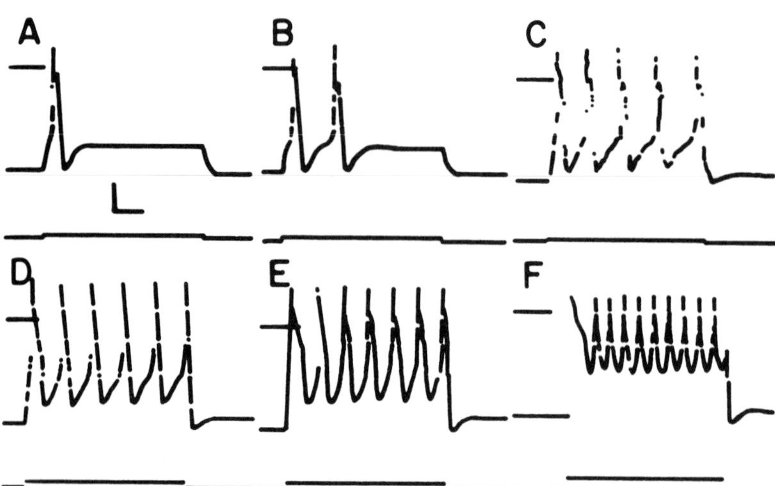

FIGURE 22-2. The effect of depolarizing current pulses of progressively greater strength on the electric activity of a quiescent canine Purkinje fiber exposed to sodium-free solution containing 16 mM calcium. *Line at top left of each figure,* zero membrane potential; *bottom traces,* the strength of the depolarizing current on an arbitrary scale, the deflection of the current trace in **F** corresponding to 2×1^{-7} A. The stronger the depolarizing pulse, the more rapid is the spontaneous activity. *Calibrations,* horizontal 2 seconds and vertical 20 mV. (Aronson RS, Cranefield PP: The effect of resting potential on the electrical activity of canine cardiac Purkinje fibers exposed to Na-free solution or to ouabain. Pflugers Arch 347:101, 1974.)

two types of automaticity is that the resting membrane potential of a fiber showing abnormal automaticity is markedly reduced from its normal level.[18]

Overdrive Suppression

Unlike normal automaticity, abnormal automaticity may not be overdrive-suppressed.[23] Therefore, even transient sinus pauses or occasional long sinus cycle lengths permit ectopic foci exhibiting abnormal automaticity to capture the heart for one or more beats. In contrast, an ectopic focus with a normal mechanism for automaticity would probably remain overdrive-suppressed during relatively short, transient sinus pauses. In addition, the low level of resting membrane potential at which abnormal automaticity occurs may block the conduction of impulses entering the abnormally automatic focus ("entrance block") and prevent it from being overdriven by the SA node.[24] This situation would lead to parasystole, an example of a dysrhythmia involving abnormalities of both conduction and automaticity.

Clinical Implications

The distinction between normal and abnormal automaticity has clinical relevance. Abnormal automaticity has been demonstrated in diseased human cardiac fibers [25–28] and can be produced by experimental interventions that mimic pathophysiologic states.[22,29,30] How anesthetics and related drugs affect abnormal forms of automaticity is unknown. In addition, because different ionic mechanisms may be involved in abnormal compared with normal forms of automaticity,[18] the response to antidysrhythmic drugs may not be the expected one. Thus, although lidocaine is effective in suppressing normal automaticity in Purkinje fibers, it is not as effective as verapamil in suppressing abnormal automaticity in these fibers.[29]

Triggered Activity and Afterdepolarizations

Triggered Activity

Triggered activity is sustained rhythmic activity initiated by automatic or stimulated action potentials, without which electrical quiescence is present (Fig. 22-3).[17,18] Thus, unlike the phenomenon of abnormal automaticity, which can occur spontaneously, triggered activity relies on the presence of a preceding action potential (depolarization) for its initiation. If the oscillation occurs before completion of myocardial repolarization (ie, during phases 2 or 3 of the action potential), it is termed an early afterdepolarization (EAD). Likewise, if the oscillation occurs after completion of repolarization (ie, during diastole—phase 4 of the action potential), it is called a delayed afterdepolarization (DAD).

Early Afterdepolarizations

Conditions that modulate ionic currents in a way that prolongs repolarization can create early afterdepolarizations (EADs) (Fig. 22-3). In other words, EADs result from a reduced repolarizing current relative to the depolarizing current.[31–33] General mechanisms that can produce EADs include: (1) a reduction in the normal repolarizing current (eg, I_K); (2) an abnormal increase of the inward current carried by sodium and/or calcium currents; and/or (3) a simultaneous increased inward and decreased outward current. EADs are most likely to arise during conditions that prolong ventricular repolarization (ie, lengthening of the QT interval and action potential). Thus, slow heart rates, decreased extracellular potassium, congenitally prolonged QT syndromes, tricyclic antidepressant or antidysrhythmic therapy (eg, quinidine or d-sotalol) therapy, left stellate ganglion stimulation and/or drugs that inhibit repolarizing currents (I_K and I_{K1}) significantly increase the risk of developing EADs and torsades de pointes. In addition, EADs have been associated with hypoxia, acidosis, and states of catecholamine excess.

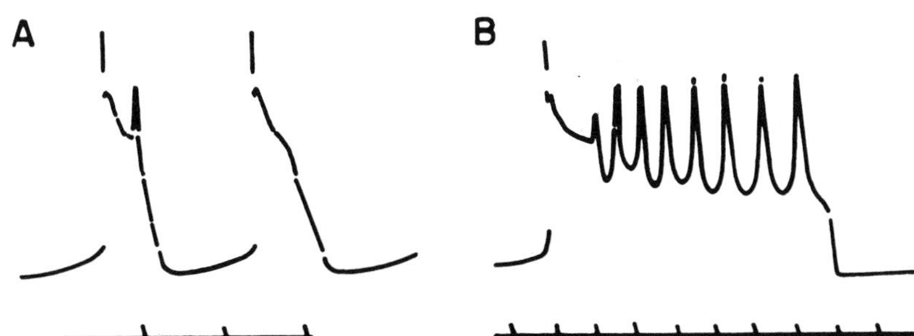

FIGURE 22-3. Early afterdepolarizations, second upstrokes, and repetitive activity in canine cardiac Purkinje fibers exposed to a 4 mM potassium chloride-containing Tyrode solution. (**A**) The two spontaneous action potentials show an early afterdepolarization, or "hump," during the repolarization phase (*right*) and a second upstroke arising from an early afterdepolarization (*left*). These action potentials were recorded while the fiber was recovering from the effects of a brief exposure to norepinephrine. (**B**) A spontaneous action potential recorded in another preparation shortly after replacement of the bicarbonate–carbon dioxide buffering system with N-2-hydroxy-ethylpiperazine-N′-2-ethanesulfonic acid. The second upstroke is followed by a "burst" of rhythmic activity arising from a low level of membrane potential. The maximum diastolic potential was −84 mV (**A**) and −87 mV (**B**). The second upstroke in **A** and the later slow-response action potentials in **B** peaked near 0 mV. *Time marks,* 1-second intervals. (Wit AL, Cranefield PF, Gadsby DC: Triggered activity. In Zipes DP, Bailey JC, Elharrar V, et al (eds): The slow inward current and cardiac arrhythmias. The Hague: Martinus Nijhoff, 1980: 437.)

More recently, a variety of drugs with markedly different structures has been found to cause torsades de pointes in humans. For example, an increase in the incidence of torsades de pointes was noted in patients receiving the highly selective H_1-histamine receptor antagonist terfenadine (SELDANE)[34,35] and the antiprotozoal drug pentamidine.[36] In the case of terfenadine, the prodysrhythmic effect of the antihistamine appears to be attributable to blockage of repolarizing potassium currents, specifically the rapidly rectifying component (I_{Kr}) of the delay rectifier current (I_K).[35] A number of other currents have also been implicated as possible mediators of EADs, such as the L-type calcium current, sodium "window" or slowly inactivating current, sodium channel exchange mechanism, and the transient inward current that is activated by high concentrations of intracellular calcium.[31–33]

A major "vulnerable parameter" of EAD-induced triggered activity is prolongation of repolarization (abnormally long action potentials or QT intervals). Thus, therapy directed at shortening these intervals should be effective in terminating (and suppressing) EADs.[32] Indeed increasing heart rate by pharmacologic (vagolytic drugs or β-adrenergic receptor agonists) or electric (pacing) therapy, increasing extracellular potassium concentration, shortening action potential duration using drugs, and/or withdrawal of inciting agents can effectively treat EADs. In addition, EADs can be suppressed by reducing inward currents (eg, blocking β- and α-adrenergic receptors) or administering magnesium.[32,33]

Delayed Afterdepolarizations

Conditions that cause intracellular calcium overload can in turn elicit an additional ryanodine-sensitive oscillatory release of calcium from the sarcoplasmic reticulum and produce delayed afterdepolarizations (DADs).[31–33] An inward, depolarizing current is responsible for the genesis of DADs and is consequently the "vulnerable parameter" to target during antidysrhythmic drug treatment.[32] DADs occur early in diastole during phase 4. Thus, unlike EADs, which develop during phase 2 or 3 of the action potential, DADs develop after completion of ventricular repolarization. Similar to EADs, the formation of DADs is not spontaneous (self-initiated) but depends on a prior depolarization. If a DAD attains threshold, it can produce a single depolarization, or if it is followed by other DADs, can cause couplets and tachydysrhythmias (eg, atrial and ventricular tachydysrhythmias). Although DADs cannot be self-initiated, they can be self-sustained.[31–33] Because reentrant dysrhythmias share many characteristics with DAD-induced triggered activity, it is very difficult to differentiate the two forms of tachydysrhythmias.

A variety of conditions can produce DADs.[31–33] They are observed in cardiac cells exposed to catecholamines, digitalis, and conditions of low extracellular potassium concentration and high extracellular calcium concentration. Several factors can increase the amplitude and/or frequency of DADs: increased heart rate, catecholamines, increased concentration of extracellular calcium, premature systoles and especially supratherapeutic concentrations of digoxin. It is not yet clear what current(s) comprise the inward current that creates a DAD. Some investigators have shown a role for the calcium-activated nonspecific cation channel (I_{NS}), whereas others have implicated the sarcolemmal Na/CA exchanger.[37–39] Regardless of the exact mechanism, a major "vulnerable parameter" of DADs is intracellular calcium overload; therapy should be directed at decreasing intracellular calcium.[32] This can be achieved by administering L-type calcium channel blockers (eg, verapamil). Likewise, DADs may be suppressed by inhibiting I_{NS} (ie, sodium channel blockers) or by increasing outward potassium currents (eg, adenosine).

Characteristics of Triggered Activity

Several features of triggered activity must be considered when postulating that a clinical dysrhythmia is due to this mechanism. First, triggered activity appears to be induced easily in a variety of fiber types and conditions, including excess digitalis and catecholamines.[8]

Second, pacing at rates faster than that of the triggered activity (overdrive pacing) may increase the amplitude and rate of sustained rhythmic activity after cessation of pacing (overdrive excitation).[40,41] Premature stimulation has a similar effect. The clinical implication is that triggered dysrhythmias may not be suppressed easily, or even worse, may be precipitated by rapid heart rates, including sinus tachycardia and rapid electronic pacing.

Third, because a single premature impulse can both initiate and terminate either triggered activity or reentrant excitation, differentiation between these two mechanisms for dysrhythmias is difficult. Fourth, small changes in the rate of stimulation of driven preparations may affect the likelihood of triggering.[42] This frequency dependence suggests that for triggering to be a cause of clinical dysrhythmia, it must occur in a protected (parasystolic) focus.

Reentrant Excitation

Under certain conditions, the propagating impulse may not dissipate after complete activation of the heart but rather persists to reexcite the atria or ventricles after the end of the refractory period. This process is termed reentrant excitation.[43] Reentrant excitation may be *random* or *ordered*, the principal distinction between the two being that the former involves impulse propagation over pathways that continuously change their size and location (eg, fibrillation), and the latter, impulse propagation over a relatively fixed reentrant pathway (AV nodal reentrant tachycardia).[18]

Requirements

The basic requirements for either kind of reentry are similar: a transient or unidirectional conduction block somewhere in the reentrant circuit; the zone of block enables an excitable pathway to persist over which the reentrant impulse returns to reexcite previously excited tissue; and wave length of the impulse in the reentrant circuit (conduction velocity × effective refractory period) is shorter than the length of the circuit so that tissue into which the impulse propagates has sufficient time to recover excitability.[44] Because of the last requirement, a critical relation exists between pathway length, conduction velocity and refractory period. Reentry can be promoted by slowing conduction, decreasing refractoriness, or a combination of the two.

Regardless of the etiology, reentrant tachydysrhythmias can be grouped into those with long of short excitable gaps.[32] With a long excitable gap, conduction is primarily impaired. That is, the circuit between the refracting tail and the crest of the wavefront is fully excitable. Under these conditions, the goal of therapy is to depress conduction; this makes it less likely for the wavefront to pass through the impaired segment. In contrast, it would be illogical to prolong the effective refracting period because it may need to be increased two- to three-fold to be effective. A short excitable gap is characterized by conduction encroaching on refractoriness. Thus, only a small segment of fully excitable tissue exists between the wavefront crest and its refractory tail. Therapy for short gap reentry is directed at prolonging the effective refractory period (ie, I_K blockers). It can be difficult clinically to differentiate between short and long excitable gap reentry. However, short gap reentry tends to be faster and not entrained by extra stimuli. The opposite is true for long gap reentry.

Causes

A number of causes are responsible for the slowed conduction and block required for reentrant excitation. The speed of conduction in cardiac fibers is dependent on both active (eg, membrane responsiveness) and passive (eg, cable properties) membrane electric properties, as well as their microanatomic structure. Examples of possible mechanisms for reentrant excitation are discussed below, but these are by no means all inclusive. The cause for reentry may vary with specific dysrhythmias and the underlying pathophysiologic conditions.

PREMATURE ACTIVATION AND INCOMPLETE REPOLARIZATION. Premature activation of the heart (external stimuli, automatic discharge) can induce reentrant excitation because impulses conduct slowly in incompletely repolarized regions of the heart. Reentry may also occur in cells with persistent low levels of resting membrane potential and resultant depressed fast responses. Depending on the level of resting membrane potential, such cells may be the site of slowing or actual conduction block.

SLOW INWARD CURRENT. Under certain conditions, the slow inward current can underlie the genesis of reentrant dysrhythmias.[17] Slow-response action potentials, as in SA and AV node cells and in depressed fast-response fibers (resting membrane potential <-60 mV), conduct quite slowly and can be the cause of unidirectional or complete conduction block.

REENTRY WITH AN ANATOMIC OBSTACLE. Reentrant excitation caused by slowed conduction and block can also occur in anatomically distinct circuits. These circuits can be formed by branching Purkinje fiber bundles, bundles of surviving muscle fibers in healed infarcts, or in fibrotic regions of the atria or ventricles. Gross anatomic circuits are also required for reentry involving accessory conduction pathways and the bundle branches.[43]

REENTRY DUE TO FUNCTIONAL, LONGITUDINAL DISSOCIATION. Reentry can also occur in contiguous pathways (Fig. 22-4), based on the observations that such pathways can undergo functional, longitudinal dissociation.[44–46] This kind of reentry, also termed reflection,[17] occurs in unbranched bundles of Purkinje fibers in which conduction is slow because of reduced resting membrane potentials. Reflection can also be caused by electrotonic transmission across a blocked segment in a single fiber.[47]

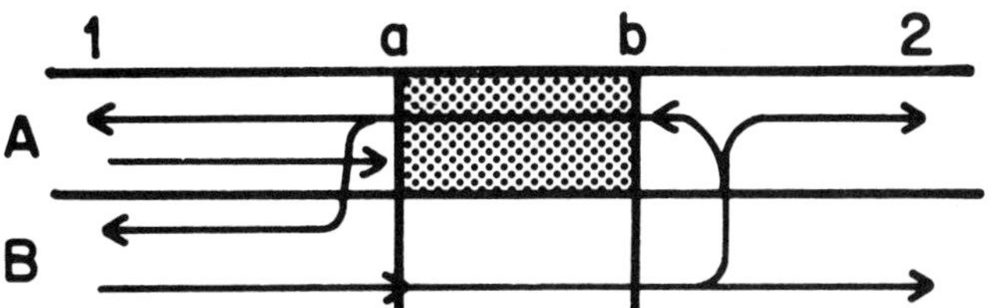

FIGURE 22-4. Reentry in contiguous pathways. Initial impulse propagation begins at site 1 in contiguous pathways A and B. It blocks at the depressed zone (*a–b, stippled*) in pathway A but propagates in pathway B to site 2. The impulse propagation also excites pathway A distal to the depressed zone and returns through the now-recovered depressed zone to reexcite tissue proximal to the zone of block (unidirectional block). (Modified from Schmidt OF, Erlanger J: Directional differences in the conduction of the impulse through heart muscle and their possible relation to extrasystolic and fibrillary contractions. Am J Physiol 87:326, 1929.)

LEADING CIRCLE CONCEPT FOR REENTRY. Studies by Allessie and colleagues have shown that, under appropriate conditions, the propagating impulse can create a functionally inactive core around which it can circulate, so that no requirement exists for an anatomically distinct tissue circuit.[48] This mechanism, the leading circle concept for reentry, probably can operate anywhere in the heart if conditions are favorable.

CAUSES OF CARDIAC DYSRHYTHMIAS

Anesthetic Action

Inhalation Agents

Because knowledge concerning the anesthetic effects on abnormal electrophysiologic mechanisms (depressed fast response, abnormal automaticity, triggering, mechanisms for reentry) is scant, a definitive statement concerning anesthetic dysrhythmic potential cannot be offered. Yet, with the exception of halothane, the modern inhalation and intravenous anesthetic agents are not considered dysrhythmic, chiefly because they are not particularly sensitizing; that is, compared with the awake state, anesthetics may reduce the dose of catecholamines required for ventricular dysrhythmias. However, this definition ignores known actions of anesthetics on normal electrophysiologic mechanisms that could be the cause of dysrhythmias during anesthesia.

PACEMAKER EFFECTS. The actions of modern inhalation agents (enflurane, halothane, isoflurane) on normal electrophysiologic mechanisms include depression of SA node automaticity,[49,50] with negligible effects (except halothane) on normal automaticity in latent pacemakers,[51–53] and depression of AV nodal conduction and refractoriness.[50,54–57]

These actions can facilitate or aggravate some dysrhythmias, including wandering atrial pacemaker, AV junctional or ventricular escape rhythms, and AV conduction block at the AV node. The consequence of these dysrhythmias can span any disturbance from partial to complete AV dyssynchrony with resulting hemodynamic impairment.

VENTRICULAR DYSRHYTHMIAS. Inhalation anesthetics, given their effects in vivo on ventricular conduction and refractoriness,[50] or on normal Purkinje fiber action potentials,[51–53,59] are unlikely to be the cause of ventricular dysrhythmias in the absence of other permissive factors, such as excess digitalis, electrolyte imbalance, and catecholamines. In particular, they (at least halothane) do not sufficiently alter the resting membrane potential of quiescent ventricular muscle or Purkinje fibers[59] to depress the fast response or activate the slow inward current. Thus, in terms of their effects on normal electrophysiologic mechanisms, the modern inhalation anesthetics should be viewed as least potentially dysrhythmic.

ABNORMAL MECHANISMS. In terms of abnormal mechanisms, little is known except by way of inference. Enflurane, halothane, and isoflurane differ with respect to potentiation of epinephrine-induced ventricular dysrhythmias (Fig. 22-5).[60] As mentioned earlier, catecholamines are among the factors that can cause loss of resting membrane potential that could be the basis for dysrhythmias due to reentrant excitation or abnormal forms of automaticity. Anesthetics may have varying effects on these abnormal mechanisms.

Intravenous Agents

The dysrhythmic potential of intravenous anesthetics (narcotics, barbiturates, nonbarbiturates) is discussed in some detail elsewhere.[6] With the exception of droperidol, little is known of the effects of the intravenous anesthetics on cardiac electrophysiologic properties. In general, none are dysrhythmogenic alone, but all can contribute to dysrhythmias because of associated central or peripheral autonomic effects, or through interactions with other drugs.

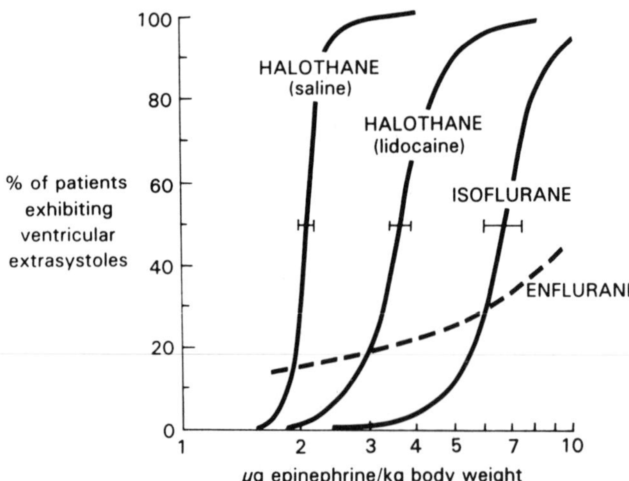

FIGURE 22-5. The results of statistical analysis suggest that the halothane and isoflurane curves (but not the enflurane curve) are parallel and that the doses effective in 50% of subjects are significantly different from each other ($P < 0.01$). *Bars,* standard deviation from the 50% effective dose. (Johnston RR, Eger EI, Wilson C: A comparative interaction of epinephrine with enflurane, isoflurane, and halothane in man. Anesth Analg 55:711, 1976.)

DROPERIDOL. Droperidol increases both antegrade and retrograde refractoriness in the accessory pathway of patients with the WPW syndrome,[61] effects that tend to reduce the rate of AV reciprocating supraventricular tachycardia and the ventricular response during atrial flutter or fibrillation in these patients. Droperidol has electrophysiologic properties in vitro similar to those of quinidine[62] and prevents halothane- and epinephrine-induced ventricular fibrillation in cats.[63] It also increases the tolerance to toxic doses of ouabain and converts ouabain-induced ventricular tachycardia to sinus or nodal rhythm in dogs.[64] Thus, droperidol is not likely to cause dysrhythmias during anesthesia and, indeed, has some rather interesting antidysrhythmic properties with potential implications for anesthetic management.

Catecholamine–Anesthetic Interaction

Catecholamines and other adrenergic agonists are among the most extensively discussed causes for dysrhythmias during anesthesia (see Fig. 22-5).[65,66] Whereas the exogenous administration of such compounds is an obvious cause for dysrhythmias, less obvious is the direct or permissive role that endogenous catecholamines play in dysrhythmias attributed to other causes, including those due to myocardial ischemia, digitalis,[67–69] hypoxia, hypercapnia, reflex-initiated, light anesthesia, electrolyte imbalance, hypermetabolic states, and surgical stress. Thus, the interaction of anesthetics with adrenergic compounds is important in the genesis of dysrhythmias. Currently, interest is focused on the effects of drugs and other factors in modifying catecholamine–anesthetic dysrhythmias. In addition, recent work on receptor mechanisms has provided insight into more effective means for prevention and treatment.

Modifying Drug Effects

POTENTIATION. Among the agents used for the induction of anesthesia, thiopental,[69–71] thiamylal,[70,72] and ketamine[73] increase the potential for epinephrine-induced dysrhythmias during halothane anesthesia. The thiopental effect extends to enflurane and isoflurane[71] and persists for as long as 4 hours after induction.[69,71] Succinylcholine,[74] cocaine,[73] and nitrous oxide[75,76] are other drugs used in anesthesia that lower the threshold for epinephrine dysrhythmias with halothane.

Drugs that affect catecholamine synthesis, reuptake, or biodegradation (eg, tyrosine, tricyclic antidepressants, monoamine oxidase inhibitors) should increase the likelihood of the interaction, although this hypothesis has yet to be documented. At least with halothane, a critical increase in heart rate and blood pressure favors the development of epinephrine dysrhythmias.[77]

PROTECTION. Lidocaine affords protection against epinephrine-induced ventricular dysrhythmias in both humans[60,78] (see Fig. 22-5) and dogs,[79] as do bupivacaine and etidocaine in dogs.[79] Among the adrenergic blocking agents, metoprolol (β_1-adrenergic receptor selective),[80] propranolol (β-nonselective),[81] and prazosin (α-selective) decrease the dysrhythmic potential of epinephrine in halothane-anesthetized dogs. Verapamil is effective against epinephrine-induced dysrhythmias with halothane.[82] Other anesthetic agents or adjuvants, pancuronium,[83] d-tubocurarine,[83] and etomidate[84,85] have been shown not to affect the production of halothane-epinephrine dysrhythmias.

Receptor Mechanisms

Because most of the myocardial receptors are of the β_1 and α_1 subclasses, the assumption has been made that the former represent the principal receptor mechanism mediating catecholamine–anesthetic dysrhythmias.[86] In addition, nonselective β-adrenergic blocking agents are known to be effective against epinephrine-anesthetic dysrhythmias.[81] However, α-adrenergic receptors possibly are also involved, because in earlier studies, nonselective α-adrenergic blocking agents had an inconsistent action in blocking catecholamine–anesthetic dysrhythmias.[65]

Maze and Smith[80] and Spiss and colleagues[87] examined the relative contribution of the α_1- and β_1-adrenergic receptors to the genesis of halothane-epinephrine dysrhythmias. The effect of prazosin (α_1-selective) was significantly greater than that of metoprolol (β_1-selective) in increasing the epinephrine dysrhythmia threshold. Furthermore, sodium nitroprusside, which causes a similar lowering of arterial pressure as prazosin, has no effect on the epinephrine threshold dose.

CLINICAL IMPLICATIONS. Blood pressure, per se, does not appear important in the genesis of epinephrine dysrhythmias. Rather convincing evidence, at least at the myocardial level, suggests that both α_1 and β_1 receptors are involved. This hypothesis has implications for both the prevention and treatment of catecholamine–anesthetic dysrhythmias. Possibly, because both α_1 and β_1 receptors are involved, a drug such as labetalol (α_1- and β_1-blocking agent, partial β_2 agonist) is a better preventive agent against catecholamine dysrhythmias than either an α- or β-blocking agent alone.

Local Anesthetic Cardiotoxicity

Mechanisms

The local anesthetics depress both conduction and excitability in nerves and cardiac tissue by selective block of the fast (sodium ion) channels. This effect is thought to be accomplished by both direct binding of the charged (dissociated) form of the local anesthetic to receptor sites within the cell, and to conformational changes in the cell membrane produced by the undissociated form. The latter action, should be more pronounced with more lipid-soluble agents, especially bupivacaine and etidocaine.[88] Either of these actions, in addition to block of the sodium ion channels, could also influence other ion-specific channels as well, particularly in the heart.

CARDIOVASCULAR RESISTANCE. The cardiovascular system is more resistant than the central nervous system to the depressant effects of local anesthetics. Whereas central nervous system toxicity is manifest as irritability and seizures, cardiotoxicity usually presents as bradycardia, AV conduction block and hypotension, or both. Sudden cardiovascular collapse, without antecedent hypoxia or evidence of central nervous system toxicity, may occur with customary clinical dosages of bupivacaine and etidocaine.[89–92] Although the toxicity associated with bupivacaine and etidocaine has prompted a flurry of animal investigation,[93–102] published data regarding the clinical incidence are unavailable.

RELATIVE TOXICITY. Taken collectively, animal reports indicate the following: bupivacaine, and possibly etidocaine, appear more cardiotoxic than lidocaine; a specific dysrhythmic effect of bupivacaine and etidocaine is present with subconvulsive or convulsive dosages, confirming the clinical impression that cardiovascular collapse and seizures can occur simultaneously; an increase in serum potassium level lowers the cardiotoxic dose of both lidocaine and bupivacaine, but does not affect the seizure dose; dysrhythmias due to cardiotoxicity are more severe with bupivacaine than with lidocaine; and dysrhythmias due to cardiotoxicity with bupivacaine occur in the absence of marked hypoxia, acidosis, hyperkalemia, or hypotension, indicating that these are not factors in the production of dysrhythmias.

BUPIVACAINE. The mechanism for increased cardiotoxicity with bupivacaine, as compared with lidocaine, probably involves increased affinity of bupivacaine for inactivated sodium ion channels in the heart.[88] Also, because bupivacaine is so tightly bound, recovery from block during diastole is slower than with lidocaine. Consequently, sodium ion channel block with bupivacaine has a greater chance to accumulate than that with lidocaine, even at physiologic heart rates. Regardless of mechanism, however, prudence might suggest the avoidance of bupivacaine altogether, or restriction of its use to situations where the possible benefit clearly outweighs the risk of cardiotoxicity, and then only with precautions to minimize the risk of intravascular absorption.

Succinylcholine

This drug has been associated with all types of cardiac dysrhythmias, including brady- and tachysupraventricular and ventricular dysrhythmias, heart block, and AV junctional rhythms. This association should not be surprising when one considers that succinylcholine stimulates all cholinergic autonomic receptors, including those located in autonomic ganglia (nicotinic) and within the SA and AV nodes and AV junctional tissues (muscarinic).[103] In addition, succinylcholine is frequently used to facilitate tracheal intubation, which by itself cause intense autonomic stimulation.

Mechanisms

Although the choline produced by hydrolysis of the initial succinylcholine dose had been thought responsible for bradycardia with repeated doses,[104] subsequent work indicates that succinylmonocholine is the major cause.[105] Bradycardia with repeated doses of succinylcholine can be at least partially blocked by atropine. In the monkey and the dog, succinylcholine lowers the threshold for epinephrine-induced ventricular dysrhythmias.[74]

An association between succinylcholine and ventricular dysrhythmias in patients receiving chronic digitalis therapy[106] must be questioned[107] however, because digitalis levels in the former study may have been excessive. Other factors, including inadequate ventilation and oxygenation, and the stress of laryngoscopy appear more important.[6]

Succinylcholine administration to patients with burns, extensive muscle trauma, certain neuromuscular disease, and closed head injuries may be associated with exaggerated potassium release and life-threatening cardiac dysrhythmias.[6,108]

Nondepolarizing Muscle Relaxants

The nicotinic receptors at the neuromuscular junction have features in common with those found in autonomic ganglia, but the two are not identical.[103,109] Hence, in view of their varying neuromuscular blocking potency, the nondepolarizing neuromuscular blocking agents, not surprisingly, vary in their potency as ganglionic blockers; ganglionic blockade is seen usually only with larger dosages.[74,103]

In addition, the nondepolarizers, which are quaternary ammonium compounds and do not cross the central nervous system blood–brain barrier, are largely devoid of stimulatory or depressant effects on central nervous system circulatory regulatory mechanisms after usual clinical doses.[103] Thus, none of the nondepolarizers is likely to cause dysrhythmias, although pancuronium can cause sinus tachycardia. The mechanism probably involves muscarinic blockade,[109,110] possibly at the vagal level.[103,110]

Associated Drug Therapy

During anesthesia and surgery, many drugs are administered for the continued management of preexisting medical disorders. Although some could cause or aggravate dysrhythmias, most often the cause is an adverse drug interaction or the result of some drug-induced physiologic derangement. Only documented interactions that either are or could be the cause for dysrhythmias are discussed here.

Aminophylline

The synthesis and release of catecholamines is increased by phosphodiesterase inhibition, the enzyme responsible for the hydrolysis of cyclic adenosine monophosphate (cAMP). Aminophylline interacts with halothane[111] but not isoflurane[112] to reduce the epinephrine dysrhythmia threshold in dogs. Clinical reports have implicated aminophylline as the cause for dysrhythmias with halothane[113,114] and pancuronium.[115] This problem may be greater with acute than with chronic aminophylline administration.[116]

Calcium Channel–Blocking Agents

Verapamil and diltiazem, particularly when used in combination with β-adrenergic receptor blocking agents such as propranolol, can cause conduction block at the AV node or hypotension and myocardial depression. In our canine model for awake-anesthetized cardiac electrophysiologic investigation,[117] clinically relevant levels of verapamil and diltiazem, but not nifedipine, produce significant additive depression to that of enflurane and halothane on AV nodal conduction time. Indeed, diltiazem or verapamil administered with any of the potent inhalation anesthetics, but especially enflurane, can be the cause for heart block and escape rhythms.[118]

The mechanism for "apparent" heart block and escape rhythms with the anesthetics and verapamil or diltiazem may not be AV block but, rather, SA block. Clinically, the likelihood of significant AV block appears remote, provided that the patient is not also receiving β-adrenergic blocking agents or excessive concentrations of the potent volatile agents were used.

Digitalis

Cardiac toxicity, manifest as dysrhythmias or worsening of heart failure, can occur in as many as 25% of patients receiving digitalis.[119] No dysrhythmia is specific for digitalis toxicity, although atrial tachycardia with block in a patient receiving chronic digitalis therapy is highly suggestive.

Many factors increase the toxicity of digitalis: hypoxia, catecholamines, hypokalemia, hypercalcemia, and acid–base imbalance.[6] Halothane,[120] enflurane,[121] ketamine,[122] droperidol,[122] droperidol–fentanyl mixtures (Innovar),[122] and d-tubocurarine[106] increase the tolerance of the heart to digitalis-induced ventricular dysrhythmias in the dog, whereas thiopental[123] and fentanyl[122] have no effect. None of these agents should be considered protective against or treatment for dysrhythmias in patients receiving digitalis. Succinylcholine,[106] neostigmine,[124] and diazepam[125] are reported to have induced ventricular dysrhythmias in these patients. However, such reports are largely anecdotal, and one must question their validity without knowledge of the status of digitalization.

β-Adrenergic Receptor Blockade

Vagal predominance with slowing of heart rate and increased AV nodal conduction time and refractoriness can result from this therapy. It may be the cause for bradydysrhythmias and heart block, particularly in patients also receiving calcium channel–blocking agents, or when the potent volatile anesthetics are used. Also, the risk of bradydysrhythmias or heart block is increased when repeated doses of succinylcholine or anticholinesterases are used in patients receiving large doses of β-blocking agents.[126,127]

Lithium

Commonly used to treat manic-depressive disorders, lithium replaces sodium ion in generating the action potential; that is, it enters the cell with depolarization but cannot be actively extruded.[128] This translocation can lead to loss of the resting membrane potential, associated T-wave changes, and QRS widening.[129] Dysrhythmias have been reported with lithium,[129,130] it merits further investigation as a cause for dysrhythmias during anesthesia.

Tricyclic Antidepressants

These agents have been implicated in the development of dysrhythmias during anesthesia in stressful situations.[131–133] Glisson and associates reported that atropine–neostigmine antagonism of neuromuscular blockade increased the frequency of ECG changes associated with lithium administration in cats pretreated with amitriptyline.[134]

Terbutaline

Chiefly a β_2-adrenergic receptor agonist, terbutaline has been implicated in dysrhythmias developing during anesthesia for cervical cerclage.[135,136] However, associated hypokalemia and some β_1-adrenergic receptor affinity could explain these cases.

Amiodarone

An antidysrhythmic and noncompetitive, nonspecific adrenergic receptor blocking drug, amiodarone has been implicated in causing an atropine-resistant bradycardia.[137] This drug has a long duration of action (elimination half-life $\geq$ 30 days) and is used for the management of supraventricular and ventricular tachydysrhythmias refractory to conventional therapy and occasionally for the treatment of angina.[138]

Cimetidine

Particularly when used in repeated intravenous doses, cimetidine has been associated with sinus arrest and dangerous ventricular dysrhythmias.[139] The mechanism may relate to block of myocardial histamine receptors, but cimetidine also reduces hepatic blood flow. Inhibition of drug-metabolizing enzymes in the liver could potentiate dysrhythmic actions of other drugs the patient might be receiving.

Electrolyte Imbalance

The dysrhythmic and ECG effects of electrolyte imbalance are discussed elsewhere,[6] and only briefly summarized here. Dysrhythmias do not result from the actions of the ions themselves, but rather to their relative excess or lack on the extracellular side of the cell membrane; hence the term *electrolyte imbalance*. Thus, a reported serum potassium level of 3.0 mEq/L is misleading unless considered within the context of the time over which the decrease occurred. Such an electrolyte abnormality developing over hours could be the cause of dysrhythmias, whereas a chronic change occurring over days would be better tolerated. Similarly, rapid correction of hypokalemia will be tolerated if the condition was acute, but not so if hypokalemia was a long-standing one.

Hyperkalemia

Unanesthetized patients with long-standing, moderate hyperkalemia (between 5.0 and 7.5 mEq/L) rarely have atrial or ventricular premature beats or disturbed AV conduction.[140] The effect of potassium ion administration on cardiac rhythm and conduction depends on myocardial integrity, the amount of potassium administered, and the initial value of and change in, especially rate of change, extracellular potassium concentration.[141]

EFFECTS. Progressive slowing of AV conduction and decrease in excitability terminate in cardiac arrest when potassium ion depolarizes ventricular fibers to the level at which they become nonexcitable. A more common event with extremes of hyperkalemia, however, is ventricular fibrillation. Lethal hyperkalemia in the anesthetic setting is rare, and most likely due to error in the amount, rate, or route of potassium administration, or to exaggerated potassium release after succinylcholine in susceptible patients.[108] Ventricular fibrillation after the central administration of potassium can be initiated by a single premature beat and may not be accompanied by any of the usual ECG manifestations of toxicity.

Finally, loss of intracellular potassium ion with a resultant increase in interstitial potassium surrounding an area of acute myocardial ischemia is generally believed responsible for dysrhythmias related to myocardial ischemia and infarction, possibly in association with other factors (loss of resting membrane potential, changes in cell membrane function).

Hypokalemia

Hypokalemia is more likely to be a cause of dysrhythmias during anesthesia than is hyperkalemia. It commonly results from respiratory or metabolic alkalosis, or the result of potassium-depleting diuretic therapy.

EFFECTS. Hypokalemia facilitates or causes dysrhythmias resulting from automaticity and reentry. It promotes the appearance of atrial and ventricular premature beats and AV conduction disturbances. Dysrhythmias due to hypokalemia are the same as those in patients with digitalis toxicity (atrial and ventricular ectopy, atrial tachycardia with block, AV junctional rhythms and ventricular tachycardia). Similar to digitalis, hypokalemia intensifies the effects of vagal stimulation.

POSTPONEMENT OF ELECTIVE SURGERY. In one study of 81 patients, none of whom was receiving digitalis therapy, who had plasma potassium levels of 3.1 mEq/L or lower, a 22% incidence of premature ventricular beats (PVBs) and 12% incidence of AV conduction disturbances were noted.[142] In another study, the incidence of PVBs was 24% in normotensive and 30% in hypertensive patients with potassium levels 3.6 mEq/L or lower.[143] In both studies the incidence of PVBs was two to three times that of other hospitalized patients, lending support to the postponement of elective surgery until the patient is rendered normokalemic.

Even minimal hypokalemia (ie, 3.0 to 3.5 mEq/L) is associated with myocardial electrical instability among patients with mild hypertension and ischemic heart disease.[144] However, controversy exists in the management of patients who are found preoperatively to have hypokalemia, especially at modest levels. Several observations underlie this controversy: normokalemia is often noted on repeat testing; less potassium supplementation than that estimated often returns the serum potassium level to normal; and dysrhythmias are usually infrequent when the patients undergo emergency procedures that cannot be delayed.

CHRONIC HYPOKALEMIA. To assess whether chronic hypokalemia per se increases the incidence of dysrhythmias during anesthesia, Vitez and colleagues monitored continuously the intraoperative ECGs of normokalemic (3.5 to 5.0 mEq/L) and hypokalemic (2.6 to 3.4 mEq/L) patients.[145] The occurrence of intraoperative dysrhythmias correlated only with the presence of preoperative dysrhythmias. However, potassium values were obtained 12 to 24 hours before surgery, abnormal potassium determinations were not repeated, many patients were receiving potassium supplementation, and two thirds of the hypokalemic patients had values in the near-normal range, 3.0 to 3.4 mEq/L.

Modification by Other Ions

In patients with hyperkalemia, the calcium concentration may be the important factor that determines the severity of the AV and intraventricular conduction disturbances, as well as vulnerability to ventricular fibrillation.[140] Coexisting hyperkalemia and hypocalcemia are common in patients with advanced renal disease.

Hypocalcemia, hyponatremia, and hypermagnesemia may be expected to aggravate disturbed conduction and the vulnerability to fibrillation with hyperkalemia. Hypercalcemia, hypernatremia, and hypomagnesemia counter the tendency of hyperkalemia to promote dysrhythmias and conduction disturbances. Although hypocalcemia augments the dysrhythmic effects of hypokalemia experimentally, this relation was not seen clinically.[142] The incidence of dysrhythmias in hypokalemic patients is similar with and without acidosis.[142]

Calcium Disorders

Only extremes of hyper- or hypocalcemia are likely to produce cardiac electrophysiologic abnormalities of clinical importance.[140] Within the range of changes in extracellular calcium ion concentration compatible with life, calcium ion has little effect on resting membrane potential. A low extracellular calcium ion concentration prolongs, and a high value shortens, action potential duration and refractoriness, changes that are dependent on heart rate and extracellular magnesium ion concentration. Low extracellular calcium concentration can cause increased dispersion of refractoriness, depress contractility, lower the threshold of excitability, and slightly decrease the slope of phase 4 depolarization in Purkinje fibers. A high extracellular calcium level has just the opposite effects on Purkinje fibers.

The level of extracellular calcium affects conduction most in slow channel fibers (SA and AV nodes, depressed fast-response fibers). Sudden deaths caused by ventricular fibrillation in patients in hyperparathyroid crisis are thought to be caused by hypercalcemia (total serum calcium >18 mEq/L). Finally, moderate hypocalcemia produced by sodium ethylenediamine tetraacetic acid may suppress atrial and ventricular PVBs.

Other Ion Disorders

Sodium ions have no dysrhythmic effects or discernible effects on the ECG independent of those of other ions.[139] Hypermagnesemia depresses AV and intraventricular conduction. In animals depression of conduction occurs at magnesium concentrations between 6 and 10 mEq/L, and cardiac arrest at levels above 30 mEq/L. In patients with toxemia of pregnancy treated with magnesium sulfate, respiratory depression occurs at serum magnesium levels above 10 mEq/L. Consequently, magnesium levels that might impair conduction or cause cardiac arrest would be unlikely except during controlled ventilation.

Acid–Base Imbalance

Metabolic and respiratory alkalosis are usually associated with changes in extracellular potassium and calcium concentrations. As a result, whether changes in extracellular pH per se cause the ECG changes and dysrhythmias seen in patients with acidosis and alkalosis is difficult to determine. They probably do not; electrolyte imbalance is a more likely cause.

Autonomic Reflexes

The term *reflex-caused dysrhythmia* is synonymous with autonomic imbalance-caused dysrhythmia.[6] With the exception of the oculocardiac reflex, autonomic imbalance resulting from laryngoscopy, traction on viscera, anorectal dilatation, periosteal stimulation, and similar stimuli is not likely to be a cause of clinically important cardiac dysrhythmias in adequately anesthetized and otherwise well-managed patients.

Sympathetic and Parasympathetic Predominance

The net result of autonomic imbalance brought about by surgical stimulation or manipulation is usually sympathetic predominance and, hence, catecholamine-mediated tachycardia and dysrhythmias. With the oculocardiac (trigeminovagal) reflex, however, the net result is vagal predominance and bradydysrhythmias or even asystole. This reflex occurs even in adequately anesthetized and well-managed patients. The term "vasovagal reflex," often used in the older literature, was considered by Katz and Bigger a "wastebasket category for a multitude of untoward events."[146] They considered the effects of vagal stimulation to be minimal in well-managed cases in the absence of electrolyte imbalance, hypoxia, and hypercapnia.

OCULOCARDIAC REFLEX. This reflex is mediated by the trigeminal (afferent arc) and vagal (efferent arc) nerves, due to stimulation of the ophthalmic branch of the trigeminal nerve. Stimulation of this branch results from traction on the extrinsic eye muscles, acute glaucoma, stretching of the eyelid muscles, and intraorbital injections or hematomas. Prolonged oculocardiac reflex activity may also be seen with orbital hemorrhage, after enucleation of the eye, and after ocular trauma.

Contrary to popular opinion, in a study of infants and children undergoing strabismus surgery, Blanc and associates found that traction on the medial rectus is not more reflexogenic than traction on the other extraocular muscles.[147] Slow gentle traction is less reflexogenic than acute, sustained traction. In addition, hypercapnia significantly augments the reflex.

Anticholinergic Prophylaxis. Prevention of the oculocardiac reflex by intravenous anticholinergics was not studied by these authors, but mentioned as deserving of further study. However, they agreed with Schwartz, who argued against the routine use of atropine for the prevention of the reflex in children.[148] Schwartz gave the following reasons: Intravenous atropine causes a high incidence of ventricular dysrhythmias; unlike bradycardia, these atropine-induced dysrhythmias may persist after release of traction on the extraocular muscles; ventricular dysrhythmias are frequently of a more disturbing nature than the bradycardia that may have been prevented. Blanc and associates recommend that if the oculocardiac reflex is elicited, the surgeon should release the traction, wait, and then continue the operation with more gentle manipulation.[147]

Conditions Associated With Dysrhythmias

Conditions and circumstances that either predispose to or are likely to be associated with serious dysrhythmias are discussed here apart from other causes of intraoperative cardiac dysrhythmias. These include long QT syndromes, mitral valve prolapse (MVP) syndrome, sympathetic imbalance disorders, and electrically susceptible patients.

Long QT Syndromes

Torsades de pointes is a specific type of ventricular tachydysrhythmia that occurs in the setting of a prolonged QT interval.[148,149] Although the morphology of various tachydysrhythmias can appear similar to that of torsades de pointes, the term should be reserved for those tachydysrhythmias associated with an abnormal TU complex (prolonged QT interval).

The abnormalities of ventricular repolarization that characterize the long QT syndromes can be divided into two groups: (1) acquired or pause-dependent long QT syndromes; and (2) congenital, idiopathic or adrenergic-dependent long QT syndromes. Acquired long QT syndromes can be caused by a number of etiologies: drugs (eg, Type Ia antidysrhythmics: quinidine, procainamide, disopyramide; tricyclic antidepressants; terfenadine; pentamidine; erthromycin, ketoconazole); dietary deficiencies (anorexia nervosa); electrolyte abnormalities (eg, hypokalemia, hypomagnesemia, hypocalcemia); and/or severe bradydysrhythmias (eg, 3° AV block, sinus node dysfunction).

The most common cause of acquired long QT syndrome is antidysrhythmic drug therapy, particularly when quinidine is used. In the acquired form, the tachydysrhythmia commences after a pause or abrupt deceleration of ventricular rhythm. A prominent U wave is created by the pause and forms the nidus for the development of the tachydysrhythmia. In contrast, the congenital (adrenergic-dependent) form of long QT syndrome is characterized by adrenergic hyperresponsiveness. These dysrhythmias are typically initiated when catecholamines levels increase such as during times of stress or fright. A family of congenital disorders is included in this category: (1) the Jervell and Lange-Nielsen syndrome,[148,150] characterized by neural deafness and an autosomal recessive inheritance pattern, and (2) the Romano-Ward syndrome[151,152] characterized by normal hearing and an autosomal dominant inheritance pattern.

Other diseases that can cause adrenergic-dependent long QT syndromes include patients with a history of mitral valve prolapse, myocardial infarction, surgery affecting the autonomic nervous system (eg, right radical neck dissection, carotid endarterectomy and truncal vagotomy) and central nervous system disorders (eg, subarachnoid hemorrhage, tumors, infection).[148,153,154]

Although the "sympathetic imbalance" hypothesis for congenital QT syndrome (excessive left- or lower-than-normal right-sided cardiac sympathetic innervation) was proposed 20 years ago,[155,156] its validity currently remains in doubt. Recent studies[158,159] have failed to demonstrate abnormal sympathetic innervation in the hearts of patients with familial long QT syndrome. Although not definitely ruling out the "sympathetic imbalance theory," these findings do suggest that an inherited defect in one or more cardiac channels responsible for ventricular repolarization may be an important mechanism ("primary myocardial" hypothesis).[160]

Patients with long QT syndromes are at significant risk for developing torsades de pointes, ventricular fibrillation, and hence, sudden death. Fortunately, new diagnostic criteria have been developed that more accurately identify patients with long QT syndrome.[161] Because the treatments are markedly different, it is very important for the anesthesiologist to identify whether a bout of torsades de pointes is pause-dependent (acquired) or adrenergic-dependent (congenital). A thorough preoperative review of the patient's history (family genetics and current drug therapy), laboratory work (electrolyte abnormalities), electrocardiograms (new and old records), and performance of a detailed physical exam (eg, presence of mitral valve prolapse) provide important information to the anesthesiologist. For example, stress-induced syncope in a young person with electrocardiographic findings of a prolonged QT interval, T wave alternans, and an impressive U wave strongly suggests congenital QT syndrome.

Therapy for pause-dependent torsades de pointes consists of increasing heart rate (overdrive pacing, vagolytic agents), eliminating the pause using the β-adrenergic agonist isoproterenol, and correcting any underlying condition. Magnesium sulfate (1–2 grams IV) may also be effective even when magnesium levels are normal. In the case of early afterdepolarization-induced torsades de pointes, calcium channel blockers may also be effective therapeutically. However, our bias is to consider using this class of drugs only after more established therapeutic modalities have failed.

Conversely, the treatment of adrenergic-dependent torsades de pointes consists of β-adrenergic blockers (ie, propranolol), or, if the rhythm is refractory to drug treatment, ablation of the left stellate ganglion. Increasing heart rate by overdrive pacing or drugs is not indicated in adrenergic-dependent torsades de pointes. Unlike its effect in pause-dependent torsades de pointes, pacing maneuvers may increase the U wave amplitude. In addition, it is not only important to differentiate the two types of torsades de pointes, it is equally important to distinguish bouts of polymorphic ventricular tachydysrhythmias unrelated to QTU abnormalities (eg, reentry) from episodes of torsades de pointes. For example, quinidine (or procainamide) may be therapeutically indicated for reentrant ventricular tachycardias but be contraindicated for torsades de pointes. Regardless of etiology, the initial therapy-of-choice for ventricular tachydysrhythmias causing hemodynamic instability is immediate DC cardioversion.

Patients with long QT syndrome who present preoperatively pose a therapeutic dilemma to the anesthesiologist. The first order of business is to search for an etiology of delayed ventricular repolarization. If the condition is congenital, there is little the physician can do to change the underlying condition. These individuals are definitely at increased risk during anesthesia and surgery because of stress-induced catecholamine release. The risk of developing torsades de pointes can be significantly reduced by proper preoperative treatment:[148,162] adequate premedication, pretreatment with β-blockers, possibly left stellate ganglion block, and avoidance of anesthetics known to facilitate catecholamine dysrhythmias.

A variety of options are available to the anesthesiologist in cases of acquired (eg, drug-induced) long QT syndrome. For example, what would be the appropriate decision if a patient scheduled for elective surgery presented with a terfenadine-induced prolongation of the QT interval? Unfortunately, specific criteria are not yet available that relate electrocardiographic findings to the likelihood of developing torsades de pointes. In several studies, it appears that the extent of QT interval prolongation poorly discriminates which patients are at greatest risk.[148,163,164] In our opinion, postponement of elective surgery should be given serious consideration, especially if the corrected (for heart rate) QT interval (QT_C) is more than 10% above normal values for age and sex. By delaying surgery and discontinuing the offending drug(s), ventricular repolarization can be normalized. In the event of emergency surgery where anesthesia must be administered in the setting of drug-induced long QT syndrome, strategies should be employed that shorten ventricular repolarization. Thus, drugs that increase heart rate or shorten repolarization will be beneficial. The equipment needed to overdrive pace should also be readily available. In the future, when detailed information about the effects of anesthetics on cardiac repolarization becomes available, more knowledgeable management decisions can be made in these patients.

Mitral Valve Prolapse Syndrome

MVP syndrome occurs in 5% to 10% of the population, and has been observed in patients of all ages and both sexes; in younger age groups, it is more common in women.[165]

SYMPTOMS. The vast majority of patients are asymptomatic. Palpitations, atypical anginal chest pain, and evidence of diminished cardiac reserve are the most common symptoms. Many of these may be related to autonomic dysfunction, which is common in these patients.

CAUSES. Any maneuver that decreases left ventricular volume (increased heart rate or contractility, reduced afterload or venous return) will cause the mitral valve to prolapse earlier in systole and increase symptoms. Just the opposite maneuvers will cause the prolapse to occur later in systole, or not at all. These points are stressed, not only because they are important to the diagnosis of MVP, but also because they are important to intraoperative management, including the prevention and management of dysrhythmias.

DYSRHYTHMIAS. A wide variety of dysrhythmias, including supraventricular and ventricular premature beats and brady- or tachydysrhythmias, and varying degrees of conduction block have been observed in these patients. Although many are of little clinical importance, life-threatening recurrent ventricular tachydysrhythmias refractory to conventional treatment have been reported. These usually are seen in patients with associated ST-segment or T-wave abnormalities in the resting ECG. Paroxysmal supraventricular tachycardia (PSVT) is the most common sustained tachydysrhythmia in patients with MVP, and may be related to the high incidence of left-sided accessory AV pathways in this condition.

ANESTHETIC MANAGEMENT. The anesthetic management of MVP has been reviewed by Krantz and colleagues.[166] In the absence of more specific, empirically-derived recommendations for anesthetic management, one should administer adequate premedication and anesthesia to reduce stress-induced catecholamine release, and avoid drugs and conditions likely to aggravate or cause dysrhythmias. For patients in whom dysrhythmias develop or who show signs of increasing mitral regurgitation in the perioperative setting, β-adrenergic blocking drugs are indicated.

Sympathetic Imbalance Disorders

Cardiovascular instability is common in patients with sympathetic dysfunction associated with orthostatic hypotension.[167,168] Dysrhythmias are likely in improperly managed patients for two reasons. Loss of sympathetic compensatory mechanisms leads to hypotension and bradycardia with inadequate myocardial perfusion, ischemia, and dysrhythmias; and exaggerated responses (denervation hypersensitivity) follows the administration of directly acting adrenergic agonists. Sympathetic hyperfunction and catecholamine-induced dysrhythmias are also common in patients with pheochromocytoma, neurofibromatosis,[169] thyrotoxicosis, tetanus,[170] and some types of chemodectoma.[171]

Electrically Susceptible Patients

Electric hazards in the intraoperative environment are reviewed elsewhere.[172,173] Microshock can be a cause of lethal dysrhythmias in electrically susceptible patients (eg, chronic central venous cannulation, invasive hemodynamic monitoring, esophageal probe, cardiac pacemakers). An electric cause should be suspected, particularly after others have been excluded and whenever a dysrhythmia recurs despite therapeutic measures.

RECOGNITION OF CARDIAC DYSRHYTHMIAS

Detection

Many cardiac dysrhythmias, some of which can cause clinically important hemodynamic impairment, are not detected chiefly because of the inability to clearly discern atrial activity. A normal QRS configuration does not necessarily establish a SA mechanism for a given beat, for it could have originated anywhere above the bifurcation of the common bundle. Without a normal atrial activation sequence, a significant reduction in cardiac output can occur, particularly in patients with marginal cardiac reserve. Similarly, supraventricular tachydysrhythmias with ventricular aberration and nonapparent atrial activity, or P waves with an uncertain relation to the QRS complex, may be easily mistaken for ventricular tachycardia. Thus, for the diagnosis of all but the most simple dysrhythmias, atrial activity must be discerned to establish its relation to the QRS complex.

Electrocardiographic Leads

Although ventricular activity is easily recognized using most conventional surface ECG leads, atrial activity is best monitored from surface leads II, aVF, and V_1. Monitoring with surface leads (eg, CB_5, MCL_1, S_5[4,5,174]) is helpful in amplifying P waves in some patients, but esophageal[175,176] or intra-atrial[169,170] leads are best for this purpose. However, esophageal and intra-atrial leads present a microshock hazard, and precautions to minimize this risk must be taken. In addition, with esophageal and intracavitary atrial monitoring, measures to minimize electrocautery interference (eg, electrocautery protection filters) are required.[178,179]

Aids to Diagnosis

Marriott suggests a five-step approach to the diagnosis of complex dysrhythmias[5]:

1. Know the possible causes. Thus, in the setting of surgical stress and light anesthesia, the appearance of premature beats with widened QRS complexes favors the diagnosis of ventricular ectopy as opposed to supraventricular ectopy with QRS aberration.
2. Study the QRS complex. If of normal duration, the rhythm is likely of supraventricular origin. However, the width of the QRS complex should be checked in several leads. Knowledge of the diagnostic morphologic features of the QRS complex may be helpful to distinguish the mechanism for tachycardia in the presence of wide QRS complexes,[5,180] other authorities attribute less importance to this relation.[181,182]
3. Look for the P wave. Seemingly apparent P waves adjacent to the QRS complex may be part of the QRS complex, or they may represent artifact. Select a lead at the start of anesthesia that shows P waves best, or use an esophageal or intra-atrial lead if the patient has a history of complex tachydysrhythmias or if they are likely to develop. A baseline ECG recording from the operating room monitor is also helpful for comparison should an arrhythmia arise.
4. Determine the relation of the P waves to the QRS complexes. Are they conducted with functional ventricular aberration? Maneuvers that increase vagal tone (carotid sinus massage, edrophonium) may be useful for this purpose. In addition,, P waves may be retrograde, hence the result of, rather than responsible for, ventricular activation.
5. Identify the primary diagnosis. The final diagnosis cannot be a secondary phenomenon, such as AV dissociation, escape, or aberration. All of these abnormalities are caused by some primary disturbance (ie, idioventricular rhythm with AV dissociation, sinus bradycardia with AV junctional or ventricular escape beats, or PSVT with ventricular aberration). Treatment of a secondary phenomenon can be dangerous. An example is the use of lidocaine to treat escape beats when atropine or pacing is indicated to increase the atrial rate.

Ventricular Aberration

The term *ventricular aberration* describes a supraventricular impulse with abnormal, bizarre intraventricular conduction. It refers to intraventricular conduction abnormalities related to changing heart rate or other electrophysiologic properties, anomalous AV conduction, metabolic disorders, electrolyte imbalance, or drug toxicity. As currently used, the term does not include fixed, organic conduction defects.

Electrophysiologic Alterations

The numerous ECG manifestations of aberration can be related to alterations in the electrophysiologic parameters affecting normal impulse propagation.[183] When these alterations are nonuniform, conduction in the ventricles may also be nonuniform, with ventricular aberration the result. More specifically, one or more of the following mechanisms may be responsible for QRS aberration: premature excitation; unequal refractoriness in the conducting tissues; preceding cycle length refractoriness; failure of restitution of the transmembrane ionic gradients during diastole; failure of the refractory period to shorten with faster heart rates; reduction in resting membrane potential due to phase 4 (diastolic) depolarization; concealed transseptal conduction with delay or block of conduction in the opposite bundle branch; diffuse depression in specialized ventricular and myocardial conduction; ventricular preexcitation (eg, bundle of Kent, Mahaim or James fibers); or predestination of ventricular conduction caused by altered intra-atrial conduction.[2,181]

QRS ABNORMALITIES. QRS aberration may result when any of the previously discussed mechanisms alter conduction in the bundle or fascicular branches, the Purkinje fibers or the ventricular myocardium. The right bundle branch (RBB) block pattern is the most common form of aberrancy and is frequently associated with left anterior fascicular block. Left bundle branch block pattern aberrancy is much less common and nearly always due to heart disease, although the latter may not be apparent.[184] Furthermore, an abnormality of in-

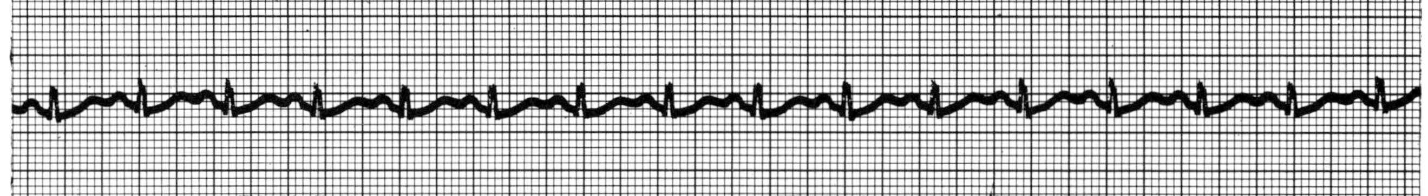

FIGURE 22-6. Sinus tachycardia at a rate of about 135 beats/minute. (Mangiola S, Ritota MC: Cardiac arrhythmias: practical ECG interpretation, 2nd ed. Philadelphia: JB Lippincott, 1982: 236.)

traventricular conduction should be suspected when both the initial and terminal portions of the QRS complex are abnormal.

Specific Dysrhythmias

The ECG features of supraventricular and ventricular dysrhythmias and heart block are briefly outlined. Their clinical features and manifestations in the perioperative setting are discussed in more detail elsewhere.[6]

Sinus Tachycardia and Bradycardia

With normal sinus rhythm (impulse formation beginning in the SA node at a rate between 60 and 100 beats/min in adults), the P waves are upright in leads I, II, and aVF, and negative in aVR, with a vector in the frontal plane of 0° to +90°. The PR interval exceeds 0.12 second and may vary slightly with changes in heart rate. Deviation from these morphologic limitations indicates a shift in the atrial pacemaker.

Sinus tachycardia is sinus rhythm at a rate exceeding 100 beats/min and normally does not exceed 180 beats/min in adults (but may be as high as 200 beats/min in trained athletes, infants and children). With advanced age, the upper limit is lower. Sinus tachycardia has a gradual onset and termination, in contrast to some other supraventricular tachydysrhythmias (Fig. 22-6). In addition, the P-P interval may vary slightly from cycle to cycle.

Sinus bradycardia is sinus rhythm at a rate less than 60 beats/min (in adults) with a PR interval exceeding 0.12 second (Fig. 22-7). Sinus bradycardia is common in young adults and trained athletes, and decreases in prevalence with advancing age.

Sinus Dysrhythmia

Sinus dysrhythmia is characterized by a phasic variation in sinus cycle length exceeding 0.12 second. Thus, the morphologic characteristics of the P wave do not vary, whereas the PR interval exceeds 0.12 second and varies little with long and short cycle length beats. With *phasic* sinus dysrhythmia, the P-P interval shortens during inspiration and lengthens during expiration (Fig. 22-8). With the *nonphasic* form, the P-P interval cycle length variation is unrelated to respiration. Phasic sinus dysrhythmia is common in young adults and well-trained individuals. The nonphasic form is more common with advanced age and may result from digitalis intoxication.

Wandering Atrial Pacemaker

Wandering atrial pacemaker is a variant of sinus dysrhythmia in which variation in morphologic features of the P wave occur, usually along with cyclical changes in the P-P interval (Fig. 22-9). It occurs in phasic and nonphasic forms and is differentiated from AV junctional rhythm with manifest P waves and AV dissociation (a secondary phenomenon) in which the P waves march back and forth through the QRS complex but remain upright. The latter dysrhythmia, often incorrectly termed "isorhythmic AV dissociation," is extremely common during anesthesia with the potent volatile agents, especially in individuals with heightened vagal tone.

Premature Atrial Beats

A premature atrial beat is associated with a premature P wave and a PR interval exceeding 0.12 second. It may be shorter in patients with ventricular preexcitation (eg, WPW). The morphologic appearance of the P wave may resemble that of sinus origin beats, but usually differs (Fig. 22-10). When a premature atrial beat occurs early in atrial diastole, its subsequent conduction through the AV node may be blocked (no associated QRS), prolonged (prolonged PR interval), or associated with ventricular aberration. Because the RBB has a longer refractory period than the left bundle branch, aberration usually has a RBB block pattern.

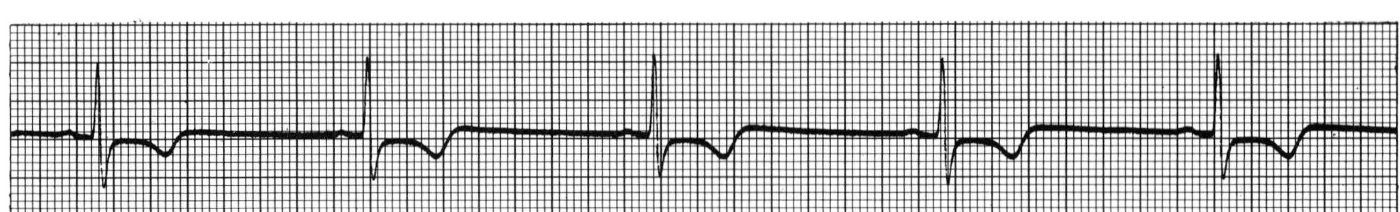

FIGURE 22-7. Sinus bradycardia at a rate of about 40 beats/minute. (Mangiola S, Ritota MC: Cardiac arrhythmias: practical ECG interpretation, 2nd ed. Philadelphia: JB Lippincott, 1982: 237.)

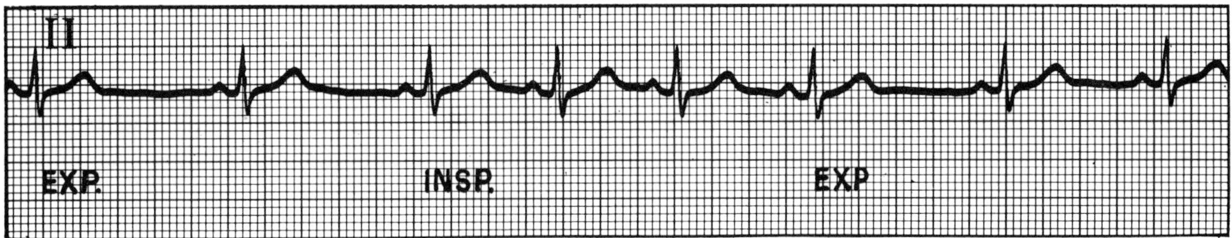

FIGURE 22-8. Sinus dysrhythmia. The rate increases with inspiration (*INSP*) and decreases during expiration (*EXP*) when it becomes more regular. (Mangiola S., Ritota MC: Cardiac arrhythmias: practical ECG interpretation. Philadelphia: JB Lippincott, 1974.)

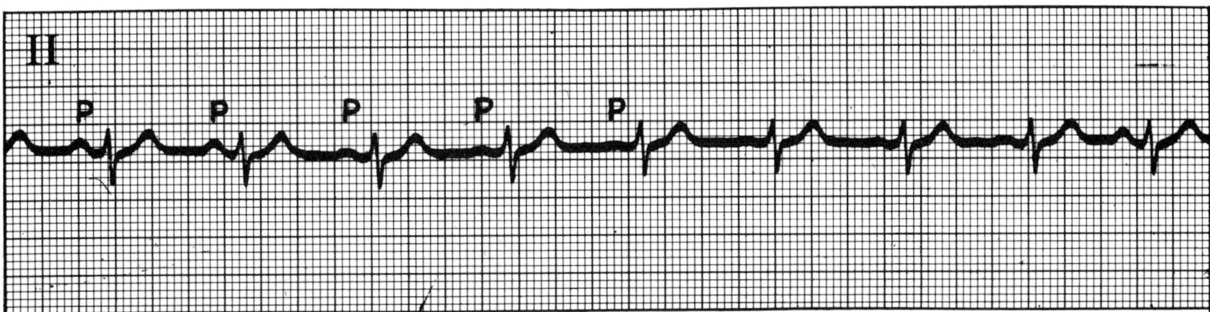

FIGURE 22-9. Wandering atrial pacemaker. The configuration of the P wave changes as the pacemaker shifts within the sinus node. (Mangiola S, Ritota MC: Cardiac arrhythmias: practical ECG interpretation. Philadelphia: JB Lippincott, 1974.)

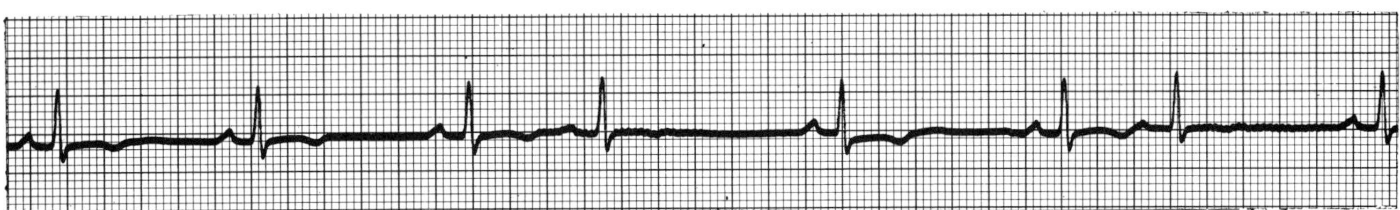

FIGURE 22-10. Sinus rhythm with two premature atrial beats (fourth and seventh). Mangiola S, Ritota MC: Cardiac arrhythmias: practical ECG interpretation, 2nd ed. Philadelphia: JB Lippincott, 1982: 237.)

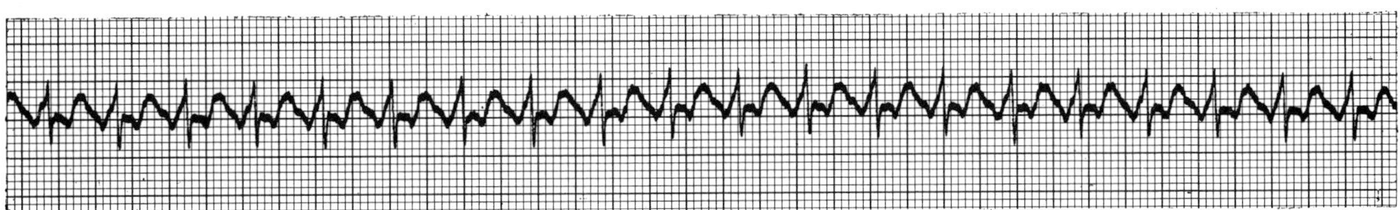

FIGURE 22-11. Atrial flutter with 2:1 conduction. (Mangiola S, Ritota MC: Cardiac arrhythmias: practical ECG interpretation, 2nd ed. Philadelphia: JB Lippincott, 1982: 240.)

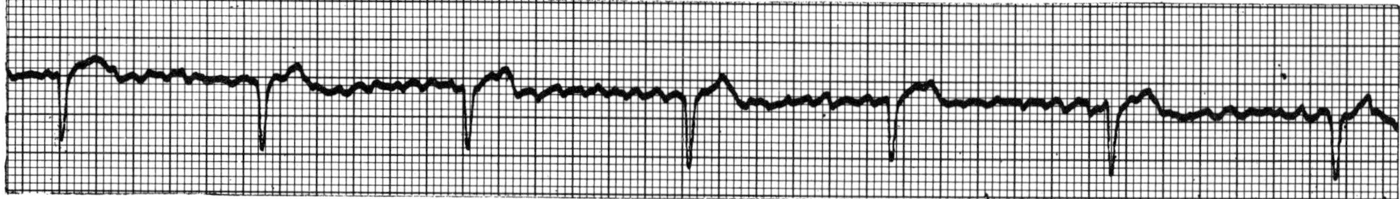

FIGURE 22-12. Atrial fibrillation with slow ventricular response. (Mangiola S, Ritota MC: Cardiac arrhythmias: practical ECG interpretation, 2nd ed. Philadelphia: JB Lippincott, 1982: 241.)

Atrial Flutter

Identical recurring flutter waves with a sawtooth appearance and no isoelectric interval between them characterize atrial flutter (Fig. 22-11). The atrial rate is usually 250 to 350 beats/min. Quinidine and related drugs (disopyramide, procainamide) may reduce it to around 200 beats/min, with the danger that the ventricles may respond in a 1:1 fashion to the slower rate. Usually the ventricular rate is half the atrial rate (see Fig. 22-11). A significantly slower rate suggests impaired AV conduction.

If the AV conduction ratio remains constant, the ventricular rhythm will be regular. If it varies, often as the result of Wenckebach AV block, the rhythm will be "regularly" irregular. Most often, an even ratio (2:1, 4:1) of flutter waves to ventricular complexes is present.[185] In children, patients with ventricular preexcitation, and occasionally those with hyperthyroidism, atrial flutter may conduct to the ventricle in a 1:1 fashion with ventricular rates as high as 300 beats/min.

Atrial flutter tends to be unstable, reverting to sinus rhythm or changing to atrial fibrillation. It responds to enhanced vagal tone (carotid sinus massage, edrophonium) by a stepwise decrease in the ventricular response. An increase in sympathetic tone may reduce the AV conduction delay and double the ventricular rate.

Atrial Fibrillation

Totally disorganized atrial activity, seen on the ECG as small, irregular baseline undulations of variable amplitude and morphologic features at a rate of from 300 to 600 beats/min characterize atrial fibrillation (Fig. 22-12). The ventricular response (usually 100 to 150 beats/min) is grossly ("irregularly") irregular due to variable conduction of the fibrillatory activity. Although atrial fibrillation may be seen in normal patients, underlying heart disease should always be suspected. Hypertensive cardiovascular disease is the most common antecedent factor.

Atrial Tachycardia

Paroxysmal atrial tachycardia, sometimes associated with AV block, is characterized by regular atrial rhythm at rates between 150 and 220 beats/min (Figs. 22-13 and 22-14). In contrast to atrial flutter, isoelectric intervals are present between P waves, which are of uniform appearance. The appearance of paroxysmal atrial tachycardia with block (Mobitz type I or II, second-degree AV block) in a patient receiving digitalis therapy strongly suggests toxicity, with or without associated hypokalemia. In the absence of digitalis, paroxysmal atrial tachycardia is usually associated with 1:1 AV conduction.

Multifocal Atrial Tachycardia

Sometimes termed chaotic atrial tachycardia or rhythm, this abnormality is characterized by atrial rates between 100 and 130 beats/min, marked variation in P-wave morphologic features (three or more types of P waves), and irregular P-P intervals. Usually, 1:1 AV conduction is present, but aberrant ventricular conduction with single or multiple beats may occur (Fig. 22-15).

Atrioventricular Junctional Beats and Rhythm

Pacemaker cells probably are not present within the AV node, but are found in the AV junctional tissues in areas adjacent to the atrium and the His (common) bundle. Hence, the term

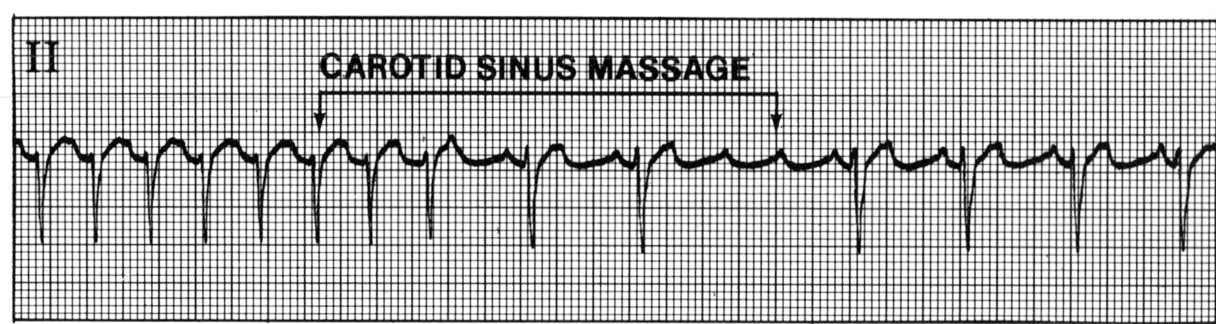

FIGURE 22-13. Paroxysmal atrial tachycardia. Carotid sinus massage increases vagal tone, depressing AV conduction and decreasing the ventricular response. (Mangiola S: Self-assessment in electrocardiography. Philadelphia: JB Lippincott, 1977.)

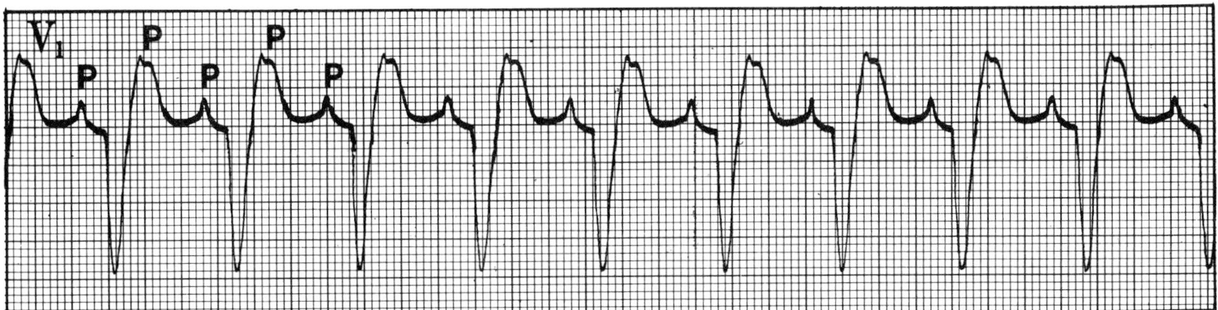

FIGURE 22-14. Paroxysmal atrial tachycardia with 2:1 block. (Mangiola S: Self-assessment in electrocardiography. Philadelphia: JB Lippincott, 1977.)

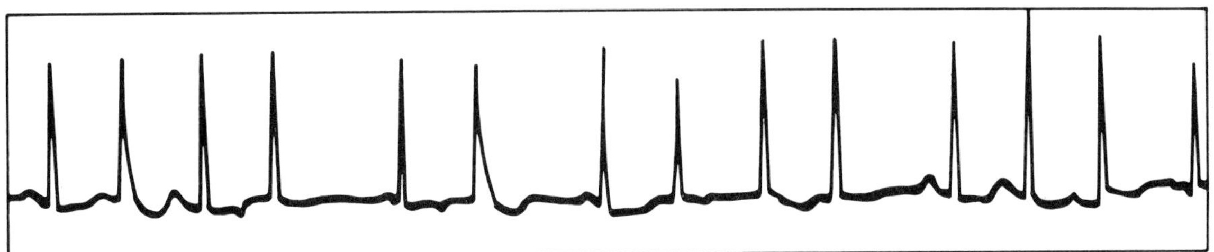

FIGURE 22-15. Multifocal atrial tachycardia in a patient with chronic obstructive pulmonary disease. Morphologic features of the P wave vary, and P–P intervals are irregular. There appears to be 1:1 AV conduction, but some QRS complexes are associated with ventricular aberration. (Atlee JL III: Perioperative cardiac dysrhythmias: mechanisms, recognition, management, 2nd ed. Chicago: Year Book Medical Publishers, 1985.)

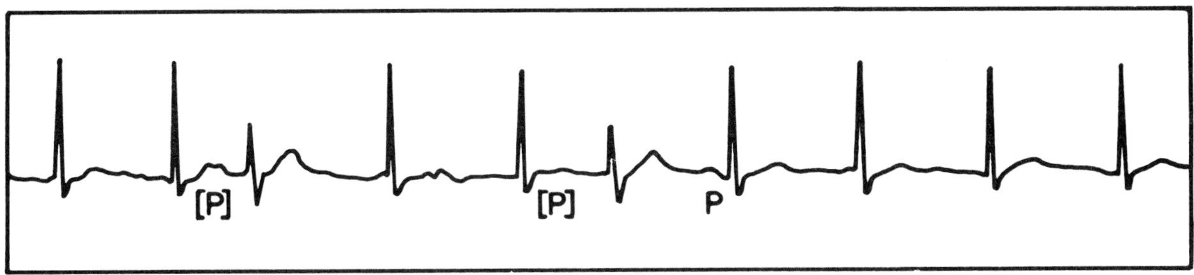

FIGURE 22-16. AV junctional rhythm with AV dissociation in a patient not receiving digitalis, β-adrenergic blocking agents, or calcium channel blocking agents. [*P*], P waves, followed by aberrant QRS complexes, that are reciprocal beats. Although the nonbracketed P wave is followed by a normal QRS interval, the short PR interval (0.10 s) suggests that this beat is of AV-junctional origin. (Atlee JL III: Perioperative cardiac dysrhythmias: mechanisms, recognition, management, 2nd ed. Chicago: Year Book Medical Publishers, 1985.)

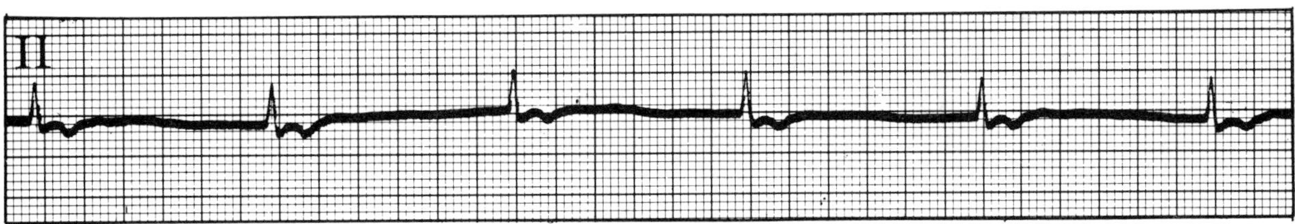

FIGURE 22-17. Junctional (nodal) rhythm. In this rhythm, the P wave most often is concealed within the QRS complex but may appear inverted in the ST segment. (Mangiola S, Ritota MC: Cardiac arrhythmias: practical ECG interpretation. Philadelphia: JB Lippincott, 1974.)

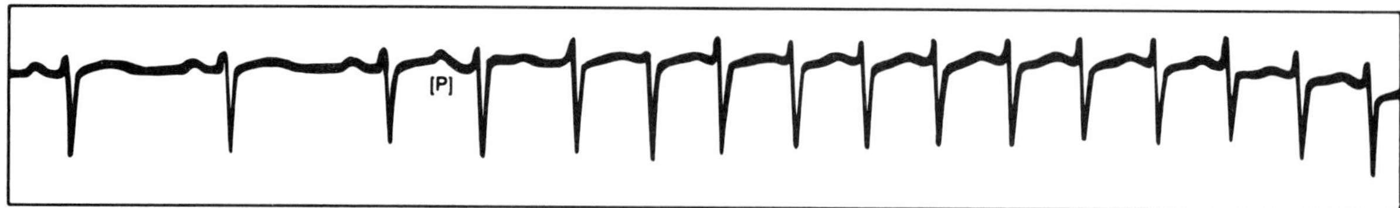

FIGURE 22-18. PSVT initiated by a premature atrial beat ([*P*]). The R–R interval during the dysrhythmia shortens over the first three beats of the tachycardia, the rate of which is 188 beats/min. (Atlee JL III: Perioperative cardiac dysrhythmias: mechanisms, recognition, management, 2nd ed. Chicago: Year Book Medical Publishers, 1985: 239.)

AV junctional is preferred for beats arising from this region as opposed to the terms "high, mid, or low nodal" used in the older literature (Fig. 22-16).

ATRIOVENTRICULAR JUNCTIONAL ESCAPE BEATS. An *AV junctional escape beat* is recognized in the ECG by a pause longer than the normal P-P interval interrupted by a QRS complex with supraventricular morphologic features. If P waves are present, they have a PR interval shorter than 0.12 second and may be antegrade (upright), absent (buried in the QRS complex), fusion complexes (with the sinus P), or retrograde (inverted and within the ST segment). Fusion P waves differ from normal sinus P waves (lower amplitude, bifid, notched, nearly isoelectric).

PREMATURE ATRIOVENTRICULAR JUNCTIONAL BEATS. *Premature AV junctional beats* are distinguished from AV junctional escape beats by their occurrence within the normal P-P interval. These beats, if unimpeded, conduct in retrograde fashion to the atria and in a typical antegrade way to the ventricles. The retrograde P wave (inverted) may occur before, during (Fig. 22-17), or after the QRS complex. It may follow the QRS complex by a fairly long interval. If the AV node, His bundle, and bundle branches are no longer refractory, the retrograde P may reactivate, in turn, the ventricle producing a *reciprocal beat* (see Fig. 22-17).

VENTRICULAR ACTIVATION. The ventricles may be activated normally (normal QRS) or conduction delayed (aberrant QRS) with both premature AV junctional and reciprocal beats. Such beats when associated with aberrant ventricular conduction may be impossible to distinguish from PVBs without His bundle electrograms. When an AV junctional focus escapes from sinus dominance, *AV junctional rhythm* occurs (see Fig. 22-17). The rate is between 35 and 60 beats/min. The ECG shows a normal QRS complex, and retrograde atrial conduction may be present (inverted P waves in ST-segment), or the QRS may be independent of atrial discharge producing AV dissociation (see Fig. 22-16).

Atrioventricular Junctional Tachycardia

This rhythm is usually of gradual onset and termination and thus often is referred to as accelerated junctional rhythm. The rate, 70 to 130 beats/min, represents tachycardia for the junctional (but not SA node) pacemakers. The QRS complexes are normal.

Enhanced vagal tone may slow, and removal of vagal tone increase, the rate of AV junctional discharge. Although the atria may be activated in a retrograde fashion, more commonly they are controlled by a sinus, atrial or second AV junctional focus resulting in AV dissociation. The ventricular rhythm in AV junctional tachycardia may be regular or irregular, often in recurring fashion. Especially important is the recognition of slowing and regularization of the ventricular rhythm in a patient with atrial fibrillation as a possible early sign of digitalis intoxication.

Atrioventricular Nodal Reentrant Tachycardia

Reentrant tachycardia involving the AV node, commonly referred to as PSVT, is characterized by its sudden onset and termination, and rates between 150 and 220 beats/min with regular rhythm (Fig. 22-18). Unless a functional ventricular aberration or a preexisting ventricular conduction defect is present, the QRS complexes are normal.

The onset of PSVT is abrupt, often after a premature atrial beat that conducts with a prolonged PR interval (see Fig. 22-18). It also terminates abruptly and is sometimes followed by a brief period of asystole or bradycardia (Fig. 22-19). The R-R interval may shorten over the course of the first few beats and lengthen over the course of the last few beats of the

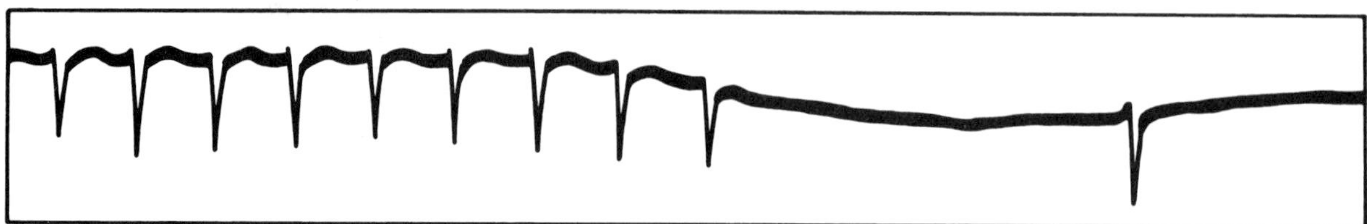

FIGURE 22-19. Termination of PSVT followed by a period of asystole lasting 1.1 sec. Asystole ends with an AV-junctional (escape) beat. (Atlee JL III: Perioperative cardiac dysrhythmias: mechanisms, recognition, management, 2nd ed. Chicago: Year Book Medical Publishers, 1985: 239.)

tachycardia. Vagal maneuvers may slow the tachycardia slightly before its termination or, if not successful in terminating the dysrhythmia, minimally slow the rate. Adenosine or verapamil administered intravenously is highly effective in terminating reentrant tachycardias involving the AV node.

Retrograde Conducting (Concealed) Pathway Reentry

The presence of an accessory pathway that conducts unidirectionally retrograde (VA conduction) but not antegrade (AV conduction), is not apparent in the surface ECG during sinus rhythm because the ventricle is not preexcited. Therefore, any ECG manifestations of ventricular preexcitation are absent, and the accessory pathway is said to be concealed.[186,187] The mechanism responsible for most tachycardias in patients with ventricular preexcitation probably involves reentry caused by antegrade conduction over the normal AV pathway and retrograde conduction over the accessory pathway; the latter, even if it only conducts in the retrograde direction, still participates in the reentrant circuit.

A tachycardia caused by this mechanism, thought to account for 30% of patients with recurrent supraventricular tachycardia referred for electrophysiologic investigation,[153] is suspected when the QRS complex is normal and a retrograde P wave occurs after the QRS complex in the ST-segment or early in the T wave. This mechanism for apparently "routine" PSVT should be understood, because therapy, which differs from that for PSVT (vagal maneuvers, edrophonium, verapamil), may require sodium channel blockers (eg, quinidine) to prolong accessory pathway refractoriness in addition to the usual treatment.

Ventricular Preexcitation

Preexcitation occurs when the atrial impulse activates, via an accessory conduction pathway, the whole or some part of the ventricles earlier than would be expected had the impulse been conducted by the normal conducting pathways. The reported incidence of preexcitation syndromes varies from 0.1 to 3.0 per thousand in apparently healthy subjects.[153]

Ventricular preexcitation syndromes include the WPW (Fig. 22-20)[188] and Lown-Ganong-Levine (LGL)[189] syndromes. Recurrent supraventricular tachydysrhythmias and ventricular preexcitation occur during normal sinus rhythm (P-R interval <0.12 second). However, with WPW, abnormal intraventricular conduction is present ("delta wave"), whereas with LGL, intraventricular conduction is normal.

The reported incidence of tachydysrhythmias in patients with ventricular preexcitation varies from 4% to 80%.[153] The most common tachycardia in these patients, *reciprocating tachycardia*, is characterized by a normal QRS, ventricular rates of from 150 to 250 beats/min (generally faster than with PSVT), and by its sudden onset and termination. Reciprocating tachycardia behaves in most respects like the tachycardia thought to be due to reentry over a retrograde (concealed) conducting pathway. Seventy to 80% of patients with ventricular preexcitation will have reciprocating tachycardia, 15% to 30% will have atrial fibrillation, and 5% atrial flutter.[151]

Premature Ventricular Beats

These beats are characterized by QRS complex having a bizarre appearance and a longer duration (>0.12 second) than QRS complexes conducted from a supraventricular focus (Fig. 22-21). Often, but not always, the T wave is large and opposite in direction to that of the major deflection of the premature QRS complex. The latter is not preceded by a premature P wave, but may be preceded by a sinus P wave occurring at its expected time. Usually, the P wave is buried in the QRS complex or, if the PVB is transmitted back to the atria, follows the QRS complex and is inverted (retrograde P wave).

If the retrograde P wave prematurely discharges the SA

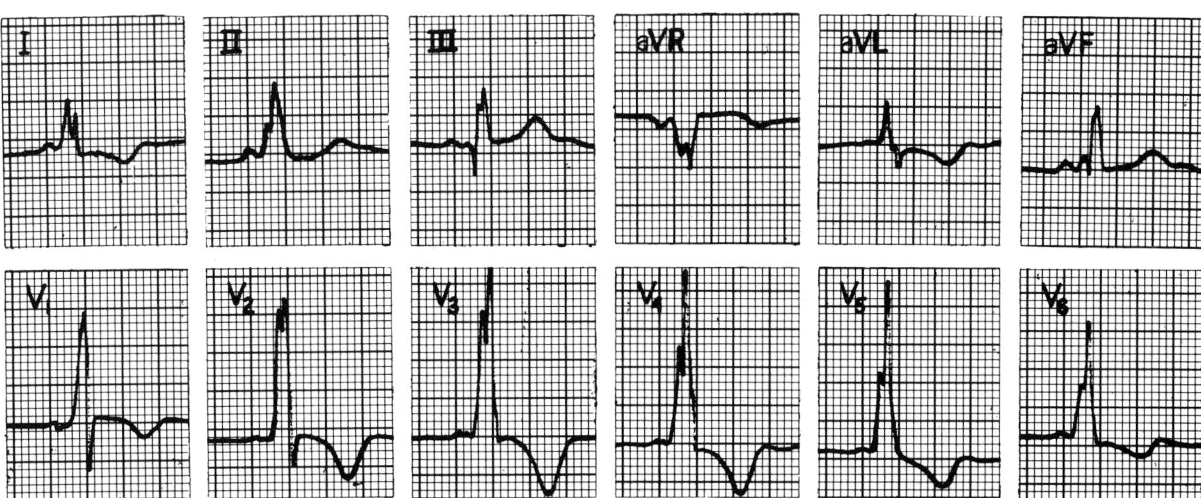

FIGURE 22-20. Wolff-Parkinson-White syndrome. The sinus (or atrial) impulse propagates to the ventricles simultaneously through both the normal AV conduction pathway and an aberrant pathway. The impulse spreads more rapidly through the aberrant pathway, reaching the ventricles earlier, causing a short PR interval and a wide QRS complex, which begins with a slurring resembling the Greek letter Δ (hence, "delta wave"). (Mangiola S, Ritota MC: Cardiac arrhythmias: practical ECG interpretation. Philadelphia: JB Lippincott, 1974.)

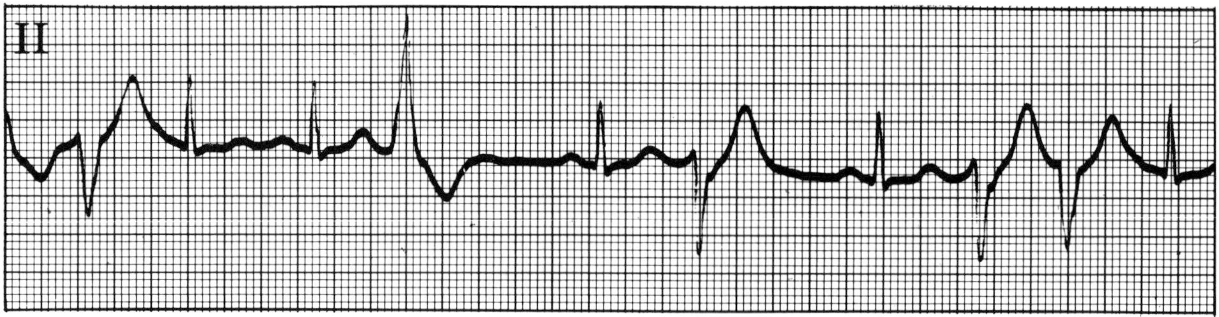

FIGURE 22-21. Sinus rhythm with frequent multifocal ventricular extrasystoles, occurring isolated ("bigeminy") or in pairs ("trigeminy"). (Mangiola S: Self-assessment in electrocardiography. Philadelphia: JB Lippincott, 1977.)

node and resets its automaticity, the pause after the PVB before the next normal beat will not be fully compensatory. More often than not, however, the pause after a PVB is fully compensatory because the retrograde and antegrade impulses collide within the AV junctional tissues. Consequently, a *fully compensatory pause* usually follows a PVB; that is, the R-R interval between normal QRS complexes on either side of the PVB is twice that of the dominant rhythm. If no compensatory pause is present, the PVB is said to be *interpolated* (R-R interval same as that of dominant rhythm). The terms bigeminy (two), trigeminy (three), quadrigeminy (four) refer to the repetitive association of PVBs with dominant beats (see Fig. 22-21). Two successive PVBs are termed a *couplet* and three, a *triplet*. Three or more PVBs in the same patient may have different morphologic characteristics, in which case they are called *multiform*.

Ventricular Tachycardia

When three or more PVBs occur in succession, ventricular tachycardia is present (Fig. 22-22). The ventricular rate is regular or slightly irregular at rates between 110 and 250 beats/min. Atrial activity may be independent of ventricular activity (AV dissociation), or the atria may be depolarized in retrograde fashion by the ventricles (ventricular–atrial association). Onset of the tachycardia may be sudden (paroxysmal) or gradual (nonparoxysmal). The morphologic appearance of the QRS may be uniform; vary in a random (multiform) or repetitive (*torsades de pointes*) fashion; alternate with each QRS complex (bidirectional ventricular tachycardia); or have a more or less stable but gradually changing contour (RBB changing to left bundle branch contour).

Ventricular tachycardia is sustained when it must be terminated because of circulatory collapse or lasts longer than 30 seconds. Finally, the ECG distinction between wide QRS tachycardias of supraventricular and ventricular origin can be extremely difficult. Certain features favor the diagnosis of one or the other of the two mechanisms (Table 22-2).

Ventricular Flutter and Fibrillation

Ventricular flutter has the ECG appearance of sine wave oscillations around the isoelectric line at a rate of 150 to 300 beats. Ventricular fibrillation is recognized by irregular undulations in the ECG baseline with no distinct QRS complexes, ST-segments or T waves (Fig. 22-23; see also Fig. 22-5). The distinction between the two is moot, because both are lethal dysrhythmias.

Heart Block

Heart block is a temporary or permanent disturbance of AV impulse conduction due to anatomic or functional impairment of conduction. It is not the same as *interference*, in which physiologic refractoriness induced by the preceding impulse affects transmission of the subsequent impulse. With *first-degree AV block*, conduction time is prolonged, but all impulses are conducted (Fig. 22-24). With *second-degree AV block*, some

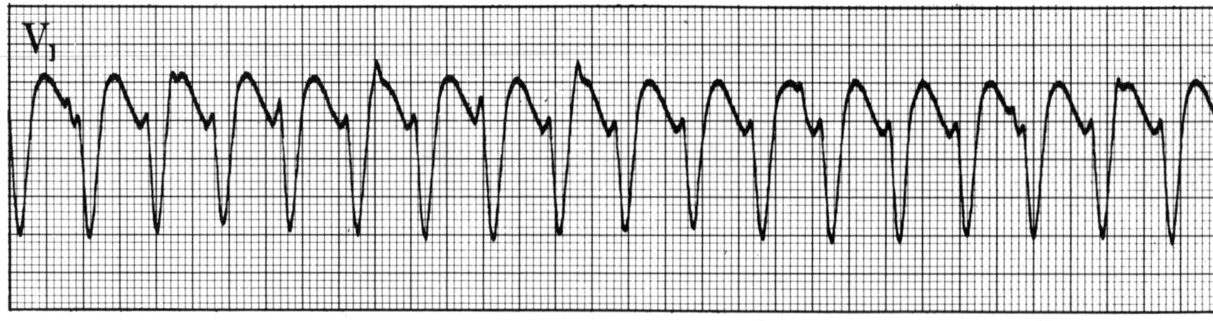

FIGURE 22-22. Ventricular tachycardia. (Mangiola S: Self-assessment in electrocardiography. Philadelphia: JB Lippincott, 1977.)

TABLE 22-2
Features of Wide QRS Tachycardias of Supraventricular and Ventricular Origin

SUPRAVENTRICULAR TACHYCARDIA
rSR′ in V_1
P and QRS linked to suggest AV activation
Onset with premature P wave
Slowing or termination by vagal maneuvers
PR interval ≤0.10 s
VENTRICULAR TACHYCARDIA
Specific QRS patterns
AV dissociation or ventricular–atrial association
Capture or fusion beats
Compensatory pause at termination of tachycardia
QRS during tachycardia similar

impulses are blocked, either with prior, progressive PR interval prolongation (Type I or Wenckebach block) (Fig. 22-25) or without PR interval prolongation (Type II or Mobitz block) (Fig. 22-26). No impulses are conducted with *third-degree or complete heart block* (Fig. 22-27).

Bundle branch and *fascicular blocks* are not dysrhythmias, but rather ECG patterns associated with conduction block in the right or left bundle branch, or fascicles (anterior or posterior) of the left bundle branch. Left anterior fascicular block frequently occurs in association with RBB block. Isolated left posterior fascicular block is much rarer than left anterior fascicular block, and even less frequently associated with RBB block. The association of either left anterior or left posterior fascicular block with RBB block is termed *bifascicular block*.

MANAGEMENT OF CARDIAC DYSRHYTHMIAS

Proper management of intraoperative dysrhythmias is based on correct diagnosis of the specific disturbance, identification and treatment of the cause, removal or correction of aggravating factors, and measures to prevent recurrences. Antidysrhythmic drugs, pacemakers, or direct-current (DC) cardioversion will be required to manage some dysrhythmias, and their efficacy will be increased by the prior institution of corrective measures. The principal causes and management of specific dysrhythmias are summarized in Table 22-3. A brief discussion of individual drugs used in dysrhythmia management, electronic pacemakers, and DC cardioversion follows.

Drugs

Mechanisms of Action

Antidysrhythmic drugs can slow the spontaneous discharge rate of a pacemaker exhibiting normal or abnormal automaticity by depressing the slope of diastolic depolarization, shifting the threshold potential toward zero, or by increasing the resting membrane potential. In general, most antidysrhythmics in the therapeutic range slow the rate of ectopic, but not SA node, pacemaker cells.

Calcium channel–blocking agents (verapamil), β-adrenergic receptor blocking agents (esmolol, propranolol), and amiodarone suppress automaticity in both ectopic and SA node pacemaker cells. Quinidine and similar drugs (procainamide, disopyramide) suppress automaticity in ectopic pacemakers, but may increase the SA node discharge rate because of their indirect (vagolytic) action.

Drug actions relating to afterdepolarizations and triggering are poorly understood. Antidysrhythmic drugs may abolish reentry or prevent its occurrence by improving or depressing conduction, increasing or decreasing refractoriness, or both. A drug that improves conduction could abolish reentry by eliminating unidirectional conduction block. Consequently, the returning impulse reenters too soon and becomes extinguished when it encounters still refractory fibers. A drug that further impairs conduction will transform an area of unidirectional block to bidirectional conduction block and thus terminate or prevent reentry.

Most antidysrhythmic drugs share the ability to prolong the effective refractory period relative to their effect on action potential duration; that is, the ratio of effective refractory period to action potential duration increases and may exceed 1.0. If a drug increases refractoriness in fibers of the reentrant pathway, they may not recover excitability in time to be depolarized by the reentrant impulse. Finally, a drug that slows conduction without producing conduction block or increasing refractoriness may promote reentrant dysrhythmias.

Adenosine

Adenosine is an endogenous nucleoside present in all body cells. Two recent reviews detail adenosine's cardiac effects.[190,191] Its mechanism of action involves activation of an inwardly rectifying potassium current ($I_{KAdo,\ Ach}$). Adenosine is about 90% to 95% effective in terminating PSVT and is currently considered to be the drug of choice for the prompt management of this dysrhythmia.[192–194] The extremely short half-life of adenosine in blood (about 10–15 sec) also makes

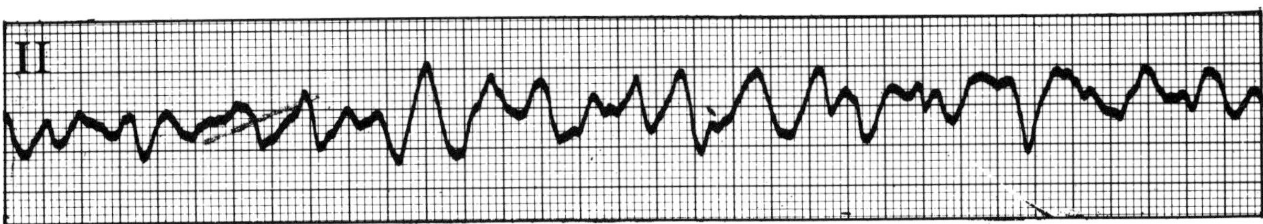

FIGURE 22-23. Ventricular fibrillation. (Mangiola S, Ritota MC: Cardiac arrhythmias: practical ECG interpretation. Philadelphia: JB Lippincott, 1974.)

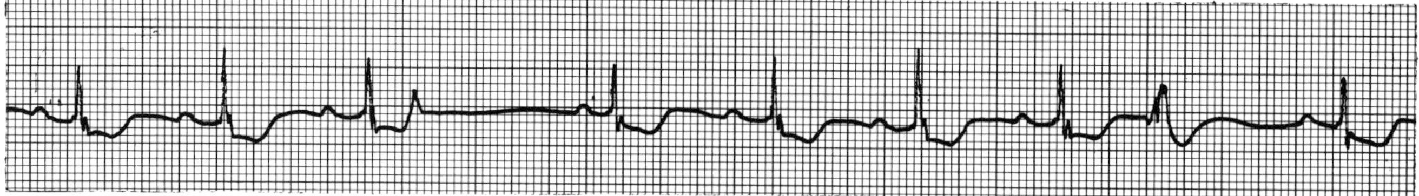

FIGURE 22-24. Sinus rhythm with first-degree AV block, one nonconducted atrial extrasystole, and one ventricular extrasystole. (Mangiola S, Ritota MC: Cardiac arrhythmias: practical ECG interpretation, 2nd ed. Philadelphia: JB Lippincott, 1982: 239.)

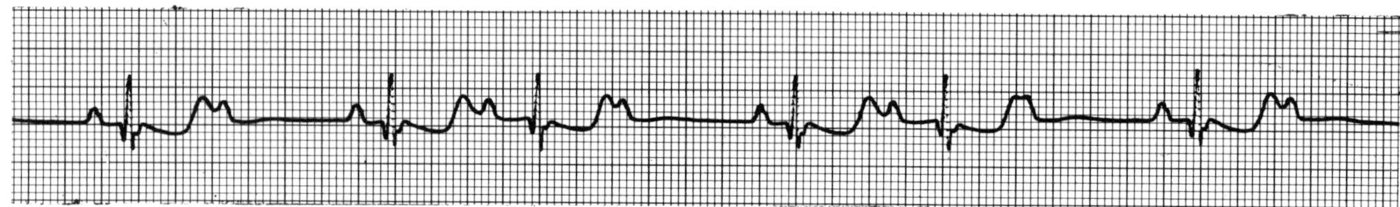

FIGURE 22-25. Sinus rhythm with second-degree AV block, type I (Wenckebach); 2:1 and 3:2 Wenckebach sequences are present. (Mangiola S, Ritota MC: Cardiac arrhythmias: practical ECG interpretation, 2nd ed. Philadelphia: JB Lippincott, 1982: 243.)

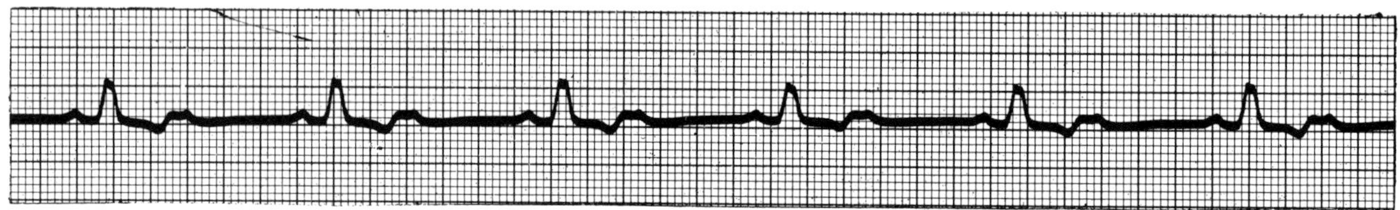

FIGURE 22-26. Sinus rhythm with 2:1 second-degree AV block and bundle branch block. (Mangiola S, Ritota MC: Cardiac arrhythmias: practical ECG interpretation, 2nd ed. Philadelphia: JB Lippincott, 1982: 243.)

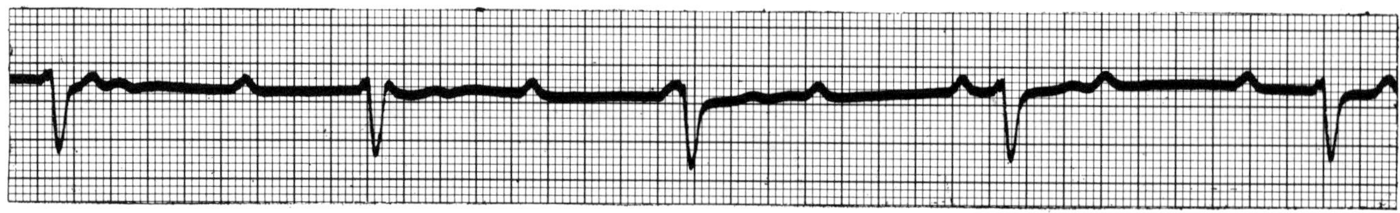

FIGURE 22-27. Sinus rhythm with third-degree (complete) AV block and idioventricular escape rhythm. (Mangiola S, Ritota MC: Cardiac arrhythmias: practical ECG interpretation, 2nd ed. Philadelphia: JB Lippincott, 1982: 244.)

TABLE 22-3
Principal Causes and Management of Dysrhythmias

DYSRHYTHMIA	CAUSE	MANAGEMENT
Sinus tachycardia	Fever, blood loss, light anesthesia, early hypoxia, hypercarbia, catecholamines	Treat cause; β blockers, narcotics, volume expansion, increase anesthesia
Sinus bradycardia	Deep anesthesia, late hypoxia, reflexes, cold, narcotics, sinus node dysfunction	Treat cause; atropine, isoproterenol, pacing
Sinus dysrhythmia	Same as those of sinus bradycardia	Same as for sinus bradycardia
Wandering atrial pacemaker	Deep anesthesia, sinus node dysfunction	Same as for sinus bradycardia
Premature atrial beats	Chronic pulmonary disease, sepsis, myocardial ischemia, central venous catheter	Treat cause; quinidine, procainamide, disopyramide if PABs provoke tachydysrhythmias; retract central catheter
Atrial flutter	Organic heart disease, atrial distension, hypertension, pulmonary embolism, metabolic conditions	Treat cause; DC cardioversion, digitalis, β blockers, verapamil, quinidine, procainamide, disopyramide
Atrial fibrillation	Same as those of atrial flutter	Same as for atrial flutter
Atrial tachycardia with or without block	Organic heart disease, cor pulmonale, digitalis toxicity, hypokalemia	Same as atrial flutter or fibrillation; phenytoin if caused by digitalis toxicity
Multifocal atrial tachycardia	Chronic pulmonary disease, diabetes, coronary artery disease	Same as atrial flutter or fibrillation
AV junctional beats and rhythm	Depressed sinus node function, enhanced automaticity in junctional pacemakers	Atropine, isoproterenol, pacing; lidocaine for premature AV junctional beats
AV junctional tachycardia	Myocarditis, inferior wall myocardial infarction, open heart surgery, digitalis toxicity	Treat cause; improve hemodynamics; consider digitalis if not already given
Sinus tachycardia	Fever, blood loss, light anesthesia, early hypoxia, hypercarbia, catecholamines	Treat cause; β blockers, narcotics, volume expansion, increased anesthesia
AV nodal reentrant tachycardia (PSVT)	Stress, anxiety, fatigue, caffeine; occasionally, organic heart disease	Sedation, reassurance, avoidance of provocative factors; vagal maneuvers, adenosine, verapamil, edrophonium, propranolol, cardioversion, digitalis, antitachycardia pacing
Reentry over a retrograde (concealed) pathway	May account for 30% of cases of "routine" PSVT; no specific causes	Quinidine, procainamide, disopyramide; otherwise, same as for PSVT
Ventricular preexcitation	Accessory conduction pathways (WPW or LGL)	Same as for reentry over a retrograde (concealed) pathway
PVBs	Multifactorial; increased incidence with advanced age	Treat cause, underlying heart disease; lidocaine and all other approved antidysrhythmics, except bretylium
VT	Digitalis toxicity, myocardial ischemia or infarction, catecholamines, quinidine, disopyramide, procainamide, long QT interval	Same as for PVBs; bretylium indicated when VT refractory to other drug management
Ventricular flutter or fibrillation	Same as those for VT	Immediate DC cardioversion; then treat as for VT
First-degree AV block	Excessive vagal tone, rapid atrial rates, deep anesthesia, narcotics, diltiazem, verapamil, β blockers	Usually none; atropine, isoproterenol
Type I AV block (Wenckebach)	Same as first-degree AV block; organic heart disease, acute inferior wall infarction	Same as for first-degree AV block; possibly temporary pacing
Type II AV block (Mobitz)	Organic heart disease, acute anterior wall infarction	Atropine and isoproterenol (temporary); pacing (definitive)
Sinus tachycardia	Fever, blood loss, light anesthesia, early hypoxia, hypercapnia, catecholamines	Treat cause; β blockers, narcotics, volume expansion, increase anesthesia
Complete AV block	Organic heart disease	Same as type II AV block .
Bundle branch and fascicular blocks	Organic heart disease	None; possibly temporary pacing when associated with first-degree or type I AV block; pacing when associated with type II AV block

PSVT, paroxysmal supraventricular tachycardia; *PVBs*, premature ventricular beats; *VT*, ventricular tachycardia.

it an extremely useful diagnostic tool (eg, in differentiation of supraventricular from ventricular dysrhythmias).

Because adenosine antagonizes the effects of catecholamines in ventricular tissue, it may also be effective in treating a small subset of ventricular tachycardias that are cAMP-dependent.[190–191] However, because it is often difficult to differentiate catecholamine-dependent episodes of ventricular tachycardia from those that are not, adenosine cannot be recommended for the routine treatment of ventricular tachycardia. Since the effects of the nucleoside are markedly enhanced in patients receiving the nucleoside uptake blocker, dipyridamole,[190] it is wise to avoid administering adenosine in these patients.

Adenosine is less effective in the presence of adenosine receptor antagonists (eg, caffeine, theophylline). In high doses, it slows conduction and interrupts reentry pathways through the AV node and restores sinus rhythm in patients with PSVT including WPW syndrome.[195] A dose of 6 to 12 mg normally is effective within 60 seconds and has minimal adverse hemodynamic effects. Although adenosine is not effective in terminating atrial fibrillation or flutter, its depressant properties on AV nodal conduction (ie, increase in AV nodal effective refractory period) will significantly reduce the ventricular rate. Adenosine is not recommended in the presence of a second or third degree heart block unless the patient has a functioning pacemaker.

Amiodarone

A benzofuran derivative, amiodarone is structurally similar to triiodothyronine and is unrelated to other antidysrhythmics. It lengthens the action potential duration and increases refractoriness in all cardiac tissues and slows conduction within the AV node and specialized conduction tissues. In addition, it depresses SA node function. Unlike other antidysrhythmic drugs (eg, d-sotalol) that prolong ventricular refractoriness by inhibiting the delayed rectifier current (I_K), amiodarone does not cause reverse use-dependence. That is, it does not preferentially prolong refractoriness at slower heart rates. Reverse use-dependence is a prodysrhythmic affect that can lead to the development of EADs and torsades de pointes.

Ideally, the effect of an antidysrhythmic drug on repolarization should be greatest at fast heart rates (use-dependent behavior). The favorable frequency-dependent actions of amiodarone on repolarization are probably attributable to its complex cardiac electrophysiologic profile. Amiodarone not only inhibits I_K but also antagonizes L-type calcium and sodium channels, as well as β-adrenergic receptors. These effects probably account for (1) the much lower incidence of drug-induced torsades de pointes with amiodarone compared to that of other Class III antidysrhythmic agents, and (2) why amiodarone can be safely used in patients with a history of Class Ia drug-induced torsades de pointes.

It is noteworthy that amiodarone produces cardiac electrophysiologic changes that resemble those produced by thyroid ablation, suggesting that its fundamental action on cardiac muscle is selective block of triiodothyroxine effects on the myocardium.[196] Amiodarone has an exceptionally long elimination half-life (>30 days) that may vary with individual patients. It is used for the treatment of supraventricular and ventricular dysrhythmias that are refractory to conventional therapy. Hii and coworkers[197] recently found that Type Ia antiarrhythmic drugs caused an increase in regional QT interval dispersion in patients who developed torsades de pointes. In contrast, chronic amiodarone therapy caused comparable maximum QT interval prolongation in patients with a history of Class Ia-induced torsades de pointes but did not increase QT interval dispersion.

Atropine

Atropine increases sinus rate and AV nodal conduction time by blocking the effects of acetylcholine on cardiac M_2–muscarinic receptors. It has little effect on automaticity, conduction time or refractoriness below the AV node. This drug is most useful for treating sinus bradycardia associated with high spinal or epidural blocks. It is also used for treating sinus bradycardia during general anesthesia. However, consider the possibility that the resulting reduction in vagal tone could unmask sympathetic hyperactivity and precipitate severe ventricular dysrhythmias.

β-Adrenergic Receptor–Blocking Drugs

Propranolol is the prototype of this class of drugs, and along with the shorter-acting β-blocking agent, esmolol, the ones most likely to be used for intraoperative dysrhythmias due to endogenous or exogenous catecholamine excess and hyperthyroid states. The mixed α_1–β_1 receptor antagonist labetalol may also be useful in the prevention and management of such dysrhythmias and is particularly useful when dysrhythmias are the result of hypertensive crises.

The antidysrhythmic effects of propranolol have been attributed to competitive β-adrenergic receptor blockade and membrane-stabilizing ("quinidine-like" or local anesthetic) properties, though the latter are not clinically important effects because they occur at levels 10 times those required to produce β receptor blockade.[198] Propranolol slows sinus rate and increases AV nodal conduction time and refractoriness, the magnitude of which effect depends on the level of underlying sympathetic tone. If heart rate is particularly dependent on sympathetic tone, or if sinus node dysfunction or impaired AV nodal conduction is present, severe bradycardia, escape rhythms or heart block may result. Propranolol is most commonly used to slow the rate of sinus tachycardia and to terminate or prevent PSVT. It may be used to reduce the ventricular rate in atrial flutter or fibrillation, but digitalis is usually preferred. Propranolol also is used for the treatment of ventricular tachydysrhythmias associated with catecholamine–excess states (cAMP–dependent), long QT syndromes (congenital or adrenergic type), and MVP syndromes.

Bretylium

Bretylium has a direct effect on the cell membrane (increased action potential duration and refractoriness in cardiac muscle and Purkinje fibers) and accumulates in sympathetic nerve terminals and ganglia where it prevents the releases of norepinephrine. In other words, bretylium causes a chemical sympathectomy. It does not antagonize, and may increase sensitivity to, the β-adrenergic receptor effects of circulating catecholamines.

A transient increase in automaticity, heart rate, contractility, and blood pressure occurs before the onset of adrenergic blockade, and is caused by the initial release of norepinephrine from the sympathetic nerve terminals. This catechol release may aggravate some dysrhythmias, particularly those caused by digitalis excess or myocardial infarction. Evidence that bretylium reduces the disparity in action potential and refractory period duration between regions of normal and ischemic or infarcted canine myocardium may account for its antifibrillatory effects in clinical myocardial infarction.

Bretylium should be used only in the treatment of life-threatening, recurrent ventricular tachydysrhythmias not responsive to conventional drugs (ie, lidocaine).[195] It sometimes is particularly effective in the treatment of ventricular fibrillation, terminating the dysrhythmia, facilitating successful DC cardioversion, and preventing recurrences.

Digitalis

Digitalis inhibits or inactivates the sodium pump (specifically, the enzyme sodium–potassium adenosine triphosphatase), with subsequent changes in intracellular sodium and potassium concentrations, and a small net increase in intracellular calcium concentration. These effects are thought to underlie the direct cardiac electrophysiologic and toxic effects of digitalis. By increasing the binding (affinity) of digoxin to the sodium–potassium ATPase pump, hypokalemia renders the patient more susceptable to the development of digitalis toxicity. In addition, hypercalcemia and a number of drugs (eg, quinidine) can potentiate the cardiac effects of digoxin.

Most of the antidysrhythmic actions of digitalis are the result of its indirect (neurally mediated) effects on the atria and AV junction.[199] Digitalis increases refractoriness and conduction time within the AV node, but not the His–Purkinje system, an effect that results from an increase in efferent vagal discharge and reflex-induced decrease in sympathetic tone. It is of potential value in the management of PSVT, atrial flutter or fibrillation, and reciprocating tachycardia in patients with ventricular preexcitation (WPW and LGL) syndromes. It is not indicated for atrial flutter or fibrillation in patients with ventricular preexcitation because it may shorten refractoriness in the accessory pathway and thereby increase the ventricular response.

Disopyramide

The electrophysiologic effects of disopyramide are similar to those of quinidine and include prolongation of the QT interval. Disopyramide exerts greater anticholinergic effects than quinidine, which apparently nullifies some of its direct depressant effects on conduction and refractoriness in the AV node.[200] Disopyramide also depresses cardiac contractability more than quinidine and procainamide. It does not appear to affect α- or β-adrenergic receptors.

The usefulness of disopyramide in treating many categories of supraventricular and ventricular dysrhythmias is not completely resolved.[195] It appears comparable to quinidine in reducing the frequency of PVBs and may prevent recurrences of ventricular tachycardia in selected patients. Its role in preventing dysrhythmias or reducing mortality in patients after acute myocardial infarction has not been established.

Edrophonium

Edrophonium sometimes terminates PSVT when carotid sinus massage has failed or is contraindicated. Because of its rapid onset and termination of action, it is preferred to neostigmine for this purpose. Anticholinesterase drugs may also be used to slow the ventricular response in atrial flutter or fibrillation.[201] Edrophonium is especially useful for this purpose when these dysrhythmias with consequent hemodynamic deteriorization appear suddenly before the institution of cardiopulmonary bypass. It should be given particularly cautiously to patients receiving digitalis, or with sinus node dysfunction and heart block, because it can produce sinus arrest and complete AV block. Because the cardiac A_1-adenosine and M_2–muscarinic cholinergic receptors are coupled to a common transduction protein ($G_{i,o}$), the same electrophysiologic effects (activation of $I_{KAdo,Ach}$) can be achieved using the ultra–short-acting nucleoside, adenosine.[190,191] Thus, the role of edrophonium in managing dysrhythmias has declined in recent years. Atropine is used to reverse the effects of edrophonium or other anticholinesterase drugs.

Flecainide

The electrophysiologic actions of flecainide are similar to those of quinidine. Consequently, it has a wide spectrum of antidysrhythmic effectiveness. Flecainide prolongs conduction in all cardiac tissues so that intra-atrial, AV nodal, His–Purkinje, and ventricular conduction times are prolonged with the potential for high degree AV block in patients with impaired conduction. It is 7 to 12 times more potent than conventional antidysrhythmics (including lidocaine) in suppressing chloroform-epinephrine ventricular dysrhythmias in mice.[202] It is used on a chronic basis to suppress PVBs and nonsustained episodes of ventricular tachycardia. Prolongation of the QT interval and ventricular tachycardia may complicate long-term therapy with flecainide.[203]* A careful risk–benefit analysis must be carried out prior to administering flecainide chronically to patients.

Isoproterenol

Isoproterenol stimulates both β_1- and β_2-adrenergic receptors and has no clinically important effects on α-adrenergic receptors. It is used to maintain adequate heart rate and cardiac output in patients with symptomatic sinus bradycardia or with advanced degrees of AV block before the insertion of a pacemaker. Isoproterenol is also useful in the management of β-adrenergic blocker poisoning and EAD-induced torsades de pointes.

* The results of the CAST study clearly demonstrated the potential prodysrhythmic effects of class Ic drugs and their adverse effects on patient morbidity and mortality.[203]

Lidocaine

Unlike quinidine and related class Ia antidysrhythmics (disopyramide, procainamide), lidocaine exerts most of its electrophysiologic effects by a direct action. It does not suppress SA node automaticity (except possibly in patients with preexisting SA node dysfunction), but does suppress both normal and abnormal automaticity in Purkinje fibers. Extracellular potassium concentration and acidosis significantly influence the electrophysiologic actions of lidocaine.[6]

Unlike the class Ia agents, which have the highest affinities for the activated state of the cardiac sodium channel, lidocaine and other class Ib drugs preferentially block the sodium channel in the inactivated state.[32,33] Thus, class Ia drugs primarily block sodium channels when they are open, whereas class Ib drugs predominantly block sodium channels when they are closed. Because the action potential duration is much shorter in atria than ventricles, the sodium channels in the atria spend much less time in the inactive state. These findings explain why lidocaine, unlike quinidine, has minimal to no effect on atrial tissue refractoriness and membrane responsiveness in normal ventricular tissue.[32,33]

Lidocaine reduces action potential duration and refractoriness in Purkinje and ventricular muscle fibers, but has no effect on these parameters in specialized atrial fibers. Its effectiveness against ventricular dysrhythmias may be related to a reduction in the temporal and spatial dispersion of refractoriness within the ventricular specialized conducting tissues and muscle. It has a narrow antidysrhythmic spectrum and is used almost exclusively for the treatment of ventricular dysrhythmias in the anesthetic setting, after myocardial infarction, or due to digitalis excess.

Phenytoin

The electrophysiologic actions of phenytoin are similar to those of lidocaine. It is particularly noted for its efficacy against dysrhythmias in patients with digitalis toxicity, including multiform PVBs, ventricular tachycardia, and atrial tachycardia with block. It is somewhat less effective against nonparoxysmal AV junctional tachycardia, and ineffective against other atrial dysrhythmias, including atrial flutter or fibrillation and PSVT. It is not particularly effective against ventricular dysrhythmias due to myocardial ischemia.[204]

Some of phenytoin's antidysrhythmic actions may be neurally mediated because it decreases efferent traffic in cardiac sympathetic nerves caused by ouabain toxicity,[204] and when injected into the central nervous system protects against digitalis-induced ventricular dysrhythmias.[206]

Procainamide

Procainamide has antidysrhythmic physiologic effects similar to those of quinidine and may also cause QT interval progression and related ventricular tachydysrhythmias. Its anticholinergic action is weaker than that of disopyramide and quinidine, but its local anesthetic potency is greater. Vasodilation with procainamide is the result of mild ganglionic blockade rather than peripheral α-adrenergic receptor blockade, as with quinidine.

The indications for procainamide and quinidine are similar, although the two drugs may not have the same effect on a particular dysrhythmia in individual patients. Procainamide is preferred to quinidine for intravenous use because it has fewer adverse hemodynamic effects. For chronic use, quinidine is preferred because of a lupus-like syndrome associated with prolonged procainamide therapy.

Tocainide

A primary amine analogue of lidocaine, tocainide is effective when given orally and has similar electrophysiologic actions.[196,207] It is not useful in the management of supraventricular tachydysrhythmias. Oral tocainide is effective initially in about 60% of patients with ventricular dysrhythmias that are refractory to quinidine, procainamide, disopyramide or propranolol, given singly or in combination.[196]

The response to lidocaine may help to predict a patient's response to tocainide for the long-term management of ventricular dysrhythmias. If lidocaine fails to suppress the dysrhythmias, tocainide has about a 60% chance of success. When tocainide is not effective alone, ventricular dysrhythmias can sometimes be controlled by combined therapy with quinidine, propranolol, or disopyramide. The use of tocainide for long-term dysrhythmia control may be limited because of adverse reactions or late treatment failures.

Quinidine

Quinidine has both direct (cell membrane) and indirect (anticholinergic) effects. It has little direct effect on sinus rate, except that it may slow the rate in patients with sinus dysfunction. However, because of its vagolytic action and reflex sympathetic stimulation resulting from peripheral vasodilation (α-adrenergic receptor blockade), an increase in sinus rate as well as enhancement of AV nodal conduction may occur.

The direct effect of quinidine is to prolong AV nodal and His–Purkinje conduction time. Quinidine suppresses normal automaticity in the His–Purkinje system, which may be a hazard in the treatment of dysrhythmias in patients with AV block. It does not affect abnormal automaticity or delayed afterpotentials in depressed Purkinje fibers, but in high doses may cause abnormal discharge in such fibers.[208]

Quinidine minimally prolongs action potential duration, but greatly increases effective refractoriness in atrial and ventricular muscle and Purkinje fibers. QT interval prolongation is minimal with therapeutic levels of quinidine, but becomes more pronounced as plasma levels are increased. Quinidine can cause ventricular tachydysrhythmias, including torsades de pointes, as a result of QT interval prolongation; these are a frequent cause of "quinidine syncope". Other potential side effects include cinchonism, gastrointestinal disturbances, and hypersensitivity reactions (eg, thrombocytopenia, fever). It is used for the treatment of supraventricular and ventricular premature beats and sustained tachydysrhythmias and is often preferred to procainamide because the dosage schedule is more convenient and therapy with procainamide is associated with drug-induced systemic lupus. Before its use in an attempt to convert atrial flutter or fibrillation (either alone or before DC cardioversion), the ventricular rate should first be slowed pharmacologically (eg, with digoxin or β-blockers).

Quinidine may be used to prevent spontaneous recurrences

of PSVT. It increases antegrade refractoriness in the normal (AV node) and accessory pathways in patients with ventricular preexcitation and therefore is useful for managing reciprocating tachycardia and atrial flutter or fibrillation in these patients (WPW, LGL syndromes). Finally, quinidine and related drugs (disopyramide, procainamide) may help to prevent the recurrence of supraventricular and ventricular tachydysrhythmias by suppressing premature beats that could initiate such dysrhythmias.

Vasopressors

In the past, methoxamine and phenylephrine, essentially pure α-adrenergic receptor agonists, have been used in the management of PSVT after failure of vagal maneuvers or edrophonium. A baroreceptor-mediated increase in vagal tone is the underlying mechanism whereby α-agonists may be effective. Currently, adenosine and verapamil are preferred and more effective. Vasopressors should not be used in patients with hypertension, hyperthyroidism, or organic heart disease. They appear useful only if PSVT is accompanied by severe hypotension.

Verapamil

At therapeutic levels, verapamil has no effect on action potential characteristics in normal fast-response fibers. In depressed fibers, it may suppress abnormal forms of automaticity as well as afterdepolarizations and triggered activity.[32] Verapamil directly decreases sinus rate, slows AV nodal conduction time, and increases antegrade AV nodal refractoriness. It does not affect atrial, His–Purkinje, or ventricular conduction time and refractoriness, nor does it affect retrograde AV nodal conduction or refractoriness, or antegrade or retrograde conduction and refractoriness in accessory conduction pathways.[209,210]

Racemic verapamil, the clinically used compound, has some local anesthetic activity, a property of its (+) stereoisomer. The (−) stereoisomer blocks the slow inward current. Because verapamil commonly causes reflex sympathetic stimulation (resulting from peripheral vasodilation), sinus rate may be minimally reduced or not at all; the depressant effect on AV nodal conduction is not eliminated.

Intravenously administered verapamil is effective in treating PSVT that does not terminate after simple vagal maneuvers. Verapamil decreases the ventricular response in patients with atrial flutter or fibrillation and may convert a small number of episodes to sinus rhythm, particularly if they are of recent onset.[210] It may accelerate the ventricular response in patients with ventricular preexcitation (WPW, LGL syndromes) and atrial flutter or fibrillation, and therefore is relatively contraindicated in these situations.[212] In patients with WPW, verapamil (particularly when administered intravenously) may accelerate ventricular rate via two mechanisms: (1) reflex sympathetic activation and (2) a reduction in the effective refractory period of the bundle of Kent. Verapamil is not usually of value in ventricular dysrhythmias, but may work in selected cases.[32,212]

NEWER CONCEPTS IN ANTIDYSRHYTHMIC DRUG CLASSIFICATION

The Vaughan Williams Classification

Twenty-five years ago, Dr. Vaughan Williams created a simple and easy to use physiologically-based classification of antidysrhythmic drugs[214,215] His original classification was subsequently modified[216] and currently groups antidysrhythmic drugs into four classes (Table 22-4)

Although this classification greatly facilitated the teaching

TABLE 22-4
Vaughan Williams Classification of Antidysrhythmic Drugs

DRUG CLASS	MECHANISM	EXAMPLES
CLASS I	Drugs with direct membrane action (ie, sodium channel blockade)	
Class Ia Depress phase 0 Slow conduction; prolong repolarization		Quinidine Porcainamide Disopyramide
Class Ib Little effect on phase 0 in normal tissues; depress phase 0 in abnormal fibers; shorten repolarization		Lidocaine Mexilitene Tocainide Phenytoin
Class Ic Markedly depress phase 0 Markedly slow conduction; slight effect on repolarization		Flecainide Encainide
CLASS II	Anti-adrenergic drugs	Propranolol Esmolol
CLASS III	Drugs that prolong repolarization	Amiodarone Bretylium Sotalol
CLASS IV	Calcium-channel blocking drugs	Diltiazem Verapamil

of antidysrhythmic drugs to students as well as the design and development of new antidysrhythmic drugs, it has several significant limitations.[32,217] Because the etiologies and dysrhythmogenic mechanisms were not integrated into this classification and the actions of antidysrhythmic drugs vary considerably in different types of dysrhythmias, the clinical efficacy of antidysrhythmic drugs could not be predicted. Other important limitations[32,216] of the Vaughan Williams classification are as follows:

1. The Vaughan Williams classification is a hybrid. Drugs in classes I and IV work by blocking channels, in class II by blocking receptors, and in class III by altering an electrophysiologic parameter (prolongation of repolarization). In addition, the Vaughan Williams classification has difficulty in placing drugs with multiple mechanisms of action. For example, amiodarone is known to have Class I, II, III, and IV activities.
2. The Vaughn Williams classification indicates antidysrhythmic effects are secondary to blockage of channels. It does not address how an antidysrhythmic drug that stimulates ionic channels could be categorized.
3. The Vaughan Williams classification is incomplete. Well-known antidysrhythmic drugs such as adenosine, digitalis, muscarinic cholinergic agonists and α-adrenergic receptor blockers are not included in this classification.
4. The Vaughan Williams classification is primarily based on the electrophysiologic effects of drugs in normal isolated cardiac tissues. It does not evaluate the efficacy of these drugs in diseased cardiac tissue or modulation of their antidysrhythmic effects by the autonomic nervous system.

The explosion of new information regarding the pathogenesis of dysrhythmias and the cellular mechanisms of antidysrhythmic agents, coupled with the shortcomings of the Vaughan Williams classification and the results of the CAST study,[217] which demonstrated the potential prodysrhythmic effects of potent sodium channel blockers, provided the impetus for a group of prominent basic and clinical scientists to meet in Sicily, Italy and propose a new antidysrhythmic drug classification entitled the Sicilian gambit[32,217] (Fig. 22-28).

The Sicilian Gambit

The Sicilian gambit, a new antidysrhythmic drug classification based on the findings of molecular biologic, basic and clinical electrophysiologic and pharmacologic studies, is the best current system of understanding and classifying antidysrhythmic drugs.[32,217] In the Sicilian gambit, an operational framework was created that emphasizes knowledge of drug action, mechanisms of dysrhythmias, autonomic influences and drug target sites. It not only focuses on the effect of antidysrhythmic drugs on receptors, ionic channels and ionic pump/carriers, but also identifies the "vulnerable parameter" which might be most accessible to drug therapy. The latter emanates from an understanding of the action of antidysrhythmogenic mechanisms in myocardial cells and the heart.

The clinical efficacy of a drug can only be predicted from information on its action at the"target level," the dysrhythmia mechanism and the weak link (or "vulnerable parameter") of the specific rhythm disorder. The vulnerable parameter is that electrophysiologic feature(s) unique to a specific dysrhythmia that may be exploited to terminate the dysrhythmia. Thus, from a clinical point of view, the following information is required: (1) the mechanism of the clinical dysrhythmias, (2) the vulnerable parameters, and (3) the ionic channel or receptor that needs to be modified in order to terminate the arrhythmias (target site). Table 22-5 lists the "vulnerable parameter(s)" associated with a variety of dysrhythmias. Likewise, a provisional listing of the major cellular mechanisms (eg, modulation of receptor, ionic channel/pump function) whereby antidysrhythmic drugs can alter the vulnerable parameter and thus terminate dysrhythmias is shown in Table 22-3.

The Sicilian gambit offers the clinician a logical and rational approach to the problem of which drug to select for the treatment of a specific dysrhythmia. It offers an opening to a new classification whereby the combined knowledge of molecular biology and basic electrophysiology is directed towards the optimal treatment of clinical arrhythmias.[32,217] The Task Force of the Working Group on Arrhythmias of the European Society of Cardiology has published an excellent detailed review of cardiac electrophysiology, the pathogenesis of dysrhythmias, and the Sicilian gambit.[32,217]

Cardiac Pacemakers

A United States national survey in 1981 indicated that the ratio of patients with pacemakers to the total population was 1:460, and that 513 new pacemaker units were implanted per million population per year.[218] With the current interest in pacemakers for the management of tachydysrhythmias[219] and ever increasing numbers of elderly patients with established indications, the number of patients with pacemakers or requiring new pacemakers continues to increase. Thus, perioperative management is of appropriate concern to anesthesiologists. The following discussion summarizes the principal complications associated with pacemakers.[6,220,221]

Pacemaker Malfunction

Five general categories occur: failure to pace, failure to sense, oversensing, pacing at an altered rate, and undesirable patient/pacemaker interactions.

FAILURE TO PACE. Failure to pace results from nondelivery of a stimulus or delivery of an ineffective stimulus. Failure to deliver a stimulus can be due to improper connection of the leads to the pulse generator; broken lead wires; electric "crosstalk" with DVI* (AV sequential) pacemakers as the result of incorrectly spaced bipolar electrodes or inadequately separated unipolar atrial and ventricular electrodes; pulse generator component failure; power source depletion; and oversensing. Delivery of an ineffective stimulus is most com-

* Inter-Society Commission for Heart Disease Pacemaker Identification Code. The first letter (A = atrium, V = ventricle, D = both chambers) designates the chamber paced, the second (A, V, or D) the chamber sensed, and the third (I = inhibited, T = triggered) the mode of response to sensed events. The letter O (none) in either the second or third positions indicates an asynchronous (atrial = AOO, ventricular = VOO, dual-chamber = DOO) pacemaker.

DRUG	CHANNELS						RECEPTORS				PUMPS	CLINICAL EFFECTS			ECG EFFECTS		
	NA										Na-K ATPase	Left ventricular function	Sinus Rate	Extracardiac	PR Interval	QRS width	JT interval
	Fast	Med.	Slow	Ca	K	I_f	α	β	M_2	P							
Lidocaine	L											→	→	M			↓
Mexiletine	L											→	→	M			↓
Tocainide	L											→	→	H			↓
Moricizine	H (I)											↓	→	L		↑	
Procainamide		H (A)			M							↓	→	H	↑	↑	↑
Disopyramide		H (A)			M				L			↓	→	M	↑↓	↑	↑
Quinidine		H (A)			M		L		L			→	↑	M	↑↓	↑	↑
Propafenone		H (A)						M				↓	↓	L	↑	↑	
Flecainide			H (A)		L							↓	→	L	↑	↑	
Encainide			H (A)									↓	→	L	↑	↑	
Bepridil	L			H	M							?	↓	L			↑
Verapamil	L			H			M					↓	↓	L	↑		
Diltiazem				M								↓	↓	L	↑		
Bretylium					H		○	○				→	↓	L			↑
Sotalol					H			H				↓	↓	L	↑		↑
Amiodarone	L			L	H		M	M				→	↓	H	↑		↑
Alinidine					M	H						?	↓	H			
Nadolol								H				↓	↓	L	↑		
Propranolol	L							H				↓	↓	L	↑		
Atropine									H			→	↑	M	↓		
Adenosine										●		?	↓	L	↑		
Digoxin									●		H	↑	↓	H	↑		↓

RELATIVE POTENCY OF BLOCK:
L = low M = moderate H = high ● = agonist ○ = agonist/antagonist
A = activated state blocker I = inactivated state blocker

FIGURE 22-28. Cellular Basis of Action of Antidysrhythmic Drugs Based on the Sicilian Gambit Classification. Shown is a brief summary of the most important effects of antidysrhythmic drugs on cardiac membrane channels, receptors and ion pumps as well as on the surface ECG, sinus rate and left ventricular function. Most of the drugs listed are currently in use in the United States; others are not yet approved. For the section on channels, receptors and pumps, the actions of drugs on the sodium (Na), calcium (Ca), potassium (K) and the pacemaker (i_f) channels are indicated. Sodium channel blockade is subdivided into three groups according to the time it takes for the sodium channel to recover from the block: 1) fast time constants (τ < 300 msec), 2) medium time constants (τ = 300–1500 msec) and 3) slow time constants (τ > 1500 msec). This parameter is measure of use dependence of the sodium channel and predicts the likelihood that a drug will decrease conduction velocity of normal sodium-dependent tissues in the heart and perhaps the propensity of a drug for causing bundle-branch block or prodysrhythmia. Drugs having larger τ values are more likely to cause these side effects. The rate constant for onset of block might be even more clinically relevant. Blockade in the inactivated (I) or activated (A) state is indicated. Drug interaction with α-, β-, muscarinic cholinergic subtype (M_2) and purinergic (P, e.g., A_1-adenosine) receptors and drug effects on the Na-K-ATPase pump are given. The absence of a symbol indicates lack of effect. The use of a question mark indicates uncertainty concerning effect. The arrows in the clinical effect and ECG section indicate direction; no quantitative differentiation has been made between weak and strong effects. The effects listed for ECG, left ventricular function, sinus rate and "extracardiac" are those that may be seen at therapeutic plasma levels. Deleterious effects that may appear with concentrations above the therapeutic range are not listed. Adapted and modified with permission from References 32 and 217.

TABLE 22-5
Classifications of Drug Actions Based on Modification of Vulnerable Parameters*

DYSRHYTHMIA	MECHANISM	VULNERABLE PARAMETER	IONIC CURRENT MOST LIKELY TO MODULATE VULNERABLE PARAMETER	REPRESENTATIVE DRUGS
	Automaticity			
Inappropriate sinus tachycardia	A. Enhanced normal automaticity	Phase-4 Depolarization (decrease)	I_f; $I_{Ca\text{-}T}$ (block) $I_{K(ACh,Ado)}$ (activate)	β-adrenergic blockers, M_2 agonists; A_1-adenosine agonists (e.g., adenosine)
Some idiopathic ventricular tachycardias				Sodium channel-blocking agents
Ectopic atrial tachycardias	B. Abnormal automaticity	Maximum diastolic potential (hyperpolarization) or	$I_{K(ACh,Ado)}$ (activate)	M_2 and A_1-adenosine agonists
		Phase 4 depolarization (decrease)	$I_{Ca\text{-}L}$; I_{Na} (block)	Calcium or sodium channel-blocking agents; M_2 and A_1-adenosine agonists
Accelerated idioventricular rhythms		Phase 4 depolarization (decrease)		Calcium or sodium channel-blocking agents
	Triggered Activity based on:			
Torsades de pointes	A. Early afterdepolarizations (EAD)	Action potential duration (shorten), or	I_K (activate)	β-adrenergic agonists, vagolytic drugs (increase rate)
		Early afterdepolarization (suppress)	$I_{Ca\text{-}L}$; I_{Na} (block)	Calcium channel blockers, Mg^{2+}, β-adrenergic blockers
Digitalis-induced dysrhythmias	B. Delayed afterdepolarizations (DAD)	Calcium overload (unload) or DAD (suppress)	$I_{Ca\text{-}L}$; (block) $I_{Ca\text{-}L}$; I_{Na} (block)	Calcium channel blockers Sodium channel blockers
Certain autonomically mediated ventricular tachycardias		Calcium overload (unload) or DAD (suppress)	$I_{Ca\text{-}L}$; (block) $I_{Ca\text{-}L}$; I_{Na} (block)	β-adrenergic blockers Calcium channel blockers Adenosine
	Reentry (Sodium channel dependent)			
Atrial flutter type I	A. Primary impaired conduction (Long excitable gap)	Conduction and excitability (depress)	I_{Na} (block)	Atrium: sodium channel blockers (except lidocaine,mexiletene and tocainide)
Circus movement tachycardia in Wolff-Parkinson-White syndrome		Conduction and excitability (depress)	I_{Na} (block)	Sodium channel blockers (except lidocaine, mexiletine and tocainide)
Sustained monomorphic ventricular tachycardia		Conduction and excitability (depress)	I_{Na} (block)	Ventricle: sodium channel blockers
Atrial flutter type II	B. Conduction encroaching on refractoriness (Short excitable gap)	Refractory period (prolong)	I_K (block)	Potassium channel blockers
Atrial fibrillation		Refractory period (prolong)	I_K (block) I_{Na} (block) (delay reactivation)	Potassium channel blockers Sodium channel blockers
Circus movement tachycardia in Wolff-Parkinson-White syndrome		Refractory period (prolong)	I_K (block)	Potassium channel blockers
Polymorphic and sustained monomorphic ventricular tachycardia		Refractory period (prolong)	I_{Na} (block)	Sodium channel blockers
Bundle branch reentry		Refractory period (prolong)	I_{Na} (block)	Sodium channel blockers
Ventricular fibrillation		Refractory period (prolong)	I_K (block)	Potassium channel blockers
	Reentry (calcium channel dependent)			
AV nodal reentrant tachycardia		Conduction and excitability (depress)	$I_{Ca\text{-}L}$ (block)	Calcium channel blockers
Circus movement tachycardia in Wolff-Parkinson-White syndrome		Conduction and excitability (depress)	$I_{Ca\text{-}L}$ (block)	Calcium channel blockers
Verapamil-sensitive ventricular tachycardia		Conduction and excitability (depress)	$I_{Ca\text{-}L}$ (block)	Calcium channel blockers

Adapted and modified with permission from Task Force of the Working Group on Arrhythmias of the European Society of Cardiology. The Sicilian gambit: a new approach to the classification of antiarrhythmic drugs based on their actions of arrhythmogenic mechanisms. Circulation 84:1831, 1991 monly due to lead dislodgment. It may also result from lead insulation failure, lead wire fracture, increased stimulation threshold as the result of drugs, electrolyte imbalance, fibrosis at the electrode site, myocardial infarction or ischemia, and improper programming of the stimulus strength.

FAILURE TO SENSE. This problem is most commonly caused by lead dislodgment. It may also be due to improper lead placement, fibrosis at the electrode site, drug effects, electrolyte imbalance, improper programming of the amplifier sensitivity, insulation defect or lead fracture, connection defect, and component failure. Sensing failure can be misdiagnosed when spontaneous activity occurs simultaneously with delivery of the pacemaker stimulus, resulting in fusion beats. A cause for apparent sensing failure is reversion to asynchronous operation in the presence of electromagnetic interference (EMI). This is a normal mode of operation for many current pacemaker models.

OVERSENSING. When a pacemaker senses signals other than the cardiac signals it is supposed to detect, it is oversensing. Ventricular sensing pacemakers may sense T waves if the pacemaker amplifier is too sensitive or if its programmed refractory period is too short. T-wave sensing may also occur in patients with large (hyperkalemia) or delayed (hypocalcemia) T waves. Atrial sensing pacemakers may sense ventricular activity if the atrial refractory period is too short of if the signals are too small to be sensed. In either case, the pacemaker will not initiate appropriate atrial refractory periods.

The ventricular amplifier in some DVI pacemakers may sense delivery of the atrial stimulus and inhibit the ventricular stimulus (crosstalk) if the pacemaker unit is used with incorrectly spaced bipolar electrodes, or if the atrial or ventricular electrodes are not separated by a suitable distance. Unipolar pacemakers may sense pectoral muscle potentials resulting in inappropriate inhibition. Myopotential inhibition can also occur with succinylcholine-induced fasciculations in patients with unipolar pacemakers.

Except for asynchronous types, all pacemakers sense voltage changes when a lead with a hairline fracture or loose connection makes intermittent contact ("make–break" signals) or when two endocardial leads come into contact, a problem similar to that produced by EMI. Although make–break signals or EMI detection may result in inhibition or triggering of pacemaker stimuli, more commonly it causes the pacemaker to revert to the asynchronous mode. With suspected cases of oversensing, converting the pacemaker to the asynchronous mode (by reprogramming or external magnet) will abolish the symptoms caused by malfunction and confirm the diagnosis.

PACING AT AN ALTERED RATE. Oversensing, rate drift as the result of aging or temperature changes, rate reduction (a feature incorporated into most pacing devices to indicate approaching power source depletion), and component failure lead to altered rate pacing. Causes of misdiagnosis of pacing at an altered rate include the presence of rate hysteresis (a long pacemaker escape interval after sensed beats to maximize the benefit of spontaneous rhythm); reprogramming of a pacemaker without proper documentation; tracking of spontaneous heart rate increases with atrial and ventricular demand (AAT, VVT); atrial synchronous (VAT, DDD), and AV universal (DDD) pacemakers; and misinterpretation of nonpacemaker artifacts in the ECG.

UNDESIRABLE INTERACTIONS BETWEEN PATIENT AND PACEMAKER. Occasionally, problems arise from hematoma or infection at the pacemaker pocket; erosion of the pulse generator through the implant site; "twiddlers" syndrome, in which patients rotate their pulse generators in their pockets leading to lead retraction, fracture or disconnections with total system failure; and diaphragmatic or pectoral muscle stimulation.

Selection of the wrong pacing mode for a given patient or changes in the patient's status after implantation can have serious consequences. Examples include patients with atrial demand pacemakers in whom AV conduction block develops or patients with atrial tracking pacemakers that detect retrograde P waves with a long RP interval after ventricular stimulation and consequently fire into the vulnerable period of the ventricle.

Electromagnetic Interference

This problem is more prone to occur with unipolar than bipolar pacemakers, because the large interelectrode distance encourages sending of extrinsic EMI and permits sensing of intrinsic EMI at the anode. If the device is not properly shielded, EMI may also enter the pulse generator directly. In addition to proper shielding, corrective measures include electronic filtration of extraneous signals and the provision of an interference mode. The latter feature permits the pacemaker to revert to a fixed rate (asynchronous mode) and preserves pacing despite strong, continuous EMI signals.

Symptomatic pacemaker inhibition by skeletal muscle potentials (myotonic inhibition) is an important problem in as many as 20% of patients with unipolar pacemakers. Weapons detection systems and microwave ovens once posed a problem for patients with pacemakers, but improvements in design and other technologic advances have largely overcome these problems. Although EMI from radios, televisions, and radio transmitters occurs, it is not an important clinical problem.

Electrocautery Units

Pacemaker output may be inhibited if the electrocautery unit is used within a few inches of the pulse generator. In addition, direct or indirect contact between the electrocautery probe and pulse generator may produce local heating and destruction of the pacemaker circuitry. Hence, the grounding plate should be located as far as possible from the pulse generator and the current path: cautery to grounding pad should not traverse the pacemaker or its lead(s). When ventricular demand pacemakers (VVI) were not programmable, an acceptable solution for electrocautery inhibition was the use of an external magnet to convert the pacemaker to the asynchronous (VOO) mode. With programmable pacemakers, a different procedure should be followed. For simple programmable units, a magnet should not be used because "phantom reprogramming" may occur.[†]

The patient's pulse should be monitored closely via the pulse oximeter's pulse plethysmograph display or by manual means, and electrocautery used only in short bursts (a few beats missed by the pulse generator will not be detrimental). For multiprogrammable units, the pacemaker should be programmed before surgery to either the VVT or VOO modes, preferably the latter, if the patient is not at risk for competing rhythms.

The risk of initiating dangerous dysrhythmias during competitive pacing will be increased by acid–base, electrolyte, or other physiologic aberrations. Universally applicable recommendation cannot be made concerning the placement of an external magnet over the pulse generator, because no consistent, industry-wide response of a pacemaker to a magnet has been developed.[6]

Direct-Current Defibrillation

Although pulse generators are relatively resistant to external DC defibrillation, they can be reprogrammed or destroyed during defibrillation. Consequently, the defibrillator paddles should be placed as far as possible from the pulse generator and the general line of the pacemaker leads. Electroconvulsive therapy presents no hazard with implanted pacemakers because the stimulating electrodes are remote from the pacemaker.

Ionizing Radiation

Although in the past ionizing radiation from diagnostic or therapeutic equipment had no effect on implanted pulse generators, this situation has changed with incorporation of computer memory operating system (CMOS) digital chips in pacemaker circuits. These circuits are extremely sensitive to ionizing radiation and may be destroyed by conventional levels of therapeutic radiation. Moreover, the radiation effect is cumulative over the life of the pacemaker. No evidence shows that routine diagnostic radiography produces radiation levels sufficient to destroy a pulse generator. However, therapeutic radiation may cause unpredictable results ranging from erratic behavior to sudden cessation of function or runaway rates. A patient who is to undergo radiation therapy should have the pulse generator carefully shielded from the radiation beam, or if this approach is not possible, repositioned before therapy.

Direct-current Cardioversion

DC cardioversion offers several advantages over drug therapy in the management of supraventricular and ventricular tachydysrhythmias. Under conditions that are usually optimal for close supervision and management, a precisely regulated amount of current can be used to restore sinus rhythm immediately and safely. In addition,, the distinction between supraventricular and ventricular tachydysrhythmias, critical for effective drug management, is less important. Finally, the time-consuming titration of drugs that may not be effective and could have adverse side effects, is not required.

TABLE 22-6
Methods for Direct-current Cardioversion

1. Blood gas, electrolyte, and metabolic imbalance should be corrected before cadioversion is attempted.
2. Digitalis need not be withheld if serum levels are not increased and hypokalemia or evidence of clinical toxicity is absent.
3. Drug therapy and other therapeutic measures directed toward recurrences increase the likelihood of successful cardioversion.
4. Paddles of adequate diameter (12 to 13 cm for adults) should be used and placed in firm contact with the chest wall (with sufficient electrode paste or gel).
5. A synchronized shock should be used for all cardioversions except those for ventricular flutter or fibrillation.
6. Shock energy should be increased to effect, with use of only the lowest effective energy levels (50–200 J).
7. Light levels of anesthesia (thiopental, methohexital, or midazolam) with assisted ventilation and supplemental oxygen should be used for most elective cardioversions.

Indications

DC cardioversion is most effective in terminating dysrhythmias presumed to be due to reentry or excitation (eg, atrial flutter or fibrillation, AV nodal reentrant tachycardia, reciprocating tachycardia in patients with ventricular preexcitation, most forms of ventricular tachycardia and flutter or fibrillation). The DC shock, by depolarizing all excitable tissue and discharging automatic foci, establishes electric homogeneity and thus temporarily interrupts the circuit(s) involved in reentry. However, the tachycardia may be reinitiated by factors that provoked it in the first place. Correction of these and institution of other therapeutic measures (including drugs; see Table 22-5) may help to prevent such recurrences.

Contraindications

DC cardioversion is not indicated for terminating tachydysrhythmias thought to be due to disordered automaticity, including parasystole, some forms of atrial tachycardia with or without block (particularly if digitalis is suspected as the cause), nonparoxysmal AV junctional tachycardia, and accelerated idioventricular rhythm. The reasons are several: the ventricular rate generally is not very fast; the patient usually is hemodynamically stable; the dysrhythmia may terminate spontaneously or with drug therapy; if digitalis is the cause, DC cardioversion could initiate life-threatening ventricular tachydysrhythmias; and if the dysrhythmia is due to enhanced automaticity, electric shock might only reset the pacemaker cycle with tachycardia resuming after attempted cardioversion.

[†] Phantom (random) reprogramming: The magnet activates a radiofrequency (RF) programming sequence; that is, programming is by RF commands, but a magnet is required to make the pacemaker receptive to programming commands. More complete discussion can be found elsewhere.[6]

Technique

Consideration of the methods and indications for DC cardioversion is provided in more detail elsewhere, as is information pertaining to the automatic implantable cardioverter–defibrillator and the perioperative treatment of patients with or undergoing implantation of one of these devices.[6,196,221–223] However, several points relating to methods for DC cardioversion are included in Table 22-6, because anesthesiologists must on occasion use this technique in the management of dysrhythmias.

REFERENCES

1. Snow J: On chloroform and other anaesthetics. London: John Churchill, 1858
2. Fisch C: Electrocardiography and vectorcardiography. In Braunwald E (ed): Heart disease: a textbook of cardiovascular disease, 2nd ed. Philadelphia: WB Saunders, 1984: 195
3. Castellanos A, Myerburg RF: The resting electrocardiogram. In Hurst JW, Logue RB, Rackley CE (eds): The heart, 6th ed. New York: McGraw-Hill, 1986: 206
4. Goldman MJ: Principles of clinical electrocardiography, 11th ed. Los Altos, CA: Lange Medical Publications, 1982
5. Marriott HJL: Practical electrocardiography, 7th ed. Baltimore: Williams & Wilkins, 1983
6. Atlee JL: Perioperative cardiac dysrhythmias: mechanisms, recognition, management, 2nd ed. Chicago: Year Book Medical Publishers, 1989
7. Weidmann S: The effect of the cardiac membrane potential and the rapid availability of the sodium-carrying system. J Physiol 127:213, 1955
8. Zipes DP: Genesis of cardiac arrhythmias: electrophysiological considerations. In Braunwald E (ed): Heart disease: a textbook of cardiovascular medicine, 2nd ed. Philadelphia: WB Saunders, 1988: 605
9. Cora E, Deroubaix E, Coulombe A: Effect of tetrodotoxin on action potentials of the conducting system in the dog. Am J Physiol 236:H561, 1979
10. Vassalle M: Electrogenic suppression of automaticity in sheep and dog Purkinje fibers. Circ Res 27:361, 1970
11. Carmeleit E, Saikawa T: Shortening of the action potential and reduction of pacemaker activity by lidocaine, quinidine, and procainamide in sheep cardiac Purkinje fibers. Circ Res 50:257, 1982
12. Brown HF, Noble SJ: Effects of adrenaline on membrane currents underlying pacemaker activity in frog atrial muscle. J Physiol 238:51P, 1974
13. Noma A, Irisawa H: Electrogenic sodium pump in rabbit sinoatrial node cell. Pflugers Arch 351:177, 1974
14. Fozzard HA: Cardiac muscle: excitability and passive electrical properties. Prog Cardiovasc Dis 19:343, 1977
15. Wit AL, Rosen MR, Hoffman BF: Electrophysiology and pharmacology of cardiac arrhythmias: II. relationship of normal and abnormal electrical activity of cardiac fibers to the genesis of arrhythmias—b. reentry: II. Am Heart J 88:798, 1974
16. Gilmour RF Jr, Zipes DP: Different electrophysiological responses of canine endocardium and epicardium to combined hyperkalemia, hypoxia and acidosis. Circ Res 46:814, 1980
17. Cranefield PF: The conduction of the cardiac impulse. Mt. Kisco, NY: Futura Publishing, 1975
18. Hoffman BF, Rosen MR: Cellular mechanisms for cardiac arrhythmias. Circ Res 49:1, 1981
19. Randall WC: Sympathetic control of the heart. In Randall WC (ed): Neural regulation of the heart. New York: Oxford University Press, 1977
20. Imanishi S, Surawicz B: Automatic activity in depolarized guinea pig ventricular myocardium: characteristics and mechanisms. Circ Res 39:751, 1976
21. Katzung BG, Morgenstern JA: Effects of extracellular potassium on ventricular automaticity and evidence for a pacemaker current in mammalian ventricular myocardium. Circ Res 40:105, 1977
22. Surawicz B: Depolarization-induced automaticity in atrial and ventricular myocardial fibers. In Zipes DP, Bailey JC, Elharrar V, et al (eds): The slow inward current and cardiac arrhythmias. The Hague: Martinus Nijhoff, 1980: 375
23. Dangman KH, Hoffman BF: Studies on overdrive stimulation of canine Purkinje fibers: maximum diastolic potential as a determinant of the response. J Am Coll Cardiol 2:1183, 1983
24. Ferrier GR, Rosenthal JE: Automaticity and entrance block induced by focal depolarization of mammalian ventricular tissues. Circ Res 47:238, 1980
25. Singer DH, Baumgarten CM, Ten Eick RE: Cellular electrophysiology of ventricular and other dysrhythmias: studies on diseased and ischemic heart. Prog Cardiovasc Dis 24:97, 1981
26. Rosen MR, Hordof AJ: The slow response in human atrium. In Zipes DP, Bailey JC, Elharrar V, et al (eds): The slow inward current and cardiac dysrhythmias. The Hague: Martinus Nijhoff, 1980: 295
27. Ten Eick RE, Singer DH: Electrophysiological properties of diseased human atrium: I. low diastolic potential and altered cellular response to potassium. Circ Res 44:545, 1979
28. Spear JF, Horowitz LN, Moore EN: The slow response in human ventricle. In Zipes DP, Bailey JC, Elharrar V, et al (eds): The slow inward current and cardiac dysrhythmias. The Hague: Martinus Nijhoff, 1980: 309
29. Elharrar V, Zipes DP: Voltage modulation of automaticity in atrial and ventricular fibers. In Zipes DP, Bailey JC, Elharrar V, et al (eds): The slow inward current and cardiac dysrhythmias. The Hague: Martinus Nijhoff, 1980: 357
30. Gilmour RF Jr, Zipes DP: Electrophysiological characteristics of rodent myocardium damaged by adrenaline. Cardiovasc Res 14:582, 1980
31. Cranefield PF, Aronson RS: In Cardiac Arrhythmias: The Role of Triggered Activity and Other Mechanisms. Mt Kisco, NY: Futura, 1988
32. Task Force of the Working Group on Arrhythmias of the European Society of Cardiology: The Sicilian gambit: A new approach to the classification of antiarrhythmic drugs based on their actions on arrhythmogenic mechanisms. Circulation 84: 1831, 1991
33. Zipes DP: Cardiac electrophysiology: promises and contributions. JACC 6:1329, 1989
34. Monohan BP, Ferguson CL, Killeavy ES, Lloyd BK, Troy J, Cantilena LR: Torsades de pointes occurring in association with terfenadine use. JAMA 264:2788, 1990
35. Salata JJ, Jurkiewicz NK, Wallace AA, Stupienski III RF, Guinosso PJ, Lynch JR JJ: Cardiac electrophysiological actions of the histamine H_1-receptor antagonists astemizole and terfenadine compared with chlorpheniramine and pyrilamine. Circ Res 76:110, 1995
36. Eisenhauer MD, Eliasson AH, Taylor AJ, Coyne PE Jr, Wortham DC: Incidence of cardiac arrhythmias during intravenous pentamidine therapy in HIV-infected patients. Chest 105:389, 1994
37. Kass RS, Tsien RW, Weingart R: Ionic basis of transient inward current induced by strophanthidin in cardiac Purkinje fibers. J Physiol (Lond) 281:209, 1978
38. Kass RS, Lederer WJ, Tsien RW, Weingart R: Role of calcium ions in transient inward currents and aftercontractions induced by strophantidin in cardiac Purkinje fibers. J Physiol 281:187, 1987
39. Eisner DA, Lederer WJ: Na-Ca exchange: Stoichiometry and electrogenicity. Am J Physiol 248:C189, 1985
40. Ferrier GR: Digitalis arrhythmias: role of oscillatory afterpotentials. Prog Cardiovasc Dis 19:459, 1977
41. Vasalle M, Cummins M, Castro C, et al: The relationship between overdrive suppression and overdrive excitation in ventricular pacemaker in dogs. Circ Res 38:367, 1976
42. Mendez C, Delmar M: Triggered activity: Its possible role in cardiac arrhythmias. In Zipes DP, Jalife J (eds): Cardiac elec-

trophysiology and arrhythmias. Orlando, FL: Grune and Stratton, 1985
43. Wit AL, Cranefield PF: Reentrant excitation as a cause of cardiac arrhythmias. Am J Physiol 235:H1, 1978
44. Mines GR: On circulatory excitations in heart muscle and their possible relation to tachycardia and fibrillations. Trans R Soc Can Surg 8:43, 1914
45. Scherf D: Studies on auricular tachycardia caused by aconitine administration. Proc Soc Exp Biol Med 64:233, 1947
46. Schmitt FO, Erlanger J: Directional differences in the conduction of the impulse through heart muscle and their possible relation to extrasystolic and fibrillary contractions. Am J Physiol 87:326, 1929
47. Antzelevitch C, Moe GK: Electronically-mediated delayed conduction and reentry in relation to 'slow responses' in mammalian ventricular conduction tissue. Circ Res 49:1129, 1981
48. Allessie MA, Bonke FIM, Schopman F: Circus movement in rabbit atrial muscle as a mechanism of tachycardia: the 'leading circle' concept—a new model of circus movement in cardiac tissue without the involvement of an anatomical obstacle. Circ Res 41:9, 1977
49. Bosnjak ZJ, Kampine JP: Effects of halothane, enflurane and isoflurane on the SA node. Anesthesiology 58:314, 1983
50. Atlee JL, Brownlee SW, Burstrom RE: Conscious state comparisons of the effects of inhalation anesthetics and autonomic blockers on specialized atrioventricular conduction in dogs. Anesthesiology 64:703, 1986
51. Reynolds AK, Chiz JF, Pasquet AF: Halothane and methoxyflurane: a comparison of their effects on cardiac pacemaker fibers. Anesthesiology 33:602, 1970
52. Pruett JK, Mote PS, Grover TE, et al: Enflurane and halothane effects on cardiac Purkinje fibers (abstract). Anesthesiology 55:A65, 1981
53. Pruett JK, Grover TE: The influence of isoflurane on canine cardiac Purkinje fiber action potentials. Fed Proc 43:1022, 1984
54. Atlee JL, Rusy BF: Halothane depression of AV conduction studied by electrograms of the bundle of His in dogs. Anesthesiology 36:112, 1972
55. Atlee JL, Alexander SC: Halothane effects on conductivity of the AV node and His-Purkinje system in the dog. Anesth Analg 56:378, 1977
56. Atlee JL, Rusy BF: Atrioventricular conduction times and atrioventricular nodal conductivity during enflurane anesthesia in dogs. Anesthesiology 47:498, 1977
57. Atlee JL, Rusy BF, Kreul JF, et al: Supraventricular excitability in dogs during anesthesia with halothane and enflurane. Anesthesiology 49:407, 1978
58. Turner LA, Zuperku EJ, Purtock RV, et al: *In vivo* changes in canine ventricular cardia conduction during halothane anesthesia. Anesth Analg 59:327, 1980
59. Hauswirth O: Effects of halothane on single atrial, ventricular and Purkinje fibers. Circ Res 24:745, 1969
60. Johnston RR, Eger EI II, Wilson C: A comparative interaction of epinephrine with enflurane, isoflurane and halothane in man. Anesth Analg 55:709, 1976
61. Gomez-Arnau J, Marquez-Montes J, Auello F: Fentanyl and droperidol effects on refractoriness of the accessory pathway in the Wolff-Parkinson-White syndrome. Anesthesiology 58: 307, 1983
62. Hauswirth O: Effects of droperidol on sheep Purkinje fibers. Naunyn Schmiedebergs Arch Pharmacol 261:133, 1968
63. Bertolo L, Novakovic L, Penna M: Antiarrhythmic effects of droperidol. Anesthesiology 37:529, 1972
64. Ivankovich AD, El-Etr AA, Janeczko GF: The effects of ketamine and Innovar anesthesia on digitalis tolerance in dogs. Anesth Analg 54:106, 1975
65. Katz RL, Epstein RA: The interaction of anesthetic agents and adrenergic drugs to produce cardiac arrhythmias. Anesthesiology 29:763, 1968
66. Katz RL, Katz GJ: surgical infiltration of pressor drugs and their interactions with volatile anesthetics. Br J Anaesth 38: 712, 1966
67. Gillis RA, Raines A, Sohn Y, et al: Neuroexcitatory effects of digitalis and their role in the development of cardiac arrhythmias. J Pharmacol Exp Ther 183:154, 1972
68. Somberg JC, Smith TW: Localization of the neurally mediated arrhythmogenic properties of digitalis. Science 204:321, 1979
69. Atlee JL, Malkinson CE: Potentiation by thiopental of halothane-epinephrine-induced arrhythmias in dogs. Anesthesiology 51:285, 1982
70. Bednarski RM, Majors LJ, Atlee JL III: Epinephrine-induced ventricular arrhythmias in dogs anesthetized with halothane: potentiation by thiamylal and thiopental. Am J Vet Res 46: 1829, 1985
71. Atlee JL, Roberts FL: Thiopental and epinephrine-induced dysrhythmias in dogs anesthetized with enflurane or isoflurane. Anesth Analg
72. Bednarski RM, Muir WW: Arrhythmogenicity of dopamine, dobutamine, and epinephrine in thiamylal-halothane anesthetized dogs. Am J Vet Res 44:2341, 1983
73. Koehntop DE, Liao JC, Van Bergen FH: Effects of pharmacologic alterations of adrenergic mechanisms by cocaine, tropolone, aminophylline, and ketamine on epinephrine-induced arrhythmias during halothane–nitrous oxide anesthesia. Anesthesiology 46:83, 1977
74. Savarese JJ, Miller RD, Lien CA, et al: Pharmacology of muscle relaxants and their antagonists. In Miller RD (ed): Anesthesia, 4th ed. New York: Churchill Livingstone, 1994: 417
75. Liu WS, Wong KC, Port JD, et al: Epinephrine-induced arrhythmias during halothane anesthesia with the addition of nitrous oxide, nitrogen or helium in dogs. Anesth Analg 61: 414, 1982
76. Roizen MF, Plummer GO, Lichtor JL: Nitrous oxide and dysrhythmias. Anesthesiology 66:427, 1987
77. Zink J, Sasyniuk BI, Dresel PE: Halothane–epinephrine–induced cardiac arrhythmias and the role of heart rate. Anesthesiology 43:548, 1975
78. Horrigan RW, Eger EI, Wilson C: Epinephrine-induced arrhythmias during enflurane anesthesia in man: a nonlinear dose-response relationship and dose-dependent protection from lidocaine. Anesth Analg 57:547, 1978
79. Chapin JC, Kushins LG, Munson ES, et al: Lidocaine, bupivacaine, etidocaine, and epinephrine-induced arrhythmias during halothane anesthesia in dogs. Anesthesiology 52:23, 1980
80. Maze M, Smith CM: Identification of receptor mechanism mediating epinephrine-induced arrhythmias during halothane anesthesia in the dog. Anesthesiology 59:322, 1983
81. Sharma PL: Effect of propranolol on catecholamine-induced arrhythmias during nitrous oxide-halothane anaesthesia in the dog. Br J Anaesth 38:871, 1966
82. Kapur PA, Flacke WE: Epinephrine-induced arrhythmias and cardiovascular function after verapamil during halothane anesthesia in the dog. Anesthesiology 55:218, 1981
83. Schick LM, Chapin JC, Munson ES, et al: Pancuronium, *d*-tubocurarine, and epinephrine-induced arrhythmias during halothane anesthesia in dogs. Anesthesiology 52:207, 1980
84. Roberts FL, Burstrom RE, Atlee JL: Effects of ketamine and etomidate on epinephrine-induced ventricular dysrhythmias in dogs anesthetized with halothane (abstract). Anesthesiology 61:A36, 1984
85. Metz S, Maze M: Halothane concentration does not alter the threshold for epinephrine-induced arrhythmias in dogs. Anesthesiology 62:470, 1985
86. Szekeres L, Papp JG: Effect of adrenergic activators and inhibitors on electrical activity of the heart. In Szekeres L (ed): Handbook of experimental pharmacology. Berlin: Springer-Verlag, 1980: 597
87. Spiss CK, Maze M, Smith CM: Alpha-adrenergic responsiveness correlates with epinephrine dose for arrhythmias during halothane anesthesia in dogs. Anesth Analg 63:297, 1984
88. Clarkson CW, Hondeghem LM: Mechanisms for bupivacaine depression of cardiac conduction: fast block of sodium chan-

nels during the action potential with slow recovery from block during diastole. Anesthesiology 62:396, 1985
89. Albright GA: Cardiac arrest following regional anesthesia with etidocaine or bupivacaine. Anesthesiology 51:285, 1979
90. Davis NL, deJong RH: Successful resuscitation following massive bupivacaine overdose. Anesth Analg 61:62, 1982
91. Rosenberg PH, Kalso EA, Tuominen MK, et al: Acute bupivacaine toxicity as a result of venous leakage under the tourniquet cuff during a Bier block. Anesthesiology 58:95, 1983
92. Conklin KA, Ziadlon-Rad F: Bupivacaine cardiotoxicity in a pregnant patient with mitral valve prolapse. Anesthesiology 58:596, 1983
93. Liu PL, Feldman HS, Covino BM, et al: Acute cardiovascular toxicity of intravenous amide local anesthetics in anesthetized ventilated dogs. Anesth Analg 61:317, 1982
94. Avery P, Redon D, Schaenzer G, et al: The influence of serum potassium on the cerebral and cardiac toxicity of bupivacaine and lidocaine. Anesthesiology 61:134, 1984
95. deJong RH, Ronfield RA, DeRosa RA: Cardiovascular effects of convulsant and supraconvulsant doses of amide local anesthetics. Anesth Analg 61:3, 1982
96. Liu P, Feldman HS, Covino BM, et al: Acute cardiovascular toxicity of intravenous amide local anesthetics in anesthetized ventilated dogs. Anesth Analg 61:317, 1982
97. Liu P, Feldman HS, Giasi R, et al: Comparative CNS toxicity of lidocaine, etidocaine, bupivacaine, and tetracaine in awake dogs following rapid intravenous administration. Anesth Analg 62:375, 1983
98. Kotelko DM, Shnider SM, Dailey PA, et al: Bupivacaine-induced cardiac arrhythmias in sheep. Anesthesiology 60:10, 1984
99. Thigpen JW, Kotelko DM, Shnider SM, et al: Bupivacaine cardiotoxicity in hypoxic–acidotic sheep (abstract). Anesthesiology 59:A204, 1983
100. Morishima HO, Pedersen H, Finster M, et al: Is bupivacaine more cardiotoxic than lidocaine? (abstract). Anesthesiology 59:A409, 1983
101. Clarkson CW, Hondeghem L, Matsubara T, et al: Possible mechanism of bupivacaine toxicity: fast inactivation block with slow diastolic recovery. Anesth Analg 63:175, 1984
102. Clarkson CW, Thigpen J, Shnider SM, et al: Bupivacaine toxicity: fast inactivation block and slow diastolic recovery. Circ Res 68:296, 1983
103. Taylor P: Agents acting at the neuromuscular junctions and autonomic ganglia. In Gilman AG, Rall TW, Nies AS, Taylor P (eds): The pharmacological basis of therapeutics, 8th ed. New York: MacMillan, 1990: 166
104. Schoenstadt DA, Whitcher CE: Observations on the mechanism of succinylcholine-induced cardiac arrhythmias. Anesthesiology 24:358, 1963
105. Yasuda I, Hirano T, Amaha K, et al: Chronotropic effects of succinylcholine and succinylmonocholine on the sinoatrial node. Anesthesiology 57:289, 1982
106. Dowdy EG, Fabian LWL: Ventricular arrhythmias induced by succinylcholine in digitalized patients. Anesth Analg 42:501, 1963
107. Bartolone RS, Tadikonda LKR: Dysrhythmias following muscle relaxant administration in patients receiving digitalis. Anesthesiology 58:567, 1983
108. Burroughs Wellcome: Anectine (succinylcholine chloride) injection, USP and Anectine (succinylcholine chloride) sterile powder Flo-Pack (package insert). Research Triangle Park, NC: Burroughs Wellcome, June 1993
109. Weiner N, Taylor P: Neurohumoral transmission: the autonomic and somatic nervous systems. In Gilman AG, Goodman LS, Rall TW, et al (eds): The pharmacological basis of therapeutics, 7th ed. New York: MacMillan, 1985: 66
110. Lee Son S, Waud DR: A vagolytic action of neuromuscular blocking agents at the pacemaker of the isolated guinea pig atrium. Anesthesiology 48:191, 1978
111. Stirt JA, Berger JM, Ricker SM, et al: Arrhythmogenic effects of aminophylline during halothane anesthesia in experimental animals. Anesth Analg 59:410, 180
112. Stirt JA, Berger JM, Sullivan SF: Lack of arrhythmogenicity of isoflurane following administration of aminophylline in dogs. Anesth Analg 62:568, 1983
113. Barton MD: Anesthetic problems with aspirin-intolerant patients. Anesth Analg 54:376, 1975
114. Roizen MF, Stevens WC: Multiform ventricular tachycardia due to the interaction of aminophylline and halothane. Anesth Analg 57:738, 1978
115. Belani KG, Anderson WW, Buckley JJ: Adverse drug interaction involving pancuronium and aminophylline. Anesth Analg 61:473, 1982
116. Prokocimer PG, Nicholls E, Gaba DM, et al: Epinephrine arrhythmogenicity is enhanced by acute, but not chronic, aminophylline administration during halothane anesthesia in dogs. Anesthesiology 65:13–18, 1986
117. Atlee JL, Dayer AM, Houge JC: Chronic recording from the His bundle in awake dog. Basic Res Cardiol 79:627, 1984
118. Atlee JL, Hamann SR, Brownlee SW, et al: Conscious state comparisons of the effects of the inhalation anesthetics and diltiazem, nifedipine, or verapamil on specialized atrioventricular conduction times in spontaneously beating dog hearts. Anesthesiology 68:519, 1988
119. Hoffman BF, Bigger JT Jr: Digitalis and allied cardiac glycosides. In Gilman AG, Goodman LS, Rall TW, et al (eds): The pharmacological basis of therapeutics, 7th ed. New York: MacMillan, 1985: 716
120. Morrow DH, Townley NT: Anesthesia and digitalis toxicity: an experimental study. Anesth Analg 49:510, 1964
121. Ivankovich AD, Miletich DJ, Grossman RK, et al: The effects of enflurane, isoflurane, fluroxene, methoxyflurane and diethyl ether anesthesia on ouabain tolerance in the dog. Anesth Analg 55:360, 1976
122. Ivankovitch AD, El-Etr AA, Janeczko GF: The effects of ketamine and Innovar anesthesia on digitalis tolerance in dogs. Anesth Analg 54:106, 1975
123. Morrow DH: Anesthesia and digitalis toxicity: VI. effect of barbiturates and halothane on digoxin toxicity. Anesth Analg 49:305, 1970
124. Ivankovich AD, Ruggiero RP, El-Etr AA, et al: Effect of neostigmine on cardiac rhythm in digitalized dogs. Anesth Analg 50:1079, 1971
125. Barrett JS, Hey EB: Ventricular arrhythmias associated with the use of diazepam for cardioversion. JAMA 214:3323, 1970
126. Sprague DH: Severe bradycardia after neostigmine in a patient taking propranolol to control paroxysmal atrial tachycardia. Anesthesiology 42:208, 1975
127. Prys-Roberts C: Hemodynamic effects of anesthesia and surgery in renal hypertensive patients receiving large doses of β-receptor antagonists. Anesthesiology 51:S122, 1979
128. Carmeliet EE: Influence of lithium ions on transmembrane potential and cation content of cardiac cells. J Gen Physiol 47:501, 1964
129. Havdala HS, Borison RL, Diamond BI: Potential hazards and applications of lithium in anesthesiology. Anesthesiology 50: 534, 1979
130. Azar I, Turndorf H: Paroxysmal left bundle branch block during nitrous oxide anesthesia in a patient on lithium carbonate: a case report. Anesth Analg 56:868, 1977
131. Tangedahi TN, Gar GT: Myocardial irritability associated with lithium carbonate therapy. N Engl J Med 287:867, 1972
132. Plowman PE, Thomas WJW: Tricyclic antidepressant and cardiac dysrhythmias during dental anaesthesia. Anaesthesia 29:576, 1974
133. Moir DC, Crooks J, Cornwell WB, et al: Cardiotoxicity of amitriptyline. Lancet 2:561, 1972
134. Glisson SN, Fajardo L, El-Etr AA: Amitriptyline therapy increases electrocardiographic changes during reversal of neuromuscular blockade. Anesth Analg 57:77, 1978
135. Ravidran R, Viegas OJ, Padilla LM, et al: Anesthetic considerations in pregnant patients receiving terbutaline therapy. Anesth Analg 59:391, 1980
136. Hurlbert BJ, Edelman JD, David K: Serum potassium levels during and after terbutaline. Anesth Analg 60:723, 1981

137. Gallagher JD, Lieberman RW, Meranze J, et al: Amiodarone-induced complications during coronary artery surgery. Anesthesiology 55:186, 1981
138. Charlier R: Cardiac actions in the dog of a new antagonist of adrenergic excitation which does not produce competitive blockade of adrenoreceptors. Br J Pharmacol 39:674, 1970
139. Lineberger AS, Sprague DH, Battaglini JW: Sinus arrest associated with cimetidine. Anesth Analg 64:554, 1985
140. Surawicz B: The interrelationship of electrolyte abnormalities and arrhythmias. In Mandel WJ (ed): Cardiac arrhythmias: their mechanisms, diagnosis, and management. Philadelphia: JB Lippincott, 1980: 83
141. Bettinger JC, Surawicz B, Bryfogle JW, et al: The effect of intravenous administration of potassium chloride on ectopic rhythms, ectopic beats, and disturbances in AV conduction. Am J Med 21:521, 1956
142. Davidson S, Surawicz B: Ectopic beats and atrioventricular conduction disturbances in patients with hypopotassemia. Arch Intern Med 120:280, 1967
143. Weaver WF, Burchell HB: Serum potassium and electrocardiogram in hypokalemia. Circulation 21:505, 1960
144. Stewart DE, Ikram H, Espiner EA, et al: Arrhythmogenic potential of diuretic-induced hypokalemia in patients with mild hypertension and ischemic heart disease. Br Heart J 54:290, 1985
145. Vitez TS, Soper LE, Wong KC, et al: Chronic hypokalemia and intraoperative dysrhythmias. Anesthesiology 63:130, 1985
146. Katz RL, Bigger JT Jr: Cardiac arrhythmias during anesthesia and operation. Anesthesiology 33:193, 1970
147. Blanc VF, Hardy JF, Milot J, et al: The oculocardiac reflex: a graphic and statistical analysis in children. Can Anaesth Soc J 30:360, 1983
148. Jackman WM, Friday KJ, Anderson JL, Aliot EM, Clark M, Lazzara R: The long QT syndromes: A critical review, new clinical observation and a unifying hypothesis. Prog Cardiovasc Dis 2:115, 1988
149. Wit AL, Rosen MR: Afterdepolarizations and triggered activity: Distinction from automaticity as an arrhythmogenic mechanism. In: Fozzard et al (eds): *The Heart and Cardiovascular System,* 2nd ed. 2113–2163, 1992
150. Curtiss EI, Heibel RH, Shaver JA: Autonomic maneuvers in hereditary QT interval prolongation (Romano-Ward syndrome). Am Heart J 95:420, 1978
151. Romano C, Gemme G, Pongiglione R: Aritmie cardiache rare dell'eta pediatrica. La Clinic Paed 45:656, 1963
152. Ward OC: A new familial cardiac syndrome in children. Journal of the Irish Medical Association 54:103, 1964
153. Zipes DP: Specific arrhythmias: Diagnosis and treatment. In Braunwald E (ed): Heart disease: a textbook of cardiovascular disease, 2nd ed. Philadelphia: WB Saunders, 1984: 683
154. Lown B: Cardiovascular collapse and sudden cardiac death. In Braunwald E (ed): Heart disease: a textbook of cardiovascular disease, 2nd ed. Philadelphia: WB Saunders, 1984: 774
155. Vincent GM, Abildskov JA, Burgess MJ: The QT interval syndromes. Progr Cardiovasc Dis 16:527, 1974
156. Schwartz PJ, Periti M, Malliani A: The long QT syndrome. Am Heart J 89:378, 1975
157. Schwartz H: Oculocardiac reflex: is prophylaxis necessary? In Mark LC, Ngai S (eds): Highlights of clinical anesthesiology. New York: Harper & Row, 1971: 111
158. Calkins H, Lehmann MH, Allman K, Wieldand D, Schwaiger M: Scintigraphic pattern of regional cardiac sympathetic innervation in patients with familial long QT syndrome using positron emission tomography. Circulation 87:1616, 1993
159. Jervell A, Lange-Nielsen F: Congenital deaf mutism, functional heart disease with prolongation of QT interval and sudden death. Am Heart J 54:59, 1957
160. Moss AJ: Molecular genetics and ventricular arrhythmias. N Engl J Med 327:885, 1993
161. Schwartz PJ, Moss AJ, Vincent GM, Crampton RS: Diagnostic criteria for the long QT Syndrome: an update. Circulation 88: 782, 1993
162. Medak R, Benumof JL: Perioperative management of the prolonged QT interval syndrome. Br J Anaesth 55:361, 1983
163. Morganroth J, Brown AM, Critz S, Crumb WJ, Kunze DL, Lacerda AE, Lopez H: Variability of the QT interval: Impact on defining drug effect and low-frequency cardiac event. Am J Cardiol 72:26B, 1993
164. Morganroth J: Relations of QT_C prolongation on the electrocardiogram to torsades de pointes: Definitions and mechanisms. Am J Cardiol 72:10B, 1993
165. Braunwald E: Valvular heart disease. In Braunwald E (ed): Heart disease: a textbook of cardiovascular disease. 2nd ed. Philadelphia: WB Saunders, 1984: 1063
166. Krantz EM, Viljoen JF, Schermer R, et al: Mitral valve prolapse. Anesth Analg 59:379, 1980
167. Stirt JA, Frantz RA, Gunz EF: Anesthesia, catecholamines, and hemodynamics in autonomic dysfunction. Anesth Analg 61:701, 1982
168. Roizen MF: Anesthetic implications of concurrent disease. In Miller RD (ed): Anesthesia, 2nd ed. New York: Churchill Livingstone, 1994: 903
169. Krishna G: Neurofibromatosis, renal hypertension, and cardiac dysrhythmias. Anesth Analg 54:542, 1975
170. Tsueda K, Oliver PB, Richter RW: Cardiovascular manifestations of tetanus. Anesthesiology 40:588, 1974
171. Newland MC, Hurlbert BJ: Chemodectoma diagnosed by hypertension and tachycardia during anesthesia. Anesth Analg 59:388, 1980
172. Hull CJ: Electrocution hazards in the operating theatre. Br J Anaesth 50:647, 1978
173. Leeming MN: Protection of the 'electrically susceptible patient.' Anesthesiology 38:370, 1973
174. Bazaral MG, Norfleet EA: Comparison of CB_5 and V_5 leads for intraoperative electrocardiographic monitoring. Anesth Analg 60:849, 1981
175. Kates RA, Zaidan JR, Kaplan JA: Esophageal lead for intraoperative electrocardiographic monitoring. Anesth Analg 61: 781, 1982
176. Brown DL, Greenberg DJ: A simple device for monitoring the esophageal electrocardiogram. Anesthesiology 59:482, 1983
177. Michenfelder JD, Terry HR, Daw EF, et al: Air embolism during neurosurgery: a new method of treatment. Anesth Analg 45:390, 1966
178. Westheimer DN: Right atrial catheter placement: use of a wire guide as the intravascular ECG lead. Anesthesiology 56: 478, 1982
179. Gesclowitz DB, Arzbaecher RC, Barr DB, et al: Electrical safety standards for electrocardiographic apparatus. Circulation 61:669, 1980
180. Wellens HJJ, Bar FW, Lie KI: The value of the electrocardiogram in the diagnosis of a tachycardia with a widened QRS complex. Am J Med 64:27, 1978
181. Pietras RJ, Mautner R, Denes P, et al: Chronic recurrent right and left ventricular tachycardia: comparison of clinical, hemodynamic, and angiographic findings. Am J Cardiol 40:32, 1977
182. Zipes DP: Diagnosis of ventricular tachycardia. Drug Ther 9: 83, 1979
183. James TN, Sherf L: Specialized tissues and preferential conduction in the atria of the heart. Am J Cardiol 28:414, 1971
184. Risch C, Zipes DP, McHenry PL: Rate dependent aberrancy. Circulation 48:714, 1973
185. Pick A, Langendorf R: Interpretation of complex arrhythmias. Philadelphia: Lea and Febiger, 1979: 127
186. Spurell RAJ, Krikler DM, Sowton E: Concealed bypasses of the atrioventricular node in patients with paroxysmal supraventricular tachycardia revealed by intracardiac electrical stimulation and verapamil. Am J Cardiol 33:590, 1974
187. Barold SS, Coumel P: Mechanisms of atrioventricular junction tachycardia: role of reentry and concealed accessory bypass tracts. Am J Cardiol 39:97, 1977
188. Wolff L, Parkinson J, White PD: Bundle branch block with

short PR interval in healthy young people prone to paroxysmal tachycardia. Am Heart J 5:685, 1950
189. Lown B, Ganong WF, Levine SA: The syndrome of short PR interval, normal QRS complex and paroxysmal rapid heart action. Circulation 5:693, 1952
190. Belardinelli L, Linden J, Berne R: The cardiac effects of adenosine. Prog Cardiovasc Dis 32:73, 1989
191. Lerman BB, Belardinelli L: Cardiac electrophysiology of adenosine: Basic and clinical concepts. Circulation 81:686, 1990
192. DiMarco JP, Miles W, Akhtar M, et al: Adenosine for paroxysmal supraventricular tachycardia: Dose ranging and comparison with verapamil. Ann Int Med 113:104, 1990
193. DiMarco JP, Sellers TD, Lerman BB, Greenberg ML, Berne RM, Belardinelli L: Diagnostic and therapeutic use of adenosine in patients with supraventricular tachyarrhythmias. J Am Coll Cardiol 6:417, 1985
194. Clarke B, Rowland E, Burnes PJ, Till J, Ward DE, Shinebourne EA: Rapid and safe termination of supraventricular tachycardia in children by adenosine. Lancet 1:299, 1987
195. Guidelines for advanced cardiac life support and emergency cardiac care. JAMA 268:2205, 1992
196. Freedberg AS, Papp JG, Williams EM: The effect of altered thyroid state on atrial intracellular potentials. J Physiol (London) 207:357, 1970
197. Hii JT, Wyse DG, Gillis AM, Duff HJ, Solylo MA, Mitchell LB: Precordial QT interval dispersion as a marker of torsades de pointes: Disparate effects of class Ia antiarrhythmic drugs and amiodarone. Circulation 86:1376, 1992
198. Zipes DP: Management of cardiac arrhythmias. In Braunwald E (ed): Heart disease: a textbook of cardiovascular disease, 2nd ed. Philadelphia: WB Saunders, 1984: 648
199. Gillis RA, Quest JA: The role of the nervous system in the cardiovascular effects of digitalis. Pharmacol Rev 31:19, 1979
200. Birkhead JS, Vaughan Williams EM: Dual effect of disopyramide on atrial and atrioventricular conduction and refractory periods. Br Heart J 39:657, 1977
201. Frieden J, Cooper JA, Grossman JI: Continuous infusion of edrophonium (Tensilon) in treating supraventricular arrhythmias. Am J Cardiol 27:294, 1971
202. Cardiac Arrhythmias Suppression Study (CAST) Investigators: Increased mortality due to encainide or flecainide in a randomized trial of arrhythmias suppression after myocardial infarction. N Engl J Med 321:406, 1990
203. Scmid JF, Seeback BD, Henrie CL, et al: Some antiarrhythmic actions of a new compound, R-818, in dogs and mice. Fed Proc 34:775, 1975
204. Peter T, Ross D, Duffield A, et al: Effect on survival after myocardial infarction of long-term treatment with phenytoin. Br Heart J 40:1356, 1978
205. Gillis RA, McClellan JR, Sauer TS, et al: Depression of cardiac sympathetic nerve activity by diphenylhydantoin. J Pharmacol Exp Ther 179:599, 1971
206. Garan H, Ruskin JN, Powell WJ Jr: Centrally mediated effect of phenytoin on digoxin-induced ventricular arrhythmias. Am J Physiol 241:H67, 1981
207. Antiarrhythmic agents. In Bennett DR (ed): AMA Drug Evaluations, 5th ed. Chicago: American Medical Association, 1983: 623
208. Zipes DP: Management of cardiac arrhythmias: pharmacological, electrical, and surgical techniques. In Braunwald E (ed): Heart disease: a textbook of cardiovascular medicine. Philadelphia: WB Saunders, 1984: 648
209. Hordof AJ, Edie R, Malm JR, et al: Electrophysiologic properties and response to pharmacologic agents of fibers from diseased human atria. Circulation 54:774, 1976
210. Spear JF, Horowitz LN, Moore EN: The slow response in human ventricle. In Zipes DP, Bailey JC, Elharrar V, et al (eds): The slow inward current and cardiac arrhythmias. The Hague: Martinus Nijhoff, 1980: 309
211. Waxman HL, Myerburg RJ, Appel R, et al: Verapamil for control of ventricular rate in paroxysmal supraventricular tachycardia and atrial or flutter: a double-blind randomized cross-over study. Ann Intern Med 94:1, 1981
212. Rinkenberger RL, Prystowsky EN, Heger, et al: Effects of intravenous and chronic oral verapamil administration in patients with supraventricular tachyarrhythmias. Circulation 62: 996, 1980
213. Singh BN, Collett JT, Chew CY: New perspectives in the pharmacologic therapy of cardiac arrhythmias. Prog Cardiovasc Dis 22:243, 1980
214. Vaughan Williams EM: Classification of antiarrhythmic drugs. In: Sandoe E, Flensted-Jensen E, Olesen K (eds): Cardiac Arrhythmias. Sweden, Astra, Sodertalje, 1981: 449
215. Vaughan Williams EM: A classification of antiarrhythmic actions reassessed after a decade of new drugs. J Clin Pharmacol 24:129, 1984
216. Harrison DA, Winkle RA, Sami M, Mason J: Encainide: a new and potent antiarrhythmic agent. In Harrison DC (ed): Cardiac Arrhythmias: A Decade of Progress. Boston; GK Hall, 1981: 315
217. Smeets JLRM: Special Issue on the Sicilian Gambit. Impulse: Advances in arrhythmology 1992 (August): 1–17, 1992
218. Parsonnet V, Furman S, Smyth NP, et al: Optimal resources for implantable cardiac pacemakers. Circulation 68:226A, 1983
219. Zipes DP: electrical therapy of cardiac arrhythmias. N Engl J Med 309:1179, 1983
220. Zaidan JR: Pacemakers. Anesthesiology 60:319, 1984
221. Platia EV: Management of cardiac arrhythmias: the nonpharmacologic approach. Philadelphia: JB Lippincott, 1987
222. Resnekov L: High-energy electrical current in the management of cardiac dysrhythmias. In Mandel WJ (ed): Cardiac arrhythmias. Philadelphia: JB Lippincott, 1980: 589
223. Banka VS: Defibrillation and electrical countershock. In Helfant RH (ed): Bellet's essentials of cardiac arrhythmias, 2nd ed. Philadelphia: WB Saunders, 1980: 352

FURTHER READING

Atlee JL III: Perioperative cardiac dysrhythmias: mechanisms, recognition, management, 2nd ed. Chicago: Year Book Medical Publishers, 1989

Complications in Anesthesiology, second edition,
edited by Nikolaus Gravenstein and Robert R. Kirby.
Lippincott-Raven Publishers, Philadelphia © 1996.

CHAPTER 23

Failure of the Peripheral Circulation

Marcel E. Durieux
David E. Longnecker

The primary role of the peripheral circulation is to deliver oxygen and other metabolic substrates to the capillaries, where the essential exchange processes between blood and tissue occur. The metabolic processes that produce energy to maintain cellular activity are primarily oxygen dependent. Although anaerobic pathways are available for energy production, they are stopgap measures that can meet the cellular energy requirements for only brief periods. Any significant impairment of peripheral circulatory function results in tissue ischemia and, potentially, in cellular damage or death.

Peripheral circulatory failure may be localized or generalized. Examples of local regional hypoperfusion include the "steal" syndromes, which result from the shunting of blood away from an organ or circulatory bed, and localized ischemia associated with specific vascular abnormalities, such as transient ischemic attack, myocardial infarction, and vascular trauma.

This chapter considers the function of the peripheral circulation, the pathophysiologic mechanisms of peripheral circulatory failure, and the therapy of these disorders. The primary emphases are on anesthetic overdose and hypovolemic shock, the types of peripheral circulatory failure encountered most commonly by the anesthesiologist. Septic shock and other causes seen less commonly in the operating room are discussed briefly.

PERIPHERAL CIRCULATION

Anatomical Considerations

The principal function of the peripheral circulation is to distribute the cardiac output to all tissues in amounts sufficient to meet the metabolic demands of those tissues. Although the rate and function of the heart and the impedance of the peripheral circulation determine the absolute amount of cardiac output, the peripheral circulation alone is responsible for the distribution of blood flow and oxygen. The peripheral circulation can be divided into four sections: conductance vessels, resistance vessels, exchange vessels, and capacitance vessels.

Conductance Vessels

Although arteries from the aorta to arterioles with a diameter of several hundred micrometers have smooth muscle in their walls, these vessels have little influence on the distribution of cardiac output to various organs. Their primary function is to act as conduits. Although obstruction of such vessels can induce regional circulatory failure, their most important role in generalized failure of the circulation occurs when they are ruptured because of disease or trauma and hypovolemia ensues.

Resistance Vessels

By far the most important determinants of vascular resistance are the small arterioles. The walls of these vessels, ranging in diameter from 10 to 50 μm, contain large amounts of smooth muscle. Alterations in the contractile state of this muscle result in arteriolar constriction or dilation and regulation of vascular resistance and blood flow. Because vascular resistance is related inversely to arteriolar caliber by approximately the fourth power of the vessel radius, small changes in arteriolar diameter produce very large changes in vascular resistance.

Exchange Vessels

The dense networks of capillaries found in almost all tissues are primarily responsible for the exchange function of the circulation. Capillaries are thin-walled endothelial tubes that permit the diffusion of oxygen and carbon dioxide between the tissues and the blood. Blood flow within the capillaries is controlled by precapillary sphincters in the terminal arterioles. Local tissue hypoxia results in dilation of arterioles and precapillary sphincters. The former reduce vascular resistance to increase overall flow, and the latter open more capillaries to increase the surface area for gas exchange. Both act to increase the delivery of oxygen to the hypoxic site.

In addition to facilitating gas exchange, the capillaries allow hydrogen ion, electrolyte, protein, and water flux between the intravascular compartment and the tissues. Solute movement across the capillary is determined by capillary permeability and by concentration gradients across the endothelial walls. Fluid movement across the capillary is determined by capillary permeability and by the balance between pressures that force fluid out of the capillary (ie, capillary hydrostatic pressure and the tissue oncotic pressure) and pressures that hold fluid in the capillary (ie, plasma oncotic pressure and tissue hydrostatic pressure). Water, solute, and gas exchange are markedly altered by peripheral circulatory failure, with effects that can be predicted easily from changes in the variables that determine their flux.

Capacitance Vessels

The major portion (approximately 70%) of the circulating blood volume is contained in the veins. Small veins act as reservoirs for blood and alterations in venous capacitance are responsible for major changes in venous return and, ultimately, for cardiac output. Large veins act primarily as conduits to return blood to the heart.

Control of the Peripheral Circulation

Microvascular control may be divided into two categories: remote and local.

Remote

NEURAL CONTROL. Neural control of the microvasculature is accomplished primarily through the autonomic nervous system, with sympathetic activation resulting in arteriolar and venular constriction. The microvascular responses to neural stimulation are not uniform among the various vascular beds. Stimulation of the sympathetic nervous system produces only minor changes in vascular resistance in the cerebral and coronary circulations, but the cutaneous, muscle, and renal circulations constrict dramatically. A gradation in response may be apparent even within a single vascular bed. In general, arterioles are more responsive than veins, and small arterioles (10 to 30 μm in diameter) are more responsive than larger arteries.

HUMORAL CONTROL. Humoral mechanisms serve as remote and local microvascular regulators. Some of the humoral agents that alter the microvasculature include epinephrine, norepinephrine, vasopressin, nitric oxide, prostaglandins, kinins, and angiotensin. The relative importance of these substances in normal circumstances is not defined completely, although their role in pathologic states, such as hypertension or hemorrhagic shock, is evident.

Local

METABOLIC CONTROL. Metabolic control implies that some local substance is responsible for moment-to-moment control of the microvasculature. Numerous substances have been implicated as mediators, including oxygen, carbon dioxide, potassium, hydrogen, adenosine, nitric oxide, phosphate, and magnesium. Although the exact role of each of these substances remains uncertain, tissue hypoxia results in the opening of arterioles and precapillary sphincters, presumably in response to local mediators.

MYOGENIC CONTROL. Local myogenic control is based on the principle that increased transmural pressure across the vascular wall stimulates vascular smooth muscle to contract and that relaxation occurs when transmural pressure decreases. Hypertension and increased microvascular flow result in arteriolar constriction to reduce flow, but hypotension causes local arteriolar dilation to restore flow. This mechanism may be responsible for the prevention of edema in the legs when humans assume the erect posture, and it contributes to the local autoregulation of blood flow in the brain and other organs.

Effects of Anesthesia

Anesthetic Overdose

Recognition of the difference between relative and absolute overdose is essential. An absolute overdose represents administration of a dose that is outside of the recommended dosage range. It may occur when, for example, a vaporizer is inadvertently left at the high setting used during induction. Much more important in the current context is relative overdose: administration of a dose that induces side effects in a particular patient because of the presence of a disease state. This occurs commonly in patients with failure of the peripheral circulation and can occur at what would otherwise be considered normal or even low dosages of the drug.

Premedication

Commonly administered premedicant drugs include the benzodiazepines and opiates. These drugs have considerable effects on the cardiovascular system when administered in absolute or relative overdoses. Barbiturates are rarely used as premedication any more. In appropriate doses, they have little effect on the cardiovascular system.

BENZODIAZEPINES. Diazepam and midazolam have relatively little direct effect on the cardiovascular system.[1] The major manifestations of an overdose—respiratory and cardiovascular depression—occur as a result of hypoxia rather than as a primary event. Therapy should therefore be directed toward correcting the ventilatory problem. The combination of narcotics and benzodiazepines can lead to pronounced synergistic cardiovascular depression through mechanisms that have not been fully elucidated. Although this effect is seen primarily after induction doses of the drugs, it should be kept in mind when combinations of narcotics and benzodiazepines are administered as premedication to patients with fragile cardiovascular stability.

OPIATES. In general, the cardiovascular effects of typical premedicant doses of fentanyl are minimal. Morphine dilates resistance and capacitance vessels, although in the supine patient, these effects are negligible.[2] However, in the erect person, venous dilation results in pooling of blood in the capacitance vessels and a consequent decrease in cardiac output and arterial pressure. The combination of morphine and proper position is a common therapeutic maneuver for the treatment of pulmonary edema; its effectiveness results from the drug's action on peripheral capacitance vessels. Orthostatic hypotension is enhanced by hypovolemia that results from dehydration or acute blood loss.

The treatment of orthostatic hypotension associated with narcotic premedication begins with awareness on the part of the clinician and with prevention. The premedicated patient should not be allowed to stand without assistance, and the dose of the drug should be reduced in patients who are potentially hypovolemic. More specific therapy should include wrapping the legs with elastic bandages and intravenous fluid therapy. Only rarely are vasopressors required to treat this problem.

General Anesthesia

BARBITURATES. Experimentally, barbiturates can depress the function of cardiac and vascular smooth muscle, but the doses required to produce these effects exceed those usually administered. More commonly, barbiturates produce only modest changes in blood pressure and blood flow. Of course, hypotension may result if these drugs are given by rapid injection, which produces quite high, but transient, plasma concentrations. These effects are seen primarily in hypovolemic patients and those with poor cardiac function. Barbiturates should be used in reduced dosage and with the utmost care in these populations. Autonomic ganglionic blockade and especially histamine release may contribute to the development of hypotension in response to barbiturates.

ETOMIDATE. Etomidate causes little cardiovascular depression when used in appropriate induction dosages. When given to patients without significant cardiac disease, changes of less than 10% occur in mean arterial pressure, pulmonary artery pressure, pulmonary capillary wedge pressure, central venous pressure, stroke volume, cardiac index, and systemic vascular resistance.[3] In patients with heart disease, these cardiovascular effects are enhanced only modestly.

OPIATES. Fentanyl, sufentanil, and alfentanil may be associated with cardiac slowing but usually have reasonably benign cardiovascular effects. Morphine, even in very large doses, is surprisingly free of cardiovascular effects, provided that two conditions are met: the patient remains supine, and ventilation is supported.[4] Nonetheless, the shorter-acting synthetic opiates largely have replaced morphine for cardiac surgery.

KETAMINE. Ketamine administration typically results in increases in heart rate, cardiac output, and arterial pressure, without significant alterations in total peripheral resistance.[5] These effects, symptoms of a relative increase in sympathetic tone, may result from ketamine's muscarinic antagonist properties.[6] However, the cardiovascular depressant effects of the drug become apparent when relative or absolute overdoses are administered. Large doses of ketamine given to animals result in little change in heart rate or cardiac output but do reduce systemic vascular resistance; the net effect is a tendency toward hypotension.

In hemorrhaged animals, ketamine decreases mean arterial pressure, cardiac output, and stroke volume.[7] The drug should therefore be used with caution in patients who are unable to mount a sympathetic response to combat its direct depressant effects, including hypovolemic trauma patients whose sympathetic systems are already fully activated. Therapy should be directed primarily at restoring myocardial performance, and a vasopressor with α- and β-adrenergic receptor activity may well be indicated.

VOLATILE AGENTS. The volatile inhalation anesthetics differ in their effects on cardiac performance and the peripheral vascular circulation. Deep halothane anesthesia in volunteers results in profound reductions in cardiac output (almost 50%) and arterial pressure but a less than 10% decrease in systemic vascular resistance.[8] Isoflurane induces less cardiac depression but more pronounced vasodilation.[7] The primary treatment of arterial hypotension resulting from anesthetic overdose consists of eliminating the drug. When pharmacologic agents are indicated, they should be selected based on the cause of the problem. The hypotension that accompanies deep levels of halothane anesthesia is best treated with intravenous administration of a β-adrenergic agonist or calcium to improve cardiac output, but overdose of isoflurane may require a peripheral vasoconstrictor.

Regional Anesthesia

Local anesthetics appear to have biphasic effects on the peripheral vasculature.[9,10] At low concentrations, they produce vasoconstriction, but at greater (clinical) concentrations, they are vasodilators. Peripheral vasodilation occurs by at least two mechanisms: direct dilation of vascular smooth muscle (cocaine is an exception) and interruption of neurally mediated adrenergic vasoconstrictor activity through chemical sympathectomy.

Because vascular resistance is decreased in the anesthetized area, superficial warmth and venodilation are early signs of regional anesthesia. Alterations in cardiac output, total peripheral resistance, and regional blood flow reflect the balance between vasodilation in the anesthetized area and compensatory vasoconstriction in nonanesthetized regions. Vascular resistance is greatly reduced and capacitance is increased in the lower extremities during spinal or epidural anesthesia, but reflex arteriolar and venous constriction occur in the upper extremities to compensate for the decreases in arterial pressure and central blood volume.

The circulatory consequences of regional anesthesia may be minimized considerably by efforts to correct the alterations in venous capacitance. Wrapping the lower extremities with elastic bandages, rapid infusion of 500 to 800 mL of a balanced salt solution immediately before induction of anesthesia, and avoidance of head-up tilt are usually effective. Vasopressors are rarely needed when these preventive measures are taken. Spinal or epidural anesthesia should not be used in hypovolemic patients, because absolute hypovolemia potentiates the additional relative hypovolemia produced by the anesthetic procedure and may result in severe reductions in venous return, cardiac output, and arterial pressure.

HEMORRHAGIC SHOCK

Pathophysiology

Tissue Perfusion

The fundamental defect in hemorrhagic shock is a reduction in effective circulating blood volume, with a resultant decrease in cardiac output. As circulating volume and arterial pressure decrease, the remote and local microvascular regulatory mechanisms are activated to restore tissue perfusion. One of the earliest homeostatic mechanisms is an increase in oxygen extraction from the blood, which increases the difference in arteriovenous oxygen content.[11] Another prompt compensatory factor is the redistribution of cardiac output to favor perfusion of essential organs.

Flow Distribution

With the onset of hemorrhage, prompt increases in vascular resistance occur in several organs, with a consequent redistribution of cardiac output (Table 23-1). The essential features of this redistribution include marked increases in vascular resistance in the renal, skeletal muscle, and cutaneous circulations. Splanchnic vascular resistance is increased modestly, and the cerebral and coronary vascular resistances are altered only slightly.[7] An absolute reduction in blood flow occurs, but the fraction of blood delivered to the brain and heart is increased at the expense of other organs.[12] Although the short-term effects of this flow distribution are valuable to maintain perfusion to the brain and myocardium, where ischemia is tolerated poorly, the long-term consequences are failure in other essential organs. With pronounced, prolonged hypovolemia, certain critical organs tend to become ischemic; these are called the target organs. Major target organs include the brain, heart, kidneys, and splanchnic viscera.

BRAIN. During moderate hypovolemia, brain perfusion is well maintained.[7] During severe hemorrhage, cerebral blood flow decreases, although the brain receives an increased proportion of cardiac output. Anesthetics modify this response considerably. Hemorrhage during ketamine anesthesia results in significant decreases in cerebral perfusion, but flows are well maintained and even increased with isoflurane.[7]

HEART. Myocardial performance ultimately declines during the terminal stages of hemorrhagic shock. This myocardial failure has been attributed to the release of a specific toxic material, called myocardial depressant factor, allegedly liberated from the splanchnic viscera during hemorrhage.[13] However, there is little evidence for its existence. The hearts of dogs in irreversible hemorrhagic shock can be transplanted into healthy recipients, with excellent survival rates.[14] Most evidence now supports the concept that myocardial failure during hemorrhage is not a primary event; it is a terminal development resulting from peripheral circulatory failure.

KIDNEYS. Renal failure is a frequent consequence of profound hemorrhagic hypotension. Hemorrhagic hypotension activates the sympathetic nervous system, and the renal vasculature is especially responsive to this activation and to humoral control. Renal vascular resistance increases promptly in response to hemorrhage. Although this response helps to maintain glomerular filtration pressure, the combination of reduced perfusion pressure and renal arteriolar constriction severely impairs renal blood flow. Unfortunately, the kidneys are quite sensitive to ischemia. As little as 10 minutes of hypotension can lead to acute renal failure in selected circumstances.[15]

SPLANCHNIC VISCERA. Splanchnic ischemia and consequent tissue hypoxia accompany prolonged hemorrhage. The prevention of splanchnic ischemia markedly enhances

TABLE 23-1
Relative Distribution of Cardiac Output and Regional Vascular Resistance During Normovolemia and During Hemorrhage

REGIONAL CIRCULATION	NORMOVOLEMIA: CARDIAC OUTPUT (%)	HEMORRHAGE	
		Vascular Resistance	*Blood Flow*
Brain	14	Slight increase	Slight reduction
Heart	5	No change	Slight reduction
Splanchnic viscera	28	Increase	Decrease
Kidney	23	Marked increase	Marked decrease
Muscle	16	Marked increase	Marked decrease
Skin	8	Marked increase	Marked decrease

the survival of hemorrhaged dogs. In one study, the mortality rate of bled dogs was reduced from 90% to 10% by cross-perfusion of the splanchnic circulation from donor dogs.[16] Necrosis of intestinal villi due to inadequacy of the oxygen supply to the gut during hemorrhage is a common finding in many species after hemorrhagic hypotension; however, this effect is not uniformly present in primates, including humans, and its exact significance is unclear.

Metabolic Alterations

IMPAIRMENT OF ENERGY PRODUCTION. A progressive decline in aerobic metabolism and a compensatory increase in anaerobic metabolism occur as tissue ischemia develops during hemorrhage. The shift to anaerobic metabolism has two important consequences: energy production is markedly impaired, and metabolic acidosis develops. Adenosine triphosphate (ATP) is the major source of energy for cellular activity. Some ATP is produced during glycolysis, the breakdown of glucose to pyruvate.

Under aerobic conditions, pyruvate enters the mitochondria and is metabolized in the citric acid cycle. The hydrogen atoms produced during the cycle are carried by reduced nicotinamide adenine dinucleotide (NADH) and $NADH_2$ to the electron transport chain, where 3 ATP molecules are produced for every 2 hydrogen atoms delivered. The final acceptor in this chain is molecular oxygen, which is converted to water. Under aerobic conditions, this pathway generates 36 ATP molecules per glucose molecule, but anaerobic glycolysis produces only 2 ATP molecules for the same amount of glucose.

LACTIC ACIDOSIS. In the absence of molecular oxygen, the final acceptor is lacking, and NADH accumulates. The citric acid cycle is blocked because of the lack of NAD^+, and pyruvate also accumulates. NADH and pyruvate then react to form lactic acid and NAD^+. Lactic acid diffuses out of the cell, and NAD^+ permits glycolysis to proceed. ATP production, however, is severely restricted, to approximately 5% of that produced by the aerobic metabolism of glucose. Lactic acid accumulation is a major source of the metabolic acidosis that accompanies prolonged hemorrhage. The severity of shock sometimes correlates closely with the concentration of lactate in the arterial blood.[17] In regions of vascular stasis, the acidosis is aggravated further by accumulation of carbon dioxide.

Besides these alterations in the composition of body fluids, which are a direct result of ischemia, several metabolic changes are brought about by the autonomic response to hemorrhage. These include an increase in the concentrations of glucose, pyruvate, and cyclic adenosine monophosphate and a decrease in the concentration of plasma free fatty acids. These changes are reduced considerably by anesthesia.[18]

Cellular Disruption

As ischemia continues, metabolism gradually deteriorates, and biologic membranes become damaged. This process results in inhibition of mitochondrial function, electrolyte shifts across the cell membrane (ie, movement of sodium and chloride into the cell and movement of potassium outward), and the release of lysosomal enzymes into the cellular interior. Membrane peroxidation leads to a chain reaction of free radical formation, which soon exhausts scavenging systems and results in severe damage to the intracellular machinery.

Hemodilution

The balance of forces that control fluid transport across the capillary endothelium is altered markedly by hemorrhagic shock. The reduced capillary hydrostatic pressure that accompanies arterial hypotension favors the net transfer of interstitial fluid into the intravascular compartment.[19] The result is a decrease in hematocrit (ie, hemodilution). The magnitude of hemodilution correlates closely with the volume deficit and is an indicator of the severity of hemorrhage.[20] Moderate hemodilution may have beneficial effects, because it improves the rheologic properties of blood and enhances perfusion. The optimal balance between oxygen carrying capacity and rheologic properties has been considered to occur at a hematocrit of 30% to 35%, although this range has been determined in animals only. Few clinical data support this concept.[21]

Ventilatory Responses

Hemorrhagic shock is a potent stimulus to respiration and results in increases of respiratory rate and minute ventilation. Airway resistance is slightly reduced, and pulmonary compliance is slightly increased during hemorrhagic shock.[22] The proportion of wasted or dead space ventilation is increased during hemorrhage and correlates directly with the decrease in pulmonary artery pressure.[23]

In uncomplicated hemorrhagic shock, the respiratory stimulation more than compensates for the increase in the proportion of dead space ventilation, and arterial carbon dioxide partial pressure is reduced to approximately 25 to 30 mm Hg. Arterial hypoxemia is rarely seen until the very late stages of hemorrhage, when generalized circulatory collapse occurs. However, patients with multiple trauma or sepsis frequently manifest arterial hypoxemia resulting from increased pulmonary shunting.[24]

Mediators

CATECHOLAMINES. The autonomic nervous system plays a key role in the response to hemorrhage. The initial response to hypovolemia is an increase in sympathetic activity, which acts as a compensatory mechanism to facilitate perfusion of vital organs (eg, brain, heart). Although the initial sympathetic activation is beneficial, prolonged increases in sympathetic activity result in major reductions in renal and splanchnic perfusion, which ultimately contribute to the patient's death. The survival times and the survival rates of hemorrhaged dogs are reduced by the continuous infusion of catecholamines during hemorrhage.[25,26] Several investigators have demonstrated a marked increase in circulating catecholamines and in plasma renin activity during hemorrhage.[27,28] Pharmacologic blockade of either system prevents the marked increase in vascular resistance that accompanies hemorrhage in animals and improves survival rates.[29-31] However, it is not certain that these findings are applicable to humans.

EICOSANOIDS. The role of eicosanoids as mediators in shock is incompletely defined. Eicosanoids are derivatives of arachidonic acid and occur in three major forms: prostaglandins and thromboxanes, which are generated from arachidonic acid by the cyclooxygenase pathway, and leukotrienes, which are produced by the lipooxygenase pathway.

Prostaglandin $F_{2\alpha}$, one of the major prostaglandins, is a potent and universal vasoconstrictor, constricting coronary arteries and the mesenteric and renal vascular beds. It is thought to play a supporting role in shock. However, thromboxane A_2 has been shown to be an important mediator in circulatory shock because it acts as a very potent vasoconstrictor and because it aggregates platelets and increases the permeability of lysosomal membranes. It may be especially damaging to the myocardium.[32] There is considerable interest in modifying its actions by means of specific thromboxane synthetase inhibitors, such as dazoxiben, or by inhibitors of the cyclooxygenase pathway, such as aspirin, indomethacin, and ibuprofen.

In contrast, other cyclooxygenase products, such as prostaglandin E_2 and prostacyclin, are potent vasodilators. These compounds are also released during hypotensive episodes, and particularly during renal ischemia. Nonsteroidal antiinflammatory drugs may block the production of such protective prostaglandins, and the production of leukotrienes by the lipoxygenase pathway may be accelerated. The role of leukotrienes in hemorrhagic shock awaits further evaluation.[33] Their biologic effects, including vasoconstriction, bronchoconstriction, and chemotaxis, suggest that they play a role in anaphylaxis.[34]

OTHER SUBSTANCES. Our understanding of the various mediators and their interactions that determine the responses of the organism to circulatory failure is still severely limited. The number of potential mediators, particularly in septic shock, has grown enormously with the discoveries of whole classes of interleukins, but their roles remain unclear.[35] Nitric oxide is a likely candidate for a role in the regulation of the peripheral vascular system during circulatory shock.[36] Novel mediators, such as the vasoconstrictive and platelet-aggregating phosphopolipid lysophosphatidate, may play important roles.[37] Although all these issues are being actively investigated, clinically applicable conclusions are premature at this time.

Diagnosis of Hemorrhagic Hypotension

Clinical Manifestations of Hypovolemia

When it occurs during surgery, hypovolemia is usually apparent, and the obvious major blood loss plus hypotension leaves little room for doubt about the diagnosis. Blood loss before or after surgery is more difficult to determine. Significant hemorrhage may occur within body cavities without obvious external bleeding; examples include hemothorax or retroperitoneal hemorrhage accompanying trauma, leaking aortic aneurysm, or postoperative hemorrhage after abdominal or thoracic surgery. Significant blood loss also may occur in the pelvis and thighs in association with fractures in these areas. The major clinical manifestations of hemorrhagic shock result from reduced blood volume and cardiac output and from consequent activation of the sympathetic nervous system in response to hypotension.

The hemodynamic manifestations may include arterial hypotension in the supine position, although hypotension is frequently a late sign of hemorrhage in the nonanesthetized patient. Orthostatic hypotension, produced by moving the patient to the sitting position, occurs frequently in patients who are normotensive in the supine position. Conscious patients often complain of intense thirst.

Sympathetic nervous system activation is manifested by tachycardia, peripheral vasoconstriction, and diaphoresis and produces the classic signs of a rapid, thready peripheral pulse and cold, clammy skin. Tachycardia is a key sign and is a compensatory mechanism that is frequently evident well before hypotension.

Monitors of Hypovolemia

Several monitors can provide valuable assistance in the diagnosis of hypovolemia and serve as variably sensitive guides to the success of therapy. Techniques include the measurement of central venous pressure, arterial pressure, heart rate, urine output, and blood gases. Measurements of pulmonary artery pressure, pulmonary artery occlusion pressure, and cardiac output also are valuable and may be especially important in patients with myocardial failure, but they are not essential to the proper care of most patients in hemorrhagic shock. Specialized pulmonary artery catheters for measurement of right ventricular ejection fraction also are available but have a limited role. Transesophageal echocardiography is finding increased application in the assessment of cardiac volume and performance during anesthesia and surgery.[38]

ARTERIAL AND VENOUS BLOOD PRESSURE. Arterial pressure should be monitored carefully during hypovolemia, but hypotension should be considered a relatively late sign of hemorrhagic shock, especially in the awake patient. In the anesthetized patient with blunted compensatory mechanisms, arterial pressure falls more rapidly in response to hemorrhage. Although oscillometric measurements are somewhat more robust, the Korotkoff sounds become vague and unreliable during profound shock, and direct measurement of arterial pressure by means of an arterial cannula and pressure transducer is useful. Direct arterial cannulation has the added advantage of providing a ready source of arterial blood for the determination of arterial oxygen and carbon dioxide partial pressures and pH.

Although arterial pressure is maintained until hypovolemia is marked, the central venous pressure decreases early during hemorrhage. Early investigations demonstrated that right atrial pressure decreases approximately 0.7 cm H_2O for each 100 mL of blood removed from a 70-kg adult.[39] Hemorrhage of 500 to 800 mL in human volunteers results in no change in arterial pressure, but central venous pressure is reduced by as much as 7 cm H_2O.

Unlike arterial pressure, the variation in the arterial waveform can be used to assess the degree of hypovolemia. A decrease in systolic pressure of more than 10 mm Hg with positive pressure ventilation indicates a 10% reduction in blood volume and is more sensitive than central venous pressure (Fig. 23-1).[40]

ORGAN PERFUSION. Monitoring of organ perfusion is indicated during hemorrhage. Although direct measurement of tissue blood flow is still an investigative technique, the pulse oximeter provides quantitative information on oxygenation and a qualitative assessment of tissue perfusion. Urine flow is also a relative indicator of tissue perfusion, especially because renal hypoperfusion and, consequently, decreased urine formation occur early during hypovolemia. The rate of urine flow is approximately 1 mL/kg/hour in normotensive, nonanesthetized humans. Although anesthesia may reduce renal blood flow and urine formation, a urine flow rate of less than 0.5 mL/kg/hour suggests poor renal perfusion. Urine flow is likely to stop during moderate to severe hemorrhagic shock.

BLOOD GAS PARTIAL PRESSURES AND pH. Measurement of arterial oxygen and carbon dioxide partial pressures and pH can be extremely valuable during hypovolemia. However, arterial blood gas values are often misleading during hemorrhage. Typically, the oxygen partial pressure remains normal, and arterial pH is near normal, but the carbon dioxide partial pressure is reduced. With severe hemorrhage, ventilation-perfusion abnormalities and anaerobic metabolism result in arterial hypoxemia and metabolic acidosis, manifested by a decrease in pH, despite hypocapnia.

Tissue hypoxia and hypercapnia always accompany hemorrhagic shock, but these alterations usually are not apparent in the arterial blood. Marked tissue hypoxia and hypercapnia have been demonstrated during hemorrhage despite normal levels of arterial blood gas values.[41] However, central venous blood gas measurements do reflect tissue hypoxia and hypercapnia.[42,43] Normal values for mixed venous oxygen and carbon dioxide partial pressures are approximately 43 and 46 mm Hg, respectively. The value for mixed venous oxygen may decrease to approximately 20 mm Hg, but that for carbon dioxide increases to 55 to 60 mm Hg during hemorrhage in the absence of major changes in arterial blood gases. Mixed venous blood gas measurements become useful monitors of the extent of the microcirculatory impairment accompanying hemorrhage.

Modified pulmonary artery catheters allowing continuous measurement of mixed venous oxygen saturation are the most practical means to accomplish this goal and may be useful during operations such as liver transplantation during which massive blood loss sometimes occurs.

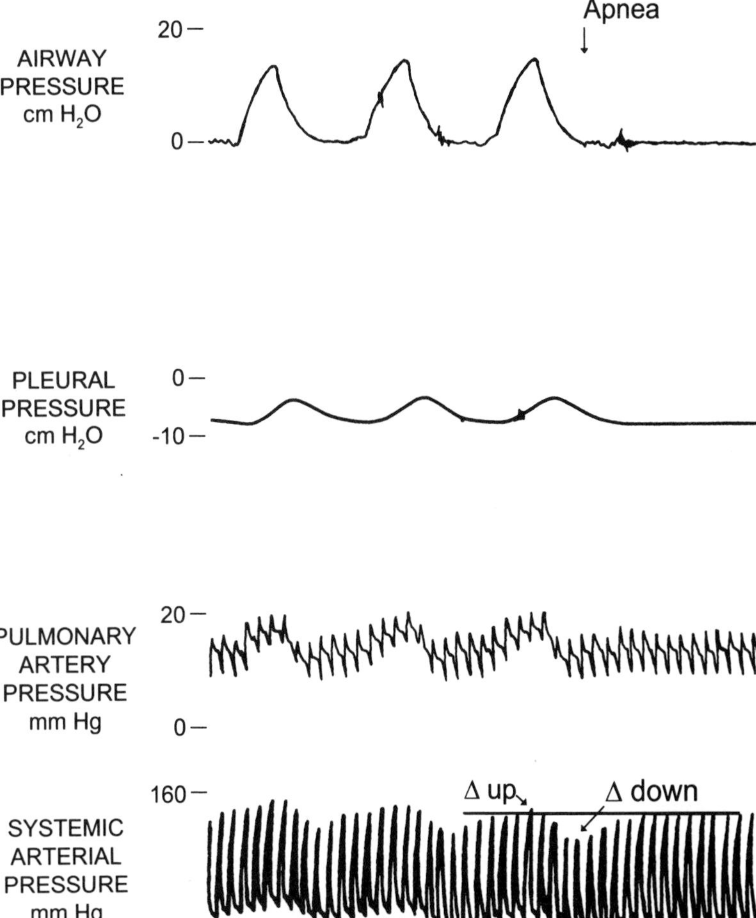

FIGURE 23-1. Continuous record from a single mechanically ventilated dog with inflated thoracic vest after bleeding of 10% of estimated blood volume. The record shows airway, pleural, pulmonary arterial, and systemic pressures. The Δ up and Δ down components of SPV are indicated relative to systolic blood pressure during a 5-s period of apnea. (Perel A, Pizov R, Cotev S: Systolic blood pressure variation is a sensitive indicator of hypovolemia in ventilated dogs subjected to graded hemorrhage. Anesthesiology 67:499, 1987)

NONINVASIVE ASSESSMENT. Pulse oximetry may be a useful monitor for the patient with hypovolemia, particularly if the plethysmographic waveform is observed (Fig. 23-2).[44] However, as peripheral perfusion falls, pulse oximetry may become nonfunctional. Measurement of the partial pressure of transcutaneous oxygen has been advocated, but it has been superseded by the more practical pulse oximetry. During high cardiac output, transcutaneous oxygen fairly accurately reflects arterial oxygen tension, but during low cardiac output, as blood flow through the skin decreases, it follows cardiac index more closely.

Capnography also may be used to assess low-output status.[45] With constant carbon dioxide production and minute ventilation, changes in end-tidal carbon dioxide partial pressure directly correlate with cardiac output.[46]

CARDIAC OUTPUT. Cardiac output is a helpful guide during hemorrhagic shock. Table 23-2 shows the relation between cardiac output and arterial pressure in hemorrhaged dogs.[47] Arterial hypotension is a late manifestation of hemorrhage, because of the accompanying increase in peripheral resistance. Balloon-tipped, flow-directed pulmonary artery catheters allow the measurement of cardiac output (by thermodilution) and the estimation of left atrial pressure during massive fluid replacement accompanying hemorrhage. However, the total cardiac output gives essentially no information regarding the distribution of blood flow and does not replace the measurements of urine flow, blood gases, or heart rate. Although this technique is not essential, it is especially valuable in patients with compromised myocardial function and superimposed hypovolemia.

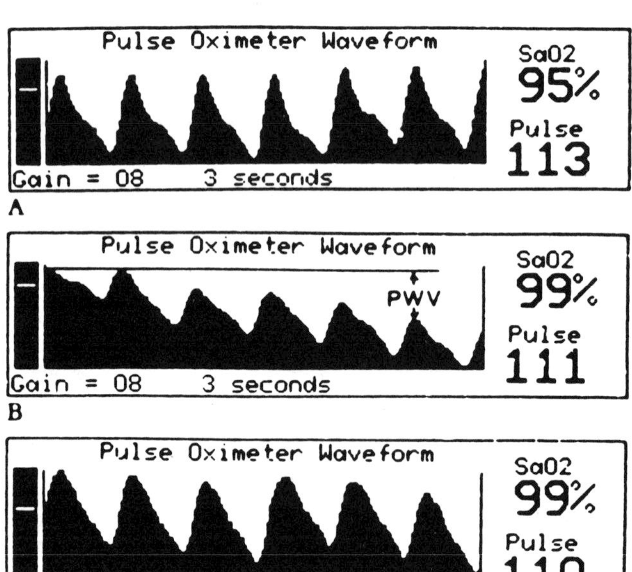

FIGURE 23-2. Pulse oximeter waveform. (A) When the patient arrived in the operating room, central venous pressure was 8 mm Hg. Little variation was seen in the waveform with positive-pressure ventilation. (B) After third-space translocation and blood loss, central venous pressure was 4 to 5 mm Hg. The pulse waveform varied with respiration. The method for measuring pulse waveform variation is shown. (C) After fluid resuscitation, central venous pressure was 8 mm Hg. The pulse waveform no longer showed significant variation with respiration. Sa_{O_2}, arterial oxygen saturation. (Partridge BL: Use of pulse oximetry as a noninvasive indicator of intravascular volume status. J Clin Monit 3:263, 1987.)

TABLE 23-2
Decreases in Cardiac Output and Arterial Pressure During Graded Hemorrhage in Dogs

BLOOD VOLUME REMOVED (%)	CARDIAC OUTPUT (%)	ARTERIAL PRESSURE (%)
10	−21	−7
20	−45	−15

Hinshaw DB, Peterson M, Huse WM, et al: Regional blood flow in hemorrhagic shock. Am J Surg 102:224, 1961.

Therapy

Goals

The essential feature in hemorrhagic shock is tissue ischemia. Ischemia results from a reduction in cardiac output and from increased peripheral vascular resistance. Therapy should be directed toward correcting both aspects. Restoration of effective circulating blood volume is the cornerstone of treatment of hemorrhagic hypotension. Although drug therapy may increase arterial pressure or cardiac output, the only really effective method of restoring arterial pressure, cardiac output, and normal distribution of blood flow requires the restoration of blood volume. Vasopressors should be regarded as temporizing measures, to be used only when absolutely essential and for the shortest possible time.

In the operating room, it is at times possible to predict the occurrence of severe hemorrhage, and in such cases, preventive measures should be taken. If major blood loss is anticipated, the monitoring techniques described previously should be applied, and the availability of sufficient replacement fluid should be ascertained. Preoperative isovolemic hemodilution has been advocated because it can decrease the amount of red cells lost with a certain volume of blood loss, and this method is probably not applied to the extent it could be.[48]

Fluids

BLOOD. Replacement fluids may be categorized according to whether they contain red blood cells, which provide the only method of carrying significant amounts of oxygen in the blood stream. Novel non–blood solutions with oxygen carrying capacity, such as the perfluoro compounds and stroma-free hemoglobin, are still in the investigative stages in the United States. Although concerns about disease transmission have made many clinicians reluctant to administer blood, it should not be withheld until tissue ischemia has occurred. Healthy patients can tolerate hemodilution to a hematocrit of 20% without difficulties if adequate intravascular volume is maintained. In patients with coronary artery disease or critical stenoses in cerebral vessels, a higher hematocrit is recommended.

The amount of blood to be replaced once the decision to transfuse has been made is difficult to recommend on an absolute basis. The adequacy of blood replacement therapy should be evaluated by the clinical signs and monitors described earlier. The goal should be to maintain the hematocrit at an acceptable level while the absence of significant systolic pressure variation and tachycardia, the restoration of central venous pressure and urine output, and the absence of tachycardia indicate that circulating volume has been restored. However, it should be remembered that the fluid losses during hemorrhage exceed the visible loss as a result of the fluid shifts that accompany hemorrhage. Fluid therapy must restore the volume of blood lost from the intravascular compartment and must replace the fluid lost to the interstitium.

Two categories of replacement fluids that do not contain red blood cells are crystalloid solutions (ie, electrolyte solutions) and colloid solutions (ie, solutions with high-molecular-weight molecules).

CRYSTALLOIDS. Crystalloid solutions may be subdivided into saline solutions and balanced salt solutions. Normal saline (0.9% NaCl) does not replace the great number of electrolytes that are contained in extracellular (ie, intravascular or interstitial) fluid. Balanced salt solutions are designed to approximate more nearly the electrolyte composition of the extracellular fluid. During acute hemorrhage, normal saline is still the initial replacement fluid of choice. It is inexpensive, has a long shelf life, and can be given with packed red blood cells. Hypertonic (≥3%) saline solutions are finding increasing use in shock resuscitation, because smaller volumes are required.[49] Their potential disadvantage is the development of hypernatremia.

COLLOIDS. Colloid solutions include those containing molecules with a molecular mass greater than 30,000 daltons. Whole blood, blood components, albumin solutions, and plasma expanders such as hydroxyethyl starch are colloids in clinical use. The relative merits of various nonsanguinous replacement fluids have not been resolved, but hemodynamic stability can be restored by crystalloid or colloid solutions. However, a larger volume of crystalloid is needed to reach the same end point. Crystalloids tend to lower the colloid oncotic pressure, but colloids increase it. Despite the theoretical value of colloid therapy, a recent consensus conference found little justification for its use.[49] Colloids are significantly more expensive than crystalloids; the per patient cost of 500 mL of albumin is approximately $200.

Interest has developed in fractionating hydroxyethyl starch (ie, hetastarch). The molecular mass of hetastarch ranges from 70,000 to 450,000 daltons. New preparations include pentastarch, with a molecular mass of 63,000 to 264,000, and pentafraction, 120,000 to 280,000 daltons. The latter compound has attracted interest, because it may be able to reduce edema formation by "plugging" the openings between endothelial cells. More research is necessary before the clinical role for pentafraction is defined.

Oxygen

Although arterial hypoxemia is uncommon in pure hemorrhagic shock, the administration of supplemental oxygen is advisable to help optimize oxygen delivery to tissues at risk and to help protect against unrecognized pulmonary problems resulting from intrapulmonary shunts or ventilation-perfusion abnormalities. This situation may occur in elderly patients, patients with chronic lung disease, and patients with associated sepsis, pulmonary contusion, or aspiration of gastric contents after multiple trauma. The head-injured patient with a decreased level of consciousness and resultant hypoventilation is at particular risk. Oxygen therapy may be initiated with a fraction of inspired oxygen of approximately 0.4; further adjustments should be based on pulse-oximetric and arterial blood gas values.

Acid-Base Regulation

The usual acid-base response to hemorrhage is metabolic acidosis with superimposed respiratory alkalosis. Generally, the resultant pH is not markedly abnormal. However, acidosis ensues if shock is prolonged. Any significant acid-base disturbance should be addressed promptly. Metabolic acidosis formerly was treated with intravenous sodium bicarbonate, therapy that is increasingly challenged because the carbon dioxide produced may increase intracellular acidosis and thereby worsen the physiologic consequences. Other alkalinizing agents such as tris buffer (Tham), dichloroacetate, and equimolar mixtures of carbonate and bicarbonate (Carbicarb) have not shown clear efficacy or superiority.

The best approach, difficult as it often is, entails treatment and correction of the underlying cause. If respiratory acidosis (ie, arterial hypercapnia) occurs, a significant pulmonary abnormality usually exists that mandates tracheal intubation and assisted ventilation.

Pharmacologic Agents

VASOPRESSORS. In general, vasopressors should not be used for the treatment of hemorrhagic shock. Occasionally, infusion of small amounts may be necessary temporarily to support myocardial and cerebral perfusion until adequate circulating volume has been restored. One of the major pathophysiologic changes during hypovolemia is the development of intense peripheral vasoconstriction; α-adrenergic vasopressors increase the mortality rate for hemorrhaged animals, but pharmacologic blockade (with adrenergic blockers) in conjunction with volume replacement improves survival.[25,26,29–31] Vasopressor therapy should take these findings into consideration.

Dopamine may be the drug of choice when a vasopressor is required. In low dosages (3 to 5 μg/kg/minute) dopamine exhibits a mild positive inotropic effect, minimal chronotropic effects, and no change in peripheral vascular resistance. Stimulation of dopaminergic receptors in the renal vasculature increases renal blood flow, a beneficial effect during hypovolemia. High dosages of dopamine (>10 μg/kg/minute) result in α-adrenergic receptor–mediated vasoconstriction in almost all circulatory beds, including the renal bed, and should be avoided whenever possible.

EXPERIMENTAL THERAPIES. The beneficial effects of opioid antagonists, such as naloxone, have been studied. In various models of shock, naloxone administration is associated with improved cardiovascular function and survival, although not with altered organ perfusion, during hemorrhage.[51] The mechanism of action has not been elucidated, but it appears that opioid systems in the brain stem and midbrain affect autonomic outflow so that sympathetic activity is inhibited during shock, an effect that is antagonized by naloxone. However, improved human survival rates have not been demonstrated.

In pharmacologic doses, protirelin (thyrotropin-releasing hormone) and T_3 (triiodothyronine) also have protective effects in hemorrhagic shock.[52,53]

STEROIDS. The use of steroids in the therapy of hemorrhagic shock has been praised and condemned during the past 25 years. In laboratory animals, steroids block the intense arteriolar constriction associated with hypotension, without producing vasodilation.[54] This effect is similar to that achieved with α-adrenergic receptor–blocking drugs but without the potential for severe hypotension resulting from arteriolar dilation.

Steroids appear to restore arteriolar diameters and vascular resistance to near-normal values, and α-adrenergic blockade changes vasoconstriction to vasodilation. The survival rates of hemorrhaged animals are improved considerably when steroids are administered shortly after the period of hemorrhage.[54] The administration of steroids also produced significant hemodynamic improvements in hypovolemic patients: cardiac output increased, and pulmonary and systemic vascular resistances decreased after steroid administration during hemorrhagic shock.[55] These findings were not reproduced by later work. In two well-controlled studies of septic shock, no efficacy was found and detrimental effects were reported.[56,57] Similarly, improved survival after hypovolemic shock, as seen in animals, has not been found in humans, even after massive doses of glucocorticosteroids.

Prevention of Renal Failure

One of the most disturbing complications of hemorrhagic shock in a patient who survives the initial hypotensive insult is subsequent development of acute renal failure. Significant hypotension markedly reduces total renal blood flow and especially renal cortical blood flow.[15]

The effects of anesthetics on renal blood flow during hemorrhage are controversial.[7,58–60] Seyde and Longnecker reported decreased renal blood flow with ketamine, isoflurane, enflurane, and halothane, compared with flow in the awake control condition, during hemorrhage in rats anesthetized before hemorrhage.[7] However, Priano, in a study using dogs anesthetized after being hemorrhaged, found no significant changes in renal blood flow during halothane anesthesia.[58] Peters and colleagues compared renal lesions histologically in anesthetized rats after hemorrhage and reported a protective effect from enflurane, methoxyflurane, and halothane, but little or no protection by ketamine.[60] Some of the differences among these results may reflect differences in experimental protocol, but more research is needed to resolve the controversy.

Although definitive data for humans are lacking, laboratory results indicate that furosemide[61] and mannitol[62] may selectively increase renal cortical blood flow. When oliguria occurs, therapy with one or both of these diuretic agents is appropriate, although proof of benefit does not exist. The intraoperative urinary output was not predictive of postoperative renal function when blood volume was maintained in patients undergoing abdominal aortic reconstruction.[63] The initial dose of furosemide is 0.5 mg/kg administered intravenously, and the dose is doubled after 30 minutes if oliguria persists. Mannitol (0.25 g/kg, intravenously) also may be administered to attempt to restore renal perfusion and urine output.

Anesthetic Management

Anesthetics differ in their hemodynamic effects during normovolemia and hypovolemia. An important cause of these differences is the influence of the anesthetics on the sympathetic nervous system.[64] Although little objective evidence has been obtained from humans to support one anesthetic technique over another, some data are available that compare various anesthetics in animals.

In severely hypovolemic patients, all general anesthetics pose significant risks. In those instances, modest doses of scopolamine or benzodiazepines should be employed to prevent recall, combined with a muscle relaxant (preferably pancuronium) to prevent reflex motor responses to surgery. In somewhat more stable patients, ketamine, etomidate, isoflurane, or narcotics may be considered.

KETAMINE. Ketamine has attracted much attention because it has been alleged to lower mortality,[65] to support blood pressure by increasing cardiac output,[58] and compared with enflurane, to reduce arteriolar constriction and tissue hypoxia in hemorrhaged animals.[66] Compared with halothane, ketamine is associated with less histologic evidence of tissue hypoxia and a smaller increase in lactate concentration.[67] Survival and histologic and biochemical data support the use of ketamine during hemorrhage. However, decreases in blood pressure and cardiac output have been reported in hemorrhaged rats anesthetized with ketamine compared with those receiving isoflurane.[7] Cardiac output has increased during ketamine anesthesia in dogs before hemorrhage but decreased after hemorrhage; systemic vascular resistance tended to rise.[68] Ketamine also increases intracranial pressure and should therefore be used with caution or not at all in patients with head trauma.

Ketamine is a direct cardiac depressant, although this effect tends to be obscured by its stimulating activity on the sympathetic system. However, if further increases in sympathetic activity cannot occur, as in hypovolemic trauma patients or those in cardiac failure, the depressant effects of ketamine may be unmasked, resulting in decreased cardiac output.

ETOMIDATE. Etomidate is a useful agent for inducing anesthesia in hypovolemic patients, particularly those with poor cardiac function. The drug depresses adrenal steroid production. However, this effect does not appear to be a problem when etomidate is used as a single bolus for induction. Increases in morbidity and mortality have only been reported after prolonged infusions. Nonetheless, steroid administration is appropriate in patients with a history of steroid use.

ISOFLURANE. Isoflurane may most closely approximate the awake state during hypovolemia in terms of its effects on blood pressure, cardiac output, and stroke volume. These findings are at odds with those of a study that found no major differences among halothane, enflurane, or isoflurane under similar circumstances.[68]

NARCOTICS. The semisynthetic narcotics, particularly fentanyl, have been used successfully. In low doses, recall is a problem in as many as 40% of patients anesthetized. Small doses of midazolam may render the patient amnestic. Larger doses of fentanyl (>20 μg/kg) may be tolerated poorly. Experience with alfentanil and sufentanil in shock is limited.

SEPTIC SHOCK

Pathophysiology

Most cases of septic shock result from bacteremia produced by gram-negative enteric bacilli. The specific shock-producing agent is believed to be an endotoxin, a lipoprotein-carbohydrate complex in the bacterial cell wall. However, several structural components of other microorganisms also can cause mediator release. The precise role of most mediators in septic shock is unknown; kinins, histamine, complement, prostaglandins, serotonin, tumor necrosis factor, and various other interleukins all have been implicated.

Septic shock may be characterized by at least two distinct stages. Early endotoxin shock, the classic hyperdynamic phase, is manifested by fever, chills, hypotension, and warmth in the extremities. Hemodynamic studies reveal a normal or increased cardiac output and a reduced systemic vascular resistance, despite hypotension. The sympathoadrenal response to this hypotension may be blunted by anesthetics. Many patients have increased pulmonary vascular resistance and evidence of pulmonary hypertension, and the mortality rate is high.

As shock progresses, vasodilation is rapidly replaced by peripheral vasoconstriction and reduced cardiac output, which characterize the hypodynamic phase. This later stage of endotoxin shock closely resembles hemorrhagic shock in most respects, including hemodynamic, respiratory, and metabolic alterations.[69] Because the phases of septic shock are associated with widely different hemodynamic profiles, a pulmonary artery catheter is recommended for monitoring and treatment.

The role of myocardial depression during sepsis is still controversial. Although most patients have increased cardiac output during the early phase of shock, a subgroup may have a decreased cardiac index.[70] In either condition, decreased perfusion of the tissues with resultant cellular damage probably occurs. In septic shock, the glucose to lactate ratio can be a useful monitor; values less than 10 indicate inadequate liver function and possible hepatocellular damage.[71]

Treatment

Elimination of the source of infection is the major goal in septic shock and is accomplished primarily by two methods: appropriate antibiotic therapy and surgical drainage of the infected site.

Because the late, severe manifestations of septic shock are almost identical to those of hemorrhagic shock, the same therapeutic principles apply in both conditions. Fluid replacement, correction of acid-base disturbance, and avoidance of potent peripheral vasoconstrictor drugs are important aspects in the management of septic shock, just as they are in hemorrhagic shock. Corticosteroids have not proven to be effective.[56,57] Large volumes of fluid often are required to correct the intravascular volume deficits associated with sequestration of fluid, fever, vomiting, and diarrhea. Because gluconeogenesis is depressed, infusions with glucose, insulin, and potassium have been suggested, but definitive evidence of their value is lacking. Therapy employing specific antagonists directed against various intercellular mediators seems to offer promise, although these drugs are still in the developmental stages.[35]

OTHER CAUSES OF PERIPHERAL CIRCULATORY FAILURE

Three less common causes of peripheral circulatory failure that may be encountered in the operating room are hypoxia, carcinoid syndrome, and the application of methylmethacrylate cement.

Hypoxia

The cardiovascular responses to hypoxia, with or without accompanying hypercapnia, are not clearly defined in humans. Of necessity, only relatively mild or brief hypoxic periods have been studied. In animals, the circulatory responses to hypoxia and hypercapnia are time and dose dependent; anesthetics significantly blunt these responses. Overall, the circulatory responses to hypoxia or hypercapnia reflect the combination of responses to the direct vascular effects of the gases plus the neural and humoral responses triggered by the changes in their concentrations through mechanisms such as carotid chemoreception.

Typically, arterial hypoxemia without hypercapnia produces tachycardia and hypertension and increases cardiac output. Total systemic and pulmonary vascular resistance is increased, although individual vascular beds may respond quite differently. The renal and skeletal muscle vasculature constricts during arterial hypoxemia,[72] but coronary and cerebral arterioles dilate.[73] These changes are consistent with the well-established physiologic principle that redistribution of blood flow during cellular hypoxia (resulting from ischemia or hypoxemia) tends to preserve essential organs at the expense of less vital ones.

Anesthesia affects these responses considerably.[74] Although brain and coronary blood flows increase during hypoxemia in awake rats, flow decreases in those anesthetized with halothane, enflurane, or isoflurane. Although hypoxemia does not alter renal, gastrointestinal, or hepatic blood flow in awake rats, decreases are seen during hypoxia in anesthetized animals. Volatile anesthetics modify the compensatory responses to hypoxemia that occur in the awake animal, resulting in decreased blood flow to vital organs.

Cardiovascular responses to hypoxia are enhanced by hypercapnia, and intestinal vasodilation also is seen when carbon dioxide tensions are elevated.[72] Hypercapnia in nonanesthetized humans and animals results in hypertension, tachycardia, and increases in cardiac output and in systemic and pulmonary vascular resistances. The fraction of cardiac output distributed to the brain and gut is enhanced by hypercapnia, but renal and skeletal muscle blood flow are reduced by vasoconstriction.[72] Hyperventilation can be identified by the monitoring of end-tidal or arterial carbon dioxide partial pressure.

Carcinoid Syndrome

Carcinoid tumors occur most commonly in the gastrointestinal tract and the bronchial tree. The tumors contain chromaffin tissue, the secretions of which include serotonin, vasoactive polypeptides such as bradykinin, and prostaglandins. The carcinoid syndrome consists of marked cutaneous flushing, hypotension, diarrhea, tachycardia, and bronchospasm. Symptoms result from the sudden release of vasoactive substances from the tumors and often are associated with stress or alcohol ingestion.

Because the treatment of this syndrome involves surgical excision of the tumors, these cases present special hazards for the anesthetist. Hypotension resulting from peripheral vasodilation may accompany anesthetic induction and operative manipulation of the tumor. Hypotension may be enhanced by the use of vasopressors, which can stimulate the release of vasoactive substances from the tumors. Pure α-adrenergic receptor agonists, such as phenylephrine, appear not to enhance tumor secretion. The principles of good anesthetic care, including careful attention to anesthetic depth and fluid balance, are cornerstones in the management of these cases.

Methylmethacrylate Cement

Arterial hypoxemia, hypotension, and even cardiac arrest have been associated with the introduction of acrylic cement into bone (especially the femoral shaft) during orthopedic surgery, usually for total hip replacement. However, investigations in animals and humans strongly suggest that the cement itself is not the cause of these respiratory and circulatory alterations.[75-77] Intravenous infusions of the monomer do not produce cardiovascular or pulmonary changes, unless the concentration of cement is many times that seen in clinical practice. The alterations appear to result from embolization produced by the high pressures occurring in the marrow cavities during implantation of the prosthesis. Possible mechanisms include fat and gas embolization and the release of tissue-thromboplastic substances.[76] The anesthetic management includes the use of high inspired oxygen concentrations and adequate fluid volume at the time of prosthetic implantation. Venting of the femoral shaft to reduce the amount of embolization is especially helpful.[77]

REFERENCES

1. Dalen JE, Evans GL, Banas JS Jr, et al: The hemodynamic and respiratory effects of diazepam. Anesthesiology 30:259, 1969
2. Drew JH, Dripps RD, Comroe JH Jr: Clinical studies on morphine: II. The effect of morphine upon the circulation of man and upon the circulatory and respiratory responses to tilting. Anesthesiology 7:44, 1946
3. Gooding J, Corssen G: Effect of etomidate on the cardiovascular system. Anesth Analg 56: 717, 1977
4. Lowenstein E, Hallowell P, Levine FH, et al: Cardiovascular response to large doses of intravenous morphine in man. N Engl J Med 281:1389, 1969
5. Tweed WA, Minuck M, Mymin D: Circulatory responses to ketamine. Anesthesiology 37:613, 1972
6. Durieux ME: Inhibition by ketamine of muscarinic acetylcholine receptor function. Anesth Analg 81:57, 1995
7. Seyde WC, Longnecker DE: Anesthetic influences on regional hemodynamics in normal and hemorrhaged rats. Anesthesiology 61:686, 1984
8. Eger EI II, Smith NT, Stoelting RK, et al: Cardiovascular effects of halothane in man. Anesthesiology 32:396, 1970
9. Johns RA, DiFazio CA, Longnecker DE: Lidocaine constricts or dilates rat arterioles in a dose-dependent manner. Anesthesiology 62:141, 1985
10. Johns RA, Seyde WC, DiFazio CA, et al: Dose-dependent effects of bupivacaine on rat muscle arterioles. Anesthesiology 65:186, 1986
11. Tung SH, Bettice J, Wang BO, et al: Intracellular and extracellular acid-base changes in hemorrhagic shock. Respir Physiol 26:229, 1976
12. Blahitka J, Rakusan K: Blood flow in rats during hemorrhagic shock: differences between surviving and dying animals. Circ Shock 4:79, 1977
13. Lefer AM: Role of a myocardial depressant factor in the pathogenesis of circulatory shock. Fed Proc 29:1836, 1970
14. Culpepper RD, Kondo Y, Hardy JO, et al: Successful orthotopic allotransplantation of hearts from dogs in irreversible shock. Surgery 77:126, 1975
15. Beck C: Disordered renal function: diagnosis. In Civetta JM, Taylor RW, Kirby RR (eds): Critical care. Philadelphia: JB Lippincott, 1988: 1315
16. Lillehei RC: The intestinal factor in irreversible hemorrhagic shock. Surgery 42:1043, 1957
17. Border G, Weil MH: Excess lactate: an index of reversibility of shock in human patients. Science 143:1457, 1964
18. Farnebo LO, Fredholm BB, Hamburger B: Cyclic AMP and metabolic substrates following hemorrhage in awake and anesthetized rats. Acta Anaesthesiol Scand 24:206, 1980
19. Haddy FJ, Scott JB, Molnar JI: Mechanism of volume replacement and vascular constriction following hemorrhage. Am J Physiol 208:169, 1965
20. Chien S, Dellenback RJ, Usami S, et al: Blood volume, hemodynamic, and metabolic changes in hemorrhagic shock in normal and splenectomized dogs. Am J Physiol 225:886, 1973
21. Archer DP: The role of bloodletting in the prevention and treatment of asthenic apoplexy. J Neurosurg Anesthesiol 6:51, 1994
22. Cahill JM, Byrne JJ: Ventilatory mechanics in hypovolemic shock. J Appl Physiol 19:679, 1964
23. Gerst PH, Rattenborg C, Holday DA: The effects of hemorrhage on pulmonary circulation and respiratory gas exchange. J Clin Invest 38:524, 1959
24. Clowes GHA Jr, Hirsch E, Williams L, et al: Septic lung and shock lung in man. Ann Surg 181:681, 1975
25. Hakstian RW, Hampson LG, Gurd FN: Pharmacologic agents in experimental hemorrhagic shock: a controlled comparison of treatment with hydralazine, hydrocortisone, and levarterenol. Arch Surg 83:335, 1961
26. Close AS, Wagner JA, Klochn RA, et al: The effect of norepinephrine on survival in experimental acute hemorrhagic hypotension. Surg Forum 8:22, 1957
27. Jakschik BA, Garland RM, Kourik JL, et al: Profile of circulating vasoactive substances in hemorrhagic shock and their pharmacologic manipulation. J Clin Invest 54:842, 1974
28. Hall RC, Hodge RL: Changes in catecholamine and angiotensin levels in the cat and dog during hemorrhage. Am J Physiol 221: 1305, 1971
29. Errington ML, Rocha E, Silva M: On the role of vasopressin and

angiotensin in the development of irreversible hemorrhagic shock. J Physiol 242:119, 1974
30. Halmagyi DFJ: Combined adrenergic receptor blockade in experimental post-hemorrhagic shock. In Forscher BK, Lillehei RC, Stubbs SS (eds): Shock in low- and high-flow states. Amsterdam: Excerpta Medica, 1972: 49
31. Errington ML, Rocha E, Silva M: On the role of vasopressin and angiotensin in the development of irreversible hemorrhagic shock. J Physiol 242:119, 1979
32. Burke SE, DiCola G, Lefer AM: Protection of ischemic cat myocardium by CGS-13080, a selective potent thromboxane A_2 synthesis inhibitor. J Cardiovasc Pharmacol 5:842, 1983
33. Bone RC: Phospholipids and their inhibitors: a critical evaluation of their role in the treatment of sepsis. Crit Care Med 20:884, 1992
34. Lefer AM: Eicosanoids as mediators of ischemia and shock. Fed Proc 44:275, 1985
35. Kashiwagi H, Suzuki H: Specific cytokine regulators and their therapeutic potentials—an overview. Int Med 31:1245, 1992
36. Anggard E: Nitric oxide: mediator, murderer, and medicine. Lancet 343:1199, 1994
37. Durieux ME, Lynch KR: Signalling properties of lysophosphatidic acid. Trends Pharmacol Sci 14:249, 1993
38. Seward JB, Khanderia BK, Edwards WD, et al: Biplanar transesophageal echocardiography: anatomic correlations, image orientation, and clinical applications. Mayo Clin Proc 65:1193, 1990
39. Gauer OH, Henry JP, Sieker HO: Changes in central venous pressure after moderate hemorrhage and transfusion in man. Circ Res 4:79, 1956
40. Perel A, Pizov R, Cotev S: Systolic blood pressure variation is a sensitive indicator of hypovolemia in ventilated dogs subjected to graded hemorrhage. Anesthesiology 67:498, 1987
41. Brantigan JW, Ziegler EC, Hynes KM, et al: Tissue gases during hypovolemic shock. J Appl Physiol 37:117, 1974
42. Halmagyi DFJ, Kennedy M, Varga D: Hidden hypercapnia in hemorrhagic hypotension. Anesthesiology 33:594, 1970
43. Lee J, Wright F, Barber R, et al: Central venous oxygen saturation in shock. Anesthesiology 36:472, 1972
44. Partridge BL: Use of pulse oximetry as a noninvasive indicator of intravascular volume status. J Clin Monit 3:263, 1987
45. Callahan M, Barton C: Prediction of outcome of cardiopulmonary resuscitation from end-tidal carbon dioxide concentration. Crit Care Med 18:358, 1990
46. Gravenstein N, Good M: Noninvasive assessment of cardiopulmonary function. In Civetta JM, Taylor RW, Kirby RR (eds): Critical care, 2nd ed. Philadelphia: JB Lippincott, 1992: 291
47. Hinshaw DB, Peterson M, Huse WM, et al: Regional blood flow in hemorrhagic shock. Am J Surg 102:224, 1961
48. Feldman JM, Roth JV, Bjoraker DG: Maximum blood savings by acute normovolemic hemodilution. Anesth Analg 8:108, 1995
49. Layon AJ, Bernards WC, Kirby RR: Fluids and electrolytes in the critically ill. In Civetta JM, Taylor RW, Kirby RR (eds): Critical care, 2nd ed. Philadelphia: JB Lippincott, 1992: 457
50. Center for Biologies; Food and Drug Administration and National Heart, Lung, and Blood Institute, Division of Blood Diseases and Resources: Workshop on assessment of plasma volume expanders. Bethesda, MD: March 25 and 26, 1991
51. Coates DP, Seyde WC, Epstein RM, et al: The influence of naloxone on regional hemodynamics in hemorrhaged rats. Circ Shock 16:173, 1985
52. Dulchavsky SA, Lucas CE, Ledgerwood AM, Grabow D, Brown TR, Bagchi N: Triiodothyronine (T_3) improves cardiovascular function during hemorrhagic shock. Circ Shock 39:68, 1993
53. Zheng D, Chen HS, Hu DY: Cardiovascular mechanisms of thyrotropin-releasing hormone against experimental hemorrhagic shock. Circ Shock 36:169, 1992
54. Altura BM, Altura BT: Peripheral vascular actions of glucocorticoids and their relationship to protection in circulatory shock. J Pharmacol Exp Ther 190:300, 1974
55. Lozman J, Dutton RE, English M, et al: Cardiopulmonary adjustments following single high dose administration of methylprednisolone in traumatized man. Ann Surg 181:317, 1975
56. Bove RC, Fisher CJ, Clemmer TP, et al: A controlled clinical trial of high dose methylprednisolone in the treatment of severe sepsis and septic shock. N Engl J Med 317:653, 1987
57. Veterans Administration Systemic Sepsis Cooperative Study Groups: Effect of high-dose glucocorticoid therapy on mortality in patients with clinical signs of systemic sepsis. N Engl J Med 317:659, 1987
58. ldvall J: Influence of ketamine anesthesia on cardiac output and tissue perfusion in rats subjected to hemorrhage. Anesthesiology 55:297, 1981
59. Priano LL: Effect of halothane on renal hemodynamics during normovolemia and acute hemorrhagic hypovolemia. Anesthesiology 63:357, 1985
60. Peters JM, Van der Meer C, Czanky JC, et al: Effects of anesthetics on mortality and kidney lesions caused by hypertension. Arch Int Pharmacodyn Ther 238:134, 1979
61. Birtch AG, Zakheim RM, Jones LG, et al: Redistribution of renal blood flow produced by furosemide and ethacrynic acid. Circ Res 21:869, 1967
62. Abbott WM, Austen WG: The reversal of renal cortical ischemia during aortic occlusion by mannitol. J Surg Res 16:482, 1974
63. Alpert RA, Roizen MF, Hamilton WF, et al: Intraoperative urinary output does not predict postoperative renal function in patients undergoing abdominal aortic revascularization. Surgery 95:707, 1984
64. Hamberger B, Bengtsson L, Jarnberg PO, et al: Anesthetic agents and sympatho-adrenal response to hemorrhage in the rat. Acta Chir Scand 520:109, 1984
65. Longnecker DE, Sturgill BC: Influence of anesthetic agent on survival following hemorrhage. Anesthesiology 45:516, 1976
66. Longnecker DE, Ross DC, Silver IA: Anesthetic influences on arteriolar diameters and tissue oxygen tension in hemorrhaged rats. Anesthesiology 57:177, 1982
67. Longnecker DE, McCoy S, Drucker WR: Anesthetic influence on response to hemorrhage in rats. Circ Shock 6:55, 1979
68. Weiskopf RB, Townsley MI, Riordan KK, et al: Comparison of cardiopulmonary responses to graded hemorrhage during enflurane, halothane, isoflurane and ketamine anesthesia. Anesth Analg 60:481, 1981
69. Rutherford RB, Balis JB, Trow RS, et al: Comparison of hemodynamic and regional blood flow changes at equivalent stages of endotoxin and hemorrhagic shock. J Trauma 16:886, 1976
70. Parker MM, Parillo JE: Septic shock, hemodynamics and pathogenesis. JAMA 250:3324, 1983
71. Schumer W: Pathophysiology and treatment of septic shock. Am J Emerg Med 2:74,1983
72. Weissman ML, Rubinstein EH, Sonnenschein RR: Vascular responses to short-term systemic hypoxia, hypercapnia, and asphyxia in the cat. Am J Physiol 230:595, 1976
73. Wyler F: Effects of hypoxia on distribution of cardiac output and organ blood flow in the rabbit. Cardiology 60:163, 1975
74. Durieux ME, Sperry RJ, Longnecker DE: Effects of hypoxemia on regional blood flows during anesthesia with halothane, enflurane or isoflurane. Anesthesiology 76: 402, 1992
75. Modig J, Busch C, Waermbaum G: Effects of graded infusions of monomethylmethacrylate on coagulation, blood lipids, respiration, and circulation. Clin Orthop 113:187, 1975
76. Modig H, Busch C, Olerud S, et al: Arterial hypotension and hypoxaemia during total hip replacement: the importance of thromboplastic products, fat embolism and acrylic monomers. Acta Anaesthesiol Scand 19:28, 1975
77. Kallos T: Impaired arterial oxygenation associated with use of bone cement in the femoral shaft. Anesthesiology 42:210, 1975
78. Gooding JM, Smith RA, Weng JT: Is methylmethacrylate safer than previously thought? Anesth Analg 59:542, 1980

Complications in Anesthesiology, second edition,
edited by Nikolaus Gravenstein and Robert R. Kirby.
Lippincott-Raven Publishers, Philadelphia © 1996.

CHAPTER 24

Perioperative Myocardial Infarction

Sandra L. Roberts
John H. Tinker

Among the most feared complications in surgery and anesthesia, myocardial infarction (MI) is also one of the earliest described.[1–4] Yet despite our awareness of the association of this complication with coronary artery disease (CAD) and certain risk factors, the incidence of MI is generally unchanged. This chapter takes an epidemiologic view, surveying the characteristics of patients most at risk for MI and the practical issues involved in reducing its incidence.

PREVALENCE OF CORONARY ARTERY DISEASE

CAD is pandemic in the United States and other well-developed countries. It is responsible for one third to one half of all deaths in the United States, or approximately 500,000 per year. One third to one half of these cases have no preceding symptoms and are classified as "sudden deaths."[5] An autopsy study of 23,996 asymptomatic persons who died of noncoronary causes revealed greater than 50% narrowing of one coronary vessel in 6.4% of men and 2.6% of women. However, after 65 years of age, 12.3% of men and 7.5% of women in this study had autopsy evidence of CAD.[6]

Studies of the prevalence of angiographically demonstrable CAD, categorized on the basis of the pattern of chest pain, indicate that almost 90% of patients with typical angina pectoris, 54% with atypical angina pectoris, and 11% with nonanginal chest pain actually have CAD confirmed at cardiac catheterization (Table 24-1).[7–12] The presence of ST-segment or T-wave abnormalities on the resting electrocardiogram (ECG) should increase the clinician's's consideration of CAD in patients with angina or atypical angina.[12]

Many patients with known or possible CAD require anesthetic care, but definitive noninvasive diagnosis of CAD is often difficult to obtain. Noninvasive techniques are expensive even when used in appropriately selected patients and may be frustratingly inconclusive if used indiscriminately. Familiarity with cardiac risk factors[13] can be valuable in guiding appropriate preoperative evaluation and in determining who is most at risk for perioperative cardiac complications.

CARDIAC RISK FACTORS IN THE GENERAL POPULATION

Increasing Age

Not unexpectedly, increasing age correlates with increasing cardiac risk. The average age at the time of a first MI is 55 years for men and 65 years for women. In the previously mentioned autopsy study of asymptomatic persons between the ages of 30 and 39 years, 1.9% of men and 0.3% of women had CAD, whereas between the ages of 60 and 69 years, 12.3% and 7.5%, respectively, had CAD.[6] Aging, of course, is not subject to individual control.

Gender

Gender is another inflexible risk factor. The chance that cardiovascular disease will develop by age 65 years is 37% for men and 18% for women.[14]

Family History

Family history is a third unchangeable, prominent risk factor. First-degree male relatives of men who died of CAD at less

This work was funded in part through National Institutes of Health grant GM 33137-03.

TABLE 24-1
Prevalence of Significant Angiographic Coronary Artery Disease in Middle-aged Patients According to Chest Pain Classifications

STUDY	YEAR	PATIENTS (no.)	ANGINA PECTORIS Typical (%)	ANGINA PECTORIS Atypical (%)	NONANGINAL CHEST PAIN (%)
Proudfit et al	1966[8]	790	89	58	10
Campeau et al	1968[9]	131	80	42	4
Friesinger and Smith	1972[10]	251	92	66	16
McConahay et al	1971[11]	100	96	42	12
Weiner et al	1979[12]	2045	85	61	13
Total (average)		**3317**	**88**	**54**	**11**

Adapted from Gibson RS, Beller GA: Should exercise electrocardiographic testing be replaced by radioisotope methods? In Rahimtoola S (ed): Controversies in coronary artery disease. Philadelphia: FA Davis, 1983:5.

than 55 years of age are 5.2 times more likely to die of coronary causes than are those without this history and 2.8 times more likely if a first-degree female relative died of coronary causes before the age of 65.[15] Women younger than 65 years who have a first-degree male relative who died of heart disease before age 55 years are 6.4 times more likely to have coronary death and 6.9 times more likely if a first-degree female relative died of heart disease.[15] A family history of early coronary deaths or undiagnosed sudden death combined with other risk factors suggests the need for a more aggressive diagnostic evaluation to establish the presence or absence of heart disease.

Personality Type

A fourth and highly controversial risk factor is personality type. Rosenman and colleagues described patients of "type A" personality as more susceptible to CAD. This personality type is characterized by a pressing sense of urgency, hostility, enhanced aggressivity, competitive drive, and chronic impatience. Type A men aged 39 to 49 years were 1.87 times more likely to have CAD compared with calmer, "type B" men; this risk increased to a 2.16 times greater likelihood for men 50 to 59 years old.[16]

Success has been reported in modifying type A behavior through counseling. These patients recovering from their first MI who received behavioral counseling had a reinfarction rate of 7.2%, whereas those who received routine postcoronary counseling had a reinfarction rate of 13%.[17] Others argue that personality, like age, family history, and gender, is not a risk factor that can be changed.

Smoking

Cigarette smoking is a coronary risk factor that is under more individual control than are the aforementioned factors. Unlike pipe or cigar smoking, cigarette smoking has been shown to increase the risk of CAD and sudden death. Thirty-seven percent of the 325,000 premature deaths per year in smokers in the United States are attributable to CAD.[18] In men 45 to 74 years of age, smoking more than 20 cigarettes per day doubles the risk of sudden death. Cessation of cigarette smoking results in the halving of one's coronary risk within 1 year.[18] Smoking combined with use of birth control pills can further increase risk, particularly in women older than 35 years.[19] For cigarette smokers, the most important way to reduce coronary risk is to stop smoking.

Hyperlipidemia

Hyperlipidemia predisposes to CAD, particularly in patients with decreased high-density lipoproteins and increased low-density lipoproteins, cholesterol, and triglycerides. In 85% of patients with hypercholesterolemia, an MI occurs by age 60 years, in contrast to its occurrence in 20% in the general population.[5] Fifty percent of men with hypercholesterolemia die of MI before the age of 60 years—a rate 15 times greater than in the general population.[15]

This risk factor may be reduced through diet modification and medication. In a large multicenter study, in men with primary hypercholesterolemia, cholestyramine treatment resulted in a 13.4% reduction in low-density lipoprotein cholesterol. The cholestyramine group showed a 24% reduction in definite CAD death and a 19% reduction in nonfatal MI. In addition, incidences were reduced by 25% for new positive exercise tests, 20% for new onset angina, and 21% for coronary artery bypass graft (CABG) surgery.[20] Treatment in this high-risk group offers definite benefit. Although the costs of this pharmacologic therapy are high, it may be even more cost-effective when combined with a variety of low-cost initiatives (eg, dietary change or cessation of smoking).[21]

Hypertension

Hypertension has long been known to accelerate atherosclerosis.[22] Systolic hypertension is associated with a five times greater risk of cardiovascular death. Medical control, coupled with sodium restriction and weight reduction where indicated, can lower this risk factor.[19] After an aggressive "systematic" antihypertensive program in one large study, 50% of patients were able to achieve normal diastolic pressures.[23] Five-year mortality from all causes was reduced by 17% in the systematic-care group compared with patients referred to community facilities for blood pressure management. Twenty-six percent fewer MI deaths occurred in the systematic-care group.[23]

Diabetes Mellitus

Diabetes is a well-known risk factor: diabetic patients have an increased incidence and earlier onset of CAD than do nondiabetic persons. For men 40 to 64 years old with blood sugar concentrations greater than the 98th percentile by the glucose tolerance test, the CAD mortality rate is approximately doubled.[24] The atherosclerotic process in these patients affects small vessels preferentially, a feature that has great relevance for the success of subsequent coronary revascularization procedures. Whether tight glucose control can materially reduce cardiac risk in this susceptible patient group is unknown and remains very controversial.

Obesity and Sedentary Lifestyle

Obesity and sedentary lifestyle are other less well-established risk factors. Of course, there may be overlap among risk factors such as obesity, hypertension, hyperlipidemia, and physical inactivity. This overlap combines with influences of both genetic and cultural heritage to make further differentiation of these traits as separate risk factors difficult. For example, assuming a risk factor of isolated systolic hypertension at 150 mm Hg, the chance that a serious cardiovascular event will occur in the next 8 years is 4.3% in men. Adding four other risk factors—cholesterol greater than or equal to 335 mg/dL, glucose intolerance, cigarette smoking, and left ventricular hypertrophy demonstrated on a resting ECG—the risk increases to 63.3%. In women, hypertension alone carries a 2.4% risk of serious cardiovascular sequelae in the next 8 years, but when it is combined with the other factors, the risk increases to 24.3%.[18]

CARDIAC RISK FACTORS AND ANESTHESIA OUTCOME

Studies of the influence of cardiac risk factors on CAD and the outcome of anesthesia have used preoperative MI as a marker to define CAD and another MI as a definable postoperative event.[13] MI is not likely to be forgotten or overlooked by the patient and is usually documented in the medical records of previous hospital admissions or demonstrated by ECG changes. The occurrence of MI is also easier to document postoperatively than is transient myocardial ischemia.

Perioperative Myocardial Infarction

Incidence

The incidence of perioperative MI (<7 days after noncardiac surgery) in all patients without a history of previous MI has been reported in the range of 0.13% to 0.66% (Table 24-2).[25-28] In patients with a previous history of MI, however, the reported incidence of perioperative MI increases to 4.3% to 15.9% (Table 24-3).[25-31] (However, in a prospective study by Rao and colleagues, the incidence was 1.9%.[31] This group is discussed below.) In patients who had MI within 3 months prior to surgery, the incidence of myocardial reinfarction perioperatively ranges from 27%[29] to 37%.[26] Surgery 3 to 6 months after MI is complicated by perioperative reinfarction 6%[30] to 54%[26] of the time. After 6 months, the incidence decreases to 4% to 6%, the same as for any patient with a previous MI.[25-31]

Thus, 6 months or more after MI, no further diminution of risk seems to occur; from this comes the commonly cited recommendation that surgery be postponed for at least 6 months after MI, when possible.

Mortality

The mortality associated with perioperative MI is substantial: 27% to 69% for patients without previous MI (see Table 24-2),[25-28] and 28% to 70% for those with previous MI (see Table 24-3).[25-31] These mortality rates are considerably higher than the 20% mortality rate for MIs not associated with surgery and anesthesia.[32] Until the report by Rao and colleagues in 1983,[31] the incidence of perioperative MI and associated mortality had remained essentially unchanged for 20 years, despite growing awareness of the high-risk status of these patients and numerous improvements in anesthetic practice.

Recent Improvements

In an attempt to alter these apparently unimprovable mortality rates, Rao and colleagues performed a retrospective analysis of their patients (group 1) and found that the incidence of

TABLE 24-2
Incidence of Perioperative Myocardial Infarction in Patients Without Previous Myocardial Infarction

STUDY	YEARS	OPERATIONS	MI RATE (%)	MORTALITY RATE (%)
Topkins and Artusio[25]	1959–1963	12,054	0.66	27
Tarhan et al[26]	1967–1968	32,455	0.13	69
von Knorring[27]	1975–1977	12,497	0.20	36
Schoeppel et al[28]	1980	928	0.40	

TABLE 24-3
Incidence of Perioperative Myocardial Infarction in Patients With Previous Myocardial Infarction

STUDY	YEARS	OPERATIONS	MI RATE (%)	MORTALITY RATE (%)
Topkins and Artusio[25]	1959–1963	658	6.5	70
Tarhan et al[26]	1967–1968	422	6.6	54
Steen et al[29]	1974–1975	587	6.1	69
von Knorring[27]	1975–1977	157	15.9	28
Eerola et al[30]	1979	111	5.4	50
Schoeppel et al[28]	1980	63	4.3	50
Rao et al[31]	1977–1982	733	1.9	36

reinfarction in their institution was consistent with that reported earlier. In 1976, they began to study a prospective group (group 2) who were treated with newer techniques such as invasive monitoring (eg, pulmonary artery pressure monitoring), pharmacologic agents (eg, increased use of β-adrenergic receptor blockers or nitroglycerin), and intensive care. They succeeded in greatly decreasing the incidence of perioperative reinfarction (Table 24-4). In addition, the mortality of reinfarction decreased from 57% in group 1 to 36% in group 2. Although their results indicate great improvement compared with those of earlier studies, attributing this improvement to a specific intervention is not valid. Table 24-5 details major diagnostic and therapeutic differences between the groups, illustrating the increased use of each treatment modality except vasopressors. However, this study for the first time lent support to a more aggressive approach, contending that the use of all available "tools" can actually lower reinfarction incidence and save lives. Verification is eagerly awaited but has yet to be published.

TABLE 24-4
Incidence of Reinfarction and Mortality in Relation to Interval From Previous Myocardial Infarction

	PATIENTS (no.)		POSTANESTHETIC REINFARCTIONS (no. [%])	
	Group 1	*Group 2*	*Group 1*	*Group 2*
INTERVAL BETWEEN MI AND ANESTHESIA (months)				
0–3	11	52	4 (36%)	3 (5.8%)*
4–6	31	86	8 (26%)	2 (2.3%)†
7–12	127	104	6 (5%)	1 (1.0%)
13–24	114	256	6 (5%)	4 (1.56%)
>25	81	235	4 (5%)	4 (1.7%)
MORTALITY			15 (57%)	5 (36%)
TOTAL	**364**	**733**	**28 (7.7%)**	**14 (1.9%)†**

Incidence of postanesthetic reinfarctions in group 2 compared with group 1:

* $P < 0.05$.

† $P < 0.005$.

Rao TL, Jacobs KH, El-Etr AA: Reinfarction following anesthesia in patients with myocardial infarction. Anesthesiology 59:499, 1983.

The study also supported the long-held belief that patients with congestive heart failure (CHF) are at increased risk[31]: patients with CHF or angina or both had higher rates of reinfarction. Patients in group 2 with CHF alone had the highest rate of reinfarction (11%) of all associated medical problems examined.[31] The risk of perioperative MI in patients with angina or CHF who have not sustained an MI is not as well documented.

Cardiac Risk Indexes

Goldman Index

Goldman and associates developed a cardiac risk index for general use in patients scheduled to undergo surgery (Table 24-6).[33] They found that a history of MI within 6 months is associated with a 14% risk of life-threatening complications (perioperative MI, pulmonary edema, or ventricular tachycardia) and a 23% risk of perioperative cardiac death. The presence of a third heart sound or jugular-vein distention was associated with a 14% incidence of life-threatening complications and a 20% incidence of cardiac death.[33] These observations suggest that CHF as a marker for perioperative cardiac disaster is as significant as a history of a recent MI.

American Society of Anesthesiologists Physical Status Classification

The accuracy of Goldman and associates' numerical cardiac risk index as a predictor of cardiac outcome has been shown in one prospective study to be no better than the American Society of Anesthesiologists' physical status classification (Table 24-7).[34] Although it was not designed to measure risk, increasing numerical values in the American Society of Anesthesiologists' physical status classification have correlated with increasing mortality (Table 24-8). Among patients undergoing abdominal aortic surgery in another study, the risk of cardiac complications increased as predicted in the group having a high cardiac risk index (38% of class 3), but the percentage of similar complications in the low-score, class 1 group (7%) was much higher than predicted (1%) by the cardiac risk index (Table 24-9).[35] The authors concluded that a risk index de-

TABLE 24-5
Hemodynamic Monitoring and Vasoactive and Cardioactive Drugs Used by Rao and Colleagues

MONITORING AND DRUGS	GROUP 1, n = 364, n (%)	GROUP 2, n = 733, n (%)
Direct arterial pressure	137 (37.6)	651 (88.8)
Pulmonary artery catheter	8 (2)	607 (82.8)
Vasodilators	24 (6.5)	584 (79.6)
Inotropic drugs	94 (25.8)	231 (31.5)
Vasopressors	114 (31.3)	21* (2.8)
β-Adrenergic blocking agents	40 (10.9)	612 (83.5)
Antidysrhythmic agents	18 (4.9)	210 (28.6)

* Use of vasopressors in group 2 compared with group 1: $P < 0.005$.

Rao TL, Jacobs KH, El-Etr AA: Reinfarction following anesthesia in patients with myocardial infarction. Anesthesiology 59:499, 1983.

veloped for the general surgical population could not be applied to patients having specific operations known to carry high risk for perioperative cardiac complications, such as abdominal aortic surgery, without specific prospective testing.[35]

Others have followed Goldman and associates' lead in using, developing, and evaluating cardiac risk indexes.[36–40] Although these indexes may facilitate similar predictions, occasionally the results are sufficiently different that the methods are questioned. It has been shown that the validity of the indexes is sensitive to differences in surveillance strategies and outcome definitions as well as differences in patient populations (eg, type of surgery).[41]

Type of Surgery

As has been suggested, different surgical procedures are associated with different degrees of cardiac risk. When evaluating any type of anesthetic risk, anesthetic-related risk should be distinguished from surgery-related risk.

Ophthalmic Surgery

A review of 10,000 ophthalmic procedures performed with local anesthesia yielded a 0% incidence of MI, despite the inclusion of 288 procedures in patients with a documented previous history of MI.[42] Thus, this procedure involves low risk, possibly because of the limited systemic physiologic trespass involved.

General, Vascular, Noncardiac Thoracic Surgery

In contrast, great-vessel, noncardiac thoracic, and upper abdominal operations are associated with increased risks of reinfarction (16%, 13%, and 8%, respectively).[29] Patients undergoing intrathoracic or upper abdominal surgery lasting longer than 3 hours have a 15.9% reinfarction rate compared with 5.9% in the same surgical group undergoing surgery lasting less than 3 hours. At least in this surgical subgroup, increased duration of surgery is associated with increased cardiac risk.[29]

TABLE 24-6
Indicators of Increased Perioperative Risk and Need for More Detailed Evaluation in High-risk Patients

CARDIOVASCULAR	PULMONARY	NEUROLOGIC
Third heart sound gallop	Chronic lung disease	Central nervous system injury
Jugular venous distention	FEV_1 <2.0 L	Carotid bruit*
MI within 6 months	Obesity	
Dysrhythmias†	Hypercapnia at rest	
Age >70 years	Age >70 years	
Emergency operation	Site of operation	
Important aortic stenosis	Smoking history	
Poor general health		

FEV_1, forced expiratory volume in 1 s.

* As a marker for ischemic heart disease.

† Other than sinus or premature atrial contractions, or premature ventricular contractions >5 min.

Modified from Goldman L, Caldera DL, Nussbaum SR, et al: Multifactorial index of cardiac risk in noncardiac surgical procedures. N Engl J Med 297:845, 1977; Tisi GM: Preoperative evaluation of pulmonary function: validity, indications, and benefits. Am Rev Respir Dis 119:293, 1979; and Wolf PA, Kannel WB, Sorlie P, et al: Asymptomatic carotid bruit and risk of stroke: the Framingham study. JAMA 245:1442, 1981.

TABLE 24-7
The American Society of Anesthesiologists Physical Status Classification

PHYSICAL STATUS	DEFINITION
1	Healthy
2	Mild systemic disease; no functional limitation
3	Severe systemic disease; definite functional limitation
4	Severe systemic disease that is constant threat to life
5	Moribund; unlikely to survive 24 h, with or without operation

Brown DL, Kirby RR: Preoperative evaluation of high-risk surgical patients. In Civetta JM, Taylor RW, Kirby RR (eds): Critical care, 2nd ed. Philadelphia: JB Lippincott, 1992:572.

Carotid Endarterectomy

Carotid endarterectomy is associated with an incidence of perioperative MI of 1.3%.[43] The long-term risk of MI after carotid endarterectomy is 15% to 36%.[44] In cases of combined carotid artery disease and CAD, the decision as to whether carotid endarterectomy or CABG should be done first is difficult. Some support exists for doing the procedures sequentially during the same general anesthetic in this high-risk patient group.[44–47]

Coronary Revascularization

The perioperative MI risk for coronary revascularization is 5.0% to 46%.[48,49] As expected, the range in these estimates may be explained by differences in diagnostic regimen. In 100 consecutive patients undergoing CABG, Fennell and colleagues found the incidence of postoperative MI to be 9% when diagnosed by 12-lead ECG, 17% by cardiac isoenzyme analysis, 19% by vector cardiography, and 25% by technetium pyrophosphate scintigraphy.[50]

MI diagnosis by ECG changes was associated with a higher mortality (30%) than that without diagnostic ECG change (2%). One factor associated with ECG-diagnosed postoperative MI was the presence of preoperative unstable angina.[50] Increased operative mortality (6.9%) is associated with decreased left ventricular function (ejection fraction <36% and abnormal wall motion) preoperatively.[51] Other factors not unexpectedly associated with an increased operative mortality include age greater than 70 years, female gender, symptoms of heart failure, left main coronary artery stenosis, and the need for emergency surgery.[52]

PREVIOUS CORONARY ARTERY BYPASS GRAFT. The influence of previous CABG on perioperative cardiac risk is an unsettled issue. The risk of perioperative MI after CABG for subsequent noncardiac surgery was reported in 1978 to be zero; the duration between CABG and subsequent surgery averaged 22 months.[53] Others have reported a post-CABG perioperative MI incidence of 1.2%.[54,55] Preliminary data by Backofen and associates, in contrast, showed an incidence of 6% perioperative MI and 16% incidence of ischemic events in 42 patients undergoing surgery an average of 33 months after CABG. Their conclusion was that CABG was not protective.[56] A graft attrition rate of 11% at 1 year and 15% at 5 years post-CABG may account for diminution of any "protective" effect over time.[57]

CLINICAL IMPLICATIONS. The preceding estimates illustrate the significance of perioperative MI as a complicating factor in anesthesia. Perioperative reinfarction has a 36%[31] to 70%[25] mortality in contrast to the 20% mortality risk associated with a nonsurgery reinfarction.[32] Either anesthesia and surgery stress patients to such a degree that further cardiac demands imposed by MI cannot be met, or the care given to this subgroup of MI patients differs from that given to other MI patients. Emphasis should be placed both on decreasing the incidence of MI and on improving the survival of patients

TABLE 24-8
Perioperative Mortality in Patients Stratified According to American Society of Anesthesiologists Classification

PHYSICAL STATUS	ANESTHETICS	DEATHS	MORTALITY RATE (%)	MORTALITY FACTOR*
1	50,703	43	0.08	—
2	12,601	34	0.27	3.4
3	3626	66	1.8	22.5
4	850	66	7.8	97.5
5	608	57	9.4	117.5

* The mortality factor was increased over that in patients of physical status 1.

Brown DL, Kirby RR: Preoperative evaluation of high-risk surgical patients. In: Civetta JM, Taylor RW, Kirby RR (eds): Critical care, 2nd ed. Philadelphia: JB Lippincott, 1992:573.

Modified from Vacanti CJ, Van Houten RJ, Hill RC: A statistical analysis of the relationship of physical status to postoperative mortality in 68,388 cases. Anesth Analg 49:564, 1970.

TABLE 24-9
Computation of the Cardiac Risk Index

CRITERION	POINTS*
Age >70 years	5
MI in previous 6 months	10
Third heart sound gallop or jugular vein distention	11
Important valvular aortic stenosis	3
Rhythm other than sinus or premature atrial contractions on last preoperative ECG	7
>5 premature ventricular contractions/min documented at any time before operation	7
Arterial oxygen tension <60 mmHg or arterial carbon dioxide tension >50 mmHg; potassium <3.0 mEq/L or bicarbonate <20 mEq/L; blood urea nitrogen >50 mg/dL or creatinine >3.0 mg/dL; abnormal serum glutamic oxaloacetic transaminase; signs of chronic liver disease; bedridden condition from noncardiac causes	3
Intraperitoneal, intrathroacic, or aortic operation	3
Emergency operation	4
	Total possible 53

* Class I risk <5 points; class II risk 6 to 12 points; class III risk >13 points.
Modified from Jeffrey CC, Kunsman J, Cullen DJ, et al: A prospective evaluation of cardiac risk index. Anesthesiology 58:462, 1983.

in whom MI does occur; both goals require an appreciation of the underlying physiologic mechanisms.

Physician Care

Slogoff and Keats demonstrated that perioperative MI varied sevenfold among cases handled by different anesthesiologists in the same institution.[58] Thus physicians caring for at-risk patients are an important factor in outcome.

PATHOPHYSIOLOGIC MECHANISMS OF MYOCARDIAL ISCHEMIA AND INFARCTION

Myocardial ischemia results from an imbalance in the supply–demand relation for myocardial perfusion and resultant oxygen delivery.

Myocardial Oxygen Supply

Regional Versus Global

The myocardial oxygen supply is determined by the blood oxygen content and coronary blood flow. Coronary blood flow is a function of coronary driving pressure across the vascular bed divided by the coronary vascular bed resistance. Coronary driving pressure is defined as the difference between the aortic diastolic pressure and the right atrial pressure, which is an acceptable definition for total myocardial perfusion.[59] However, regional perfusion is altered by the gradient between coronary perfusion pressure and intraventricular end-diastolic pressure. Length of diastolic filling time also affects total coronary perfusion: as heart rate increases total coronary perfusion decreases.

Optimization

Some supply factors are more easily controlled by the anesthesiologist than others. Oxygen content may be ensured by adequate hematocrit preoperatively combined with appropriate airway management and optimal delivered oxygen concentrations. Maintenance of satisfactory coronary blood flow requires adequate diastolic pressure and, for cases in which the left ventricle is particularly at risk, monitoring of pulmonary artery occlusion pressure as an indicator of left ventricular end-diastolic pressure (LVEDP). Attempts to decease the latter should be made when necessary to optimize the relation between aortic diastolic pressure and LVEDP. Coronary vascular resistance may be lowered by the anesthetic regimen or by the administration of coronary vasodilators such as nitroglycerin or calcium-channel blocking agents.

Myocardial Oxygen Demand

Myocardial oxygen demand is a function of systolic wall tension, contractility, heart rate, and metabolic level of the heart. Systolic wall tension is set by the aortic systolic blood pressure (afterload), LVEDP (preload), and ventricular volume.[58] Metabolic needs of the myocardium, in addition to a minimal baseline level of precursors required to maintain cellular integrity, are increased by activation of the sympathetic nervous system and the resultant increased levels of catecholamines. Increasing contractility and heart rate also increase oxygen demand. Heart rate and LVEDP are of particular importance because they affect myocardial oxygen demand and supply simultaneously. As heart rate or LVEDP increases, myocardial oxygen demand increases and supply decreases.

Afterload

Anesthesiologists can decrease systolic blood pressure in an effort to decrease oxygen demand, but must not drop diastolic blood pressure to such a degree that coronary perfusion pressure is threatened. Also, should the well-intended lowering of systolic pressure result in tachycardia or increased sympathetic tone, the resultant increased oxygen demand could well exceed the previous myocardial oxygen demand at the higher systolic blood pressure.

Preload

Preload may be altered by changing patient position or by administering nitroglycerin, again striving to avoid hypotension. Appropriate heart rate management has the dual effect of decreasing demand and, by prolonging diastolic perfusion pressure, increasing supply. Avoiding sympathetic stimulation can lower metabolic demands as well.

Preexisting Myocardial Compromise

Significant hypoxemia or hypotension may result in ischemia and MI in a normal heart. This clinical presentation is more likely in an operating or emergency room than in a coronary care unit. Most instances of perioperative ischemia, however, are in patients with preexisting myocardial compromise.

Patients with CAD may have plaque-induced changes in coronary resistance that make increases in cardiac demand impossible to meet. This sequence can result in classical exertion-related angina. The idea of a slowly growing atherosclerotic plaque occluding a passive, nonresponsive conduit is an inaccurate oversimplification and explains only a limited number of cardiac patients' histories. Though plaque accumulation may play a role, other mechanisms including coronary vasospasm, platelet aggregates, and the overall metabolic status of the heart in combination or alone probably induce most ischemic events.

Thrombosis

Formation

Thrombosis has been strongly associated with MI since Herrick's classic 1912 description of MI and its appearance postmortem.[59,60] Indeed, "coronary thrombosis" has became synonymous with MI. About 90% to 99% of transmural MIs greater than 6 hours old have associated coronary thrombosis.[61] Whether the thrombosis formation triggers an MI or vice versa is still unclear.

PLATELET AGGREGATION. The theory of thrombus as a cause of infarct describes increased platelet aggregation as a trigger to thrombus formation. Patients with acute MI and patients with unstable angina have increased platelet aggregability.[62,63] Synthesis of thromboxane A_2, a powerful vasoconstrictor and platelet aggregator, occurs in platelets and is released during platelet aggregation. Prostacyclin, a potent vasodilator and inhibitor of platelet aggregation, is produced within the vascular endothelium. Atherosclerotic endothelium has decreased levels of prostacyclin production, resulting in an arterial area at risk for platelet aggregation and clot formation. Hyperlipidemia, diabetes, and cigarette smoking, all established coronary risk factors, also increase platelet aggregation.[64]

Thrombolysis

Early MI therapy aimed at intracoronary thrombolysis has used systemic or intracoronary thrombolysis. Mathey and colleagues reported successful recanalization in 73% of patients with acute coronary occlusion using intracoronary streptokinase. They believed the increased left ventricular ejection fraction in most of the patients in whom recanalization had been performed successfully indicated myocardial salvage, even though 80% of this group showed ECG and enzyme changes consistent with MI.[65]

Rentrop and associates recanalized 22 of 29 patients with a similar technique and, in 18 of the 19 patients who underwent repeat angiography three weeks later, the vessels remained patent.[66] The long-term outcome of this approach has not been determined, particularly in comparison with angioplasty, medical management, or emergent CABG. The application of thrombolytic agents both in the face of an acute MI and in chronic preventive management of CAD is an exciting clinical application of a theoretical concept. Currently used agents include streptokinase, urokinase, and tissue plasminogen activator. Whether the latter agent, which is many times more expensive, confers sufficient additional benefit to justify the cost, is a source of ongoing debate.

Coronary Artery Spasm

Coronary artery spasm as a possible cause of myocardial ischemia has been recognized since Prinzmetal described variant angina in the 1950s and hypothesized that it is due to a temporary increase in tone in a narrowed vessel.[67] The mechanism responsible for vasospasm is not well understood. Levels of thromboxane A_2 and its inactive metabolite have been elevated in patients with Prinzmetal angina.[68]

Another proposed mechanism for spasm is excessive α-adrenergic receptor stimulation. An imbalance of α- versus β-receptor tone in the epicardial coronaries could result in a slight change of resistance that would materially decrease coronary perfusion in these high-flow vessels. The calcium-channel blocking agents have become a valuable therapeutic tool in the management of patients with variant angina, and in those with mixed classical and variant angina.

RELEVANCE OF CARDIAC CATHETERIZATION DATA

Right and Left Dominance

Catheterization reports often describe a patient's circulation in terms of right- or left-dominance. This categorization describes the arterial supply source to the sinoatrial node. If the blood supply to the sinoatrial node is interrupted as it might be with an MI involving the dominant artery, the patient may require a pacemaker. With either right or left dominance, an MI may result in necrosis of a critical amount of myocardial tissue. An important prognostic factor is the presence of left main CAD in combination with a left-dominant circulation; operative mortality is 25% compared with 5.7% with severe left main disease and a right-dominant circulation.[52] No data exist for this high-risk group having noncardiac surgery.

Collateral Circulation

Collateral circulation is also often demonstrated on catheterization. The blood supply to the normal human heart is end-arterial. In cases of trauma, anomalous coronary arteries, or in some cases of CAD, anastomotic channels between arterial beds open, allowing cross-perfusion. This collateral pattern of supply has been described as being capable of back filling a traumatically severed left anterior descending coronary artery.[69] Distal refill through these vessels is often demonstrable through catheterization.

The developmental prerequisites of these collateral pathways are not known. Their functional significance is debated, and their response to pharmacologic manipulation of coronary resistance (eg, coronary steal with isoflurane vasodilation) is not well understood. For those cases in which a large myocardial area apparently depends on refill via collateral circulation, particular attention should be paid to maintaining coronary perfusion pressure.

PREOPERATIVE EVALUATION

The Anesthesiologist's Assessment

Cardiac risk factors, as previously discussed, should be sought carefully in every adult patient, in addition to the topics usually covered in the anesthesiologist's preoperative visit (see Table 24-6).

Chest Pain

Obtaining information about chest pain can yield surprising results. If a patient has a history of reflux esophagitis or refers to "just a little heartburn, Doc," do not assume that clinically important CAD is excluded. Twenty-two percent of men with chest pain assessed as "nonanginal" have CAD confirmed on catheterization.[12] Reflux esophagitis and CAD are common occurrences and can coexist, and both patients and physicians are eager to attribute chest pain to the less-threatening diagnosis. In patients with known CAD, particular attention should be given to recent changes in chest pain patterns or physical functioning. In particular, unstable angina or new-onset angina is an indication for evaluation and treatment before any elective noncardiac surgery.

Symptoms of Heart Failure

These are important prognostic factors, and may have the highest correlation with perioperative myocardial morbidity and mortality.[31,34,40] Severe orthopnea may prevent the patient from lying flat for transport or for central venous cannulation. New or worsening heart failure should also be evaluated and treated before any noncardiac elective surgery.

Electrocardiographic Abnormalities

The ECG is not a reliable screening test for occult CAD.[70] A normal ECG should not allay a previously serious consideration of CAD and should not dissuade one from seeking cardiologic consultation.

The Cardiologist's Role

Every patient deserves optimal medical management in preparation for the unavoidable stresses of anesthesia and surgery. Postponement of elective surgery for adequate cardiac evaluation and management can be lifesaving. Potential benefits for the patient easily outweigh the inconvenience for all involved. The same attention should be given to patients with equivocal chest pain and multiple cardiac risk factors.

Questions To Be Addressed

Cardiology consultants should answer the following questions. Does this patient have significant CAD and, if so, is medical treatment optimal? How impaired is the patient's myocardial contractility? Is any further evaluation recommended to help answer these questions? What are specific recommendations for medical management pre- and postoperatively?

This thoughtful consultation is a far cry from the request to "clear for surgery" often issued; little wonder that the latter, loosely worded request usually results in nebulous, unhelpful responses. As anesthesiologists, we have a responsibility to educate cardiologist colleagues regarding our needs.[71,72] A thorough cardiology consultation can help to plan surgical scheduling relative to the patient's evaluation or medical conditioning and preoperative and postoperative management. A poor consultation is a waste of everyone's time and the patient's money, and may actually complicate anesthetic management.

Recommendations Not To Be Made

The occasional consultant practice of specifically dictating anesthetic technique is particularly unacceptable. The often stated "would recommend spinal due to heart disease" has no support in the literature, and the cardiologist giving this advice certainly is not speaking from actual clinical experience. Dictating specific anesthetic agents or technique is no more appropriate for the cardiologist than is dictating what instruments the surgeon may use.

Exercise Tolerance

Traditional

The exercise tolerance test is especially helpful in the initial evaluation of an asymptomatic patient with multiple risk factors, or in a patient believed to have nonanginal chest pain. Although an exercise tolerance test cannot absolutely exclude the presence of CAD, the ability of a patient to tolerate this controlled stress test without cardiac symptoms or changes suggests similar ability to tolerate the occasionally incompletely controlled stresses involved in surgery, anesthesia, and recovery.

In evaluating patients with chest pain, the specificity of an exercise tolerance test is 89% but the sensitivity is only 69%.[72] A false-negative result is more likely in a patient who later is shown to have single-vessel disease. In a population with no chest pain, the exercise tolerance test yields a 47%[73] to 63%[74] false-positive rate.

Thallium 201 Imaging

With a thallium 201 exercise scan, sensitivity and specificity values are above 90% when quantitative image interpretation is used.[75] Unlike traditional exercise testing, thallium 201 exercise scanning maintains a sensitivity of 80% in patients with single-vessel disease and may yield meaningful results even in patients who are unable to attain 85% of maximum predicted heart rate. In the patient unable to perform exercise, it is possible to mimic this pharmacologically by the coadministration of a coronary vasodilator such as dipyridamole (Persantine) or adenosine.

Thallium 201 imaging is demanding, is more costly, and takes longer. Adequate evaluation of an asymptomatic patient may require ECG and thallium 201 exercise testing to exclude CAD. In an excellent review of these tests, Gibson and Beller conclude that an asymptomatic patient with both a negative exercise ECG and exercise thallium 201 scan has less than a 1% incidence of clinically important CAD.[75]

Another benefit of thallium 201 imaging is that a positive result provides more detailed information about the extent of coronary involvement than does a positive ECG exercise test. This information can guide the decision whether to undertake cardiac catheterization in a patient with newly diagnosed CAD before a trial of medical management.

Coronary Revascularization and Elective Surgery

In patients with known CAD and worsening symptoms, or viable myocardium at risk (eg, a thallium 201 scan that demonstrates delayed redistribution of myocardial blood flow), coronary revascularization before elective surgery should be considered. Some of these patients will have already undergone cardiac catheterization and will have been judged not to be candidates for CABG. This group, after optimal medical management is achieved, may proceed with elective surgery. The patient whose symptoms are becoming more severe, and who has not been evaluated with catheterization, requires completion of a diagnostic workup before being subjected to the additional stress of elective surgery. As was discussed previously, some evidence suggests that CABG may provide a "protective" quality for subsequent surgeries.

In high-risk surgical groups, such as those undergoing aortic aneurysm resection, attention must be given to reducing the patient's MI risk even if a preceding CABG is required. Emergency CABG surgery is associated with a higher mortality,[52,76] part of which is due to inability to achieve preoperative stabilization. In critically ill patients, the possible benefits of emergency surgery outweigh the obvious risks inherent in going to the operating room ill-prepared. This statement does not hold true for elective cases. Optimal anesthetic and surgical management intra- and postoperatively may not be able to compensate for deficiencies in preoperative care.

Laboratory Studies

Further preoperative assessment should assure adequate hematocrit and hemoglobin. Hypokalemia, if chronic, appears to be relatively well tolerated in patients not receiving chronic digitalis therapy.[77] If a foreign body such as a cardiac valve or prosthetic hip is to be placed, a complete blood count and urinalysis should verify the patient to be free of active infection.

Renal function should be assessed especially before procedures that may jeopardize it, such as those involving nearby aortic cross-clamping. Preoperative ECG assessment can guide lead selection in the operating room and provide a valuable baseline for possible postoperative comparison. If an exercise tolerance test shows ST-segment changes in a particular lead, the same lead should be monitored intraoperatively.

Long-Term Medications

After adequate cardiac evaluation and optimal medical management, every attempt is made to preserve the patient's cardiac stability. Medications, including antihypertensives, β-adrenergic receptor blockers, and calcium-channel antagonists, particularly when prescribed for control of angina, should be continued through the morning of surgery. Nitrates, including topical preparations, are continued as well. If cardiopulmonary bypass is planned, the anesthesiologist may opt to remove topical nitrates because of possible alteration of uptake with skin temperature and perfusion changes. Diuretics, when given for CHF, should be continued.

Digitalis

Digoxin is a possible exception to continuing medication until time of surgery. If the drug was started recently for heart failure or for atrial fibrillation, it is best continued. However, patients receiving digoxin chronically for unclear reasons usually can have their morning-of-surgery or even day-before-surgery dose omitted. In these individuals with no well-documented need for the drug, the risks of toxicity and possible interactions with hypokalemia may outweigh the ill-defined benefits.

Preanesthetic Sedation

Adequate anxiety relief should be provided when necessary. Patients vary in their need for preoperative sedation; the type and amount should be tailored to the individual. In some cases, bedtime sedation the night before surgery is welcome. If nighttime sedation is provided, the patient must be assisted if he or she arises in the early hours.

When invasive monitors are to be placed before induction, most patients better tolerate these unpleasant and potentially painful procedures with some sedation and pain medication. Dosages generally need to be reduced for elderly or debilitated individuals. For those with CAD that is unstable or high risk (such as left main CAD), sedation should be aimed at preventing preoperative tachycardia while maintaining perfusion pressure.

Intraoperative Patient Monitoring

Monitoring decisions also should be made at the time of the preoperative evaluation. This approach allows adequate discussion with the patient and also provides time to evaluate possible cannulation sites. Decisions should be guided by the patient's innate physiologic risk state and degree of surgical risk. The risks of a particular modality should be outweighed by its benefits. Low-risk monitors such as multiple-lead ECG, pulse oximetry, capnography, precordial or esophageal stethoscope, temperature monitoring, and noninvasive blood pressure monitoring should be used liberally, as indicated.

Electrocardiography

Multiple lead ECG monitoring with a recording or memory option is invaluable. Any intraoperative changes in ST-segment location can be compared with a previously obtained baseline for confirmation, and this modality can then be used to follow effects of treatment. Monitoring lead V_5 is the single most helpful lead for detecting ischemia.[78] The second most sensitive lead is V_4 (Fig. 24-1). If only a three-lead system is available, placing the right arm lead on the upper manubrium, the left arm lead at the fifth intercostal space, and the ground lead in the left leg position with the lead selection switch set on Lead I yields a CM_5 view (central manubrium to V_5 lead) that has been shown to be sensitive to anterior-lateral ischemic changes in exercise testing.[79]

Intra-arterial Catheterization

Intra-arterial monitoring is a high-yield, low-risk procedure,[80] and is helpful for cases in which wide swings in blood volume, pressure, or both are anticipated; frequent arterial blood gas measurements are needed to follow respiratory or metabolic status; and noninvasive methods of blood pressure monitoring are difficult or impossible.

Central Venous Pressure

Monitoring of central venous pressure allows central access that is helpful when continuous infusion drugs will be needed. The central venous pressure may accurately reflect LVEDP and, therefore, left ventricular contractility in those patients with good contractility.[81] The complications of placement vary with expertise, site, and technique of insertion. The incidence of pneumothorax ranges from 0.2% to 4.7%; carotid puncture occurs in about 2%.[82]

Pulmonary Artery Pressure

Pulmonary artery pressure monitoring is not without risk. A reported series of 6245 patients who received pulmonary artery catheters included a 0.5% incidence of pneumothorax, a 72% incidence of arrhythmias, and a 0.07% incidence of a bundle branch block as well as a 2% incidence of carotid punctures and 0.08% incidence of RV or PA perforations.[83]

For patients with known ventricular impairment, a pulmonary artery catheter is indicated if surgery involves large intravascular volume shifts or myocardial stress. Pulmonary artery catheters may also enhance detection of myocardial ischemia,[84] and may be indicated for patients with unstable angina or known critical CAD, left main, or severe three-vessel disease. Continuous monitoring of mixed-venous oxygen saturation by reflectance spectrophotometry is helpful in patients who are septic, particularly in the stormy postoperative period.

Transesophageal Echocardiography

Transesophageal echocardiography is increasingly popular and in the minds of many clinicians provides as much or even more useful information than does pulmonary artery catheterization.[85,85] Its most useful applications include not only detection of segmental wall motion abnormalities indicative of ischemia[86] but also actual observation of changes of left ventricular end-diastolic volume, contractility, and occurrence of intracardiac air.

INTRAOPERATIVE CONSIDERATIONS

Intraoperative goals should focus on maintaining blood pressure and heart rate within preoperative angina-free limits. Tachycardia particularly must be avoided. In most patients, a target maximum heart rate of 70 beats/min or less is a desirable goal.

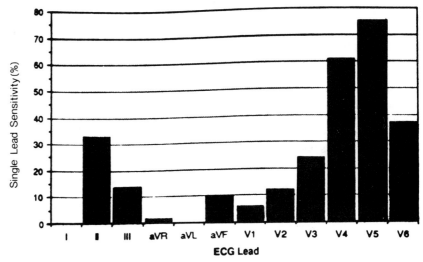

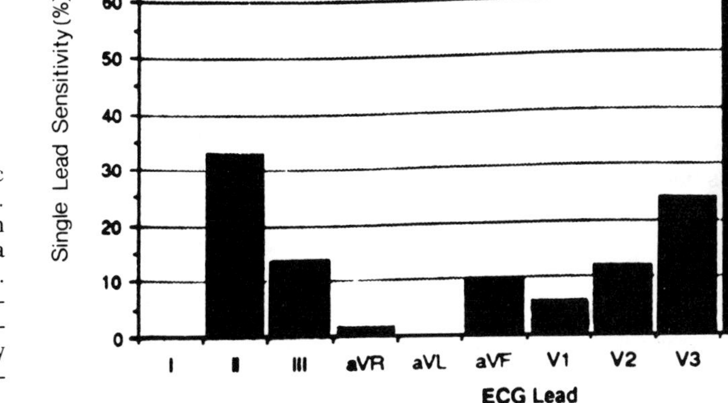

FIGURE 24-1. The distribution of ischemic ST-segment changes in each of the 12 leads. The estimated sensitivity was calculated from the number of changes in a single lead as a percentage of the total number of episodes. Sensitivity was highest in lead V_5 (75%). (London MJ, Hollenberg M, Wong MG, et al: Intraoperative myocardial ischemia localization by continuous 12-lead electrocardiography. Anesthesiology 69:237, 1988.)

General Anesthesia

Insufficient depth of anesthesia can result in tachycardia after surgical stimulation. In normal volunteers, isoflurane and especially desflurane contribute to tachycardia.[87] This phenomenon appears to be particularly evident if the inspired concentration is abruptly increased. Sympathetic hyperactivity resulting in tachycardia and hypertension has been shown to occur with desflurane administration as well.[88] If ECG, pulmonary artery pressures, or transesophageal echocardiography indicates early ischemia, rate slowing through β-adrenergic receptor blockade should be implemented unless it is contraindicated (eg, active asthma). If reattaining a normal preinduction rate does not relieve ischemia, nitroglycerin should be infused intravenously, with carefully adjustment of dosage to avoid lowering perfusion pressure precipitously.

Myocardial Contractility

Myocardial contractility is an especially important consideration. Subnormal (less than 40%) left ventricular ejection fraction suggests that further anesthetic-induced myocardial depression may be poorly tolerated. Among volatile agents, halothane is the most depressant. In patients with intermittent outflow obstruction caused by muscular hypertrophy, such as idiopathic subaortic stenosis, this agent may be used advantageously to depress contractility, thereby maintaining the patency of the outflow path. However, in patients with symptomatic heart failure, halothane is best avoided or used with caution.

The most severely impaired patients may benefit from a short-acting narcotic–oxygen–relaxant technique. However, Rao and associates found the highest incidence of group 2 reinfarction to be in the narcotic–nitrous oxide–oxygen–relaxant group.[31] Using small amounts of volatile anesthetic to supplement a narcotic–oxygen–relaxant technique to maintain an acceptable blood pressure also helps to ensure amnesia, a continued concern with narcotic "anesthesia."

Regional Anesthesia

Regional anesthesia can be used as long as the patient is protected from tachycardia and hypotension. To avoid tachycardia, we suggest not using epinephrine-containing test doses of local anesthetics. Large volume loads, commonly recommended as prophylaxis against sympathectomy-induced hypotension, may not be well tolerated in patients with borderline heart failure. A continuous regional technique, either epidural or spinal, that enables gradual increase in the level of anesthesia (with concurrent, controlled sympathectomy-induced blood pressure changes), appears preferable to a single-injection spinal technique in CAD patients. However, this hypothesis has not been proven.

Muscle Relaxants

Atracurium or vecuronium provide excellent relaxation for short procedures. Atracurium occasionally causes sufficient histamine release to result in hypotension and tachycardia. Metocurine, a muscle relaxant that provides stable hemodynamic conditions,[89] also may cause profound hypotension as a result of histamine release. Both atracurium and metocurine should be given slowly with careful observation of the patient's blood pressure response.

Pancuronium, though relatively free of histamine release, can cause profound tachycardia that may induce ischemia in CAD patients. Thomsen and associates reported that a mixture of 4 mg metocurine and 1 mg pancuronium is associated with a lower incidence of ECG-indicated ischemia than pancuronium alone.[90] Total doses in the mix were 0.108 mg/kg metocurine and 0.027 mg/kg pancuronium. In this study, one case of a marked pancuronium-induced tachycardia occurred. Whether pancuronium can induce changes without an associated tachycardia has not been demonstrated.

POSTOPERATIVE CONSIDERATIONS

Postoperative management of patients with known or possible CAD should include the same degree of vigilance as that of pre- and intraoperative care. Often everyone breaths a sign of relief once the surgical procedure itself is completed without complication. This relief is premature, however, because the most common time for perioperative MI is on the 3rd or 4th postoperative day.[29,31]

Consideration should be given to placing the patient in an intensive care setting, or at least monitoring the patient postoperatively with ECG telemetry, particularly if the surgical procedure is associated with a high incidence of MI.[31] If intensive care is not indicated or possible, perhaps the "routine" postoperative regimen should be continued for longer than 24 hours.

Activity levels should be returned to normal at a slower pace than in patients without CAD. Postoperative pain management should be designed to avoid tachycardia and excess sympathetic stimulation as well as to improve postoperative comfort.

TREATMENT OF PERIOPERATIVE MYOCARDIAL ISCHEMIA

In the event that ischemia is detected perioperatively, an adequate myocardial oxygen supply must be assured. Inadequate oxygenation and falling red blood cell volume are easily and quickly assessed.

Hypotension

Hypotension, another possible cause of ischemia, requires correction of the underlying cause. If the patient is hypovolemic, intravascular volume replacement is promptly instituted. If hypotension is due to impairment by surgical retractors of inferior vena caval blood return or due to ill-timed release of an aortic cross-clamp, the surgeon must be informed of the situation and correction made. Gradual release of major vessel cross-clamps, with adequate warning to allow volume infusion and discontinuation of volatile anesthetics and vasodilator infusions, works best to maintain stable hemodynamic function.

Tachycardia

If tachycardia is the culprit, it must be treated promptly. Adequate volume status should be assured before instituting β-adrenergic receptor blockade in a tachycardiac patient. In hypovolemic patients the tachycardia may be essential to maintaining adequate perfusion of vital organs. If tachycardia is due to inadequate anesthesia, then further supplementation is indicated. If it is due to isoflurane,[88] reduction in dose, change to another volatile anesthetic, or narcotic supplementation (eg, fentanyl or sufentanil) may lower the rate. As was noted previously, pancuronium can induce profound tachycardia that, if associated with ischemia, may necessitate β-adrenergic blockade and consequent avoidance of further pancuronium.

Neurologically Induced Electrocardiographic Changes

Changes consistent with ischemia can have a neurologic etiology. Subarachnoid hemorrhage, meningitis, and intracranial space-occupying tumors are associated with ST-segment changes that suggest ischemia.[91] In such patients, cardiac enzyme studies may be needed to exclude MI. If ischemic changes persist despite maintenance of heart rate and blood pressure within a nonischemic preoperative range, nitroglycerin should be given intravenously. One possible limitation for this therapy is the patient with increased intracranial pressure, in which case nitroglycerin may cause a further increase.[92–94] Should that scenario become manifest and administration of β-blocking agents is not feasible or is inadequate, intracranial pressure monitoring is then also instituted to detect this side effect.

Miscellaneous Considerations

If the patient was responsive to calcium-channel blocking agents preoperatively, sublingual nifedipine may be instituted, although it may be necessary to counter possible resulting blood pressure decreases. If ischemia persists, the surgeon should be informed in an effort to minimize further surgical time and arrangements made for appropriate postoperative cardiac care until MI can be excluded. If MI is supported by ECG changes immediately postoperatively, or if the patient is hemodynamically unstable, intensive care unit placement is indicated.

For the patient with MI, cardiac care is more crucial to survival than every other tenet of postoperative care. Forcing patients in pain with intraoperative ischemia or possible MI to get out of bed and walk on the evening of surgery, often without telemetry or even pulse rate monitoring, courts disaster. Those with perioperative MI are at high risk for mortality and require optimal medical management coupled with judicious integration of necessary surgical care throughout the entire length of their hospital stay.

REFERENCES

1. Wilson LB: Fatal postoperative embolism. Ann Surg 56:809, 1912
2. Sprague HB: Heart in surgery. Surg Gynecol Obstet 49:54, 1929
3. Butler S, Feeley N, Levine SA: Patient with heart disease as a surgical risk. JAMA 95:84, 1930
4. Randall OS, Orr TG: Post-operative coronary occlusion. Ann Surg 92:1014, 1930
5. Sokolow M, McIlroy M (eds): Clinical cardiology, 3rd ed. Los Altos, CA: Lange Medical Publications, 1981: 131
6. Diamond GA, Forester JC: Analysis of probability as an aid in the clinical diagnosis of coronary artery disease. N Engl J Med 300:1350, 1979
7. Gibson RS, Beller GA: Should exercise electrocardiographic testing be replaced by radioisotope methods? In Rahimtoola S (ed): Controversies in coronary artery disease. Philadelphia: FA Davis, 1983: 5
8. Proudfit WL, Shirey EK, Sones FM: Selective cine coronary arteriography correlation with clinical findings in 1000 patients. Circulation 33:901, 1966
9. Campeau L, Bourassa MG, Bois MS, et al: Clinical significance of selective coronary cine arteriography. Can Med Assoc J 99: 1063, 1968
10. Friesinger GC, Smith RF: Correlation of electrocardiographic studies and arteriographic findings with angina pectoris. Circulation 46:1173, 1972
11. McConahay DR, McCallister BD, Smith R: Postexercise electrocardiography: correlations with coronary arteriography and left ventricular hemodynamics. Am J Cardiol 28:1, 1971
12. Weiner DA, Ryan TJ, McCabe CH, et al: Exercise stress testing: correlations among history of angina, ST-segment response, and prevalence of coronary artery disease in the Coronary Artery Surgery Study (CASS). N Engl J Med 301:230, 1979
13. Haagensen R, Steen PA: Perioperative myocardial infarction. Br J Anaesth 61:24, 1988
14. Kannel WB, McGee D, Gordon T: A general cardiovascular risk profile: the Framingham Study. Am J Cardiol 38:46, 1976
15. Slack J: Risk factors in coronary heart disease. Lancet 1:366, 1977
16. Rosenman RH, Brand RJ, Sholtz RI, et al: Multivariate prediction of coronary heart disease during 8.5 year follow-up in the Western Collaborative Group Study. Am J Cardiol 37:903, 1976
17. Friedman M, Thorensen C, Gill J, et al: Alteration of type A behavior and reduction in cardiac recurrences in post myocardial infarction patients. Am Heart J 108:237, 1984
18. Kannel WB: Update on the role of cigarette smoking in coronary artery disease. Am Heart J 101:319, 1981
19. Crawley IS, Walter PF, Hurst JW: Atherosclerotic coronary heart disease. In Chung EK (ed): Quick reference to cardiovascular diseases, 3rd ed. Philadelphia: JB Lippincott, 1987: 1
20. Lipid Research Clinics Program: The Lipid Research Clinics Coronary Primary Prevention Trial results: I. Reduction in incidence of coronary heart disease. JAMA 251:351, 1984
21. Kinosian BP, Eisenberg JM: Cutting into cholesterol: cost-effective alternatives for treating hypercholesterolemia. JAMA 259:2249, 1988
22. Lober PH. Pathogenesis of coronary sclerosis. Arch Pathol 55: 357, 1953
23. Hypertension Detection and Follow-up Program Cooperative Group: Five-year findings of the Hypertension Detection and Follow-up Program: 1. Reduction in mortality of persons with high blood pressure, including mild hypertension. JAMA 242: 2562, 1979
24. Fuller JH, McCartney P, Jarret J, et al: Hyperglycemia and coronary heart disease: the Whitehall Study. Journal of Chronic Diseases 32:721, 1979
25. Topkins MJ, Artusio JF: Myocardial infarction and surgery, a five year study. Anesth Analg 42:716, 1964
26. Tarhan S, Moffitt EA, Taylor WF, et al: Myocardial infarction after general anesthesia. JAMA 220:1451, 1972
27. Knorring J von: Postoperative myocardial infarction: a prospective study in a risk group of surgical patients. Surgery 90: 55, 1981
28. Schoeppel SL, Wikinson C, Waters J, et al: Effects of myocardial infarction on preoperative cardiac complications. Anesth Analg 62:493, 1983
29. Steen PA, Tinker JH, Tarhan S: Myocardial reinfarction after anesthesia and surgery. JAMA 239:2566, 1978

30. Eerola M, Eerola R, Kaukinen S, et al: Risk factors in surgical patients with verified preoperative myocardial infarction. Acta Anaesthesiol Scand 24:219, 1980
31. Rao TL, Jacobs KH, El-Etr AA: Reinfarction following anesthesia in patients with myocardial infarction. Anesthesiology 59:499, 1983
32. Norris R, Barnaby P, Brandt P, et al: Prognosis after recovery from first acute infarction: determinants of reinfarction and sudden death. Am J Cardiol 53:408, 1984
33. Goldman L, Caldera D, Nussbaum SR, et al: Mutifactorial index of cardiac risk in noncardiac surgical procedures. N Engl J Med 297:845, 1977
34. Waters J, Wilkinson C, Golmon M, et al: Evaluation of cardiac risk in noncardiac surgical patients (abstract). Anesthesiology 55:A343, 1981
35. Jeffrey CC, Kunsman J, Cullen D, et al: A prospective evaluation of cardiac risk. Anesthesiology 58:462, 1983
36. Zeldin RA: Assessing cardiac risk in patients who undergo noncardiac surgical procedures. Can J Surg 27:402, 1984
37. Gerson MC, Hurst JM, Hertzberg VS, et al: Cardiac prognosis in noncardiac surgery. Ann Intern Med 103:832, 1985
38. Detsky AS, Abrams HB, McLaughlin JR, et al: Predicting cardiac complications in patients undergoing non-cardiac surgery. J Gen Intern Med 1:211, 1986
39. Detsky AS, Abrams HB, Forbach N, et al: Cardiac assessment for patients undergoing noncardiac surgery: a multifactorial clinical risk index. Arch Intern Med 246:2131, 1986
40. Goldman L: Assessment of the patient with known or suspected ischaemic heart disease for non-cardiac surgery. Br J Anaesth 61:38, 1988
41. Charlson ME, Ales KL, Simon R, et al: Why predictive indexes perform less well in validation studies: is it magic or methods? Arch Intern Med 147:2155, 1987
42. Backer CL, Tinker JH, Robertson DM, et al: Myocardial reinfarction following local anesthesia for ophthalmic surgery. Anesth Analg 59:257, 1980
43. Nunn DB: Carotid endarterectomy: analysis of 234 operative cases. Ann Surg 182:733, 1975
44. Okies EJ, MacManus Q, Starr A: Myocardial revascularization and carotid endarterectomy: a combined approach. Ann Thorac Surg 23:560, 1977
45. Urshel HC, Razzuk MA, Gardner MA: Management of concomitant occlusive disease of the carotid and coronary arteries. J Thorac Cardiovasc Surg 72:829, 1976
46. Hertzer NR, Loop FD, Taylor PC, et al: Staged and combined surgical approach to simultaneous carotid and coronary vascular disease. Surgery 84:803, 1978
47. Rice PL, Plfarre R, Sullivan HG, et al: Experience with simultaneous myocardial revascularization and carotid endarterectomy. J Thorac Cardiovasc Surg 79:922, 1980
48. Manley JC, Johnson WD: Effects of surgery on angina (pre and post infarction) and myocardial function (failure). Circulation 46:1208, 1972
49. Shrank JP, Slabaugh TK, Beckwith JR: The incidence and clinical significance of ECG-VCG changes of myocardial infarction following aortocoronary saphenous vein bypass surgery. Am Heart J 87:46, 1974
50. Fennell WH, Chua KG, Cohen L, et al: Detection, prediction, and significance of perioperative myocardial infarction following aortocoronary bypass. J Thoracic Cardiovasc Surg 78:244, 1979
51. Alderman EL, Fisher LD, Litwin P, et al: Results of coronary artery surgery in patients with poor left ventricular function (CASS). Circulation 68:785, 1983
52. Kennedy JW, Kaiser GC, Fisher LD, et al: Clinical and angiographic predictors of operative mortality from the Collaborative Study in Coronary Artery Surgery (CASS). Circulation 63:793, 1981
53. Maher LJ, Steen PA, Tinker JH, et al: Perioperative myocardial infarction in patients with coronary artery disease with and without aorta-coronary artery bypass grafts. J Thorac Cardiovasc Surg 76:533, 1978
54. Crawford SE, Morris GC, Howell JF, et al: Operative risk in patients with previous coronary artery bypass. Ann Thorac Surg 26:215, 1978
55. Prorok JJ, Trostle D: Operative risk of general surgical procedures in patients with previous myocardial revascularization. Surg Gynecol Obstet 159:214, 1984
56. Backofen JE, Schauble JF, Baughman KL, et al: Does previous coronary artery bypass surgery protect from ischemia during subsequent anesthesia? Abstracts of the Sixth Annual Meeting of the Society of Cardiovascular Anesthesiologists, 1984: 142
57. Frick HM, Harjola PT, Valle M: Persistent improvement after coronary bypass surgery: ergometric and angiographic correlations at 5 years. Circulation 67:491, 1983
58. Slogoff S, Keats AS: Does perioperative myocardial ischemia lead to postoperative myocardial infarction? Anesthesiology 62: 107, 1985
59. Kaplan JA: Hemodynamic monitoring. In Kaplan JA (ed): Cardiac anesthesia, 2nd ed. New York: Grune and Stratton, 1987: 179
60. Brest A, Goldberg S: Thrombosis: historical aspects. In Goldberg S (ed): Coronary artery spasm and thrombosis. Philadelphia: FA Davis, 1983: 6
61. Oliva P: The role of coronary spasm in acute myocardial infarction. In Goldberg S (ed): Coronary artery spasm and thrombosis. Philadelphia: FA Davis, 1983: 46
62. Sevenri CG, Gensini GF, Abbate R, et al: Increased fibrinopeptide A formation and thromboxane A production in patients with ischemic heart disease: relationships to coronary pathoanatomy, risk factors, and clinical manifestations. Am Heart J 101:185, 1981
63. Hirsh PD, Hillis LD, Campbell WB, et al: Release of prostaglandins and thromboxane into the coronary circulation in patients with ischemic heart disease. N Engl J Med 304:685, 1981
64. Hillis LD, Hirsh PD, Campbell WB, et al: Interactions of the arterial wall, plaque, and platelets in myocardial ischemia and infarction. In Goldberg S (ed): Coronary artery spasm and thrombosis. Philadelphia: FA Davis, 1983: 31
65. Mathey DG, Kuck K-H, Tilsner V, et al: Nonsurgical coronary artery recanalization in acute transmural myocardial infarction. Circulation 63:489, 1981
66. Rentrop P, Blanke H, Karsch R, et al: Selective intracoronary thrombolysis in acute myocardial infarction and unstable angina pectoris. Circulation 63:307, 1981
67. Weintraub WS, Helfaut RH: Coronary artery spasm: historical aspects. In Goldberg S (ed): Coronary artery spasm and thrombosis. Philadelphia: FA Davis, 1983: 3
68. Lewy RI, Smith BJ, Silver MJ, et al: Detection of thromboxane B in peripheral blood of patients with Prinzmetal's angina. Prostaglandins Med 5:243, 1979
69. Carleton RA, Boyd T: Traumatic laceration of the anterior descending coronary artery treated by ligation without myocardial infarction: report of a case with review of the literature. Am Heart J 56:136, 1958
70. Benchimol A, et al: Resting electrocardiogram in major coronary artery disease. JAMA 224:1489, 1973
71. Choy JJ: An anesthesiologist's philosophy on 'medical clearance' for surgical patients. Arch Intern Med 147:2090, 1987
72. Limacher LC, Robbins WC: Cardiology consultation. In Kirby RR, Gravenstein N (eds): Clinical anesthesia practice. Philadelphia: WB Saunders, 1994:125
73. Froelicher VF, Yanowitz F, Tompson AJ, et al: The correlation of coronary angiography and the electrocardiographic response to maximal treadmill testing in 76 asymptomatic men. Circulation 48:597, 1973
74. Borer JS, Brensike JF, Fedwood DR, et al: Limitations of the electrocardiographic response to exercise in predicting coronary artery disease. N Engl J Med 293:367, 1975
75. Gibson RS, Beller GA: Should exercise electrocardiographic testing be replaced by radioisotope methods? In Rahimtoola S (ed): Controversies in coronary artery disease. Philadelphia: FA Davis, 1983: 8
76. Mears JH, Plitt K, Tinker JH: Coronary artery bypass: are there legitimate emergencies? (abstract). Anesthesiology 55:A22, 1981
77. Vitez TS, Soper LE, Soper PG: Chronic hypokalemia does not increase anesthetic dysrhythmias. Anesth Analg 61:221, 1982
78. London MJ, Hollenberg M, Wong MG, et al: Intraoperative

myocardial ischemia: localization by continuous 12-lead electrocardiography. Anesthesiology 69:237, 1988

79. Blackburn H, Taylor H, Okamoto N, et al: Standardization of the exercise electrocardiogram. In Karvonen M, Barry A (eds): Physical activity and the heart. Springfield, IL: CC Thomas, 1967: 101
80. Slogoff S, Keats AS, Arlund BS: On the safety of radial artery cannulation. Anesthesiology 59:42, 1983
81. Mangano DT: Monitoring pulmonary arterial pressure in coronary artery disease. Anesthesiology 53:364, 1980
82. Otto CW: Central venous pressure monitoring. In Blitt CD (ed): Monitoring in anesthesia and critical care medicine. New York: Churchill Livingstone, 1985: 121
83. Shah LB, Rao TLK, Laughlin S, et al: A review of pulmonary artery catheterization in 6,245 patients. Anesthesiology 61:27, 1984
84. Kaplan JA, Wells PH: Early diagnosis of myocardial ischemia using the pulmonary artery catheter. Anesth Analg 60:789, 1981
85. Seward JB, Khanderia BK, Edwards WB, et al: Biplanar transesophageal echocardiography: anatomic correlations, image orientation, and clinical applications. Mayo Clin Proc 65:1193, 1990
86. Clements FM, de Bruijn NP: Perioperative evaluation of regional wall motion by transesophageal two-dimensional echocardiography. Anesth Analg 66:249, 1987
87. Weiskopf RB, Moore MA, Eger EI, et al: Rapid increase in desflurane concentration is associated with greater transient cardiovascular stimulation than with rapid increase in isoflurane concentration in humans. Anesthesiology 80:1035, 1994
88. Ebert T, Muzzi M: Sympathetic hyperactivity during desflurane anesthesia in healthy volunteers: a comparison with isoflurane. Anesthesiology 79:444, 1993
89. Savarese JJ, Miller RD, Lien CA, Caldwell JE: Pharmacology of muscle relaxants and their antagonists. In Miller RD (ed): Anesthesia, 4th ed. New York: Churchill Livingstone, 1991:417
90. Thomson IR, Putnins CL: Adverse effects of pancuronium during high-dose fentanyl anesthesia for coronary artery bypass grafting. Anesthesiology 62:708, 1985
91. Hersch C: Electrocardiographic changes in subarachnoid hemorrhage, meningitis, and intracranial space-occupying lesions. Br Heart J 26:785, 1964
92. Cottrell JE, Gupta B, Rappaport H, et al: Intracranial pressure during nitroglycerin-induced hypotension. J Neurosurg 53:309, 1980
93. Cottrell JE, Patel K, Turndorf J, et al: Intracranial pressure changes induced by sodium nitroprusside in patients with intracranial mass lesions. J Neurosurg 48:329, 1978
94. Gagnon R, Marsh ML, Smith RW, et al: Intracranial hypertension caused by nitroglycerin. Anesthesiology 51:86, 1979

FURTHER READING

Brown DL, Kirby RR: Preoperative evaluation of high-risk surgical patients. In Civetta JM, Taylor RW, Kirby RR (eds): Critical care. Philadelphia: JB Lippincott, 1992: 571

Goldman L: Assessment of the patient with known or suspected ischemic heart disease for non-cardiac surgery. Br J Anaesth 61:38, 1988

Haagensen R, Steen PA: Perioperative myocardial infarction. Br J Anaesth 61:24, 1988

Mangano DT: Beyond CK-MP: Biochemical markers for perioperative myocardial infarction (editorial). Anesthesiology 81:1317, 1994

McGough EK: Cardiovascular system. In Gravenstein N (ed): Manual of complications during anesthesia. Philadelphia: JB Lippincott, 1991: 181

Prys-Roberts C: Anaesthetic considerations for the patient with coronary artery disease. Br J Anaesth 61:85, 1988

Reiz S: Myocardial ischaemia associated with general anaesthesia: a review of clinical studies Br J Anaesth 61:68, 1988

Complications in Anesthesiology, second edition, edited by Nikolaus Gravenstein and Robert R. Kirby. Lippincott-Raven Publishers, Philadelphia © 1996.

CHAPTER 25

Complications of Deliberate Hypotension

The deliberate induction of hypotension during surgery (variously termed "controlled hypotension," "induced hypotension," "hypotensive anesthesia," and "deliberate hypotension") is a limited but popular anesthetic technique affording a dry operative field. In the past 40 years, studies of deliberate hypotension during scoliosis surgery,[1] hip replacement,[2–6] portocaval shunting, radical cancer surgery,[7] craniotomy, and rhinoplasty[8] have described its benefits, including reduced blood loss, shortened operating time, lessened hematoma formation, and reduced scarring.

With increasing concern regarding hepatitis, the acquired immunodeficiency syndrome, and other diseases that may be transmitted through transfusion, the technique has generated renewed interest. Nevertheless, its use has been criticized by some physicians, who consider it an unjustified "physiologic trespass," with risks out of proportion to any possible benefits. This chapter reviews the incidence, recognition, and avoidance of complications associated with this technique.

INCIDENCE OF COMPLICATIONS

Mortality

Shortly after the cardiovascular effects of ganglionic blocking agents were described in the late 1940s, Enderby reported the use of pentolinium as a hypotensive agent during general anesthesia.[9] Concern about the risks of deliberate hypotension prompted Hampton and Little to circulate a questionnaire, the results of which were summarized in 1953.[10] Overall mortality was 96 in 27,930 cases, a rate of 0.34%; in 0.24%, death was thought to be related to anesthesia or hypotension. Subsequent series suggest that the mortality rate may now be lower (Table 25-1).[11–16] Several studies of patients undergoing prostatectomy suggest that mortality rates do not differ between procedures with or without deliberate hypotension.[17–21]

Morbidity

Nonfatal complications are more common. Hampton and Little[10] reported an incidence of 3.3%, with reactionary hemorrhage, delayed awakening, blurred vision, oliguria, anuria, and persistent hypotension occurring more frequently. Noteworthy in Little's series[11] was the observation that no major complications occurred in patients whose systolic pressure was maintained at greater than 80 mm Hg.

Most complications appear related to inadequate perfusion of major organs, and risks probably are increased by vascular disease, preexisting hypertension, hypocapnia, very low arterial pressure (systolic pressure <70 mm Hg), severe anemia, hypovolemia, and careless monitoring.[22] Although modern methods of monitoring and postoperative care would be expected to occasion fewer complications than those of the 1950s, no evidence supports this belief.

EFFECTS ON ORGAN SYSTEMS

The physiologic mechanisms responsible for the decreased arterial blood pressure produced by deliberate hypotension are diverse and often complex. Not unexpectedly, the effects of this technique on organ systems may differ. Moreover, the various pharmacologic agents and adjunctive maneuvers used to produce deliberate hypotension differ in their regional hemodynamic and microvascular actions, even within a single organ system. Therefore, generalizations about unqualified deliberate hypotension are tenuous, if not frankly unreliable. Safe use of this technique requires meticulous attention to blood pressure monitoring and control. Approaches to monitoring and the organ-specific effects are described in the following sections. Differential drug effects are described afterwards.

The Nervous System

Injury

In general, injury to the central nervous system from institution of deliberate hypotension reflects impaired cerebral perfusion, which leads progressively to imbalances in cellular metabolic supply and demand, metabolic acidosis, derangement in cellular membrane permeability, and eventual cell

TABLE 25-1
Mortality Associated With Deliberate Hypotension

STUDY	YEARS	PATIENTS (no.)	MORTALITY RATE (%)
Hampton and Little[10]	1950–1953	27,930	0.34
Enderby[12]	1950–1960	9107	0.10
Larson[13]	1958–1964	13,264	0.10
Enderby[14]	1960–1976	9256	0.02
Enderby[15]	1950–1979	20,558	0.04
Pasch and Huk[16]	1977–1984	1802	0.06

death.[23,24] The symptoms may be mild and transient (eg, yawning, confusion, or fainting) or severe (eg, loss of intellect, convulsions, paralysis, or death).[25] Adjunctive maneuvers used with pharmacologic agents may impair cerebral perfusion and include patient positioning with head-up tilt,[26] hypocapnia from hyperventilation,[27,28] and hypoxemia due to increased pulmonary shunting.[29]

Of the complications reported by Hampton and Little in 27,930 patients, the incidence of central nervous system injury, consisting of cerebral and retinal artery thrombosis, constituted 0.02%.[10] No prospective controlled studies of cerebral complications are available.

Neuropsychological Changes

Coinciding with increasing emphasis on ambulatory care, investigators have studied neuropsychological changes associated with anesthesia. In one study, a battery of psychological tests failed to identify differences in performance between young adults undergoing maxillofacial surgery during deliberate hypotension and those receiving normotensive anesthesia.[30] This report corroborated Eckenhoff's early work, which had found no changes in mental acuity related to the technique.[31] However, general anesthesia per se is associated with subtle, transient impairment of memory and learning related specifically to the storage of new information; this defect is present for at least 24 hours.[30]

Preexisting Disease

Patient-related factors may have an adverse influence. Chronic hypertension increases the risk of cerebral ischemia from induced hypotension because the brain's capacity to maintain normal cerebral blood flow (CBF) despite changes in blood pressure (eg, its ability to autoregulate) is impaired.[31] Thus, mildly hypertensive patients with mean arterial pressure (MAP) of 113 mm Hg tolerate reductions in MAP to 42% of baseline, whereas more severely hypertensive patients (MAP of 180 mm Hg) manifest signs of cerebral ischemia at a MAP of 90 mm Hg.[25,32] In one series, awake normotensive patients showed evidence of ischemia when MAP was 36% of baseline.[25]

Adequacy of Cerebral Perfusion

Because all approaches to deliberate hypotension can reduce cerebral perfusion substantially, the adequacy of cerebral perfusion is of great interest. In any patient who is in a head-elevated position it is especially important to reference the blood pressure to brain level as opposed to heart level. A reliable, readily available means to assess cerebral function during hypotension and to predict good outcome after hypotension is still being sought. Psychometric testing, usually a sensitive indicator of cerebral function, has not proven to be useful in distinguishing normotensive patients from patients whose MAP is decreased to as low as 56% of the normal level.[26,30,33,34]

Monitoring of Cerebral Function

ELECTROENCEPHALOGRAPHY. Electroencephalography (EEG) has been proposed as a means of monitoring cerebral function during hypotension and carotid endarterectomy.[35–37] Most data from animal and human studies suggest that for a cerebral ischemic event to result in a clinically apparent neurologic deficit, a critical amount of time must elapse before derangement or extinction of the EEG occurs.[38]

Animal models of focal and global ischemia have been used to define thresholds for CBF depression and derangement of EEG activity.[36,39–42] Although the models used different species and methods, electric abnormalities were not consistently evident until CBF fell below a critical value that may have corresponded to the particular model's lower limit of autoregulatory capacity.

In normotensive humans without central nervous system lesions, autoregulation of CBF usually fails at an MAP of less than 60 mm Hg.[43] However, a study of healthy young volunteers subjected to an MAP of 59 mm Hg showed so much variability in the EEG power spectra, with and without hypotension, that the monitoring was concluded to be insensitive.[30] Abnormal states, such as hypertension, subarachnoid hemorrhage, or the presence of brain tumors, may raise the autoregulatory threshold and thus increase the risk of these patients for ischemia when hypotension is induced.[32]

EEG monitoring remains attractive because of its advantages, which include direct measurement of spontaneous cortical electric activity; rapidity of indication of change, usually within 20 to 40 seconds, of a cerebral insult; and noninvasiveness. The disadvantages of this technique include its lack of specificity; its high susceptibility to artifact; cumbersome equipment; lack of information from subcortical structures; possible encroachment on the surgical field during neurosurgical procedures; and possible inability to monitor the desired cerebral region. It also is susceptible to changes induced by anesthetic drugs (Table 25-2).

Current EEG techniques do not provide additional clinically important information on cerebral function in normal patients unless MAP is lower than the normal autoregulatory range (ie, <60 mm Hg). However, EEG monitoring may be used increasingly in instances in which MAP must be decreased below autoregulatory limits, such as in cerebral aneurysm clipping, and in known chronically hypertensive patients undergoing a procedure in which some reduction in cerebral perfusion pressure is necessary, such as carotid endarterectomy.[44]

SOMATOSENSORY EVOKED POTENTIALS. Somatosensory evoked potentials (SSEPs) also are used for cerebral function monitoring during hypotension,[45,46] aneurysm clipping,[47,48] and carotid endarterectomy.[35,49] In addition to detecting changes in cortical activity, the SSEPs reflect changes in subcortical, brain stem, and spinal cord function.[45,46,50–53] As the name implies, this monitoring technique involves application of a rapid, repetitive stimulus to an extremity or to the spinal cord to elicit electric activity. The changes produced by anesthetic agents in SSEPs are less severe than are those produced in EEG activity.[38,54] The SSEP changes that do occur essentially are limited to the cortical response, with preservation of all subcortical ones (eg, cervical). However, because the SSEP method requires repetition of a stimulus over time to produce a response, the EEG can give more rapid information when an abrupt ischemic event occurs.

SSEP monitoring has been used successfully in clinical investigations to signal encroachment on brain and spinal cord function during intracranial, carotid artery, and some spinal cord procedures. However, like the EEG, SSEP monitoring can be insensitive to important clinical events.[55–57] During intracranial aneurysm resection and major spinal cord surgery, SSEP monitoring is an important tool in the intraoperative detection and management of cerebral compromise in some patients. Its usefulness in monitoring spinal cord integrity also is of great value.

TABLE 25-2
Electroencephalographic Changes Associated With Anesthetic Drugs

INCREASED FREQUENCY
Barbiturates (low dose)
Benzodiazepines (low dose)
Etomidate (low dose)
Nitrous oxide (30% to 70%)
Inhalation agents (<1 MAC)
Ketamine
DECREASED FREQUENCY, INCREASED AMPLITUDE
Barbiturates (moderate dose)
Etomidate (moderate dose)
Narcotics
Inhalation agents (>1 MAC)
DECREASED FREQUENCY, DECREASED AMPLITUDE
Barbiturates (high dose)
ELECTRICAL SILENCE
Barbiturates (coma dose)
Etomidate (high dose)
Isoflurane (2 MAC)

MAC, minimum alveolar concentration.

Bendo AA: Monitoring the nervous system. Problems in Anesthesia 7: 115, 1993.

The Heart

The heart is less likely to be damaged by hypotension than is the brain, for two reasons: hypotension reduces the work load of the heart and thus its oxygen requirements, and electrocardiographic monitoring is a reasonably sensitive indicator of reversible ischemia. Hampton and Little's series found a 0.27% incidence of major cardiovascular events (eg, cardiac arrest, acute myocardial infarction) and a 0.079% mortality rate.[11] Enderby reported only one such event, occurring 20 hours postoperatively, among 9107 hypotensive anesthetics.[12]

Hypocapnia

Some evidence suggests that to protect the myocardium, hypocapnia should be avoided. During halothane-induced hypotension in dogs, myocardial oxygen consumption decreases in proportion to the decrease in blood flow. This balance is disturbed by hypocapnia, which causes a further decrease in coronary flow without a proportional decrease in oxygen consumption. Reduction of MAP to 55% of control values is accompanied by a reduction of myocardial blood flow to 47% and oxygen consumption to 55% of control values. Subsequent hypocapnia, to an arterial carbon dioxide partial pressure of 26 mm Hg, causes a further reduction of blood flow to 38% of control values without any concomitant decrease in oxygen consumption.[58]

Moderate Hypotension

Moderate hypotension caused by spinal anesthesia also may have little harmful effect on myocardial oxygenation. In one study, spinal anesthesia to a T4 dermatomal level caused a decrease in MAP from 120 to 62 mm Hg, with an associated decrease in coronary blood flow from 153 to 74 mL/100 g/min.[59] In only one of six subjects did coronary sinus oxygen content decrease; a decrease in myocardial oxygen extraction was statistically insignificant. The patients were, however, extremely sensitive to blood volume changes: a loss of 70 mL of blood was reported to result in "vascular collapse" and myocardial ischemia.

Coronary blood flow may increase during moderate hypotension induced by sodium nitroprusside (SNP), but at more profound levels of hypotension, flow decreases.[60] Flow in superior mesenteric and femoral arteries follows a similar course.[61] Hypotension-induced reflex tachycardia causes further decreases in coronary blood flow because of decreased diastolic filling time. Resultant increases in oxygen demand, with concomitant decreases in oxygen supply, pose a particular threat to patients with coronary artery disease.[62]

These patients are at potentially greater risk because hypotensive agents may not influence regional myocardial perfusion and oxygen consumption favorably. In a dog model with a single severe coronary artery stenosis sufficient to prevent an increase in coronary blood flow, hypotension (MAP of 50 mm Hg) was produced with halothane, trimethaphan camsylate, or SNP. In normal portions of the myocardium, reductions in subendocardial blood flow, subepicardial blood flow, and myocardial oxygen consumption were similar. However, in myocardium affected by the stenosis, perfusion was reduced, with resultant myocardial ischemia.[63]

Electrocardiographic Changes

A variety of electrocardiographic changes can occur during induced hypotension, all apparently reversible. Rollason and colleagues reported major changes, consisting of decreased P-wave voltage, ST-segment elevation or depression, and T-wave alterations, in about half of the cases studied. Other minor changes in the QRS and QT intervals and PQ and ST segments brought the total incidence of transient changes to almost 80%. Most major changes appeared to result from rapid induction of hypotension rather than from the depth of hypotension or the agent used.[64,65]

The Lungs

Dead Space

No complications of hypotensive anesthesia specifically involve the lungs. When the head-up position is used, physiologic dead space increases,[66,67] probably because of a decrease in pulmonary artery pressure and an enlarged zone 1 (the areas of the lungs that are ventilated but poorly perfused). Thus, measurement of the end-tidal partial pressure of carbon dioxide may not accurately reflect its arterial partial pressure. A comparison of the end-tidal with the arterial carbon dioxide partial pressure by blood gas analysis allows the clinician to determine the extent of the arterial–to–end-tidal carbon dioxide partial pressure gradient to guide subsequent ventilation settings. These patients may require higher than predicted minute volumes to achieve satisfactory alveolar ventilation. However, this approach exacerbates the increase of dead space. If cardiac output is maintained by increasing the intravenous fluid infusion rate, no change in physiologic dead space occurs.[68,69]

Arterial Oxygenation

Arterial oxygenation may be impaired during hypotension induced by a variety of agents, including inhalation anesthetics and direct vasodilators.[70-72] Not all investigators have found this impairment with SNP,[73,74] and nitroglycerin may not produce an increase in pulmonary arteriovenous shunt either.[29] Inspired concentrations of oxygen should be increased if pulse oximetry or arterial blood gas analysis demonstrates a decrease in hemoglobin oxygen saturation or a decrease in oxygen partial pressure, respectively.

The Splanchnic Organs

No reports of ischemia of the liver or the bowel during induced hypotension have been published, but no systematic studies have been performed. Most anesthetic agents decrease splanchnic blood flow more than they reduce oxygen consumption.[75] Mild hypotension induced by SNP increases superior mesenteric artery flow in chloralose-anesthetized dogs; more severe hypotension decreases it.[61] A similar effect occurs when SNP is given to halothane-anesthetized dogs.[76]

The clearance of indocyanine green dye from plasma can be used as an index of hepatic function. When hypotension is induced by SNP or epidural blockade in dogs anesthetized with halothane, no change in clearance occurs, suggesting no change in hepatic excretory function or hepatic blood flow.[77] One report of adynamic ileus after deliberate hypotension with SNP has been published.[78]

The Kidneys

Most anesthetics, except perhaps neuroleptic agents, reduce renal blood flow, resulting in transient decrease in renal function, with diminished filtration rates and electrolyte excretion. The changes can usually be explained by systemic hypotension, catecholamine release, or the release of antidiuretic hormone. They revert to normal upon discontinuation of the agent.

Hypotension produced by halothane and trimethaphan reduces glomerular filtration rate and filtration fraction during mannitol-induced diuresis; a less consistent decline is seen in effective renal plasma flow.[79] Hypotension with 2% halothane causes diminished renal blood flow, but apparently no intrarenal shunting; the ratio of renal blood flow to cardiac output remains constant.[80] Hypotension with SNP and halothane produces a greater decrease in renal blood flow than in iliac, celiac, or mesenteric blood flow. These other vascular beds probably are further dilated by SNP, whereas the renal vascular bed is limited in its capacity to so respond.[76] In one study, endogenous creatinine clearance fell from 106 to 41 mL/min during hypotension induced with halothane and SNP.[81]

Many practitioners measure the urine output and give diuretics to maintain an adequate flow output during the period of hypotension. No evidence shows that this treatment is beneficial, and some evidence suggests that it is unnecessary.[82] As with other organ systems, the renal effects of different hypotensive techniques deserve further study.

The Gravid Uterus

Although deliberate hypotension is rarely, if ever, used in the pregnant patient (cerebral aneurysm clipping is an exception), the same hypotensive agents are commonly used to treat the hypertension that is part of severe preeclampsia and eclampsia. Two major additional concerns unique to the pregnant patient arise. First, uterine perfusion must be sufficient to maintain normal fetal oxygenation and acid–base regulation. Second, these hypotensive agents may cause fetal toxicity.

Because uterine blood vessels have no autoregulatory

mechanism, maternal arterial pressure is the chief determinant of uterine perfusion.[83] Monitoring of fetal heart tones with external Doppler ultrasound is a useful indicator of fetal well-being throughout the second and third trimesters of pregnancy[84–89] and should be instituted in those rare circumstances in which deliberate hypotension is used.

Pharmacologic Agents

Pharmacologic agents used to induce deliberate hypotension may affect the fetus as well as the mother. The association between teratogenicity and the administration of inhalational agents during the first trimester has been inconclusive in humans and animals.[90,91] Ganglionic blocking agents such as trimethaphan should be used with caution in pregnant patients because of a decrease in pseudocholinesterase activity,[92–94] which slows inactivation of the drug and prolongs succinylcholine-induced paralysis.[95,96] Autonomic blockade may interfere with the ability of capacitance vessels to compensate for the effects of uterine compression on venous return.

β-Adrenergic receptor blockade with propranolol decreases umbilical blood flow and blocks the β-receptors of the fetal sympathetic nervous system in animals.[97,98] Hypoglycemia, bradycardia, acidosis and apnea have been observed in newborns whose mothers received propranolol therapy during pregnancy and uncomplicated deliveries.[99–103] Nitroglycerin administered during delivery apparently has no adverse maternal or fetal effects.[104,105] Hydralazine has frequently been used to treat pregnancy-induced hypertension without apparent ill effects.[106]

SODIUM NITROPRUSSIDE. Numerous case reports and animal studies indicate that SNP may be used safely, without cyanide toxicity (discussed below), during pregnancy when it is administered at a dosage of less than 3 μg/kg/min.[107–110] However, these studies do not specifically address the question of how long SNP may be chronically administered without development of fetal toxicity. In pregnant ewes, fetal death resulted from cyanide toxicity when mean rates of 25 $\mu g/kg^{-1}/min^{-1}$ were used for 60 minutes to maintain a 20% reduction in MAP. Animals given a lower dose showed no fetal toxicity.[108] Intrauterine death occurred in three severely hypotensive patients between 22 and 25 weeks gestation after 36 hours of SNP infusion; however, information regarding total SNP dose, rate of administration, fetal monitoring, and maternal toxicity is unavailable.[111]

SNP aggravates the hypertension-induced reduction in uterine blood flow in pregnant sheep with renal hypertension.[112] Good maternal and fetal outcome have been reported in patients who received SNP for as long as 8 hours for control of hypertension.[113] A 57-kg woman at 20 weeks gestation received a total of 90 mg of SNP within 48 hours without untoward effects on mother or fetus.[110] Shoemaker and Meyers described a case in which SNP was administered at a rate of 3.9 μg/kg/min over a 15-h period to a severely preeclamptic patient at 24 weeks gestation before delivery of a stillborn infant.[114] The mother manifested no signs of cyanide intoxication, and fetal liver cyanide levels were well below the toxic range, suggesting that fetal circulatory compromise was a contributing factor.

Several clinical reports have demonstrated the safe use of SNP during profound hypotension in pregnant patients for cerebral aneurysm clipping.[87,109,110] The drug may not be appropriate for chronic control of gestational hypertension, but it is suitable in the short term to control hypertension during pregnancy, provided that one adheres to recommended dosage limits and monitors the mother for SNP toxicity.

COMPLICATIONS DUE TO PHARMACOLOGIC AGENTS

Hypotensive agents conveniently can be classified as inhalation, short-acting intravenously administered, or long-acting intravenously administered. The effects of short-acting agents are rapid, profound, and controllable; these agents do not produce postoperative hypotension. On the other hand, they require constant intraoperative blood pressure monitoring and regulation of infusion rate to obtain the desired level of hypotension.

Long-acting agents may require somewhat less attention to pressure monitoring, fluid replacement, and anesthetic depth because their hypotensive effects are usually less profound. They may prove to be less troublesome in an operation requiring prolonged duration of hypotension, but their effects extend into the postoperative period.

Inhalation Agents

The potent inhalation anesthetic agents, halothane, enflurane, isoflurane, and desflurane all produce mild to moderate levels of hypotension in a dose-related fashion. Complications from these agents are generally related to cardiovascular depression[115] and impaired organ perfusion at higher dosages.[116] Cardiovascular depression may be minimized by decreasing the dosage of a given agent by combining its use with that of intravenously administered agents.

Halothane

In high doses, halothane causes profound myocardial, baroreceptor, and cardiac conducting system depression, that may result in cardiovascular instability and impair organ perfusion.[117] Its relatively high blood and tissue solubility not only prolong its elimination but also render its hypotension somewhat less readily alterable than that achieved with short-acting, intravenously administered agents or other inhalation agents. Halothane generally decreases the cerebral metabolic oxygen requirement, but increases CBF in a dose-dependent fashion, which may be detrimental to patients with decreased intracranial compliance.[116,118,119]

Enflurane

In addition to the characteristics noted for halothane, enflurane produces a greater decrease in systemic vascular resistance (SVR) than halothane, especially in nonstimulated surgical patients.[116,120,121] Reflex tachycardia is greater than with halothane, because less depression of the cardiac conducting system and baroreceptors occurs. A high dose of enflurane (>2.5%) can result in seizure activity, particularly during hyperventilation (arterial carbon dioxide partial pressure >2.5).[122,123]

Isoflurane

Isoflurane is associated with the least depression of myocardial and conducting systems of the three common potent inhalation agents, but the greatest decrease in SVR at higher doses.[116,124,125] It has been used as the sole hypotensive agent for cerebral aneurysm clipping, without evidence of adverse effects at a MAP of 50 mm Hg.[126] Although both CBF and intracranial pressure increase in patients at risk, the increases are less than with halothane or enflurane at equipotent doses.[116,127] Furthermore, isoflurane, 2% to 4%, produces major reductions in cerebral metabolism and EEG activity in humans, effects that may be protective during severe hypotension.[125,127–129] Although isoflurane lowers the cerebral metabolic oxygen requirement without affecting CBF, its use may be followed by hyperemia characterized as increased CBF without change in the cerebral oxygen requirement.[127] Isoflurane may cause undesirable tachycardia at higher doses, necessitating co-administration of a β-adrenergic receptor–blocking agent.

Desflurane

Desflurane appears to have hypotensive properties similar to those of isoflurane but with more rapid onset and offset.[130] It also may possess cerebral protective properties. In general, its effects on systemic, coronary, renal, hepatic, and cerebral circulation are strikingly similar to isoflurane.[131]

Short-acting Intravenously Administered Agents

A variety of agents are available that act on many parts of the circulation (Table 25-3).

Trimethaphan Camsylate

With actions rather similar to the ganglionic-blocking agent pentolinium, which is no longer available in the United States, trimethaphan camsylate decreases both arteriolar and venular tone. Reflex sympathetic activation, present with other hypotensive agents, is blunted by its inherent ganglionic blockade. In addition to ganglionic blockade, it produces histamine release and bronchoconstriction.

Because trimethaphan is inactivated by serum cholinesterase, its clinical effect may be prolonged in patients with abnormal, deficient, or blocked cholinesterase. For example, through its inhibition of plasma cholinesterase, neostigmine may retard the metabolism of trimethaphan. Moreover, large dosages (eg, infusions at >5 mg/min) of trimethaphan can cause neuromuscular block, manifesting as respiratory muscle weakness that is not antagonized by neostigmine.[132]

Trimethaphan causes pupillary dilatation through blockade of the ciliary ganglion. Thus, eye signs that are otherwise valuable in assessing postoperative neurologic status may be obscured for hours.

Sodium Nitroprusside

A direct-acting dilator of both veins and arterioles, sodium nitroprusside (SNP) is the most commonly used adjunctive hypotensive agent for the acute control of blood pressure. It has high potency, rapid onset, and short duration of action. Its cardiac effects, such as on heart rate and stroke volume, are variable, depending on the anesthetic circumstances in which it is used.

Not unexpectedly, the most immediate danger associated with SNP is overdose, with profound hypotension. This complication can best be avoided by continuous direct arterial blood pressure monitoring and close attention to the infusion rate with delivery via an infusion pump rather than by gravity. Long-term toxicity has been reported in one uremic patient: hypothyroidism was caused by the metabolic product thiocyanate, which inhibits thyroid function.[133] This type of toxicity is unlikely to be important in anesthetic practice.

In clinical concentrations, SNP is a potent inhibitor of platelet aggregation,[134] but increased bleeding has not been

TABLE 25-3
Intravenous Hypotensive Agents

DRUG	DOSE	COMMENTS
Hydralazine	5- to 10-mg boluses	Arteriolar dilator; initial effect in 3 to 5 min, peak in 20 min
Phentolamine	0.5- to 2-mg boluses; 2.5 to 10 μg/kg/min	α-Blocker, therapy for hypertension after topical or infiltrated phenylephrine
Propranolol	0.5 to 1 mg intravenously, up to 0.1 mg/kg	Nonselective β-blocker
Esmolol	500-μg/kg loading dose; 50 to 300 μg/kg/min	Nonselective, short-acting β-blocker
Labetalol	5 to 20 mg; repeat as necessary	Nonselective β-blocker with some α-blocker activity
Trimethaphan	1- to 5-mg bolus; 10 to 100 μg/kg/min	Ganglionic blocker; tachyphylaxis common
Nifedipine	20 mg sublingually	Calcium-channel blocker
SNP	0.5 μg/kg/min to start; titrate to effect	Specific arteriolar dilator; potential for cyanide toxicity
Nitroglycerin	25- to 200-μg bolus; 1 to 4 μg/kg/min	Primary capacitance vessel dilator; decreased preload

reported. In physiologic conditions, nitroprusside can react with therapeutic secondary amines to form potentially carcinogenic n-nitrosoamines[135]; the significance of this finding awaits further study. Nitroprusside use is somewhat limited in patients with intracranial masses because the resultant cerebral dilatation can result in intracranial hypertension.[136,137] Thus, it is best avoided during induction of anesthesia for intracranial tumor surgery and should only be used after the cranium is opened.

CYANIDE TOXICITY. An especially serious problem is cyanide poisoning after SNP metabolism.

SNP ($Na_2Fe(CN)_5NO \cdot 2H_2O$), contains 44% cyanide by weight. Figure 25-1 summarizes the known pathways through which SNP is broken down in the body.

SNP is degraded in a two-step process, the first of which is a nonenzymatic reaction occurring in the presence of hemoglobin. The substituted radical receives an electron from the heme group of hemoglobin to yield five cyanide ions, as well as nitric acid and methemoglobin (see Fig. 25-1, reaction *a*). This reaction is complete within a few minutes in hemoglobin solutions but has a half-time of about 20 minutes with intact human erythrocytes in vitro.[138]

Released cyanide, the amount of which is directly related to the dose of SNP infused, can combine with cytochrome oxidase, resulting in inhibition of intracellular electron transfer and thus cellular respiration (see Fig. 25-1, reaction *d*). Anaerobic metabolism increases and leads to metabolic acidosis, which allows the observant practitioner to detect this cellular toxicity.

In ordinary clinical circumstances, cyanide toxicity is prevented by several detoxification mechanisms. The most important of these is the second part of the two-step degradation of SNP: An enzymatic reaction of four of the five cyanide ions with thiosulfate produces thiocyanate (see Fig. 25-1, reaction *b*); this irreversible reaction is catalyzed by the enzyme rhodanase, found in liver and other tissues. Thiocyanate is excreted in the urine but, at high serum concentrations, inhibits gastric acid secretion and thyroid function.[139] Thiocyanate is degraded slowly back to cyanide by thiocyanate oxidase (see Fig. 25-1, reaction *c*). Several other minor protective mechanisms exist to help prevent cyanide toxicity. The remaining cyanide ion readily binds to methemoglobin (see Fig. 25-1, reaction *g*), producing cyanmethemoglobin. Although SNP can cause the formation of cyanmethemoglobin in human erythrocytes in vitro, methemoglobin concentrations are not elevated in patients receiving SNP infusions.[140] Some cyanide diffuses out of erythrocytes and is metabolized in the liver and kidney to thiocyanate, which is excreted in the urine. Additional minor pathways exist for the excretion or detoxification of cyanide (see Fig. 25-1, reaction *e*), but they are not thought to be of clinical importance.

Great interest focuses on the circumstances in which cyanide is released apart from SNP overdose. Some investigators have questioned whether cyanide is released in vivo, noting that photodegradation occurs in vitro and, once infused, a photo-degraded solution might account for cyanide levels detected in blood.[141] Yet, no significant degradation occurs in vitro for 24 hours if the recommended 5%-dextrose solution is protected from light[142]; degradation takes even longer in fresh electrolyte solutions.[143] In an elegant study of the effect of potassium cyanide or SNP on cytochrome oxidase activity in mice, similar depression of enzyme activity was noted, but the effect of SNP required time, suggesting that in vivo degradation does occur.[144]

Clinical doses of SNP are capable of yielding toxic amounts

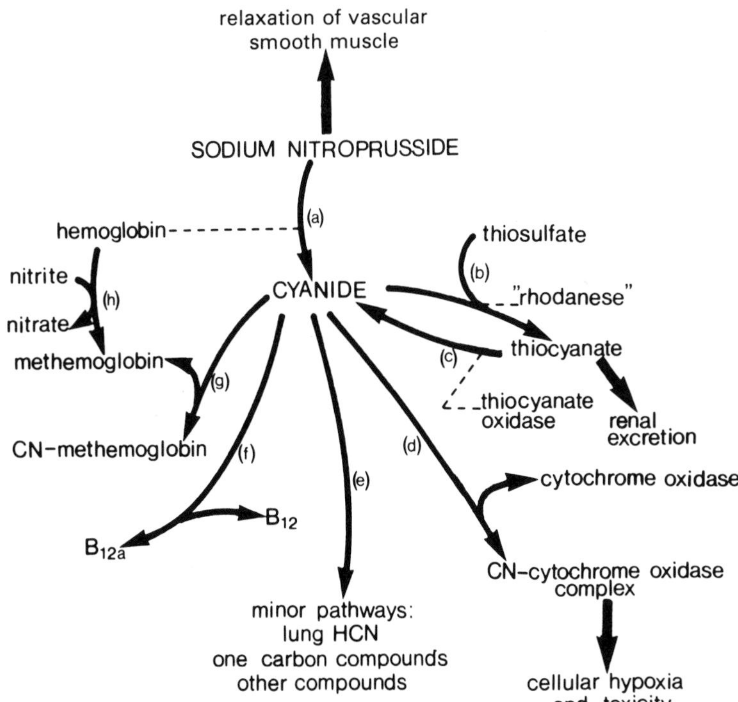

FIGURE 25-1. Breakdown, toxicity, and detoxification of SNP and cyanide (*CN*) in the body.

of cyanide. An absorbed dose of as little as 24 mg of cyanide may be fatal to humans.[145] One ampule of 50 mg of SNP contains 22 mg (835 μmol) of cyanide. In fatal cases of SNP intoxication, adults usually received more than 400 mg and children more than 300 mg. Yet many other patients have received large doses without reported toxicity. Therefore, great variation in tolerance must occur among individuals, perhaps because of differing rates of breakdown of SNP or detoxification of cyanide.

Therapy. The recommended therapy for cyanide poisoning is administration of nitrite, which oxidizes the Fe^{2+} of hemoglobin to form methemoglobin (see Fig. 25-1, reaction *h*) and shifts the equilibrium of reaction g toward the relatively stable and nontoxic cyanmethemoglobin.

Another effective method is to give hydroxocobalamin, vitamin B_{12} (see Fig. 25-1, reaction *f*).[146] However, the dose form and current availability of B_{12} make this an impractical method at present. Because an abnormality of rhodanase or a deficiency of thiosulfate may limit the rate of detoxification (see Fig. 25-1, reaction *b*), cyanide toxicity is rationally treated with thiosulfate.

CLINICAL RECOMMENDATIONS. SNP may be contraindicated in patients with conditions that affect cyanide metabolism: impaired liver function, low plasma concentration of B_{12}, chronic cyanide intoxication, tobacco amblyopia, or Leber's optic atrophy.[147–149] Others have speculated that some patients may have small bodily reserves of thiosulfate, limiting the rate of cyanide detoxification.[150] Based on the forgoing metabolic considerations and the clinical experience reported in the literature, recommendations for use of SNP[151–166] are summarized in Table 25-4.

The guidelines available are not entirely satisfactory because of the anecdotal nature of most reports of SNP toxicity in humans. Those in Table 25-4 are based on sound theoretical grounds and some animal experiments. Overall experience with SNP is favorable. The number of cases of toxicity is small in relation to its frequent use, but SNP must be given only by physicians who are aware of and ready to treat the possible complications.

Adenosine and Adenosine Triphosphate

Adenosine and adenosine triphosphate are both rapidly acting, short-lived vasodilators that can be infused.[167,168] Their advantages over SNP include the lack of tachycardia, tachyphylaxis, and rebound hypertension; also, recovery is more rapid.[168,169] Clinical action is terminated so rapidly that administration via central rather than peripheral veins is suggested. Their disadvantages include increases in CBF and metabolism, possibly causing increased intracranial pressure when the dura is closed[167,170]; impaired cerebrovascular reactivity[171]; atrioventricular block[169,172]; and metabolic acidosis.[168,173–175] When used in coronary artery disease patients, ST segment changes similar to coronary steal–induced ischemia may result.[176]

Nitroglycerin

Acting more on capacitance than resistance vessels, nitroglycerin tends to reduce preload and thus cardiac output. As a result, the patient's sensitivity to the drug may be more dependent upon the adequacy of blood volume than is the case with other vasodilators. Although no apparent toxicity is associated with nitroglycerin, this drug may prolong neuromuscular blockade produced by pancuronium (but not that resulting from other relaxants).[177,178]

Esmolol

Esmolol is a short-acting β-adrenergic blocking agent whose activity rapidly dissipates upon discontinuation. Unlike many

TABLE 25-4
Recommendations for Use of Sodium Nitroprusside

1. ***Limit the dose.*** Estimates of the maximum allowable dose range from 1.5 to 3 mg/kg, but even 1 mg/kg may be too much. Chronic nitroprusside administration should not exceed 0.5 mg/kg/h.
2. ***Measure acid–base status hourly.*** If metabolic acidosis begins to develop, SNP should be discontinued and sodium bicarbonate and specific antidotes given.
3. ***Be prepared to give antidotes for cyanide poisoning.*** All should be given intravenously.
   - Sodium nitrite: 10 ml of a 3% solution for adults, 0.2 ml/kg for children
   - Sodium thiosulfate: 150 mg/kg body weight, as a 25% solution
   - Hydroxocobalamin (B_{12}): 5 mol/mol SNP, or 1 g/50 mg SNP
4. ***Consider prophylactic administration of sodium thiosulfate or hydroxocobalamin.*** These antidotes may be given with SNP.
5. ***Supplement SNP with adjuvant agents.*** SNP requirement can be reduced by propranolol in a dosage sufficient to slow heart rate during deliberate hypotension. The underlying mechanism may be suppression by propranolol of SNP-induced renin release. Similarly, captopril, an inhibitor of angiotensin I–converting enzyme, also reduces the required dose of SNP. Clonidine attenuates the baroreceptor-mediated, sympathetic activity that accompanies SNP-induced hypotension, thereby reducing the SNP dosage requirement. Not unexpectedly, adding or increasing the concentration of a potent inhalation anesthetic also decreases the SNP requirement.

Data from references 151–166.

other β-adrenergic blocking agents, it does not significantly increase bronchospasm. Thus, it may be used effectively in patients with chronic obstructive lung disease.

Long-Acting Intravenously Administered Agents

A variety of vasoactive agents (see Table 25-3) can be used to supplement the hypotensive actions of the potent inhalation anesthetics.

Hydralazine

Hydralazine is a direct vasodilator that can be administered orally or intravenously to produce mild to moderate reductions in blood pressure.[179] Combined with the potent inhalation agent enflurane, hydralazine produces a stable level of hypotension without tachyphylaxis or rebound hypertension.[180] The increase in organ perfusion due to reduced vascular resistance is generally beneficial, but patients with diffusely impaired cerebral autoregulation may experience a detrimental increase in intracranial pressure.[180,181]

Phentolamine and Phenoxybenzamine

Phentolamine and phenoxybenzamine are α-adrenergic receptor blocking agents that are longer in onset and duration than the previously described short-acting agents. Complications may result from excessive dose or prolonged duration of action. A parenteral form of phenoxybenzamine is not available in the United States.

Propranolol

A β-adrenergic receptor blocking agent, propranolol is often used to blunt the tachycardia resulting from profound levels of hypotension obtained with SNP or high concentrations of isoflurane.[157] It is also effective in attenuating the rebound hypertension that accompanies the abrupt discontinuation of SNP.[158] Complications include myocardial depression, excessive bradycardia, bronchospasm in susceptible patients, masked hypoglycemia, and unopposed α-adrenergic receptor activity.[182]

Labetalol

Labetalol combines α- and β-adrenergic receptor antagonist properties lasting 30 to 60 minutes.[183] It is less potent than either phentolamine or propranolol, and the decreases in blood pressure that can be safely achieved with labetalol alone are limited. It can worsen bronchial asthma, congestive heart failure, heart block greater than first-degree, and bradycardia.

Calcium Channel-Blocking Agents

Nifedipine, verapamil, and diltiazem have been used to produce moderate reductions in blood pressure.[184–188] Their onsets and durations of action vary, but none is as easily adjusted as SNP. All three agents have been shown to produce increases in intracranial pressure[185,189,190] making them generally unsuitable for use before opening of the dura in neurosurgery performed in patients with space-occupying lesions. Nicardipine appears to be as effective as SNP for induced hypotension when infused intravenously but may act as a slight myocardial depressant, as seen in a study of hypotensive anesthesia in total hip arthroplasty.[191]

REFERENCES

1. McNeil TW: DeWald RL, Juo KN, et al: Controlled hypotensive anesthesia in scoliosis surgery. J Bone Joint Surg Am 56:1167, 1974
2. Mallory TH: Hypotensive anesthesia in total hip replacement. JAMA 224:248, 1973
3. Davis NJ, Jennings JJH, Harris WH: Induced hypotensive anesthesia for total hip replacement. Clin Orthop 101:93, 1974
4. Amaranath L, Cascorbi HF, Singh-Amaranath AV, et al: Relation of anesthesia to total hip replacement and control of operative blood loss. Anesth Analg 54:641, 1975
5. Thompson GE, Miller RD, Stevens WC, et al: Hypotensive anesthesia for total hip arthroplasty: a study of blood loss and organ function (brain, heart, liver, and kidney). Anesthesiology 48:91, 1978
6. Modig J, Karlstrom G: Intra- and post-operative blood loss and haemodynamics in total hip replacement when performed under lumbar epidural versus general anaesthesia. Eur J Anaesth 4:345, 1987
7. Boyan CP: Hypotensive anesthesia for radical pelvic and abdominal surgery. Arch Surg 67:803, 1953
8. Eckenhoff JE, Rich JC: Clinical experience with deliberate hypotension. Anesth Analg 45:21, 1966
9. Enderby GEH: Controlled circulation with hypotension drugs and posture to reduce bleeding in surgery: preliminary results with pentamethonium iodide. Lancet 1:1145, 1950
10. Hampton LJ, Little DM Jr: Complications associated with the use of 'controlled hypotension' in anesthesia. Arch Surg 67: 549, 1953
11. Little DM: Induced hypotension during anesthesia and surgery. Anesthesiology 16:320, 1955
12. Enderby GEH: A report on mortality and morbidity following 9,107 hypotensive anaesthetics. Br J Anaesth 33:109, 1961
13. Larson AG: Deliberate hypotension. Anesthesiology 25:682, 1964
14. Enderby GEH: Hypotensive anaesthesia. In Gray TC, Nunn JF, Utting JE (eds): General anaesthesia, 4th ed, vol 2. London: Butterworths, 1980: 1149
15. Enderby GEH: Safe hypotensive anaesthesia. In Hypotensive anaesthesia. London: Churchill Livingstone, 1985: 262
16. Pasch T, Huk W: Cerebral complications following induced hypotension. Eur J Anaesth 3:299, 1986
17. Bodman RI: Dangers of hypotensive anaesthesia. Proc R Soc Med 57:1184, 1964
18. Way GL, Clarke HL: An anaesthetic technique for prostatectomy. Lancet 2:888, 1959
19. Baker AH: Prostatectomy without a catheter. Proc R Soc Med 57:1179, 1964
20. Boreham P: Retropubic prostatectomy with hypotensive anaesthesia. Proc R Soc Med 57:1181, 1964
21. Rollason WN, Hough JM: A study of hypotensive anaesthesia in the elderly. Br J Anaesth 32:276, 1960
22. Lindop MJ: Complications and morbidity of controlled hypotension. Br J Anaesth 47:799, 1975
23. Nilsson L, Siesjo BK: The effect of deep halothane hypotension upon labile phosphates and upon extra- and intracellular lactate and pyruvate concentrations in the rat brain. Acta Physiol Scand 81:508, 1971
24. Siesjo BK: Cerebral circulation and metabolism. J Neurosurg 60:883, 1984
25. Finnerty FA, Witkin L, Fazekas JF: Cerebral hemodynamics during cerebral ischemia induced by acute hypotension. J Clin Invest 33:1227, 1954

26. Eckenhoff JE, Enderby GEH, Larson A, et al: Human cerebral circulation during deliberate hypotension and head-up tilt. J Appl Physiol 18:1130, 1963
27. Levin RM, Zadigian ME, Hall SC: The combined effect of hyperventilation and hypotension on cerebral oxygenation in anaesthetized dogs. Can Anaesth Soc J 27:264, 1980
28. Harp JR, Wollman H: Cerebral metabolic effects of hyperventilation and deliberate hypotension. Br J Anaesth 45:256, 1973
29. Casthely PA, Cottrell JE, Lear E: Intrapulmonary shunting during induced hypotension. Anesth Analg 61:231, 1982
30. Townes BD, Dikmen SS, Bledsoe SW, et al: Neuropsychological changes in a young, healthy population after controlled hypotensive anesthesia. Anesth Analg 65:955, 1986
31. Hoffman WE, Miletich DJ, Albrecht RF: The influence of aging and hypertension on cerebral autoregulation. Brain Res 214: 196, 1981
32. Strandgaard S: Autoregulation of cerebral blood flow in hypertensive patients: the modifying influence of prolonged antihypertensive treatment on the tolerance to acute, drug-induced hypotension. Circulation 53:720, 1976
33. Robertson GS, Cordiner CM: A comparison of mental function in relation to hypotensive and normotensive anaesthesia in the elderly. Br J Anaesth 43:561, 1971
34. Eckenhoff JE, Compton JR, Larson A, et al: Assessment of cerebral effects of deliberate hypotension by psychological measurements. Lancet 2:711, 1964
35. McPherson RW, Johnson RM, Graf M: Intraoperative neurological monitoring during carotid endarterectomy: electroencephalogram versus somatosensory evoked potential (abstract). Anesthesiology 59:A368, 1983
36. Jones TH, Chiappa KH, Young RL, et al: EEG monitoring for induced hypotension for surgery of intracranial aneurysms. Stroke 10:292, 1979
37. Ferguson GG, Ganache FW, Farrah J, et al: Physiological monitoring during carotid endarterectomy: evidence that an internal shunt is not necessary. J Cereb Blood Flow Metab1: S530, 1981
38. Prior PF: EEG monitoring and evoked potentials in brain ischemia. Br J Anaesth 57:63, 1985
39. Dong WK, Bhedsoe SW, Eng DY, et al: Profound arterial hypotension in dogs: brain electrical activity and organ integrity. Anesthesiology 58:61, 1983
40. Astrup J, Symon L, Branston NM, et al: Cortical evoked potential and extracellular K^+ and H^+ at critical levels of brain ischemia. Stroke 8:51, 1977
41. McDowall DG: Induced hypotension and brain ischemia. Br J Anaesth 57:110, 1985
42. Brierley JB, Brown AW, Excell BJ, et al: Brain damage in the *Rhesus* monkey resulting from profound arterial hypotension: I. its nature, distribution and general physiologic correlates. Brain Res 13:68, 1969
43. Lassen NA: Cerebral blood flow and oxygen consumption in man. Physiol Rev 39:183, 1959
44. Silbert BS, Koumoundouros E, Davies MJ, et al: Comparison of the processed electroencephalogram and awake neurologic assessment during carotid endarterectomy. Anaesth Intensive Care 17:298, 1989
45. Grundy BL: Intraoperative monitoring of sensory-evoked potentials. Anesthesiology 58:72, 1983
46. Grundy BL, Nash CL, Brown RH: Deliberate hypotension for spinal fusion: prospective randomized study with evoked potential monitoring. Can Anaesth Soc J 29:452, 1982
47. Schramm J, Koht A, Schmidt G, et al: Surgical and electrophysiologic observations during clipping of 134 aneurysms with evoked potential monitoring. Neurosurgery 26:61, 1990
48. Friedman WA, Chadwick GM, Verhoeven FJS, et al: Monitoring of somatosensory evoked potentials during surgery for middle cerebral artery aneurysms. Neurosurgery 29:83, 1991
49. Markand ON, Dilhey RS, Moorthy SS, et al: Monitoring of somatosensory evoked responses during carotid endarterectomy. Arch Neurol 41:375, 1984
50. Grundy BL, Nelson PB, Doyle E, et al: Intraoperative loss of somatosensory-evoked potentials predicts loss of spinal cord function. Anesthesiology 57:321, 1982
51. Branston NM, Ladds A, Symon L, et al: Comparison of the effects of ischemia on early components of the somatosensory evoked potential in brainstem, thalamus, and cerebral cortex. J Cereb Blood Flow Metab 4:68, 1984
52. Sato M, Pawlik G, Umbach C, et al: Comparative studies of regional CNS blood flow and evoked potentials in the cat. Stroke 15:9, 1984
53. McPherson RW, Szymanski J, Rogers MC: Somatosensory evoked potential changes in position-related brainstem ischemia. Anesthesiology 61:88, 1984
54. Ganes T, Lundar T: The effect of thiopentone on somatosensory evoked responses and EEGs in comatose patients. J Neurol Neurosurg Psychiatry 46:509, 1983
55. Ginsburg HH, Shetter AG, Raudzens PA: Postoperative paraplegia with preserved intraoperative somatosensory evoked potentials. J Neurosurg 63:296, 1985
56. Levy WJ Jr, York DH: Evoked potentials from the motor tracts in humans. Neurosurg 12:422, 1983
57. Lesser RP, Raudzens P, Luders H, et al: Postoperative neurological deficits may occur despite unchanged intraoperative somatosensory evoked potentials. Ann Neurol 19:22, 1986
58. Vance JP, Smith G, Thorburn J, et al: The combined effect of halothane-induced hypotension and hypocapnia on canine myocardial blood flow and oxygen consumption. Br J Anaesth 47:824, 1975
59. Hackel DB, Sancetta SM, Kleinerman J: Effect of hypotension due to spinal anesthesia on coronary blood flow and myocardial metabolism in man. Circulation 13:92, 1956
60. Tountas CJ, Georgopoulos AJ, Kyriakou KV: The effect of sodium nitroprusside on coronary circulation. Bull Soc Int Chir 23:267, 1964
61. Ross G, Cole PB: Cardiovascular action of sodium nitroprusside in dogs. Anaesthesia 28:400, 1973
62. Loeb HS, Sandje A, Croke RP, et al: Effects of pharmacologically-induced hypertension on myocardial ischemia and coronary hemodynamics in patients with fixed coronary obstruction. Circulation 57:41, 1978
63. Hickey RF, Verrier ED, Baer RW, et al: A canine model of acute coronary artery stenosis: effects of deliberate hypotension. Anesthesiology 59:226, 1983
64. Rollason WN, Dundas CR, Milne RG: ECG and EEG change during hypotensive anaesthesia. Proc III Congr Mund Anaesth 1:106, 1964
65. Rollason WN, Hough JM: Some electrocardiographic studies during hypotensive anaesthesia. Br J Anaesth 31:66, 1959
66. Askrog VF, Pender JW, Eckenhoff JE: Changes in physiological dead space during deliberate hypotension. Anesthesiology 25: 744, 1964
67. Eckenhoff JE, Enderby GEH, Larson A, et al: Pulmonary gas exchange during deliberate hypotension. Br J Anaesth 35:750, 1963
68. Khambatta JH, Stone JG, Matteo RS: Effect of sodium nitroprusside-induced hypotension on pulmonary deadspace. Br J Anaesth 54:1197, 1982
69. Suwa K, Hendley-Whyte J, Bendixen HH: Circulation and physiologic deadspace changes on controlling the ventilation of dogs. J Appl Physiol 21:1855, 1966
70. Arkin DB, Wahrenbrock EA: Hypoxemia following nitroprusside administration: effect of cardiac output and pulmonary autoregulation (abstract). In Abstracts of Scientific Papers, Annual Meeting of the American Society of Anesthesiologists, 1975: 161
71. Mookherjee S, Keighley JFH, Warner RA, et al: Hemodynamic, ventilatory and blood gas changes during infusion of sodium nitroferricyanide (nitroprusside): studies in patients with congestive heart failure. Chest 72:273, 1977
72. Colley PS, Cheney FW: Sodium nitroprusside increases Q_s/Q_t in dogs with regional atelectasis. Anesthesiology 47:338, 1977
73. Parson NL, Sullivan SF: Effect of sodium nitroprusside hypotension on pulmonary blood/gas distribution (abstract). In Ab-

stracts of Scientific Papers, Annual Meeting of the American Society of Anesthesiologists, 1975: 75

74. Stone JG, Khambatta HJ, Matteo RS: Pulmonary shunting during anesthesia with deliberate hypotension. Anesthesiology 45: 508, 1976
75. Price HL, Pauca AL: Effects of anesthesia on the peripheral circulation. Clinical Anesthesia 7:74, 1969
76. Bagshaw RJ, Cox RH, Campbell KB: Sodium nitroprusside and regional arterial haemodynamics in the dog. Br J Anaesth 49: 735, 1977
77. Salam ARA, Drummond GB, Bauld HW, et al: Clearance of indocyanine green as an index of liver function during cyclopropane anaesthesia and induced hypotension. Br J Anaesth 48:231, 1976
78. Chen JW, Rafii A, Keenan RL: Adynamic ileus following induced hypotension. JAMA 253:633, 1985
79. Pannacciuli E, Quarto DePalo FM, Trazzi R, et al: Renal function changes in controlled hypotension. Minerva Anestesiol 36:625, 1970
80. Engelman RM, Guy HH, Smith SJ, et al: The effect of hypotensive anesthesia on renal hemodynamics. J Surg Res 18: 293, 1975
81. Behnia R, Siqueira EB, Brunner EA: Sodium nitroprusside-induced hypotension: effect on renal function. Anesth Analg 57:521, 1978
82. Albert RA, Roizen MF, Hamilton WK, et al: Intraoperative urinary output does not predict postoperative renal function in patients undergoing abdominal aortic revascularization. Surgery 95:709, 1984
83. Ladner C, Brinkman CR, Weston P, et al: Dynamics of uterine circulation in pregnant and nonpregnant sheep. Am J Physiol 218:257, 1970
84. Trierweiler MW, Freeman RK, James J: Baseline FHR characteristics as indicator of fetal status during antepartum period. Am J Obstet Gynecol 125:618, 1976
85. Lee CY, Deloreto PC, O'Lane JM: A study of FHR acceleration patterns. Obstet Gynecol 45:142, 1975
86. Schifrin BS, Dame L: Fetal heart rate patterns. JAMA 219: 1322, 1972
87. Aitken RR, Drake CG: A technique of anesthesia with induced hypotension for surgical correction of intracranial aneurysms. Clin Neurosurg 21:107, 1974
88. Nochimson DJ, Turbeville JS, Terry JE, et al: The nonstress test. Obstet Gynecol 51:429, 1978
89. Sampson MB, Mudaliar NA, Léle AS: FHR variability as indicator of fetal status. Postgrad Med 67:207, 1980
90. Levinson G, Shnider SM: Anesthesia for surgery during pregnancy. In Shnider SM, Levinson G (eds): Anesthesia for obstetrics, 2nd ed. Baltimore: Williams & Wilkins, 1987: 188
91. Wright RG, Shnider SM: Fetal and neonatal effects of maternally administered drugs. In Shnider SM, Levinson G (eds): Anesthesia for obstetrics, 2nd ed. Baltimore: Williams & Wilkins, 1987: 536
92. Wetstone JH, LaMotta RV, Middlebrook L, et al: Studies of cholinesterase activity. Am J Obstet Gynecol 76:480, 1958
93. Pritchard JA: Plasma cholinesterase activity in normal pregnancy and eclamptogenic toxemias. Am J Obstet Gynecol 70: 1083, 1955
94. Friedman MM, Lapan B: Variations of enzyme activities during normal pregnancy. Am J Obstet Gynecol 82:132, 1961
95. Poulton TJ, James FM III, Lockridge O: Prolonged apnea following trimethaphan and succinylcholine. Anesthesiology 50: 54, 1979
96. Shnider SM: Serum cholinesterase activity during pregnancy, labor and the puerperium. Anesthesiology 26:335, 1963
97. Oakes GK, Walker AM, Ehrenkranz RA, et al: Effect of propranolol infusion on the umbilical and uterine circulations of pregnant sheep. Am J Obstet Gynecol 126:1038, 1976
98. Joelsson I, Barton MD: The effect of blockade of the β-receptors of the sympathetic nervous system of the fetus. Acta Obstet Gynaecol Scand Suppl 3:75, 1969
99. Habib A, McCarthy JS: Effects on the neonate of propranolol administered during pregnancy. J Pediatr 91:808, 1977
100. Gladstone GR, Hordof A, Gersony WM: Propranolol administration during pregnancy: effects on the fetus. J Pediatr 86: 962, 1975
101. Fiddler GI: Propranolol and pregnancy. Lancet 2:722, 1974
102. Reed RL, Cheney CB, Fearon RE, et al: Propranolol therapy throughout pregnancy: a case report. Anesth Analg 53:214, 1974
103. Cottrill CM, McAllister RG, Gettes L, et al: Propranolol therapy during pregnancy, labor, and delivery: evidence for transplacental drug transfer and impaired neonatal drug disposition. J Pediatr 91:812, 1977
104. Snyder SW, Wheeler AS, James FM III: The use of nitroglycerin to control severe hypertension of pregnancy during caesarean section. Anesthesiology 51:563, 1979
105. Wheeler AS, James FM, Meis PJ, et al: Effects of nitroglycerin and nitroprusside on the uterine vasculature of gravid ewes. Anesthesiology 53:390, 1980
106. Berkowitz RL: The management of hypertensive crises during pregnancy. In Berkowitz RL (ed): Critical care of the obstetric patient. New York: Churchill Livingstone, 1983: 309
107. Ellis CS, Wheeler AS, James FM, et al: Fetal and maternal effects of sodium nitroprusside used to counteract hypertension in gravid ewes. Am J Obstet Gynecol 143:766, 1982
108. Naulty J, Cefalo RC, Lewis PE: Fetal toxicity of nitroprusside in the pregnant ewe. Am J Obstet Gynecol 139:708, 1981
109. Donchin Y, Amirav B, Sahar A, et al: Sodium nitroprusside for aneurysm surgery in pregnancy. Br J Anaesth 50:849, 1978
110. Rigg D, Mcdonogh A: Use of SNP for deliberate hypotension during pregnancy. Br J Anaesth 53:985, 1981
111. Goodlin RC: Fetal and maternal effects of sodium nitroprusside. Am J Obstet Gynecol 146:350, 1983
112. Lieb SM, Zugaib M, Nuwayhid B, et al: Nitroprusside-induced hemodynamic alternations in normotensive and hypertensive pregnant sheep. Am J Obstet Gynecol 139:925, 1981
113. Stempel JE, O'Grady JP, Morton MJ, et al: Use of SNP in complications of gestational hypertension. Obstet Gynecol 60: 533, 1982
114. Shoemaker CT, Meyers M: Sodium nitroprusside for control of severe hypertensive disease of pregnancy: a case report and discussion of potential toxicity. Am J Obstet Gynecol 149:171, 1984
115. Brown BR Jr,Crout JR: A Comparative study of the effects of five general anesthetics on myocardial contractility: I. isometric contractions. Anesthesiology 34:236, 1971
116. Eger EI II: Isoflurane: a review. Anesthesiology 55:559, 1981
117. Prys-Roberts C, Lloyd JW, Fisher A, et al: Deliberate profound hypotension induced with halothane: studies of haemodynamics and pulmonary gas exchange. Br J Anaesth 46:105, 1974
118. Eger EI II, Smith NT, Stoelting RK, et al: Cardiovascular effects of halothane in man. Anesthesiology 32:396, 1970
119. Keykhah MM, Welsh FA, Harp JR: Cerebral energy levels during trimethaphan-induced hypotension in the rat: effects of light versus deep halothane anesthesia. Anesthesiology 50:36, 1979
120. Calverley RK, Smith NT, Jones CW, et al: Ventilatory and cardiovascular effects of enflurane anesthesia during spontaneous ventilation in man. Anesth Analg 57:610, 1978
121. Newberg LA, Milde JH, Michenfelder JD: Systemic and cerebral effects of isoflurane-induced hypotension in dogs. Anesthesiology 60:541, 1984
122. Neigh JL, Garman JK, Harp JR: The electroencephalographic pattern during anesthesia with Ethrane: effects of depth of anesthesia, P_aCO_2, and nitrous oxide. Anesthesiology 35:482, 1971
123. Lebowitz MH, Blitt CD, Dillon JB: Enflurane-induced central nervous system excitation and its relation to carbon dioxide tension. Anesth Analg 51:355, 1972
124. Blitt CD, Raessler KL, Wightman MA, et al: Atrioventricular conduction in dogs during anesthesia with isoflurane. Anesthesiology 50:210, 1979

125. Newberg LA, Milde JH, Michenfelder JD: The cerebral metabolic effects of isoflurane at and above concentrations that suppress cortical electrical activity. Anesthesiology 59:23, 1983
126. Madsen JB, Cold GE, Hansen ES, et al: Cerebral blood flow and metabolism during isoflurane-induced hypotension in patients subjected to surgery for cerebral aneurysms. Br J Anaesth 59:1204, 1987
127. Cucchiara RF, Theye RA, Michenfelder JD: The effects of isoflurane on canine cerebral metabolism and blood flow. Anesthesiology 40:571, 1974
128. Newberg LA, Michenfelder JD: Cerebral protection by isoflurane during hypoxemia or ischemia. Anesthesiology 59:29, 1983
129. Newberg LA, Milde JH, Michenfelder JD: Systemic and cerebral effects of isoflurane-induced hypotension in dogs. Anesthesiology 60:541, 1984
130. Milde LN, Milde JH: The cerebral and systemic hemodynamic and metabolic effects of desflurane-induced hypotension in dogs. Anesthesiology 74:513, 1991
131. Warltier DC, Pagel PS: Cardiovascular and respiratory actions of desflurane: is desflurane different from isoflurane? Anesth Analg 75:S17, 1992
132. Dale RC, Schroeder ET: Respiratory paralysis during treatment of hypertension with trimethaphan camsylate. Arch Intern Med 136:816, 1976
133. Nourok DS, Glasscock RJ, Solomon DH, et al: Hypothyroidism following prolonged sodium nitroprusside therapy. Am J Med Sci 248:129, 1964
134. Saxon A, Kattlove HE: Platelet inhibition by sodium nitroprusside, a smooth muscle inhibitor. Blood 47:957, 1976
135. Park JW, Means GE: Formation of N-nitrosoamines from sodium nitroprusside and secondary amines. N Engl J Med 313: 1547, 1985
136. Cottrell JE, Patel K, Turndorf H, et al: Intracranial pressure changes induced by sodium nitroprusside in patients with intracranial mass lesions. Neurosurg 48:329, 1978
137. Marsh ML, Shapiro HM, Smith RW, et al: Changes in neurologic status in intracranial pressure associated with sodium nitroprusside administration. Anesthesiology 51:336, 1979
138. Vesey CJ, Cole P, Simpson P: Changes in cyanide concentrations induced by sodium nitroprusside (SNP). Br J Anaesth 48: 268, 1976
139. Davenport HW: The inhibition of carbonic anhydrase and of gastric acid secretion by thiocyanate. Am J Physiol 129:505, 1940
140. Smith RP, Carleton RA: Nitroprusside and methemoglobinemia. N Engl J Med 294:502, 1976
141. Bisset WIK, Butler AR, Glidewell C, et al: Sodium nitroprusside and cyanide release: reasons for reappraisal. Br J Anaesth 53: 1015, 1981
142. Ikeda S, Schweiss JF, Frank PA, et al: *In vitro* cyanide release from sodium nitroprusside. Anesthesiology 66:381, 1987
143. Ikeda S, Frank PA, Schweiss JF, et al: *In vitro* cyanide release from sodium nitroprusside in various intravenous solutions. Anesth Analg 67:360, 1988
144. Norris JC, Hume AS: *In vivo* release of cyanide from sodium nitroprusside. Br J Anaesth 59:236, 1987
145. Gettler AO, Baine JO: Toxicity of cyanide. Am J Med Sci 195: 182, 1938
146. Posner MA, Tobey RE, McElroy H: Hydroxocobalamin therapy of cyanide intoxication in guinea pigs. Anesthesiology 44:157, 1976
147. Vesey CJ, Cole PV, Linnell JC, et al: Some metabolic effects of sodium nitroprusside in man. Br Med J 2:140, 1974
148. Vesey CJ, Cole PV: Nitroprusside and cyanide. Br J Anaesth 47:1115, 1975
149. Wilson J: Leber's hereditary optic atrophy: a possible defect of cyanide metabolism. Clin Sci (Colch) 29:505, 1965
150. Davies DW, Greiss L, Kadar D, et al: Sodium nitroprusside in children: observations on metabolism during normal and abnormal responses. Can Anaesth Soc J 22:553, 1975
151. Vesey CJ, Cole P, Simpson P: Sodium nitroprusside in anaesthesia. Br Med J 3:229, 1975
152. Michenfelder JD, Tinker JH: Cyanide toxicity and thiosulfate protection during chronic administration of sodium nitroprusside in the dog: correlation with a human case. Anesthesiology 47:441, 1977
153. Posner MA, Rodkey FL, Tobey RE: Nitroprusside-induced cyanide poisoning: antidotal effect of hydroxocobalamin. Anesthesiology 44:330, 1976
154. Lutie F, Dusoleil P, DeMontgros J: Action de l'hydroxocobalmine à dose massive dans l'intoxication aigue au cyanure. Arch Mal Prof 32:683, 1972
155. Done AK: Clinical pharmacology of systemic antidotes. Clin Pharmacol Ther 2:750, 1961
156. Cottrell JE, Casthely P, Brodie JD, et al: Prevention of nitroprusside-induced cyanide toxicity with hydroxocobalamin. N Engl J Med 298:809, 1978
157. Bedford RF, Berry FA, Longnecker DE: Impact of propranolol on hemodynamic responses and blood cyanide levels during nitroprusside infusion: a prospective study in anesthetized man. Anesth Analg 58:466, 1979
158. Khambatta HJ, Stone JG, Khan E: Propranolol abates nitroprusside-induced renin release. Anesthesiology 51:S74, 1979
159. Marshall WK, Bedford RF, Arnold WP, et al: Effects of propranolol on the cardiovascular and renin-angiotensin systems during hypotension produced by sodium nitroprusside in humans. Anesthesiology 55:277, 1981
160. Khambatta JH, Stone JG, Khan E: Propranolol alters renin release during nitroprusside-induced hypotension and prevents hypertension on discontinuation of nitroprusside. Anesth Analg 60:569, 1981
161. Vidt DG, Bravo EL, Fouad FM: Captopril. N Engl J Med 306: 214, 1982
162. Woodside J, Garner L, Bedford RF, et al: Captopril reduces the dose requirements for sodium nitroprusside induced hypotension. Anesthesiology 60:413, 1984
163. Jennings GL, Gelman JS, Stockigt JR, et al: Accentuated hypotensive effect of sodium nitroprusside in man after captopril. Clin Sci (Colch) 61:521, 1981
164. Woodside J, Garner L, Bedford RF, et al: Captopril reduces the dose requirement for sodium nitroprusside-induced hypotension. Anesthesiology 60:413, 1984
165. Fahmy NR, Gavras HP: Captopril decreases nitroprusside requirements and prevents rebound hypertension following cessation of nitroprusside infusion in humans (abstract). Anesthesiology 59:A359, 1983
166. Bloor BC, Finander LS, Flacke WE, et al: Effect of clonidine on sympathoadrenal response during sodium nitroprusside hypotension. Anesth Analg 65:469, 1986
167. Forrester T, Harper AM, MacKenzie ET, et al: Effect of adenosine triphosphate and some derivatives on cerebral blood flow and metabolism. J Physiol 296:343, 1979
168. Kassell NF, Boarini DJ, Olin JJ, et al: Cerebral and systemic circulatory effects of arterial hypotension induced by adenosine. J Neurosurg 58:69, 1983
169. Owall A, Lagerkranser M, Sollevi A: Effects of adenosine-induced hypotension on myocardial hemodynamics and metabolism during cerebral aneurysm surgery. Anesth Analg 67:228, 1988
170. Van Aken H, Puchstein CH, Anger C, et al: Changes in intracranial pressure and compliance during adenosine triphosphate-induced hypotension in dogs. Anesth Analg 63:381, 1984
171. Van Aken H, Puchstein C, Fitch W, et al: Haemodynamic and cerebral effects of ATP-induced hypotension. Br J Anaesth 56: 1409, 1984
172. Belardinelli L, Belloni FL, Rubio R, et al: Atrioventricular conduction disturbances during hypoxia: possible role of adenosine in rabbit and guinea pig heart. Circ Res 47:684, 1980
173. Gonzalez-Miranda F, Juarez JB, Santos ML, et al: Adenosine/ATP and induced hypotension. Anesth Analg 63:538, 1984
174. Newberg LA, Milde JH, Michenfelder JD: Cerebral and systemic effects of hypotension induced by adenosine or ATP in dogs. Anesthesiology 62:429, 1985
175. Fukunaga AF, Hung JH, Blooz BC, et al: ATP-induced prolonged arterial hypotension in the anesthetized dog. Anesth Analg 63: 213, 1984
176. Zäll S, Milocco I, Ricksten S-E: Effects of adenosine on myo-

cardial blood flow and metabolism after coronary artery bypass surgery. Anesth Analg 73:689, 1991
177. Glisson SN, Sanchez MM, El-Etr AA, et al: Nitroglycerin and the neuromuscular blockade produced by gallamine, succinylcholine d-tubocurarine and pancuronium. Anesth Analg 59: 117, 1980
178. Gold MR, Dec GW, Cocca-Spofford D, et al: Esmolol and ventilatory function in cardiac patients with COPD. Chest 100: 1215, 1991
179. Koch-Weser J: Hydralazine. N Engl J Med 293:320, 1976
180. James DJ, Bedford RF: Hydralazine for controlled hypotension during neurosurgical operations. Anesth Analg 61:1016, 1982
181. Overgaard J, Skinhoj E: A paradoxical cerebral hemodynamic effect of hydralazine. Stroke 6:402, 1975
182. Shand DG: Propranolol. N Engl J Med 293:280, 1975
183. Richards DA, Prichard BNC: Clinical pharmacology of labetalol. J Clin Pharm 8(suppl 2):89S, 1979
184. Zimpfer M, Fitzal S, Tonczar L: Verapamil as a hypotensive agent during neuroleptanaesthesia. Br J Anaesth 53:885, 1981
185. Mazzoni P, Giffin JP, Cottrell JE, et al: Intracranial pressure during diltiazem-induced hypotension in anesthetized dogs. Anesth Analg 64:1001, 1985
186. Kates RA, Zaggy AP, Norfleet EA, et al: Comparative cardiovascular effects of verapamil, nifedipine, and diltiazem during halothane anesthesia in swine. Anesthesiology 61:10, 1984
187. Pederson OL, Christensen NJ, Ramsch KD: Comparison of acute effects of nifedipine in normotensive and hypertensive man. Cardiovasc Pharmacol 2:357, 1980
188. Sodeyama O, Ikeda K, Matsuda I, et al: Nifedipine for control of postoperative hypertension (abstract). Anesthesiology 59: A18, 1983
189. Bedford RF, Dacey R, Winn HR, et al: Adverse impact of a calcium entry-blocker (verapamil) on intracranial pressure in patients with brain tumors. J Neurosurg 59:800, 1983
190. Giffin JP, Cottrell JE, Hartung J, et al: Intracranial pressure during nifedipine-induced hypotension. Anesth Analg 62:1078, 1983
191. Bernard JM, Pinaud M, François T, et al: Deliberate hypotension with nicardipine or nitroprusside during total hip arthroplasty. Anesth Analg 73:341, 1991

FURTHER READING

Adams AP: Techniques of vascular control for deliberate hypotension during anesthesia. Br J Anaesth 47:777, 1975

Larson AG: Deliberate hypotension. Anesthesiology 25:682, 1964

Lindop MJ: Complications and morbidity of controlled hypotension. Br J Anaesth 47:799, 1975

McGough EK: Cardiovascular system. In Gravenstein N (ed): Manual of complications during anesthesia. Philadelphia: JB Lippincott, 1991:181

Miller ED Jr: Deliberate hypotension. In Miller RD (ed): Anesthesia, 4th ed. New York: Churchill Livingstone, 1994:1481

Ornstein E: Deliberate hypotension in anesthesia and surgery. Problems in Anesthesia. Philadelphia: JB Lippincott, 1993

Complications in Anesthesiology, second edition,
edited by Nikolaus Gravenstein and Robert R. Kirby.
Lippincott-Raven Publishers, Philadelphia © 1996.

CHAPTER 26

Anesthesia–Related Trauma Caused by Patient Malpositioning

Beverley A. Britt
Nancy Joy
Margot B. Mackay

There are many hazards and pitfalls of positioning an anesthetized patient. An understanding of the peripheral nervous system and the physiology of the respiratory and cardiovascular systems is essential to avoid potentially injury-producing positions. Meticulous care must be taken while moving a patient into the desired surgical position to ensure that the change is carried out in a slow and gentle manner; to ascertain that all pressure points caused by surgical and anesthetic apparatus are padded thoroughly, especially when situated over bony prominences; and to ensure that the patient is not contorted into any positions that strain the nerves, tendons, or ligaments in a way that the patient would not tolerate if awake.

Incorrect positioning of a patient during anesthesia may cause trauma to nerves, spinal cord, eyes, skin, muscles, tendons, ligaments, and appendages and may produce malfunctioning of the respiratory and cardiovascular systems. Although these events have been observed since the introduction of ether and many of the causes and remedies have been understood for decades, patient malpositioning continues to constitute a significant source of postanesthetic complications.[1–11]

HISTORY

Early investigators blamed nerve palsies on the toxic properties of the anesthetic agent used. In 1894, Budinger was the first to recognize that most postoperative neuropathies were caused by malpositioning with consequent nerve stretching and compression. His findings were verified by Krumm,[11] Garriques,[8] and Horsley.[10] Clausen in 1942[12] and Ewing in 1950[13] emphasized the importance of avoiding nerve stretching during anesthesia. Since then, additional publications on this subject have continued to appear.[1–4,6,14–19]

NERVE TRAUMA

Causes

Several factors contribute to peripheral nerve injuries.[20–40]

Ischemia of the Vasa Nervorum

The principal cause of most peripheral nerve injuries in anesthetized patients is ischemia of the intraneural vasa nervorum.[20–22] This problem results primarily from stretching of the nerve and secondarily from compression of a nerve already rendered vulnerable by stretching. Stretching and compression are likely to occur in anesthetized patients for two reasons. First, muscle tonus is reduced, especially when muscle relaxants are used, and susceptibility to unnatural positions is increased.[12] Second, with perceptive powers no longer intact, the patient is unable to complain of postural insults that normally would not be tolerated.[9] Even in conscious patients, abduction of the arm to more than 90° in a steep Trendelenburg position becomes intolerable after a few minutes, and the radial pulse disappears in 83% of volunteers so positioned.[6,23] Just 30 to 40 minutes of anesthesia in an unfavorable position may be sufficient to result in nerve palsy.[6]

Congenital Anomalies

Some congenital anomalies increase nerve vulnerability to injury during anesthesia. The brachial plexus is particularly susceptible to injury with preexisting hypertrophy of the scalenus anterior,[12,15,16] hypertrophy of the scalenus medius, a cervical rib,[12] anomalous derivation of the plexus (higher or lower than normal),[12] or abnormal slope of the shoulder.[2]

Preexisting Disease

Patients with diabetes mellitus are especially vulnerable to irreversible nerve injury during anesthesia. Jones described a diabetic patient in whom, after anesthesia, an ulnar nerve palsy developed and progressively became worse.[27] Malposition during anesthesia stresses the nerves and the blood vessels, permitting hematoma formation in patients who have blood dyscrasias (eg, factor VIII deficiency) and in patients who are receiving anticoagulant therapy.[28–32] These hematomas can exacerbate nerve injuries induced directly by malposition. Other conditions that predispose to nerve palsies during anesthesia are anemia, hypotension, electrolyte imbalances,[33] and arteriosclerosis.[8]

Hypothermia

More than 30 minutes of hypothermia may be followed by peripheral neuropathy.[24] With surface cooling, far lower temperatures (3°C to 5°C) are recorded peripherally than in the core (27°C to 31°C).[35,36] Even minimal concomitant stretching or compression exaggerates the likelihood of hypoxia within nerve cells.[37]

Tourniquet Compression

A tourniquet has been reported occasionally to cause damage to the nerves over which it was applied if the pressure was excessive or prolonged or if the patient had diabetes mellitus.[38] However, when the tourniquet is not applied for an excessive period, if it is properly positioned, and if the patient is healthy, neuropathy after tourniquet application is extremely unlikely, because no stretching occurs. Compression is dissipated around the entire circumference of the limb and is exerted through an abundance of soft tissues and not directly against a hard, bony point.

Radial nerve palsy has been associated with use of an automatically cycled blood pressure machine.[39] The injury may have resulted from the mechanical effects of differential pressure exerted at the distal edge of the cuff and not from ischemia. In very thin patients, the use of these monitors has been recommended only when the intervals between sequential measurements are not brief.[40]

Differential Diagnosis

Before a peripheral nerve injury is suspected to be the result of an error in positioning by the anesthesiologist before or during anesthesia, several other diagnoses must be excluded.[24]

Trauma Before Hospitalization

When patients arrive in the operating room, they may already have nerve injuries, which remain undiagnosed before anesthesia. This situation is most likely in cases of injuries that are extremely painful or life threatening; the comparatively painless nerve lesion goes unnoticed by the patient and surgeon until the postoperative period.

Blood Dyscrasias

Neuropathies that are caused entirely by compression from hematomas resulting from preexisting blood dyscrasias or excessive therapeutic anticoagulation may become evident in the immediate postoperative period. Frequently, the sciatic,[28,32] median,[30,31] and femoral[32,41] nerves are injured. Injury to the femoral nerve may be caused in the retroperitoneal area by formation of a hematoma that compresses it as it descends between the iliac and psoas muscles.[42]

Misplacement of Needles

Injuries caused by malposition of the patient during anesthesia should be differentiated from those caused by needles inserted by personnel other than anesthesiologists. Palsy may result from direct probing with a needle; chemical irritation by injected drugs (eg, calcium chloride, sodium bicarbonate, diazepam, chlorpromazine, norepinephrine); bacterial contamination; or local hematoma formation caused by perforation of an adjacent blood vessel.[43,44]

Spinal Anesthesia

The low cerebrospinal fluid pressure that accompanies a dural leak is probably the cause of the cranial nerve palsies that have been observed after spinal anesthesia.[45,46] The result is presumed to be descent of the medulla and pons, with secondary stretching of the cranial nerves.[47–51] Paralysis of every cranial nerve except the tenth has been reported, but in 90% of the cases, the sixth nerve is affected. The incidence is probably greater than reports indicate, because a slight paresis is overlooked when the patient complains only of slight blurring of vision that clears up in a few days. In advanced cases, diplopia is preceded by severe headache, stiff neck, nausea, dizziness, and photophobia. The time of onset of the palsy varies and can begin up to 21 days postoperatively, and recovery may not be complete for as long as 2 years.[52]

Surgical Manipulation

Overstrenuous use of surgical instruments such as retractors or obstetric forceps may compress and stretch nerves to the point of causing neuropraxia and occasionally to the point of causing permanent injury (Fig. 26-1). Nerves, particularly those in the neck, may be severed by surgical scalpel blades or scissors.

Toxic Effect of General Anesthetics

Damage to the nervous system may be produced by direct toxic action of the degradation products of anesthetics or by

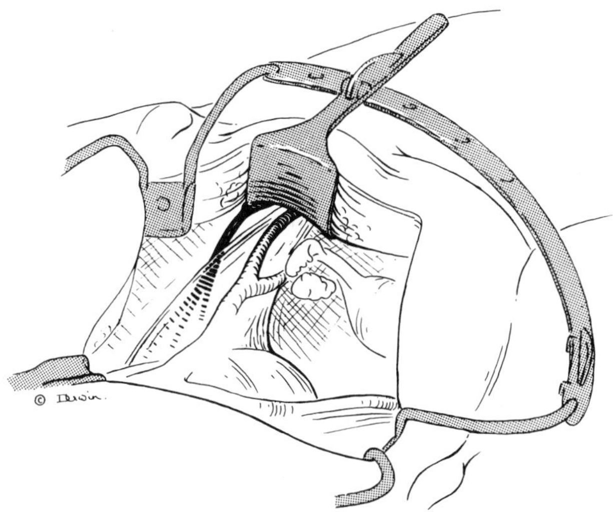

FIGURE 26-1. The femoral nerve is compressed and laterally deflected by the leg of a self-retaining retractor. (Britt BA, Gordon RA: Peripheral nerve injuries associated with anaesthesia. Can Anaesth Soc J 11:514, 1964.)

other impurities they may contain. When chloroform was used, phosgene was produced following exposure of the agent to heat. In the presence of heat and alkali, trichloroethylene decomposed to form dichloroacetylene, which was converted by heat to phosgene and carbon monoxide.[52–54] Soda lime triggered each of these reactions, because carbon dioxide absorption by soda lime is an exothermic reaction. These agents were extremely toxic to the central nervous system and to the cranial nerves but are no longer problematic because they are not currently used.

UPPER EXTREMITY NEUROPATHIES

Branches of Roots of the Brachial Plexus

Damage to branches of the roots of the brachial plexus during anesthesia are rare but have occurred. The most common is injury to the long thoracic nerve of Bell arising from the 5th to 7th cervical nerve roots, with resultant paralysis of the ipsilateral latissimus dorsi. Severe pain in the region of the shoulder and winging of the scapula result.[55] The affected shoulder is lower than the normal shoulder, and because of inability to stabilize the shoulder, use of the arm is limited. This injury may be associated with dislocation of the shoulder joint and is attributed to abrupt movement of the arm away from the torso during the anesthetic. It is one of the few peripheral nerve injuries for which really efficacious therapy is available in the form of pectoralis major muscle transfer with a fascia lata graft and placement of a ligament augmentation device to the inferior angle of the scapula.

Brachial Plexus Neuropathies

Mechanisms of Injury

For two reasons, the brachial plexus is the most susceptible to damage of all nerve groups from malpositioning during anesthesia.[1,2,4–7,9–13,23,35,44,56–63] First, it has a relatively long, mobile, and superficial course in the axilla between two firm points of fixation: the vertebrae and prevertebral fascia above; and the axillary fascia below (Fig. 26-2). Second, it lies in proximity to a number of freely movable bony structures.

STRETCHING. Stretching is usually the chief cause of injury.[10,15,64,65] Compression plays only a secondary role, acting as a fulcrum or stabilizing point and compelling the nerves

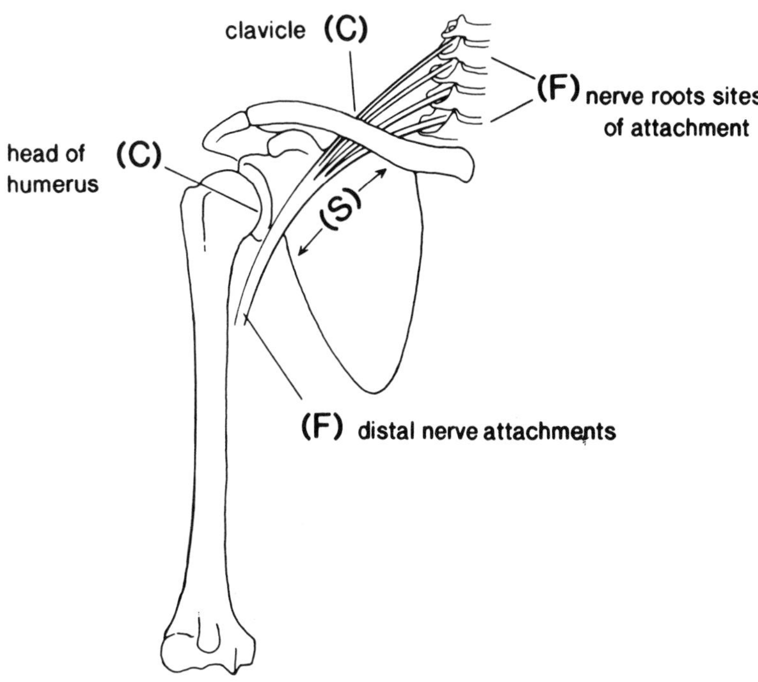

FIGURE 26-2. Brachial plexus injury. Positioning may stretch (*S*) the plexus between points of fixation (*F*), increasing the likelihood of compression injury at several sites (*C*). (Mahla ME: Nervous system. In Gravenstein N (ed): Manual of complications during anesthesia. Philadelphia: JB Lippincott, 1991: 384.)

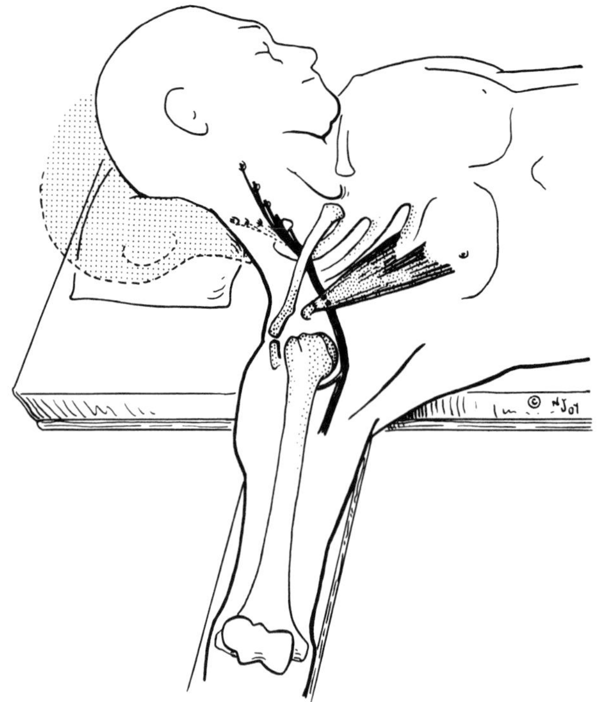

FIGURE 26-3. Dorsal extension and lateral flexion of the head to the opposite side stretch the brachial plexus. (Britt BA, Gordon RA: Peripheral nerve injuries associated with anaesthesia. Can Anaesth Soc J 11:514, 1964.)

to traverse a greater than normal distance around this fulcrum. Damage to the plexus is produced by an increase in the distance between the points of fixation above and below. For example, dorsal extension and lateral flexion of the head to the opposite side in the supine (Fig. 26-3) or lateral (Fig. 26-4) position widens the angle between the head and shoulder tip and stretches the plexus.[1,10,12,66] Stretching may also occur when the arm is abducted on an arm board (Fig. 26-5).

Stretching is worse when the body is in the Trendelenburg position but can occur even in the supine position if the degree of stretching is great enough. If possible, the arm should not be abducted with patients in the Trendelenburg position. The arm ought not to be abducted to greater than 60° when patients are supine. We think that previous recommendations allowing abduction up to 90° are too lax.[67,68]

Stretching may also occur when the patient is positioned prone on MacKay, Hall, Wilson, or similar frames with the arms abducted, often also extended, and the forearms flexed. To prevent brachial plexus injury in the prone position, the arms should be kept as close as possible to the patient's side, with the forearms flexed and pronated and with the hands placed on either side of the patient's head.

Stretching is aggravated when the forearm and hand are supinated. We know of a patient who suffered a brachial plexus injury after undergoing anesthesia in the supine horizontal position, during which the forearm and hand were supinated and the arm was only abducted to 30°. When the arm is abducted, the forearm and hand should always be pronated.

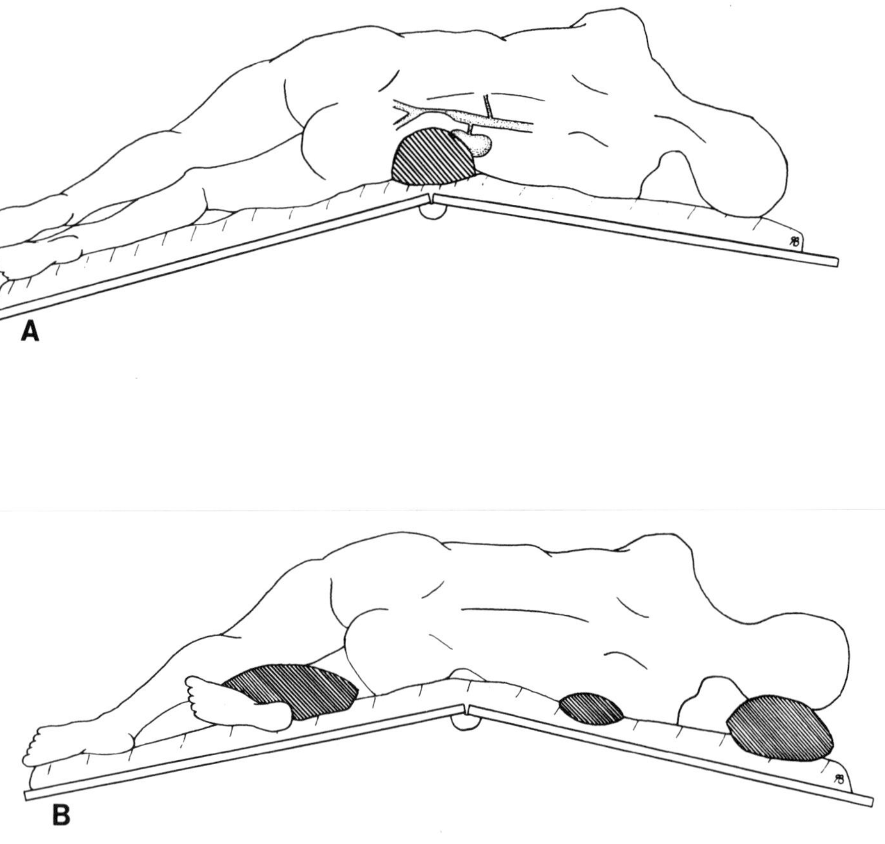

FIGURE 26-4. (A) Incorrect lateral nephrectomy position. The top leg lies directly over the bottom leg, so that bony prominences are directly opposing each other, with inadequate padding between them. Inadequate support under the head permits excessive lateral flexion of the head. A lack of padding behind the rib cage leaves the head of the humerus directly under the thorax. The high kidney rest constricts the inferior vena cava. Consequently, the brachial plexus is compressed. (B) Correct lateral nephrectomy position. The bottom leg is flexed more than the top leg, so that bony prominences are opposed by soft muscles. Padding between the legs is ample. A pillow prevents excessive lateral flexion of the head. Padding behind the lower rib cage permits slight posterior tilting of the upper part of the rib cage, so that the humeral head is anterior to the thorax, thus preventing compression of the brachial plexus. Use of a small or no kidney rest ensures free flow of blood through the inferior vena cava.

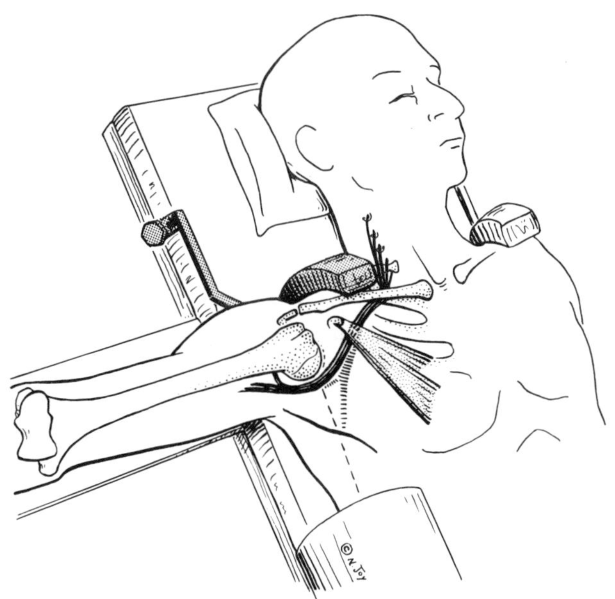

FIGURE 26-5. Placement of shoulder rests too medially and abduction of the arm in the Trendelenburg position cause deviation and compression of the plexus between the depressed clavicle and first rib. (Britt BA, Gordon RA: Peripheral nerve injuries associated with anaesthesia. Can Anaesth Soc J 11:514, 1964.)

McAlpine and Seckel advocated a position in which the forearm was supinated.[18] However, we have found, by cadaver dissection, that stretching is actually increased by supination but decreased by pronation. Presumably, McAlpine and Seckel made their recommendation to avoid compression of the ulnar nerve at the elbow behind the medial epicondyle. However, if the forearm and hand are fully rather than partially pronated, the medial tip of the medial condyle presses against the arm board while the posterior surface of the medial epicondyle, with its adherent ulnar nerve, faces posteriorly and is free of pressure from the arm board. The superiority of the pronated position over the supinated position can be easily confirmed in an awake individual by fully abducting the arm and observing that the degree of discomfort is greater in the supinated than in the pronated positions.

SAGGING OF THE ARM. Permitting the arm to sag off the side of the table and become abducted, externally rotated, and dorsally extended, especially if it is at an angle of more than 60° to the table, considerably elongates the plexus.[1,12]

PINCHING. The plexus also may be pinched between the clavicle and first rib. When shoulder braces are used to prevent the patient from slipping downward in the Trendelenburg position but are placed too far medially, they depress the clavicle caudally and posteriorly into the retroclavicular space.[1,7,12] The plexus must then travel a convoluted S-shaped course, increasing the distance between the proximal and distal points of fixation. If the patient's arm also is abducted on an arm board, stretching becomes extreme (see Fig. 26-5).

CAUDAL DEPRESSION. The plexus may be depressed caudally if it is stretched over the head of the humerus with the patient in the Trendelenburg position and the arm abducted on an arm board. The shoulder braces in this case are placed too far laterally and ride over the humeral head, which is driven downward into the axilla, carrying the plexus with it (Fig. 26-6).[13,66] In the Trendelenburg position, if shoulder braces are used, they should be padded well and placed over the acromii, not over the clavicles or the heads of the humeri. Better still, shoulder braces should not be used at all. Slipping can be prevented by the use of a ribbed mattress.[69,70] If possible, the arms should be kept close to the patient's sides with a metal arm guard or a draw sheet (Fig. 26-7).[61] Care must be taken to ensure that the ulnar nerve at the elbow is not in contact with the bed or the arm guard. If a metal arm guard is used, its inner side must be well padded. If a draw sheet is used, obese surgeons should be deterred from using the patient's arm as a resting place for their abdomens. A steep Trendelenburg position must be discouraged.[71].

POSTERIOR DEVIATION. The plexus may be deviated posteriorly by the tendon of the pectoralis minor or even by the tip of the coracoid process in obese patients undergoing open cholecystectomy. This circumstance occurs when a gallbladder rest has been inserted, and the head of the humerus on the same side is allowed to sag down off the operating table mattress onto an arm board that is not padded up to the level of the mattress. The entire shoulder girdle is depressed posteriorly and laterally in relation to the rib cage. The attachment of the pectoralis minor tendon to the coracoid process and, with it, the brachial plexus are deviated in the same direction (Fig. 26-8).[2]

ARM SUSPENSION. Intraneural ischemia is likely when the patient is in the lateral position with an arm suspended

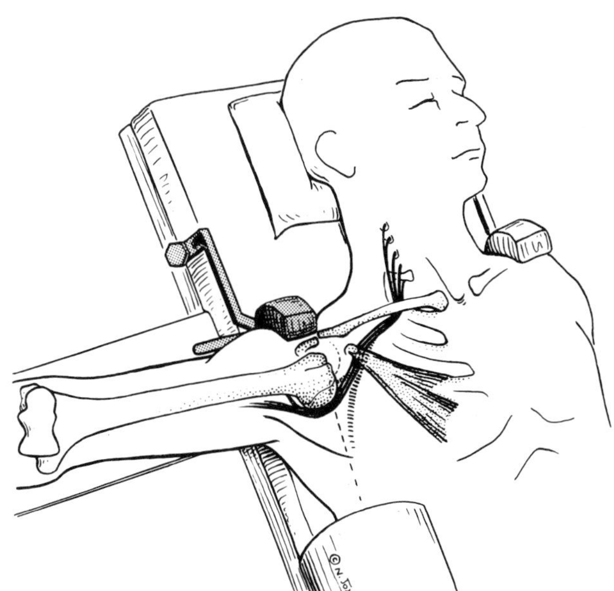

FIGURE 26-6. Placement of shoulder rests too far laterally and abduction of the arm in Trendelenburg position cause deviation of the brachial plexus below the head of the humerus, which has been forced down into the axilla. (Britt BA, Gordon RA: Peripheral nerve injuries associated with anaesthesia. Can Anaesth Soc J 11:514, 1964.)

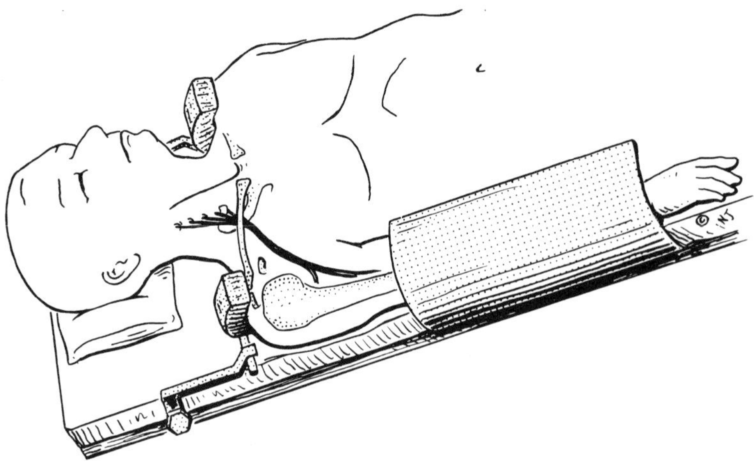

FIGURE 26-7. Correct placement of the patient and supports in the Trendelenburg position. The arms are at the sides and are protected by a well-padded metal arm guard or draw sheet. Shoulder rests are placed over the acromioclavicular joint. (Britt BA, Gordon RA: Peripheral nerve injuries associated with anaesthesia. Can Anaesth Soc J 11:514, 1964.)

from an ether screen, causing the extremity to be abducted to more than 90°, with the forearm pronated. Pronation twists the ulnar, radial, and median nerves into a more circuitous course, and gravity accentuates intraneural ischemia (Fig. 26-9). In the lateral position, a suspended arm should be abducted to less than 90°, and the forearm must be supinated slightly to preclude brachial plexus injury.[15]

EXTREME ABDUCTION. Extreme abduction without anterior arm flexion, so the hands rest beside, above, or behind the head, along with supination of the forearms, induces extreme plexus stretching. The patient may be supine for a cardiac operation (Fig. 26-10) or flexed prone (ie, jackknife) on an orthopedic frame for spinal surgery (Fig. 26-11).[59] In either of these positions, anterior flexion and abduction of the arms must be minimized (Figs. 26-12 and 26-13).

WRIST SUSPENSION. Suspension of a patient by the wrists to prevent slipping in an extreme Trendelenburg position has been reported by some investigators to heighten plexus tension. Clausen believed that the first rib became a fulcrum over which the plexus rubbed when anticephalad traction was placed on the abducted arm.[12] Ewing disputed this interpretation.[13] In our experience with cadaver dissection, a significant increase in the tension of the plexus in such a position does not occur, nor does the first rib in any way compress the plexus.

COMPRESSION. Compression appears to play a predominant role in traumatizing the brachial plexus when the patient is in the lateral position with the lower shoulder and arm directly under the rib cage.[72,73] This injury can be prevented by ensuring that, in the lateral position, the entire lower hu-

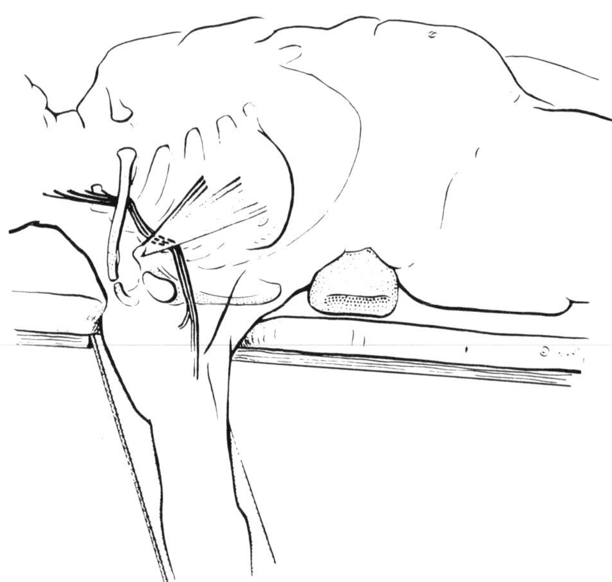

FIGURE 26-8. In the obese patient, abduction of the arm and insertion of a gall bladder rest stretches and shifts the tendon of the pectoralis minor backward, thus causing posterior deviation of the brachial plexus. (Britt BA, Gordon RA: Peripheral nerve injuries associated with anaesthesia. Can Anaesth Soc J 11:514, 1964.)

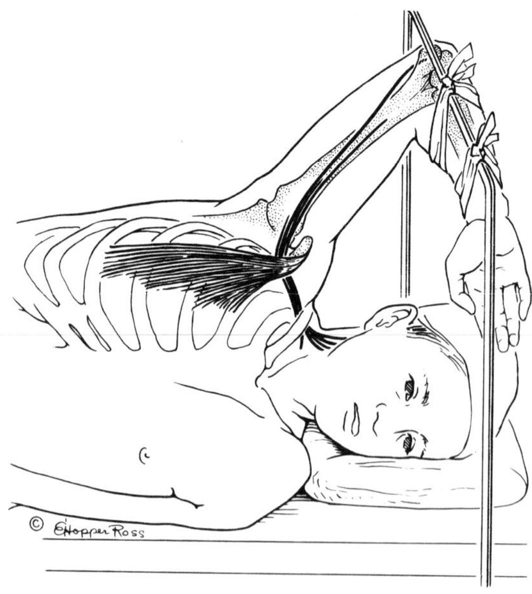

FIGURE 26-9. Suspension of the arm from an ether screen, resulting in extreme abduction of the arm and pronation of the forearm, deviates the brachial plexus posteriorly, behind the tendon of the pectoralis minor. (Britt BA, Gordon RA: Peripheral nerve injuries associated with anaesthesia. Can Anaesth Soc J 11:514, 1964.)

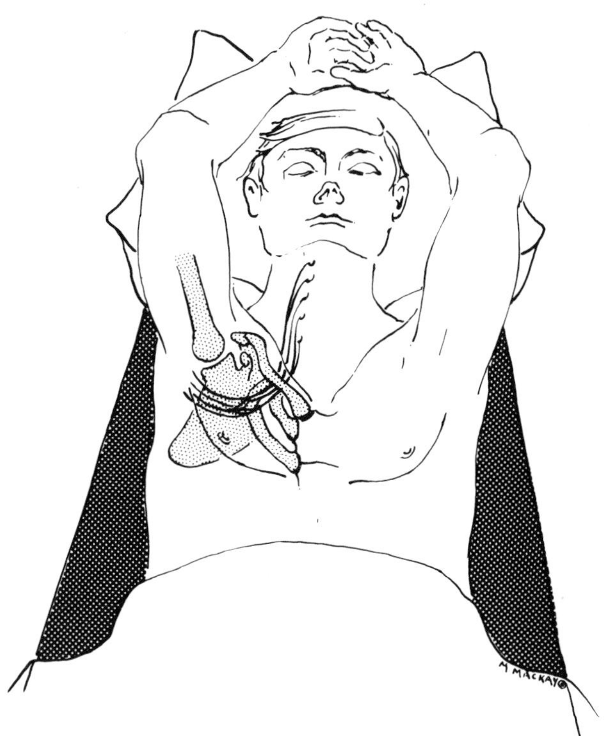

FIGURE 26-10. Incorrect "arms-up" position for open heart surgery. Extreme abduction and anterior flexion of the arms radically stretches the brachial plexus behind the clavicle and tendon of the pectoralis minor and below the head of the humerus.

merus, including the humeral head, is positioned anterior to the rib cage.

NEEDLE MISPLACEMENT. Needles misplaced by anesthesiologists may be responsible for injury to the brachial plexus. Palsy has resulted from irritation during cannulation of the internal jugular vein and regional anesthesia of the plexus by the axillary[74] and supraclavicular routes.[44] Damage has followed percutaneous angiography performed by the Seldinger technique through the axillary artery.[56,76–77] In some cases, a particularly uncooperative adult or child is anesthetized for this procedure or is anesthetized shortly thereafter, and determination of the exact mechanism of the injury is difficult.

Clinical Features

Characteristically, shoulder pain and tenderness in the supraclavicular area beginning one to several days postoperatively are prominent features. If the entire plexus is involved, the arm hangs flaccid, and the skin of the whole limb is numb. The upper roots (C5 to C7) only may be injured, with consequent internal rotation of the arm, extension of the forearm, and pronation of the hand (ie, Erb's palsy). More rarely, the lower roots, C8 and T1, also may be affected, with loss of flexion of the fingers, paralysis of the hand muscles, and perhaps Horner's syndrome (ie, Klumpke's paralysis).

Involvement may be confined chiefly to one of the cords. With posterior cord damage, loss of arm abduction and pa-

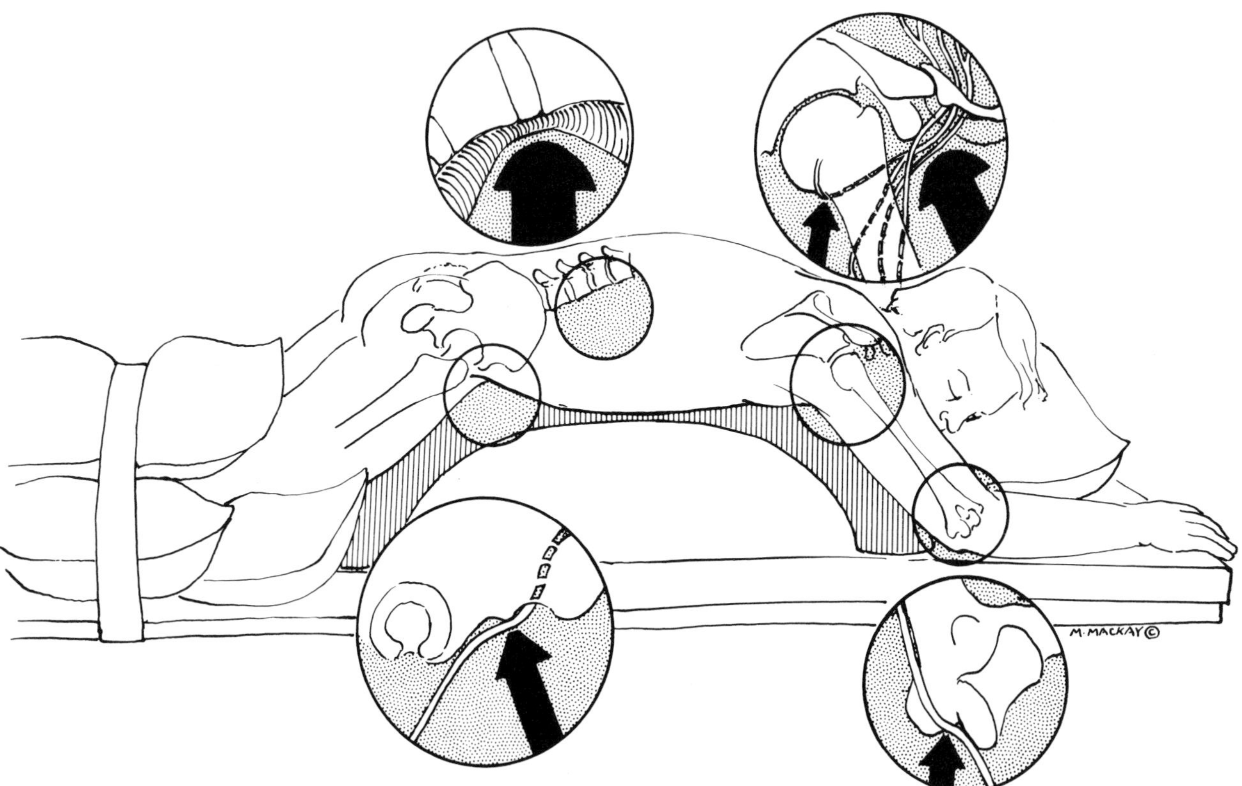

FIGURE 26-11. Incorrect flexed prone position. Abduction and anterior flexion of the arms stretch the brachial plexus. Inadequate padding of the elbows compresses the ulnar nerve. A bolster under the anterosuperior and inferior iliac spine compresses the anterolateral femoral nerve of the thigh. Improper padding under the cheek and forehead permits compression of the lower eyelid. Exaggerated upward convexity of the orthopedic frame constricts the inferior vena cava, especially in obese patients.

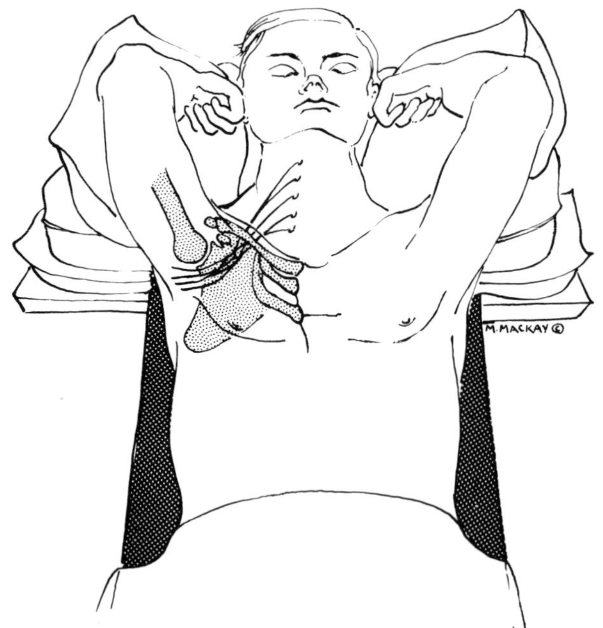

FIGURE 26-12. Correct "arms-up" position for open heart surgery. Arms are abducted and anteriorly flexed to less than 90°.

ralysis of the extensors of the elbow, wrist, and fingers are seen. With lateral cord involvement, paralysis of the flexors of the elbow and wrist occur. With medial cord injury, the lesion is similar to that affecting the lower roots. Wide retraction of the sternum during sternotomy and long cardiopulmonary bypass pump runs seem to predispose to neuropraxia of the medial cord.[78] Compression of the medial cord between the soft tissues about the clavicle and first rib during sternal retraction can also occur.[78] During retraction after longitudinal splitting of the sternum, the first rib can only rotate upward because of its dorsal articulations.[78] At the same time, if the patient is positioned with a rolled towel between the scapulae, the acromion and lateral clavicle are displaced inferiorly and backward.[78] When the sternum is then split and retracted, the first rib is forced upward, thereby encroaching on the space through which the plexus exits.[78] Posturing the shoulders forward helps to prevent such injury.[78]

Determining exactly which area of the skin is numb may be very difficult, because of extensive overlapping in the distribution of cutaneous nerves. A simple method is to test the dorsum of the first web space for posterior cord damage, the palmar pad of the distal phalanx of the index finger for lateral cord palsy, and the palmar pad of the distal phalanx of the little finger for medial cord anesthesia.

Circumflex Nerve

Circumflex nerve injury has been reported in a patient who was placed in the Trendelenburg position. The patient's arm, at right angles to the body, was allowed to press against the vertical portion of a metal ether screen.[58,79] In such cases, the nerve is compressed between bone and metal as it circles lateral to the neck of the humerus (Fig. 26-14). The force of gravity on the patient in the head-down position undoubtedly accentuates the pressure. This injury causes an inability to abduct the arm and a loss of sensation over the upper half of the lateral aspect of the arm.

Radial Nerve

The radial nerve may be injured as it traverses the brachium if the arm is permitted to slip off the side of the operating table. When the patient is in the Trendelenburg position, the arm tends to be pushed up against the ether screen (Fig. 26-15), squeezing the nerve between the screen and the spiral groove. Clinically, wristdrop, an inability to extend the metacarpophalangeal joints, and weakness of abduction of the thumb are prominent features. The dorsal surface of the lateral three and one-half fingers and adjacent hand show various degrees of numbness, dryness, increased warmth, and redness.

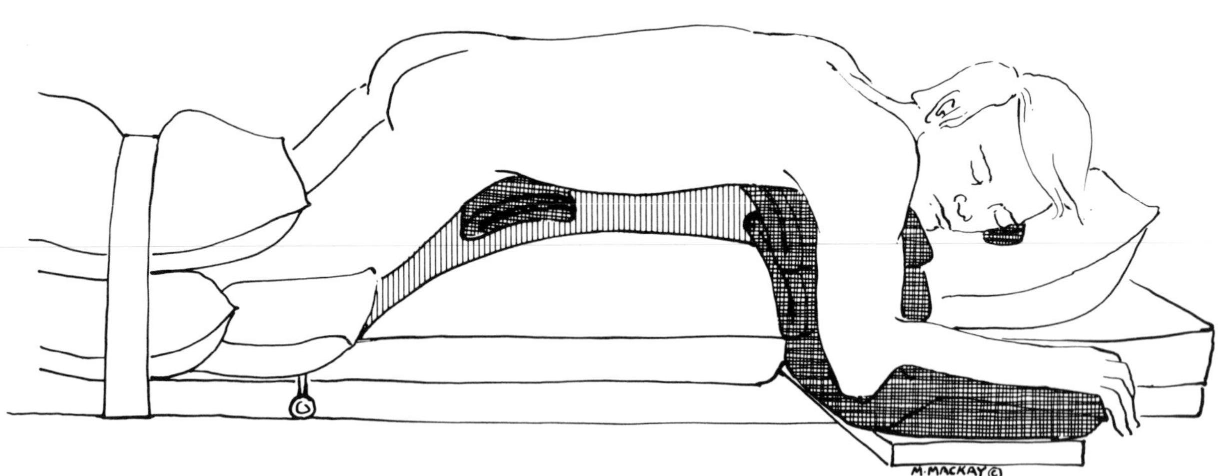

FIGURE 26-13. Correct flexed prone position. Arms are abducted and anteriorly flexed to less than 90°. The elbows, groin, and lower face and forehead are well padded. Upward convexity of the orthopedic frame is minimal.

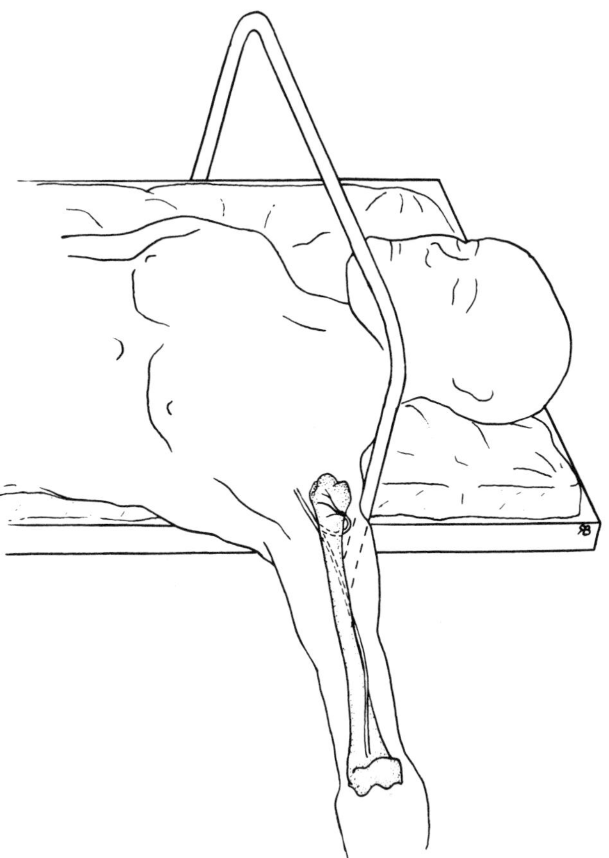

FIGURE 26-14. Abduction of the arm against an ether screen in the Trendelenburg position pinches the circumflex nerve.

Premedication distal to, rather than into, the deltoid muscle may damage the radial nerve in the spiral groove.[80] Infusion of thiopental into a vein passing up the lateral side of the wrist has injured the underlying superficial radial nerve, producing numbness of the dorsum of the thenar web. Radial nerve injury has also been reported following use of an automatically cycled blood pressure cuff positioned near the elbow in an active parturient.[81] We believe the patient's movements may have contributed by causing longer and more frequent inflation cycles.

Median Nerve

The median nerve, lying adjacent to the medial cubital and basilic veins in the antecubital fossa, may be traumatized during injection into or cannulation of an antecubital vein (Fig. 26-16).[82] The inability to appose the thumb and little finger, weakness of thumb abduction, and loss of flexion of the distal phalanx of the index finger occur. Eventually, the thenar eminence becomes flattened. Sensation and sweating are diminished on the palmar surface of the lateral three and one-half digits and adjacent palm.

Ulnar Nerve

Mechanisms of Injury

COMPRESSION. The ulnar nerve can be compressed against the posterior aspect of the medial epicondyle of the humerus.[15,16,83,84] Compression may result from the sharp edge

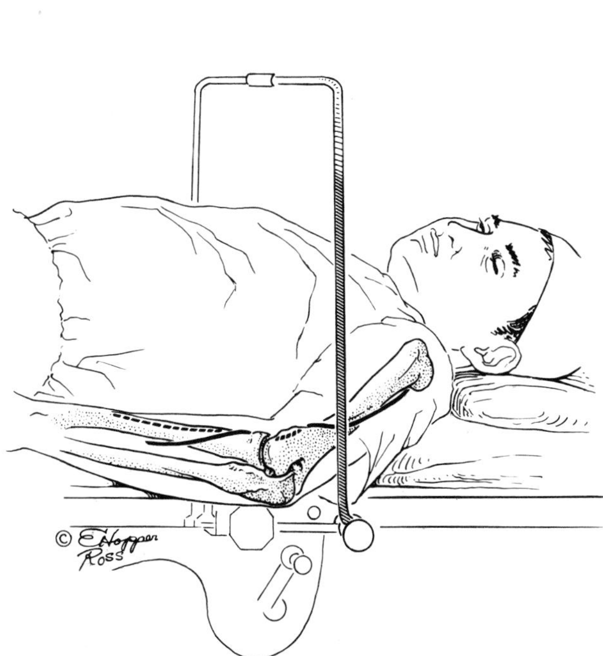

FIGURE 26-15. When the arm of the patient in the Trendelenburg position slips off the table and against the ether screen, the radial nerve is pinched. (Britt BA, Gordon RA: Peripheral nerve injuries associated with anaesthesia. Can Anaesth Soc J 11:514, 1964.)

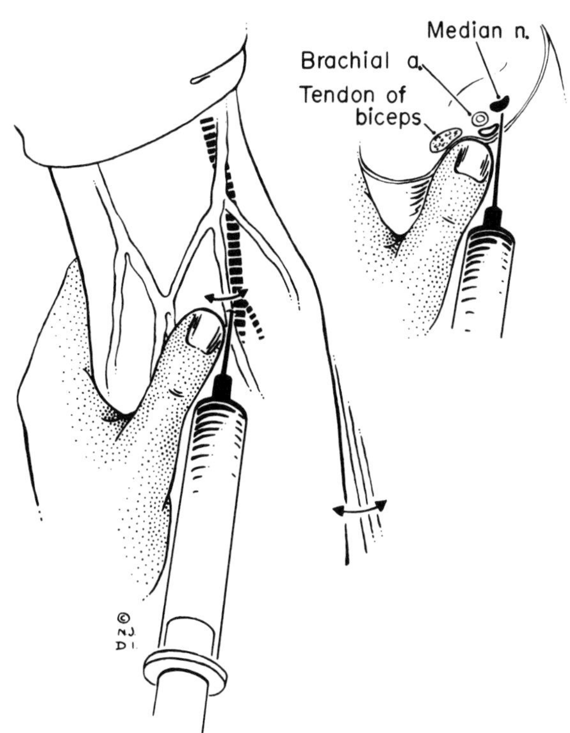

FIGURE 26-16. The median nerve is traumatized by a misplaced needle during attempted puncture of a vein in the antecubital fossa. (Britt BA, Gordon RA: Peripheral nerve injuries associated with anaesthesia. Can Anaesth Soc J 11:514, 1964.)

of the table if the elbow is allowed to slip just slightly over its side. This sequence may occur if the draw sheet used to keep the arm at the patient's side is tucked between mattress and table, rather than between patient and mattress. In the adducted position, failure to use protective arm guards may permit compression of the nerve by the surgeon, particularly by an obese surgeon or by a surgeon with a beeper on the side of her or his pants.[85] In this same position, keeping the forearm and hand supinated may also result in an ulnar nerve palsy.[86]

STRETCHING. We have observed stretching-induced ulnar nerve palsies when the arm was abducted between 60° and 90° on an arm board in the horizontal supine position with the patient supine or prone on a frame. Alvine[86] made similar observations of three patients whose arms were abducted between 45° and 70°. In these cases, the mechanism of injury is much the same as for brachial plexus damage in similar positions; the ulnar nerve is simply an extension of the brachial plexus. Stretching of any part of the brachial plexus is always associated with stretching of its peripheral extensions. The claim of McAlpine and Seckel[18] that the forearm and hand should be supinated is not supported by these cases. Full pronation of the arm is safe for the ulnar nerve for the reasons described in the section on brachial plexus injury, but when the forearm and hand are supinated, stretching of the ulnar nerve is considerably increased.

FLEXION. Injuries to the ulnar nerve also have been reported after operations in which the patient's arm was folded across the abdomen or chest with extreme elbow flexion.[87] The stretching of the nerve around the medial epicondyle of the humerus by acute flexion of the elbow and the pressure exerted by the weight of the arm itself apparently are sufficient to produce ischemia. This problem may occur because the ulnar nerve pursues a more medial course in more then 20% of people than that described in anatomy texts and passes behind the posteriorly projecting tip of the epicondyle, rather than in the more protected groove (Fig. 26-17).

ABDUCTION. If, in the lateral decubitus position, the upper arm is abducted above the patient's head, an ulnar nerve palsy may ensue.[86] In the prone position, the ulnar nerve may be damaged when the arm is abducted and the forearm is flexed, stretching the ulnar nerve over the ulnar condyle and leaving it vulnerable to compression.[88]

TOURNIQUET. The ulnar nerve may be injured by a thick, rigid tourniquet[38] or by an automatic blood pressure cuff,[89] particularly when either is placed too low and compression is maintained for too long.

Contributing Factors

The largest published series identifies male gender, extremes of body habitus, and prolonged hospitalization as risk factors associated with an increased incidence of postoperative ulnar neuropathy.[90] A more detailed description of efforts taken to avoid this complication in each case is important to improve our understanding of the etiologic factors and to assist in medicolegal defense or settlement when a claim results.

Clinical Features

Signs of an ulnar nerve injury may be observed immediately after awakening from the anesthetic but usually are not detected for at least 1 day and often not for several postoperative days.[90,91] If the injury has occurred as the nerve passes posterior to the medial epicondyle, there may be pain at the elbow. Grip on the ulnar side of the fist is weak, as is flexion of the interphalangeal joints of the medial two digits. Flexion of the metacarpophalangeal and proximal interphalangeal joints, extension of the distal interphalangeal joints, and abduction and adduction of the medial four digits, when extended, are impaired. An inability to abduct or appose the little finger occurs. Sensory and autonomic loss affect both surfaces of the medial one and one-half fingers and adjacent hand. Eventually, the intrinsic hand muscles, except for the thenar em-

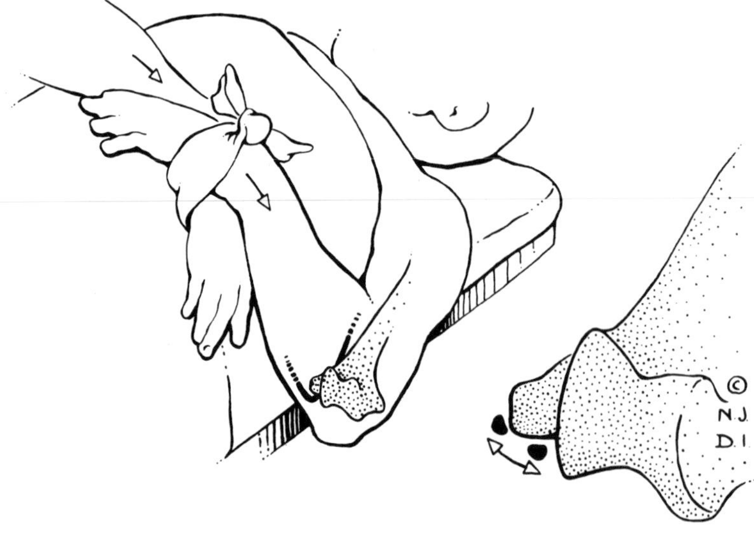

FIGURE 26-17. When the elbow slips off of the side of the table, the ulnar nerve is squeezed between the sharp edge of the table and the medial epicondyle of the humerus. The anomalous course of the ulnar nerve behind the tip of the medial epicondyle (*arrows*) predisposes it to injury. (Britt BA, Gordon RA: Peripheral nerve injuries associated with anaesthesia. Can Anaesth Soc J 11:514, 1964.)

TABLE 26-1
Prevention of Brachial Plexus Injuries

1. Do not abduct the arm to more than 60°.
2. Keep the forearms and hands fully pronated.
3. In the prone position and during open heart surgery, keep abduction of the arms to less than 45°, and keep forearms flexed so the hands are beside the head.
4. Minimize combinations of lateral flexion of the head and abduction and dorsal extension of the contralateral arm.
5. Avoid steep Trendelenburg positions.
6. Avoid downward pressure on the head of the humerus or on the clavicle.
7. In the lateral, partial prone, or prone position, minimize compression between the lateral thorax and the head of the humerus with a roll placed under and against the lateral thorax and not in the axilla.

inence, become wasted, and contractures develop, resulting in a characteristic claw-like hand.

Musculocutaneous Nerve

The musculocutaneous nerve is particularly vulnerable to injury when the arm is externally rotated and abducted to 90° for prolonged periods.[92] The nerve is stretched as it passes over the head of the humerus, the prominence of the curve. The coracobrachialis muscle may also play a major role in the mechanism of injury, because the nerve may be injured as it travels through the tunnel in the coracobrachialis muscle.[92]

The lateral cutaneous nerve of the forearm, a terminal branch of the musculocutaneous nerve, has been damaged by a traumatic intravenous injection into the antecubital area, with resultant hematoma formation (Britt BA: unpublished data), with numbness and pain down the lateral aspect of the upper two thirds of the forearm.

Table 26-1 summarizes our recommendations for the prevention of brachial plexus injuries.

LOWER EXTREMITY NEUROPATHIES

Lower extremity anatomy and the mechanism of nerve injuries are illustrated in Figure 26-18.

Sciatic Nerve

Two situations can cause injury to the sciatic nerve: the lateral and lithotomy positions.

In a thin, emaciated patient who is lying on a poorly padded table in the lateral position, the sciatic nerve may be squeezed as it escapes from under cover of the piriformis when the opposite buttock is elevated, as during hip arthroplasty or thoracoabdominal incisions.

A patient in the lithotomy position can sustain sciatic nerve damage if the thighs and legs are externally rotated (Fig. 26-19) or if the knees are extended (Fig. 26-20).[60] Both of these positions increase the distance between the points of fixation of the sciatic nerve, in the sciatic notch proximally and in the neck of the fibula distally. To reduce stretch of the sciatic nerve, external rotation of the thighs and knees must

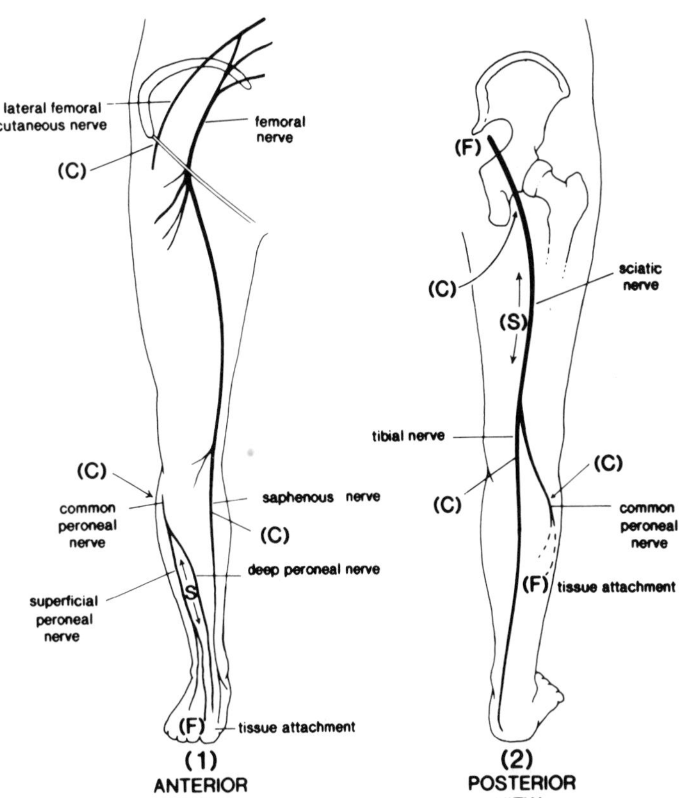

FIGURE 26-18. Lower-extremity nerve injuries. (1) Anterior view. The lateral femoral cutaneous nerve may be compressed (C) between an external appliance and the iliac spine. The common peroneal nerve may be compressed (C) between the head of the fibula and an external appliance. Pressure against the medial aspect of the upper one third of the tibia may compress (C) the saphenous nerve. The superficial and deep peroneal nerves may be stretched (S) if the foot is plantar-flexed. *F*, point of fixation. (2) Posterior view. The sciatic nerve may be stretched (S) between its fixation points (*F*) by flexion of the hip without flexion at the knee. It also may be compressed (*C*) at the ischial tuberosity. The common peroneal nerve may be compressed as shown in the anterior view. The tibial nerve is susceptible to compression (C) at the popliteal fossa. (Mahla ME: Nervous system. In Gravenstein N (ed): Manual of complications during anesthesia. Philadelphia: JB Lippincott, 1991: 388.)

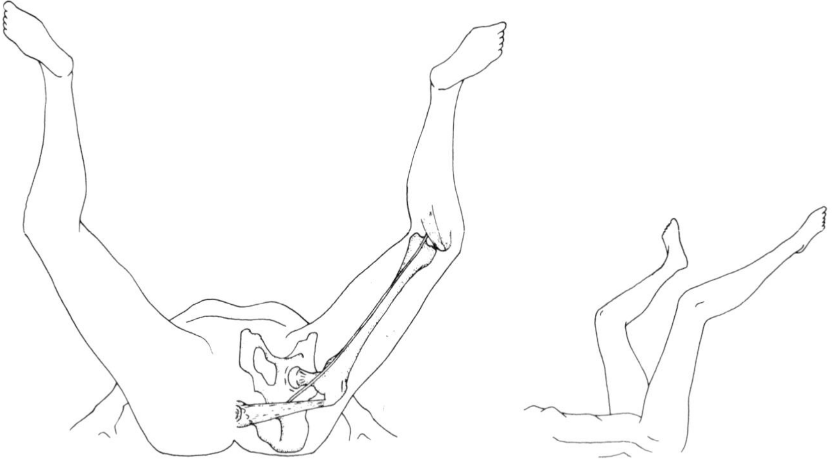

FIGURE 26-19. Incorrect lithotomy position. Extreme external rotation of the hips stretches the sciatic nerve.

be minimal, and the knees should be flexed (Fig. 26-21). Care should be exercised by assistants to avoid leaning on the inner aspect of the leg or thigh.[93] Failure to flex the knees in the sitting position may also stretch the sciatic nerve, with unfortunate consequences.

Femoral Nerve

In the early 1900s, the reported incidence of femoral neuropathy after childbirth was 4.7%.[94] Although the condition is rare today, it still occurs as a result of prolonged lithotomy position with a combination of flexion, abduction, and external rotation of the thighs.[95,96] This forces the femoral nerve into an 80° to 90° angulation on the inguinal ligament.[96] Pressure on the nerve is continuous while this posture is maintained.[93]

Warner and Martin identified a body mass index (kg/m^2) of less than 20, lithotomy position for more than 4 hours, and history of smoking within 30 days of the procedure as major risk factors for the development of a persistent neuropathy of the lower extremity.[95] Pressure placed on the legs by surgeons during lower pelvic and perineal surgery are probably contributing factors. Clinically, all muscles below the knee and perhaps the hamstrings are paralyzed. During gynecologic laparotomy, the femoral nerve has been damaged by pressure and lateral deflection of the leg of a self-retaining retractor (see Fig. 26-1).[97]

Examination reveals an inability to flex the hip and the knee as a result of quadriceps femoris palsy. Sensation and autonomic function are lost over the anterior aspect of the thigh, the medial and anteromedial sides of the calf, and the medial side of the foot.

Common Peroneal Nerve

The common peroneal nerve is the most frequently damaged nerve in the lower limb,[98] although injuries to it are not as common as those to the brachial plexus. It may be compressed against the head of the fibula in the lithotomy position, in which case it is stretched by flexion of the hips and knees.[99]

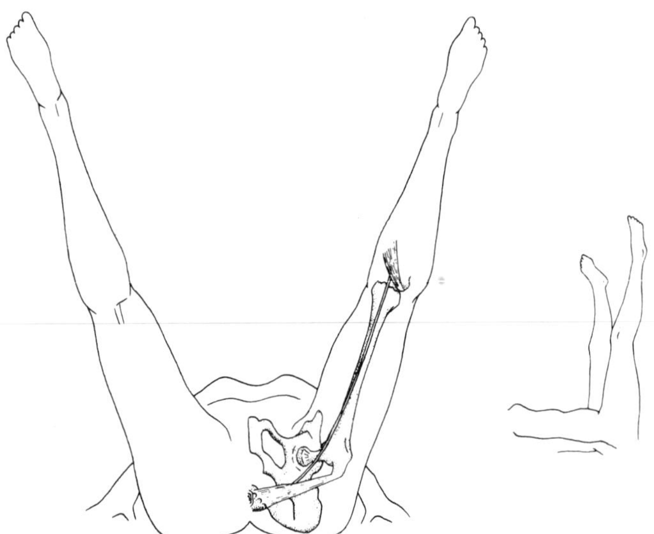

FIGURE 26-20. Incorrect lithotomy position. Extension of the knees stretches the sciatic nerve.

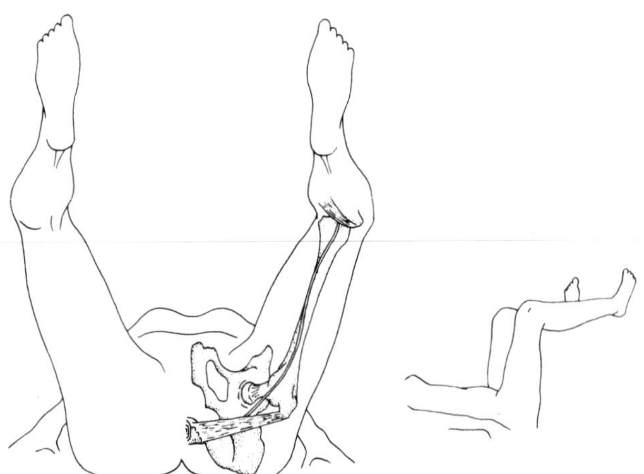

FIGURE 26-21. Correct lithotomy position. External rotation of the hips is minimal. The knees are flexed.

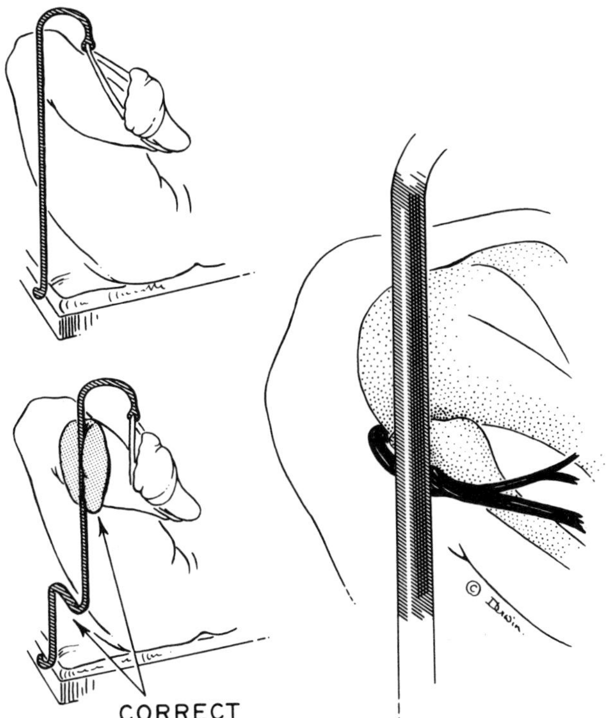

FIGURE 26-22. In the lithotomy position, the common peroneal nerve is compressed (*right*) between the fibula and the vertical metal brace when padding is inadequate (*top left*). (Britt BA, Gordon RA: Peripheral nerve injuries associated with anaesthesia. Can Anaesth Soc J 11:514, 1964.)

The neck of the fibula rubs against the vertical metal brace, from which the supporting foot strap is slung, or against a curved metal support under the knee, pinching the already overstretched nerve (Fig. 26-22).

The common peroneal nerve, like the sciatic nerve, can be stretched in the lithotomy position when the knees are extended or the thighs and legs are externally rotated.[98] Damage may also follow undue, prolonged pressure against the nerve by a poorly padded table when the patient is in the lateral position.[79] In the supine position, similar injury may be produced by hard knee rolls. An improperly applied tourniquet may lead to neuropathy, particularly if it is of the thick and hard variety or, most commonly, if it is not calibrated properly and overinflated.[100]

The physical findings are footdrop, loss of dorsal extension of the toes, inability to evert the foot,[99] and numbness of the lateral and anterolateral aspects of the calf and medial half of the dorsum of the foot.

Anterior Tibial (Deep Peroneal) Nerve

Footdrop and anesthesia of the dorsum of the foot proximal to the first and second toes may occur if the feet are left plantarflexed for extended periods during anesthesia. This position increases the distance that the anterior tibial nerve must travel over the anterior surface of the ankle joint (see Fig. 26-18). That portion of the nerve lying between its origin lateral to the head of the fibula above and the superior and inferior extensor retinacula below is stretched (Fig. 26-23). Patients in the sitting position should have a foot support under their feet, and patients in the prone position should have a roll placed under the anterior aspect of their ankles to maintain the feet in the dorsiflexed (extended) position.

Posterior Tibial Nerve

The posterior tibial nerve may be injured when the legs of a patient in the lithotomy position are placed on Bierhoff stirrups that support the posterior aspect of the knee. If undue weight is borne by the popliteal fossa, through which this nerve passes, weakness of plantar flexion of the foot and anesthesia of the toes, sole, and lateral aspect of the foot result.[72]

Saphenous Nerve

The saphenous nerve can be compressed against the medial tibial condyle if the foot is suspended lateral to the vertical brace (Fig. 26-24).[9] Paresthesia develops along the medial and anteromedial sides of the calf. In the lithotomy position, ample padding should always be placed between the legs and vertical metal braces.

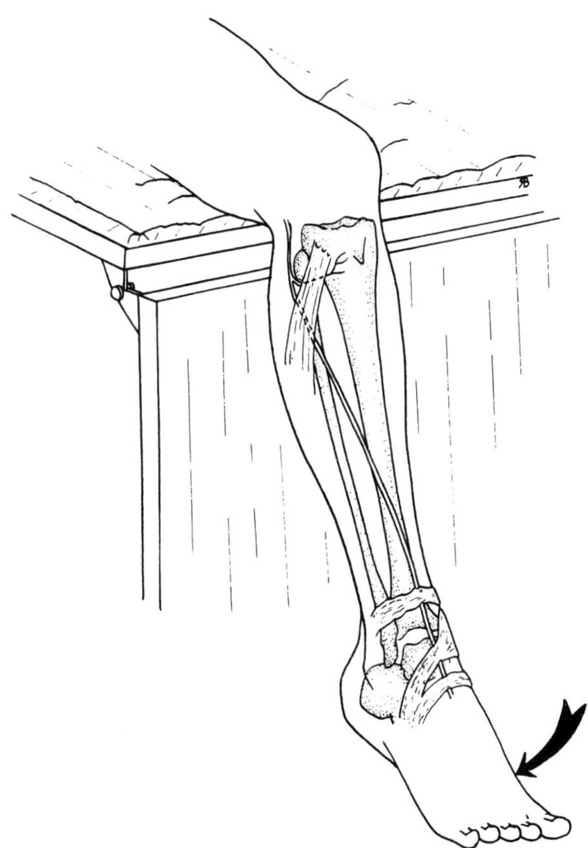

FIGURE 26-23. Plantar flexion of the foot in the sitting or prone position stretches the anterior tibial nerves.

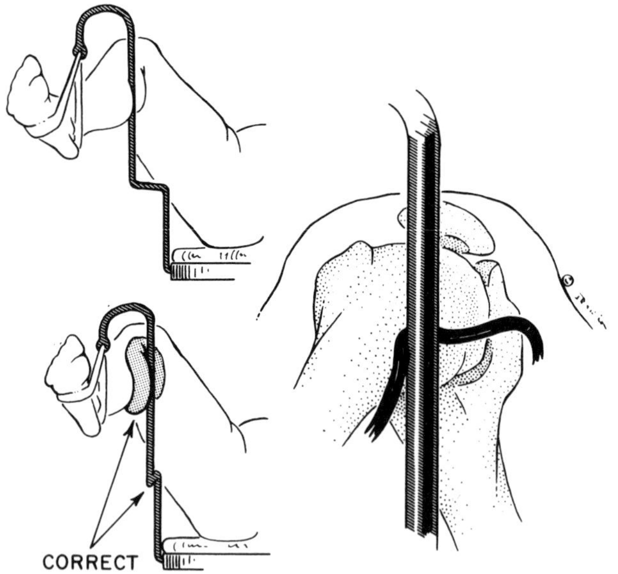

FIGURE 26-24. In the lithotomy position, the saphenous nerve is pinched (*right*) between the medial condyle of the tibia and the vertical metal brace when padding is inadequate (*top left*). (Britt BA, Gordon RA: Peripheral nerve injuries associated with anaesthesia. Can Anaesth Soc J 11:514, 1964)

Lateral Femoral Cutaneous Nerve of the Thigh

In the flexed-prone position, the lateral femoral cutaneous nerve of the thigh can be damaged by hard bolsters. The nerve is pinched between the bolster and the ilium as it passes behind the inguinal ligament medial to the anterosuperior spine (see Fig. 26-11). The injury is characterized by anesthesia of the lower, lateral portion of the anterior aspect of the thigh. Injury to this nerve also has been reported during laparoscopic cholecystectomy with the patient in a steep reverse Trendelenburg position when a restraining strap was placed across the upper thighs.[101]

Pudendal Nerve

The pudendal nerve may be pressed against the ischial tuberosity by traction of both legs against a poorly padded orthopedic post.[102] The nerve may also be damaged in anesthetized obese patients by acute flexion of the thigh to the groin.[103] A resultant loss of perineal sensation and incontinence of feces may occur. An outward swing of the legs occurs with walking.[103]

Obturator Nerve

Obturator nerve palsy with paralysis of the abductors and numbness over the medial side of the thigh has been observed in a patient after an epidural anesthetic (Gordon RA: personal communication). This patient had undergone a difficult forceps delivery, and the obstetrician recalled that he had had to "pull harder" on the forceps than he had ever done before.

Table 26-2 summarizes suggestions to aid in the prevention of lower extremity nerve injuries.

CRANIAL NERVES AND BRANCHES OF CRANIAL NERVES

Supraorbital Nerve

The supraorbital nerve can be compressed by the connector of an endotracheal tube if padding is insufficient (Fig. 26-25). The injury results in photophobia, numbness of the forehead, and pain in the eye.

Facial Nerve

The facial nerve may be pinched between the anesthesiologist's fingers and the ascending ramus of the mandible if unusual or sustained forward pressure is required to maintain a clear airway (Fig. 26-26).[104] The corner of the mouth sags; saliva drools; chewing is difficult; and the affected side of the face is smoother than normal because of the loss of muscle tone.

The buccal branch of the facial nerve can be impaired by pressure from a head strap that is applied too tightly or too long or from excessive and prolonged pressure by fingers against the angles and body of the mandible.[105] This complication is especially likely to occur if the course of the nerve is superficial to the parotid gland. Injury is characterized by loss of function of the orbicularis oris muscle (Fig. 26-27).[52]

Recurrent Laryngeal and Superior Laryngeal Nerve

Mechanisms of Injury

INTUBATION. The vocal cords can be paralyzed during the process of intubation because of damage to the recurrent laryngeal nerve, superior laryngeal nerve, or both. Prolonged intubation raises the possibility of vocal cord damage.[106] The damage may be caused by trauma during repeated intubation attempts by the laryngoscope blade or the stylet. Most commonly, damage is to either or both of the anterior and posterior branches of the recurrent laryngeal nerve, but sometimes, the superior laryngeal nerve is injured.[107] Usually, there are associated hematomas.[108] Arytenoid dislocation, laryngeal laceration and edema, and pseudomembrane and granuloma formation also may occur.[109,110] In some cases, arytenoid dislocation may occur without vocal cord paralysis.[111]

CUFF. Injury may also be caused by endotracheal tube cuff problems. For instance, the cuff may be situated too high,

TABLE 26-2
Prevention of Lower Extremity Nerve Injuries

1. In the lithotomy position, avoid external rotation of the hips and extension of the knees.
2. Avoid compression of lateral head of the fibula and medial condyle of the tibia against the stirrups or other sharp objects.
3. Keep feet dorsiflexed.
4. Avoid compression against the popliteal fossa.
5. Avoid pressure on the anterior superior iliac spine, and pad this area in the prone position.

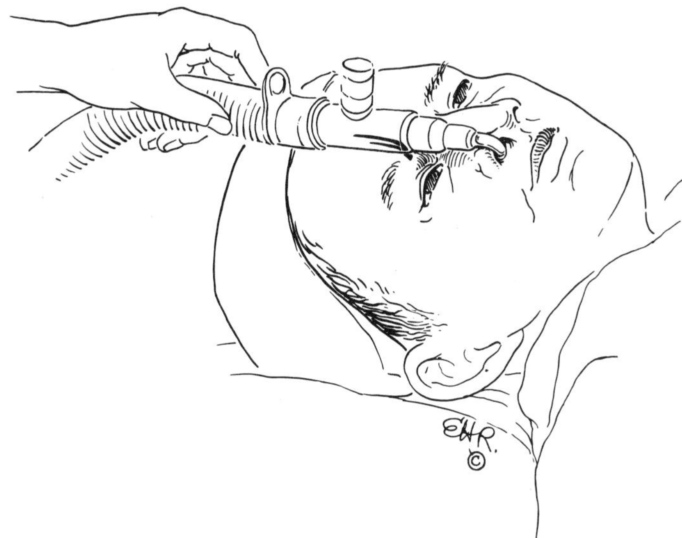

FIGURE 26-25. The supraorbital nerve is squeezed between the metal connectors and the bony forehead when padding is insufficient. (Britt BA, Gordon RA: Peripheral nerve injuries associated with anaesthesia. Can Anaesth Soc J 11:514, 1964.)

with resultant compression of the anterior branch of the laryngeal nerve between the cuff and the lamina of the thyroid bone.[112–116] Overinflating the cuff or using a cuff that inflates irregularly, rigidly, and with high pressure increases the likelihood of such injury.[112,116,117]

Nitrous oxide is 34 times more soluble than nitrogen.[118–121] Nitrous oxide infuses into the cuff much more rapidly than nitrogen diffuses out of the cuff. Consequently, if the cuff is not deflated periodically during a long operation, it may become hyperinflated and cause extreme pressure on the recurrent laryngeal nerve. Vocal cord paralysis may also develop when the endotracheal tube is gas sterilized in ethylene oxide and then not aerated adequately.[122,123]

Cuff-induced vocal cord paralysis may also include paralysis of the muscles of the tongue due to damage to the hypoglossal nerve. In this situation, known as Tapia's syndrome, the cuff pressure occurs just at the point at which the vagal and the hypoglossal nerves cross each other.[124] To prevent cuff damage to the vocal cords, the cuff should be positioned midway between the carina and the vocal cords, should have low pressure and not be overinflated, should be periodically deflated, and should not be reused.

Shin[125] has reported a high incidence of lower serum albumin in patients suffering from recurrent laryngeal nerve paralysis due to overinflated cuffs. Other factors include decreased elasticity of the trachea and surrounding tissues,

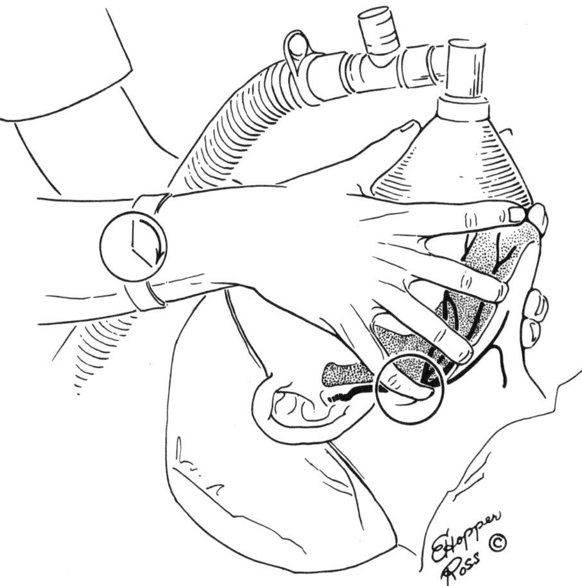

FIGURE 26-26. The facial nerve is pinched between the finger and ascending ramus of the jaw when unusual forward pressure is applied. (Britt BA, Gordon RA: Peripheral nerve injuries associated with anaesthesia. Can Anaesth Soc J 11:514, 1964.)

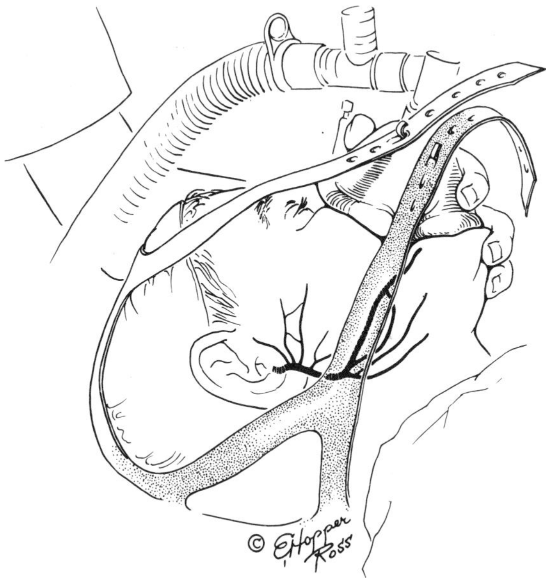

FIGURE 26-27. The buccal branch of the facial nerve is injured by a mask strap that is fitted too tightly. (Britt BA, Gordon RA: Peripheral nerve injuries associated with anaesthesia. Can Anaesth Soc J 11:514, 1964.)

anomalous distribution of the laryngeal nerves, and the influence of muscle relaxants.[126]

TUBES. The posterior branch of the recurrent laryngeal nerve may be compressed by a centrally positioned esophageal stethoscope or nasogastric tube.[127,128]

Differential Diagnosis

Vocal cord paralysis due to an error in positioning of an endotracheal tube or in the inflation of the cuff should be differentiated from paralysis due to heat from the use of electrocautery;[129] direct trauma to one of the laryngeal nerves or the vagus nerve by a surgeon during an anterior cervical fusion, a thyroidectomy, or a thoracic procedure;[130–136] stretching of the right recurrent laryngeal nerve around the right subclavian artery while this vessel is being retracted during open heart surgery;[137,138] a previously existing asymptomatic laryngeal nerve palsy; or intracranial pathology.[135] However, many cases of recurrent laryngeal nerve or superior laryngeal nerve paralysis have occurred during anesthesia for procedures unrelated to the neck or chest and so cannot possibly be the result of surgical trauma.[106,139,140] If the paralysis is bilateral, one or both of the arytenoids is dislocated, or local mucosa or soft tissue damage exists, the cause is related to intubation rather than surgical trauma.[141–143]

Clinical Features

Unilateral recurrent laryngeal nerve paralysis, paralysis of the posterior and lateral cricoarytenoids, interarytenoids, and thyroarytenoids results in the injured vocal cord resting in the medial position and the normal cord being abducted to provide a marginal to adequate airway. During phonation, tensing and lengthening of the paralyzed cords results from the contraction of both cricothyroid muscles (supplied by the superior laryngeal nerve).[107] The speaking voice is initially hoarse but then becomes almost normal. Efforts to sing, however, are severely impaired.

Bilateral recurrent laryngeal nerve paralysis causes both cords to be in the medial position, producing severe respiratory distress, inspiratory and expiratory stridor, and cyanosis. Tracheotomy is required to relieve the respiratory distress. If only the anterior branches of the recurrent laryngeal nerve are injured (ie, paralysis of lateral cricoarytenoids and thyroarytenoids), the cords are fixed in the intermediate position and are shortened and relaxed. The voice is hoarse. If only the posterior branches of the recurrent laryngeal nerve are damaged (ie, paralysis of posterior cricoarytenoids and interarytenoids), the vocal cords are in spasm. Signs and treatment are the same as for palsy of the entire recurrent laryngeal nerves.

Complete unilateral superior and recurrent laryngeal nerve paralysis leads to the affected cord being motionless and bowed in the lateral position and provides a better airway than with simple recurrent laryngeal nerve paralysis.[107] During phonation, faint adduction of the posterior commissure area results from contraction of the bilaterally innervated interarytenoids.[107] The voice is breathy and raspy, and the singing voice is affected.

Combined complete bilateral superior and recurrent laryngeal nerve injury causes aphonia and an extremely weak, breathy, and barely audible voice.[107] Both cords are motionless and bowed in the lateral or intermediate position. The airway is adequate, but aspiration may be severe enough to require tracheotomy.

Unilateral superior laryngeal nerve paralysis results in the affected cord being shorter than normal, the epiglottis being tilted to the affected side, and the posterior commissure being shifted to the normal side.[107] The voice is breathy and raspy. The singing voice is impaired.

Bilateral superior laryngeal nerve paralysis causes both cords to be shortened and bowed and to fail to lengthen and tense during phonation.[107] The epiglottis overhangs the anterior portion of the larynx, making visualization of the endolarynx difficult. Initially, the voice becomes lower, weaker, breathy, and hoarse, and speech lacks inflection. After compensation, the speaking voice sounds normal, but the singing voice is severely compromised.

Treatment

Vocal cord paralysis is treated by Gelfoam paste injection to produce temporary rehabilitation.[144] More permanent repair can be achieved with Teflon or fat injection[144–146] or by lateralizing procedures to produce longer-lasting effects. Lateralizing surgery, however, leads to further weakening of the voice.

Prognosis

A neuropraxic injury, in which function is lost without anatomic damage, usually recovers spontaneously within 6 weeks. In contrast, an axonotmetic injury that has axonal disruption but preservation of the nerve sheath results in regeneration of the nerve from the point of injury at the rate of 1 mm per day and a corresponding recovery of function. A neurotmetic lesion disrupts the axon and sheath. The nerve degenerates distally and cannot heal normally. Most position-related injuries are neuropraxic in nature.

Recovery from a peripheral nerve injury may require a few days, weeks, or months; otherwise, permanent weakness, wasting, and sensory and autonomic loss may be the result.

OTHER TRAUMATIC INJURIES

Eyes

Mechanisms of Injury

Damage to the eyes has the most serious consequences for the patient. Pressure against the globe, especially during controlled or accidental hypotension, promotes thrombosis of the central retinal artery, with permanent blindness on awakening from the anesthetic. Disorganization may affect the entire globe.

Such pressure is more likely to occur in the prone position. This is the position in which controlled hypotension is often used, as during spinal fusion or Harrington rod insertion. Walkup reports two cases of unilateral blindness after pressure on the eye; a horseshoe headrest had been used for pulmonary resection in the prone position.[147] We know of a similar complication produced by this type of headrest during a neurosurgical procedure. Eyeball compression also has resulted from the pressure produced by a frontal bone flap that was turned down over the face and inadvertently into one or both eyes. Pressure against a headrest is more likely to occur when the patient partially rouses and moves during the anesthetic. The most common cause of blindness from an eye injury associated with anesthesia was patient movement during ophthalmologic surgery, as reported in a closed claims analysis.[148]

Gillan reported that blindness may be caused entirely by hypotension during anesthesia, without any compression against the eyeball.[149] On other occasions, blindness followed a combination of hypotension and pressure by endotracheal tube connectors or the anesthesiologist's hands.[150,151]

Clinical Features

Sometimes on examination within the first 24 hours, the eyes and eyelids may appear entirely normal, especially if the examiner is not expert and meticulous. However, the pupil more commonly is dilated and reacts consensually but not directly to light. The cornea is slightly hazy, and the lids are often edematous. The retinal arterioles are dilated, and the venules are engorged. The macula and the retina surrounding the optic disc are edematous. If the damage is severe, a cherry red spot may exist in the fovea. The patient may complain of pain in the region of the eye. After several days, the optic disc becomes pearly white. The arterioles narrow to white threads. The macula and peripapillary retina may become diffusely pigmented, and faint radical scarring may appear in the fovea.[152]

Spinal Cord

Compression and actual disruption of the cervical spinal cord, with subsequent quadriplegia, has been observed after anesthesia. The cause appears to be excessive extension or flexion of the head, often associated with spondylitic spurs. This gross distortion can occur during a tonsillectomy in which a Boyle-Davis mouth gag suspended from a Mayo stand is adjusted so high that the patient's occiput is lifted (Fig. 26-28). These patients may also have retropharyngeal abscesses or hematomas that may exacerbate the severity of the neurologic deficit. In the correct tonsillectomy position, use of a doughnut-shaped support under the head prevents dorsal extension (Fig. 26-29). Quadriplegia may also occur after a posterior fossa procedure during which the patient's neck was acutely flexed.[153]

Cauda equina syndrome has been reported after continuous spinal anesthesia administered through microcatheters.[154] Eleven cases occurred since 1989, leading the United States Food and Drug Administration to order withdrawal of the catheters from the market. Subsequently, the role of microcatheters in causing this complication has been questioned, focusing instead on the possibilities of maldistribution of drug within the cerebrospinal fluid and inappropriate drug dose.[155,156]

Appendages

In the lithotomy position with the arms resting at the patient's side, fingers have been severed. As the foot of the table is rolled back up at the end of surgery, the digits become crushed if care is not taken to keep them out of the progressively narrowing gap between the main portion and the foot of the table (Fig. 26-30).

The ear may be necrosed by a head strap or by being folded forcibly between the patient's head and a hard pillow during a long operation (Fig. 26-31),[156] and the nose may be crushed by the elbow of a leaning surgeon when the head is completely covered by surgical drapes.

The tongue can be grossly lacerated and require sutures if the mouth gag is incorrectly positioned during electroshock therapy (Fig. 26-32). The gag should be placed so that its flanges lie between the lips and the teeth.

Parotid gland obstruction and swelling has been reported as a complication of dislocation of the temporomandibular joint, prolonged lateral decubitus positioning during surgery, or both.[156]

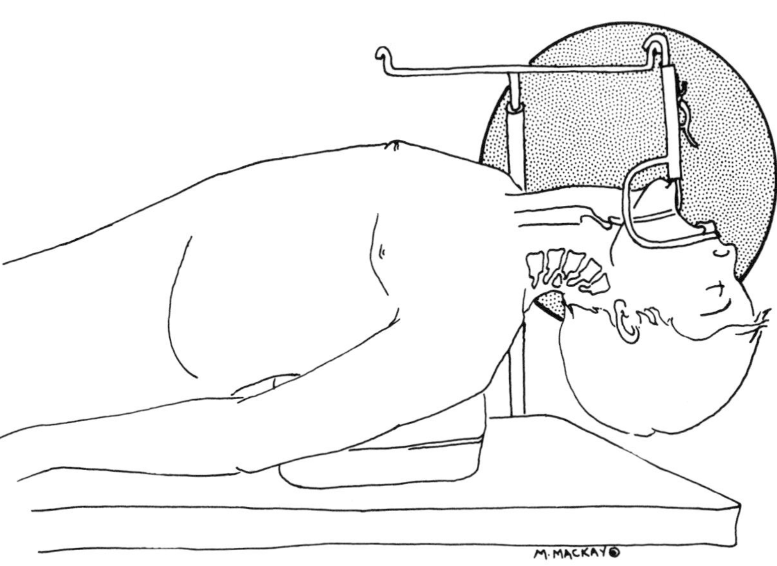

FIGURE 26-28. Incorrect tonsillectomy position. Suspension of a Boyle-Davis mouth gag from a Mayo stand placed too high induces extreme dorsal extension of the head. This distortion, when associated with spondylitic spurs, retropharyngeal abscesses, or hematomas, can disrupt the spinal cord.

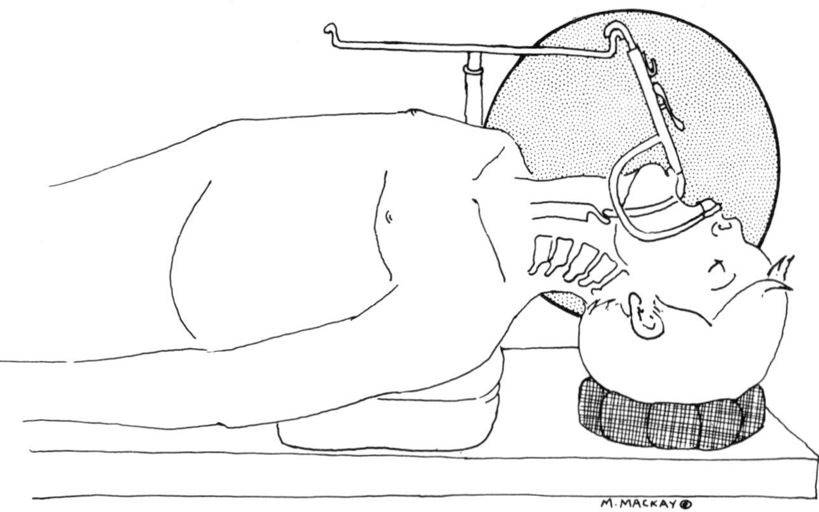

FIGURE 26-29. Correct tonsillectomy position. The posterior aspect of the head is supported by a doughnut-shaped pillow. The Mayo stand is sufficiently low to prevent excessive dorsal extension of the head.

Teeth

Because patients value their teeth, metal objects must be positioned gently within the mouth. During a laryngoscopy or tracheal intubation, if a tooth, crown, or bridge is chipped, loosened, or knocked out—even if it is discolored, misshapen, decayed, or loose—the anesthesiologist will promptly discover the high value attached to that tooth! The value is correspondingly greater if the tooth happens to be healthy or belongs to a child whose jaw development is incomplete.[157] When a tooth is knocked out or chipped, the tooth fragments must be located and recovered, employing radiologic examination and bronchoscopy, if necessary.[158]

Skin and Mucosa

Excessive pressure over a localized area of skin with resulting ischemia and even localized gangrene is a frequent complication. This complication continues to occur, with an incidence of more than 1 of every 100 patients despite careful padding of pressure points and attention to avoiding skin traction. Because it is impractical to rotate a patient's position routinely during lengthy procedures, no completely reliable preventive measure exists for this complication. Skin damage is worsened if the patient is hypotensive and the ischemic area is wet and macerated with water, sterilizing solution, or electrode jelly.

The skin may be burned when the cautery pad is malpositioned, the electrosurgical unit (ESU) is defective, or backpack-type electrocardiogram (ECG) electrodes are used and become wet with blood or irrigating fluids. We observed a patient who underwent anesthesia in the supine position

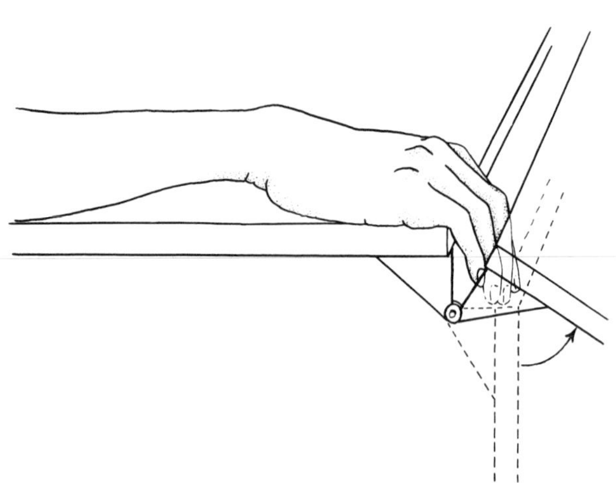

FIGURE 26-30. When the patient is in the lithotomy position with arms to the side, the fingers may be pinched as the foot of the table is rolled up (*arrow*).

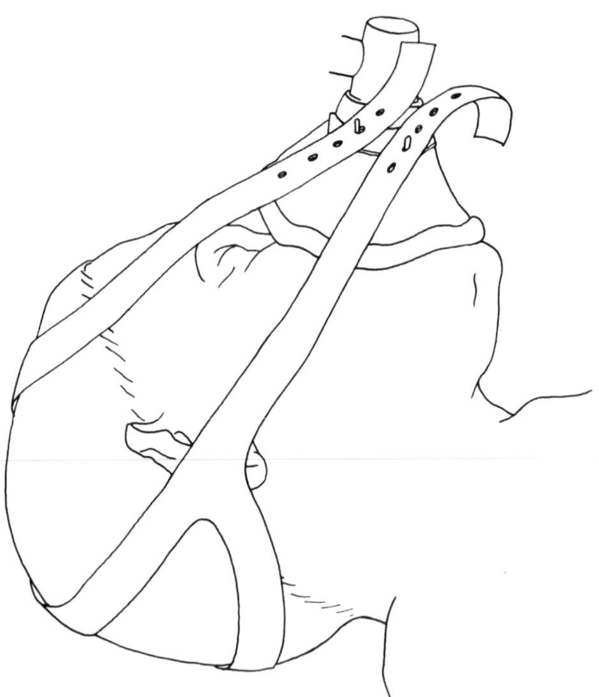

FIGURE 26-31. An ear is necrotized when it is buckled under a tightly fitted mask strap.

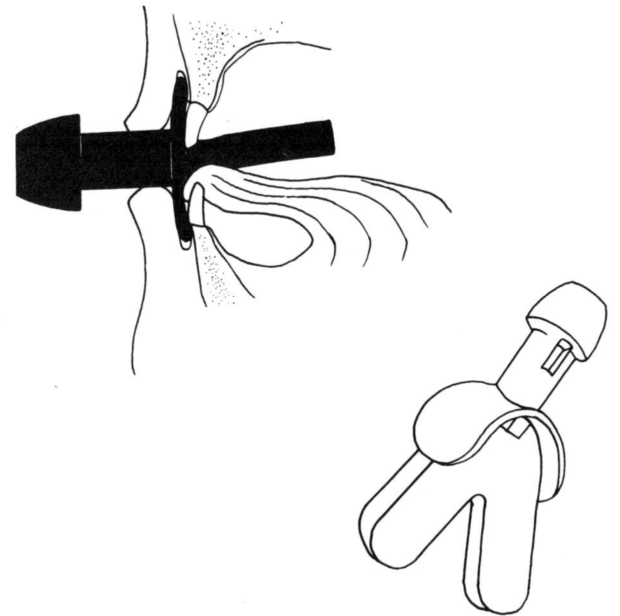

FIGURE 26-32. Incorrect positioning of a mouth gag (*top*) during electroconvulsive therapy results in laceration of the tongue by the teeth (*bottom*).

for a knife wound to the neck. A cautery pad was placed on the thigh. The backpack-type ECG electrodes became thoroughly wet with irrigating solutions. The ESU was defective. Because the ECG electrodes lay closer to the site of the cautery application than did the cautery pad, the current escaped to ground from the ECG electrodes rather than the cautery pad. The patient sustained third-degree burns that required skin grafting.

Scalp

Insufficiently padded headrests placed posterior to the ears to maintain the patient in a sitting or semisitting position during a neurosurgical procedure are liable to cause ischemia of the underlying skin. Hypotension that accompanies this position is a contributory factor. The end result may be permanent baldness of the ischemic areas. Examination of scalp biopsy specimens from these bald spots reveals "obliterative vasculitis."[156] These unsightly cosmetic defects tend to cause marked dissatisfaction among affected patients. A soft foam pad placed underneath the patient's head is highly recommended.

Face

Facial skin may be damaged by an inadequately padded support when the patient is in the prone position. The "catcher face mask" type of support is particularly at fault. These supports are used to maintain the eyes free of pressure, but skin ischemia may ensue, especially in the area of the chin, if great care is not taken to provide substantial padding. Periodic elevation or repositioning of the patient's face on the support during lengthy procedures helps to prevent this complication.

Mouth and Throat

Care must be taken when positioning an endotracheal tube to ensure that it does not exert undue pressure on the angle of the mouth. This problem is seldom brought to the anesthesiologist's attention by the patient, because the only complaint is that of marked tenderness at the corner of the mouth.[72] Pressure from an endotracheal tube over a prolonged period can cause enough necrosis of the tongue to require surgical excision of part of the tongue.[159] Maintaining the head in a position of acute flexion during anesthesia can result in airway-obstructing supraglottic edema.[160]

Groin

Bolster-type orthopedic frame posts used to support patients during spinal surgery must be well padded to prevent pressure necrosis of skin in the groin. The knees must also be padded amply in this position.[94]

Buttocks

In patients whose buttocks have rested in a pool of alcoholic sterilizing or iodine-based solution through a long operation, a pressure sore in this area may develop. Pressure sores also may develop on the apposing surfaces of the legs, particularly over the medial tibial condyles and medial malleoli when the patient is lying in the lateral nephrectomy position without pillows between the legs (see Fig. 26-4*A*, *B*). The heels of very tall people require padding or a table extension, because they are likely to sag over the end of the mattress onto the hard edge of the lower end of the table.[156]

Ligaments and Tendons

Stress, strains, and stretches of the back are most likely to occur when the position is extreme, when muscle relaxation is profound, and when the duration of the operation is long.[9,50,66] This combination of factors is common. Postoperative low backache occurs in 12% to 37% of all patients anesthetized in the supine, lithotomy, prone, and lateral nephrectomy positions.[156,161]

Supine Position

Anesthesia relaxes paraspinal muscles. In the supine position, the convexity of the lumbar spine flattens, and tension is applied to the interlumbar and lumbosacral ligaments. Moreover, the legs lie perfectly flat on the table (unlike the legs of the conscious patient), stretching the ligaments and muscles of the lower spine.[50]

Lithotomy Position

In the lithotomy position, rotation of the pelvis flattens the convexity of the lumbar spine to an even greater degree and puts great tension of these ligaments.[156] Postoperatively, minor stretch is interpreted as pain, soreness, or stiffness localized to the lumbosacral area or radiating down the sciatic nerve.[72] Such discomfort may last from a few days to several months. To avoid such injury, the knees should be flexed slightly in the supine position. In the lithotomy position, small pillows should be placed at the side of and slightly under the hips, and the legs should be placed in the stirrups or removed from them at the same time.[156]

Cervical Movement

Whiplash injury to the cervical area is another anesthetic complication. It can be avoided by supporting the patient's head and shoulders as a unit during turning to ensure that the head is turned at the same speed and in the same direction as the torso. In this way, undue tension on the cervical ligaments is avoided. Prevention of markedly unnatural head torsion (ie, lateral flexion and extension) also lowers the incidence of whiplash injury.

RESPIRATORY EFFECTS

The single most important effect of posture on respiration is mechanical interference with chest movement. Interference with chest movement results from kidney, lateral, prone, jackknife, Trendelenburg, reverse Trendelenburg, and gallbladder positions.[162] The result is limitation of lung expansion, leading to progressive closure of the alveoli and abnormal distribution of inspired air.[50] Pulmonary compliance may also be reduced because of increased stasis of blood in the lungs.[163] The longer the time an adverse surgical posture is maintained, the greater are the deleterious effects of respiratory muscle fatigue and hypoventilation. Frank postoperative atelectasis may follow.

Obesity, which constitutes a major hazard in anesthesia, grossly exaggerates respiratory insufficiency induced by unnatural postures.[156] The lateral nephrectomy, flexed-prone (ie, jackknife), and Trendelenburg[71] positions cause the greatest decreases in ventilation in the spontaneously breathing, anesthetized patient, and the reverse Trendelenburg and gallbladder position lead to more modest impairments of ventilation.[50,156,162]

Any position that compresses the abdomen, preventing diaphragmatic descent, is inadvisable. During prone positioning with rolls, bolsters, or padded frames, the anesthesiologist should palpate the abdomen to ensure its freedom from pressure.

CIRCULATORY EFFECTS

The untoward effects of surgical posture on the circulatory system can occur suddenly and, unlike neuropathies, are obvious during rather than after anesthesia. Anesthesia causes pooling of blood in the dependent portion of the peripheral vasculature because of dilatation of blood vessels,[164] direct depression of the myocardium (to a lesser extent), and inhibition of reflex compensatory mechanisms. Gravity and external obstruction of blood vessels further exacerbate pooling and sludging of blood.

The degree to which a patient tolerates these effects depends on his or her cardiovascular reserve. When the latter is reduced by heart disease, decreased blood volume, or peripheral vascular decompensation, the patient is at a disadvantage in some surgical postures, especially if moved into these positions rapidly rather than slowly.[50,156]

Supine Position

The supine position usually has fewer deleterious effects on the circulation than does any other position. It can be hazardous, however, when a large abdominal mass, such as a tumor, gravid uterus, or the contents of a large hernia sac recently returned to the abdomen, squeezes the inferior vena cava, aorta, or both sufficiently to impede blood flow. Venous return to the heart and arterial blood pressure are reduced.[50,165–167]

Lithotomy Position

An abdominal mass may also obstruct the inferior vena cava when the patient is in the lithotomy position.[156] This problem is especially dramatic after hypotension has been induced by an epidural anesthetic (Fig. 26-33). During labor, such hypotension can be treated by placing a roll under the right hip, which tilts the uterus to the left and away from the inferior vena cava.

A rare complication of prolonged lithotomy position under general anesthesia is lower extremity compartment syndrome.[168] Postoperative epidural analgesia is said to obscure this diagnosis, but a case report suggests this observation is incorrect.[169] However, a high index of suspicion should be maintained for patients at risk. The subject of compartment syndrome has been reviewed extensively by Martin.[170]

Trendelenburg Position

By decreasing arterial flow to the legs and increasing venous return from them, the Trendelenburg position engorges the blood vessels of the thorax and mediastinum, raises cerebrospinal fluid pressure in the cranial vault, and compresses brain tissue.[71] Pressure of the viscera on the diaphragm lowers stroke volume and cardiac output and increases the work of breathing.[50,156] Some of these harmful effects can be attenuated by positive-pressure ventilation.

Flexed-Prone Position

The flexed-prone position causes pooling of blood in the dependent cephalad half of the body and in the legs. The abdominal contents are compressed dorsally, obstructing the inferior vena cava (see Fig. 26-11).[156] In obese patients, a large panniculus of abdominal fat further obstructs the inferior vena cava.[50] Hypotension and increased venous bleeding at the wound site in the lumbar area of the back occurs because blood is forced to return from the legs to the heart by way of collateral veins that course cephalad through the paravertebral area.

This complication can be mitigated by refraining from too-marked dorsal flexion of the torso (see Fig. 26-13). Quadriceps bolsters and long rolls placed vertically under the lateral part of each side of the body cause less flexion than does the

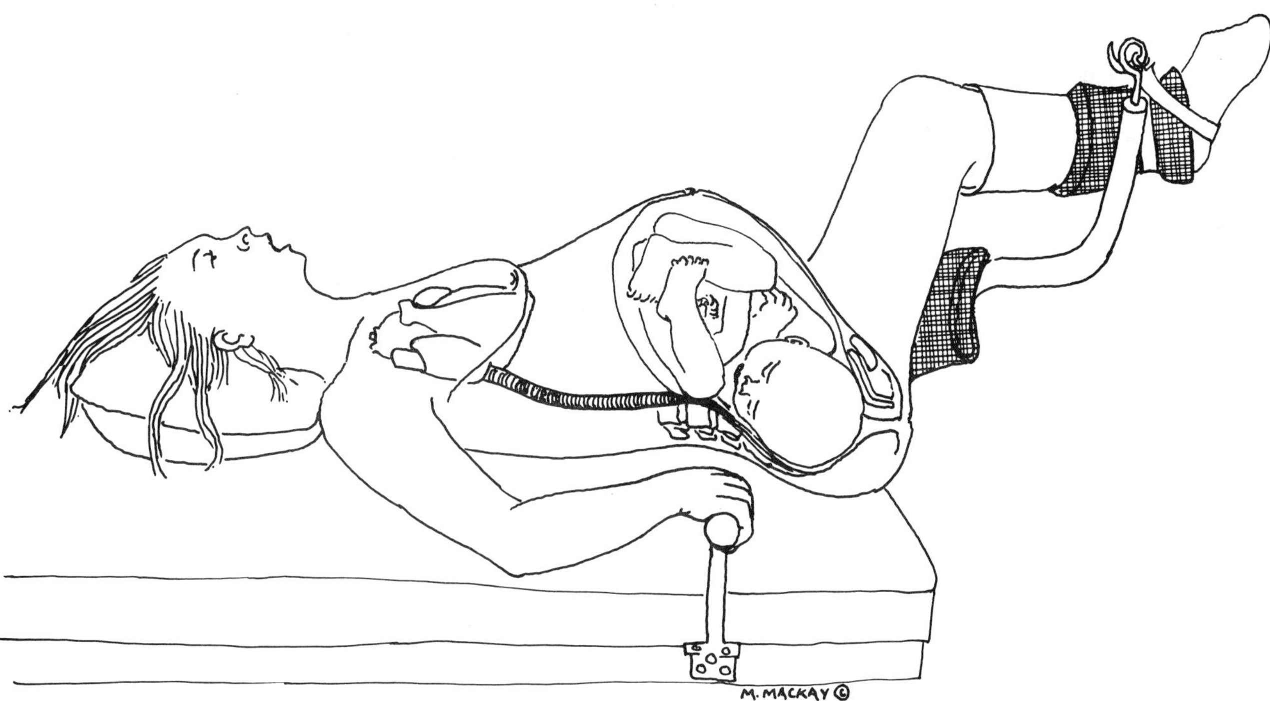

FIGURE 26-33. An abdominal mass compresses the inferior vena cava in the supine or lithotomy position. Compression is relieved by a roll inserted under the right hip.

MacKay frame. However, the bolsters can exert excessive pressure in the groin and obstruct the femoral artery.

Lateral Nephrectomy Position

Like the flexed-prone position, the right and, less often, the left lateral nephrectomy positions cause pooling of blood in the lower half of the body.[156,171] Marked compression of the inferior vena cava occurs. Exaggeration of this position with a high kidney rest can precipitate cardiovascular collapse (see Fig. 26-4*A, B*). The left lateral nephrectomy position puts pressure on the lower chest, which may shift the position of the heart sufficiently to interfere with cardiac action.[50,156]

Sitting and Reverse Trendelenburg Positions

Cerebral Perfusion and Oxygenation

The sitting and reverse Trendelenburg positions lower blood pressure and cerebral blood flow. Consequently, oxygenation of the brain tissues may be endangered if a hyperventilation technique is used or if the intracranial vasculature is already compromised by preexisting disease.[172] These positions are also associated with marked stasis of blood in the lower part of the body, possibly with thrombus formation. The latter may embolize to the lungs postoperatively.[50,156,173,174] Wrapping the legs with sequential compression stockings during the operation may help to prevent pulmonary emboli. Pads should be placed behind the buttock rather than bandaged to the leg, where they would further exacerbate venous stasis of the leg.

Bleeding

In the sitting position, sagging of the cerebellar hemispheres potentially stretches and tears superior and inferior cerebellar veins that communicate with adjacent venous sinuses. After such a tear, continuous bleeding from the superior surface of the cerebellum occurs after excision of a posterior fossa mass.

Air Embolization

In the sitting position, venous pressure in the cranium is below atmospheric pressure. A tear in a vein can allow a fatal air embolus to be sucked in through the vessel to the heart. This complication is most likely to occur during inspiration if the patient is breathing spontaneously. Sequelae are minimized through prompt diagnosis and treatment. Diagnosis is aided by the use of an esophageal stethoscope, a precordial Doppler device, continuous capnography, or transesophageal echocardiography. Treatment consists of obstruction of the open veins to prevent further air entry; movement of the patient into the recumbent left lateral position, thereby inhibiting movement of more air into the entry site and into the heart; ventilation with 100% oxygen; an attempt to aspirate air from the region of the right atrial–superior vena cava junction through a central venous catheter if one is in place; and support of the blood pressure.[172,174–178]

Unnatural Head Positions

Extreme extension or lateral flexion of the head sufficient to induce tension of the neck muscles, as in the supine position during thyroidectomy or in the lateral position with insufficient support under the head, may permit obstruction of venous return from the head, resultant elevation of the intracerebral blood pressure, and plethora and edema of the superficial blood vessels.[72] Sufficient extension of the head may occur in an aged patient with a prominent dorsal kyphosis lying on a gallbladder rest, producing compression of the vertebral artery with resultant cerebral ischemia.

Pressure Against Arteries

Extreme pressure against the carotid artery with consequent compression and stretching of the carotid artery between the fingers and the transverse processes of the cervical vertebrae during difficult ventilation with a mask, particularly when there is extreme hyperextension or lateral flexion of the head, has induced a dissecting aneurysm of the carotid artery, leading to an embolic-type stroke several hours or even days later.[179,180]

Litigation

Of interest to anesthesiologists is the possibility that an injury resulting from positioning trauma may result in litigation. In 1990, the American Society of Anesthesiologists closed claims study reviewed 227 cases of alleged anesthesia-related nerve damage.[91] Ulnar neuropathy was the most frequent, representing one third of all injuries (Table 26-3); next most frequent were injuries of the brachial plexus (23%) and the lumbosacral nerve roots (16%). The reviewers suggested that the standard of care had been met significantly more often in claims involving nerve damage than in claims not involving nerve damage. They concluded that nerve damage was a significant source of anesthesia-related claims but that the exact mechanism of injury often was unclear, particularly with respect to ulnar nerve injuries. Mechanisms commonly described usually were not apparent in the claim files analyzed.[18,181,182] This conclusion also was reached independently by Stoelting.[183]

We disagree strongly with these opinions. In many of these cases, the standard of care was said to allow the arm to be abducted to 90° and to keep the forearm and hand supinated in accordance with published data.[67,68] We have determined that the brachial plexus or the ulnar nerve can be injured in some patients, particularly if the procedure is long or preexisting abnormalities such as diabetes mellitus are present. Based on our experience, abduction of the arm to greater than 60° and supination rather than pronation of the hand are the culprits. As long as what we view as lax standards for positioning patients during anesthesia prevail, positional trauma will continue to occur.

TABLE 26-3
The American Society of Anesthesiologists Closed Claims Study of 277 Nerve Injuries

NERVE INJURIES	NUMBER OF CLAIMS
Ulnar	77
Brachial Plexus	53
Lumbosacral	36
Spinal cord	13
Sciatic	11
Median	9
Radial	6
Femoral	6
Multiple	5
Other	11

Data from Kroll, DA, Caplan RA, Posner K, et al: Nerve injury associated with anesthesia. Anesthesiology 73:202; 1990

REFERENCES

1. Dhuner KG: Nerve injuries following operations: a survey of cases occurring during a six-year period. Anesthesiology 289: 11, 1950
2. Kiloh LG: Brachial plexus lesions after cholecystectomy. Lancet 258:103, 1950
3. Lincoln JF, Sawyer HP Jr: Complications related to body positions in surgical procedures. Anesthesiology 22:800, 1961
4. Magendie J, Bergouignan M, Royyere R, et al: Troubles sensitive-moteurs du plexus brachial dus a certains positions sur la table d'operation. Bordeaux Chir October, 1949, p. 133
5. Shaw WM: Prevention of brachial plexus paralysis. Anesthesiology 14:206, 1953
6. Westin B: Prevention of upper limb nerve injuries in Trendelenburg position. Acta Chir Scand 108:61, 1954
7. Budinger K: Über Lähmungen nach Chloroformnarkosen. Arch Klin Chir 47:121, 1894
8. Garriques H: Anesthesia paralysis. Am J Med Sci 113:81, 1897
9. Slocum HC, O'Neal KC, Allen CR: Neurovascular complications from malposition on the operating table. Surg Gynecol Obstet 86:729, 1948
10. Horsley V: On injuries to peripheral nerves. Practitioner 113: 131, 1898
11. Krumm F: Editorial on narcosis paralysis. Ann Surg 25:203, 1897
12. Clausen EG: Postoperative "anesthetic" paralysis of the brachial plexus: a review of the literature and report of nine cases. Surgery 12:933, 1942
13. Ewing MR: Postoperative paralysis in the upper extremity: report of five cases. Lancet 1:99, 1950
14. Brahams D: Ulnar nerve injury after general anesthesia and intravenous infusion. Lancet 2:1306, 1984
15. Britt BA, Gordon RA: Peripheral nerve injuries associated with anaesthesia. Can Anaesth Soc J 11:514, 1964
16. Britt BA, Joy N, MacKay MB: Positioning trauma. In Orkin FK, Cooperman LH (eds): Complications in anesthesiology. Philadelphia: JB Lippincott, 1982: 646
17. Martin JT (ed): Positioning in anesthesia and surgery, 2nd ed. Philadelphia: WB Saunders, 1987
18. McAlpine FS, Seckel BR: Complications of positioning: the peripheral nervous system. In Martin JT (ed): Positioning in anesthesia and surgery, 2nd ed. Philadelphia: WB Saunders, 1987: 303
19. Wey JM, Guinn GA: Ulnar nerve injury with open-heart surgery. Ann Thorac Surg 39:358, 1985
20. Denny-Brown D, Brenner C: Lesion in peripheral nerve resulting from compression by spring clip. Arch Neurol Psychiatry 52:1, 1944
21. Denny-Brown D, Doherty M: Effects of transient stretching of peripheral nerves. Arch Neurol Psychiatry 54:116, 1945
22. Sunderland S: Blood supply of the nerves of the upper limb in man. Arch Neurol Psychiatry 53:91, 1945
23. Wright IS: The neurovascular syndrome produced by hyperabduction of the arms. Am Heart J 29:1, 1945
24. Staal A: The entrapment neuropathies. In Vinken PJ, Bruyn GW (eds): Handbook of clinical neurology: diseases of the nerves, part 1, vol 7. New York: Elsevier, 1971: 285
25. Pommerenke WT, Risteen WA: Scalenus anticus syndrome as

a complication after gynecologic operations. Am J Obstet Gynecol 47:395, 1944
26. Turney HG: Post anaesthetic paralysis. Clin J 14:185, 1899
27. Jones HD: Ulnar nerve damage following general anaesthetic: a case possibly related to diabetes mellitus. Anaesthesia 22: 471, 1967
28. Patten BM: Neuropathy induced by hemorrhage. Arch Neurol 21:381, 1969
29. Cordingley FT, Crawford GPM: Ulner nerve palsy in a haemophiliac due to intraneural haemorrhage. Br Med J 289:18, 1984
30. Hartwell SW, Kurtay M: Carpal tunnel compression caused by hematoma associated with anticoagulant therapy: report of a case. Cleve Clin Q 33:127, 1966
31. Macon WL, Futrell JW: Median-nerve neuropathy after percutaneous puncture of the brachial artery in patients receiving anticoagulants. N Engl J Med 288:1396, 1973
32. Parkes JD, Kidner PH: Peripheral nerve and root lesions developing as a result of hematoma formation during anticoagulant treatment. Postgrad Med J 46:146, 1970
33. Bartholomew LG, Scholz DA: Reversible postoperative neurological symptoms: a report of five cases secondary to water intoxication and water depletion. JAMA 162:22, 1956
34. Delorme EJ: Hypothermia. Anaesthesia 11:221, 1956
35. Stephens JW: Neurological sequelae of congenital heart surgery. Arch Neurol 7:459, 1962
36. Stephens J, Appleby S: Polyneuropathy following induced hypothermia. Trans Am Neurol Assoc 80:102, 1955
37. Swan H, Virtue RW, Blout SG, et al: Hypothermia in surgery. Ann Surg 142:382, 1955
38. Eckhoff NL: Tourniquet paralysis. Lancet 3:343, 1931
39. Bickler PE, Schapera A, Bainton C: Acute radial nerve injury from use of automated blood pressure monitor. Anesthesiology 73:186, 1990
40. Schaer HM: Peripheral nerve injury and automatic blood pressure measurement. Anesthesiology 75:381, 1991
41. Kounis NG, Macauley MB, Ghorbal MS: Iliacus hematoma syndrome. Can Med Assoc J 112:872, 1975
42. Butterfield WC, Neviaser RJ, Roberts MP: Femoral neuropathy and anticoagulants. Ann Surg 176:58, 1972
43. Johnson PS, Greifenstein FE: Brachial plexus block anesthesia. J Mich State Med Soc 53:1329, 1955
44. Wooley EJ, Vandam LD: Neurological sequelae of brachial plexus nerve block. Ann Surg 194:53, 1959
45. Cappe BE: Prevention of postspinal headache with a 22-gauge pencil-point needle and adequate hydration. Anesth Analg 39: 462, 1960
46. Enhorning G, Westin B: Aspects on the technique in giving spinal analgesia. Acta Chir Scand 108:69, 1954
47. Gilbert RGB, Brindle GF: Spinal surgery and anesthesia. Int Anesthesiol Clin 4:863, 1966
48. Atkinson RS, Rushman GB, Lee JA: A synopsis of anaesthesia, 8th ed. Bristol: John Wright & Sons, 1977: 453
49. Sixth nerve palsy after spinal analgesia (letter). Br Med J 4: 842, 1952
50. Little DM Jr: Posture and anaesthesia. Can Anaesth Soc J 7: 2, 1960
51. Sadove MS, Levin MJ, Rant-Sejdinaj I: Neurological complications of spinal anaesthesia. Can Anaesth Soc J 8:405, 1961
52. Conway C: Neurological and ophthalmic complications of anaesthesia. In Churchill-Davidson HD (ed): A practice of anaesthesia, 4th ed. London: Lloyd-Luke, 1978: 1021
53. Carden S: Hazards in the use of the closed circuit technique for trilene anaesthesia. Br Med J 1:319, 1944
54. Humphrey JH, McClelland M: Cranial nerve palsies with herpes following general anaesthesia. Br Med J 1:315, 1944
55. Foo CL, Swann M: Isolated paralysis of the serratus anterior. J Bone Joint Surg [Br]65B:552, 1983
56. Dudrick S, Masland W, Mishkin M: Brachial plexus injury following axillary artery puncture. Radiology 88:271, 1967
57. DeForest HP: Krumm on narcosis paralysis. Ann Surg 25:203, 1897
58. Halstead AE: Anesthesia paralysis. Surg Gynecol Obstet 6:201, 1908
59. Jackson L, Keats AS: Mechanism of brachial plexus palsy following anesthesia. Anesthesiology 26:190, 1965
60. Nicholson MJ, Eversole UH: Nerve injuries incident to anesthesia and operation. Anesth Analg 36:19, 1957
61. Petrick EC: Paralysis of the brachial plexus following elective surgical procedures. Anesth Analg 34:119, 1955
62. Raffian AW: Postoperative paralysis of the brachial plexus. Br Med J 3:149, 1950
63. Wood-Smith FF: Postoperative brachial plexus paralysis. Br Med J 2:1115, 1952
64. Gerdy P, quoted in Clausen EG: Postoperative "anesthetic" paralysis of the brachial plexus: a review of the literature and report of nine cases. Surgery 12:933, 1942
65. Stevens J: Brachial plexus paralysis. In Codman EA (ed): The shoulder. Boston: T Todd Company, 1934
66. Brown C, cited by Garriques H: Anesthesia paralysis. Am J Med Soc 113:81, 1897
67. Leffert RD: Postanesthetic brachial plexus palsy. In Leffert RD (ed): Brachial plexus injuries. New York: Churchill Livingston, 1985
68. Leffert RD: Brachial plexus injuries. N Engl J Med 291:1059, 1974
69. Hewer CL: Maintenance of Trendelenburg position by skin friction. Lancet 1:522 1953
70. Hewer CL: Latest pattern of non slip mattress. Anaesthesia 8: 198, 1953
71. Inglis JM, Brook BN: Trendelenburg tilt: obsolete position. Br Med J 2:343, 1956
72. Costley DO: Peripheral nerve injury. Int Anesthesiol Clin 10: 189, 1972
73. Wisconsin Anesthesia Study Commission of the Wisconsin Society of Anesthesiologists: crush syndrome. Wis Med J 57:185, 1958
74. Selander D, Edshage S, Wolff T: Paresthesiae or no paresthesiae? Nerve lesions after axillary blocks. Acta Anaesthesiol Scand 23:27, 1979
75. Seldinger SI: Catheter replacement of the needle in percutaneous arteriography. Acta Radiol 39:368, 1953
76. Carroll SE, Wilkins WW: Two cases of brachial plexus injury following percutaneous arteriograms. Can Med Assoc J 102: 861, 1970
77. Staal A, Van Voorthuisen AE, Van Dijk LM: Neurological complications following arterial catheterization by the axillary approach. Br J Radiol 39:115, 1966
78. Seyfer AE, Grammer NY, Bogumill GP, et al: Upper extremity neuropathies after cardiac surgery. J Hand Surg 10A:16, 1985
79. Ellul JM, Notermans SLH: Paralysis of the circumflex nerve following general anesthesia for laparoscopy. Anesthesiology 41:520, 1974
80. Mazzia VDB: Radial nerve palsy from intramuscular injection. NY State J Med 62:1674, 1962
81. Bickler PE, Schapera A, Bainton CR: Acute radial nerve injury from use of an automatic blood pressure monitor. Anesthesiology 1990;73:186
82. Pask EA, Robson JG: Injury to the median nerve. Anaesthesia 9:94, 1954
83. Wood DA: Injuries to nerves during anesthesia. Calif West Med 53:267, 1940
84. Cameron MGP, Stewart OJ: Ulnar nerve injury associated with anaesthesia. Can Anaesth Soc J 22:253, 1975
85. Zylicz Z, Nuyten FJJ, Notermans SLH, et al: Postoperative ulner neuropathy after kidney transplantation. Anaesthesia 39: 1117, 1984
86. Alvine FG, Schurrer ME: Postoperative ulnar-nerve palsy. Are there predisposing factors? J Bone Joint Surg 69A:255, 1987
87. Ekerot L: Postanesthetic ulnar neuropathy at the elbow. Scand J Plast Reconstr Surg 11:225, 1977
88. Rabon RJ, Zakov ZN, Meyers SM, et al: Ulnar nerve mononeuropathies after face-down positioning. Am J Ophthalmol 102: , 1986

89. Sy WP: Ulnar nerve palsy possibly related to use of automatically cycled blood pressure cuff. Anesth Analg 60:687, 1981
90. Warner MA, Warner ME, Martin JT: Ulnar neuropathy: Incidence, outcome, and risk factors in sedated or anesthetized patients. Anesthesiology 81:1332, 1994
91. Kroll DA, Caplan RA, Posner K, et al: Nerve injury connected with anesthesia. Anesthesiology 73:202, 1990
92. Dundore DE, Delisa JA: Musculocutaneous nerve palsy: an isolated complication of surgery. Arch Phys Med Rehabil 60:130, 1979
93. Burkhart FL, Caly JW: Sciatic and peroneal nerve injury: a complication of vaginal operations. Obstet Gynecol 28:99, 1966
94. Vargo MM, Robinson LR, Micholas JJ, et al: Postpartum femoral neuropathy: relic of an earlier era. Arch Phys Med Rehabil 71:591, 1990
95. Warner MA, Martin JT: Lower extremity neuropathies associated with the lithotomy position abstract). Anesthesiology 79:A1075, 1993
96. Hopper CL, Baker JB: Bilateral femoral neuropathy complicating vaginal hysterectomy. Analysis of contributing factors in 3 patients. Obstet Gynecol 32:543, 1968
97. Ruston FG, Politi VL: Femoral nerve injury from abdominal retractors. Can Anaesth Soc J 5:428, 1958
98. Sunderland S: Relative susceptibility to injury of medial and lateral popliteal divisions of sciatic nerve. Br J Surg 41:300, 1953
99. Garland H, Moorhouse D: Compressive lesions of the external popliteal (common peroneal) nerve. Br Med J 4:1373, 1952
100. Monroe MC: The arterial tourniquet. In Gravenstein N (ed): Manual of complications during anesthesia. Philadelphia: JB Lippincott, 1991: 663
101. Johnston RV, Lawson NW, Nelson WH: Lower extremity neuropathy after laparoscopic cholecystectomy. Anesthesiology 77: 835, 1992
102. Lembcke W: Rare nerve paralysis due to pressure while lying on an extension table: two cases. Chirurgie 17:264, 1947
103. Goldstein PJ: The lithotomy position. Surgical aspects: obstetrics and gynecology. In Martin JT (ed): Positioning in anesthesia and surgery, 2nd ed. Philadelphia: WB Saunders, 1987
104. Bernsen PLJA: Peripheral facial nerve paralysis after local upper dental anaesthesia. Eur Neurol 33:90, 1993
105. Fuller JE, Thomas DV: Facial nerve paralysis after general anesthesia. JAMA 162:645, 1956
106. Lim EK, Chia KS, Ng BK: Recurrent laryngeal nerve palsy following endotracheal intubation. Anesth Intensive Care 15: 342, 1987
107. Ward PH, Berci G, Calcaterra TC: Superior laryngeal nerve paralysis: an often overlooked entity. Trans Am Acad Ophthamol Otolaryngol 84:78, 1977
108. Peppard SB, Dickens JH: Laryngeal injury following short-term intubation. Ann Otol Rhinol Laryngol 92:327, 1983
109. Komorn RM, Smith CP, Erwin JR: Acute laryngeal injury with short-term endotracheal anesthesia. Laryngoscope 83:683, 1973
110. Jackson C: Contact ulcer granuloma and other laryngeal complications of endotracheal anesthesia. Anesthesiology 14:425, 1953
111. Quick CA, Merwin GE: Arytenoid dislocation. Arch Otolaryngol 104:267, 1978
112. Baraka A, Hemady K, Yamut F, et al: Postoperative paralysis of phrenic and recurrent laryngeal nerves. Anesthesiology 55: 78, 1981
113. Gibbin KP, Egginton JJ: Bilateral vocal cord paralysis following endotracheal intubation. Br J Anaesth 53:1091, 1981
114. Cavo JW Jr: True vocal cord paralysis following intubation. Laryngoscope 95:1352, 1985
115. Nuutinen J, Karja J: Bilateral vocal cord paralysis following general anesthesia. Laryngoscope 91:83, 1981
116. Brandwein M, Abramson AL, Shikowitz MJ: Bilateral vocal cord paralysis following endotracheal intubation. Arch Otolaryngol 112:877, 1986
117. Knowlson GTG, Bassett HFM: The pressures exerted on the trachea by endotracheal inflatable cuffs. Br J Anaesth 42:834, 1970
118. Stanley HT, Kawamura R, Graves C: Effects of nitrous oxide on volume and pressure of endotracheal tube cuffs. Anesthesiology 41:256, 1974
119. Eger EIII, Saidman LJ: Hazards of nitrous oxide anesthesia in bowel obstruction and pneumothorax. Anesthesiology 26:61, 1965
120. Dohi S, Okubo N, Kondo Y: Pulmonary oedema after airway obstruction due to bilateral vocal cord paralysis. Can J Anaesth 38:492, 1991
121. Minuck M: Unilateral vocal-cord paralysis following endotracheal intubation. Anesthesiology 45:448, 1976
122. Cunliffe AC, Wesley F: Hazards from plastics sterilized by ethylene oxide. Br Med J 1:575, 1967
123. Holley HS, Gildea JE: Vocal cord paralysis after tracheal intubation. JAMA 215:281, 1971
124. Gelmers HJ: Tapia's syndrome after thoracotomy. Arch Otolaryngol 109:622, 1983
125. Shin T, Nozoe I, Maeyama T, et al: Recurrent laryngeal nerve paralysis caused by endotracheal intubation. Hiroshima J Anaesth 21:39, 1975
126. Yamashita T, Harada Y, Ueda N, et al: Recurrent laryngeal nerve paralysis associated with endotracheal anesthesia. J Otorhinolaryngol Soc Jpn 11:62, 1968
127. Friedman M, Toriumi DM: Esophageal stethoscope. Another possible cause of vocal cord paralysis. Arch Otolaryngol 115: 95, 1989
128. Sofferman RA, Haisch CE, Kirchner JA, et al: The nasogastric tube syndrome. Laryngoscope 100:962, 1990
129. Hockauf H, Sailer R: Postoperative recurrent nerve palsy. Head Neck Surg 4:380, 1982
130. Bulger RF, Rejowski JE, Beatty RA: Vocal cord paralysis associated with anterior cervical fusion: considerations for prevention and treatment. J Neurosurg 62:657, 1985
131. Rueff FL, Mohr KU: Nil nocere! Rekürrensschädigung bei Kropfoperationen. Befunde-Kriterien-Indikationen auf grund der Ergebnisse bei 1596 Operierten. Munchener Medizinische Wochenschrift 112:437, 1970
132. Baranyai L, Madarasz G: Recurrent nerve paralysis following lung surgery. J Thorac Cardiovasc Surg 46:531, 1963
133. Blomstadt B, Rydmark K-E: Paralysis of the recurrent laryngeal nerve following thyroidectomy. A study of paralyses occurring postoperatively. Acta Otolaryngol 52:150, 1960
134. Salem MR, Wong AY, Barangan VC, et al: Postoperative vocal cord paralysis in pediatric patients. Br J Anaesth 43:696, 1971
135. Chaten FC, Lucking SE, Young ES, et al: intracranial pathology causing postextubation vocal cord paralysis. Pediatrics 87:39, 1991
136. Maartensson H, Terins J: Recurrent laryngeal nerve palsy in thyroid gland surgery related to operations and nerves at risk. Arch Surg 120:475, 1985
137. Horn KL, Abouav J: Right vocal-cord paralysis after open-heart operation. Ann Thorac Surg 27:344, 1979
138. Casthely PA, Labagnara J: Hoarseness and vocal cord paralysis following coronary artery bypass surgery. J Cardiothorac Vasc Anesth 6:263, 1992
139. Hahn FW, Martin JT, Lillie JC: Vocal cord paralysis with endotracheal intubation. Arch Otolaryngol 192:226, 1970
140. Renault J, Wesoluch M, Souron R: Laryngeal paralysis after intratracheal intubation. Ann Fr Anesth Reanim 4:75, 1985
141. Nicholls BJ, Packham RN: Arytenoid cartilage dislocation. Anaesth Intensive Care 14:196, 1986
142. Blanc VF, Tremblay NAG: The complications of tracheal intubation: a new classification with a review of the literature. Anesth Analg 53:202, 1974
143. Kambic V, Radsel Z: Intubation lesions of the larynx. Br J Anaesth 50:587, 1978
144. Schramm VL, May M, Lavorato AS: Gelfoam paste injection for vocal cord paralysis: temporary rehabilitation of glottic incompetence. Laryngoscope 88:1268, 1978
145. Lewy RB: Experience with vocal cord injection. Ann Otol 85: 440, 1976

146. Montgomery WW: Laryngeal paralysis Teflon injection. Ann Otolaryngol 88:647, 1978
147. Walkup HE, Murphy JD, Steen NC: Retinal ischemia with unilateral blindness, a complication occurring during pulmonary resection in the prone position. J Thorac Surg 23:174, 1952
148. Gild WM, Posner KL, Caplan RA, Cheney FW: Eye injuries associated with anesthesia. A closed claims analysis. Anesthesiology 76:204, 1992
149. Gillan JG: Two cases of unilateral blindness following anaesthesia with vascular hypotension. Can Med Assoc J 69:294, 1953
150. Givner I, Jaffe N: Occlusion of the central retinal artery following anesthesia. Arch Ophthalmol 43:197, 1950
151. Barron DW: Supraorbital neuropraxia. Anaesthesia 10:374, 1955
152. Hollenhorst RW, Svien HJ, Benoit CF: Unilateral blindness occurring during anesthesia for neurosurgical operations. Arch Ophthalmol 52:819, 1954
153. Standefer M, Bay JW, Trusso R: The sitting position in neurosurgery: a retrospective analysis of 488 cases. Neurosurgery 14:649, 1984
154. Rigler ML, Drasner K, Krejcie TC, et al: Cauda equina syndrome after continuous spinal anesthesia. Anesth Analg 72: 275, 1991
155. Peyton P: Cauda equina syndrome and continuous spinal anesthesia. Anesthesiology 78:214, 1993
156. Drasner K: Cauda equina syndrome and continuous spinal anesthesia. Anesthesiology 78:215, 1993
157. Canadian Medical Protective Association: The 66th annual report, 1967
158. Wasmuth CE: Anesthesia and the law. Springfield: Charles C. Thomas, 1961: 22
159. Bagenyi J, Barankay A: Report on a partial necrosis of the tongue caused by an endotracheal tube. Anaesthesist 24:136, 1975
160. Bennett RL, Lee TS, Wright BD: Airway-obstructing supraglottic edema following anesthesia with the head positioned in forced flexion. Anesthesiology 54:78, 1981
161. Brown EM, Elman DS: Postoperative backache. Anesth Analg 40:683, 1961
162. Wood-Smith FF, Horne GM, Nunn JF: Effect of position on ventilation of patients anaesthetized with halothane. Anaesthesia 16:340, 1961
163. Kaneko K, Milic-Emili J, Dolovich MB, et al: Regional distribution of ventilation and perfusion as a function of body position. J Appl Physiol 21:767, 1966
164. Canadian Medical Protective Association: The 73rd annual report, 1974
165. Yaster M, Buck JR, Dudgeon DL, et al: Hemodynamic effects of primary closure of omphalocele/gastroschisis in human newborns. Anesthesiology 69:84, 1988
166. Eckstein KL, Marx GF: Aortocaval compression and uterine displacement. Anesthesiology 40;92, 1974
167. Grennell HJ, Vanderwater SL: The supine hypotensive syndrome during conduction anaesthesia for the near term gravid patient: case reports. Can Anaesth Soc J 8:417, 1961
168. Lydon JC, Spielman FJ: Bilateral compartment syndrome following prolonged surgery in the lithotomy position. Anesthesiology 60:236, 1984
169. Montgomery CJ, Ready LB: Epidural opioid analgesia does not obscure diagnosis of compartment syndrome resulting from prolonged lithotomy position. Anesthesiology 75:541, 1991
170. Martin JT: Compartment syndromes: concepts and perspectives of the anesthesiologist. Anesth Analg 75:275, 1992
171. Malatinsky J, Kadlic T: Inferior vena caval occlusion in the left lateral position: a case report. Br J Anaesth 46:165, 1974
172. Tindall GT, Craddock A, Greenfield JC: Effects of the sitting position on blood flow in the internal carotid artery of man during general anesthesia. J Neurosurg 26:383, 1967
173. Ward RJ, Danziger FA, Bonica JJ, et al: Cardiovascular effects of change of posture. Aerospace Med 37:257, 1966
174. Hodgson DC: Venous stasis during surgery. Anaesthesia 19: 96, 1964
175. Hunter AR: Air embolism in the sitting position. Anaesthesia 4:467, 1962
176. Marshall BM: Air embolus in neurosurgical anaesthesia, its diagnosis and treatment. Can Anaesth Soc J 12:255, 1965
177. Michenfelder JD, Miller RH, Gronert GA: Evaluation of an ultrasonic device (Doppler) for the diagnosis of venous air embolism. Anesthesiology 36:164, 1972
178. Gildenberg PL, O'Brien RP, Britt WJ, et al: The efficacy of Doppler monitoring for detection of venous air embolism. J Neurosurg 54:75 1981
179. Leopjarvi M, Tarkka M, Leinonen A, Kallanranta T: Spontaneous dissection of the internal carotid artery. Acta Chir Scand 154:559, 1988
180. Stringer WL, Kelly DL Jr: Traumatic dissection of the extracranial internal carotid artery. Neurosurgery 6:123, 1980
181. Dornett WHL. Compression neuropathies: medical aspects and legal implications. Int Anesthesiol Clin 24:20, 1986
182. Dawson DM, Krarup C: Perioperative nerve lesions. Arch Neurol 46:1355, 1989
183. Stoelting RK: Postoperative ulnar nerve palsy—is it a preventable complication? Anesth Analg 76:7, 1993

Complications in Anesthesiology, second edition,
edited by Nikolaus Gravenstein and Robert R. Kirby.
Lippincott-Raven Publishers, Philadelphia © 1996.

CHAPTER 27

Increased Intracranial Pressure

Jerry D. Levitt

Increased intracranial pressure (ICP) is a common finding in patients with a wide variety of neoplastic, congenital, vascular, metabolic, infectious, and traumatic lesions of the central nervous system. Inappropriate anesthetic management can increase brain damage and make neurologic surgery more difficult or impossible. Appropriate anesthetic drugs and techniques can reduce ICP, maintain cerebral perfusion, and expedite the surgical procedure. This chapter considers how anesthetic drugs and techniques influence ICP and how they may ameliorate or aggravate ICP if it is abnormal.

ANATOMIC AND PATHOPHYSIOLOGIC FEATURES

The skull is an almost rigid box that in an adult contains about 1400 g of brain tissue, 110 mL of cerebrospinal fluid (CSF),[1] and 130 mL of blood.[2] As a general rule, cranial capacity is fixed; any increase in the volume of one component leads to an increase in ICP unless the volume of one of the other components decreases reciprocally.

Cerebrospinal Fluid

In normal circumstances, ICP results from the production and absorption of CSF. About 70% of CSF production occurs in the choroid plexus of the lateral ventricles; the balance is derived from the brain interstitial fluid. In an adult, CSF is produced at a rate of 0.4 mL/min; this rate is constant at ICPs less than 20 mm Hg.[3] It flows from the lateral ventricles through the foramina of Monro to the third ventricle, then through the aqueduct of Sylvius to the fourth ventricle, and finally through the foramina of Luschka and Magendie into the spinal and cerebral subarachnoid spaces.

Absorption occurs through unidirectional tubules in the arachnoid villi into the large dural venous sinuses.[4] The rate of CSF absorption varies directly with the pressure gradient between the subarachnoid space and the dural sinuses, and absorption ceases when the gradient is less than 5 mm Hg. Although this circulation clears particulate material and large molecules from the brain, CSF is not simply an ultrafiltrate of plasma; rather, it is a fluid, the chemical composition of which is narrowly regulated.[3]

Intracranial Pressure

Normal Variations

ICP is the hydrostatic pressure of the CSF within the ventricular system or in the subarachnoid space over the cerebral hemispheres. ICP values greater than 15 cmH_2O (11 mm Hg) usually are considered abnormal. The instantaneous value of ICP reflects each heart beat and the respiratory cycle. Increases of about 2 mm Hg occur with each cardiac cycle because of an increase in cerebral blood volume (CBV) with arterial pulsation. Changes in ICP during the respiratory cycle are similar to the changes in central venous pressure with respiration. During spontaneous ventilation, ICP decreases by a few millimeters of mercury with inspiration and increases at the onset of expiration. With intermittent positive-pressure ventilation, ICP increases with inspiration.

Response to Mass Lesions

The ICP response to a mass lesion depends on the nature of the lesion, its location, and its rate of expansion. The conventional representation of the intracranial volume–ICP curve is shown in Figure 27-1. The form of this curve originally was derived from experiments in which the ICP of six monkeys was recorded during the constant, slow inflation of a supratentorial extradural balloon with saline.[5] The curve has three phases. In the first, little change in ICP occurs as the balloon is inflated. In the second, increase in balloon volume causes larger increases in ICP. In the third, the baseline ICP is elevated, and small increases in volume cause very large increases in ICP.

In these experiments, the balloon was inflated at the rate of 1 mL/h, and phase 2 of the curve was reached when the volume increase was 5 mL. Injection of the 8th mL of saline

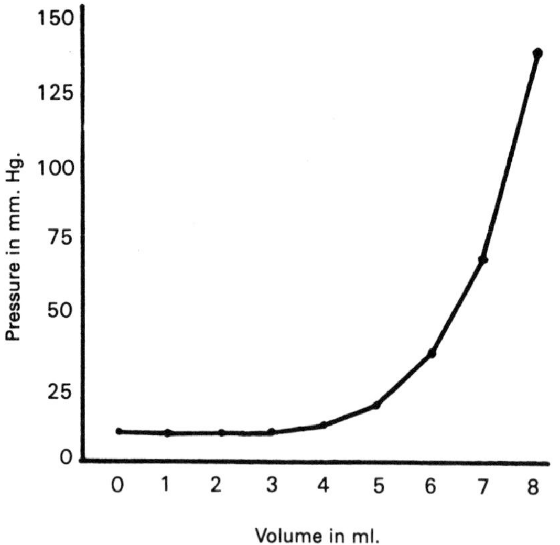

FIGURE 27-1. The intracranial volume–ICP curve. This curve was compiled from the ICP responses of six monkeys in which a supratentorial extradural balloon was inflated. (Langfitt TW: Increased intracranial pressure. Clin Neurosurg 16:436, 1969.)

produced a 70-mm Hg increase in pressure. This curve is relevant clinically because the course of patients with expanding lesions seems similar but is different in time scale. For example, in a patient with a slowly growing meningioma, phase 2 might not be reached for many years, whereas an intracranial hemorrhage could reach phase 2 in much less than 1 hour.

Compensatory Mechanism

Several mechanisms exist by which volume compensation occurs during the initial phase of a mass lesion expansion. CSF is translocated through the foramen magnum into the spinal subarachnoid space. When any increase in ICP occurs, the absorption of CSF increases. These mechanisms lead to a decrease in the size of the ventricular system, if obstruction does not prevent the flow of CSF from the third or fourth ventricle. As ICP increases further, thin-walled cerebral veins are compressed, reducing cerebral venous blood volume and providing additional spatial compensation for the expanding mass.

Phase 2 is reached when these compensatory mechanisms are exhausted. As the volume of the mass lesion increases, obstruction of CSF channels may occur. In addition, chronically increased ICP eventually leads to compression of dural sinuses and increased dural venous pressure,[6] reducing the pressure gradient across the arachnoid villi and decreasing CSF absorption.

Intracranial Elastance and Compliance

Eventually, as ICP increases, small changes in volume lead to progressively greater changes in ICP. The function that describes this property is called *elastance of the CSF space* and is defined as follows[7]:

$$E_{CSF} = \frac{dP}{dV}$$

where E_{CSF} = elastance of the CSF space; dP = immediate change in ICP with a small change in intracranial volume; and dV = change in intracranial volume. The reciprocal of elastance, *intracranial compliance* (C_{CSF}), is the change in volume that results in a unit change in ICP:

$$C_{CSF} = \frac{1}{E_{CSF}} = \frac{dV}{dP}$$

Determination of Compliance Changes

Conventionally, C_{CSF} is said to decrease as a mass lesion expands—that is, as the patient's status moves to the right on the intracranial volume–ICP curve (see Fig. 27-1). If ICP is monitored by a catheter in a lateral ventricle, C_{CSF} may be measured by injecting a small volume of saline (as much as 1 mL) or by withdrawing a similar volume of CSF and recording the change in ICP.[8] A change in ICP greater than 2 mm Hg/mL indicates decreased C_{CSF}.

Without injecting or withdrawing fluid, one can observe the change in ICP with each heart beat as an indication of C_{CSF}. The increase in intracranial blood volume that occurs with arterial pulsation is analogous to saline injection; an increase in the ICP pulse pressure indicates a decrease in C_{CSF}. Cerebral vasodilation induced by hypercapnia, hypoxia, volatile anesthetics, and other interventions discussed later also increases CBV. Similarly, the ICP responses to these alterations depend on C_{CSF}.

Mathematical models to describe the volume–pressure relations of the intracranial contents have been analyzed. Some investigators have attempted to verify their models by comparing experimental results with computer predictions.[7,9] These experiments suggest that evaluation of C_{CSF} or elastance of the CSF space alone will not predict how close a patient's status is to decompensation. However, the rate of return of ICP to baseline after a saline injection can be evaluated.[10] This decrease reflects CSF absorption and may be a better predictor of a patient's capacity for further spatial compensation.

Finally, investigators have stated that elastance of the CSF space is itself a function of ICP; therefore, its calculation does not provide any more clinically useful information than does measurement of ICP.[11] In the presence of a normal ICP, C_{CSF} testing can demonstrate how near a patient's status is to phase 2 on the volume–ICP curve (see Fig. 27-1). When ICP is increased, one can assume that C_{CSF} is decreased.

CONSEQUENCES OF INCREASED INTRACRANIAL PRESSURE

The effects of increased ICP depend on the magnitude of the pressure and on the nature of the lesion. In general, five consequences within the cranium are recognized as a result of increased ICP:

1. A decrease in *cerebral perfusion pressure* (CPP) that may cause cerebral ischemia. Ordinarily, CPP equals

mean arterial pressure (MAP) minus cerebral venous pressure. However, in the presence of increased ICP, CPP equals MAP minus ICP. Brain blood flow is maintained until CPP decreases to less than 50 mm Hg in a previously normotensive patient. Patients with chronic hypertension require a higher CPP. Uncontrolled ICP leading to cerebral ischemia is a common cause of brain death after head injury.

2. *Regional* ischemia in an area of the brain already subjected to pressure from a mass lesion.
3. A state of *vasomotor paralysis,* in which cerebral blood flow (CBF) becomes a passive function of MAP. In this state, arterial hypertension leads to increased CBV and cerebral edema, which further increase ICP.
4. Any of the brain herniation syndromes illustrated in Figure 27-2.[12]
5. Neurologic dysfunction caused by distortion of the brain in the presence of a space-occupying lesion.

The falx cerebri and the tentorium cerebri are rather rigid; an expanding lesion or localized brain edema results first in a local ICP increase. In general, a pressure gradient exists between the affected and adjacent intracranial compartments. Increases in CBV as a result of volatile anesthetic administration can magnify these pressure gradients and cause brain distortion or herniation.

Increased ICP causes systemic changes, the most important of which involve the cardiovascular and pulmonary systems.[13–15] These include hypertension, bradycardia and other dysrhythmias, and electrocardiographic changes similar to those occurring with myocardial infarction. Neurogenic pulmonary dysfunction ranges from slight ventilation–perfusion mismatch to florid neurogenic pulmonary edema.

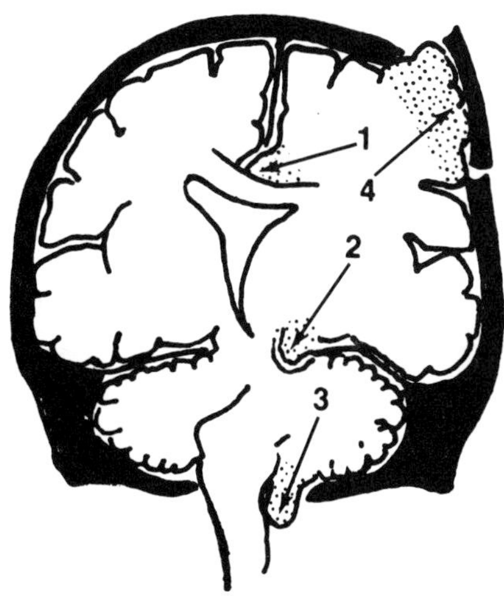

FIGURE 27-2. Brain herniations. *1,* Cingulate. The cingulate gyrus and a portion of the affected hemisphere are displaced beneath the falx, causing pressure on the anterior cerebral artery and vein. 2, Temporal, tentorial, or uncal. The medial aspect of the temporal lobe is displaced through the tentorial notch, compressing the oculomotor (third cranial) nerve and the midbrain, causing ipsilateral pupillary dilatation. *3,* Cerebellar or tonsillar. The cerebellar tonsils are displaced through the foramen magnum, compressing the cervicomedullary junction and causing respiratory and then cardiac arrest. *4,* Transcalvarial. Brain tissue herniates through an operative or traumatic opening in the cranium. (Fishman RA: Brain edema. N Engl J Med 293:706, 1975.)

CEREBRAL BLOOD FLOW AND INTRACRANIAL PRESSURE

Any anesthetic drug or technique that increases CBF is capable of increasing ICP. CBF is regulated by the cross-sectional area of the cerebral arterioles. An increase in CBF generally leads to an increase in CBV and an increase in ICP. The extent of the increase in ICP depends on the magnitude of the blood volume increase and the patient's "position" on the intracranial volume–ICP curve. CBF is regulated by several factors, including chemical (arterial carbon dioxide partial pressure [Pa_{CO_2}] and arterial oxygen partial pressure [PaO_2]), metabolic (cerebral metabolic rate of oxygen consumption [CMR_{O_2}]), autoregulatory, and neurogenic changes. Many anesthetic drugs also affect CBF.

Chemical Regulation

Hydrogen Ion

Although other mechanisms may be involved, the final common pathway of chemical regulation of CBF is believed to be the hydrogen ion concentration of the brain interstitial space. Increased hydrogen ion concentration (acidosis) causes vasodilatation, whereas decreased concentration causes vasoconstriction.[16]

Arterial Partial Pressures of Carbon Dioxide and Oxygen

In the Pa_{CO_2} range of 20 to 60 mm Hg, CBF varies directly with Pa_{CO_2} and changes by a factor of at least 3 (20 to 60 mL/100 g/min) (Fig. 27-3).[17,18] Changes in PaO_2 at levels greater than 50 mm Hg affect CBF very little; as arterial oxygen partial pressure decreases below this value, a large, progressive increase in CBF occurs.[19] Tissue lactic acid is believed to mediate this response.

Metabolic Regulation

Normally, cortical blood flow is coupled to neuronal activity on a milliliter-by-milliliter and second-to-second basis.[20] Opening the eyes, for example, increases blood flow in the visual cortex. Probably through metabolic regulation, seizures and painful stimulation increase CBF. The mediator of this response is not known, but local hypoxia and hydrogen ion concentration do not seem to be involved.

Autoregulation

Limits

Through autoregulation, CBF normally remains constant over a CPP range of 50 to 130 mm Hg (Fig. 27-4).[21] Below the lower limit of autoregulation, cerebrovascular resistance is minimal and CBF is a function of arterial pressure. As CPP

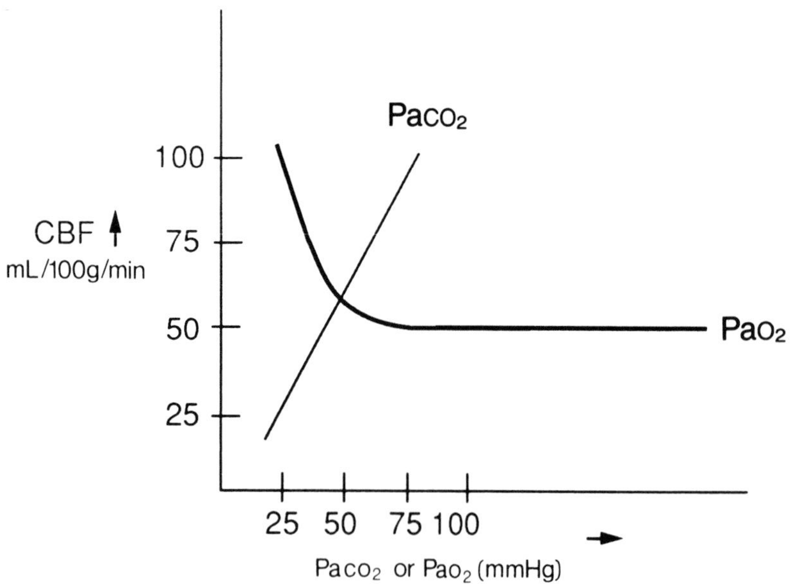

FIGURE 27-3. Effects of Pa_{CO_2} or Pa_{O_2} on CBF. (Mahla ME: Nervous system. In Gravenstein N (ed): Manual of complications during anesthesia. Philadelphia: JB Lippincott, 1991: 401.)

is increased toward the upper limit of autoregulation, the cerebral vessels constrict maximally until the "breakthrough point" is reached. CBF then increases as the arterial pressure increases. These high flows are associated with opening of tight junctions in the vascular endothelium and with vasogenic cerebral edema.[22]

Time Course

Autoregulatory changes in cerebrovascular tone require as long as 2 minutes to complete. Therefore, sudden changes in blood pressure may change CBF and ICP temporarily. Head trauma, hypoxia, hypercapnia, tumors, some drugs, and increased ICP may produce a state of "vasomotor paralysis," in which CBF varies with blood pressure in the range in which autoregulation normally occurs.

Up-regulation

In patients with chronic hypertension, the lower and upper limits of autoregulation are higher than in normal subjects. This characteristic affords some protection against hypertensive cerebral edema but renders the brain more sensitive to ischemic damage during hypotension.

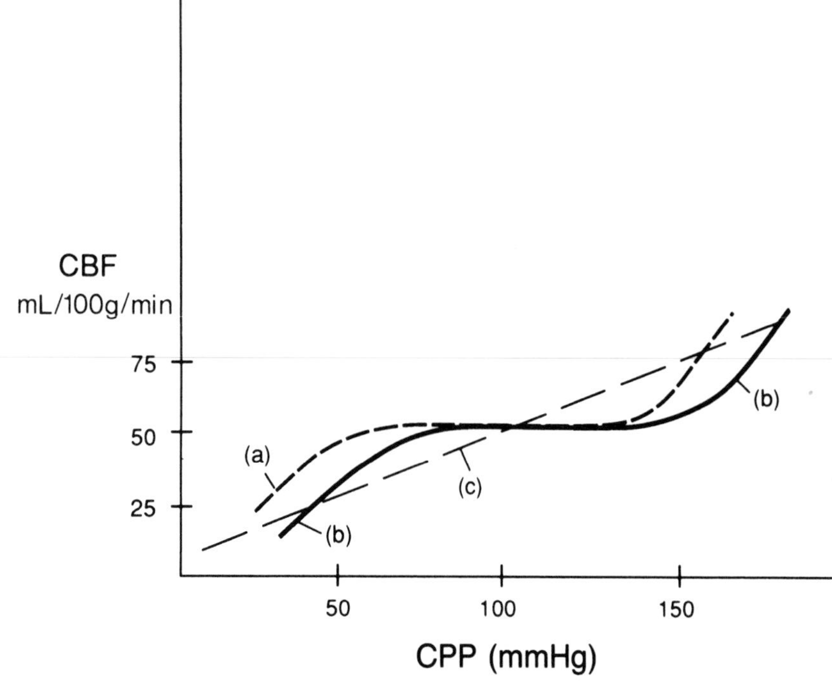

FIGURE 27-4. *a*, Autoregulation of CBF under normal conditions between MAPs of approximately 60 to 130 mmHg (CBF versus control). Changes associated with hypertension (*b*) and faulty autoregulation (*c*), in which blood flow changes primarily with CPP. (Mahla ME: Nervous system. In Gravenstein N (ed): Manual of complications during anesthesia. Philadelphia: JB Lippincott, 1991: 399.)

Neurogenic Regulation

Neurogenic mechanisms have been thought to exert little influence on resting CBF. Stimulation or interruption of the cervical sympathetic chain reduces or increases CBF by only about 10%. However, hypovolemic hypotension (shock) reduces CBF, whereas a similar level of induced hypotension does not.[23] Stimulation of the cervical sympathetic chain reduces CBF during hypercapnia.[24]

Research in baboons suggests that the increase in CBF during hypoxia is a function of carotid body chemoreceptor activity.[25] Similarly, the cerebrovascular response to hypercapnia may be mediated by a catecholamine system that originates in the locus ceruleus in the brain stem. In rats, sedative doses of diazepam block the response to hypercapnia.[26] The clinical implications of these observations are unknown.

ANESTHETIC AND ADJUNCTIVE DRUGS

Drug-induced hypercapnia increases CBF and ICP. In this discussion of drug effects, it is assumed that ventilation is controlled; the changes in ICP that occur during normocapnia and hypocapnia are considered. The discussion is limited to drugs currently in use.

Inhalation Anesthetics

Halothane

CBF and ICP increase with administration of halothane. In patients without intracranial pathologic lesions, these increases are small and of no clinical importance. In 13 normocapnic patients who had space-occupying intracranial lesions and who were anesthetized with nitrous oxide, the addition of 1% halothane caused a mean increase in ICP of 20 mm Hg.[27] The ICP of one patient in that series increased by 37 mm Hg, whereas that of most of the others was still increasing when the halothane was discontinued after 10 minutes.[27]

These and similar findings and the observation of massive brain swelling during some neurosurgical procedures in which halothane anesthesia was used have prompted anesthesiologists to question whether halothane has any place in neurosurgical anesthesia. On the other hand, for years halothane was the principal anesthetic for neurosurgical patients. One group reported that hyperventilation with nitrous oxide and oxygen to a Pa_{CO_2} of less than 30 mm Hg for 10 minutes, followed by restriction of inspired halothane concentration to 0.5%, prevents dangerous increases in ICP.[28] When halothane was administered at the same time as hyperventilation was begun, some patients had large increases in ICP, but in every case the ICP returned to its pre-halothane level within 30 minutes. If halothane is used, certain precautions should be observed for patients with intracranial pathologic lesions (Table 27-1).

Halogenated agents may be most useful in neurosurgical patients whose oxygen saturation decreases with nitrous oxide anesthesia and in patients with intracranial aneurysms, in whom control of blood pressure is usually more important than control of ICP.

TABLE 27-1
Precautions When Halogenated Agents Are Administered to Patients With Intracranial Pathologic Lesions

1. Hyperventilate the patient and limit the halothane concentration to 0.5% or isoflurane concentration to 1.0%.
2. Do not administer halogenated agents to patients with clear evidence of increased ICP (eg, papilledema, large masses, midline shift, or severe injury) unless ICP is measured or the bone flap has been removed and the brain is in view.
3. Be prepared to discontinue halogenated agents if brain swelling increases or is not controlled by hyperventilation or osmotic diuretics.

Methoxyflurane

At inspired concentrations of 0.5% and 1.5%, methoxyflurane causes dose-related increases in ICP in patients with space-occupying lesions.[27] Methoxyflurane might be useful at lower concentrations, but this possibility has not been investigated.

Enflurane

An early study in humans suggested that enflurane has no effect on CBF.[29] This work was criticized because of possible masking of an effect by anesthetic-induced systemic blood pressure reduction. In a subsequent study in which blood pressure was supported with phenylephrine, enflurane was found to cause large increases in CBF.[30] This finding suggests that enflurane can increase ICP.

I have observed alarming brain swelling when enflurane was administered to a neurosurgical patient to reduce blood pressure. Because the electroencephalographic (EEG) seizure activity that occurs during enflurane anesthesia is potentiated by hypocapnia and because enflurane increases CSF production,[31] this drug may be less useful than halothane for patients with increased ICP. Nevertheless, some have advocated its use.[32]

Isoflurane

Several properties of isoflurane suggest that it might have a lesser effect on ICP than the other halogenated anesthetics. An early study in humans demonstrated that isoflurane is a less potent cerebral vasodilator than is halothane,[30] and a later study showed intact autoregulation at 1 minimum alveolar concentration (MAC) in the cat.[33] In dogs, hypotension induced by isoflurane at an inspired concentration of 2.5% reduces CMR_{O_2} to 40% and CBF to 60% of control values. The greater reduction in CMR_{O_2} relative to CBF maintained a normal cerebral energy state, as measured by brain adenosine triphosphate, lactate, and phosphocreatine concentrations.[34] Also in dogs, isoflurane does not increase CSF formation (as does enflurane) or decrease CSF absorption (as does halothane).[35,36]

CEREBROSPINAL FLUID PRESSURE. The first study of CSF pressure measured in the lumbar area during isoflurane anesthesia in humans was misinterpreted. Purportedly, it demonstrated that if isoflurane is administered at less than

1% inspired concentration and if the patient's lungs are hyperventilated to a Pa_{CO_2} of less than 30 mm Hg, no increase in ICP occurs.[37] In fact, one of the patients in the "normocapnic" group had a Pa_{CO_2} of 27 mm Hg because of chronic hyperventilation. When isoflurane was administered, this patient's CSF pressure increased precipitously and remained elevated until further hyperventilation reduced Pa_{CO_2} to 23 mm Hg.[37] The proper interpretation of this study is not that the patient should be ventilated to a $PaCO_2$ less than 30 mm Hg when isoflurane is administered in the presence of a mass lesion, but rather that the target $PaCO_2$ should be 7 to 10 mm Hg less than the patient's resting $PaCO_2$. Another study concluded that isoflurane was suitable for neurosurgical anesthesia in patients with mass lesions both at normocapnia and at hypocapnia,[38] but further experience with isoflurane has demonstrated that it increases ICP and decreases CPP in some patients.

CEREBRAL PERFUSION PRESSURE. In a later study of 14 patients with brain tumors whose lungs were ventilated to a Pa_{CO_2} of 26 mm Hg with nitrous oxide–oxygen, 6 sustained increased ICP and decreased CPP when 1.1% isoflurane as added to the anesthetic.[39] Those 6 patients all had midline shift of brain structures evident on preoperative computed tomographic scans of the head, whereas only 1 of the other 8 patients had a shift. In a very similar study, ICP (measured through ventricular cannulas) increased when isoflurane was added to an etomidate–nitrous oxide–oxygen anesthetic.[40] In 4 of 10 patients, ICP increased to above preanesthetic levels, and in 8 of 10 patients, CPP decreased to less than 50 mm Hg. Of interest, when isoflurane was discontinued and 100 to 200 mg meperidine was administered, ICP decreased and CPP increased in every case.

CLINICAL IMPLICATIONS. Isoflurane is the most useful of the halogenated anesthetics for patients with intracranial pathologic lesions, but it must be administered with care. The same precautions suggested for the use of halothane (see Table 27-1) should be observed for isoflurane. Isoflurane, with or without nitrous oxide, has been used both as the anesthetic and as the hypotensive agent during clipping of cerebral aneurysms. Brain swelling was not a problem in these cases: neurosurgeons reported excellent operating conditions and no complications related to the anesthetic technique.[41,42]

Desflurane

In normocapnic dogs desflurane is a potent dilator of the cerebral vasculature,[43] but the response of CBF to hyperventilation is preserved in the presence of up to 1.5 MAC desflurane.[44] In patients undergoing craniotomy for intracranial mass lesions, desflurane and isoflurane at concentrations of 1.0 and 1.5 MAC were found to have similar effects on CBF at $PaCO_2$ of 25 mm Hg. With both anesthetics the response of CBF to $PaCO_2$ was preserved.[45] However, in hyperventilated adult patients with supratentorial mass lesions and mass effect seen on CT-scan, 1 MAC desflurane in 50% oxygen and 50% nitrogen, increased lumbar CSF pressure from a mean of 11 mm Hg to 18 mm Hg at the time of dural opening. Under the same conditions 1 MAC isoflurane did not increase lumbar CSF pressure.[46]

Clearly desflurane causes dose-dependent decreases in cerebrovascular resistance and $CMRO_2$ and may increase ICP in susceptible patients. As with isoflurane the cerebrovascular response to hypocapnia is usually maintained.[47] Desflurane is probably safe to use in patients with decreased intracranial compliance if the guidelines in Table 27-1 are observed.

Sevoflurane

In hypocapnic dogs, at end-tidal concentrations up to 1.5 MAC sevoflurane did not increase ICP. However, MAP was observed to decrease considerably.[48] In patients given sevoflurane 1.5% (.88 MAC) in 33% N_2O and 33% argon, the response of CBF to $PaCO_2$ was preserved as was autoregulation.[49] Sevoflurane appears to be similar in its cerebrovascular effects to isoflurane and desflurane.

Nitrous Oxide

In a study of 12 patients with intracranial pathologic lesions, induction of anesthesia with 66% nitrous oxide in oxygen increased ICP by a mean of 27 mm Hg in the absence of changes in MAP or Pa_{CO_2}. Hyperventilation to a Pa_{CO_2} of 29 mm Hg reduced ICP to control levels in all cases.[50] In two reports in which nitrous oxide was not associated with increases in CBF or ICP, short-acting barbiturates had been used to induce anesthesia.[51,52] Two studies of dogs initially anesthetized with 0.1% to 0.2% halothane in 60% to 70% nitrogen in oxygen demonstrated increases in CBF and CMR_{O_2} when nitrous oxide was substituted for the nitrogen.[53,54]

Precautions

Clearly, nitrous oxide can increase ICP. This increase can be prevented by previous barbiturate administration and treated by hyperventilation. Few anesthesiologists would use only nitrous oxide to induce anesthesia in an alert patient, but some might attempt this approach in a lethargic or drowsy patient. If increased ICP or intracranial mass lesion is a possibility, a barbiturate should be used for induction, with hyperventilation to a Pa_{CO_2} of 30 mm Hg or less.

Tension Pneumocephalus

During intracranial procedures—notably, posterior fossa explorations in the sitting position—loss of CSF and brain shrinkage may lead to an accumulation of intraventricular or subdural air, a condition called *pneumocephalus*. Nitrous oxide diffuses into a closed air cavity faster than nitrogen diffuses out, producing in some conditions *tension pneumocephalus*.[55]

This complication is most likely to occur if nitrous oxide is introduced or increased in concentration after dural closure.[56] If the concentration of nitrous oxide is stable, ICP usually does not increase. Withdrawal of nitrous oxide causes a rapid decrease in ICP.[56,57] In the immediate postoperative period, changes in Pa_{CO_2}, arterial and venous pressures, CBV, brain edema, and CSF formation may contribute to tension pneumocephalus if intracranial air is present.[57] An intraventricular catheter is useful for diagnosis and treatment.

Intravenous Agents

Barbiturates

Thiopental, 1.5 to 3.0 mg/kg, in bolus doses causes rapid intraoperative reduction of ICP in neurosurgical patients. This effect occurs both in patients with chronically increased ICP during anesthetic induction and in those with ICP increases caused by painful stimulation, such as tracheal intubation.[58]

THERAPEUTIC COMA. Pentobarbital coma has been used over periods of several days or weeks to control ICP in patients with severe head injury[59] or Reye's syndrome.[60] The dose is 3 to 5 mg/kg initially followed by hourly administration to maintain a blood barbiturate concentration of about 3 mg/dL. At institutions where continuous EEG monitoring is available, maintenance of a burst-suppression EEG pattern, rather than the barbiturate concentration in blood, is used to determine appropriate dosing. These techniques are used only in cases in which ventilation is controlled. Their efficacy in improving survival has not been substantiated.

CEREBRAL BLOOD FLOW AND CEREBRAL METABOLIC RATE OF OXYGEN CONSUMPTION. Barbiturates cause dose-related decreases in CBF and $CMRo_2$. Sedative doses are without effect, but light thiopental anesthesia results in a 35% decrease in CBF and $CMRo_2$; deep thiopental anesthesia decreases them by 50%.[61] After a dose of barbiturate sufficient to silence the EEG, additional administration causes no further reduction in CBF and $CMRo_2$.[62] Probably the primary effect of barbiturates is to reduce neuronal activity and oxygen demand; metabolic regulation then reduces CBF proportionally. Barbiturates also may constrict cerebral vessels directly, but in either case the resulting decrease in CBF reduces ICP.

MANAGEMENT OF INCREASED INTRACRANIAL PRESSURE. Barbiturates play a key role in the treatment of patients with increased ICP. First, they can be used to attenuate the ICP response to tracheal intubation and other painful manipulations in the emergency care of head-injured patients and in the induction of anesthesia in patients with increased ICP.[63] Second, they can be used to treat increases in ICP that occur intraoperatively.[58] Third, they are useful for the long-term management of increased ICP in patients in intensive care units.[64–67]

Benzodiazepines

DIAZEPAM. Diazepam, 0.5 mg/kg, administered intravenously to induce anesthesia reduces lumbar CSF pressure in patients without pathologic brain lesions.[68] This finding is consistent with a study of comatose head-injured patients in whom 15 mg diazepam decreased CBF and $CMRo_2$ by 25%.[69] However, in a study of paralyzed and ventilated rats, sedative doses of diazepam reduced CBF but not $CMRo_2$.[70] When 70% nitrous oxide was added, both CBF and $CMRo_2$ decreased by 40%.

Although diazepam can decrease ICP, two precautions should be observed in its use. First, it has an extremely long half-life in plasma, and because its metabolism also produces centrally active metabolites, if given before surgery it may result in a somnolence postoperatively. Physostigmine has been used, with unpredictable success, to reverse the somnolence.[71] However, flumazenil, a specific benzodiazepine antagonist released in 1992, is preferable for this purpose. If a benzodiazepine is antagonized, this should be done by a technique analogous to antagonism of narcotic effect with naloxone. Small titrated amounts such as 0.1 mg should be used rather than bolus administration, which risks abrupt awakening, anxiety reactions, and the associated increases in ICP. Second, patients with intracranial pathologic lesions may be very sensitive to depressant drugs, and respiratory arrest has occurred after intravenously administered diazepam.[72] This complication is particularly serious in a patient with increased ICP.

MIDAZOLAM. In a dose of 0.15 mg/kg, midazolam reduces CBF 32% in human volunteers.[73] In rats, this effect is antagonized only slightly by nitrous oxide.[74] In patients with normal ICPs who are undergoing craniotomy for brain tumors, 0.32 mg/kg midazolam for induction with 0.1 mg/kg before tracheal intubation is followed by changes in ICP and MAP similar to those occurring after thiopental administration.[75] Midazolam may be most useful for the induction of anesthesia in patient with decreased C_{CSF} and heart disease. A residual effect of midazolam may be reversed with flumazenil.

Midazolam, 0.15 mg/kg IV, given to patients with severe head injury who were sedated and paralyzed resulted in small, non-significant changes in ICP. However, patients whose ICP was less than 18 mm Hg were more likely to have an increase in ICP. CPP decreased to less than 50 mm Hg in one third of the patients.[76]

Etomidate

This agent reduces ICP[77] and has been used for induction of anesthesia and for prolonged control of ICP in head-injured patients.[78] The discovery that etomidate inhibits corticosteroid synthesis has tempered enthusiasm for infusion. Induction of anesthesia with 0.3 mg/kg etomidate does not cause clinically significant adrenocortical suppression and is hemodynamically innocuous.[79] However, except for more rapid awakening, etomidate seems to offer no advantage over midazolam.

Propofol

In patients with severe brain injury who were sedated with an opioid and ventilated to $Paco_2$ 30–35 mm Hg, 2 mg/kg propofol followed by an infusion of 150 μg/kg/min reduced ICP from 11.3 mm Hg mean to 9.5 mm Hg. CPP was reduced, but not to critical levels. The ICP of all patients was less than 15 mm Hg before propofol was infused.[80]

Propofol/fentanyl anesthesia was found to be an acceptable anesthetic for adults undergoing elective surgical removal of a supratentorial mass lesion. In one study, ICP measured through the first burr hole, brain swelling, arterial blood pressure, and immediate recovery were compared in patients receiving anesthetics consisting of propofol/fentanyl, thiopental/isoflurane/nitrous oxide, and thiopental/fentanyl/nitrous oxide with low-dose isoflurane. Immediate recovery was 5 minutes faster in the last group. Otherwise the differences among the techniques were clinically insignificant.[81] Propofol reduces $CMRO_2$ and CBF similarly to barbiturates. Propofol infusion is especially useful in neuroanesthesia in situations where it is desirable to avoid nitrous oxide, for example, when cortical evoked potentials are monitored.

Narcotics

MORPHINE. At normocapnia in humans, morphine causes no change in ICP.[82] The effects of morphine on CBF and $CMRO_2$ in humans are not known with certainty. A study in which 3 mg/kg morphine and 70% nitrous oxide were given to normocapnic volunteers showed no change from awake control subjects in either CBF or $CMRO_2$.[83] However, in this study, any effect of morphine in reducing CBF and $CMRO_2$ possibly was masked by the opposing effects of nitrous oxide (discussed above).

FENTANYL AND SUFENTANIL. Moderate-dose fentanyl, 5 to 20 μg/kg, with nitrous oxide–oxygen has been used extensively for neurosurgical anesthesia and does not increase ICP. High-dose fentanyl, $\geqslant$100 μg/kg,[84] and sufentanil, $\geqslant$20 μg/kg,[85] have been used with 100% oxygen for neuroanesthesia. However, these high-dose narcotic techniques require a naloxone infusion after the procedure if postoperative mechanical ventilation is not desired. High-dose sufentanil is associated with high-voltage, slow δ waves in humans[86] and, in the rat, with seizure activity.[87] Also in rats, cortical blood flow and oxygen consumption are reduced by high-dose sufentanil, but glucose utilization increases markedly in the amygdala and hippocampus, suggesting that the seizure activity reflects subcortical rather than cortical activity.[88]

Concern has been raised about the use of sufentanil in neuroanesthesia because in dogs ventilated at normocarbia with 30% oxygen in nitrogen, 10 to 200 μg/kg sufentanil caused a marked increase in CBF. However, this effect lasted only 20 minutes and was not accompanied by increased ICP. $CMRO_2$ was decreased.[89] In another study in which dogs were anesthetized with isoflurane/nitrous oxide, 20 μg/kg sufentanil caused a 35% to 40% decrease in both $CMRO_2$ and CBF.[90]

In unpremedicated normocapnic patients without intracranial pathologic lesions, the infusion of sufentanil (mean dose 1.7 μg/kg) or fentanyl (mean dose 16 μg/kg) increased middle cerebral arterial blood flow velocity by about 25% as measured by transcranial Doppler ultrasonography. No significant differences were noted between the results with fentanyl or sufentanil.[91] In ten patients with head trauma who were sedated with propofol, paralyzed and ventilated to a $PaCO_2$ of 35 to 35 mm Hg, the injection of sufentanil, 1 μg/kg followed by an infusion of 0.005 μg/kg/min resulted in an increase in ICP of 9 $\pm$ 7 mm Hg (+53%), which lasted 15 minutes. MAP decreased 25%, resulting in decreased CPP. Cerebral autoregulation in response to the decreased CPP may be the mechanism for the increased ICP.[92] In 9 patients with severe head trauma who were paralyzed and ventilated, 3.0 μg/kg fentanyl or 0.6 μg/kg sufentanil given over 1 minute caused statistically significant increases in ICP of 8 $\pm$ 2 mm Hg and 6 $\pm$ 1 mm Hg respectively. MAP decreased about 10 mm Hg with each opioid.[93]

Although sufentanil seems capable of increasing ICP briefly in susceptible patients given bolus doses, clinical experience and experimental evidence[94] have shown no difference in operating conditions or outcome among patients given alfentanil, fentanyl or sufentanil.

ALFENTANIL. In normocapnic patients with intracranial mass lesions anesthetized with 70% nitrous oxide the addition of 5 μg/kg fentanyl caused no change in lumbar CSF pressure (CSFP), but the addition of 50 μg/kg alfentanil increased CSFP from a mean of 9.5 mm Hg to a mean of 13.0 mm Hg.[95] In another study, alfentanil, up to 50 μg/kg, was found to be neither a cerebral vasodilator nor a vasoconstrictor and caused no clinically significant increase in intracranial pressure in neurosurgical patients maintained with low-dose isoflurane and nitrous oxide.[96] Similarly, 70 μg/kg alfentanil, given over 9 minutes to pediatric patients with hydrocephalus anesthetized with oxygen, nitrous oxide, and isoflurane, and ventilated at normocapnia did not increase intracranial pressure. However, because of a marked reduction in MAP, CPP became marginal.[97] Increases in ICP following alfentanil in adequately ventilated patients are clinically insignificant.

Droperidol

In a study of nine normocapnic patients who had been given muscle relaxants and whose lungs were ventilated with nitrous oxide, 5 mg droperidol and 100 μg fentanyl administered intravenously resulted in a mean reduction in ICP from 23 to 18 mm Hg.[98] Although MAP decreased, no significant change in CPP resulted. The mechanism for this reduction in ICP was suggested by a study in which dogs' lungs were ventilated at normocapnia with nitrous oxide.[99] Droperidol, 0.3 mg/kg, caused a persistent 40% decrease in CBF, with little change in $CMRO_2$. Fentanyl, 6 μg/kg, reduced both CBF and $CMRO_2$ by 45%, but both returned to control levels in 30 minutes. When droperidol and fentanyl were given together, the initial decreases in CBF and $CMRO_2$ were similar to those occurring after droperidol alone.

These studies suggest that droperidol is a potent, long-acting cerebral vasoconstrictor that should be useful in anesthetic management in cases of increased ICP. However, in another study of nine patients with intracranial pathologic lesions who were anesthetized with barbiturate and nitrous oxide, 7.5 to 12.5 mg droperidol increased ICP in four, although the mean ICP of the group did not change. CPP decreased in all patients after droperidol administration and decreased further when 200 to 300 μg fentanyl was injected.[100]

Two precautions should be taken in the use of droperidol for patients with intracranial pathologic lesions. First, the sedative properties of droperidol may last 18 hours and affect neurologic function postoperatively. This effect may be antagonized with physostigmine.[101] Second, because droperidol reduces CBF out of proportion to $CMRO_2$, it may critically decrease CPP.[100] When droperidol is used, drugs that decrease $CMRO_2$ (eg, barbiturates) also should be administered.

Ketamine

Increased CBF and alarming increases in ICP have followed ketamine administration in patients with intracranial disease.[102,103] The increase in CBF is not related to a global increase in $CMRO_2$. Although ketamine has been used in neuroradiologic applications, its use in neuroanesthesia cannot be recommended.

Muscle Relaxants

Succinylcholine

When succinylcholine is administered to patients with intracranial pathologic lesions to facilitate tracheal intubation, large increases in ICP can result.[104] Previously this response was believed to be caused by increases in intra-abdominal, intrathoracic, and venous pressures that occur with succinylcholine-induced fasciculations. However, a study in anesthetized dogs presented strong evidence that ICP increases because of cerebral activation that follows succinylcholine-induced afferent muscle spindle stimulation.[105] In dogs[105] and humans,[106] the ICP increase can be prevented by previous complete nondepolarizing neuromuscular blockade. Administration of a "defasciculating" dose of metocurine and probably other nondepolarizing blocking drugs before succinylcholine prevents increased ICP,[107] but this subject has not been confirmed by a controlled study.

When administered to patients with any of a variety of neurologic lesions, including head injury,[108] succinylcholine can cause dysrhythmias and cardiac arrest as a result of acute hyperkalemia.[109,110] Although the increase in serum potassium can be modified by previous administration of a nondepolarizing blocking agent,[111,112] some anesthesiologists prefer to avoid the use of succinylcholine in neurosurgical cases. In patients in whom airway management is not anticipated to be difficult, one can administer an "intubating dose" of a nondepolarizing neuromuscular blocking drug after induction of anesthesia. However, in the emergency treatment of a head-injured patient, the urgency of establishing an airway may override concerns about succinylcholine administration.

d-Tubocurarine

Intubating doses of d-tubocurarine administrated rapidly may increase ICP[113] and decrease MAP, by means of histamine release; as a result, CPP is reduced. The ICP response lasts less than 2 minutes and can be prevented by thiopental administration,[63] but the hypotension may persist.

Pancuronium

Pancuronium does not release histamine, but may cause tachycardia and hypertension, especially after an intubating dose, unless a narcotic or β-blocking agent is administered concurrently. These hemodynamic changes are undesirable in patients with decreased C_{CSF} or cerebral aneurysms.

Vecuronium and Atracurium

Vecuronium, 0.1 mg/kg, has no effect on ICP or MAP in neurosurgical patients anesthetized with fentanyl–nitrous oxide–oxygen.[114] An intubating dose of atracurium, 0.5 mg/kg, administered rapidly after induction of anesthesia with thiopental–nitrous oxide–oxygen has no effect on ICP, MAP, or CPP.[115,116] In halothane-anesthetized dogs, large doses of atracurium are followed by EEG changes consistent with cerebral arousal, presumably caused by laudanosine, a metabolite of atracurium. These changes are not accompanied by increases in CBF, $CMRO_2$, or ICP and are probably of no consequence in clinical anesthesia.

For tracheal intubation, the available neuromuscular blocking agents that should have the least effect on ICP if the patients' lungs are adequately ventilated are atracurium or vecuronium. After intubation, the prolonged duration of pancuronium may be a convenience in maintaining paralysis. Small doses of pancuronium seldom cause tachycardia or hypertension.

Doxacurium, pipecuronium, and rocuronium are not believed to increase ICP.

HYPOTENSIVE AGENTS

The combination of induced hypotension and hyperventilation appears to be safe as long as MAP does not decrease below the lower limit of autoregulation.[117]

Sodium Nitroprusside

Sodium nitroprusside (SNP) is a direct dilator of the cerebral vasculature and interferes with CBF autoregulation.[118] ICP increases and CPP decreases when this drug is administered to patients with intracranial mass lesions.[119] These patients should probably not receive SNP before the dura is open.

The increase in ICP occurs only at the start of the SNP infusion; ICP returns to baseline when MAP is reduced to 70% of its initial value.[120] In one study, ICP did not increase in hyperventilated patients,[120] but in another, all patients' lungs were hyperventilated and the increase in ICP occurred nonetheless.[119] Another report suggests that interference with autoregulation persists after SNP hypotension is terminated; thus, an abrupt increase in MAP during that period may cause large increases in CBF.[121]

This problem is aggravated by the rebound arterial hypertension that may follow discontinuation of SNP. Increased plasma renin activity and catecholamines are responsible. It can be prevented by administration of 0.5 mg propranolol, titrated to effect for patients in whom it is indicated, before hypotension is induced.[122,123] Propranolol pretreatment also reduces the dose of SNP required to induce hypotension, lessening the possibility of cyanide toxicity. SNP is most useful for inducing profound hypotension during surgery for aneurysms or arteriovenous malformations and for controlling bleeding during dissections of vascular tumors.

Nitroglycerin

Nitroglycerin is a potent cerebral vasodilator when injected into the cerebral circulation of the goat,[124] but another early study suggested that it might be useful in neuroanesthesia when infused intravenously.[125] However, nitroglycerin clearly increases lumbar CSF pressure (and presumably increases ICP also) in normal humans.[126] In anesthetized, hyperventilated patients undergoing craniotomy, nitroglycerin increases ICP markedly and reduces CPP to less than 40 mm Hg.[127] It should not be used in patients with decreased C_{CSF} unless ICP is monitored or the brain is visible.

Trimethaphan

A short-acting ganglionic-blocking drug with some direct vasodilating properties, trimethaphan causes no vasodilatation when injected directly into the cerebral vasculature of the goat.[124] In a group of neurosurgical patients rendered hypotensive with trimethaphan, mean ICP did not change, but two patients had modest ICP increases of 9.3 and 5.7 mm Hg.[120] Within the autoregulatory range, trimethaphan seems less likely than SNP to cause increases in ICP. Because trimethaphan causes prolonged pupillary dilation, which may confuse a neurologic examination, it is seldom used, in spite of its lack of effect on ICP.

Bolus doses of trimethaphan, 3 to 5 mg, control blood pressure when necessary during the induction of anesthesia, and constant infusion produces moderate decreases in blood pressure during neurosurgery. Profound hypotension induced by trimethaphan in dogs may cause more disturbance of cerebral metabolism than does similar hypotension produced by SNP, if the dose of the latter can be kept at less than 1 mg/kg.[128] However, SNP, compared with trimethaphan, may cause more disruption of the blood–brain barrier.[129]

Hydralazine

Hydralazine is used commonly to control hypertension in postoperative neurosurgical patients, although it may increase ICP.[130] During craniotomy, 10 to 30 mg intravenous hydralazine increased ICP slightly in four of eight patients with brain tumors who were anesthetized and hyperventilated.[131] Hydralazine should be used with caution when the brain is not visible or when ICP is not being measured. In July 1993, the manufacturer announced that this drug would no longer be produced in parenteral form. It is unknown how long available supplies will last or when a lyophilized version will become available. At this time a shortage does not appear imminent.

Adenosine

Adenosine triphosphate and its active metabolite, adenosine, have been used for induced hypotension in humans. In dogs, adenosine triphosphate increases ICP in animals in normal condition and in those with intracranial hypertension[132]; C_{CSF} is reduced in both groups. Profound hypotension (MAP 40 to 50 mm Hg) with adenosine triphosphate or adenosine reduces CPP to the extent that the oxygen requirement of the brain is not met and anaerobic metabolism occurs.[133] These drugs seem to offer no advantages over other hypotensive agents.

Nifedipine

Nifedipine, a calcium-channel blocking agent, administered in doses that reduce MAP by 40%, causes similar increases in ICP in the cat.[134]

Labetalol

A more promising drug is labetalol, a combined α- and β-adrenergic blocking agent. In dogs, labetalol reduces MAP without increasing ICP or reducing C_{CSF}.[135] In neurosurgical patients, labetalol is useful for control of blood pressure and as an adjunct to other drugs in induced hypotension. However, its duration of action is too long for it to be used alone for inducing profound hypotension.

Esmolol

Esmolol has been used for inducing hypotension in patients undergoing craniotomy for removal of arteriovenous malformations. It caused a marked decrease in cardiac output. There was no indication of unsatisfactory operating conditions, and a beta-adrenergic blocking agent is not expected to increase intracranial pressure.[136]

EFFECTS OF ANESTHETIC TECHNIQUES ON INTRACRANIAL PRESSURE

Maneuvers performed during anesthesia and intensive care can influence ICP and CPP by effecting changes in Pa_{O_2} and Pa_{CO_2}, cerebral venous drainage, CMR_{O_2}, and systemic blood pressure.

Oxygenation and Ventilation

Abnormal pulmonary findings range from mild hypoxemia to fulminant pulmonary edema.[137] Hypoxia and hypercapnia increase CBF, CBV, and, in susceptible patients, ICP. Both problems can result from the hypoventilation that follows respiratory obstruction or insufficient manual or mechanical ventilation. Because control of the airway may be lost temporarily when anesthesia is induced, patients with increased ICP should be encouraged to hyperventilate while oxygen is administered immediately before anesthetic induction. Ventilation should be interrupted for only the briefest periods necessary for tracheal intubation, suctioning, and positioning.

Patients with increased ICP may require a higher than expected fraction of inspiratory oxygen to prevent hypoxia because of neurogenic pulmonary edema. During induced hypotension, both the inspired oxygen fraction and minute ventilation may need to be increased because of the increase in ventilatory dead space[138] and ventilation–perfusion mismatch[139] that occur with this technique. Frequent blood gas determinations or the continuous measurement of end-tidal carbon dioxide and blood hemoglobin oxygen saturation by pulse oximetry are important in management.

Cerebral Venous Drainage

Impediment to venous drainage from the brain increases ICP by engorging cerebral veins.[140,141] Maneuvers that impede cerebral venous drainage include any extreme positioning of a patient's head and neck[141]; the increasing of intrathoracic (and venous) pressure; and placement of the patient in a head-down position. Head position is critically important because the head-up position modifies the transmission of intrathoracic venous pressure into the intracranial compartment.

Airway Pressure

Positive End-Expiratory Pressure

Positive end-expiratory pressure (PEEP) increases ICP in some patients with severe head injuries. MAP and CPP decrease and neurologic deterioration sometimes occurs.[142] Of interest, the magnitude of the increase in ICP frequently exceeds the level of PEEP applied. The application of PEEP probably increases ICP only in patients with decreased C_{CSF}.[143] Some investigators have found no increase in ICP after the application of very high levels of PEEP.[144] Nevertheless, ICP monitoring is indicated in comatose head-injured patients who are treated with PEEP.

Coughing

Coughing can increase ICP. The abrupt increase in intraabdominal and intrathoracic pressures is transmitted by the epidural veins to the spinal subarachnoid space, where it initiates a pressure wave that rises to the foramen magnum.[145] Lumbar CSF pressures in excess of 100 mm Hg have been recorded. When a patient "bucks" on an endotracheal tube, the same mechanism probably acts in concert with impeded cerebral venous drainage to increase ICP.

Clinical Implications

Patients with increased ICP should be maintained in a head-up position, more so if PEEP is necessary. The head and neck should be kept in a neutral position, and the ventilatory pattern adjusted to minimize mean airway pressure while still preventing atelectasis. Coughing, straining, and bucking should be prevented by the administration of adequate doses of nondepolarizing muscle relaxants.

Cerebral Metabolic Rate of Oxygen Consumption

Regional CBF is coupled to regional $CMRO_2$ through metabolic regulation of CBF. Therefore, factors that increase brain activity increase CBV and ICP in susceptible patients. Anxiety has been shown to increase CBF,[146] and pain is known to increase ICP.[147] Adequate anesthesia, usually in the form of barbiturates and narcotics, should precede potentially painful stimulation, such as laryngoscopy, tracheal intubation, surgical incision, endotracheal suctioning, or application of a head clamp. Of interest is the observation that ICP can increase after painful stimulation even when MAP does not increase.[147]

Blood Pressure

Hypertension

MAP, when above the upper limit of autoregulation, increases CBV and ICP and promotes cerebral edema. In a normal brain, these changes occur at a MAP greater than 130 mm Hg, but a diseased brain is more vulnerable.[148] Cerebral ischemia, and in some patients, head injury, cause diffuse hyperemia that may represent impaired autoregulation. Any increase in MAP may increase ICP and cerebral edema.

Luxury Perfusion

Intracranial mass lesions and infarcts may be surrounded by an area of hyperemia that has been called "luxury perfusion" and that represents regional vasomotor paralysis (see Fig. 27-4).[5] Hypertension can increase the blood volume in these areas, promote edema formation, and cause a local increase in ICP. Of course, hypertension also can increase ICP by causing bleeding from an intracranial aneurysm or arteriovenous malformation.

Clinical Implications

The blood pressure of patients with intracranial pathologic lesions should be controlled. During surgery, control may be achieved by adequate anesthesia with barbiturates, narcotics, or inhalational agents. If these are not sufficient, a hypotensive drug, as described earlier, may be used, with care taken not to reduce CPP to less than 50 mm Hg. After a period of profound hypotension, autoregulation may be impaired for 1.5 hours.[121,149] Thus, blood pressure control should be continued postoperatively for patients treated intraoperatively with deliberate hypotension.

Regional Anesthesia

Regional anesthesia should be used for patients with increased ICP only if the perceived benefits outweigh the problems associated with control of ventilation and CMR_{O_2} during general anesthesia. Few studies are available on which to base practice. In general, dural puncture is contraindicated in patients with increased ICP because of the possibility of brain stem herniation after the loss of spinal CSF. A study of epidural anesthesia demonstrated dramatic transient increases in ICP in two patients 2 and 4 weeks after head injury.[150] Epidural anesthesia should not be used in patients with increased ICP unless the advantages are clear, as in severe preeclampsia. Extradural injection should be performed very slowly to minimize the increase in ICP.[150]

PREOPERATIVE CONSIDERATIONS

Patients at Risk

Patients with head trauma, large space-occupying lesions, rapidly enlarging lesions, recent hemorrhage, or hydrocephalus are likely to have increased ICP. The computed tomographic scan of the head is valuable to identify these conditions. Signs of acutely increased ICP may be limited to altered consciousness and a herniation syndrome. In chronic conditions, papilledema and radiographic changes consisting of a "beaten silver" appearance of the cranial vault and erosion of the posterior clinoids of the sella turcica may be seen. When ICP has increased sufficiently to cause medullary ischemia, the Cushing triad (systemic hypertension, bradycardia, and respiratory irregularities) may appear.[151]

Measurement of Intracranial Pressure

ICP is measured most commonly through an intraventricular catheter, a subdural catheter, or a subarachnoid bolt connected by a fluid path to an electronic pressure transducer external to the patient.[152,153] By convention, ICP is referenced to the level of the external auditory meatus. The intraventricular catheter is introduced into a lateral ventricle through a burr hole and passes through the substance of the brain, whereas the subdural catheter lies between the dura and the arachnoid on the surface of the brain. The bolt is simply screwed into a drill hole in the skull after a small incision is made in the dura.

Comparative Features

CSF can be drained from the intraventricular catheter but not from the bolt or the subdural catheter. The intraventricular catheter is therefore a therapeutic as well as a diagnostic tool. Also, saline can be injected into the catheter systems to calculate C_{CSF}. Less commonly, ICP is measured by a non–fluid-coupled system with an implanted pressure transducer in the epidural or subdural space. Because of ICP gradients and problems of placement, values reported by the various systems may differ, especially when ICP is increased greatly.[154] Recording the ICP on slowly moving paper simplifies recognition of pressure waves but is not necessary for adequate monitoring.

Measurement of pressure in the spinal subarachnoid space does not provide information about ICP if obstruction to CSF flow is present. Furthermore, in the presence of a mass lesion, loss of CSF from a lumbar puncture may lead to brain stem herniation. Clinically, the lumbar space is not used for continuous measurement of CSF pressure, but it has been used to do so experimentally.

Indications

At present, no consensus exists concerning the indications for ICP monitoring. In an alert patient, changes in the level of consciousness, headache, the computed tomographic scan, magnetic resonance imaging (MRI), and signs elicited by neurologic examination should provide adequate warning of increasing ICP. ICP monitoring provides important management information for patients with impaired consciousness, especially those being treated for hydrocephalus or for cerebral edema resulting from trauma, mass lesion, or infarct. Should these patients come to surgery, intraoperative monitoring eliminates any speculation about the effects on ICP and CPP of drugs, manipulations, ventilation, MAP changes, and position.

Characteristics

Lundberg, in 1960, was the first to perform long-term monitoring of ICP in patients with intracranial pathologic lesions.[155] He described A, B, and C waves; the clinical significance of the B and C waves is uncertain. Lundberg's A waves, which are now called *plateau waves*, consist of abrupt increases in ICP to greater than 50 mm Hg lasting 5 to 20 minutes. Plateau waves, which occur only when C_{CSF} is severely decreased, have been studied in animal models.[156] The waves seem to be initiated by a decrease in CPP. Some degree of cerebral ischemia then leads to an increase in systemic arterial blood pressure, which increases CPP and terminates the wave. In some cases, ICP increases to the level of systemic blood pressure, and blood flow to the brain ceases. This event is called a *terminal wave* and is followed rapidly by brain death.

Infection

Infection is a serious complication of ICP monitoring. In one clinical study the infection rate was 7.5% for the subarachnoid bolt, 14.9% for the subdural catheter, and 21.9% for the intraventricular catheter.[157]

INTRAOPERATIVE DIAGNOSIS

Because many of the cardiopulmonary signs of intracranial hypertension are nonspecific, this complication is unlikely to be diagnosed intraoperatively in a patient in whom it was not considered before operation. Hypertension and bradycardia may not appear because of the administration of anesthetic and adjunctive drugs.

Cardiorespiratory Changes

Respiratory irregularities will not be seen if the patient's lungs are ventilated mechanically or manually. A large alveolar–arterial oxygen partial pressure gradient may be an expression of neurogenic pulmonary edema resulting from intracranial hypertension.[137,158] Because of other, more likely causes of a large alveolar–arterial oxygen partial pressure gradient during anesthesia, this change cannot be considered an important sign.

Pupillary Changes

Similarly, the ocular signs of transtentorial herniation may be obscured by anesthesia. Trimethaphan administration or very deep halothane anesthesia can dilate the pupils widely and render them unresponsive. However, unilateral pupillary dilatation during anesthesia, particularly in a patient with a supratentorial mass lesion, is evidence of transtentorial herniation in the absence of other obvious cause.

Electrocardiographic Changes

The electrocardiograms of nonanesthetized patients can show prominent U waves, ST-segment elevation and depression, notched T waves, and shortening or prolongation of the QT interval in association with increased ICP.[159]

Physical Appearance

During a neurosurgical procedure, ICP becomes zero when the dura is open (although regional increases not detected by conventional monitoring may still be present). If the dura is tense before being opened, ICP is probably increased. If the brain itself is tense or herniates through the dural opening, it is obviously swollen. The causes of a swollen brain in an open skull are the same as the causes of increased ICP in a closed skull: mass lesion, hydrocephalus, edema, or increased blood volume.

TREATMENT

Intracranial hypertension occurs in many different circumstances. The treatment indicated depends on the urgency of the situation. For example, an oral corticosteroid can be used to treat increased ICP in a patient with a brain tumor and papilledema but without other neurologic signs. On the other hand, controlled hyperventilation and intravenous mannitol might be lifesaving for a patient whose pupils are dilated after a head injury. In addition to the specific therapies discussed, general measures should be observed (Table 27-2).

Hyperventilation

Hyperventilation reduces Pa_{CO_2}, CBF, and CBV by chemical regulation. In an adult, a 10-mm Hg decrease in Pa_{CO_2} can reduce CBV by about 5.6 mL.[18] In a patient with decreased C_{CSF}, this small decrease in CBV can cause a large decrease in ICP. During hyperventilation, the arterioles in relatively normal areas of the brain constrict and "make room" for a mass lesion. Hyperventilation may be less effective in diffuse lesions. In healthy humans, the effect of sustained hyperventilation on CBF diminishes dramatically after 4 hours, probably because of compensatory changes in CSF and blood acid–base status.[160] The time course of these changes in head-injured patients is not known. The effect of hyperventilation is very rapid, and this treatment alone may reverse a herniation syndrome. Reduction of Pa_{CO_2} to less than 20 mm Hg may worsen cerebral hypoxia and is not recommended.[161]

Osmotic Agents

Many agents when administered in hypertonic solution increase plasma osmolality and, in the presence of an intact blood–brain barrier, cause the movement of water from the brain to the plasma, thereby decreasing brain bulk. Intravenous mannitol is in common use. In the past, urea was administered but now is seldom used because of a "rebound" increase in ICP about 12 hours after administration. When the blood urea concentration is high, some urea diffuses across the blood–brain barrier and enters the intracellular space. When the blood urea concentration decreases as a result of renal excretion, blood osmolality becomes lower than that of the brain, and water diffuses into the brain.

Mannitol

This most commonly used osmotic agent is administered intravenously as a 20% or 25% solution. The usual acute dose is 1 to 1.5 g/kg, although as little as 0.25 g/kg is effective in head-injured patients.[162] The dose usually is given over a 10-minute period. More rapid administration can cause hypotension by increasing blood flow to skeletal muscle.[163]

MANAGEMENT. The cerebral dehydrating effect depends on the osmotic gradient between the brain and plasma and not on the volume of the diuresis. The effect is maximal in 45 minutes and lasts for 4 or 5 hours. If ICP must be controlled for a prolonged period, mannitol can be administered in repeated doses or as a continuous infusion,[164] but fluid and electrolyte losses should be replaced and the plasma osmolality used as a guide.

POTENTIAL PROBLEMS. At a plasma osmolality of greater than 310 mOsm/kg, the blood–brain barrier threshold for mannitol is exceeded, and mannitol gradually accumulates in the brain.[165] At a plasma osmolality of greater than 350 mOsm, renal failure and progressive systemic acidosis occur.[164] If ICP cannot be controlled with mannitol at a plasma osmolality of less than 310 mOsm/kg, another technique (barbiturate coma, for example) should be added to the treatment.

Mannitol is a carbohydrate that is not metabolized. It has no inherent toxicity, but the increase in intravascular volume that occurs after acute administration and preceding the diuresis may precipitate congestive heart failure in susceptible patients. Fluid and electrolyte abnormalities may follow profound diuresis.

TABLE 27-2
General Measures to Treat Increased Intracranial Pressure and Intraoperative Brain Swelling

- Ensure adequate ventilation and oxygenation to prevent hypoxia and hypercapnia.
- Ensure unimpeded cerebral venous drainage by elevating the head, placing the neck in a neutral position, correcting obstructions in the breathing circuit, and providing adequate muscular relaxation.
- Ensure that adequate sedation or narcosis precedes potentially painful stimulation.
- Discontinue halogenated anesthetic agents and substitute barbiturates or narcotics.
- Control systemic arterial pressure to provide an adequate CPP and to minimize formation of cerebral edema.
- Consider discontinuing nitrous oxide and substituting additional narcotic or propofol.
- Consider CSF drainage.

Glycerol

Glycerol, 1.5 g/kg, is administered orally or by nasogastric tube.[166] Attempts to use glycerol intravenously have resulted in hemolysis and hemoglobinuria.[167] Glycerol is metabolized and therefore may be the osmotic agent of choice for patients with renal failure and increased ICP.[168]

Loop Diuretic Agents

Furosemide, 1 mg/kg, is as effective as mannitol, 1 g/kg, in reducing brain volume during elective craniotomy for patients with no signs of increased ICP.[169] The decreases in serum sodium and potassium concentrations are small, and presumably there is no increase in intravascular volume. Therefore furosemide may be safer than mannitol for patients who are susceptible to congestive heart failure.[169]

Furosemide also has been shown to decrease ICP after head trauma in patients treated previously with a corticosteroid and mannitol.[170] The mechanism of action of furosemide on ICP is not known with certainty, but probably it is not limited to the diuretic effect.[171] Furosemide is known to reduce CSF production in animals[171,172] and may also prevent swelling of glial cells through inhibition of ion transport.[170] It has not been tested for the ability to treat herniation syndromes or to decrease severe intracranial hypertension in the absence of other agents. In a dose of 0.3 mg/kg, furosemide is used principally as an adjunct to mannitol. Although the combination provides greater brain shrinkage than does mannitol alone, it may result in marked water and electrolyte diuresis.[173]

Barbiturates

Elective Surgery

Barbiturates reduce ICP more rapidly than do any other drugs. Thiopental, for example, is effective within 1 minute after intravenous administration. For elective craniotomy, the induction of anesthesia with 5 mg/kg thiopental, followed by 0.1 mg/kg pancuronium, nitrous oxide, a second dose of thiopental (2.5 mg/kg), and topical anesthesia to the larynx prevents increased ICP after tracheal intubation.[174] However, in patients given 3 mg/kg thiopental, succinylcholine, and nitrous oxide, 1.5 mg/kg lidocaine given intravenously is more effective in preventing increased ICP than is 160 mg lidocaine given intratracheally.[175] In this setting, the most effective combination may be a second dose of barbiturate and intravenous lidocaine, but use of this combination has not been reported.

Emergency Surgery

For emergency situations such as head injury, in the absence of hypovolemia or other contraindications, administration of a barbiturate should precede tracheal intubation. Additional barbiturate may be given during subsequent diagnostic and surgical procedures and in the intensive care unit, if hyperventilation, administration of a steroid or mannitol, and surgical decompression do not control ICP.[64] However, barbiturates may be no more effective than "conventional" therapy in controlling ICP, and the use of barbiturates does not seem to improve outcome. Mortality and morbidity in cases of head injury[65,176] or Reye's syndrome[66,67] are not changed by barbiturate administration. Similarly, thiopental (as much as 30 mg/kg) did not improve outcome in a randomized study of comatose survivors of cardiac arrest.[177]

Corticosteroids

Steroids reduce the amount of edema surrounding intracranial lesions preoperatively and diminish the edema that occurs in manipulated neural tissue postoperatively.[178]

Dexamethasone

Dexamethasone is most commonly chosen for treating intracranial hypertension, in part because it lacks mineralocorticoid activity. It is administered intravenously in a dosage of as much as 10 mg every 6 hours. The well-known potential side effects of steroid therapy include gastrointestinal hemorrhage, susceptibility to infection, hyperglycemia, adrenal suppression, and psychosis.[179] Several hours are required for steroids to reduce ICP, and the full effect may not occur before 24 hours. Therefore, they are not useful in the emergency treatment of intracranial hypertension.

Although some studies have shown a beneficial effect of high-dose dexamethasone in head-injured patients,[180,181] controlled studies have failed to demonstrate that steroids lower ICP or improve outcome.[182–184] Available information suggests that glucocorticoids are no longer indicated for severe head trauma and actually may worsen outcome when used in the presence of increased ICP.[184]

Cerebrospinal Fluid Drainage

Lumbar CSF drainage is used occasionally to improve access to aneurysms of the circle of Willis. Because of the danger of herniation of the cerebellar tonsils, lumbar drainage seldom is performed when ICP is increased. Intracranial hypertension resulting from obstructive hydrocephalus can be treated by draining CSF through a burr hole with a catheter placed in a lateral ventricle. Increased ICP from cerebral edema can be treated similarly, but withdrawal of CSF may lead to collapse of the ventricular system.

Hypothermia

Hypothermia reduces ICP, probably by reducing CBF and CMR_{O_2}. When hypothermia is used to decrease ICP in the absence of barbiturates, the maximum effect is achieved at temperatures below 27°C.[185] At these temperatures, hypotension and ventricular fibrillation are common, and management is complicated by changes in the viscosity, coagulability, and acid–base status of the blood.

Shapiro and colleagues[186] found that hypothermia to 30°C further reduced the ICP of patients treated with pentobarbital coma for intracranial hypertension. These investigators allow the temperatures of similar patients to drift between 33°C and 35°C.[59] However, no clinical data demonstrate that the outcome of patients treated with barbiturates and mild hypothermia is better than that of patients treated with barbiturates alone.

Prolonged hypothermia (1 to 3 days) introduces additional problems that include progressive reduction in cardiac output and oxygen consumption with severe metabolic acidosis upon rewarming. In animal models, hemodynamic collapse and death ensue.[187,188]

Fluid Management

The argument has been advanced that when autoregulation is impaired and blood–brain barrier disruption has occurred, isotonic fluid administration increases brain edema and ICP. Colloid therapy (albumin, plasma protein fractions, or hydroxyethyl starch) is thought by some investigators to establish osmotic gradients favorable to the shift of water from the brain to the intravascular space. However, studies have not confirmed this hypothesis,[189,190] and some colloids (such as hydroxyethyl starch) may be associated with increased bleeding.[191] In the absence of shock, maintenance of euvolemia or slight dehydration, through the use of isotonic fluids, appears to be appropriate.[191,192]

REFERENCES

1. Tourtellotte WW, Shorr RJ: Cerebrospinal fluid. In: Youmans JR (ed): Neurological Surgery. 2nd ed. Philadelphia: WB Saunders, 1982:426.
2. Hedlund S, Nylin G: Cerebral flood flow and circulation time, studied with labelled erythrocytes. Arch Int Pharmacodyn Ther 139:503, 1962
3. Plum F, Siesjö BK: Recent advances in CSF physiology. Anesthesiology 42:708, 1975
4. Cutler RWP, Page L, Galicich J, et al: Formation and absorption of cerebrospinal fluid in man. Brain 91:707, 1968
5. Langfitt TW: Increased intracranial pressure. Clin Neurosurg 16:436, 1969
6. Shulman K, Yarnell P, Ransohoff J: Dural sinus pressure in normal and hydrocephalic dog. Archives of Neurosurgery 10: 575, 1964
7. Sullivan HG, Miller JD, Becker DP, et al: The physiological basis of intracranial pressure change with progressive epidural brain compression. J Neurosurg 47:532, 1977
8. Miller JD, Garibi J, Pickard JQ: Induced changes of cerebrospinal fluid volume. Arch Neurol 28:265, 1973
9. Marmarou A, Shulman K, Rosende RM: A non linear analysis of the cerebrospinal fluid system and intracranial pressure dynamics. J Neurosurg 48:332, 1978
10. Marmarou A, Shulman K, Lamorgese J: Compartmental analysis of compliance and outflow resistance of the cerebrospinal fluid system. J Neurosurg 43:523, 1975
11. Sklar FH, Elashvili I: The pressure-volume function of brain elasticity: physiological considerations and clinical applications. J Neurosurg 47:670, 1977
12. Fishman RA: Brain edema. N Engl J Med 293:706, 1975
13. Matjasko MJ: Peripheral sequelae of acute head injury. In Cottrell JE, Turndorf H (eds): Anesthesia and neurosurgery. St Louis: CV Mosby, 1980: 211
14. Miner ME, Allen SJ: Cardiovascular effects of severe head injury. In Frost EAM (ed): Clinical anesthesia in neurosurgery. Woburn, MA: Butterworths, 1984: 367
15. Messick JM Jr, Newberg LA, Nugent M, et al: Principles of neuroanesthesia for the nonneurosurgical patient with CNS pathophysiology, Anesth Analg 64:143, 1985
16. Wahl M, Deetjen P, Thurau K, et al: Micropuncture evaluation of the importance of perivascular *p*H for the arteriolar diameter on the brain surface. Pflugers Arch 316:152, 1970
17. Reivich M: Arterial PCO_2 and cerebral hemodynamics. Am J Physiol 206:25, 1964
18. Grubb RL, Raichle ME, Eichling JO, et al: The effects of changes in $PACO_2$ on cerebral blood volume, blood flow, and vascular mean transit time. Stroke 5:630, 1974
19. Kogure K, Scheinberg P, Reinmuth OM, et al: Mechanisms of cerebral vasodilatation in hypoxia. J Appl Physiol 29:223, 1970
20. Ingvar DH, Lassen NA (eds): Brain work: the coupling of function, metabolism, and blood flow in the brain. Copenhagen: Munksgaard, 1975
21. Lassen NA, Christensen MS: Physiology of cerebral blood flow. Br J Anaesth 48:719, 1976
22. Johansson B, Strandgaard S, and Lassen NA: On the pathogenesis of hypertensive encephalopathy: the hypertensive 'break through' of autoregulation of cerebral blood flow with forced vasodilation, flow increase, and blood-brain barrier damage. Circ Res 34(suppl I):I-167, 1974
23. Fitch W, Ferguson GG, Sengupta D, et al: Autoregulation of cerebral blood flow during controlled hypotension. Stroke 4: 324, 1973
24. James IM, Millar RA, Purves MJ: Observations on the extrinsic neural control of cerebral blood flow in the baboon. Circ Res 25:77, 1969
25. Ponte J, Purves MJ: The role of the carotid body chemoreceptor and carotid sinus baroreceptors in the control of cerebral blood vessels. J Physiol (Lond) 237:315, 1974
26. Berntman L, Dahlgren N, Siesjö BK: Cerebral blood flow and oxygen consumption in the rat brain during extreme hypercarbia. Anesthesiology 50:299, 1979
27. Jennett WB, Barker J, Fitch W, et al: Effect of anaesthesia on intracranial pressure in patients with space-occupying lesions. Lancet 1:61, 1969
28. Adams RW, Gronert GA, Sundt TM, et al: Halothane, hypocapnia, and cerebrospinal fluid pressure in neurosurgery. Anesthesiology 37:510, 1972
29. Wollman H, Smith AL, Hoffman JC: Cerebral blood flow and oxygen consumption in man during electroencephalographic seizure patterns induced by anesthesia with ethrane. Federation Proceedings 28:356, 1969
30. Murphy FL, Kennell EM, Johnstone RE, et al: The effects of enflurane, isoflurane, and halothane on cerebral blood flow and metabolism in man (abstract). Anesthesiology 41(suppl): A61, 1974
31. Artru AA, Nugent M, Michenfelder JD: Enflurane causes a prolonged and reversible increase in the rate of csf production in the dog. Anesthesiology 57:255, 1982
32. Moss E, Dearden NM, McDowall DG: Effects of 2% enflurane on intracranial pressure and cerebral perfusion pressure. Br J Anaesth 55:1083, 1983
33. Todd MM, Drummond JC: A comparison of the cerebrovascular and metabolic effects of halothane and isoflurane in the cat. Anesthesiology 60:276, 1984
34. Newberg LA, Milde JH, Michenfelder JD: Systemic and cerebral effects of isoflurane-induced hypotension in dogs. Anesthesiology 60:276, 1984
35. Artru AA: Isoflurane does not increase the rate of csf production in the dog. Anesthesiology 60:193, 1984
36. Artru AA: Effects of enflurane and isoflurane on resistance to reabsorption of cerebrospinal fluid in dogs. Anesthesiology 61: 529, 1984
37. Adams RW, Cucchiara RF, Gronert GA, et al: Isoflurane and cerebrospinal fluid pressure in neurosurgical patients. Anesthesiology 54:97, 1981
38. Campkin TV: Isoflurane and cranial extradural pressure: a study in neurosurgical patients. Br J Anaesth 56:1083, 1984
39. Grosslight K, Foster R, Colohan AR, et al: Isoflurane for neuroanesthesia: risk factors for increases in intracranial pressure. Anesthesiology 63:533, 1985
40. Belopavlovic M, Buchthal A: Effect of isoflurane on intracranial pressure in patients with intracranial mass lesions. In Miller JD, Teasdale GM, Rowan JO, et al (eds): Intracranial pressure VI: Proceedings of the Sixth International Symposium on In-

tracranial Pressure, Glasgow, Scotland, June 9 to 13, 1985. Berlin: Springer-Verlag, 1986: 725
41. Lam AM, Gelb AW: Cardiovascular effects of isoflurane-induced hypertension for cerebral aneurysm surgery. Anesth Analg 62: 742, 1983
42. Newman B, Gelb AW, Lam AM: The effect of isoflurane-induced hypotension on cerebral blood flow and cerebral metabolic rate for oxygen in humans. Anesthesiology 64:307, 1986
43. Lutz LH, Milde JH, Milde LN: The cerebral functional, metabolic, and hemodynamic effects of desflurane in dogs. Anesthesiology 73:125, 1990
44. Lutz LJ, Milde JH, Milde LN: The response of the canine cerebral circulation to hyperventilation during anesthesia with desflurane. Anesthesiology 74:504, 1991
45. Ornstein E, Young WL, Fleischer LH, Ostapkovich N: Desflurane and isoflurane have similar effects on cerebral blood flow in patients with intracranial mass lesions. Anesthesiology 79:498, 1993
46. Muzzi DA, Losasso TJ, Dietz NM, Faust RJ, Cucchiara RF, Milde LN: The effect of desflurane and isoflurane on cerebrospinal fluid pressure in humans with supratentorial mass lesions. Anesthesiology 76:720, 1992
47. Young WL: Effects of desflurane on the central nervous system. Anesth Analg 75 (4 Suppl):S32, 1992
48. Takahashi H, Murata K, Ikeda K: Sevoflurane does not increase intracranial pressure in hyperventilated dogs. Br J Anaesth 71: 551, 1993
49. Kitaguchi K, Ohsumi H, Kuro M, Nakajima T, Hayashi Y: Effects of sevoflurane on cerebral circulation and metabolism in patients with ischemic cerebrovascular disease. Anesthesiology 79:704, 1993
50. Henriksen HT, Jörgensen PB: The effect of nitrous oxide on intracranial pressure in patients with intracranial disorders. Br J Anaesth 45:486, 1973
51. Wollman H, Alexander SC, Cohen PJ, et al: Cerebral circulation during general anesthesia and hyperventilation in man. Anesthesiology 26:329, 1965
52. Phirman JR, Shapiro HM: Modification of nitrous oxide–induced intracranial hypertension by prior induction of anesthesia. Anesthesiology 46:150, 1977
53. Theye RA, Michenfelder JD: The effect of nitrous oxide on canine cerebral metabolism. Anesthesiology 29:1119, 1968
54. Sakabe T, Kuramoto T, Inove S, et al: Cerebral effects of nitrous oxide in the dog. Anesthesiology 48:195, 1978
55. Artru AA: Nitrous oxide plays a direct role in the development of tension pneumocephalus intraoperatively. Anesthesiology 57:59, 1982
56. Pandit UA, Mudge BJ, Keller TS, et al: Pneumocephalus after posterior fossa exploration in the sitting position. Anaesthesia 37:996, 1982
57. Skahen S, Shapiro HM, Drummond JC, et al: Nitrous oxide withdrawal reduces intracranial pressure in the presence of pneumocephalus. Anesthesiology 65:192, 1986
58. Shapiro HM, Galindo A, Wyte SR, et al: Rapid intraoperative reduction of intracranial pressure with thiopentone. Br J Anaesth 45:1057, 1973
59. Marshall LF, Smith RW, Shapiro HM: The outcome with aggressive treatment in severe head injuries: II. Acute and chronic barbiturate administration in the management of head injury. J Neurosurg 50:26, 1979
60. Marshall LF, Shapiro HM, Rauscher A, et al: Pentobarbital therapy of intracranial hypertension in metabolic coma: Reye's syndrome. Crit Care Med 6:1, 1978
61. Smith AL: Barbiturate protection in cerebral hypoxia. Anesthesiology 47:285, 1977
62. Michenfelder JD: The interdependency of cerebral functional and metabolic effects following massive doses of thiopental in the dog. Anesthesiology 41:231, 1974
63. Moss E, Powell D, Gibson RM, et al: Effects of tracheal intubation on intracranial pressure following induction of anaesthesia with thiopentone or althesin in patients undergoing neurosurgery. Br J Anaesth 50:353, 1978
64. Marsh ML, Marshall LF, Shapiro HM: Neurosurgical intensive care. Anesthesiology 47:149, 1977
65. Miller JD: Barbiturates and raised intracranial pressure. Ann Neurol 6:189, 1979
66. Rockoff MA, Marshall LF, Shapiro HM: High-dose barbiturate therapy in humans: a clinical review of 60 patients. Ann Neurol 6:194, 1979
67. Trauner DA: Treatment of Reye's syndrome. Ann Neurol 7:2, 1980
68. Nayak MM, Bali IM, Singh H, Batra YK: Cerebrospinal fluid pressure changes during the induction phase of anesthesia. Canadian Anaesthetists Society Journal 27:464, 1980
69. Cotev S, Shalit MN: Effects of diazepam on cerebral blood flow and oxygen uptake after head injury. Anesthesiology 43:117, 1975
70. Carlsson C, Hägerdal M, Kaasik AE, et al: The effects of diazepam on cerebral blood flow and oxygen consumption in rats and its synergistic interaction with nitrous oxide. Anesthesiology 45:319, 1976
71. Larson GF, Hurlbert BJ, Wingard DW: Physostigmine reversal of diazepam-induced depression. Anesth Analg 56:348, 1977
72. Hall SC, Ovassapian A: Apnea after intravenous diazepam therapy. JAMA 238:1052, 1977
73. Forster A, Juge O, Morel D: Effects of midazolam on cerebral blood flow in human volunteers. Anesthesiology 56:453, 1982
74. Hoffman WE, Miletich DJ, Albrecht RF: The effects of midazolam on cerebral blood flow and oxygen consumption and its interaction with nitrous oxide. Anesth Analg 65:729, 1986
75. Griffen JP, Cottrell JE, Shwiry B, et al: Intracranial pressure, mean arterial pressure, and heart rate following midazolam or thiopental in humans with brain tumors. Anesthesiology 60: 491, 1984
76. Papazian L, Albanese J, Thirion X, Perrin G, Durbec O, Martin C: Effect of bolus doses of midazolam on intracranial pressure and cerebral perfusion pressure in patients with severe head injury. Br J Anaesth 71:267, 1993
77. Moss E, Power D, Gibson RM, et al: Effect of etomidate on intracranial pressure and cerebral perfusion pressure. Br J Anaesth 51:347, 1979
78. Dearden NM, McDowall DG: Comparison of etomidate and althesin in the reduction of increased intracranial pressure after head injury. Br J Anaesth 57:361, 1985
79. Duthie DJ, Fraser R, Nimmo WS: Effect of induction of anaesthesia with etomidate on corticosteroid synthesis in man. Br J Anaesth 57:156, 1985
80. Pinaud M, Lelausque JN, Chetanneau A, Fauchoux N, Menegalli D, Souron R: Effects of propofol on cerebral hemodynamics and metabolism in patients with brain trauma. Anesthesiology 73:404, 1990
81. Todd MM, Warner DS, Sokoll MD, Maktabi MA, Hindman BJ, Scamman FL, Kirschner J: A prospective, comparative trial of three anesthetics for elective supratentorial craniotomy—Propofol/fentanyl, isoflurane/nitrous oxide, and fentanyl/nitrous oxide. Anesthesiology 78:1005, 1993
82. Witzner SW, McCoy GT, Binder LS: Effects of morphine, levallorphan, and respiratory gases on increased intracranial pressure. Anesthesiology 24:291, 1963
83. Jobes DR, Kennell EM, Bush GL, et al: Cerebral blood flow and metabolism during morphine-nitrous oxide anesthesia in man. Anesthesiology 47:16, 1977
84. Shupak RC, Harp JR, Stevenson-Smith W, et al: High-dose fentanyl for neuroanesthesia. Anesthesiology 58:579, 1983
85. Shupak RC, Harp JR: Comparison between high-dose sufentanil-oxygen and high-dose fentanyl-oxygen for neuroanaesthesia. Br J Anaesth 57:375, 1985
86. Bovill JG, Sebel PS, Wauquier A, et al: Electroencephalographic effects of sufentanil anaesthesia in man. Br J Anaesth 54:45, 1982
87. Keykhah MM, Smith DS, Carlsson C, et al: Influence of sufentanil on cerebral metabolism and circulation in the rat. Anesthesiology 63:274, 1985
88. Young ML, Smith DS, Greenberg J, et al: Effects of sufentanil

on regional cerebral glucose utilization in rats. Anesthesiology 61:564, 1984
89. Milde LN, Milde JH, Gallagher WJ: Effects of sufentanil on cerebral circulation and metabolism in dogs. Anesth Analg 70: 138, 1990
90. Werner C, Hoffman WE, Baughman VL, Albrecht RF, Schulte J: Effects of sufentanil on cerebral blood flow, cerebral blood flow velocity, and metabolism in dogs. Anesth Analg 72:177, 1991
91. Trindle MR, Dodson BA, Rampil IJ: Effects of fentanyl versus sufentanil in equianesthetic doses on middle cerebral artery blood flow velocity. Anesthesiology 78:454, 1993
92. Albanese J, Durbec O, Viviand X, Potie F, Alliez B, Martin C: Sufentanil increases intracranial pressure in patients with head trauma. Anesthesiology 79:493, 1993
93. Sperry RJ, Bailey PL, Reichman MV, Peterson JC, Petersen PB, Pace NL: Fentanyl and sufentanil increase intracranial pressure in head trauma patients. Anesthesiology 77:416, 1992
94. From RP, Warner DS, Todd MM, Sokoll MD: Anesthesia for craniotomy: a double-blind comparison of alfentanil, fentanyl, and sufentanil. Anesthesiology 73:896, 1990
95. Jung R, Shah N, Reinsel R, Marx W, Marshall W, Galicich J, Bedford R: Cerebrospinal fluid pressure in patients with brain tumors: impact of fentanyl versus alfentanil during nitrous oxide-oxygen anesthesia. Anesth Analg 71:419, 1990
96. Mayberg TS, Lam AM, Eng CC, Laohaprasit V, Winn HR: The effect of alfentanil on cerebral blood flow velocity and intracranial pressure during isoflurane-nitrous oxide anesthesia in humans. Anesthesiology 78:288, 1993
97. Markovitz BP, Duhaime AC, Sutton L, Schreiner MS, Cohen DE: Effects of alfentanil on intracranial pressure in children undergoing ventriculoperitoneal shunt revision. Anesthesiology 76:71, 1992
98. Fitch W, Barker J, Jennett WB, et al: The influence of neuroleptanalgesic drugs on cerebrospinal fluid pressure. Br J Anaesth 41:800, 1969
99. Michenfelder JD, Theye RA: Effects of fentanyl, droperidol, and innovar on canine cerebral metabolism and blood flow. Br J Anaesth 43:630, 1971
100. Misfeldt BB, Jörgensen PB, Spotoft H, et al: The effects of droperidol and fentanyl on intracranial pressure and cerebral perfusion pressure in neurosurgical patients. Br J Anaesth 48: 963, 1976
101. Bidwai AV, Cornelius LB, Stanley TH: Reversal of innovar-induced postanesthetic somnolence and disorientation with physostigmine. Anesthesiology 44:249, 1976
102. Shapiro HM, Wyte SR, Harris AB: Ketamine anaesthesia in patients with intracranial pathology. Br J Anaesth 44:1200, 1972
103. Takeshita H, Okuda Y, Sari A: The effects of ketamine on cerebral circulation and metabolism in man. Anesthesiology 36: 69, 1972
104. Sondergard W: Intracranial pressure during general anesthesia. Dan Med Bull 8:18, 1961
105. Lanier WL, Milde JH, Michenfelder JD: Cerebral stimulation following succinylcholine in dogs. Anesthesiology 64:551, 1986
106. Minton MD, Grosslight K, Strit JA, et al: Increases in intracranial pressure from succinylcholine: prevention by prior nondepolarizing blockade. Anesthesiology 65:165, 1986
107. Stirt JA, Grosslight KR, Bedford RF, Vollmer D: "Defasciculation" with metocurine prevents succinylcholine-induced increases in intracranial pressure. Anesthesiology 67:50, 1987
108. Stevenson PH, Brich AA: Succinylcholine-induced hyperkalemia in a patient with a closed head injury. Anesthesiology 51:89, 1979
109. Cooperman LH, Strobel GE, Kennell EM: Massive hyperkalemia after administration of succinylcholine. Anesthesiology 32:161, 1970
110. Cowgill DB, Mostello LA, Shapiro HM: Encephalitis and a hyperkalemic response to succinylcholine. Anesthesiology 40: 409, 1974
111. Weintraub HD, Heisterkamp DV, Cooperman LH: Changes in plasma potassium concentration after depolarizing blockers in anesthetized man. Br J Anaesth 41:1048, 1969
112. Konchigeri HN, Tay CH: Influence of pancuronium on potassium efflux produced by succinylcholine. Anesth Analg 55:474, 1976
113. Tarkkanen L, Laitenen L, Johansson G: Effects of *D*-tubocurarine on intracranial pressure and thalamic electrical impedance. Anesthesiology 40:247, 1974
114. Rosa G, Sanfilippo M, Vilardi V, et al: Effects of vecuronium bromide on intracranial pressure and cerebral perfusion pressure. Br J Anaesth 58:437, 1986
115. Minton MD, Strit JA, Bedford RF, et al: Intracranial pressure after atracurium in neurosurgical patients. Anesth Analg 64: 1113, 1985
116. Rosa G, Orfei P, Sanfilippo M, et al: The effects of atracurium besylate (Tracrium) on intracranial pressure and cerebral perfusion pressure. Anesth Analg 65:381, 1986
117. Artie AA, Katz RA, Colley PS: Autoregulation of cerebral blood flow during normocapnia and hypocapnia in dogs. Anesthesiology 70:288, 1989
118. Ivankovich AD, Miletich DJ, Albrecht RF, et al: Sodium nitroprusside and cerebral blood flow in the anesthetized and unanesthetized goat. Anesthesiology 44:21, 1976
119. Cottrell JE, Patel K, Turndorf H, et al: Intracranial pressure changes induced by sodium nitroprusside in patients with intracranial mass lesions. J Neurosurg 48:329, 1978
120. Turner JM, Powell D, Gibson RM, et al: Intracranial pressure changes in neurosurgical patients during hypotension induced with sodium nitroprusside or trimethaphan. Br J Anaesth 49: 419, 1977
121. Keaney NP, McDowall DG, Turner JM, et al: The effects of profound hypotension induced with sodium nitroprusside on cerebral blood flow and metabolism in the baboon. Br J Anaesth 45:639, 1973
122. Khambatta HJ, Stone JG, Khan E: Propranolol alters renin release during nitroprusside-induced hypotension and prevents hypertension on discontinuation of nitroprusside. Anesth Analg 60:569, 1981
123. Fahmy NR: Rebound arterial hypertension following discontinuation of sodium nitroprusside: aetiology and prevention. In Heuser D, McDowall DG, Hempel V (eds): Controlled hypotension in neuroanaesthesia. New York: Plenum Press, 1985: 21
124. Ivankovich AD, Sheth DJ, Shulman M, et al.: Autoregulation of cerebral blood flow during infusion of trimethaphan or nitroglycerin in the goat. Abstracts of Scientific Papers, Annual Meeting of the American Society of Anesthesiologists, 1978: 77
125. Chestnut JS, Albin MS, Gonzalez-Abola E, et al: Clinical evaluation of intravenous nitroglycerin for neurosurgery. J Neurosurg 48:704, 1978
126. Dohi S, Matsumoto M, Takahashi T: The effects of nitroglycerin on cerebrospinal fluid pressure in awake and anesthetized humans. Anesthesiology 54:511, 1981
127. Cottrell JE, Gupta B, Rappaport H, et al: Intracranial pressure during nitroglycerin-induced hypotension. J Neurosurg 53:309, 1980
128. Michenfelder JD, Theye RA: Canine systemic and cerebral effects of hypotension induced by hemorrhage, trimethaphan, halothane, or nitroprusside. Anesthesiology 46:188, 1977
129. Ishikawa T, Funatsu N, Okamoto K, et al: Cerebral and systemic effects of hypotension induced by trimethaphan or nitroprusside in dogs. Acta Anaesthesiol Scand 26:643, 1982
130. Overgaard J, Skinhoj E: A paradoxical cerebral hemodynamic effect of hydralazine. Stroke 6:402, 1975
131. James DJ, Bedford RF: Hydralazine for controlled hypotension during neurosurgical operations. Anesth Analg 61:1016, 1982
132. Van Aken H, Puchstein C, Anger C, et al: Changes in intracranial pressure and compliance during adenosine triphosphate-induced hypotension in dogs. Anesth Analg 63:381, 1984
133. Newberg LA, Milde JH, Michenfelder JD: Cerebral and sys-

temic effects of hypotension induced by adenosine or atp in dogs. Anesthesiology 62:429, 1985

134. Griffin JP, Cottrell JE, Hartung J, et al: Intracranial pressure during nifedipine-induced hypotension. Anesth Analg 62:1078, 1983

135. Van Aken H, Puchstein C, Hidding J: The use of labetalol in producing deliberate hypotension and its effects on intracranial pressure in dogs. Acta Anaesthesiol Belg 33:5, 1982

136. Ornstein E, Young WL, Ostapkovich N, Matteo RS, Diaz J: Deliberate hypotension in patients with intracranial arteriovenous malformations: esmolol compared with isoflurane and sodium nitroprusside. Anesth Analg 72:639, 1991

137. Demling R, Riessen R: Pulmonary dysfunction after cerebral injury. Crit Care Med 18:768, 1990

138. Eckenhoff JE, Enderby GEH, Larson A, et al: Pulmonary gas exchange during deliberate hypotension. Br J Anaesth 35:750, 1963

139. Wildsmith JAW, Drummond GB, MacRae WR: Blood gas changes during induced hypotension with sodium nitroprusside. Br J Anaesth 47:1205, 1975

140. Cuypers J, Matakas F, Potolicchio SF Jr: Effect of central venous pressure on brain tissue and brain volume. J Neurosurg 45:89, 1976

141. Hulme A, Cooper R: The effects of head position and jugular vein compression (JVC) on intracranial pressure (ICP): a clinical study. In Beks JWF, Bosch DA, Brock M (eds): Intracranial pressure III. Proceedings of the Third International Symposium on Intracranial Pressure held at the University of Groningen, June 1–3, 1976. Berlin: Springer-Verlag, 1976: 259

142. Shapiro HM, Marshall LF: Intracranial pressure responses to peep in head-injured patients. J Trauma 18:254, 1978

143. Apuzzo MLJ, Weiss MH, Petersons V, et al: Effect of positive end expiratory pressure ventilation on intracranial pressure in man. J Neurosurg 46:227, 1977

144. Frost EM: Effects of positive end expiratory pressure on intracranial pressure and compliance in brain-injured patients. J Neurosurg 47:195, 1977

145. Williams B: Cerebrospinal fluid pressure changes in response to coughing. Brain 99:331, 1976

146. Kety SS: Circulation and metabolism of the human brain in health and disease. Am J Med 8:205, 1950

147. Shapiro HM, Wyte SR, Harris AB, et al: Acute intraoperative intracranial hypertension in neurosurgical patients: mechanical and pharmacologic factors. Anesthesiology 37:399, 1972

148. Alexander SC, Lassen NA: Cerebral circulatory response to acute brain disease: implications for anesthetic practice. Anesthesiology 32:60, 1970

149. Keaney NP, Pickerodt VW, McDowall DG, et al: Cerebral circulatory and metabolic effects of hypotension produced by deep halothane anaesthesia. J Neurol Neurosurg Psychiatry 36:898, 1973

150. Hilt H, Gramm HJ, Link J: Changes in intracranial pressure associated with extradural anaesthesia. Br J Anaesth 58:676, 1986

151. Langfitt TW: Increased intracranial pressure and the cerebral circulation. In Youmans JR (ed): Neurological Surgery 2nd ed. Philadelphia: WB Saunders, 1982:861

152. McDowall DG: Monitoring the brain. Anesthesiology 45:117, 1976

153. Shapiro HM: Monitoring in neurosurgical anesthesia. In Saidman LJ, Smith NT (eds): Monitoring in anesthesia. New York: John Wiley & Sons, 1978: 171

154. Marmarou A: Progress in the analysis of intracranial pressure dynamics. In Miller JD, Teasdale GM, Rowan JO, et al (eds): Intracranial pressure VI: Proceedings of the Sixth International Symposium on Intracranial Pressure, Glasgow, Scotland, June 9 to 13, 1985. Berlin: Springer-Verlag, 1986: 781

155. Lundberg N: Continuous recording and control of ventricular fluid pressure in neurosurgical practice. Acta Psychiatr Scand Suppl 36:I-193, 1960

156. Rosner MJ, Becker DP: Origin and evolution of plateau waves: experimental observations and a theoretical model. J Neurosurg 60:312, 1984

157. Aucoin PJ, Kotilainen HR, Gantz NM, et al: Intracranial pressure monitors: epidemiologic study of risk factors and infections. Am J Med 80:369, 1986

158. Parks LK, Bergman NA: Hypoxia as a manifestation of neurogenic pulmonary dysfunction. Anesthesiology 45:93, 1976

159. Jachuck SJ, Ramani PS, Clark F, et al: Electrocardiographic abnormalities associated with raised intracranial pressure. British Medical Journal 1:294, 1975

160. Raichle ME, Posner JB, Plum F: Cerebral blood flow during and after hyperventilation. Arch Neurol 23:394, 1970

161. Cold GE: Does acute hyperventilation provoke cerebral oligemia in comatose patients after acute head injury? Acta Neurochir (Wien) 96:100, 1989

162. Marshall LF, Smith RW, Rauscher LA, et al: Mannitol dose requirements in brain-injured patients. J Neurosurg 48:169, 1978

163. Coté CJ, Greenhow DE, Marshall BE: The hypotensive response to rapid administration of hypertonic solutions in man and in the rabbit. Anesthesiology 50:30, 1979

164. Becker DP, Vries JK: The alleviation of increased intracranial pressure by the chronic administration of osmotic agents. In Brock M, Dietz H (eds): Intracranial pressure: experimental and clinical aspects. Berlin: Springer-Verlag, 1972: 309

165. Silber SJ, Thompson N: Mannitol induced central nervous system toxicity in renal failure. Investigative Urology 9:310, 1972

166. Cantore G, Guidetti B, Virno M: Oral glycerol for the reduction of intracranial pressure. J Neurosurg 21:278, 1964

167. Hägnevik K, Gordon E, Lins LE, et al: Glycerol-induced haemolysis with haemoglobinuria and acute renal failure. Lancet 1:75, 1974

168. Arieff AI, Lazarowitz VC, Guisado R: Experimental dialysis disequilibrium syndrome: prevention with glycerol. Kidney Int 14:270, 1978

169. Cottrell JE, Robustelli A, Post K, et al: Furosemide- and mannitol-induced changes in intracranial pressure and serum osmolality and electrolytes. Anesthesiology 47:28, 1977

170. Cottrell JE, Marx W, Marlin A, et al: Furosemide reduces increased intracranial pressure after head trauma. Abstracts of Scientific Papers, Annual Meeting of the American Society of Anesthesiologists, 1978:161

171. Pollay M, Roberts PA, Hisey B, et al: The effect of fursemide on intracranial pressure and cerebrospinal fluid formation. In Miller JD, Teasdale GM, Rowan JO, et al (eds): Intracranial pressure VI: Proceedings of the Sixth International Symposium on Intracranial Pressure, Glasgow, Scotland, June 9 to 13, 1985. Berlin: Springer-Verlag, 1986: 597

172. McCarthy KO, Reed DJ: The effect of acetazolamide and furosemide on cerebrospinal fluid production and choroid plexus carbonic anhydrase activity. J Pharmacol Exp Ther 189:194, 1974

173. Schettini A, Stahurski B, Young HF: Osmotic and osmotic-loop diuresis in brain surgery: effects on plasma and csf electrolytes and ion excretion. J Neurosurg 56:679, 1982

174. Unni VK, Johnston RA, Young HS, et al: Prevention of intracranial hypertension during laryngoscopy and endotracheal intubation: use of a second dose of thiopentone. Br J Anaesth 56:1219, 1984

175. Hamill JF, Bedford RF, Weaver DC, et al: Lidocaine before endotracheal intubation: intravenous or laryngotracheal? Anesthesiology 55:578, 1981

176. Ward JD, Becker DP, Miller JD, et al: Failure of prophylactic barbiturate coma in the treatment of severe head injury. J Neurosurg 62:383, 1985

177. Brain Resuscitation Clinical Trial I Study Group: Randomized clinical study of thiopental loading in comatose survivors of cardiac arrest. N Engl J Med 314:397, 1986

178. Maxwell RE, Long DM, French LA: The clinical effects of a synthetic gluco-corticoid used for brain edema in the practice of neurosurgery. In Reulen HJ, Schürmann K (eds): Steroids and brain edema. Heidelberg: Springer-Verlag, 1972: 219

179. Marshall LF, King J, Langfitt TW: The complications of high-dose corticosteroid therapy in neurosurgical patients: a prospective study. Ann Neurol 1:201, 1977

180. Gobiet W, Bock WJ, Liesegang J, et al: Treatment of acute cerebral edema with high dose of dexamethasone. In Beks JWF, Bosch DA, Brock M (eds): Intracranial pressure III. Proceedings of the Third International Symposium on Intracranial Pressure held at the University of Groningen, June 1–3, 1976. Berlin, Springer-Verlag, 1976: 232
181. Faupel G, Reulen HJ, Muller D, et al: Double-blind study on the effects of dexamethasone on severe closed head injury. In Pappius HM, Reulen W (eds): Dynamics of brain edema. Berlin: Springer-Verlag, 1986: 337
182. Gudeman SK, Miller JD, Becker DP: Failure of high-dose steroid therapy to influence intracranial pressure in patients with severe head injury. J Neurosurg 51:301, 1979
183. Saul TG, Ducker TB, Salcman M, et al: Steroids in severe head injury: a prospective randomized clinical trial. J Neurosurg 54:596, 1981
184. Dearden NM, Gibson JS, McDowall DG, et al: Effect of high-dose dexamethasone on outcome from severe head injury. J Neurosurg 64:81, 1986
185. Rosomoff HJ, Shulman K, Raynor R, et al: Experimental brain injury and delayed hypothermia. Surg Gynecol Obstet 110:27, 1960
186. Shapiro HM, Wyte SR, Loeser J: Barbiturate-augmented hypothermia for reduction of persistent intracranial hypertension. J Neurosurg 40:90, 1974
187. Steen PA, Soule EH, Michenfelder JD: Detrimental effect of prolonged hypothermia in cats and monkeys with and without regional cerebral ischemia. Stroke 10:522, 1979
188. Steen PA, Milde JH, Michenfelder JD: The detrimental effects of prolonged hypothermia and rewarming the dog. Anesthesiology 52:224, 1980
189. Wisner D, Busche F, Sturmond, et al: Traumatic shock and head injury. J Surg Res 46:49, 1989
190. Ducey JP, Mozingo DW, Lamiell JM, et al: A comparison of the cerebral and cardiovascular effects of complete resuscitation with isotonic and hypertonic saline, hetastarch, and whole blood following hemorrhage. J Trauma 29:1510, 1989
191. Shackford SR: Fluid resuscitation in head injury. J Intensive Care Med 5:59, 1990
192. Morse ML, Milstein JM, Haas JE, et al: Effect of hydration on experimentally induced cerebral edema. Crit Care Med 13: 563, 1985

FURTHER READING

Hayak DA, Veremakis C: Physiologic concerns during brain resuscitation. In Civetta JM, Taylor RW, Kirby RR (eds): Critical care. Philadelphia: JB Lippincott, 1992: 1449

Lanier WL, Weglinski MR: Intracranial Pressure. In: Cucchiara RF, Michenfelder JD (eds): Clinical Neuroanesthesia. New York, Churchill Livingstone, 1990:77

Lassen NA, Christensen MS: Physiology of cerebral blood flow. Br J Anaesth 48:719, 1976

Mahla M: Nervous system. In Gravenstein N (ed). Manual of complications during anesthesia. Philadelphia: JB Lippincott, 1991: 383

McPherson RW, Kirsch JR, Traystmen RJ: Optimal anesthetic techniques for patients at risk of cerebral ischemia. In Weinstein PR, Faden AI (eds); Protection of the brain from ischemia. Baltimore: Williams & Wilkins, 1990: 237

Messick MJ Jr, Newberg LA, Nugent M, et al: Principles of neuroanesthesia for the non-neurosurgical patient with CNS pathophysiology. Anesth Analg 64:143, 1985

Complications in Anesthesiology, second edition,
edited by Nikolaus Gravenstein and Robert R. Kirby.
Lippincott-Raven Publishers, Philadelphia © 1996.

CHAPTER 28

Ophthalmologic Complications

Kathryn E. McGoldrick

Providing optimal anesthesia care in ophthalmic surgery presents several unique challenges. The anesthesiologist must be well versed in the numerous, often complex, interactions between ocular disease and anesthetic effects to prevent serious complications.[1] This chapter surveys general considerations in ophthalmic anesthesia; specific complications; ocular complications that may occur during nonophthalmic surgery; and, finally, ocular complications that may occur as a result of prematurity, oxygen therapy, or both.

OPHTHALMIC SURGERY

General Considerations

Apart from many of the routine concerns in anesthetic administration such as overall safety, appropriate selection of anesthetic technique and drugs, and drug interactions, additional considerations are particularly important in ophthalmic surgery (Table 28-1). Moreover, the requirement in ophthalmic surgery that the anesthesiologist be positioned remote from the patient's airway creates certain logistic inconveniences. Communication and rapport among the physicians caring for these patients are particularly important if the anesthesiologist is to meet the necessary exacting conditions (see Table 28-1).

Just as ocular drugs can have dramatic ramifications in their interaction with anesthetics, so also can anesthetic drugs and methods affect intraocular dynamics. Factors such as ocular pathologic lesions, anesthetic depth, arterial carbon dioxide partial pressure, pupillary size, change in extraocular muscle tone, hydration, and use of adjuvant drugs such as muscle relaxants interact to determine the overall effect of anesthesia on the eye.[2,3]

In addition, the anesthesiologist must be aware of the anesthetic implications of congenital and metabolic diseases with ocular manifestations. Diabetes mellitus, for instance, often involves ocular complications. The anesthesiologist must be knowledgeable about the systemic disturbances affecting these patients. Furthermore, many ophthalmic patients are at the extremes of age—from premature infants to nonagenarians, and hence, special age-related considerations, such as altered pharmacokinetics, apply. In addition, the incidence of malignant hyperthermia is thought by some to be greater in persons with ocular muscle disturbances such as ptosis or strabismus.

Choice of Anesthetic Technique

The choice of anesthetic technique, principally between local and general anesthesia, must be individualized (Table 28-2). Germane considerations include the nature and duration of the surgical procedure, coagulation status, the patient's ability to communicate and cooperate, and the surgeon's personal preference. Of course, local anesthesia is not an ideal choice for patients who are deaf or speak a foreign language and those who have problems such as claustrophobia, excessive anxiety, or confusion. Other relative contraindications include chronic coughing, tremors, and an inability to lie flat.

Available data do not demonstrate a major difference in ocular complications such as iris prolapse or vitreous loss among anesthetic techniques for cataract surgery.[4] Local anesthesia has proven to be a safe technique for patients with certain types of cardiovascular disease.[5]

Local Anesthesia

If the patient is mature and cooperative and the surgeon is compassionate and communicative, local anesthesia should provide satisfactory conditions for almost any ophthalmic operation of reasonable length. Techniques involve facial, retrobulbar, and peribulbar blocks.[6] In most institutions, when local anesthesia is elected the ophthalmologist administers the local or regional block. The anesthetist or anesthesiologist is present to monitor the patient's electrocardiogram, vital signs, and hemoglobin oxygen saturation by pulse oximeter and to administer sedation as needed. However, one should not be lulled into a false sense of security regarding the safety of local anesthesia. The physiologic trespass involved with this technique is not always less than that with general anesthesia, and thus it is not a priori safer or better.

TABLE 28-1
Conditions Required for Safe Ophthalmic Surgery

- Stillness and fixation of the eye (akinesia)
- Profound analgesia
- Minimal bleeding
- Avoidance or obtundation of the oculocardiac reflex
- Prevention of intraocular hypertension
- Smooth emergence uncomplicated by vomiting, coughing, or retching

RETROBULBAR BLOCK. Retrobulbar block carries several attendant risks (Table 28-3), including the risk of retrobulbar hemorrhage and proptosis as well as the possibility of direct intravascular injection and the associated central nervous system and cardiovascular complications of excessive drug levels. A recent study of 12,500 consecutive retrobulbar blocks documented an incidence of retrobulbar hemorrhage of 0.44%.[5] Acquired vascular disease was a significant risk factor. Of particular interest, however, was the finding that the eventual outcome in the 55 affected persons was no different than in the control group.

Other hazards include unintended intraocular injection (scleral perforation), retinal vascular occlusion, inadequate block of muscles with compression of the globe and extrusion of intraocular contents, and penetration of the optic nerve.[6] Temporary or permanent diplopia, ptosis, or both may occur and are speculated to result from myotoxic effects of the local anesthetics.[7]

However, the etiology of postoperative ptosis may be multifactorial. That local anesthetic myotoxicity cannot be isolated as the sole factor is underscored by the observation that postsurgical ptosis is seen in patients who received general anesthesia.

Accidental Central Neuraxial Injection. An initially insidious but potentially lethal complication also arises when the local anesthetic gains access to cerebrospinal fluid as a result of perforation of the meningeal sheaths that surround the optic nerve. Symptoms range from drowsiness, contralateral blindness, and inappropriate shivering to more severe complications such as progressive respiratory depression, apnea, hemiplegia, aphasia, seizure, unconsciousness, and cardiopulmonary arrest. A typical case report describes the gradual onset of unconsciousness and apnea over the course of 7 minutes without accompanying seizure or cardiovascular collapse in a patient who received a retrobulbar injection of 6 to 8 mL of 0.75% bupivacaine.[8] A prospective series of 3123 retrobulbar blocks performed with an equal volume of 4% or 2% lidocaine mixed with 0.75% bupivacaine (total volume 10 mL) suggests that the incidence of respiratory arrest is significantly higher with the mixture containing 4% lidocaine (0.79% for 4% versus 0.09% for 2%).[9] In a prospective series of 6000 consecutive retrobulbar blocks, the incidence of symptoms suggesting local anesthetic spread to the brain was 0.27%, with life-threatening complications occurring in 0.13% of patients.[10] However, the incidence and severity of symptoms in this and another series[11] was unrelated to the dose or choice of local anesthetic.

TABLE 28-2
Choice of Anesthetic Technique for Ophthalmic Surgery: Factors to Consider

- Nature and duration of procedure
- Coagulation status
- Cooperation and ability to speak and hear
- Claustrophobia
- Anxiety
- Confusion
- Chronic cough or tremors
- Ability to lie flat
- Surgeon's and patient's preference

TABLE 28-3
Complications of Retrobulbar Block

- Hemorrhage
- Proptosis
- Intravascular injection
- Scleral perforation
- Retinal vascular occlusion
- Compression of globe and extrusion of vitreous
- Penetration of optic nerve
- Diplopia or ptosis
- Central nervous system injection
  - Paralysis
  - Cardiorespiratory arrest
  - Death

In all series, the serum levels of the local anesthetics were well below those usually associated with local anesthetic–induced central nervous system toxicity. Onset usually occurs very shortly after administration of the block but may be delayed as long as 40 minutes. Thus, anesthesia personnel and ophthalmologists should be alerted to the rare occurrence of accidental brain stem anesthesia after retrobulbar block. Practitioners skilled in airway maintenance and ventilatory support must be immediately available whenever retrobulbar nerve block is used.

Prevention involves using a block needle no longer than 3 cm[12] and performing the block with the eye in neutral gaze, or looking inferonasally, to render the optic nerve sheath less vulnerable to penetration.[13] (The traditional Atkinson position of superonasal gaze during needle placement for retrobulbar block places the optic nerve in closer proximity to the advancing needle, where the needle tip can pierce the meningeal sheath surrounding the optic nerve, allowing local anesthetics to spread throughout the central nervous system.[14])

Vasoconstrictors. Vasoconstrictors (eg, epinephrine 1: 200,000) are often mixed with local anesthetic agents to reduce vascular uptake of the injected drug and thereby prolong anesthesia. Ophthalmologists frequently inquire whether this practice is safe in patients with cardiovascular disease. Donlon and Moss emphasize that the release of endogenous catecholamines as a result of erratic analgesia may far exceed the relatively minute amount of exogenous catecholamine injected. They state that epinephrine, 0.06 mg, (12 mL of

1:200,000 solution) results in some systemic uptake but no untoward clinical effects.[15] Ocular perfusion, however, may be reduced with epinephrine-containing solutions.

FACIAL NERVE BLOCKS. A separate facial nerve block is performed in conjunction with retrobulbar block to achieve akinesia of the eyelids. This is necessary during intraocular surgery to prevent squeezing of the lids that could result in expulsion of intraocular contents. A variety of approaches can be used to block the facial nerve after it exits the skull through the stylomastoid foramen. Moving distally to proximally to the foramen, the techniques include the van Lint, Atkinson, O'Brien, and Nadbath-Rehman methods. Although each has advantages and disadvantages, the Nadbath-Rehman approach can potentially produce the most serious systemic consequences. With this approach, a 27-gauge, 12-mm needle is inserted between the mastoid process and the posterior border of the mandibular ramus. Owing to the proximity of the jugular foramen (10 mm medial to the stylomastoid foramen) to the injection site, ipsilateral paralysis of cranial nerves IX, X, and XI can occur, producing hoarseness, dysphagia, pooling of secretions, agitation, respiratory distress,[16] and laryngospasm.[17] Moreover, because the Nadbath-Rehman block produces complete hemifacial akinesia that interferes with oral intake, this approach is not recommended for outpatients.

PERIBULBAR BLOCK. Because the complications of retrobulbar block can be both vision-threatening and life-threatening, alternative approaches have been developed. Since the late 1980s, peribulbar block has become popular. With this technique anesthetic solution is not injected into the muscle cone, but rather deposited outside it, and a separate facial nerve block is usually superfluous, owing to diffusion of local anesthetic into the lid. Onset is typically slower than with retrobulbar block and forward pressure on the eyeball caused by the relatively large amount of anesthetic necessary can be a problem to the surgeon. However, optic nerve injury and central spread of anesthetic agent are exceedingly rare, if not unheard of, with peribulbar block. Globe perforation, however, can occur.

TOPICAL ANESTHESIA. Recently, in an attempt to avoid serious complications, ophthalmologists have been returning to a technique that was popular during the early 1900s—the use of topical anesthetic agents, employed particularly when the surgical incision is being made through clear cornea. Patient selection, however, is critical and should be limited to cooperative patients who can control their eye movements. Patients with small pupils who may require significant iris manipulation or those who need large scleral incisions may be contraindicated for topical anesthesia.

Sedation

Local anesthesia and heavy sedation with a variety of narcotics, tranquilizers, and hypnotic agents usually proves unsatisfactory. This heavy-handedness is to be condemned because of the unpredictability of pharmacologic actions in elders and because of the risks of excessive sedation (respiratory depression, airway obstruction, hypotension, mental aberrations, "startle" responses, and protracted recovery time). Inadequate sedation likewise should be avoided because hypertension and tachycardia are undesirable, especially in patients with coronary artery disease. The goal is a calm, cooperative, *aware* patient who will not move suddenly during delicate intraocular surgery. Patients with arthritis or orthopedic deformities must be positioned meticulously and comfortably padded. All patients must have adequate ventilation about the face and must be kept warm.

Continuous monitoring of the electrocardiogram is essential for detection of the oculocardiac reflex, typically manifested as bradydysrhythmia or tachydysrhythmia, or asystole triggered by manipulation of the retrobulbar muscles. Continuous monitoring by pulse oximetry of the hemoglobin oxygen saturation is similarly essential to ensure the adequacy of oxygenation and to infer that of ventilation.

Increased Intraocular Pressure

Ophthalmic surgery may be classified as extraocular, intraocular, or mixed. For a purely extraocular procedure, such as strabismus correction or ptosis repair, the conduct of surgery is virtually unaffected by intraocular pressure (IOP). During vitrectomy, a closed intraocular procedure, the surgeon manometrically controls IOP by a watertight infusion entry site through the pars plana. Nonetheless, control of IOP is critical for "open" procedures as glaucoma drainage, traditional intracapsular cataract extractions, corneal transplantation, and repair of penetrating eye injuries.

Practical Considerations

IOP normally varies between 10 and 22 mm Hg; a level greater than 25 mm Hg is considered abnormal. During anesthesia, an increase in IOP can lead to permanent loss of vision. If the IOP is already elevated, a further increase can precipitate an acute episode of glaucoma. Should penetration of the globe occur when the IOP is excessively high, rupture of a blood vessel with subsequent hemorrhage may follow. Once the globe has been entered, IOP becomes atmospheric, and any sudden pressure increase can result in prolapse of the lens and iris as well as loss of vitreous. Hence, without proper control of IOP, permanent injury is a likely consequence.[18] Obviously, sudden movement by the patient or coughing on the endotracheal tube during intraocular surgery can result in blindness.

Factors of Importance

IOP is influenced principally by the factors listed in Table 28-4.

AQUEOUS HUMOR. The major determinant is fluid content, especially the aqueous humor. Two thirds of the aqueous humor is formed in the posterior chamber in an active secretory process involving carbonic anhydrase and the cytochrome oxidase systems. Formation of the remaining one third occurs in the anterior chamber by simple filtration through the anterior surface of the iris. Aqueous humor flows from the posterior chamber through the pupillary aperture and into the

TABLE 28-4
Factors Controlling Intraocular Pressure

- Fluid content (especially aqueous humor)
- Intraocular blood volume (venous obstruction)
- External pressure (venous congestion of orbital veins associated with coughing and vomiting, orbital tumor, or contraction of orbicularis oculi muscle)
- Mydriasis

anterior chamber, where it exits through Fontana's spaces to enter Schlemm's canal. A network of connecting venous channels eventually leads to the superior vena cava and the right atrium. Hence, obstruction of blood flow at any site from the eye to the right side of heart impedes aqueous drainage and concomitantly elevates IOP.

INTRAOCULAR BLOOD VOLUME. IOP is influenced significantly by intraocular blood volume, determined mainly by vessel dilatation or contraction in the spongy layers of the choroid plexus. Although changes in arterial or venous pressure can influence IOP secondarily, excursions in arterial pressure have less effect than do venous fluctuations. In chronic arterial hypertension, ocular pressure returns to a normal level after a period of adaptation effected by compression of choroidal vessels as a result of high IOP. Thus, a feedback mechanism decreases the total blood volume, keeping the IOP constant in patients with systemic hypertension.[19]

IMPEDIMENT OF VENOUS DRAINAGE. If venous return from the eye is impeded at any site from Schlemm's canal to the right atrium, the IOP rises markedly as a consequence of increased intraocular blood volume, distention of orbital vessels, and obstruction of aqueous drainage. Coughing, straining, or vomiting greatly elevate venous pressure and increase IOP by 40 mm Hg or more. The harmful implications of these actions cannot be overemphasized.

LARYNGOSCOPY AND TRACHEAL INTUBATION. IOP also can be increased by laryngoscopy and tracheal intubation, even when there is no visible response to intubation, but especially when the patient coughs.[20] Laryngeal topical anesthesia may attenuate but not totally eliminate this increase in IOP associated with intubation.[21]

Dynamics of Aqueous Humor Flux

OSMOTIC PRESSURE. The most important determinant of aqueous humor formation is the difference in osmotic pressure between aqueous and plasma, as illustrated by the following equation:

$$IOP = K\,([IOP_{aq} - OP_{pl}] + CP)$$

where K = coefficient of outflow; OP_{aq} = osmotic pressure of aqueous humor; OP_{pl} = osmotic pressure of plasma; and CP = capillary pressure. That a small change in plasma solute concentration can markedly affect the formation of aqueous humor and, consequently, IOP is the rationale for using hypertonic solutions such as mannitol to lower IOP.

AQUEOUS OUTFLOW. Fluctuations in aqueous outflow can dramatically change IOP. The most important factor determining the outflow of aqueous humor is the diameter of Fontana's spaces, as illustrated by an equation based on Hagen-Poiseuille's Law[22]:

$$A = \frac{r^4 \times (IOP - P_v)}{8\eta L}$$

where A = volume of aqueous outflow per unit of time; r = radius of Fontana's spaces; P_v = venous pressure; η = viscosity; and L = length of Fontana's spaces.

With mydriasis, Fontana's spaces narrow; resistance to outflow increases; and IOP rises. Because mydriasis is a threat in both narrow- and wide-angle glaucoma, conjunctivally applied miotic agents, such as pilocarpine hydrochloride, are often efficacious preoperatively in patients with glaucoma. Concern that parenteral atropine should not be given to patients with glaucoma is invalid. Atropine in the dose range used clinically has no effect on IOP in either open- or closed-angle glaucoma. When 0.4 mg atropine is given parenterally to a 70-kg person, approximately 0.0001 mg is absorbed by the eye.[23]

Similarly, aqueous outflow is exquisitely sensitive to changes in venous pressure. Because an elevation in venous pressure increases the volume of ocular blood and decreases aqueous outflow, IOP increases considerably. Therefore, in addition to preoperative instillation of miotic agents, other anesthetic recommendations for patients with glaucoma include perioperative avoidance of venous congestion and of excessive hydration. In addition, hypotensive episodes are best avoided because purportedly these patients are vulnerable to development of retinal artery thrombosis.

Effects of Anesthetic Techniques and Adjuvant Drugs

INHALATION AGENTS. Several agents and techniques affect IOP (Table 28-5). Inhalation agents are said to cause dose-related decreases in IOP.[24] The precise mechanisms responsible for this purported decrease remain to be established, but hypothesized causes include depression of a central ner-

TABLE 28-5
Effects of Anesthetic Agents, Techniques, and Adjuvant Drugs on Intraocular Pressure

DECREASED IOP
Inhalational agents
Barbiturates, propofol, etomidate, narcotics
Neuroleptic agents
Nondepolarizing muscle relaxants (unless alveolar hypoventilation occurs)
Hyperventilation
Hypothermia
INCREASED IOP
Ketamine (questionable)
Hypoxemia
Hypercapnia
Succinylcholine

vous system control center probably located in the diencephalic region,[19] reduction of aqueous humor production, facilitation of aqueous humor outflow, or relaxation of extraocular muscle tension.[23]

The concept of dose-related decreases in IOP has been questioned by investigators who maintain that if patients are well sedated before baseline measurements are obtained, the introduction of inhalation agents will not change IOP.[25] The latter idea has not been widely promulgated.

CENTRAL NERVOUS SYSTEM DEPRESSANT AGENTS. Central nervous system depressant agents in general decrease IOP. Sedative doses of barbiturates lower IOP; thiopental reduces IOP in normal[20] and glaucomatous eyes.[24] Propofol also reduces IOP and, despite its proclivity to produce pain and muscle movement, etomidate markedly reduces IOP.[27] Neuroleptanalgesia produces a 12% decrease in IOP in normocapnic patients.[28] Intramuscular morphine produces a small decrease in IOP in normal and glaucomatous eyes, presumably by facilitating aqueous outflow.[29]

KETAMINE. Ketamine is an exception to the tendency of central nervous system–depressant drugs to reduce IOP. Administered intravenously or intramuscularly, ketamine initially was said to increase IOP significantly, as measured by indentation tonometry.[30] In more recent studies using applanation tonometry and diazepam–meperidine preanesthetic medication, ketamine produced no change in IOP when given to adults[31] and a 25% decrease when given intramuscularly to children.[32] However, ketamine's propensity to trigger nystagmus and blepharospasm makes it a suboptimal agent for many types of ophthalmic evaluations or surgery.

HYPOVENTILATION AND TEMPERATURE. Hypercapnia and hypoxia increase IOP, whereas hyperventilation reduces it.[33] These effects appear to be associated with changes in intracranial pressure consequent to vasodilatation or vasoconstriction. Hypothermia is thought to lower IOP by means of decreased formation of aqueous humor as well as vasoconstriction.

Muscle Relaxants

Nondepolarizing Neuromuscular Blocking Agents. Nondepolarizing neuromuscular blocking agents exert both direct and indirect effects on IOP. For example, d-tubocurarine, given in paralyzing doses, directly decreases IOP by relaxing the extraocular muscles,[34] as do equivalent doses of other nondepolarizing agents such as gallamine[33] and pancuronium.[34,35] However, if paralysis of the respiratory muscles is associated with alveolar hypoventilation and attendant hypercapnia, secondary effects may supervene to elevate IOP.

SUCCINYLCHOLINE. Succinylcholine, in contradistinction to nondepolarizing relaxant agents, increases IOP. Lincoff and colleagues,[36] in 1955, were the first to report extrusion of vitreous after succinylcholine administration intraoperatively in the presence of an open eye. An average peak IOP increase of 8 mm Hg occurs 1 to 4 minutes after intravenous administration, and a return to baseline occurs within 7 minutes.[21] Postulated mechanisms for the hypertensive effect of succinylcholine include tonic contraction of extraocular muscles,[23] choroidal vascular dilatation, and relaxation of orbital smooth muscle.[37] A recent study suggests that the ocular hypertensive effect may be primarily the result of the cycloplegic action of succinylcholine producing a deepening of the anterior chamber and increased outflow resistance.[38]

Numerous techniques have been claimed to prevent succinylcholine-induced increase in IOP. None of these methods consistently and reliably blocks this hypertensive response although some attenuation may result. Prior administration of acetazolamide[39] or of propranolol[40] has been said to abolish succinylcholine-induced increases in IOP.

The efficacy of pretreatment with nondepolarizing agents is highly controversial. Using indentation tonometry, Miller and associates reported that pretreatment with small doses of curare or gallamine prevented the increase.[41] However, Meyers's group, using the more sensitive applanation tonometer, could not consistently block the ocular hypertensive response when testing similar pretreatment methods.[42] To confuse the matter further, a "self-taming" dose of succinylcholine was claimed to be protective,[43] but Meyers and coworkers refuted this claim in a controlled study in which applanation tonometry was used.[44] Lidocaine pretreatment, 1 to 2 mg/kg administered intravenously, may attenuate the hemodynamic response to laryngoscopy,[45,46] but this pretreatment may be ineffective in preventing the ocular hypertensive response after succinylcholine administration or intubation.[47]

Although succinylcholine, given without pretreatment, is contraindicated in patients with penetrating ocular wounds and should not be given for the first time after the eye has been opened, the admonition that this agent be used only with great reluctance in ophthalmic surgery no longer seems rational. Clearly, in normal conditions, any increase in IOP after succinylcholine is administered is dissipated before surgery is begun. Of relevance, however, is Jampolsky's caveat that succinylcholine be avoided in patients undergoing a second operation for strabismus because the result of the forced duction test does not return to normal until 30 minutes after administration of the drug.[48]

ANESTHETIC MANAGEMENT OF OPEN EYE INJURY

Repair of a penetrating eye injury in the presence of a full stomach presents special challenges. The selected anesthetic approach must balance the risk of pulmonary aspiration against the risk of blindness resulting from elevated IOP and extrusion of ocular contents. Preoperative prophylaxis against aspiration may include the use of histamine H_2 receptor antagonists to reduce gastric acid production and to increase gastric pH[49,50]; metoclopramide to stimulate peristalsis and enhance gastric emptying; and nonparticulate antacids.

Induction

Use of a barbiturate, nondepolarizing relaxant technique frequently is suggested as the method of choice for emergency repair of an open eye injury, because the nondepolarizing relaxant pancuronium, 0.15 mg/kg, has been shown to decrease IOP.[51] Despite its widespread acceptance, this technique has associated disadvantages, not the least of which is risk of aspiration and death during the relatively long period, varying from 75 seconds[51] to 2.5 minutes,[52] that the airway is unprotected. A premature attempt at intubation results in coughing, straining, and a marked increase in IOP; cardiovascular side effects may include detrimental tachycardia, hypertension, and increased sympathetic tone. Furthermore, the prolonged duration of action of high-dose pancuronium may necessitate postoperative ventilation if the operation is unexpectedly short. Other nondepolarizing relaxants, such as atracurium and vecuronium, have shorter durations of action; vecuronium has minimal cardiovascular effects, and atracurium does not accumulate in plasma. However, in equipotent doses, these drugs have an onset of action similar to that of pancuronium.[53,54]

Succinylcholine offers the distinct advantages of rapid onset, excellent conditions for intubation, and short duration of action. After pretreatment with a nondepolarizing relaxant and an induction dose of thiopental (eg, at least 4 mg/kg), succinylcholine causes only minimal increases in IOP above baseline.[55] Although the acceptability of this method has been vociferously debated, published case reports do not document loss of intraocular contents resulting from its application in this challenging setting.[56,57] On completion of surgery and return to spontaneous respiration, an awake extubation is performed with the patient in a head-down lateral position.

Rocuronium,[58] with its purportedly rapid onset, may prove to be a useful nondepolarizing relaxant in this setting. However, additional data are needed before rocuronium can be recommended in this situation.

THE OCULOCARDIAC REFLEX

Causes

Initially described in 1908 by Aschner and Dagnini, the oculocardiac reflex consists of cardiac slowing in response to pressure on the globe and traction on the conjunctiva, orbital structures, or extraocular muscles. It also may be triggered by a retrobulbar block,[59] ocular trauma, and direct pressure on tissue remaining in the orbital apex after enucleation.[60]

This reflex may appear during local or general anesthesia, irrespective of depth, but hypercapnia or hypoxemia is said to increase its incidence and severity. The afferent limb is the trigeminal nerve, and the efferent limb is the vagus. Although sinus bradycardia is the most common manifestation, other dysrhythmias include junctional rhythm, atrioventricular block, ventricular bigeminy, wandering pacemaker, idioventricular rhythm, and asystole. The reported incidence of the reflex varies considerably, from 16% to 82%.[59–61] Commonly, the reports citing a higher incidence involve children because they have increased vagal tone.

Despite controversy surrounding the incidence and prophylaxis of the reflex, continuous monitoring of the electrocardiogram by the anesthesiologist is mandatory during eye surgery to discover ominous rhythm derangements.

Prevention and Treatment

Several methods to obtund or abolish the reflex have been advocated, but none has proven entirely effective, and each introduces some hazards. Anticholinergic agents such as atropine, scopolamine, or glycopyrrolate given intramuscularly are ineffective for prophylaxis against this reflex.[62–64] However, atropine administered intravenously within 30 minutes before surgery is said to reduce the incidence of the reflex; reports differ concerning timing and dose.[62] Some argue that the administration of intravenous atropine is associated with more ominous and more refractory dysrhythmia.[65] Atropine may be considered a potential myocardial irritant; virtually every possible dysrhythmia[66,67] and numerous conduction defects[68]—including ventricular tachycardia, ventricular fibrillation, and left bundle branch block—have been observed after intravenous atropine administration.

The possible protective value of retrobulbar block is acknowledged, but its disadvantages include stimulation of the reflex arc by the block, retrobulbar hemorrhage, and optic nerve damage, among other complications.

Adults

Many anesthesiologists concur that prophylactic measures, replete with their inherent hazards, are not usually indicated in adults.[69] Should a dysrhythmia occur, the initial approach is to ask the surgeon to stop manipulation. Then the patient's ventilatory status is quickly assessed. Heart rate and rhythm often return to baseline values within 20 seconds. Furthermore, with repeated manipulation, bradycardia is less likely to recur, probably because of fatigue of the oculocardiac reflex at the level of the cardioinhibitory center.[70] If the initial occurrence of the reflex is especially dramatic or if the reflex persistently recurs, atropine should be given intravenously, after the surgeon stops manipulation.

Children

Currently advocated practice for children undergoing surgery of the extraocular muscles is to administer 0.02 mg/kg atropine intravenously before beginning surgery.[69,71] In their report, Meyers and Tomeldan enthusiastically recommended intravenously administered anticholinergic agents as a prophylactic measure for children having correction of strabismus; they favored glycopyrrolate over atropine because, they claimed, the former causes less tachycardia.[72] Glycopyrrolate also does not cross the blood–brain barrier.

DRUG INTERACTIONS: ANESTHETIC IMPLICATIONS

The potential for drug interactions in ophthalmologic anesthesiology is great. Eyedrops and other medications used in the treatment of glaucoma and other ophthalmic conditions can exert undesirable systemic effects. Although medication tends to be absorbed slowly from the conjunctival sac, absorption is more rapid from mucosal surfaces. Therefore, absorption can be minimized by putting pressure on the inner canthus of the eye, thus occluding the nasolacrimal duct, for a few minutes after each instillation. Nasolacrimal duct occlusion is important in small children, who are highly susceptible to the toxic effects of certain drugs.

Anticholinesterase Agents

Long-acting anticholinesterase agents, such as echothiophate iodide, prolong the action of succinylcholine. Used in long-term glaucoma therapy, this miotic agent is absorbed into the systemic circulation after instillation into the conjunctival sac. Resultant pseudocholinesterase activity may be less than 5% of normal activity and requires 4 to 6 weeks to return to normal after discontinuation of the drug.[73]

Cocaine

Cocaine was first used as a local anesthetic by Koller in 1884. It is the only local anesthetic that inherently produces vasoconstriction and shrinkage of mucous membranes, yet it has limited topical use in the eye because of potential corneal injury. Cocaine as a nasal spray or in a nasal pack during dacryocystorhinostomy is popular. It inhibits catecholamine uptake at the nerve terminal and potentiates stimulation of the sympathetic nervous system.[74] Rapid absorption from mucosal surfaces results in plasma concentrations similar to those after direct intravenous injection.[74] The customary maximum dose in clinical practice is 200 mg for a 70-kg adult (approximately 3 mg/kg); a lethal dose is approximately 1 g. However, systemic reactions can occur after a dose as small as 20 mg.

Meyers reported two cases of cocaine toxicity during dacryocystorhinostomy.[75] She emphasizes that cocaine is contraindicated in hypertensive patients or in patients receiving adrenergic receptor agonists such as epinephrine and phenylephrine. Drugs such as halothane that sensitize the myocardium to catecholamines also are probably best avoided.

Physicians planning to use cocaine or another potent vasoconstrictor before dacryocystorhinostomy should carefully consider possible contraindications. Doses of dilute solutions should be calculated and administered with meticulous care so that toxic levels are avoided. Should serious cardiovascular effects occur, then labetalol offers the advantage of both α- and β-blockade. Previously propranolol had been used to control cocaine-induced hypertension,[76] but more recently a lethal hypertensive exacerbation was ascribed to unopposed α-stimulation following propranolol.[77]

Epinephrine

Topical ocular epinephrine (eg, 2% solution) has been noted to cause hypertension, angina, tachycardia, other dysrhythmias, and nervousness.[78] Of interest to ophthalmologists is the report of possible denervation supersensitivity to topical epinephrine after long-term therapy.[79]

Phenylephrine

Phenylephrine ophthalmic solution produces pupillary dilation and capillary decongestion. Although systemic effects after topical application of a judicious dose are uncommon,[80] severe hypertension, headache, and bradycardia may occur.[78,81,82] Patients with coronary artery disease are susceptible to severe ischemia, dysrhythmias, and myocardial infarction after administration of 10% phenylephrine eyedrops; patients with cerebral aneurysms may have cerebral hemorrhage.[83,84] Whether absorption is mainly from the conjunctiva or the nasal mucosa after drainage through the tear ducts is unclear. Certainly, phenylephrine should not be given topically after eye surgery has begun and venous channels are patent.

Children are especially vulnerable to overdose and manifest a dramatic response to phenylephrine eyedrops. Hence, the use of a 2.5% solution of phenylephrine is recommended in infants and elders. The frequency of application should be strictly limited.

Atropine

Atropine eye drops are used as a mydriatic and cycloplegic agent. Sufficient systemic absorption can occur to result in cardiac dysrhythmias, such as supraventricular tachycardia and atrial fibrillation.[85]

Timolol

Timolol, a nonselective β-adrenergic receptor blocking agent, is a drug topically administered for glaucoma and appears to be accepted better by patients than are many alternative drugs. Because significant conjunctival absorption may occur, timolol should be used with caution, if at all, for patients with known contraindications (asthma, congestive heart failure, or heart block greater than first degree) to systemic β-adrenergic receptor blocking agents.

Chronic, stable asthma has been reported occasionally to become uncontrollable after the administration of timolol eyedrops.[86] Severe sinus bradycardia developed in a patient with a variety of cardiac conduction defects after timolol eyedrops.[87] Furthermore, timolol has been implicated in the exacerbation of myasthenia gravis[88] and in the occurrence of postoperative apnea in neonates and young infants.[89,90]

Severe bronchospasm was reported in an elderly woman taking metoprolol when acetylcholine was injected into the anterior chamber for miosis during cataract extraction.[91] Because acetylcholine is widely used for this application, the anesthesiologist and ophthalmologist should be aware of potential complications in patients with bronchospastic or severe coronary artery disease.

Betaxolol

Betaxolol is a relatively recent addition to the list of topical agents used for glaucoma. In contrast to timolol, betaxolol is a selective β_1-blocker and has fewer systemic effects. Although betaxolol has produced only minimal effects in patients with mild to moderate obstructive airways disease, the drug is contraindicated in those patients with congestive heart failure and greater than first-degree heart block.

Intraocular Sulfur Hexafluoride and Nitrous Oxide

During repair of a detached retina, the ophthalmologist may inject intraocular air or sulfur hexafluoride into the vitreous to assist reattachment mechanically.[92] If used in the presence of nitrous oxide, the injected bubble can enlarge and cause a marked and rapid increase in IOP, which reaches a maximum value within 24 minutes.[83] In the presence of 70% nitrous oxide, 1 mL of air increases in volume to 2.85 mL within 1 hour; this expansion is even greater when the poorly diffusible sulfur hexafluoride is used. The resultant increase in IOP can compromise retinal circulation.

Stinson and Donlon recommended discontinuation of nitrous oxide 15 minutes before sulfur hexafluoride injection to prevent marked increase in the size of the intravitreous gas bubble.[93] The patient can then breathe almost 100% oxygen (admixed with a low concentration of volatile anesthetic) for the remainder of the procedure without material alteration in intravitreous gas dynamics. Wolf and colleagues demonstrated that during ventilation with oxygen, the volume of the intravitreal sulfur hexafluoride bubble increases by 35%, whereas the volume of the intravitreal air bubble decreases by 13%.[94] They recommend that if a patient requires anesthesia after intravitreal gas injection, administration of nitrous oxide be avoided for 5 days after air injection and for 10 days after sulfur hexafluoride injection.[94]

Systemic Ophthalmic Drugs

In addition to the aforementioned topical therapies, some ophthalmic drugs used systemically can cause complications. Mannitol, for example, can produce hypokalemia and hyponatremia that may be associated with dysrhythmias.[95] Hypotension, hypertension, angina, congestive heart failure, and renal failure also have been reported. Acetazolamide, a sulfonamide derivative, exerts its ocular antihypertensive effect by inhibiting carbonic anhydrase and, hence, secretion of aqueous humor. However, renal carbonic anhydrase also is affected, so bicarbonate diuresis with significant loss of water, sodium, and potassium occurs with chronic use. Thus, the status of patients receiving long-term acetazolamide treatment can be acidotic, hyponatremic, and hypokalemic. Persons with chronic lung disease may be especially vulnerable to the development of severe acidosis with the use of acetazolamide.

Fluorescein Angiography

Ophthalmologists frequently use fluorescein angiography to study ocular circulatory dynamics, sometimes while the patient is anesthetized for an ophthalmic surgical procedure. Among 55 patients who had a history of allergy or other untoward response to drugs or injections and for whom monitoring by an anesthesiologist was requested by the ophthalmologist, several symptoms were reported after injection of the dye; these included nausea (4 patients); pruritus or urticaria (2); chest pressure (2); severe hypertension (1); hypotension with bradycardia (2); hypotension with convulsion (1); and hypotension with bradycardia, loss of consciousness, and airway obstruction (1).[96]

Although nausea is the most frequent complication, deaths have been officially attributed to fluorescein angiography, often following myocardial infarction. According to Jannuzzie and colleagues,[97] the death rate is approximately 1 per 222,000. Despite extensive investigations, the pathophysiologic mechanisms(s) involved in serious reactions to fluorescein remain undetermined.

CONGENITAL AND METABOLIC DISEASES: OCULAR AND ANESTHETIC IMPLICATIONS

Many congenital and metabolic diseases are associated with ocular pathologic lesions and have important anesthetic implications. A partial list includes such syndromes as Crouzon's, Apert's, Goldenhar's (oculoauriculovertebral dysplasia), Sturge-Weber, Marfan's, Lowe's (oculocerebrorenal syndrome), Down (trisomy 21), Wagner-Stickler's, and Riley-Day's (familial dysautonomia). Other entities in this category are sickle cell disease and homocystinuria. Because discussion of these diseases is beyond the scope of this chapter, the reader is referred to other literature.[98] However, a brief review of homocystinuria is appropriate.

Homocystinuria

Pathogenesis

Homocystinuria, an inborn error of sulfur amino acid metabolism, results in the excretion of large amounts of urinary homocystine. It is associated with various abnormalities but most commonly with a deficiency of cystathionine β-synthase.[99] Though rare, homocystinuria is generally considered the second most common inborn error of amino acid metabolism, ranking behind phenylketonuria. Various stigmata are associated with the disease, but ocular findings often include myopia and ectopia lentis. The lens may subluxate into the anterior chamber, producing pupillary block glaucoma that requires surgical intervention.

Complications

In affected patients, the incidence of thromboembolic complications is high and is linked with a high mortality.[100] If untreated, homocystinuria may result in an intraoperative mortality rate as high as 50%. Abnormal amounts of homocystine irritate the vascular intima, fostering thrombolic nidus formation and increased platelet adhesiveness.[101] In addition to thromboembolic dangers, homocystinuric patients are also at risk for hypoglycemic convulsions resulting from hyperinsulinemia thought to be triggered by hypermethionemia.[102]

Treatment includes preoperative intervention to restrict homocystine levels and to prevent aberrancy in platelet function. The former goal is accomplished by a low-methionine, high-cystine diet and administration of vitamins B_6 and B_{12} and folic acid. The latter objective is achieved by administering acetylsalicylic acid and dipyridamole.[103]

Perioperative Management

With proper perioperative treatment, homocystinuric patients can have a smooth course. In addition to careful dietary and drug therapy, proper management includes prevention of hypoglycemia and practical measures to maintain adequate circulation. The latter includes the use of dextran 40 and intraoperative wrapping and manipulation of the extremities (eg, with sequential-inflation TED® stockings). Specific elements of anesthetic management include selection of techniques and drugs that favor high peripheral blood flow, reduction of vascular resistance, maintenance of cardiac output, rapid postanesthetic recovery, and early ambulation.[104]

HAZARDS IN EMERGENCE

At the time of tracheal extubation, the anesthesiologist is always concerned about potentially serious problems such as pulmonary aspiration, laryngospasm, and airway obstruction. The ocular anesthesiologist is, in addition, very eager to prevent coughing, retching, and vomiting to avoid deleterious increases in IOP that can compromise surgical outcome. Furthermore, because many ophthalmic procedures, such as strabismus repair and cataract extraction, are now performed in the ambulatory setting, the practical consequences of intractable, debilitating nausea and vomiting become obvious.

Nausea and Vomiting

With the possible exceptions of surgery for strabismus or retinal detachment and cryosurgery, ophthalmic operations are associated with little pain. Hence, routine preoperative use of opioids, which have a potential emetic side effect, is not advocated. Rather, preanesthetic medication should be selected with a view toward sedation, amnesia, and antiemesis. Rational choices include a benzodiazepine for its sedative–hypnotic effect or the phenothiazine promethazine or the antihistamine hydroxyzine for their sedative, antiemetic properties.

Vomiting after eye muscle surgery is distressingly common, giving credence to the existence of an oculogastric reflex. Abramowitz and colleagues reported that the prophylactic intravenous administration of 0.075 mg/kg droperidol given 30 minutes before termination of surgery reduced the frequency and severity of vomiting from 85% to 43% in children undergoing strabismus repair.[105] Furthermore, they observed no significant prolongation of recovery time due to sedation with this medication. More recently, the administration of the same dose of droperidol at induction of anesthesia, before manipulation of the eye, has reduced the incidence of vomiting after strabismus surgery to a clinically more acceptable level of approximately 10%.[106] Ondansetron, a new serotonin antagonist, is an extremely effective antiemetic agent.[107,108] In one study an intravenous dose of 8 mg was administered 10 minutes before induction.[108] Preoperative prophylactic administration was found to be superior to that achieved with droperidol and metoclopramide in the prevention of postoperative vomiting.

Coughing

Coughing on the endotracheal tube may be attenuated by the intravenous administration of 1.5 to 2 mg/kg lidocaine before extubation. On completion of surgery, after resumption of spontaneous respiration, the endotracheal tube is removed while the patient is still deeply anesthetized in a lateral position with the operated eye uppermost.

OCULAR COMPLICATIONS DURING NONOPHTHALMIC ANESTHESIA

Corneal Abrasion

Corneal abrasion caused by the surgical drapes, anesthetic mask, or the anesthetist's fingers is the most common ocular complication of general anesthesia. In most instances, however, the mechanism of injury is not known (Table 28-6).[18] Corneal abrasion can be avoided by selection of proper mask size and by care in laryngoscopy, intubation, and positioning. The corneal epithelium also can be damaged through drying while it remains exposed to room air for a lengthy period. Application of adhesive tape over the closed lids affords corneal protection. Some anesthesiologists routinely apply an ophthalmic ointment, although no evidence exists that doing so is more effective than merely taping the lids shut.

Iatrogenic superficial ocular damage also can occur as a result of chemical injury from spillage of solutions during skin preparation. One case report described chemical conjunctivitis from glutaraldehyde on an anesthesia mask.[109] Again, with meticulous attention to detail, these complications are preventable. The patient having corneal abrasion usually reports the sensation of a foreign body in the eye, tears, photophobia, and pain that is exacerbated by ocular movement and blinking. While recovering from anesthesia, however, the patient may describe only diffuse pain. An immediate ophthalmologic consultation is advisable. Treatment consists of putting the injured eye to rest by patching and applying antibiotic ointment. Healing usually occurs within 24 hours. Permanent sequelae are possible, although they are not nearly as common as those resulting from movement-related injuries during intraocular surgery (Fig. 28-1).

Thermal Injury

The potential for thermal injury to the cornea or retina from certain laser beams requires that the patient's eyes be pro-

TABLE 28-6
Mechanisms of Perioperative Eye Injury

MECHANISM OF INJURY	ALL EYE INJURIES (n = 71) n (%)	CORNEAL ABRASION (n = 25) n (%)
Patient movement	21 (30)	0
Chemical injury	9 (13)	1 (4)
Direct trauma	6 (8)	4 (16)
Pressure on eye	2 (3)	0
Other	3 (4)	0
Unknown	30 (42)	20 (80)

Gild WM, Posner KL, Caplan RA, et al: Eye injuries associated with anesthesia. Anesthesiology 76:205, 1992.

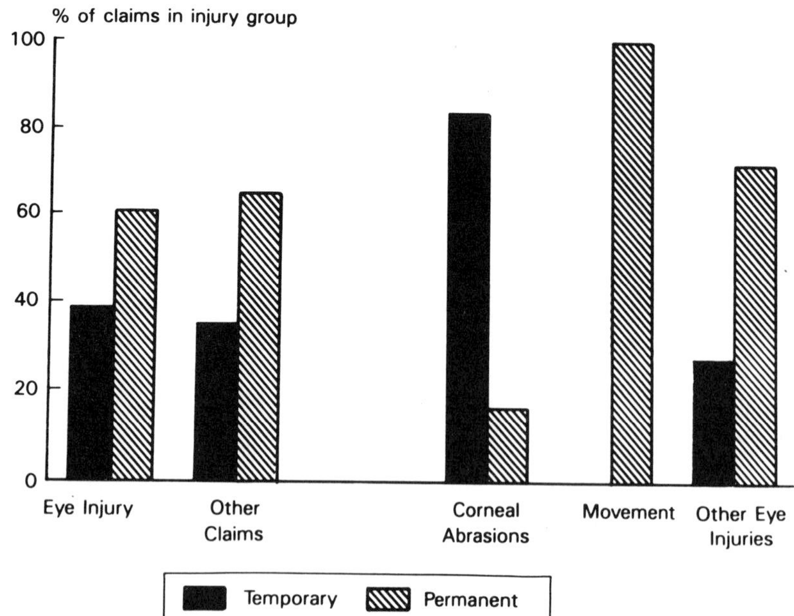

FIGURE 28-1. Severity of injury. Distribution of temporary and permanent injuries in eye injury claims compared with claims for other injuries. Permanent injuries in non–eye injury claims included 36% deaths and 28% other permanent injuries. There were no deaths among the cases of eye injury. Patient movement was alleged to be the mechanism of injury in all cases of vitreous loss or hemorrhage. (Legend modified from Gild WM, Posner KL, Caplan RA, et al: Eye injuries associated with anesthesia: a closed claims analysis. Anesthesiology 76:204, 1992.)

tected with moist gauze pads and metal shields and that operating room personnel wear protective glasses.[100a] These goggles must be appropriately tinted for the specific wavelength they are intended to block. Clear goggles are acceptable with the carbon dioxide laser, whereas the argon, Nd-YAG, or Nd-YAG-KTP lasers require goggles that are tinted orange, green, and orange-red, respectively.

Retinal Hemorrhage

After anesthesia, mild visual symptoms such as diplopia or photophobia are common.[111] Dhamee and colleagues reported a 7% to 14% incidence of benign, ephemeral visual disturbances after gynecologic procedures.[112] By contrast, loss of vision postoperatively is rare, though extremely disturbing. Recognized causes of serious visual symptoms in the postoperative period include acute corneal epithelial edema,[113] central retinal hypoperfusion with occipital infarction,[114] and Valsalva hemorrhagic retinopathy involving the macula.[115]

Retinal Venous Hemorrhage

Valsalva retinopathy refers to retinal hemorrhages, occurring in otherwise healthy persons, attributable to hemodynamic changes resulting from protracted vomiting or "stormy" emergence from anesthesia.[115] These venous hemorrhages are usually self-limiting, and complete resolution can be expected in a few days to a few months.

Retinal venous hemorrhages also are associated with a spectrum of diseases such as cystic fibrosis,[116] chronic obstructive lung disease,[117] migraine headache,[118] and battered child syndrome.[119] They are noted in a relatively large segment of high-altitude climbers,[120] in some of whom the visual impairment may be permanent.[121]

The majority of cases of retinal hemorrhage are asymptomatic; no visual changes are reported unless the macula is involved. (Indeed, 20% to 40% of neonates delivered vaginally have retinal venous hemorrhages.[122]) As with Valsalva retinopathy, complete recovery is the norm. However, should massive hemorrhage or optic atrophy develop as a result of bleeding into the optic nerve, permanent visual impairment may ensue.[123] In some cases of massive hemorrhage, vitrectomy may be helpful.

Retinal Ischemia

Arterial Bleeding

Retinal bleeding may also arise primarily from the arterial circulation. When this bleeding occurs after extraocular trauma, funduscopic examination typically discloses cotton-wool exudates, a sign of ischemia[124] known as Purtscher's retinopathy. This pathologic condition has a poor prognosis, with the majority of victims sustaining permanent visual impairment.[125] Thus, Purtscher's retinopathy should be part of the differential diagnosis when a trauma patient reports post-anesthetic vision loss.

Trauma, Embolism, and Intraocular Hypertension

Direct trauma to the eye by pressure exerted with an improperly fitting anesthetic mask can cause compression of the central retinal artery and resultant ischemia of the retina or optic nerve. This complication is especially apt to occur during hypotensive episodes. Retinal ischemia and infarction also may be caused by embolism during cardiac surgery.[126] As noted above, an increase in IOP sufficient to compromise retinal blood supply can occur if, during surgery to correct retinal detachment, more than 40% of the vitreous is replaced with sulfur hexafluoride and nitrous oxide is administered.

Acute Glaucoma

Anticholinergic Drugs

As is well known, atropine and scopolamine, when placed into the conjunctival sac, are mydriatic agents. Hence, the *topical* application of these drugs is contraindicated in patients with glaucoma. Concern was voiced several decades ago that acute glaucoma might be precipitated or exacerbated as a result of the pupillary dilatation produced by the perioperative use of anticholinergic drugs given parenterally. However, these drugs given *systemically* in the usual preanesthetic doses have no effect on pupil size or IOP in normal eyes[127] or in glaucomatous eyes.[128] Moreover, the use of atropine–neostigmine mixtures has minimal effects on pupil size and IOP when given intravenously to antagonize neuromuscular blockade.[129]

Precipitating Events

Acute angle-closure glaucoma caused by pupillary block is a multifactorial disease for which the risk factors include genetic predisposition,[130] shallow anterior chamber depth,[131] increased lens thickness,[131] small corneal diameter,[131] female gender,[131] and increasing age.[130] Although precipitating events in persons at risk are little comprehended, emotional factors have been believed to be causative, because psychological stress produces mydriasis.[132] A 1985 study found nine cases of acute angle-closure glaucoma occurring after spinal or general anesthesia among the 913 records reviewed.[133] No evidence suggested that the type of anesthetic agent, duration of the procedure, intraoperative blood pressure, or total amount of parenteral fluids administered predisposed patients to acute angle-closure glaucoma.

Preventive Measures

Acute angle-closure glaucoma is a serious and relatively unrecognized complication of surgical anesthesia. Nonophthalmic surgeons and anesthesiologists should become aware of this complication because delay in diagnosis can compromise the prognosis. Fazio and colleagues recommend that preoperative evaluation include a careful ocular history and a penlight examination to exclude a shallow anterior chamber.[133] Patients deemed to be at increased risk should have a preoperative ophthalmic evaluation as well as perioperative instillation of a miotic agent such as pilocarpine. Postoperatively, patients at risk should be observed closely for pain, blurred vision, or red eye. The pupil can be "mid-dilated" and oval, rather than round, in shape. Tonometric measurement of IOP should be performed promptly if any of these signs develop.

OCULAR COMPLICATIONS OF PREMATURITY AND OXYGEN THERAPY

Retinopathy of Prematurity

Retrolental fibroplasia (RLF) is a complex disorder the etiology of which has not been fully explained. The notion that increased arterial oxygen partial pressure (Pa_{O_2}) is completely responsible for RLF has been discarded during the past few years. We now know that the disease is multifactorial and that in some very small infants, despite meticulous monitoring of blood gases, it is not totally preventable.[134–137] The term "retinopathy of prematurity" (ROP) is used to describe all phases of retinal changes observed in premature infants; the traditional term, "RLF," describes not the acute phase of this disorder but rather the later cicatricial changes that involve the eyes of only the most severely affected infants.

Incidence

Acute retinal changes develop in approximately 45% of premature neonates with a birth weight of less than 1000 g.[138,139] In 80% to 90% of this group, the acute retinal changes regress spontaneously,[132] but in the remaining 10% to 20%, cicatricial changes develop in the retina and can lead to blindness.[140] The timing and progression of the acute proliferative lesions to severe cicatricial involvement are difficult to predict and are probably influenced by factors other than perinatal oxygen exposure alone.

Low gestational age and birth weight of less than 1000 g exert great influence on the incidence of retinopathy. Flynn states, "Acute RLF is simply so prevalent in lower–birth-weight infants (less than or equal to 1000 g) that no acquired risk factor, surgical or medical disease, or therapy significantly affected the outcome."[141]

Role of Oxygen

Sporadic cases of retinopathy of prematurity have been reported in premature neonates who received little or no supplemental oxygen. Patz asserts that these rare cases can still be explained on the basis of the effects of oxygen.[142] The fetus lives with a low Pa_{O_2} due, in part, to the normal admixture of venous and arterial blood. After birth, with lung expansion and closure of the ductus arteriosus and the foramen ovale, the Pa_{O_2} in the normal premature neonate increases rapidly even without supplemental oxygen. Possibly, a sensitive premature retina responds to this sudden increase in retinal Pa_{O_2} with irreversible retinal arterial and arteriolar vasoconstriction and vaso-obliteration.

Gestational Age

Of note, ROP has also been reported in full-term infants. In 1928, Mann proposed that the retina is fully vascularized after 8 months gestation.[143] Subsequently, however, Cogan demonstrated that the temporal retina normally is incompletely vascularized even in full-term infants and that the anterior temporal portion becomes fully vascularized only during the first few weeks of life.[144] Moreover, Brockhurst and Chishti described six patients with typical findings of RLF[145]; none of the patients had received supplemental oxygen therapy after birth, and three patients were full-term.

All of the cases occurring in full-term babies showed major involvement of the temporal peripheral retina. The propensity for ROP to occur in the temporal quadrant also supports the concept of oxygen susceptibility of immature retinal vessels because the anterior temporal region is the last zone of the retina to become completely vascularized.

Recommendations for Oxygen Administration

Even in the full-term infant, oxygen therapy should be limited to specific clinical indications and not administered indiscriminately. When supplemental oxygen must be administered to an infant whose postconception age is less than 44 weeks for respiratory therapy or general anesthesia, the physician should strive to keep the Pa_{O_2} within a normal range to minimize the likelihood of ocular injury. An oxygen–air blender is often useful in accomplishing this goal. Transcutaneous oxygen monitors are not accurate when exposed to surgical stresses; nitrous oxide and inhalational agents; electric currents in electrocautery; and changes in skin blood flow. The pulse oximeter is much more reliable for this application during anesthesia.

In 1976, the American Academy of Pediatrics recommended that the Pa_{O_2} of the newborn be kept between 60 and 100 mm Hg.[146] More recently, Bucher and colleagues suggest maintaining the oxygen saturation at 93% to 95% to avoid hyperoxia.[147] Nonetheless, adherence to these guidelines does not guarantee a safe outcome for vision. Although controversial, it has been argued that carbon dioxide, bright light in the hospital nursery, and vitamin E deficiency may be three additional factors in the pathogenesis of ROP.[148] Despite scrupulous, continuous monitoring of Pa_{O_2} in premature neonates, retinopathy of prematurity probably still will occur; it is a disease that tantalizes experts with many unanswered questions.

REFERENCES

1. McGoldrick KE: Current concepts in anesthesia for ophthalmic surgery. Anesthesiology Review 7:7, 1980
2. Rosen DA: Anesthesia in ophthalmology. Can Anaesth Soc J 9:545, 1962
3. McGoldrick KE: Pediatric anesthesia for ophthalmic surgery. In Bruce RA, McGoldrick KE, Oppenheimer P (eds): Anesthesia for ophthalmology. Birmingham, AL: Aesculapius, 1982: 51
4. Lynch S, Wolf GL, Berlin I: General anesthesia for cataract surgery: a comparative review of 2217 consecutive cases. Anesth Analg 53:909, 1972
5. Edge KR, Martin J, Nicoll JMV: Retrobulbar hemorrhage after 12,500 retrobulbar blocks. Anesth Analg 76:1019, 1993
6. Feibel RM: Current concepts in retrobulbar anesthesia. Surv Ophthalmol 30: 102, 1985
7. Rainin EA, Carlson BM: Postoperative diplopia and ptosis: a clinical hypothesis based on the mycotoxicity of local anesthetics. Arch Ophthalmol 103:1377, 1985
8. Chang J-L, Gonzalez-Abola E, Larson CE, et al: Brain stem anesthesia following retrobulbar block. Anesthesiology 61:789, 1984
9. Whittpenn JR, Rapoza P, Sternberg P Jr, et al: Respiratory arrest following retrobulbar anesthesia. Ophthalmology 93:867, 1986
10. Nicoll JMV, Acharya PA, Ahlen K, et al: Central nervous system complications after 6000 retrobulbar blocks. Anesth Analg 66: 1298, 1987
11. Javitt JC, Addiego R, Friedberg HL, et al: Brain stem anesthesia after retrobulbar block. Ophthalmology 49:718, 1987
12. Katsev DA, Drews RC, Rose B: An anatomic study of retrobulbar needle path length. Ophthalmology 96:1221, 1989
13. Liu C, Youl B, Moseley I: Magnetic resonance imaging of the optic nerve in extremes of gaze: implications for the positioning of the globe for retrobulbar anaesthesia. Br J Ophthalmol 76: 728, 1992
14. Unsöld R, Stanley JA, DeGroot J: The CT-topography of retrobulbar anesthesia. Graefes Arch Clin Exp Ophthalmol 217: 125, 1981
15. Donlon JV, Moss J: Plasma catecholamine levels during local anesthesia for cataract operations. Anesthesiology 51:471, 1979
16. Wilson CA, Ruiz RS: Respiratory obstruction following the Nadbath facial nerve block. Arch Ophthalmol 103:1454, 1985
17. Cofer HF: Cord paralysis after Nadbath facial nerve block. Arch Ophthalmol 104:337, 1986
18. Gild WM, Posner KL, Caplan RA: Eye injuries associated with anesthesia: a closed claims analysis. Anesthesiology 76:204, 1992
19. Adler FH: Physiology of the eye: clinical application, 5th ed. St. Louis: CV Mosby, 1970: 249
20. Joshi C, Bruce DL: Thiopental and succinylcholine: action on intraocular pressure. Anesth Analg 54:471, 1975
21. Pandey K, Badola RP, Kumar S: Time course of intraocular hypertension produced by suxamethonium. Br J Anaesth 44: 191, 1972
22. Hill DW: Physics applies to anesthesia, 4th ed. Woburn, MA: Butterworths, 1980: 172
23. Duncalf D, Foldes FF: Effect of anesthetic drugs and muscle relaxants on intraocular pressure. Int Anesthesiol Clin 13:21, 1973
24. Al-Abrak MH, Samuel JR: Further observation on the effects of general anesthesia on intraocular pressure in man: halothane with nitrous oxide and oxygen. Br J Anaesth 46:756, 1974
25. Ausinsch B, Braves SA, Munson ES, et al: Intraocular pressure in children during isoflurane and halothane anesthesia. Anesthesiology 42:167, 1975
26. Deroeth A, Schwartz H: Aqueous humor dynamics in glaucoma. Arch Ophthalmol 55:755, 1956
27. Thompson MF, Brock-Utne JG, Bean P, et al: Anaesthesia and intraocular pressure: a comparison of total intravenous anaesthesia using etomidate with conventional inhalational anaesthesia. Anaesthesia 37:758, 1982
28. Ivankovich AD, Lose HJ: Influence of methoxyflurane and neuroleptanesthesia on intraocular pressure in man. Anesth Analg 48:933, 1969
29. Mirakhur RK, Shepherd WFI, Darrah WK: Propofol and thiopentone: effects on intraocular pressure associated with induction of anaesthesia and tracheal intubation (facilitated with suxamethonium). Br J Anaesth 59:431, 1987
30. Yoshikawa R, Murai Y: Effect of ketamine on intraocular pressure in children. Anesth Analg 50:199, 1971
31. Peuler M, Glass DD, Arena JF: Ketamine and intraocular pressure. Anesthesiology 5:575, 1975
32. Ausinch B, Rayborn RL, Munson ES: Ketamine and intraocular pressure in children. Anesth Analg 55:773, 1976
33. Duncalf D, Weitzner SW: Ventilation and hypercapnia on intraocular pressure in children. Anesth Analg 43:232, 1963
34. Agarwal LP, Mathur SP: Curare in ocular surgery. Br J Ophthalmol 36:603, 1952
35. Litwiller RW, Difazio CA, Rushia EL: Pancuronium and intraocular pressure. Anesthesiology 42:750, 1975
36. Lincoff HA, Ellis CH, Devoe AG, et al: Effect of succinylcholine on intraocular pressure. Am J Ophthalmol 40:501, 1955
37. Bjork A, Halldin M, Wahlin A: Enophthalmus elicited by succinylcholine. Acta Anaesthesiol Scand 1:41, 1957
38. Kelly RE, Dinner M, Turner LS, et al: Succinylcholine increases intraocular pressure in the human eye with the extraocular muscles detached. Anesthesiology 79:948, 1993
39. Carballo AS: Succinylcholine and acetazolamide in anesthesia for ocular surgery. Can Anaesth Soc J 12:486, 1965
40. Kaufman L: General anaesthesia in ophthalmology. Proc R Soc Med 60:1275, 1967
41. Miller RD, Way WL, Hickey RF: Inhibition of succinylcholine-induced increased intraocular pressure by nondepolarizing muscle relaxants. Anesthesiology 29:123, 1968
42. Meyers EF, Krupin T, Johnson M, et al: Failure of nondepolarizing neuromuscular blockers to inhibit succinylcholineinduced increased intraocular pressure: a controlled study. Anesthesiology 48:149, 1978
43. Verma RS: 'Self-taming' of succinylcholine-induced fasciculations and intraocular pressure. Anesthesiology 50:245, 1979
44. Meyers EF, Singer P, Otto A: a controlled study of the effect of succinylcholine self-taming on intraocular pressure. Anesthesiology 53:72, 1980

45. Stoelting RK: Circulatory changes during direct laryngoscopy and tracheal intubation. Anesthesiology 47:381, 1977
46. Stoelting RK: Blood pressure and heart rate changes during short duration laryngoscopy for tracheal intubation: influences of viscous or intravenous lidocaine. Anesth Analg 57:197, 1978
47. Smith RB, Babinski M, Leano N: Effect of lidocaine on succinylcholine-induced rise in intraocular pressure. Can Anaesth Soc J 26:482, 1979
48. Jampolsky A: Strabismus: surgical overcorrections. Highlights in Ophthalmology 8:78, 1965
49. Williams JG: H_2 receptor antagonists and anaesthesia. Can Anaesth Soc J 30:264, 1983
50. Dobb G, Jordan MJ, Williams JG: Cimetidine in prevention of pulmonary acid aspiration syndrome. Br J Anaesth 51:967, 1979
51. Brown EM, Krishnaprasad D, Smiler BG: Pancuronium for rapid induction technique for tracheal intubation. Can Anaesth Soc J 26:489, 1979
52. Goudsouzian NG, Liu LMP, Cote CJ: Comparison of equipotent doses of nondepolarizing muscle relaxants in children. Anesth Analg 60:862, 1981
53. Savarese JJ: New neuromuscular blocking drugs are here. Anesthesiology 55:1, 1981
54. Basta SJ, Ali HH, Savarese JJ, et al: Clinical pharmacology of atracurium besylate (BW 33A): a new nondepolarizing muscle relaxant. Anesth Analg 61:723, 1982
55. Konchigeri HN, Lee YE, Venugopal K: Effect of pancuronium on intraocular pressure changes induced by succinylcholine. Can Anaesth Soc J 26:479, 1979
56. McCammon RL: Anesthesia for operations on the eye. In International Anesthesia Research Society Review Course Lectures, 1984. Cleveland: International Anesthesia Research Society, 1984: 109
57. Libonati MM, Leahy JJ, Ellison N: Use of succinylcholine in open eye surgery. Anesthesiology 62:637, 1985
58. Levy JH, Davis GK, Duggan J, et al: Determination of the hemodynamics and histamine release of rocuronium (Org 9426) when administered in increased doses under N_2O/O_2–sufentamil anesthesia. Anesth Analg 78:318, 1994
59. Berler DR: Oculocardiac reflex. Am J Ophthalmol 56:954, 1963
60. Kirsch RE, Samet PM Kugel V, et al: Electrocardiographic changes during ocular surgery and their prevention by retrobulbar injection. Arch Ophthalmol 58:348, 1957
61. Bosomworth PP, Ziegler CH, Jacoby J: Oculocardiac reflex in eye muscle surgery. Anesthesiology 19:7, 1958
62. Taylor C, Wilson FM, Roesch R, et al: Prevention of the oculocardiac reflex in children: comparison of retrobulbar block and intravenous atropine. Anesthesiology 24:646, 1963
63. Mirakhur RK, Clarke RSJ, Dundee JW, et al: Anticholinergic drugs in anaesthesia: a survey of their present position. Anaesthesia 33:133, 1978
64. Blanc VF, Hardy JF, Milot J: Oculocardiac reflex: a graphic and statistical analysis in infants and children. Can Anaesth Soc J 30:360, 1983
65. Ratz RL, Bigger JT: Cardiac arrhythmias during anesthesia and operation. Anesthesiology 33:193, 1970
66. Horgan J: Atropine and ventricular tachyarrhythmias. JAMA 223:693, 1973
67. Massumi RA, Mason DT, Amsterdam EA, et al: Ventricular fibrillation and tachycardia after intravenous atropine for treatment of bradycardias. N Engl J Med 287:336, 1972
68. McGoldrick KE: Transient left bundle branch block during local anesthesia. Anesthesiology Review 8:36, 1981
69. Schwartz H: Oculocardiac reflex: is prophylaxis necessary? In Mark LC, Ngai SH (eds): Highlights of clinical anesthesiology. New York: Harper & Row, 1971: 111
70. Moonie GT, Rees DI, Elton D: Oculocardiac reflex during strabismus surgery. Can Anaesth Soc J 11:621, 1964
71. Steward DJ: Anticholinergic premedication for infants and children. Can Anaesth Soc J 30:325, 1983
72. Meyers EF, Tomeldan SA: Glycopyrrolate compared with atropine in prevention of the oculocardiac reflex during eye muscle surgery. Anesthesiology 51:350,1979
73. Deroeth A, Detbarn W, Rosenberg P, et al: Effect of phospholine iodide on blood cholinesterase levels of normal and glaucoma subjects. Am J Ophthalmol 59:586, 1965
74. Ritchie JM, Greene NM: Local anesthetics. In Gilman AG, Goodman LS, Rall TW, et al (eds): The pharmacological basis of therapeutics, 7th ed. New York: Macmillan, 1985: 302
75. Meyers EF: Cocaine toxicity during dacryocystorhinostomy. Arch Ophthalmol 98:842, 1980
76. Rappolt RT, Gay GR, Inaba DS: Propranolol: a specific antagonist to cocaine. Clinical Toxicology 10:26 5, 1977
77. Ramosa E, Sacchetti AD: Propranolol-induced hypertension in treatment of cocaine intoxication. Ann Emerg Med 14:112, 1985
78. Lansche RR: Systemic effects of topical epinephrine and phenylephrine. Am J Ophthalmol 49:95, 1966
79. Flach AJ, Kramer SG: Supersensitivity to topical epinephrine after long term epinephrine therapy. Arch Ophthalmol 98:482, 1980
80. Brown MM, Brown GC, Spaeth GL: Lack of side effects from topically administered 10% phenylephrine eye drops: a controlled study. Arch Ophthalmol 98:487, 1980
81. Cass E, Kadar D, Stein HA: Hazards of phenylephrine topical medications in persons taking propranolol. Can Med Assoc J 120:1261, 1979
82. Solosko D, Smith RB: Hypertension following 10% phenylephrine ophthalmic. Anesthesiology 36:187, 1972
83. Adler AG, McElwain GE, Martin JH: Coronary artery spasm induced by phenylephrine eye drops. Arch Intern Med 141: 1384, 1981
84. Van Der Spek AFL, Hantler CB: Phenylephrine eyedrops and anesthesia. Anesthesiology 64:812, 1986
85. Merli GJ, Weitz H, Martin JH, et al: Cardiac dysrhythmias associated with ophthalmic atropine. Arch Intern Med 146:45, 1986
86. Jones FL, Eckberg NL: Exacerbation of asthma by timolol. N Engl J Med 301:270, 1979
87. Kim JW, Smith PH: Timolol-induced bradycardia. Anesth Analg 59:301, 1980
88. Shavitz SA: Timolol and myasthenia gravis. JAMA 242:1612, 1979
89. Olson RJ, Bromberg BB, Zimmerman TJ: Apneic spells associated with timolol therapy in a neonate. Am J Ophthalmol 88: 120, 1979
90. Bailey PL: Timolol and postoperative apnea in neonates and young infants. Anesthesiology 61:622, 1984
91. Rasch D, Holt J, Wilson M, et al: Bronchospasm following intraocular injection of acetylcholine in a patient taking metoprolol. Anesthesiology 59:583, 1983
92. Fineberg E, Machemer R, Sullivan P, et al: Sulfur hexafluoride in owl monkey vitreous cavity. Am J Ophthalmol 79:67, 1975
93. Stinson TW, Donlon JV: Interaction of SF_6 and air with nitrous oxide. Anesthesiology 51:S16, 1979
94. Wolf GL, Capuano C, Hartung J: Effect of nitrous oxide on gas bubble volume in the anterior chamber. Arch Ophthalmol 103: 418, 1985
95. Berry AJ, Peterson ML: Hyponatremia after mannitol administration in the presence of renal failure. Anesth Analg 60:165, 1981
96. Meyers EF: Fluorescein angiography complications. Anesthesiology Review 7:25, 1980
97. Yannuzzi LA, Rohrer KT, Tindel LF, et al: Fluorescein angiography complication survey. Ophthalmology 93:611, 1986
98. McGoldrick KE: Anesthetic implications of congenital and metabolic diseases. In Bruce RA, McGoldrick KE, Oppenheimer P (eds); Anesthesiology for ophthalmology. Birmingham, AL: Aesculapius, 1982: 139
99. Mudd SH, Levy HL: Disorders of transsulfuration. In Stanbury JB, Fredrickson DS, et al (eds): Metabolic basis of inherited disease, 5th ed. New York: McGraw-Hill, 1980: 522
100. Brown BR Jr, Walson PD, Taussig LM: Congenital metabolic diseases in pediatric patients: anesthetic implications. Anesthesiology 43:197, 1975

101. McDonald L, Bray C, Love F, et al: Homocystinuria, thrombosis, and the blood platelets. Lancet 1:745, 1964
102. Holmgren G, Falkmer S, Hambraeus L: Plasma insulin content and glucose tolerance in homocystinuria. Uppsala Journal of Medical Science 78: 215, 1975
103. Harker LA, Slichter SJ, Scott CR, et al: Homocystinemia: vascular injury and arterial thrombosis. N Engl J Med 291:537, 1974
104. McGoldrick KE: Anesthetic management of homocystinuria. Anesthesiology Review 8:42, 1981
105. Abramowitz MD, Epstein BS, Friendly DS, et al: Effect of droperidol in reducing vomiting in pediatric strabismic outpatient surgery. Anesthesiology 55:A329, 1981
106. Lerman J, Eustis S, Smith DR: Effect of droperidol pretreatment on postanesthetic vomiting in children undergoing strabismus surgery. Anesthesiology 65:322, 1986
107. Scuderi P, Wetchler B, Yung-Fong S, et al: Treatment of postoperative nausea and vomiting after outpatient surgery with the 5-HT_3 Antagonist ondansetron. Anesthesiology 78:15, 1993
108. Alon E, Himmelsehr: Ondansetron in the treatment of postoperative vomiting: a randomized double-blind comparison with droperidol and metoclopramide. Anesth Analg 75:561, 1992
109. Murray WJ, Ruddy MP: Toxic eye injury during induction of anesthesia. South Med J 78:1012, 1985
110. Kalhan SB, Cascorbi HF: Anesthetic management of laser microlaryngeal surgery. Anesthesiology Review 8:23, 1981
111. Conway C: Neurological and ophthalmic complications of anesthesia. In Churchill-Davidson HC (ed): A practice of anaesthesia, 5th ed. Chicago: Year Book Medical, 1984: 793
112. Dhamee MS, Ghandi SK, Munshi CA, et al: Anesthetic techniques for laparoscopy: morbidity after outpatient anesthesia. Anesthesiology Review 13:15, 1986
113. Richardson RB, McBride CM, Berkely RG, et al: An unusual ocular complication after anesthesia. Anesthesiology 43:357, 1975
114. Givner I, Jaffe N: Occlusion of the central retinal artery following anesthesia. Arch Ophthalmol 43:197, 1950
115. Devoe AG, Norton EWD, Kearns TP, et al: Valsalva hemorrhagic retinopathy: discussion. Trans Am Ophthalmol Soc 70: 307, 1972
116. Rimsza ME, Hernried LS, Kaplan AM: Hemorrhagic retinopathy in a patient with cystic fibrosis. Pediatrics 62:336, 1978
117. Austen FK, Carmichael MW, Adams RD: Neurologic manifestations of chronic and pulmonary insufficiency. N Engl J Med 257:579, 1957
118. Victor DI, Welch RB: Bilateral retinal hemorrhages and disk edema in migraine. Am J Ophthalmol 84:555, 1977
119. Mushin AS: Ocular damage in the battered-baby syndrome. British Medical Journal 3:402, 1971
120. McFadden DM, Houston CS, Sutton JR, et al: High-altitude retinopathy. JAMA 245:581, 1981
121. Shults WT, Swan KC: High altitude retinopathy in mountain climbers. Arch Ophthalmol 93:404, 1975
122. Jain IS, Singh YP, Grupta SL, et al: Ocular hazards during birth. J Pediatr Ophthalmol Strabismus 17:14, 1980
123. Madsen PH: Traumatic retinal angiopathy. Ophthalmologica 165:453, 1972
124. McLeod D: Reappraisal of the retinal cotton-wool spot. J R Soc Med 74:682, 1981
125. Teichmann KD, Gronemeyer U: Unilateral morbus purtscher with poor visual outcome. Ann Ophthalmol 13:1295, 1981
126. Gutman FA, Zegarra H: Ocular complications in cardiac surgery. Surg Clin North Am 51:1095, 1971
127. Cozanitis DA, Dundee JW, Buchanan TAS: Atropine versus glycopyrrolate. Anesthesia 34:236, 1979
128. Schwartz H, De Roeth A, Papper EM: Pre-anesthetic use of atropine in patients with glaucoma. JAMA 165:144, 1951
129. Rawstron RE, Hutchinson BR: Pupillary and circulatory changes at the termination of relaxant anesthesia. Br J Anaesth 35:795, 1963
130. Drance SM: Angle-closure glaucoma among canadian eskimos. Can J Ophthalmol 8:252, 1973
131. Alsbirk PH: Angle-closure glaucoma surveys in greenland eskimos. Can J Ophthalmol 8:260, 1973
132. Inman WS: Emotion and acute glaucoma. Lancet 2:1188, 1929
133. Fazio DT, Bateman JB, Christensen RE: Acute angle-closure glaucoma associated with surgical anesthesia. Arch Ophthalmol 103:360, 1985
134. McGoldrick KE: Factors influencing development of retrolental fibroplasia. Anesth Analg 60:539, 1981
135. Merritt JC, Sprague DH, Merritt WE, et al: Retrolental fibroplasia: a multifactorial disease. Anesth Analg 60:109, 1981
136. Sacks LM, Schaffer DB, Anday EK, et al: Retrolental fibroplasia and blood transfusion in very low-birth-weight infants. Pediatrics 68:770, 1981
137. Hammer ME, Mullen PW, Ferguson JG, et al: Logistic analysis of risk factors in acute retinopathy of prematurity. Am J Ophthalmol 102:1, 1986
138. Flynn JT: Acute proliferative retrolental fibroplasia: evolution of the lesion. Graefes Arch Klin Exp Ophthalmol 195:101, 1975
139. Kingham JD: Acute retrolental fibroplasia. Arch Ophthalmol 95:39, 1977
140. Flynn JT, Cassady J, Essner D, et al: Fluorescein angiography in retrolental fibroplasia: experience from 1969-1977. Ophthalmology 86:1700, 1979
141. Flynn JT: Oxygen and retrolental fibroplasia: update and challenge. Anesthesiology 60:397, 1984
142. Patz A: Role of oxygen in retrolental fibroplasia. Trans Am Ophthalmol Soc 66:940, 1968
143. Mann I: Development of the human eye. New York: Macmillan, 1928
144. Cogan DG: Development and senescence of human retinal vasculature. Transactions of the Ophthalmological Society of the United Kingdom 83:465, 1963
145. Brockhurst RJ, Chishti MI: Cicatricial retrolental fibroplasia: its occurrence without oxygen administration and in full-term infants. Graefes Arch Klin Exp Ophthalmol 195:128, 1975
146. American Academy of Pediatrics recommendations on oxygen use. Pediatrics 57(suppl):635, 1976
147. Bucher HU, Fanconi S, Baeckert P, et al: Hyperoxemia in newborn infants: detection by pulse oximetry. Pediatrics 84:226, 1989
148. Biglan AW, Brown D, Reynolds JD, et al: Risk factors associated with retrolental fibroplasia. Ophthalmology 91:1504, 1984

FURTHER READING

McGoldrick KE: Anesthesia for ophthalmic and otolaryngologic surgery. Philadelphia: WB Saunders, 1992: 176–302

Complications in Anesthesiology, second edition,
edited by Nikolaus Gravenstein and Robert R. Kirby.
Lippincott-Raven Publishers, Philadelphia © 1996.

CHAPTER 29

Awareness During Anesthesia

Marc Goldberg

Awareness during general anesthesia is undesired, unanticipated, patient wakefulness during surgery or recall afterward. In addition to being unexpected, awareness may be accompanied by anxiety and pain. In 1845, one of the first attempted demonstrations of general anesthesia, a dental extraction performed under nitrous oxide administered by Horace Wells, failed as the patient cried out in pain.[1] With the advent of ether and chloroform anesthesia, no further reports of awareness during general anesthesia appeared for 60 years. Crile began to encourage the use of nitrous oxide–oxygen for general anesthesia to avoid the cardiovascular depressant effects of ether in patients with shock.[2] He later reported that in 1908, although it has been performed with "complete nitrous oxide–oxygen anesthesia," a woman was able fully to describe her abdominal operation. Crile subsequently learned to supplement nitrous oxide–oxygen with morphine, atropine, and scopolamine.

Awareness during anesthesia became commonly reported only after the introduction of neuromuscular blocking drugs into anesthetic practice. Before the first clinical use of curare by Griffith and Johnson in 1942,[3] lack of patient movement and adequate muscle relaxation during surgery could be provided only by deep (stage 3) inhalational anesthesia. Curare allowed the dissociation of movement and relaxation from amnesia and analgesia. Until 1947, practitioners thought that curare might have central nervous system sedative effects. Smith and colleagues[4] demonstrated that a subject, one of the authors, could be paralyzed by curare, appear anesthetized, and yet have complete wakefulness and subsequent recall. They concluded that "if curare is to be used properly as an adjuvant in anesthesia, its inability to depress the central nervous system [should] be kept clearly in mind."

Winterbottom's case report in 1950[5] of awareness during a nitrous oxide–oxygen general anesthetic was the most prominent early report to call attention to this complication. Many subsequent reports have confirmed that awareness during anesthesia does occur, that it is more common in certain types of patients and operations, that it is often detectable and preventable, and that it may have long-lasting psychological sequelae.

INCIDENCE

The reported incidence of awareness during anesthesia depends on the type of anesthesia, the strength of the stimulus, and the timing and persistence of attempts to elicit recall. When a simple postoperative interview 12 to 48 hours after surgery is used, the reported incidences range from 0% to 7%.[6–10] Clifton and associates did not differentiate types of anesthetic or operation; 5 of 100 patients recalled dreams during surgery, and 1 had "vague" awareness.[6]

Hutchinson reported eight instances of recall or bad dreams in a series of 656 patients.[7] Use of a large dose of muscle relaxant, not supplemented by potent inhalation anesthetic agents, was significantly related to recall in this series. Urbach and Edelist reported one instance of awareness in 350 outpatient procedures but did not identify the type of anesthetic used.[8]

Fishburne and coworkers[9] described a retrospective series of 153 patients who received nitrous oxide (66% to 71%) oxygen–succinylcholine infusion and 0.1 mg fentanyl intravenously for laparoscopy. Patient response to a mailed questionnaire was 94%. Five percent of responding patients recalled conversation; 2% recalled tracheal intubation or extubation; and 1% recalled pain during the procedure. The rate of awareness during general anesthesia for trauma surgery has been reported to be 28%.[10]

Preoperative Medication

Taub and Eisenberg compared the addition of preoperative 10 mg morphine (Roosevelt technique) or morphine and diazepam pre- and intraoperatively with nitrous oxide–oxygen and curare (Liverpool technique).[11] Five percent of the group receiving the latter regimen had recall, as did 10% of those who received the Roosevelt technique. No patients who had morphine (13 to 20 mg) and diazepam (20 to 40 mg) did so. Patients in all three groups dreamed; the Liverpool and Roosevelt techniques resulted in frightening dreams, whereas patients who received morphine and diazepam reported neutral dreams.

Sensory Stimuli

Several studies have delivered specific sensory stimuli during anesthesia and assessed recall. Terrell and associates played a tape recording of nonstressful or mildly stressful messages during anesthetics of all types.[12] Recall of either type of message postoperatively could not be elicited, with or without hypnosis as an aid. However, the sample population in this study, 37 patients, was small. Brice and colleagues, using a nitrous oxide–oxygen and curare technique, exposed 57 patients to music during surgery.[13] Only 1 of 57 had vague intraoperative recall; however, 44% recalled dreaming. Patients who moved during surgery were more likely to have dreamed.

Nonstressful stimuli are rarely recalled during anesthesia. In contrast, Levinson investigated recall after a nitrous oxide–oxygen–ether anesthesic (concentration not recorded) during which the anesthetist had said loudly, "Just a moment. I don't like the patient's colour. Much too blue. His lips are very blue. I'm going to give a little more oxygen."[14] None of the ten patients was able to recall this statement in the awake state, but four recalled those words exactly during hypnosis, and four others awoke from hypnosis with great anxiety. This small study, not likely to be repeated for ethical reasons, demonstrated that certain sounds may be heard during general anesthesia and stored in the subconscious.

A small minority of anesthesiologists deny that recall during anesthesia exists ("[In] 20 years of practice of anesthesia I have never yet suffered the mortification of discovering that a patient supposedly under general anesthesia was in fact awake"),[15] but given the large number of case reports of vivid recall,[16–22] it is clear that awareness does occur.

In one case report, "a medically qualified lady" described her experience of awareness during cesarean section as follows:

> I gradually became aware of a mental haze [and] understood my predicament: that I was lying there intubated, my abdomen split open. . . . I made a massive effort to move my nonexistent right foot [and] a voice said, 'She's moving her toes; it's time you got her to sleep.' I remained in this state, continuously filled with fear. . . . [T]he pain I felt [was comparable to] the pain of a tooth drilled without local anesthetic—when the drill hits a nerve. Multiply this pain . . . [and] then pour a steady stream of molten lead into it. . . . I could not stand the pain for a split second longer. The last memory I have is of trying to jerk my trunk off the left-hand side of the table. I did not go unconscious; the pain did not stop. From then onward there is a long period of amnesia until I woke up in bed.[21]

PHARMACOLOGIC MECHANISMS OF AWARENESS

Potent Inhalational Agents

Sedation (sleep) and amnesia are integral components of general anesthesia. They may be provided by inhalational anesthetics or parenterally administered agents. When the potent halogenated anesthetics halothane, enflurane, isoflurane, and methoxyflurane are used, amnesia and sleep occur at a lower minimum alveolar concentration (MAC) (0.4 to 0.6 MAC)[23,24] than is required for inhibition of patient movement after stimulation (1.0 to 1.5 MAC).[25] In almost all patients, low concentrations of these agents are sufficient to prevent intraoperative awareness and recall. However, Bahl and Wadwa[21] and Saucier and colleagues[22] reported a halothane anesthetic that resulted in patient awareness, even though no intraoperative signs of inadequate anesthesia were noted. Bahl and Wadwa's patient was paralyzed throughout surgery; Saucier's group was not but did not move with stimulation. Awareness may occur with the halogenated agents, even though tachycardia, hypertension, lacrimation, mydriasis, sweating, and spontaneous movement are absent.

Nitrous Oxide–Relaxant

Awareness is more likely to occur during nitrous oxide–relaxant techniques, depending on whether adjuvant sedatives or narcotics are used. This technique, which "consists of heavy curarization with minimal narcosis,"[5] depends on delivery of a high concentration of nitrous oxide (70% to 75%),[14] near-total neuromuscular blockade, and hyperventilation. However, even a high concentration of nitrous oxide provides only 0.55 to 0.65 MAC[26]; it is more effective as an analgesic than as an amnesic agent in clinically used concentrations.

Frumin[27] described a series of 171 patients who received nitrous oxide–oxygen–succinylcholine as an anesthetic, with a small dose of narcotic for premedication. Eight patients, whose nitrous oxide concentration ranged from 50% to 61%, had recall of surgery. One patient who received 71% nitrous oxide had recall. Fifty patients in whom the degree of neuromuscular blockade was decreased deliberately were able on command to open their eyes and shake their heads "yes" or "no." Although no patient recalled these requests, many had intraoperative dreams or nightmares.

Agarwal and Sikh[28] analyzed 138 nitrous oxide–oxygen–curare anesthetics, and in no instance was "pain during surgery or awareness" reported. However, five of their patients were "restless" immediately after reversal of neuromuscular blockade; perhaps these patients were restless—or awake—during surgery, if not totally paralyzed. In addition, Agarwal and Sikh questioned their patients no later than 4 to 8 hours after surgery. Recall may be elicited more comprehensively with interviews 24 to 72 hours postoperatively,[12] or at the first follow-up visit to the surgeon.[29,30] Because nitrous oxide is a relatively impotent anesthetic, profound paralysis is required to prevent patient movement with this technique. This degree of paralysis makes patient awareness very difficult to detect.

Hyperventilation

Hyperventilation has three effects that cause an apparent deepening of nitrous oxide–relaxant anesthetics.[31] It causes a more rapid increase in alveolar nitrous oxide concentration; decreases ventilatory drive, thus relaxing the abdominal musculature; and decreases cerebral blood flow. When the effect of hyperventilation on MAC is assessed rigorously, it is found to decrease MAC only when combined with mild hypoxia.[32]

An early description of nitrous oxide–relaxant techniques actually suggests the use of 75% nitrous oxide[14] during intra-abdominal surgery, which may result in hypoxemia.[33] Such high concentrations of nitrous oxide are rarely used in modern anesthetic practice.

Narcotics and Sedatives

Narcotics[34,35] and sedatives[36] decrease MAC in a dose-dependent manner, thus making awareness less likely during nitrous oxide–relaxant anesthetics. The maximum potentiation of MAC, as much as 60% to 80%, is achieved with high doses of narcotics.[35] Diazepam[37] and lorazepam,[38] given in sufficient doses, 10 to 15 mg orally or 3 to 4 mg intramuscularly or intravenously, are very effective in preventing recall. Scopolamine is less so. Perhaps the most effective benzodiazepine to assist in providing amnesia is midazolam; in healthy young volunteers, 0.07 mg/kg midazolam given as an infusion at 0.5 mg per minute resulted in amnesia in all cases.[39] Although not practical for routine use, these investigators observed that the β:α ratio on the electroencephalogram was quite specific for identifying the amnesic state. Of note, the subjects were volunteers and the study did not involve evident noxious stimuli, which are a common part of intraoperative anesthesia.

Summary

From a pharmacologic viewpoint, awareness is most likely during unsupplemented nitrous oxide–relaxant techniques, less likely with parenteral adjuvants, and least likely with even small doses of potent inhalational anesthetic agents. A variety of mechanical or human errors can result in awareness during anesthesia.

FACTORS PREDISPOSING TO AWARENESS

Mechanical Problems

Waters summarized some mechanical problems that can lead to awareness.[40] These include ventilation with oxygen for a prolonged period after administration of an ultra–short-acting induction agent; onset of surgery before sufficient wash-in of anesthetic gases to the breathing circuit or before significant alveolar uptake; failure of the nitrous oxide or halogenated anesthetic gas supply; failure of the anesthesia machine to deliver anesthetic gases into anesthetic circuits; and failure of ventilators to deliver gas because of circuit leaks or disconnections.

Inhibition of Reflexes

To these problems may be added syringe swap, or failure to administer the intended parenteral adjuvant; treatment of autonomic signs of inadequate anesthesia with drugs inhibiting autonomic reflexes (eg, esmolol or labetalol); and treatment of movement during anesthesia with muscle relaxants, without determining if the patient is awake.

Type of Surgical Procedure

Certain types of operations pose a greater risk of awareness than the average. These include cesarean section and cardiac, emergency (trauma), and neonatal operations.

Cesarean Section

The reported incidence of awareness during cesarean section is 4% to 20%; pain during anesthesia and emotional distress represent common causes of obstetric malpractice claims (Table 29-1).[41–47] Awareness seems to be less common after emergency cesarean section.[46]

Concerns regarding adequate fetal oxygenation; transplacental passage of sedatives, narcotics, and inhalational anesthetics; and uterine hypotonia and vascular spasm have made nitrous oxide–oxygen 50%–60%–thiopental relaxant the preferred general anesthetic technique for cesarean section.

TABLE 29-1
Maternal Injuries in Obstetric Claims Compared With Similar Injuries in Nonobstetric Claims

INJURY	OBSTETRIC CLAIMS (n = 241) % (n)	NONOBSTETRIC CLAIMS (n = 2106) % (n)
Death (mother or infant)	26 (62)	37 (777)*
Headache	19 (45)	2 (32)*
Nerve damage (mother or infant)	12 (28)	16 (334)
Pain during anesthesia	11 (27)	1 (14)*
Brain damage (mother or infant)	9 (21)	14 (288)
Emotional distress	9 (22)	3 (68)†
Back pain	9 (22)	1 (21)*
Aspiration pneumonitis	5 (12)	1 (28)†

The most common maternal injuries in the obstetric anesthesia claims are shown in order of decreasing frequency. Percentages are based on the total records in each group. Some records, especially those with a fatal outcome, had more than one injury and are represented more than once. Cases involving brain damage include only patients who were alive when the file was closed.

* $P \leq 0.01$ vs obstetric claims.

† $P \leq 0.05$ vs obstetric claims.

Chadwick HS for the Subcommittee on Obstetric Anesthesia and Perinatology: Obstetric anesthesia closed claims update. ASA Newsletter 57:13, 1993.

Withholding of potent inhalation anesthetics or anesthetic adjuvants until umbilical cord clamping causes the increase in the incidence of awareness.

Potent Inhalational Agents

Several modifications of this technique have been proposed to decrease awareness and dreaming. Low concentrations of the potent inhalational anesthetics halothane,[43,48,49] enflurane,[48] isoflurane,[48] and methoxyflurane reduce the incidence of awareness during cesarean section to 0% to 4%, depending on the concentration used. Latto and Waldron compared the effects of 0.2% halothane with 0.65% halothane.[49] The lower concentration was effective in preventing awareness but not dreaming; unpleasant dreams were suppressed by the higher concentration.

Sedatives and Narcotics

Intravenously administered sedatives and narcotics also may decrease the incidence of awareness. Haram and colleagues compared thiopental and diazepam for induction of anesthesia.[45] Twelve percent of patients having a thiopental induction, but no patient having diazepam induction, remembered surgery. Neonatal Apgar scores did not differ between the thiopental and the diazepam groups. However, Turner and Wilson found that preoperative diazepam increased the incidence of unpleasant recall.[50] Abouleish and Taylor administered morphine and diazepam after delivery[46]; this technique decreased the incidence of recall to 4%.

Ketamine

Ketamine has been used for anesthetic induction for cesarean section. It has been associated with both decreased[51,52] and increased[53] awareness during surgery.

Summary

Potent inhalational anesthetics in concentrations sufficient to cause amnesia but less than the dose causing uterine relaxation are the most effective means of preventing awareness during cesarean section performed with general anesthesia. These concentrations (halothane 0.5%, enflurane 1.0%, and isoflurane 0.75%) are not associated with adverse neonatal outcome, as assessed by Apgar and early neonatal neurobehavioral scores, fetal blood gas partial pressure values, lactate concentration, or acid–base balance.[48]

Cardiac Surgery

Narcotics in high doses have been reported as the primary anesthetic agents for cardiac surgery since 1969, when the use of 0.5 to 3.0 mg/kg morphine plus a muscle relaxant, with or without supplementation, was instituted.[54] The rationale for this technique was as follows:

> Morphine produces profound analgesia without consistently causing loss of consciousness, in contrast to true 'anesthesia.' . . . The priorities of anesthetic practice dictate that preservation of respiratory and circulatory integrity and provision of suitable conditions for operation take precedence over the provision of absolute patient comfort.[55]

Fentanyl, in a dose of 50 to 150 μg/kg, has been reported to provide complete anesthesia.[56] Sufentanil, five to ten times as potent as fentanyl, also might be expected to produce anesthesia. With high-dose fentanyl (after lorazepam premedication), Sebel and coworkers noted a characteristic electroencephalographic change thought to be indicative of unconsciousness.[57]

Narcotics alone do not seem to be sufficient to produce anesthesia in all patients.[58–60] Elderly patients require a smaller dose of fentanyl for unconsciousness than do young patients.[56] However, multiple case reports have documented intraoperative awareness or recall after 75 to 100 μg/kg fentanyl.[61–63] Risk factors include a history of alcoholism or drug abuse and administration of two high-dose narcotic anesthetics within a short period.

Narcotics do not act on all of the central nervous system sites affected by general anesthetics.[62] The technique perhaps is more accurately portrayed as narcotic "analgesia" rather than narcotic anesthesia. The period after rewarming during preparation for separation from cardiopulmonary bypass—when the anesthetics have been intravenously diluted by the bypass circuit volume, the volatile agents have been cleared, and benzodiazepines and narcotics have been bound to the oxygenator—appears to be a particularly vulnerable time. Supplementation with adjunctive sedatives, especially during this period and most especially if additional muscle relaxants have been administered, makes awareness less likely when a high-dose narcotic technique is used.

Trauma Surgery

Patients who have sustained trauma also are more likely to experience intraoperative awareness. Although they may have conditions that reduce MAC (anemia, hypovolemia, hypothermia, hypotension, or acute alcoholic intoxication),[31] because of hemodynamic instability, these patients often receive little or no agent other than a muscle relaxant.

Bogetz and Katz studied the incidence of recall in a group of trauma patients.[10] Amnesic preoperative agents were deliberately avoided. The condition of 37 of 54 patients was stable enough to allow administration of an anesthetic for tracheal intubation and throughout surgery; only 11% had recall. Fourteen other patients, more severely injured, did not receive an anesthetic during intubation or for at least 20 minutes during surgery. Six (43%) of these patients recalled surgery. The severity of injury did not effectively predict recall or lack thereof. Bogetz and Katz suggested that to prevent recall totally, all trauma patients should receive an amnesic agent.

Neonatal Surgery

As with trauma surgery and, to a lesser extent, cesarean section and cardiac surgery, a reluctance to provide true anesthesia for neonates, especially those born prematurely, has been pervasive in anesthesiologic practice. Rather than administer cardiorespiratory depressant drugs to these tiny patients who already have cardiovascular instability, many anesthesiologists have provided only oxygen (or perhaps nitrous oxide) and muscle relaxation.

This practice was defended in part by the belief that pain perception increases with age and that neonates do not perceive pain or perceive it only minimally. However, research conducted throughout the 1980s documents that conventional anesthetic drugs are well tolerated[64–67] and that sensory pathways and brain centers necessary for pain perception are well developed late in gestation.[68] Moreover, neonates respond to painful stimuli with metabolic, hormonal, and cardiorespiratory changes similar to those observed in adults.

Neonates receiving only nitrous oxide and muscle relaxant anesthesia for major surgery experience potentially harmful stress responses (eg, increased plasma epinephrine, norepinephrine, and cortisol levels) compared with those receiving nitrous oxide supplemented by fentanyl,[69] sufentanil,[70] or halothane.[71] Thus, no valid rationale exists to deny these patients anesthesia and analgesia for surgery and other invasive procedures.

DETECTION AND PREVENTION

Detection of awareness during anesthesia is difficult.[72] Signs of light anesthesia, such as hypertension, tachycardia, sweating, lacrimation, mydriasis, and movement may be absent. Several mechanical or monitoring techniques that have been proposed but that have been found to have little reliability include electroencephalography[57,73] and other electroencephalographic wave analyses (the cerebral function monitor,[74] the power spectral array, and the compressed spectral array); the isolated forearm technique,[75] in which a tourniquet prevents muscle relaxant from reaching one forearm, thus allowing communication with the patient; surface electromyography; esophageal contractility; and the time to correct response, a retrospective method that examines how quickly after withdrawal of nitrous oxide the patient makes the correct response to a verbal stimulus.[76]

The most accurate clinical method to detect intraoperative awareness is to refrain from fully paralyzing the patient and then to give specific verbal commands (eg, "open your eyes"). Awareness and possible recall are suggested by positive responses. Unless the possibility of patient awareness is considered, many instances will be undetected. Other methods of preventing awareness, though not absolutely reliable, include the use of amnesic doses of potent inhalational anesthetic agents or intravenously administered sedative drugs.

SEQUELAE

Intraoperative awareness may result in vague somatic symptoms. Blacher described a "traumatic neurosis" syndrome consisting of repetitive nightmares, generalized irritability and anxiety, a preoccupation with death, and difficulty discussing the symptoms and operative experience.[77] In the six patients described, these symptoms persisted long enough to come to psychiatric attention but promptly resolved after discussion of the anesthetic experience.

For patients who have a greater than average risk of intraoperative awareness, frank preoperative discussion of its possibility and of plans to detect it should help to decrease the psychological discomfort and postoperative sequelae of this complication.[60] If awareness is suspected during surgery or discovered postoperatively, the patient must be given the opportunity to discuss and understand it. Psychiatric consultation should be obtained, if necessary.

REFERENCES

1. Parkhouse J: Awareness during surgery. Postgrad Med 36:674–677, 1960
2. Crile G. George Crile, an autobiography. Philadelphia: JB Lippincott, 1947: 197
3. Griffith HR, Johnson GE: The use of curare in general anesthesia. Anesthesiology 3:418, 1942
4. Smith AM, Brown HO, Toman JPE, et al: The lack of cerebral effects of D-tubocurarine. Anesthesiology 8:1, 1947
5. Winterbottom LH: Insufficient anaesthesia. British Medical Journal 1:247, 1950
6. Clifton PJ: Expectations and experiences of anaesthesia in a district general hospital. Anaesthesia 39:281, 1984
7. Hutchinson R: Awareness during surgery: a study of its incidence. Br J Anaesth 33:463, 1960
8. Urbach GM, Edelist G: An evaluation of the anaesthetic techniques used in an outpatient unit. Can Anaesth Soc J 24:401, 1977
9. Fishburne JI, Fulghum MS, Hulka JF, et al: General anesthesia for outpatient laparoscopy with an objective measure of recovery. Anesth Analg 53:1, 1974
10. Bogetz MS, Katz JA: Recall of surgery of major trauma. Anesthesiology 61:6, 1984
11. Taub HA Eisenberg L: A comparison of memory under three methods of anaesthesia with nitrous oxide and curare. Can Anaesth Soc J 22:298, 1975
12. Terrell RK, Sweet WO, Gladfelter JH, et al: Study of recall during anesthesia. Anesth Analg 48:86, 1969
13. Brice DD, Hetherington RR, Utting JE: A simple study of awareness and dreaming during anaesthesia. Br J Anaesth 42:535, 1970
14. Levinson BW: States of awareness during general anaesthesia. Preliminary communication. Br J Anaesth 37:544, 1965
15. Leaming HL: Awareness during anaesthesia. British Medical Journal 4(674):51, 1969
16. Anonymous: On being aware. Br J Anaesth 51:711, 1979
17. Si RL: Consciousness during general anesthesia. Anesth Analg 48:363, 1969
18. Marx GF: Pain and awareness during surgical anesthesia. New York State Journal of Medicine 67:2623, 1967
19. Tunstall ME: On being aware by request: a mother's unplanned request during the course of a Caesarean section under general anesthesia. Br J Anaesth 52:1049, 1980
20. Tantisira B, McKenzie R: Awareness during laparoscopy under general anesthesia: a case report. Anesth Analg 53:373, 1973
21. Bahl CP, Wadwa S: Consciousness during apparent surgical anaesthesia: a case report. Br J Anaesth 40:289, 1968
22. Saucier N, Walts LF, Moreland JR: Patient awareness during nitrous oxide, oxygen and halothane anesthesia. Anesth Analg 62:239, 1983
23. Stoelting RK, Longecker DE, Eger EI II. Minimum alveolar concentration in man on awakening from methoxyflurane, halothane, ether and fluroxene anesthesia: MAC awake. Anesthesiology 33:5, 1970
24. Eger EI II: Isoflurane: a review. Anesthesiology 55:559 1981
25. Saidman LJ, Eger EI II, Munson ES, et al: Minimum alveolar concentration of methoxyflurane, halothane, ether and cyclopropane in man: correlation with theories of anesthesia. Anesthesiology 28:994, 1967
26. Eger EI II: MAC. In Eger EI II (ed): Nitrous oxide. New York: Elsevier, 1985: 57
27. Frumin MJ: Clinical use of a physiological respirator producing nitrous oxide amnesia–analgesia. Anesthesiology 18:290, 1957
28. Agarwal G, Sikh SS: Awareness during anaesthesia: a prospective study. Br J Anaesth 49:835, 1977
29. Mainzer J: Awareness, muscle relaxants and balanced anaesthesia. Can Anaesth Soc J 26:386, 1979

30. Blacher RS: Awareness during surgery. Anesthesiology 61:1, 1984
31. Eger EI II: Minimum alveolar concentration. In Eger EI II (ed): Anesthetic uptake and distribution. Baltimore: Williams & Wilkins, 1974: 7
32. Cullen DJ, Eger EI II: The effect of extreme hypocapnia on the anesthetic requirement (MAC) of dogs. Br J Anaesth 43:339, 1971
33. Benumof JL: Respiratory physiology and respiratory function during anesthesia. In Miller RD (ed): Anesthesiology. New York: Churchill Livingstone, 1981: 709
34. Murphy MR, Hug CC: The enflurane sparing effect of morphine, butorphanol, and nalbuphine. Anesthesiology 57:489, 1982
35. Lake CL, Di Fazio CA, Moscick JC, et al: Reduction in halothane MAC: comparison of morphine and alfentanil. Anesth Analg 64: 807, 1985
36. Perisho JA, Buechel DR, Miller RD: The effect of diazepam (Valium) on minimum alveolar anaesthetic requirement in man. Can Anaesth Soc J 18:536, 1971
37. Duncan AW, Barr AM: Diazepam premedication and awareness during general anaesthesia for bronchoscopy and laryngoscopy. Br J Anaesth 45:1150, 1973
38. Pandit SK, Heisterkamp DV, Cohen PJ: Further studies of the anti-recall effect of lorazepam: a dose-time-effect relationship. Anesthesiology 45:495, 1976
39. Veselis RA, Reinsel R, Algesan R, et al: The EEG as a monitor of midazolam amnesia: changes in power and topography as a function of amnesic state. Anesthesiology 74:866, 1991
40. Waters DJ: Factors causing awareness during surgery. Br J Anaesth 40:259, 1968
41. Famewo CE: Awareness and dreams during general anaesthesia for Caesarean section: a study of incidence. Can Anaesth Soc J 23:636, 1976
42. Wilson J, Turner DJ: Awareness during Caesarean section under general anaesthesia. British Medical Journal 1(639):280, 1969
43. Morgan BM, Aulakh JM, Barker JP, et al: Anaesthesia for Caesarean section: a medical audit of junior anaesthetic staff practice. Br J Anaesth 55:885, 1983
44. Magno R, Selstam U, Karlsson K: Anesthesia for Caesarean section: II. effects of the induction-delivery interval on the respiratory adaptation of the newborn in elective Cesarean section. Acta Anaesthesiol Scand 19:250, 1975
45. Haram K, Lund T, Sagen N, et al: Comparison of thiopentone and diazepam as induction agents of anaesthesia for Caesarean section. Acta Anaesthesiol Scand 25:470, 1981
46. Abouleish E, Taylor FH: Effect of morphine-diazepam on signs of anesthesia, awareness, and dreams of patients under N_20 for Cesarean section. Anesth Analg 55:702, 1976
47. Chadwick HS for the Subcommittee on Obstetric Anesthesia and Perinatology: Obstetric anesthesia closed claims update. ASA Newsletter 57:13, 1993
48. Warren TM, Datta S, Ostheimer GW, et al: Comparison of the maternal and neonatal effects of halothane, enflurane and isoflurane for Cesarean delivery. Anesth Analg 62:516, 1983
49. Latto IP, Waldron BA: Anaesthesia for Caesarean section: analysis of blood concentrations of halothane using 0.2% or 0.65% halothane with 50% nitrous oxide in oxygen. Br J Anaesth 49(4): 371, 1977
50. Turner DJ, Wilson J: Effect of diazepam on awareness during Caesarean section under general anaesthesia. British Medical Journal 1(659):736, 1969
51. Digh-Nielson J, Holasek J: Ketamine as induction agent for Caesarean section. Acta Anaesthesiol Scand 26:139, 1982
52. Schultetus RR, Hill CR, Dharamraj CM, et al: Wakefulness during Cesarean section after anesthetic induction with ketamine, thiopental, or ketamine and thiopental combined. Anesth Analg 65:723, 1986
53. Ellingson A, Haram K, Sagen N: Ketamine and diazepam as anaesthesia for forceps delivery: a comparative study. Acta Anaesthesiol Scand 21:37, 1977
54. Lowenstein E, Hallowell P, Levine FH, et al: Cardiovascular response to large doses of intravenous morphine in man. N Engl J Med 281:1389, 1969
55. Lowenstein E: Morphine 'anesthesia': a perspective. Anesthesiology 35:563, 1971
56. Stanley TH, Webster LR: Anesthetic requirements and cardiovascular effects of fentanyl-oxygen and fentanyl-diazepam-oxygen anesthesia in man. Anesth Analg 57:411, 1978
57. Sebel PS, Bovill JG, Wauquier A, et al: Effects of high-dose fentanyl anesthesia on the electroencephalogram. Anesthesiology 55:203, 1981
58. Bailey PL, Wilbrink J, Zwanikken P: Anesthetic induction with fentanyl. Anesth Analg 64:48, 1985
59. Mark JB, Greenberg LM: Intraoperative awareness and hypertensive crisis during high-dose fentanyl-diazepam-oxygen anesthesia. Anesth Analg 62:698, 1983
60. Mummaneni N, Tao TLK, Montoya A: Awareness and recall with high-dose fentanyl-oxygen anesthesia. Anesth Analg 59: 948, 1980
61. Hilgenberg JC: Intraoperative awareness during high-dose fentanyl-oxygen anesthesia. Anesthesiology 54:341, 1981
62. Wong KC: Narcotics are not expected to produce unconsciousness and amnesia. Anesth Analg 62:625, 1983
63. Bovill JG, Sevel PS, Stanley TH: Opioid analgesics in anesthesia: with special reference to their use in cardiovascular anesthesia. Anesthesiology 61:731, 1984
64. Robinson S, Gregory GA: Fentanyl-air-oxygen anesthesia for ligation of patent ductus arteriosus in preterm infants. Anesth Analg 60:331, 1981
65. Hickey PR, Hansen DD: Fentanyl- and sufentanil-oxygen-pancuronium anesthesia for cardiac surgery in infants. Anesth Analg 63:117, 1984
66. Freisen RH, Henry DB: Cardiovascular changes in preterm neonates receiving isoflurane, halothane, fentanyl, and ketamine. Anesthesiology 64:238, 1986
67. Singleton MA, Rosen JI, Fisher DM: Plasma concentrations of fentanyl in infants, children and adults. Can J Anaesth 34:152, 1987
68. Anand KJS, Hickey PR: Pain and its effects in the human neonate and fetus. N Engl J Med 317:1321, 1987
69. Anand KJS, Sippell WG, Aynsley-Green A: Randomized trial of fentanyl anaesthesia in preterm babies undergoing surgery: Effects on the stress response. Lancet 1:243, 1987
70. Anand KJS, Hickey PR: Halothane-morphine compared with high-dose sufentanil for anesthesia and postoperative analgesia in neonatal cardiac surgery. N Engl J Med 326:55, 1992
71. Anand KJS, Sippell WG, Schofield NM, et al: Does halothane anaesthesia decrease the metabolic and endocrine stress response of newborn infants undergoing operation? British Medical Journal 296(6623):668, 1988
72. Robson JG: Measurement of depth of anaesthesia. Br J Anaesth 41:785, 1969
73. Tinker JH, Sharbrough FW, Michenfelder JD: Anterior shift of the dominant EEG rhythm during anesthesia in the Java monkey: correlation with anesthetic potency. Anesthesiology 46:252, 1977
74. Prior PE, Maynard DE, Brierly JB: EEG monitoring for the control of anaesthesia produced by the infusion of althesin in primates. Br J Anaesth 50:993, 1978
75. Tunstall ME: Detecting wakefulness during general anaesthesia for Caesarean section. British Medical Journal 1(6072):1321, 1977
76. Cormack RS: Awareness during surgery: a new approach. Br J Anaesth 51:1051, 1979
77. Blacher RS: On awakening paralyzed during surgery: a syndrome of traumatic neurosis. JAMA 234:67, 1975

FURTHER READING

Ghoneim MM, Block RI: Learning and consciousness during general anesthesia. Anesthesiology 76:279, 1992

Rosen M, Lunn JN (eds): Consciousness, awareness and pain in general anesthesia. London: Butterworths, 1987

Complications in Anesthesiology, second edition,
edited by Nikolaus Gravenstein and Robert R. Kirby.
Lippincott-Raven Publishers, Philadelphia © 1996.

CHAPTER 30

Postoperative Emotional Responses

Henry Rosenberg
Marc Goldberg

Badger, discussing his personal experience after open heart surgery, stated the following:

> It is the utter helplessness of recovery that seeks a humanizing of relationships with those around you. Were it possible for the recovery room residents to see and know their patients preoperatively, much confidence would be instilled into these patients.[1]

That personality changes may occur after surgery is well known, having been first described by Dupuytren in 1834.[2] The initial discussions of disorientation, combativeness, depression, and other inappropriate behavior that develops postoperatively usually ascribed these problems to sepsis or drug toxicity.[3–6] However, with the development of psychiatry, clinicians began to realize that in addition to organic causes, emotional upheavals after surgery often are rooted in the complex reactions of the mind–body scheme that occur with stress in general and consequent to surgery and anesthesia in particular.

At first, many physicians believed that postoperative psychosis was a distinct, clinically definable entity with a specific cause.[7,8] By the 1940s, however, the fallacy of such a view was apparent. In the 1950s, when open heart surgery began to be performed extensively, the high incidence (as great as 70%) of "postcardiotomy" delirium prompted intense study and reflection about postoperative emotional changes. "Postoperative psychosis," like "postpartum psychosis," was recognized as a multifactorial syndrome in terms of etiology, manifestation, and prognosis.[9,10]

The role of anesthetic agents and the anesthesiologist in the occurrence and manifestations of postoperative personality changes is difficult to evaluate because anesthesia is only one of several emotionally charged interventions in the surgical period.

CLINICAL PRESENTATION

Timing

In general, disruptive or disturbing behavior changes in adults occur immediately on emergence from anesthesia or after a lucid interval of 24 to 48 hours (often first in the intensive care unit).[9,10] Less overt but just as disturbing personality changes, such as depression, bad dreams, and, in children, regressive behavior, may last from days to weeks after surgery. The form and severity of these changes are varied.

Postanesthetic Excitement

Postanesthetic excitement as it occurs on emergence from anesthesia is "usually characterized by restlessness, disorientation, crying, moaning, or irrational talking. In its extreme form there is wild thrashing about together with shouting or screaming."[11] Although several studies have examined the possible causes of emergence excitement, more subtle personality changes such as quiet confusion, depression, and other affective disorders occurring in the recovery room have received little comment.[12]

Psychological Changes

In contrast, postoperative psychological changes beginning after a lucid interval have been the subject of many comments and studies. The changes that may occur at this time are varied and include dementia, neurotic emotional responses, and psychotic behavior.[7,13] Brain syndrome is a sensory defect, consisting of disorientation; impairment of memory, judgment, and intellectual functions; illusions*; and lability of affect. The syndrome is usually reversible, especially when associated with a correctable toxic or metabolic cause.

Neurotic and Psychotic Responses

Neurotic emotional responses can take the form of an anxiety state, depression, and conversion reaction (conversion of anxiety into bodily symptoms). Psychotic behavior may be expressed as psychotic depression, with suicidal tendencies, manic depressive reactions, schizophrenic reactions, hallucinations, and grossly inappropriate behavior and moods. Only rarely do these syndromes become severe enough to require psychiatric hospitalization.[14] More often they may be controlled by psychotherapy, minor and major tranquilizers, and correction of organic problems.

Withdrawal

Yet another mode of expression of personality change is a hypokinetic, withdrawn state, which is often described after sudden major catastrophes. This type of reaction usually is evident soon after the operation and may persist for an indeterminate length of time.[1,10]

Diagnostic and Therapeutic Implications

These reactions pose severe problems in nursing care and may jeopardize recovery. Often they are manifestations of the patient's inability to cope with the psychological stress imposed by the threat of loss of life and limb or change in body image, or the stress of sensory deprivation.[15] However, behavioral changes also may be the result of or aggravated by physiologic insults. Of course, preoperative identification of vulnerability to this type of psychological reaction is important in management.

Psychological and emotional problems extending into the late postoperative period (after discharge) are of concern as well, especially with the increasing popularity of outpatient surgery. These problems may take the form of recurring bad dreams, the experience of déjà vu, inability to concentrate, diminution of attention span, general malaise, and regressive behavior. These symptoms have been shown to follow even brief surgical procedures.[16] The patient's attitude toward subsequent surgery is influenced by these experiences.

Although evaluation of the etiology of postoperative and postanesthetic responses is complex, certain organic and psychological factors are known to predispose patients to emotional problems. A working knowledge of these factors is essential for prevention and treatment. Because most studies deal with observations in the post-anesthesia care unit (PACU) during emergence from anesthesia or with observations beginning 24 or more hours postoperatively, the discussion below generally follows that division.

* The misinterpretation of sensory stimuli is termed an *illusion*. *Hallucinations*, in contrast, are responses to nonexistent external stimuli.

IMMEDIATE EMOTIONAL RESPONSES TO ANESTHESIA AND SURGERY

Only 3% to 5% of patients exhibit emergence excitement, according to studies performed when cyclopropane and diethyl ether were still in general use.[11,17,18] More subtle changes were found by Winkelstein and coworkers in a far greater percentage of patients.[12] Winkelstein's group observed that patients awakening from general anesthesia (thiopental followed by halothane, cyclopropane, ether, or nitrous oxide) were lucid but exhibited a lack of concern about the surgical procedure and a lack of appropriate affective responses. Although patients undergoing procedures with spinal anesthesia showed a more appropriate affect, the investigators nevertheless attributed the changes after general anesthesia to psychogenic rather than pharmacologic factors.

Operative Site

Eckenhoff and associates retrospectively evaluated 14,000 surgical procedures in patients 3 years old or older and found that tonsillectomy, thyroid surgery, and circumcision were most frequently associated with emergence excitement (Table 30-1).[11] In general, surgery on the airway, the breast, or the organs of reproduction, as well as procedures associated with strong emotional significance, are likely to be accompanied by a high incidence of emergence excitement.

Intrathoracic and upper abdominal operations were most often accompanied by emergence excitement, according to the surveys of Smessaert and colleagues,[18] Coppolino,[17] and Knox and colleagues.[14] The discrepancies may be related to influences that were not controlled, such as premedication and anesthetic agents.

Anesthetic Drugs

Inhalational Agents

Clearly, the inhalation agents that were most often associated with emergence delirium are cyclopropane and ether. Thiopental, nitrous oxide, and narcotics are least often implicated. Halothane, enflurane, and isoflurane are intermediate.[11]

Smessaert and colleagues found that with a barbiturate–anticholinergic premedication, delirium was present in 2% of patients anesthetized with diethyl ether, 4% of those anesthetized with cyclopropane, 2.5% of those anesthetized with cyclopropane–ether, and 1% of those anesthetized with thiopental–nitrous oxide.[18] The incidence of emergence excitement varied among the anesthetic agents and regimens.

James studied the cognitive abilities of healthy volunteers after cyclopropane, given for a minimum of 20 minutes at a concentration of 20–40%.[19] He found impairment of a variety of mental performance tests as late as 1 week after exposure to cyclopropane.

A more recent evaluation of the effects of 4.4 to 7.2 hours of halothane or isoflurane anesthesia, again in healthy male volunteers not undergoing surgery, disclosed transient, subtle intellectual deficits and mood changes.[20] Subjective dysphoric complaints persisted for as long as 8 days. Halothane was associated with more complaints than was isoflurane. This

TABLE 30-1
Operations and Emergence Excitement

OPERATION	ALL PATIENTS (no.)	PATIENTS WITH EXCITEMENT (no.)	INCIDENCE (%)
Tonsillectomy	406	67	16.5
Thyroid	406	55	13.5
Circumcision	82	9	11.0
Hysterectomy	1157	90	7.8
Perineal plastic	299	21	7.0
Abdominal wall	502	35	7.0
Eye	83	5	6.0
Breast	915	55	6.0
Upper abdominal	1006	51	5.1
Extremity	1055	50	4.7
Face	737	29	3.9
Intrathoracic	608	23	3.8
Transurethral resection	187	7	3.7
Dilation and curettage	2554	72	2.9
Neck	232	6	2.6
Appendectomy	119	4	3.4
Dental	303	7	2.3
Intracranial	181	3	1.7
Spinal fusion	266	4	1.5
Other	1196	61	5.1

Eckenhoff JE, Kneale DH, Dripps RD: The incidence and etiology of postanesthetic excitement. Anesthesiology 22:667, 1961.

difference was thought to be related to the greater fat solubility of halothane compared with isoflurane, the metabolites of halothane, or both. Indeed, bromide levels after prolonged halothane anesthesia may attain levels known to cause behavioral changes.[21]

Ketamine

Ketamine is associated with a high incidence of emotional reactions during the period spent in the PACU and possibly for long periods after its administration. In the PACU, vivid dreams, often unpleasant, are common; their incidence ranges from 9% to more than 40%[10,22] Droperidol and the benzodiazepines purportedly mitigate these reactions,[23] although uniform agreement concerning their effectiveness has not been reached.[24]

Apparently, the more psychologically stressful the surgical procedure, the more likely it is that an unpleasant emotional reaction will occur. Krestow found that 30 of 50 patients undergoing therapeutic abortions had unpleasant dreams, and 17 of them subsequently rejected ketamine for other procedures.[24] However, Garfield and coworkers, studying soldiers in a burn ward undergoing skin grafts and minor orthopedic procedures, found a low incidence of unpleasant dreams and a more ready acceptance of the agent.[25] Several case reports also have incriminated ketamine as the cause of recurrent bad dreams, experiences of déjà vu, and dysphoric reactions for weeks postoperatively.[26,27]

Lack of Anesthesia: Awareness and Recall

Others have implicated the lack of anesthesia in the production of personality changes.[28,29] Predisposing factors are listed in Table 30-2. In several cases in which muscle relaxants and light anesthesia were used, patients recalled fragments of conversation and noises in the operating room. They were aware of being unable to move or talk intraoperatively. Whereas preoperatively these patients had displayed only appropriate signs of anxiety, postoperatively they were expressionless, mute, and apathetic, or sometimes excited and hallucinating. Harrowing repetitive dreams and fantasies for several days were common.

Many other emotional changes have been reported within the first 24 hours postoperatively (Table 30-3). Further studies are also needed regarding the relation between intraoperative awareness and psychological changes postoperatively.[30,31]

TABLE 30-2
Lack of Anesthesia: Predisposing Factors in Intraoperative Awareness or Recall

1. Hemodynamic instability precluding anesthetic administration
2. Failed or inappropriate delivery of inhaled agents or failed delivery of adequate dose of intravenous agent
3. Use of high doses of narcotics without supplemental concomitant barbiturates, benzodiazepines, inhaled agents, or nitrous oxide
4. Factors resulting in lower than expected levels of anesthetic agent in the brain:
   A. Obesity
   B. Chronic use of medications that induce tolerance to anesthetics or induce metabolism of anesthetics

Mahla ME: Nervous system. In Gravenstein N (ed): Manual of complications during anesthesia. Philadelphia: JB Lippincott, 1991: 393.

TABLE 30-3
Subjective Changes in the First 24 Hours after Surgery in 18 Patients

PATIENTS (%)	SUBJECTIVE CHANGE
82	Decreased desire to smoke
78	Weakness
78	Fatigue, listlessness, or decreased energy
72	Sore throat
67	Decreased ability to think and concentrate
61	Poor coordination
61	Dizziness, particularly when standing
50	Nausea with motion
44	Abnormal thoughts or depression
39	Vomiting with motion
39	Poor appetite
33	Increased cough or sputum production
28	Nervousness and restlessness
28	Sleep disturbances
28	Nausea without motion
22	Smell of odor of cyclopropane intermittently
22	Vomiting without motion
6	Taste of cyclopropane

James FM: The effects of cyclopropane anesthesia without operation on mental functions of normal man. Anesthesiology 30:264, 1969.

Preanesthetic Medication

Premedication also influences the incidence of emotional reactions on emergence from anesthesia. In both adults[16,32] and children,[22] barbiturate–anticholinergic premedication (especially scopolamine) is associated with a high incidence of excitement. Addition of a narcotic to this combination or administration of a narcotic shortly before the termination of the procedure results in a smoother, calmer awakening. Pain due to the surgery itself or prolonged immobilization leading to muscle soreness is believed to be an important contributing factor in the production of emergence excitement.[11]

Preanesthetic drugs reported to be associated with emergence excitement or delirium include the phenothiazines[33] and anticholinergic agents.[34] In cases in which scopolamine has been implicated as a cause of delirium, physostigmine, the tertiary amine cholinesterase inhibitor, in a dose of 1 to 2 mg intravenously, dramatically and rapidly reverses the delirium.[35,36] Even when delirium occurs several hours after scopolamine, the response to physostigmine may be dramatic. Clinical doses of atropine can cause prolonged disorientation and sedation in older patients.[37] These reactions also are responsive to physostigmine.

Age and Gender

Gender does not appear to influence the incidence of emergence delirium. Age, however, is a more significant factor. Eckenhoff and associates found that younger, more vigorous patients were more often excited in the recovery room; aged patients rarely displayed emergence excitement.[11]

Other Factors

A host of other factors influence the appearance of emergence excitement. Drug-dependent patients, particularly alcoholic patients, may display the first signs of withdrawal after the abstinence enforced by surgery.[38] The duration of anesthesia also is related to emergence excitement. A significantly increased incidence of delirium occurs with procedures that last for more than 4 hours.[7] This observation may be related to the complexity of the surgery, to the likelihood of fluid shifts,[39] or perhaps to the dysphoria that Davison and coworkers showed was likely to occur after 4 to 8 hours of anesthesia.[20] In open heart surgery, pump time rather than operative time is correlated with emotional upset.[32] Patients may unconsciously register auditory stimuli during apparently adequate general anesthesia.[40] When hypnotized to elicit recall, some patients have exhibited an anxiety reaction in response to the same alarming stimuli heard during surgery.[41] The relation between unconscious recall and postoperative emotional distress is unknown.

Important organic causes of behavioral disorders are hypoxia, hypercapnia, electrolyte disorders, and acid–base changes (Table 30-4).[42,43] Electrolyte changes that may occur postoperatively and lead to behavioral changes are hyponatremia (eg, after transurethral surgery), hypochloremia (eg, after intestinal drainage), and hyperosmolarity.

Patients undergoing emergency surgery also are more likely to be excited postoperatively.[44] The same is true of patients with preexisting delirium or organic brain syndrome.[45] Per-

TABLE 30-4
Organic Causes of Postoperative Disturbances of Consciousness

CEREBRAL
Trauma: primary or secondary (edema, conditioning)
Elimination of cerebral cortex
Dysfunction of sleep-wake regulation
RESPIRATORY
Hypoxemia and hypercapnia (compensated respiratory acidosis)
Decompensated respiratory acidosis and alkalosis
HEMODYNAMIC
Diminished arterial oxygen content (anemia or hypoxemia)
Diminished cardiac output (hypovolemia, circulatory collapse, heart and vascular insufficiency, or pulmonary embolism)
Circulatory arrest (Adams-Stokes syndrome; syncope, asystole, or ventricular fibrillation)
INFECTIOUS (Toxic)
Inflammation
Endogenous intoxication (burns or ileus)
Bacterial endotoxin, peritonitis, empyema, or septicemia
Exogenous intoxication
Iatrogenic (anesthesia or drugs)
METABOLIC
Hydration
Electrolyte disturbance
Acid–base imbalance
Hepatorenal collapse
Endocrine imbalance

Kaufer C: Etiology of consciousness disturbances in surgery. Minn Med 51:1509, 1968.

sonality and psychological makeup are important determinants in the expression of emotional problems. Their role is discussed below.

Treatment

The treatment of excitement and delirium in the PACU consists of verification that the patient is adequately oxygenated and ventilated, and restraint; once these measures are established, small doses of intravenous narcotics are administered, combined with repetitive reassurance, orientation, and explanation.[11] Physostigmine may be used if the patient has been given a centrally active anticholinergic. Flumazenil has been found effective in reversing the effects of benzodiazepines.[46]

EMOTIONAL CHANGES 24 HOURS OR MORE AFTER SURGERY

On occasion, despite uneventful awakening from anesthesia, disorientation, confusion, and psychotic behavior become manifest 24 to 48 hours after surgery. Although anesthetic concentrations may persist at low levels for several days postoperatively and may alter behavior as above, the anesthetic agent is of lesser consideration in the evaluation of these behavioral disturbances. Prolonged cognitive and psychomotor impairment, though rare, is a serious problem when it occurs. Risk factors are listed in Table 30-5.

Open Heart Surgery

Patients having open heart procedures are particularly susceptible to psychiatric and emotional problems that develop after the lucid interval. The incidence of postoperative emotional changes ranges from 30% to 70%, depending on the series.[47–56]

TABLE 30-5
Perioperative Risk Factors for Postoperative Cognitive and Psychomotor Impairment

PREOPERATIVE

1. Advanced age
2. Drug or alcohol abuse
3. Preexisting neurologic abnormalities
4. Preexisting cognitive or psychologic impairment
5. Other diseases (eg, porphyria, preeclampsia, or multiple sclerosis)

PERIOPERATIVE

1. Type of operation (eg, open heart surgery)
2. Inadequate cerebral oxygen supply caused by hypotension or reduction of arterial oxygen content
3. Hypoglycemia or hyperglycemia
4. Electrolyte abnormalities
5. Type of anesthetic agents
6. Type of adjuvant drugs
7. Intraoperative awareness

Mahla ME: The nervous system. In Gravenstein N (ed): Manual of complications during anesthesia. Philadelphia: JB Lippincott, 1991: 722.

Emboli, Hypoxia, and Hypoperfusion

Tufo and colleagues believe that neurologic deficits from cerebral emboli, hypoxia, and hypoperfusion are responsible for most if not all behavioral changes after open heart surgery.[49,50] In their studies, delirium and abnormal neurologic signs were demonstrated to have high positive correlation with long pump runs and the duration during bypass of a mean perfusion pressure less than 50 mm Hg. Widespread use of high-flow, low pressure cardiopulmonary bypass casts doubt on this pressure threshold as a causative factor, providing that bypass flow is adequate.

Air Embolism

Intracardiac entrapment of air during open valve, cardiac aneurysm, and transplant procedures as well as during repairs of congenital anomalies[51] is another cause of postcardiopulmonary bypass neurologic dysfunction. Psychomotor and neurologic dysfunction is much more common when the left ventricle has been opened for valve repair. Nussmeier and associates demonstrated that barbiturate infusion sufficient to maintain electroencephalographic silence provides protection against the neurologic dysfunction after valve surgery.[46]

Coronary Artery Bypass

The incidence of postoperative emotional problems has been shown to be low in patients undergoing coronary artery bypass procedures.[56] This low incidence may be the result of improvements in operative technique or a difference in the personalities of patients with coronary artery disease compared with patients with rheumatic heart disease. However, even when similar surgical populations were compared, an overall decline in the incidence of postcardiotomy delirium was noted.[52] This finding was associated with shorter pump runs and changes in intensive care procedures.

Support

Psychiatric support and increased sensitivity to patients' adjustment to the unnatural environment of the intensive care unit can significantly reduce the incidence of postcardiopulmonary bypass delirium.[22,52,53] In studies of this type of support, intensive care nurses were trained to communicate with their patients, explain procedures, and ensure appropriate sleep–wake cycles; clocks, calendars, and radios provided contact with reality. Psychiatric support was provided by preoperative exploration of patients' fears, fantasies, and expectations regarding surgery. The resultant reduction in emotional disturbances was impressive.[54,55]

General Surgery

After general surgery, patients most likely to experience gross personality difficulties 24 to 48 hours after surgery are older patients,[57] 6-month-old to 5-year-old children,[58,59] people with preexisting personality disturbances,[57] addicted or habitual drug users, and people who have little support from family and friends.[57]

A recent prospective evaluation identified a 9% incidence of postoperative delirium after major elective noncardiac surgery (Table 30-6).[60] Factors that correlated independently with postoperative delirium were age 70 years or more; self-reported alcohol abuse; poor cognitive status; poor functional status; markedly abnormal preoperative serum sodium, potassium, or glucose levels; and history of noncardiac thoracic or aortic aneurysm surgery.[60]

Organic Factors

Again, organic factors are not to be overlooked. Medical and surgical complications must always be considered in patients showing mental deterioration over a short period. Mild confusion, illusions, and disorientation often precede significant medical or surgical problems by 12 to 24 hours.[10,57] Some element of postoperative disturbance is attributable to the transient decreased mental acuity caused by general anesthesia. Several studies have demonstrated impairment of motor and verbal skills for as long as 4 days postoperatively.[19,20,61,62]

Aging

Although patients more than 70 years old are less likely to exhibit emergence excitement,[11] they frequently undergo emotional deterioration postoperatively.[62] Factors that may be involved are inadequate ability to cope with unfamiliar surroundings and situations,[8] exposure to numerous new medications, and cardiovascular and respiratory changes in this age group. In particular, immobility is not well tolerated. Changes in mental status and orientation may be induced by sedatives and narcotics and often precipitate confusion and delirium. The treatment for these states is frequently the withdrawal of these medications rather than administration of additional drugs.[63]

Nonetheless, from the psychological standpoint, elders tolerate elective surgery well.[64,65] In a detailed study of psychological and social deterioration in patients older than 65 years, Simpson and associates found a low incidence of psychological deterioration attributable to surgery and anesthesia.[66] They concluded that "anesthesia has no effect on the physical activity, mental ability, personality or social integration" in this age group when they are studied several months after surgery.

TABLE 30-6
Bivariate Correlates of Postoperative Delirium in the Derivation Set

RISK FACTOR	ALL PATIENTS No.	PATIENTS WITH DELIRIUM No. (%)	RELATIVE RISK	*P**
Age (years)				
≥70	360	55 (15)	3.4	<0.001
<70	516	23 (4)		
Alcohol abuse				
Yes	40	8 (20)	2.4	0.01
No	828	70 (8)		
TICS score				
<30	127	30 (24)	3.7	<0.001
≥30	732	47 (6)		
SAS class				
IV	70	12 (17)	2.1	0.01
I, II, or III	802	65 (8)		
Preoperative sodium, potassium, and glucose levels†				
At least one markedly abnormal	34	8 (24)	2.8	0.002
None markedly abnormal	842	70 (8)		
White blood count				
$>12 \times 10^9$/L	41	8 (20)	2.3	0.02
$\leq 12 \times 10^9$/L	813	70 (9)		
Type of surgery‡				
Aortic aneurysm	35	16 (46)	6.2	<0.001
All other noncardiac	841	62 (7)		
Type of surgery‡				
Noncardiac thoracic	82	13 (16)	1.9	0.02
All other noncardiac	794	65 (8)		

SAS, Specific Activity Scale; *TICS*, telephone interview for cognitive status.

* Two-sided significance level from χ^2 test.

† Markedly abnormal levels were defined as follows: sodium <130 or >150 mM, potassium <3.0 or >6.0 mM, and glucose <3.3 or >16.7 mM (<60 or >300 mg/dL).

‡ Procedure categories were not mutually exclusive: 17 patients were classified as having procedures in more than one category. For example, patients undergoing thoracic aortic aneurysm surgery were included in both the aortic aneurysm and the noncardiac thoracic groups.

Marcantonio ER, Goldman L, Mangione CM: A clinical prediction rule for delirium after elective noncardiac surgery. JAMA 271:134, 1994.

Children

In children, personality changes may occur after surgery or after merely the experience of hospitalization.[67] Nightmares, bed-wetting, fear of strangers, fear of the dark, temper tantrums, aggressive behavior, and fears of separation are some of the common symptoms. They are most likely to follow surgery in children 6 months to 4 years old, in whom separation anxiety figures prominently in psychic development.

The incidence of behavior disturbances in children appears to be related to the efficacy of premedication and preoperative preparation in reducing anxiety and in particular to the smoothness of induction of anesthesia.[58,68] The following have been suggested to reduce anxiety and achieve smooth induction: narcotic–barbiturate premedication[33]; intensive psychological preparation of the child by the anesthesiologist and by the parents[69]; induction of anesthesia with an ultra–short-acting barbiturate rather than a gas[59]; and minimization of hospitalization, primarily through day surgery programs.[59] Premedication with midazolam, for instance 0.5 mg/kg orally 10 to 30 minutes preoperatively, is particularly effective.[59]

Other Problems

A variety of other procedures are associated with postoperative emotional problems: orthopedic procedures, especially in older people (because of low tolerance of immobilization),[7,44] plastic surgery (because of disappointment that occurs when surgery fails to correct problems), cancer surgery,[70] vasectomy,[71] and ophthalmic surgery (because of lack of sensory input).[72]

Medications used after surgery have been associated with postoperative delirium. Marcantonio and Juarez and coworkers investigated risk factors for postoperative delirium among a group of patients at risk.[73] All patients considered had one or more of the following risk factors: advanced age; poor cognitive function; self-reported alcohol abuse; markedly abnormal serum sodium, potassium or glucose levels; aortic aneurysm surgery; or noncardiac thoracic surgery. Patients given meperidine had almost twice the incidence of postoperative delirium compared to patients given other narcotics. Both the intravenous (patient-controlled analgesia) and epidural routes of meperidine administration more frequently resulted in delirium. Long-acting benzodiazepines (diazepam, chlordiazepoxide, and flurazepam) had a stronger association with delirium than shorter acting sedatives. Marcantonio and Juarez recommended against the use of meperidine in favor of other narcotics, and for minimization of the use of long-acting benzodiazepines.

PRE-EXISTING EMOTIONAL PROBLEMS

As already indicated, attitudes, fears, ego strengths, and emotional makeup affect the patient's emotional responses to surgery and anesthesia. Titchner and colleagues found that 86% of 200 surgical patients displayed psychological symptoms or behavior disturbance to the extent that a psychiatric illness could be diagnosed preoperatively.[45] Their sample was drawn from a low socioeconomic group of deprived and underprivileged people, many from broken homes. Corman and colleagues also noted the same trends in a similar population.[73]

Predictability

The incidence of postoperative psychosis or disorders was 22% in Titchner's group's study[45] and 39% in that of Corman's group.[73] When reactions did occur, they often were explainable "in the light of the dynamic life history of the patient."[73] However, not all neurotic people have emotional upsets postoperatively. Indeed, psychotic persons often show temporary improvement in their behavior after surgery. Abram and Gill, both psychiatrists, were unable to predict accurately a patient's postoperative psychological course based on preoperative interviews.[74]

Predisposition

On a statistical basis, certain psychiatric factors were found significantly more frequently in patients manifesting postoperative delirium (Table 30-7).[44] Titchner and coworkers found that alcoholic persons, patients entering the hospital in delirium, immobilized aged patients, and aged and lonely patients were at greatest risk for psychological aberrations after surgery.[45,57,75] Their findings also showed that close attention and emotional support by family, friends, and hospital personnel were of value in the prevention of psychotic reactions. Another study has found the same to be true of patients with cancer.[69]

Preoperative Preparation

A detailed psychiatric evaluation of 26 patients undergoing routine surgical procedures led Janis to conclude that a certain amount of preoperative anxiety and tension is imperative for psychological stability postoperatively.[76] This "work of worrying" alerts the patient's psychological defenses to the im-

TABLE 30-7
Psychiatric Factors That Influence Postoperative Problems

	NO DELIRIUM (no. = 60)	DELIRIUM (no. = 57)
Factor	*No. (%)*	*No. (%)*
Alcoholism*	2 (3)	15 (26)
Depression†	6 (10)	35 (61)
Family history of psychosis†	1 (2)	7 (12)
Gastrointestinal disorder	13 (22)	24 (42)
Insomnia†	7 (12)	19 (33)
Organic brain syndrome*	0 (0)	22 (38)
Paranoid personality†	2 (3)	11 (19)
Postoperative psychosis*	3 (5)	14 (24)
Psychiatric treatment†	2 (3)	11 (19)
Psychosis†	1 (2)	7 (12)
Retirement problems†	3 (5)	12 (21)

* Statistically significant: $P < 0.01$.
† Statistically significant: $P < 0.05$.
Morse FM, Litin EM: Postoperative delirium: a study of etiologic factors. Am J Psychiatry 126:388, 1969.

pending stress. Inadequate time for this worrying predisposes patients undergoing emergency surgery to postoperative delirium. Neurotic persons, although their defenses may be weaker than those of normally adjusted patients, nevertheless also activate psychological defenses before surgery.

Deutsch observed the following more than 50 years ago.

> [T]he factor of greatest importance for the successful conquest of operation anxiety and its results is the amount of preoperative preparation; that is, whether the operation was performed as an emergency without the patient having a chance to prepare himself or whether . . . the patient had an opportunity for a longer or shorter time of inner preparation. In the first case we have to expect a psychic shock reaction in the patient and its influence on the postoperative situation. The conditions developed in such a shock reaction are very closely related to the so-called traumatic neuroses, which usually are called forth by serious accidents, unexpected attacks, train wrecks, and other situations of sudden and unheralded invasions of danger. . . . Symptoms developed in such a condition are those of general irritability, sleeplessness, anxiety dreams and nightmares, attacks of anxiety with cardiac and respiratory distress, with vasomotor and secretory disturbances.[77]

Anxiety

Janis found that patients who showed no anxiety before major surgery and patients who displayed great anticipatory fear were most liable to have behavior problems postoperatively.[76] Patients who show no anxiety must be made aware of the reality of surgery; otherwise, they may be angry, hostile, and resentful postoperatively. Patients who show great anxiety need to have their emotional excitement mitigated. Several investigators have warned physicians to take these cautions especially with patients who claim to have no fears regarding impending surgery.[13,79] Although full therapeutic results may not be achieved in a short time, a realistic exploration of the events surrounding surgery and anesthesia is usually helpful. Preoperative psychiatric consultation may be indicated when the emotional preparations for surgery seem grossly unrealistic.

THE PREOPERATIVE VISIT

The value of the anesthesiologist's preoperative visit has been widely emphasized.[79,80] The visit is of importance from a physiologic as well as psychological point of view. Several studies show that preoperative psychological preparation reduces the incidence of postoperative emotional disturbance in the patient undergoing cardiac surgery.[52,54,55] Thus, intensive preparation by nurses, anesthesiologists, surgeons, and psychiatrists may be used. This preparation usually consists of detailed descriptions of mechanical ventilation, monitoring, and physiotherapy procedures as well as psychiatric interviews. The interviews are directed toward exploring anxieties and fantasies, providing realistic explanations, and correcting misconceptions. These procedures dramatically reduce the incidence of postcardiotomy psychosis.

Children

Jackson, an anesthesiologist, showed that after honest, detailed preoperative explanation to 5-, 6-, and 7-year-old children, a mask induction of anesthesia was rarely stormy or complicated.[68] However, follow-up evaluation of problems in the recovery room and delayed abnormal behavior were not explored. Eckenhoff, however, showed that postoperative behavior problems were more likely to occur in children who had had a stormy induction of anesthesia.[58]

Adults

In adults undergoing general surgery, Egbert and colleagues evaluated the preoperative visit.[79] They found that a preoperative discussion of "the patient's condition, the time of operation, and the nature of the anesthetic, informing the patient about what would happen the next day as well as questioning him about previous experiences with anesthetics" in combination with pentobarbital and atropine premedication (producing calmness and drowsiness), "adequately" prepared 71% of patients.[80] In contrast, only 48% of patients receiving pentobarbital without an interview and 35% receiving atropine without an interview were adequately prepared. Psychological benefits were noted for as long as 18 hours after interview. Again, however, postoperative behavior was not investigated. In a subsequent study, Egbert also found that detailed preoperative instructions concerning maneuvers to relieve pain decreased morphine requirements postoperatively.[80] Kolouch commented on the use of preanesthetic posthypnotic suggestion to promote a speedy, uneventful recovery from surgery.[81]

Effect on Postoperative Emotional Response

No study directly documents the effect of a "routine" preanesthetic visit on postoperative emotional response. However, on the basis of the evidence cited as well as the comments of psychiatrists,[4,31,66] the anesthesiologist may exert significant beneficial effects on a patient's postoperative emotional responses. Too often it is assumed that the surgeon discusses and assesses the patient's attitudes toward surgery. Even if this were the case, most patients have specific questions and fears concerning anesthesia. More than 92% of patients interviewed postoperatively by Sheffer and Greifenstein feared anesthesia (Table 30-8).[65] Sometimes patients voiced specific apprehensions: 43% desired complete withdrawal from the environment during surgery; 29% found general anesthesia unpleasant; 15% were distressed by spinal anesthesia and 11% by regional or local anesthesia. Often, however, the fears were displayed by various changes in behavior before surgery (see Table 30-8). Almost all patients expressed a "healthy active interest and curiosity" in the anesthetic, but in most cases "the attitudes revealed that the anesthetists failed to establish rapport with [them]."[65] Most patients desired not only information but reassurance as well.

Goals

What can the anesthesiologist reasonably hope to accomplish in the brief preoperative visit? Direct answers to the patients' questions are of great value. Most patients are concerned about the type of anesthesia (general, spinal, or other); induction of anesthesia; the extent of pain and the plan and options to minimize it; a state of wakefulness; the chance of arousal

TABLE 30-8
Incidence of Conversion Symptoms

CHANGE	PATIENTS (no.)
MOTOR	
Restlessness	35
Pacing the floor	16
Muscle tension	18
Compulsive biting	7
Tapping of fingers	14
Compulsive hair rubbing	12
Total	**102**
AUTONOMIC	
Loss of appetite	13
Urinary frequency	23
Increased sweating	36
Total	**72**

Sheffer MB, Greifenstein FE: The emotional response of patients to surgery and anesthesia. Anesthesiology 21:502, 1960.

during anesthesia; the possibility that they might say things that would embarrass them; and the chance of not awakening from anesthesia.

These are meaningful questions and are loaded with emotional significance. Anesthesia is equated on a subconscious or conscious level with death.[4,13] As such, even though many patients ask these questions in a jocular tone, they are to be answered honestly. Even though the questions may not be expressed directly, they are of concern to all patients and may be answered as part of the description of the events that will occur before, during, and after surgery. The physician may reassure the patient by describing the events surrounding surgery and anesthesia, including details like scrub suits, intravenous cannulation, the number of people in the operating room, the circumstances on awakening from anesthesia, oxygen administration, pain, the monitoring of "vital signs," and the PACU. Other supportive or predictive statements thereby attain added weight.

Above all, though, the anesthesiologist's goal should be to establish a relationship with the patient and to present himself or herself as a person who is interested in the patient as a human being.[13] In some hospitals, a PACU nurse visits the patient before surgery to give further psychological anchoring for the transition from clouded consciousness to arousal. All patients, particularly those at greatest risk for postoperative psychiatric disturbance, should if possible be encouraged to voice their fears and concerns. Correction of misapprehensions and unrealistic expectations regarding anesthesia and particularly arousal from anesthesia is of unquestioned value.

The Postanesthesia Care Unit and Beyond

Optimally, the anesthesiologist's support should continue in the PACU and postoperatively. Although the patient's affect on emergence may be blunted, "a salutary influence" is created by continuation of the physician–patient relationship.[12] Even in the case of recovery from ketamine, for which it has been recommended that patients be left undisturbed until fully awake, Garfield and coworkers found that most patients appreciated reassurance and human contact during emergence.[25] An early postoperative visit may permit the patient to discuss unpleasant experiences and allow the clinician to explain any untoward events and answer any remaining questions concerning anesthesia. Perhaps explanation of fears and anxieties during this time can prevent them from transforming into psychological defense mechanisms that may be reactivated during similar stressful situations in the future.

For patients who experience repetitive nightmares and preoccupation with death postoperatively, the possibility that they were aware during anesthesia should be strongly considered. These patients often are reluctant to discuss their awareness because of fear that they might be thought insane. However, Blacher has shown that direct discussion of their awareness during anesthesia often reduces the symptoms dramatically (see Chapter 29).[28]

REFERENCES

1. Badger TL: The physician-patient in the recovery and intensive care units. Arch Surg 109:359, 1974
2. Dupuytren B: Clinical lectures of surgery. Lancet 2:919, 1834
3. Miller HH: Acute psychoses following surgical procedures. British Medical Journal 1:558, 1939
4. Straker M: Surgical procedures and neurotic illness. Can Med Assoc J 65:128, 1951
5. Cobb S, McDermott NT: Postoperative psychosis. Med Clin North Am 22:569, 1938
6. Savage GH: Insanity following the use of anaesthetics in operations. British Medical Journal 2:1199, 1887
7. Morse RM, Litin EM: The anatomy of a delirium. Am J Psychiatry 128:143, 1971
8. Oltman JE, Friedman S: The role of operative procedure in the etiology of psychosis. Psychiatr Q 17:405, 1943
9. Baxter S: Psychological problems of intensive care. Br J Hosp Med 11:875, 1966
10. Katz NM, Agle DP, DePalma RG, et al: Delirium in surgical patients under intensive care. Arch Surg 104:310, 1972
11. Eckenhoff JE, Kneale DH, Dripps RD: The incidence and etiology of postanesthetic excitement. Anesthesiology 22:668, 1961
12. Winkelstein C, Blacher RS, Meyer BC: Psychiatric observations on surgical patients in the recovery room. New York State Journal of Medicine 65:865, 1965
13. Schnaper N: Postanesthetic (postoperative) emotional responses. Anesthesiology 22:674, 1961
14. Knox JWD, Bovill JG, Clarke RSJ, et al: Clinical studies of induction agents: XXXVI. ketamine. Br J Anaesth 42:875, 1970
15. Zubek VP: Effects of prolonged sensory and perceptual deprivation. Br Med Bull 20:38, 1964
16. Fahy A, Marshall M: Postanaesthetic morbidity in out-patients. Br J Anaesth 41:433, 1969
17. Coppolino CA: Incidence of postanesthetic delirium in a community hospital: a statistical survey. Mil Med 128:238, 1963
18. Smessaert A, Schehr CA, Artusio JF: Observations in the immediate post-anaesthesia period: II. mode of recovery. Br J Anaesth 332:181, 1960
19. James FM: The effects of cyclopropane anesthesia without surgical operation on mental functions of normal man. Anesthesiology 30:264, 1969
20. Davison LA, Steinhelber JC, Eger EI II, et al: Psychological effects of halothane and isoflurane anesthesia. Anesthesiology 43:313, 1975
21. Johnstone RE, Kennel EM, Behar MG, et al: Increased serum bromide concentrations after halothane anesthesia in man. Anesthesiology 42:598, 1975
22. Kornfeld DS: Open heart surgery and the psyche. JAMA 213:1343, 1970

23. Sadove MS, Hartano S, Redlin T, et al: Clinical study of droperidol in the prevention of the side effects of ketamine anesthesia: a progress report. Anesth Analg 50:526, 1971
24. Krestow M: The effect of post-anaesthetic dreaming on patient acceptance of ketamine anaesthesia: a comparison with thiopentone-nitrous oxide anaesthesia. Can Anaesth Soc J 21:385, 1974
25. Garfield JM, Garfield FB, Stone JG, et al: A comparison of psychological responses to ketamine and thiopental–nitrous oxide–halothane anesthesia. Anesthesiology 36:329, 1972
26. Fine J, Finestone SC: Sensory disturbances following ketamine anesthesia: recurrent hallucinations. Anesth Analg 52:428, 1973
27. Meyers EF, Charles P: Prolonged adverse reactions to ketamine in children. Anesthesiology 49:39, 1978
28. Blacher RS: Awareness during surgery. Anesthesiology 61:1, 1984
29. Bogetz MS, Katz JA: Recall of surgery for major trauma. Anesthesiology 61:6, 1984
30. Cheek DB: Further evidence of persistence of hearing under chemoanesthesia: detailed case report. Am J Clin Hypn 7:55, 1964
31. Terrell RK, Sweet WO, Gladfelter JM, et al: Study of recall during anesthesia. Anesth Analg 48:86, 1969
32. Nadelson T: The psychiatrist in the surgical intensive care unit: I. postoperative delirium. Arch Surg 111:113, 1976
33. Freeman A, Bachman L: Pediatric anesthesia: an evaluation of preoperative medication. Anesth Analg 38:429, 1959
34. Tune LE, Holland A, Folstein MF, et al: Association of postoperative delirium with raised serum levels of anticholinergic drugs. Lancet 26:651, 1981
35. Bernards W: Case history number 74: reversal of phenothiazine induced coma with physostigmine. Anesth Analg 52:938, 1973
36. Greene LT: Physostigmine treatment of anticholinergic-drug depression in postoperative patients. Anesth Analg 50:222, 1971
37. Smith DS, Orkin FK, Gardner SM, et al: Prolonged sedation in the elderly after intraoperative atropine administration. Anesthesiology 51:348, 1979
38. Mays ET, Ransdell HT, DeWeese BM: Metabolic changes in surgical delirium tremens. Surgery 67:780, 1970
39. McMurrey JD, Law SW: Postoperative changes in electrolyte balance. Anesthesiology 22:819, 1961
40. Bennett HL, Davis HS, Giannini JA: Nonverbal response to intraoperative conversation. Br J Anaesth 57:174, 1985
41. Levinson BW: States of awareness during general anaesthesia. Br J Anaesth 37:544, 1965
42. Atlschule MD: Postoperative psychosis. Surg Clin North Am 49: 677, 1969
43. Kaufer C: Etiology of consciousness disturbances in surgery. Minn Med 51:1509, 1968
44. Morse RM, Litin EM: Postoperative delirium: a study of etiologic factors. Am J Psychiatry 126:388, 1969
45. Titchner JL, Zwerling I, Gottschalk L, et al: Psychosis in surgical patients. Surg Gynecol Obstet 102:59, 1956
46. Ghouri AF, Ruiz MA, White PF: Effect of flumazenil on recovery after midazolam and propofol sedation. Anesthesiology 81:333, 1994
47. Nussmeier NA, Arlund C, Slogoff S: Neuropsychiatric complications after cardiopulmonary bypass: cerebral protection by a barbiturate. Anesthesiology 64:165, 1986
48. Gilman S: Cerebral disorders after open heart surgery. N Engl J Med 272:489, 1965
49. Tufo HM, Muslin H, Ostfeld AM: Central nervous system: complications in the surgical patient. Dis Mon 1968 (November)
50. Tufo HM, Ostfeld AM, Shekelle R: Central venous system: dysfunction following open-heart surgery. JAMA 212:1333, 1970
51. Hickey PR, Hansen DD, Norwood WI, et al: Anesthetic complications in surgery for congenital heart disease. Anesth Analg 63:657, 1984
52. Abram HS: Psychotic reactions after cardiac surgery: a critical review. Seminars in Psychiatry 3:70, 1971
53. Heller SS, Frank KA, Malm JR, et al: Psychiatric complications of open heart surgery. N Engl J Med 283:1015, 1970
54. Layne OL Jr, Yudofsky SC: Psychosis in cardiotomy patients: the role or organic and psychiatric factors. N Engl J Med 284: 518, 1971
55. Lazarus HR, Hagens JH: Prevention of psychosis following open heart surgery. Am J Psychiatry 124:1190, 1968
56. Rabiner CJ, Willner AE, Fishman J: Psychiatric complications following coronary bypass surgery. J Nerv Ment Dis 160:342, 1975
57. Titchner JL, Levine M: Surgery as a human experience. New York: Oxford University Press, 1960
58. Eckenhoff JE: Relationship of anesthesia to postoperative personality changes in children. Am J Dis Child 86:587, 1951
59. Feld LH, Negus JB, White PF: Clinical investigations: oral midazolam preanesthetic medication in pediatric outpatients. Anesthesiology 73:831, 1990
60. Marcantonio ER, Goldman L, Mangione CM: A clinical prediction rule for delirium after elective noncardiac surgery. JAMA 271:134, 1994
61. Flatt JR, Burnell PC, Hobbes A: Effects of anaesthesia on some aspects of mental functioning of surgical patients. Anaesth Intensive Care 12:315, 1984
62. Millar HR: Psychiatric morbidity in elderly surgical patients. Br J Psychiatry 138:17, 1981
63. Patkin M: Postoperative confusion. Med J Aust 2:559, 1973
64. Brander P, Kjellberg M, Tammisto T: The effects of anaesthesia and general surgery on geriatric patients. Annales Chirurgiae et Gynaecologiae Fenniae 59:138, 1970
65. Sheffer MB, Greifenstein FE: The emotional responses of patients to surgery and anesthesia. Anesthesiology 21:502, 1960
66. Simpson BR, Williams M, Scott JF, et al: The effects of anaesthesia and elective surgery on old people. Lancet 2:887, 1961
67. Vernon DTA, Schulman JL, Foley JM: Changes in children's behavior after hospitalization. Am J Dis Child 111:581, 1966
68. Jackson K: Psychologic preparation as a method of reducing the emotional trauma of anesthesia in children. Anesthesiology 12: 293, 1951
69. Abrams RD, Funisinger JE: Guilt reactions in patients with cancer. Cancer 6:474, 1953
70. Wolfers H: Psychological aspects of vasectomy. British Medical Journal 4:297, 1970
71. Preu PW, Gueda F: Psychoses complicating recovery from extraction of cataract. Archives of Neurology and Psychiatry 38: 818, 1937
72. Quinlan DM, Kimball CP, Osborne F: The experience of open heart surgery: IV. assessment of disorientation and dysphoria following cardiac surgery. Arch Gen Psychiatry 31:241, 1974
73. Marcantonio ER, Jaurez G, et al: The relationship of postoperative delirium with psychoactive medications. JAMA 272:1518, 1994
74. Abram HS, Gill BF: Predictions of postoperative psychiatric complications. N Engl J Med 265:1123, 1961
75. Zwerling I, Titchner J, Gottschalk L, et al: Personality disorder and the relationships of emotion aid surgical illness in 200 surgical patients. Am J Psychiatry 112:270, 1955
76. Janis IL: Psychological stress. New York: John Wiley & Sons, 1958:376
77. Deutsch H: Some psychoanalytic observations in surgery. Psychosom Med 4:105, 1942
78. Schnaper N: What preanesthetic visit? Anesthesiology 22:486, 1961
79. Egbert LD, Battit GE, Turndorf H, et al: The value of the preoperative visit by an anesthetist. JAMA 185:553, 1963
80. Egbert LD, Battit GE, Welch CE, et al: Reduction in postoperative pain by encouragement and instruction in patients. N Engl J Med 270:825, 1964
81. Kolouch FT: Role of suggestion in surgical convalescence. Arch Surg 85:304, 1962

Complications in Anesthesiology, second edition,
edited by Nikolaus Gravenstein and Robert R. Kirby.
Lippincott-Raven Publishers, Philadelphia © 1996.

CHAPTER 31

Prolonged Emergence and Failure to Regain Consciousness

J. Kenneth Denlinger

Although many factors are known to prolong anesthetic effects, most reports of prolonged emergence in humans are anecdotal. This chapter categorizes the various causes of postoperative coma and cites clinical reports of prolonged emergence. Metabolic disturbances, such as the hyperosmolar syndrome, are reviewed in detail because anesthesia may mask the cerebral manifestations of these potentially lethal disturbances and thereby delay their recognition.

THE MECHANISM OF CORTICAL AROUSAL

Reticular Activating System

Classic studies by Magoun showed that wakefulness depends on diffuse cortical activation by the reticular formation of the brain stem.[1] Cortical arousal and focus of attention elicited by afferent sensory stimuli are mediated by the reticular activating system. Barbiturates produce early depression of this multisynaptic ascending pathway.[2] Certain metabolic disorders associated with central nervous system (CNS) depression, such as hypoglycemia and hypoxia, also result in early depression of auditory evoked potentials in the reticular formation of the brain stem when cortical evoked potentials are minimally depressed.[3] Selective vulnerability of the reticular activating system to certain anesthetic and metabolic disturbances may be related to the multisynaptic nature of this ascending pathway. According to this concept, functional depression of a neural pathway is directly proportional to the number of synapses in that pathway.[4]

Cortical Neural Pathways

Although selective depression of the reticular activating system may be of significance in the delayed awakening of some patients after anesthesia, many other cortical and subcortical neural pathways also are involved. General anesthesia is produced by a variety of neurophysiologic mechanisms. For example, ether produces early cortical depression, and ketamine results in neural excitation at the cortical and subcortical levels.[5,6] Thus, the neurophysiologic mechanism of prolonged narcosis after anesthesia is drug dependent and may involve neural stimulation or depression at the cortical or subcortical levels.

Cortical Neurotransmitters

Connecting the cortical neural pathways are synapses that represent drug-modifiable control points. Neurotransmitters are the endogenous agents that effect neural transmission, and include cholinergic substances, amino acids, and monoamines, all of which may be influenced by anesthetic management.

Acetylcholine

Although acetylcholine is not the primary excitatory cortical neurotransmitter, the ascending cholinergic arousal system may be the pharmacologic equivalent of the reticular activating system.[7] Stimulation of this neural pathway at the level of the midbrain causes cortical electroencephalographic (EEG) arousal and acetylcholine release. Direct application of acetylcholine to acetylcholine-sensitive cortical neurons results in prolonged excitation, a pharmacologic effect that is potentiated by anticholinesterases and blocked by atropine in experimental animals.[8]

Although atropine is capable of producing CNS depression in humans when it is given in massive doses or when the subject is elderly,[9] the central anticholinergic syndrome occurs more frequently after premedicant doses of scopolamine. Physostigmine is chosen as the pharmacologic antagonist because this anticholinesterase readily crosses the blood–brain

TABLE 31-1
Differential Diagnosis of Prolonged Recovery and Failure to Regain Consciousness

PROLONGED DRUG ACTION
Overdose
Increased central sensitivity
Age
Biologic variation
Metabolic effects
Decreased protein binding
Delayed anesthetic excretion
Anesthetic redistribution
Decreased hepatic metabolism, drug interaction, and biotransformation
METABOLIC ENCEPHALOPATHY
Hepatic, renal, endocrinologic, and neurologic disorders
Hypoxia and hypercapnia
Acidosis
Hypoglycemia
Hyperosmolar syndrome
Electrolyte imbalance (sodium ion, calcium ion, or magnesium ion)
Hypothermia and hyperthermia
Neurotoxic drugs
NEUROLOGIC INJURY
Cerebral ischemia
Intracranial hemorrhage
Cerebral embolus
Hypoxia and cerebral edema

barrier, in contrast to its analogue, neostigmine, which possesses a quaternary amine group and therefore penetrates the blood–brain barrier poorly.[10]

γ-Aminobutyric Acid

The major inhibitory neurotransmitter in the brain is γ-aminobutyric acid, which hyperpolarizes neurons by opening chloride ion channels; this opening, in turn, decreases the likelihood of depolarization by excitatory stimuli.[11] A single neural membrane protein contains the γ-aminobutyric acid recognition sites, the chloride channel, and several drug recognition sites. Among the latter is a benzodiazepine receptor that, on occupation by diazepam, enhances γ-aminobutyric acid–mediated inhibitory neurotransmission, leading to the familiar anticonvulsant and sedative effects of benzodiazepines.[11] Believed to act at the same receptor, the specific benzodiazepine antagonist flumazenil reverses the sedation and respiratory depression associated with the use of benzodiazepines.[12] Baclofen, a γ-aminobutyric acid derivative, has been associated with delayed arousal after general anesthesia.[13]

DIFFERENTIAL DIAGNOSIS OF POSTOPERATIVE COMA

Failure to awaken promptly after general anesthesia may be related to any of three causes: prolonged action of anesthetic drugs, metabolic encephalopathy, or neurologic injury (Table 31-1). Certain operations may be associated with prolonged cognitive impairment, motor impairment, or both (Table 31-2).

Prolonged Action of Anesthetic Drugs

Overdose

Delayed awakening after general anesthesia is most commonly caused by anesthetic overdose. Overdose can occur when anesthetics are administered for the wrong reason. For example, increased perfusion pressure during cardiopulmonary bypass or intraoperative hypertension caused by a catecholamine-secreting tumor might be treated with large doses of barbiturate in an attempt to deepen anesthesia. Failure to use specific vasodilators or adrenergic blocking agents in such circumstances can lead to anesthetic overdose and delayed recovery.

TABLE 31-2
Operations With Increased Risk of Cognitive or Motor Impairment

OPERATION	INCIDENCE (%)	MECHANISM(S) (If Known)
Cataract extraction	0.3–15.9	Anticholinergic drugs,* preexisting psychiatric or organic brain disease, sensory deprivation
Transurethral prostate surgery	Variable	Hyponatremia† caused by absorption of irrigant solution
Carotid endarterectomy	1–4	Embolism, hypoperfusion, infarction
Open ventricle	28.9‡	Particulate, air embolism, cerebral hypoperfusion
Coronary artery bypass	0.9–5.2§	Particulate, air embolism, cerebral hypoperfusion, infarction, preexisting cerebral vascular disease

* Summers WK, Reich TC: Delirium after cataract surgery: review and two cases. Am J Psychiatr 136: 386, 1979.

† Level of hyponatremia at which patients become symptomatic varies from patient to patient and also depends on how rapidly hyponatremia develops.

‡ Nussmeier NA, Arlund C, Slogoff S: Neuropsychiatric complications after cardiopulmonary bypass: cerebral protection by a barbiturate. Anesthesiology 64:165, 1986.

§ Farhat SM, Schneider RC: Observations on the effect of systemic blood pressure on intracranial circulation in patients with cerebrovascular insufficiency. Neurosurgery 27:441, 1967.

Mahla M: Nervous system. In Gravenstein N (ed): Manual of complications during anesthesia. Philadelphia: JB Lippincott, 1991:407.

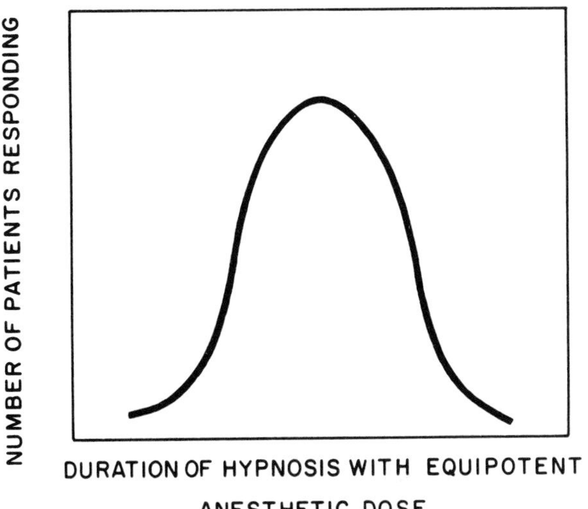

FIGURE 31-1. Biologic variation in central sensitivity to anesthetic action.

Increased Central Nervous System Sensitivity

The duration of the hypnotic effect of a general anesthetic agent depends on the concentration of anesthetic in the brain and the sensitivity of the brain receptor site to that anesthetic. Biologic variation in sensitivity is expressed by the bell-shaped Gaussian curve, which relates the number of responding patients to the duration of hypnotic effect (Fig. 31-1). Sensitivity of the brain to hypnotic drug action may be influenced by several physiologic and pharmacologic factors.

Circadian rhythm affects the halothane anesthetic requirement in rats: the minimum alveolar concentration is decreased 10% to 14% during the inactive phase of a cycle induced by alternating periods of light and darkness.[14] Cyclic variation also may apply to the duration of hypnotic effect in anesthetized humans. Anesthetic requirements are reduced by advanced age, hypothermia, and hypothyroidism.[15,16] These factors also probably increase the duration of hypnotic drug action, in part by increasing CNS sensitivity.

Reserpine, methyldopa, and chronic administration of d-amphetamine reduce anesthetic requirement in experimental animals.[17] However, significant prolongation of anesthesia has not been reported in humans after the use of catecholamine-depleting drugs. Although variation in CNS sensitivity is a valid explanation for some cases of prolonged emergence from anesthesia, this diagnosis usually is made by exclusion and cannot be substantiated until all other factors that influence drug action and level of consciousness have been considered. Another phenomenon is that of "differential awakening," which Cucchiara describes as a focal manifestation of delayed awakening.[18] He theorizes that this phenomenon may occur as a consequence of trapping of anesthetics in injured or relatively underperfused areas of the brain; increased sensitivity to anesthetic effects in injured parts of the brain; or reliance on secondary pathways after recovery from injury, pathways that are functional only in a completely awake state.[18]

Decreased Protein Binding

Drugs that compete with barbiturates for common binding sites increase barbiturate action and duration by displacement of barbiturate from plasma protein. For example, the administration of sodium acetrizoate (a radiographic contrast material) increases the duration of pentobarbital narcosis by this mechanism.[19] Thiopental concentration in the brain and heart after intravenous administration is markedly increased by pretreatment with sulfadimethoxine, a drug that undergoes extensive protein binding.[20] Hypoproteinemia may prolong the duration of barbiturate anesthesia by a reduction in the delivery of barbiturate to the liver.[21] Normal and pathophysiologic states associated with changes in plasma proteins are listed in Table 31-3 and are described further in a comprehensive review.[22]

Delayed Anesthetic Excretion

The decrease in brain anesthetic concentration, evidenced clinically by emergence or awakening from anesthesia, depends on factors similar to those that govern anesthesia uptake

TABLE 31-3
States Associated With Changes in Concentrations of Plasma Proteins

DECREASED ALBUMIN	INCREASED α-ACID GLYCOPROTEIN	DECREASED α-ACID GLYCOPROTEIN
Thermal burns	Thermal burns	Neonatal age
Renal disease	Crohn's disease	Oral contraceptives
Hepatic disease	Renal transplantation	Pregnancy
Inflammatory disease	Infection	
Nephrotic syndrome	Trauma	
Cardiac failure	Chronic pain	
Postoperative period	Myocardial infarction	
Malnutrition	Postoperative period	
Malignancy	Malignancy	
Neonatal age	Rheumatoid arthritis	
Advanced age	Ulcerative colitis	

Adapted from Wood M: Plasma drug binding: implications for anesthesiologists. Anesth Analg 65:786, 1986.

and distribution. The solubility of an anesthetic agent is directly proportional to the effect of anesthetic duration on the speed of recovery. Clinical experience has shown that emergence from anesthesia is slow when high concentrations of soluble agents are used for long surgical procedures. If the agent is highly fat soluble, an anesthetic reservoir is provided by the fat stores from which the agent is released after termination of anesthesia.

Increased cardiac output delays emergence from anesthesia by reducing anesthetic clearance from the brain in the early phases of recovery. Postoperative hypoventilation also delays emergence from anesthesia, by decreasing the alveolar–venous blood anesthetic partial pressure gradient. Stoelting and Eger compared the effect of a fourfold variation in ventilation on the rate of decrease of alveolar concentration for three anesthetic agents of differing solubilities.[23] The effect of increasing ventilation was found to be greatest for halothane, an agent of moderate solubility, whereas it had a less significant effect for nitrous oxide and methoxyflurane.

Anesthetic Redistribution

Awakening after a single intravenous dose of thiopental depends primarily on redistribution of this drug in lean body tissue.[24] In fact, redistribution may be the major factor responsible for the termination of hypnotic action of all clinically useful barbiturates as well as other hypnotic drugs, such as diazepam and midazolam.[25] However, considerable experimental evidence suggests that hepatic metabolism may be of some importance in the duration of sleep produced by a single intravenous dose of thiopental. Gross alteration in hepatic function (such as by hepatectomy or portal vein diversion) is associated with significantly prolonged barbiturate sleeping time in animals.[20] Although controversy surrounds the clinical importance of metabolism in recovery after a single intravenous dose of barbiturate,[24,26] the metabolic effect is significant when multiple doses of barbiturate or other intravenous hypnotic drugs are administered over a prolonged period. Saturation of body tissues limits the magnitude of redistribution and thus prolongs the CNS action of an otherwise short-acting agent.

Decreased Hepatic Metabolism: Microsomal Enzyme Formation and Biotransformation

Extremes of age, malnutrition, hypothermia, and simultaneous administration of several drugs that are detoxified by the hepatic microsomal system (eg, ethanol and barbiturates) are associated with decreased hepatic metabolism and prolonged anesthetic emergence. Alteration in hepatic microsomal metabolism has been demonstrated to influence the uptake and elimination of methoxyflurane in rats.[27] Monoamine oxidase inhibitors also inhibit hepatic microsomal enzymes. The mechanism by which monoamine oxidase inhibitors potentiate the effects of narcotics, barbiturates, and other sedative drugs has not been established, however.[28] Bis-[*p*-nitrophenyl] phosphate prolongs the anesthetic action of propanidid by inhibition of the hepatic enzyme system responsible for rapid hydrolysis of this agent.[29]

KETAMINE. The combination of ketamine with various tranquilizers for the purpose of reducing hallucinatory phenomena on emergence may delay anesthetic emergence. Early evidence suggested that hepatic biotransformation of ketamine plays an important role in the termination of its CNS action even after a single intravenous dose.[30] Ketamine may differ from thiopental in this respect; therefore, some degree of caution is advised when ketamine is administered to patients with gross hepatic dysfunction. Because the halothane anesthetic requirement is significantly reduced 6 hours after ketamine administration in the rat,[31] ketamine cannot be regarded as a short-acting agent and may contribute to prolonged recovery from anesthesia.

HALOTHANE. Biotransformation of halothane is associated with release of free bromide ion in concentrations sufficient to produce postoperative drowsiness and lethargy in humans.[32,33] Preoperative ingestion of bromide-containing drugs, impaired renal function, and hepatic enzyme induction are factors that may predispose patients to increases in bromide concentration in the postoperative period. Increased plasma bromide concentration may have contributed to one case of prolonged coma after successful repair of an intracranial aneurysm.[32]

CIMETIDINE AND RANITIDINE. Cimetidine and ranitidine impair the hepatic microsomal oxidation of some drugs, raising the possibility that sedatives and other CNS depressants may have a greater or more prolonged effect when used in combination with one of these two agents. However, at least in healthy volunteers, no clinically important interaction occurs between these histamine H_2–receptor antagonists and the benzodiazepines diazepam and midazolam.[34]

Metabolic Encephalopathy

Numerous systemic metabolic disturbances resulting in CNS depression can occur in the postanesthetic period and must be distinguished from residual effects of anesthesia. Metabolic encephalopathy often increases the sensitivity of the brain to depressant drugs.

Liver Disease

In patients with severe liver disease and a history of hepatic coma, EEG slowing and CNS depression develop after the administration of small doses of morphine, whereas in healthy volunteers or patients without a history of hepatic coma, EEG changes do not develop.[35] Narcotics have been implicated as a causative factor in many cases of hepatic coma and should be used with caution in patients with severe liver disease. Although barbiturate sleeping time is markedly prolonged in animals after hepatectomy or drug-induced hepatic damage, studies in patients with severe liver disease have not shown increased sensitivity to single or multiple doses of thiopental.[20,36] Enhanced CNS penetration of cimetidine in patients with liver disease results in mental confusion that may be mistaken for hepatic encephalopathy.[37]

Kidney Disease

Prolongation of barbiturate anesthesia has been reported in patients with renal failure and azotemia.[38] This effect probably results from enhanced CNS sensitivity to barbiturates, although other factors, such as decreased protein binding, electrolyte disturbances, and acid–base imbalance, also may be involved. Increased sensitivity to hypnotic drugs in uremic patients has been suggested to result from changes in the permeability of the blood–brain barrier.[39]

Endocrine and Neurologic Disorders

Hypothyroidism is associated with decreased anesthetic requirements in animals.[40] Clinical reports have suggested that unconsciousness may be prolonged in the postanesthetic period in patients with severe adrenal insufficiency.[41–43] Delayed emergence after thiopental anesthesia has been reported in a patient with Huntington's chorea, although this patient responded normally to subsequent nitrous oxide–ether anesthesia.[44]

Hypoxia and Hypercapnia

Postoperative respiratory failure may result in prolonged emergence from anesthesia. Hypoventilation not only causes respiratory acidosis and hypoxia but also retards excretion of inhalation anesthetics. Carbon dioxide narcosis in the absence of hypoxia may occur in patients with severe chronic lung disease who receive high concentrations of inspired oxygen. Studies in dogs indicate that carbon dioxide produces narcosis primarily by inducing cerebral tissue acidosis.[45] However, narcosis frequently is observed in patients with respiratory failure who have less severe hypercapnia. This discrepancy may be explained by factors other than hypercapnia, such as concomitant hypoxia, drug therapy, and cerebrovascular disease.

Cerebrospinal Fluid Acidosis

Clinical studies in patients with cerebral acidosis from various causes have shown that confusion, delirium, or coma invariably occurs when cerebrospinal fluid pH decreases to 7.25 or less (hydrogen ion concentration ⩾56 nM/L).[46] Cerebrospinal fluid acidosis and CNS depression are more severe when hypercapnia is acute, because carbon dioxide diffuses rapidly into the extracellular fluid of the brain, whereas bicarbonate ion crosses the blood–brain barrier much more slowly.

The combination of acute respiratory acidosis and chronic metabolic alkalosis may be associated with profound cerebral acidosis and coma, despite a normal arterial pH. In a comatose patient with pneumonia and chronic lung disease, during mechanical ventilation with 40% inspired oxygen, Bulger and coworkers obtained the following measurements[47]: cerebrospinal fluid pH 7.15 (hydrogen ion concentration 71 nM/L), arterial pH 7.45 (hydrogen ion concentration 36 nM/L), arterial carbon dioxide partial pressure 72 mm Hg, and arterial oxygen partial pressure 63 mm Hg. Ventilation was increased; the patient's mental status steadily improved as a result; and the pH of the cerebrospinal fluid returned to a normal value.

A paradoxical increase in cerebral acidosis with progressive deterioration in level of consciousness has been reported in diabetic patients with severe ketoacidosis who are given therapeutic doses of sodium bicarbonate.[48] The increase in arterial pH produced by bicarbonate administration results in decreased alveolar ventilation, producing an increase of arterial and brain carbon dioxide partial pressures. The net result is a decrease in brain pH, while arterial pH is increasing.

Measurement of the pH of cerebrospinal fluid is of value in explaining why some patients with serum acidosis are awake and alert, whereas others with similar serum pH values are stuporous or comatose. That systemic acidosis per se does not invariably cause coma is substantiated by arterial pH measurements of 6.8 (hydrogen ion concentration 158.0 nM/L), obtained in two laboratories independently, in a patient who was fully alert and oriented.[46] Severe metabolic acidosis in this patient resulted from chronic bicarbonate loss from the gastrointestinal tract. Concurrent cerebrospinal fluid measurements were as follow: pH 7.36 (hydrogen ion concentration 44 nM/L), arterial carbon dioxide partial pressure 15 mm Hg, and bicarbonate 8.5 mEq/L.

Hypoglycemia

Although anesthesia and surgical stress usually increase blood glucose concentration, dangerous hypoglycemia can occur intraoperatively in rare instances, such as manipulation of insulin-producing tumors of the pancreas or retroperitoneal carcinomas.[49] Fatal postoperative hypoglycemic coma has been reported in diabetic patients given insulin or chlorpropamide preoperatively.[50,51]

DRUG INTERACTIONS. Several unusual drug interactions also predispose to hypoglycemia. Salicylates, sulfonamides, and ethanol have known hypoglycemic effects. Propoxyphene has been reported to produce severe hypoglycemia manifested by hemiparesis and confusion.[52] The hypoglycemic action of tolbutamide and chlorpropamide is enhanced in patients who receive chloramphenicol.[53,54] The combination of chlorpromazine and orphenadrine also has been reported to produce hypoglycemic coma.[55]

LIVER DYSFUNCTION. Severe liver dysfunction can contribute to hypoglycemia by impairment of gluconeogenesis. Aldrete and colleagues reported several instances of severe hypoglycemia after hepatic transplantation; arterial hypotension, loss of consciousness, and metabolic acidosis resulted.[56]

The Hyperosmolar Syndrome

Clinical reports of hyperosmolar, hyperglycemic, nonketotic coma in the perioperative period have established this syndrome as a cause of prolonged unconsciousness after general anesthesia.[57–59] Because of the 40% to 60% mortality rate in patients with this disorder, early recognition and treatment are especially important.

PREDISPOSING FACTORS. Approximately half of these patients have no history of diabetes mellitus, but in most cases a severe concomitant illness, such as sepsis, pneumonia, pancreatitis, uremia, cerebrovascular accident, or large-surface area burns, is present. Severe dehydration, exacerbated by the osmotic diuretic effect of hyperglycemia, contributes to the hyperosmolarity. Administration of hypertonic solutions (eg, solutions given in hyperalimentation or mannitol) also may lead to hyperosmolarity.

As might be expected, this disorder can occur after peritoneal dialysis, hemodialysis, and cardiac surgery. Factors that tend to increase blood sugar concentration, such as massive steroid therapy and intravenous administration of dextrose, also may precipitate it. Marked hyperglycemia has been observed during extracorporeal circulation and profound hypothermia in infants.

Although not directly implicated as a causative factor, the hyperglycemic response to surgical stress and certain anesthetic agents may be an important consideration. However, hyperglycemia by itself is insufficient for coma; cellular dehydration relating to changes in the serum sodium concentration must also be present.[60]

DIAGNOSIS. The diagnosis of hyperosmolar, hyperglycemic, nonketotic coma is confirmed by a blood glucose concentration greater than 600 mg/dL and increased serum osmolality in the absence of ketoacidosis.[61] The serum osmolality reflects the number of osmotically active substances, principally sodium (and its accompanying anions), urea, and glucose.

Because the brain is relatively permeable to both urea and glucose, the ion of particular interest is sodium. Hypernatremia is not consistently a feature of the syndrome. However, hyperglycemia, by recruiting a substantial volume of sodium-poor fluid from the intracellular space, results in an artifactual reduction of the measured serum sodium value.

"Correction" of the serum sodium concentration has been suggested to adjust for this dilutional effect: the measured serum sodium concentration is multiplied by 1.3 to 1.6 mM for every 5.56 mM (100 mg/dL) increment in the serum glucose concentration.[60] Typically, the corrected serum sodium concentration is high in this syndrome. Azotemia and hypokalemia also are common.

CLINICAL COURSE AND MANAGEMENT. Although this disorder may develop slowly over a period of several days, a case described in the immediate postanesthetic period was characterized by a very rapid, fulminant course. Regular insulin, 50 U intravenously, has been recommended as the initial step in reducing blood glucose; the dose of subsequent insulin administration depends on the rate of decrease in blood glucose concentration.[62] Excessively rapid reduction in blood glucose may precipitate hypovolemic shock and cerebral edema.

Large quantities of 0.45% saline usually are required to correct dehydration, and hypovolemic shock may be corrected with saline and albumin. Potassium supplementation also is required, because large amounts of potassium are cotransported intracellularly when glucose utilization is increased. Coma that accompanies the hyperosmolar syndrome is thought to result from cerebral intracellular dehydration. Damage to intracranial "bridging" veins and subsequent subdural hematoma formation may occur as a result of brain shrinkage.

Brain edema may occur during treatment if the blood glucose concentration is allowed to decrease too rapidly. Water diffuses intracellularly along a gradient established by decreased extracellular glucose and increased intracellular sorbitol concentration.[63] Caution therefore must be exercised in the reduction of blood glucose.

Electrolyte Imbalance

Severe electrolyte disturbance in the postoperative period can contribute to prolonged emergence from anesthesia. Dilutional hyponatremia may result from water absorption during transurethral prostate surgery. Coma, hemiparesis, and other alarming neurologic sequelae can accompany water intoxication or hyponatremia because of inappropriate release of antidiuretic hormone triggered by surgical stress.

One report describes a series of 15 healthy women in whom symptomatic hyponatremia (108 mEq/L) developed about 2 days after elective surgery, with concomitant seizures, respiratory arrest, and severe brain damage.[64] Although a specific cause is unclear, concern regarding the rate at which the hyponatremia is corrected is widespread. Rapid correction has been associated with brain damage allegedly attributable to central pontine myelinolysis, although this condition is rare. Persistent hyponatremia presents the risk of continued seizures and possible brain damage. Based on analyses of reported cases, the serum sodium concentration probably should be increased by a maximum of 2 mEq/L per hour, to 128 to 132 mM.[65]

Likewise, severe hypercalcemia and hypermagnesemia produce CNS depression and can lead to coma. The hypocalcemia of hypoparathyroidism is frequently associated with mental changes, diffuse EEG abnormalities, and increased intracranial pressure.

Hypothermia and Hyperthermia

Hypothermia can contribute to prolonged postoperative unconsciousness by reducing the rate of biotransformation of depressant drugs, by increasing the solubility of inhalation anesthetics, or by directly affecting the brain (cold narcosis). Anesthetic requirements in dogs are decreased by 50% when body temperature is decreased from 38°C to 28°C.[66] However, moderate hypothermia alone (30°C to 32°C) does not produce loss of consciousness in normal humans.[67] Delayed emergence from general anesthesia was described in an elderly patient with diabetes insipidus, in whom moderate hypothermia (32°C) had developed; the authors of the report speculated that the hypothalamic endocrine disease was associated with impaired thermoregulation.[68] Severe hyperthermia (>40°C), in contrast, does result in loss of consciousness ("heat stroke").

Neurotoxic Drugs

CNS depression can result from the toxic effect of certain drugs. For example, some cancer chemotherapeutic agents, such as L-asparaginase and vincristine, frequently produce

CNS depression and EEG changes.[69] Though rare in patients emerging from anesthesia, the toxic potential of chemotherapeutic agents must be considered in the differential diagnosis. Radiologic contrast material injected in the subarachnoid space also has been associated with postoperative neurotoxicity.[70]

Neurologic Injury

Failure to regain consciousness after general anesthesia may result from neurologic damage caused by cerebral ischemia, hemorrhage, or embolism.

Cerebral Ischemia

The safety of deliberate, controlled hypotension in most patients without cerebrovascular disease has been well substantiated.[50] Satisfactory recovery of consciousness has been reported in patients undergoing deliberate hypotension with a brachial blood pressure of 40 to 65 mm Hg and with the head tilted upward by 27° for periods of as long as 90 minutes. Measurement of jugular venous oxygen partial pressure in patients without cerebrovascular disease who were undergoing deliberate hypotension induced by a combination of ganglionic blockade, head-up tilt, positive airway pressure, and halothane revealed no evidence of cerebral hypoxia.[71]

However, in rare cases, prolonged unconsciousness resulting from ischemic brain damage has complicated the technique of deliberate hypotension.[72] Brierley and Cooper reported pathologic brain lesions in a previously healthy 45-year-old woman who had prolonged postoperative unconsciousness and organic dementia after deliberate hypotension was used during anesthesia.[73] Hypotension is more likely to produce cerebral ischemia in patients with cerebrovascular disease. Thus, it can be particularly harmful in diabetic or hypertensive patients and in the elderly.

Obstruction of blood flow in the vertebral or carotid circulation may occur when the anesthetized patient is positioned improperly (eg, with extremes of cervical flexion, extension or rotation, or carotid compression from retractors or other mechanical apparatuses).[74] One study suggested that a carotid bruit in patients undergoing coronary artery bypass surgery is associated with a fourfold increased risk of stroke or transient ischemia.[75]

Hemorrhage

Intracranial hemorrhage with an expanding supratentorial hematoma can produce loss of consciousness by brain stem compression and herniation. Hypertension evoked by laryngoscopy and tracheal intubation can result in cerebral hemorrhage during anesthesia. Cerebral hemorrhage is also a feared complication in patients who require thrombolytic therapy or anticoagulation for extended periods (eg, during prolonged extracorporeal circulation).

Cerebral Embolism

AIR. Failure to regain consciousness after cardiac surgery may result from cerebral embolism. Intravenous infusion of very small amounts of air is dangerous in patients with a right-to-left shunt and should be avoided especially in children with congenital cyanotic heart disease (ie, a right-to-left shunt). Entrainment of air into the circulation may occur at any of many sites during cardiac surgery, and meticulous care is required to prevent this complication.

PARTICULATE MATTER. Other sources of cerebral embolus in the patient undergoing cardiac surgery include calcified mitral and aortic valves, atherosclerotic plaques at the cannulation site, left atrial or ventricular thrombus, and bacterial endocarditis. Even irrigation of radial arterial cannulas can result in retrograde brachial arterial flow and cause cerebral embolism.[76] Arterial cannulas should be irrigated by continuous heparinized infusion and flushed slowly with 1 or 2 mL of saline to prevent this complication.

CNS depression accompanying fat embolism typically occurs 12 to 48 hours after fracture of a long bone or massive tissue trauma. Therefore, fat embolism can present as prolonged unconsciousness after general anesthesia for reduction of skeletal fractures.[77] Fat embolism also has been reported after closed-chest cardiac massage and after massive corticosteroid therapy. Jones and colleagues described a patient who was receiving massive doses of steroids as immunosuppressive therapy after renal transplantation; the patient did not regain consciousness after general anesthesia for laparotomy.[78] Coma and death in this patient were attributed to systemic fat embolism, probably from corticoid-induced fatty liver.

CARDIOPULMONARY BYPASS. Clinical experience indicates that anesthetic requirements are markedly reduced after cardiopulmonary bypass. Lack of pulsatile blood flow, disruption of the blood–brain barrier; microembolism of air, fibrin, thrombus, calcium, or fat; and hypoperfusion of the brain all are factors that may contribute to cerebral depression in the postperfusion period. Removal of particulate material by microfiltration may reduce the incidence of embolic complications. Use of barbiturates to produce an isoelectric EEG during open-ventricle procedures also has been shown to be efficacious.[79,80] Continuous monitoring of arterial perfusion pressure and EEG or transcranial Doppler or transesophageal echocardiography may allow earlier detection of cerebral ischemia or emboli.

Hypoxia

In the past, the most common cause of postoperative unconsciousness was the delivery of hypoxic gas mixtures during induction of anesthesia with nitrous oxide. Today, cerebral hypoxia remains an important hazard, despite technologic improvements in anesthesia delivery systems and oxygen monitoring devices. When intraoperative hypoxia is believed to be the cause of prolonged postoperative unconsciousness and when other structural, metabolic, and pharmacologic causes have been reasonably excluded by clinical and laboratory examination, neurologic consultation should be obtained for further evaluation and an organized approach to therapy. Serial EEG evaluation may be of some value in establishing the likelihood of recovery.[81] Deliberate hypothermia seems to reduce cerebral edema and prevent further cerebral damage if instituted promptly. Even though the patient may seem to recover fully, neurologic deterioration has been reported days to weeks postoperatively.[82] The cause of this delayed postanoxic encephalopathy is unknown.

CLINICAL EXAMINATION AND TREATMENT

Because of the many and varied causes of prolonged postoperative unconsciousness, a systematic approach to clinical examination is mandatory. Consideration of the patient's drug history and preexisting systemic disease and of the nature of the operative procedure frequently allows the anesthesiologist to determine the most likely causes of prolonged CNS depression. Intelligent action may then be taken to make or exclude a specific diagnosis. The importance of a thorough preoperative medical history and physical examination is emphasized by the following clinical narrative:

> Unilateral pupillary dilatation was observed in a young, healthy patient who remained unconscious following cardiotomy for repair of an atrial septal defect. Because of the unequal pupil size as well as unconsciousness in the early postoperative period, this patient was feared to have suffered cerebral embolism or hemorrhage. However, no other focal neurologic signs were present, and the patient awakened within a reasonable period of time. Careful examination of the hospital record revealed that anisocoria had been present since birth.

A thorough knowledge of the patient's preoperative physical findings would have obviated the cause for concern.

When the patient remains unconscious in the postanesthesia care unit and there is no obvious explanation for the CNS depression, careful assessment of ventilation and oxygenation is of immediate importance. Measurements of minute ventilation, arterial blood gas partial pressures, pH, and blood glucose concentration should be obtained promptly. Body temperature should be measured and circulatory function assessed to evaluate cerebral perfusion. Additional laboratory studies may indicate the presence of previously undiagnosed hepatic, renal, or endocrine disease. Measurement of serum electrolyte (including calcium and magnesium) concentrations and of osmolarity should be considered. The changes in EEG patterns are of some diagnostic value in predicting the likelihood of eventual recovery.[81]

Systemic metabolic encephalopathy produces loss of consciousness with or without focal neurologic signs. For example, insulin coma in the diabetic patient may present as hemiplegia that is accompanied by the signs of a unilateral upper motor neuron lesion; as a result, cerebral vascular accident may be diagnosed, incorrectly. Treatment with intravenous administration of glucose in this case results in rapid arousal and disappearance of the abnormal neurologic signs.

Plum and Posner reported dissimilar neurologic signs accompanying successive instances of hypoglycemic coma in one patient.[83] Explanations for this variation in neurophysiologic response to a metabolic insult in an individual patient are speculative, at best. Focal neurologic signs accompanying prolonged recovery from anesthesia must therefore be interpreted in the context of anesthetic drug action and metabolic effects on the CNS.

CNS depression produced by narcotics and anticholinergic drugs may be reversed by the use of specific drug antagonists. Narcotic-induced somnolence can be excluded from the differential diagnosis by titrated administration of naloxone (20- to 40-μg boluses). Prolonged unconsciousness produced by the anticholinergic action of scopolamine also may be excluded, by administration of physostigmine. Although scopolamine may have been administered many hours previously, physostigmine, in an equal dose, administered intravenously, sometimes produces striking arousal.[84] This dose of physostigmine rarely produces other side effects. However, atropine should be available to treat bradycardia, should it occur from increased vagal tone. Flumazenil specifically antagonizes somnolence to benzodiazepines[13]; it is titrated to effect in 0.1–0.2-mg increments. Because of the tremendous interpatient variability in benzodiazepine sensitivity, flumazenil merits consideration in patients who have received a benzodiazepine and manifest otherwise unexplained CNS depression.

The value of specific drug antagonists such as naloxone, physostigmine, and flumazenil in the evaluation and treatment of postoperative CNS depression is well established. The use of nonspecific analeptic agents, however, is to be discouraged, because their diagnostic benefits are probably outweighed by the attendant risks (eg, convulsion or relapse into unconsciousness).

REFERENCES

1. Magoun HW: The waking brain. Springfield, IL: Charles C Thomas, 1964: 74
2. French JD, Verzeano M, Magoun HW: A neural basis for the anesthetic state. Arch Neurol Psychiatry 69:519, 1953
3. Arduini A, Arduini MG: Effect of drugs and metabolic alterations on brain stem arousal mechanism. J Pharmacol Exp Ther 110: 76, 1954
4. Larabee MG, Posternak JM: Selective action of anesthetics on synapses and axons in mammalian sympathetic ganglia. J Neurophysiol 15:91, 1952
5. Darbinjan TM, Golovchinsky VB, Plehotkina ST: The effects of anesthetics on reticular and cortical activity. Anesthesiology 34: 219, 1971
6. Ferrer-Allado T, Brechner VL, Dymond A, et al: Ketamine-induced electroconvulsive phenomena in the human limbic and thalamic regions. Anesthesiology 38:333, 1973
7. Krnjevic K: Central cholinergic pathways. Fed Proc 28:113, 1969
8. Krnjevic K: Chemical transmission and cortical arousal. Anesthesiology 28:100, 1967
9. Smith DS, Orkin FK, Gardner SM, et al: Prolonged sedation in the elderly after intraoperative atropine. Anesthesiology 51:348, 1979
10. Duvoisin RC, Katz R: Reversal of central anticholinergic syndrome in man by physostigmine. JAMA 206:1963, 1968
11. Snyder SH: Drug and neurotransmitter receptors: new perspectives with clinical relevance. JAMA 261:3126, 1989
12. Amrein R, Hetzel W: Pharmacology of dormicum (midazolam) and anetate (flumazenil). Acta Anaesthesiol Scand Suppl 34:6, 1990
13. Gomar C, Carrero EJ: Delayed arousal after general anesthesia associated with baclofen. Anesthesiology 81:1306, 1994
14. Munson ES, Martucci RW, Smith RE: Circadian variations in anesthetic requirement and toxicity in rats. Anesthesiology 32: 507, 1970
15. Eger EI II: MAC. In Eger EI II (ed): Anesthetic uptake and action. Baltimore: Williams & Wilkins, 1974: 1

16. Jacobs JR, Reves JG, Marty J: Aging increases pharmacodynamic sensitivity to the hypnotic effects of midazolam. Anesth Analg 80:143, 1995
17. Miller RD, Way WL, Eger EI II: The effects of alpha-methyldopa, reserpine, guanethidine and iproniazid on minimum alveolar anesthetic requirement (MAC). Anesthesiology 29:1153, 1968
18. Cucchiara RF: Differential awakening. Anesth Analg 75:467, 1992
19. Lasser EC, Elizondo-Martel G, Granke RC: Potentiation of pentobarbital anesthesia by competitive protein binding. Anesthesiology 24:665, 1963
20. Ghonein MM, Pandya HB, Kelley SE: Binding of thiopental to plasma proteins: effects on distribution in the brain and heart. Anesthesiology 45:635, 1976
21. Saidman LJ: Uptake, distribution and elimination of barbiturates. In Eger EI II (ed): Anesthetic uptake and action. Baltimore: Williams & Wilkins, 1974: 264
22. Wood M: Plasma drug binding: implications for anesthesiologists. Anesth Analg 65:786, 1986
23. Stoelting RK, Eger EI II: The effects of ventilation and anesthetic solubility on recovery from anesthesia. Anesthesiology 30:290, 1969
24. Price HL, Kovnat PJ, Safer JN, et al: The uptake of thiopental by body tissues and its relation to the duration of narcosis. Clin Pharmacol Ther 1:16, 1960
25. Way WL, Trevor AJ: Sedative-hypnotics. Anesthesiology 34:170, 1971
26. Saidman LJ, Eger EI II: The effect of thiopental metabolism on duration of anesthesia. Anesthesiology 27:118, 1966
27. Berman ML, Lowe HJ, Bochantin J, et al: Uptake and elimination of methoxyflurane as influenced by enzyme induction in the rat. Anesthesiology 38:352, 1973
28. Schmidt KF, Roth RH Jr: Interaction of psychotropic drugs with agents employed in clinical anesthesia. Clinical Anesthesia 3: 60, 1967
29. Boyce JR, Wright FJ, Cervenko FW, et al: Prolongation of anesthetic action by BNPP (bis-[p-nitrophenyl]phosphate). Anesthesiology 45:629, 1976
30. Cohen ML, Chan S, Way WL, et al: Distribution in the brain and metabolism of ketamine in the rat after intravenous administration. Anesthesiology 39:370, 1973
31. White PF, Johnston RR, Pudwill CR: Interaction of ketamine and halothane in rats. Anesthesiology 42:179, 1975
32. Tinker JH, Gandolfi AJ, Van Dyke RA: Elevation of plasma bromide levels in patients following halothane anesthesia. Anesthesiology 44:194, 1976
33. Johnstone RE, Kennell EM, Behar M, et al: Increased serum bromide concentration after halothane anesthesia in man. Anesthesiology 42:598, 1975
34. Greenblatt DJ, Locniskar A, Scavone JM, ET AL: Absence of interaction of cimetidine and ranitidine with intravenous and oral midazolam. Anesth Analg 65:176, 1986
35. Laidlaw J, Read AE, Sherlock S: Morphine tolerance in hepatic cirrhosis. Gastroenterology 40:389, 1961
36. Haselhuhn DH: The use of pentothal in the presence of severe hepatic disease. Anesth Analg 36:73, 1957
37. Schentag JJ, Cerra FB, Calleri GM, et al: Age, disease, and cimetidine disposition in healthy subjects and chronically ill patients. Clin Pharmacol Ther 29:737, 1984
38. Dundee JW, Richards RK: Effect of azotemia upon the action of intravenous barbiturate anesthesia. Anesthesiology 15:333, 1954
39. Freeman RB, Sheff MG, Maher JF, et al: The blood-cerebrospinal fluid barrier in uremia. Ann Intern Med 56:233, 1962
40. Babad AA, Eger EI II: The effects of hyperthyroidism and hypothyroidism on halothane and oxygen requirements in dogs. Anesthesiology 29:1087, 1968
41. Salam AA, Davies DM: Acute adrenal insufficiency during surgery. Br J Anaesth 46:619, 1974
42. Morss HL, Baillie TW: A case of postoperative respiratory insufficiency and prolonged unconsciousness. Br J Anaesth 30:19, 1958
43. Dundee JW: Anaesthesia and surgery in adrenocortical insufficiency. Br J Anaesth 29:166, 1957
44. Davies DD: Abnormal response to anesthesia in a case of Huntington's chorea. Br J Anaesth 38:490, 1966
45. Eisele JH, Eger EI II, Muallem M: Narcotic properties of carbon dioxide in the dog. Anesthesiology 28:856, 1967
46. Posner JB, Plum F: Spinal-fluid *p*H and neurologic symptoms in systemic acidosis. N Engl J Med 277:605, 1967
47. Bulger RJ, Schrier RW, Arend WP, et al: Spinal-fluid acidosis and the diagnosis of pulmonary encephalopathy. N Engl J Med 274:433, 1966
48. Ohman JL Jr, Marliss EB, Aoki TT, et al: The cerebrospinal fluid in diabetic ketoacidosis. N Engl J Med 284:283, 1971
49. Schnelle N, Molnar GD, Ferris DO, et al: Circulating glucose and insulin in surgery for insulinomas. JAMA 217:1072, 1971
50. Enderby GEH: A report on mortality and morbidity following 9,107 hypotensive anaesthetics. Br J Anaesth 33:109, 1961
51. Schen RJ, Khazzam AS: Postoperative hypoglycemic coma associated with chlorpropamide. Br J Anaesth 47:899, 1975
52. Wiederholt IC, Genco M, Foley JM: Recurrent episodes of hypoglycemia induced by propoxyphene. Neurology 17:703, 1967
53. Christensen LK, Skovsted L: Inhibition of drug metabolism by chloramphenicol. Lancet 2:1397, 1969
54. Petitpierre B, Fabre J: Chlorpropamide and chloramphenicol. Lancet 1:789, 1970
55. Buckle RM, Guillebaud J: Hypoglycemic coma occurring during treatment with chlorpromazine and orphenadrine. Br Med J 4: 599, 1967
56. Aldrete JA, Levine DS, Gingrich TF: Experience in anesthesia for liver transplantation. Anesth Analg 48:802, 1969
57. Bedford RF: Hyperosmolar hyperglycemic non-ketotic coma following general anesthesia: report of a case. Anesthesiology 35:652, 1971
58. Wulfson HD, Dalton B: Hyperosmolar hyperglycemic nonketotic coma in a patient undergoing emergency cholecystectomy. Anesthesiology 41:286, 1974
59. Toker P: Hyperosmolar hyperglycemic non-ketotic coma: a case of delayed recovery from anesthesia. Anesthesiology 41:284, 1974
60. Daugirdas JT, Kronfol NO, Tzamaloukas AH, et al: Hyperosmolar coma: cellular dehydration and the serum sodium concentration. Ann Intern Med 110:855, 1989
61. Arieff AI, Carroll HJ: Non-ketotic hyperosmolar coma with hyperglycemia: clinical features, pathophysiology, renal function, acid-base balance, plasma-cerebrospinal fluid equilibria and the effects of therapy in 37 cases. Medicine (Baltimore) 51:73, 1972
62. Gerich JE, Martin MN, Recant L: Clinical and metabolic characteristics of hyperosmolar non-ketotic coma. Diabetes 20:228, 1971
63. Clements RS, Blumenthal SA, Morrison AD, et al: Increased cerebrospinal-fluid pressure during treatment of diabetic ketosis. Lancet 2:671, 1971
64. Arieff AL: Hyponatremia, convulsions, respiratory arrest, and permanent brain damage after elective surgery in healthy women. N Engl J Med 314:1529, 1986
65. Narins RG: Therapy of hyponatremia: does haste make waste? N Engl J Med 314:1573, 1986
66. Eger EI II, Saidman LJ, Brandstater B: Temperature dependence of halothane and cyclopropane anesthesia in dogs: correlation with some theories of anesthetic action. Anesthesiology 26:764, 1965
67. Cooper KE, Kenyon JR: A comparison of temperatures measured in the rectum, oesophagus, and on the surface of the aorta during hypothermia in man. Br J Surg 44:616, 1957
68. Johnston KR, Vaughan RS: Delayed recovery from general anaesthesia. Anaesthesia 43:1024, 1988
69. Weiss HD, Walker MD, Wiernik PH: Neurotoxicity of commonly used antineoplastic agents. N Engl J Med 291:75, 127, 1974
70. Karl HW, Talbott GA, Roberts TS: Intraoperative administration of radiologic contrast agents: potential neurotoxicity. Anesthesiology 81:1068, 1994
71. Eckenhoff JE, Enderby GEH, Larson A, et al: Human cerebral

circulation during deliberate hypotension and head-up tilt. J Appl Physiol 18:1130, 1963

72. Miller R, Tausk HC: Prolonged anesthesia associated with hypotension induced by trimethaphan. Anesthesiology Reviews 1: 36, 1974
73. Brierley JB, Cooper JE: Cerebral complications of hypotensive anesthesia in a healthy adult. J Neurol Neurosurg Psychiatry 25:24, 1962
74. Toole JF: Effects of change of head, limb and body position on cephalic circulation. N Engl J Med 279:307, 1968
75. Read GL, Singer DE, Picard EH, et al: Stroke following coronary artery bypass surgery. N Engl J Med 319:1246, 1988
76. Lowenstein E, Little JW III, Lo HH: Prevention of cerebral embolism from flushing radial-artery cannulas. N Engl J Med 285: 1414, 1971
77. Patrick RT, Devloo RA: Embolic phenomena of the operative and postoperative period. Anesthesiology 22:715, 1961
78. Jones JP Jr, Engleman EP, Najarian JS: Systemic fat embolism after renal homotransplantation and treatment with corticosteroids. N Engl J Med 273:1453, 1965
79. Nussmeier NA, Arlund C, Slogoff S: Neuropsychiatric complications after cardiopulmonary bypass: cerebral protection by a barbiturate. Anesthesiology 64:165, 1986
80. Metz S, Slogoff S: Thiopental sodium by single bolus dose compared to infusion for cerebral protection during cardiopulmonary bypass. J Clin Anesth 2:226, 1990
81. Binnie CD, Prior PF, Lloyd DSL, et al: Electroencephalographic prediction of fatal anoxic brain damage after resuscitation from cardiac arrest. Br Med J 4:265, 1970
82. Plum F, Posner JB, Hain RR: Delayed neurological deterioration after anoxia. Arch Intern Med 110:56, 1962
83. Plum F, Posner JB: The diagnosis of stupor and coma, 2nd ed. Philadelphia: FA Davis, 1972: 39, 176
84. Hill GE, Stanley THE, Sentker CR: Physostigmine reversal of postoperative somnolence. Can Anaesth Soc J 24:707, 1977

FURTHER READING

Harmel MH (ed): Neurologic considerations. Clinical Anesthesia 3: 1, 1978

Mahla M: Nervous system. In Gravenstein N (ed): Manual of complications during anesthesia. Philadelphia: JB Lippincott, 1991: 383

Plum F, Posner JB: The diagnosis of stupor and coma, 3rd ed. Philadelphia: FA Davis, 1981

Complications in Anesthesiology, second edition,
edited by Nikolaus Gravenstein and Robert R. Kirby.
Lippincott-Raven Publishers, Philadelphia © 1996.

CHAPTER 32

Acute Adrenocortical Insufficiency and Etomidate

R. Lee Wagner

Adrenocortical insufficiency (Addison's disease) is rare. However, etomidate, an intravenous hypnotic, has been associated with adrenocortical insufficiency and death and has been shown to suppress adrenocortical function even in subanesthetic concentrations.[1–4] This chapter discusses the physiology of the adrenal cortex and the effect of etomidate on adrenocortical function, reviews the clinical presentation and management of acute adrenocortical insufficiency (Addison's disease), and provides recommendations for the safe use of etomidate.

RELEVANT BIOCHEMISTRY AND PHYSIOLOGY OF THE ADRENOCORTICAL HORMONES

Biochemistry

Synthesis

Synthesis of all corticosteroids begins with cholesterol, composed of a four-ring steroid with a long side chain (Fig. 32-1).[5] The side chain is first lysed by a cleavage enzyme to yield pregnenolone. Subsequent reactions in the glucocorticoid pathway yield 17-hydroxypregnenolone, 17-hydroxyprogesterone, 11-deoxycortisol, and the final product, cortisol. The mineralocorticoid pathway differs in that pregnenolone is converted directly into progesterone and then through intermediates to the principal mineralocorticoids, corticosterone and aldosterone. Identification of separate pathways is an artificial distinction, both because crossover points are numerous and because some products have both glucocorticoid and mineralocorticoid activity.

Figure 32-1 also depicts the principal enzymes involved in corticosteroid synthesis, all of which are of the cytochrome P450 family. Of these, cholesterol side chain cleavage enzyme ($P450_{scc}$) and 11β-hydroxylase ($P450_{11\beta}$) are both integral components of the inner membrane of the mitochondrion and the reactions they catalyze occur at that site. The cholesterol side chain cleavage enzyme catalyzes the first (and rate-limiting) step of all steroidogenesis. 11β-hydroxylase catalyzes some of the final reactions producing cortisol and aldosterone, but is not needed for the production of androgens and estrogens. All other P450 family steroidogenic enzymes are located on endoplasmic reticulum.[6]

Regulation of Glucocorticoid and Mineralocorticoid Production

Stress and other neural stimuli cause release of corticotropin releasing hormone (CRH) from the hypothalamus into the pituitary stalk. CRH then mediates the production and release of adrenocorticotropic hormone (ACTH) from the anterior pituitary into the circulation. ACTH acts as the principal acute stimulus to steroid hormone biosynthesis by facilitating the action of $P450_{scc}$ as it converts cholesterol to pregnenolone. In addition, ACTH seems to have a long term stimulatory and regulatory effect at many places in the steroidogenic pathway.[6]

Cortisol, the final product of the glucocorticoid pathway, exerts feedback inhibition both on CRH release in the hypothalamus and ACTH release in the anterior pituitary.

Aldosterone synthesis is regulated primarily by angiotensin II as the final product of the juxtaglomerular apparatus-renin-angiotensin feedback loop which regulates body fluid volume. Increased serum potassium levels are a second important stimulus to aldosterone production.

Unlike some other hormone systems, there is no storage pool of adrenocortical hormones in the body. Once synthesized, products are released into the bloodstream. The elimination half-life of cortisol in plasma is approximately 80 minutes.[7] This suggests that if hormone synthesis is blocked, it might be several hours before a cortisol deficiency state is achieved. Cortisol is metabolized primarily by the liver.

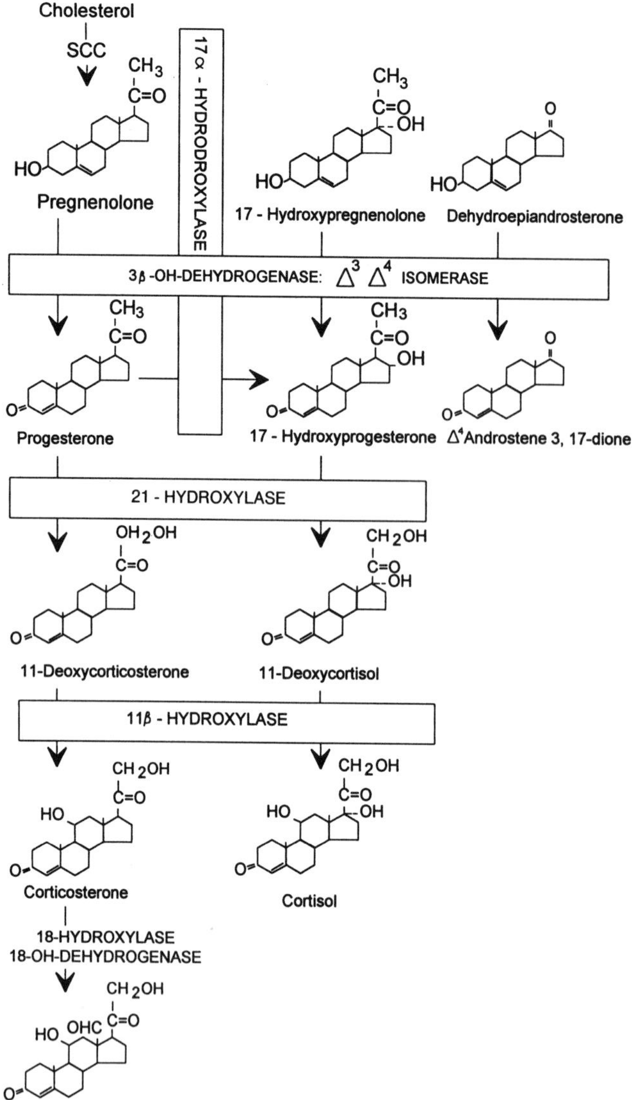

FIGURE 32-1. Pathways of glucocorticoid and mineralocorticoid biosynthesis. *Shaded bars,* probable sites of enzyme blockade by etomidate; *ovals,* enzymes having glucocorticoid activity; *hexagons,* enzymes having mineralocorticoid activity. *SCC,* cholesterol side chain–cleavage enzyme. (Modified from Harding BW: Synthesis of adrenal cortical steroids and mechanism of ACTH effects. In DeGroot LJ, Cahill GF Jr, Odell WD, et al (eds): Endocrinology, vol 2. New York, Grune & Statton, 1979: 1135.)

Once released into the circulation, cortisol is transported primarily by corticosteroid-binding globulin (CBG). Cortisol binds to specific receptors inside glucocorticoid target cells in multiple organs, activating the receptor to bind to DNA of the cell nucleus and altering the transcription rate of specific gene production of mRNA and ultimately, protein products.[8] This mode of action and sequence of events may take hours to produce visible change in the physiologic function of target tissues and explains the long delay in effect seen when glucocorticoids are used pharmacologically.

ACTH Stimulation Test

Because serum cortisol levels vary widely throughout the day, simple measurements of serum cortisol are of limited value in assessing adrenocortical function. The principal test for adrenocortical hypofunction is the ACTH stimulation test. A stimulating dose of ACTH is given, and serum cortisol measurements are made 30 or 60 minutes later and compared with baseline cortisol levels before the stimulation. The normal adrenal cortex responds with a burst of cortisol production as is discussed later.

Glucocorticoid and Mineralocorticoid Physiology

The physiology of adrenocortical hormones is highly complex and involves almost every homeostatic mechanism of the body. This chapter highlights only a few pertinent actions and refers the reader to standard endocrine texts for a more complete survey.[9,10] While glucocorticoid and mineralocorticoids are discussed as if they are separate entities, in actual function there is significant overlap.

Glucocorticoid Physiology

With regard to the cardiovascular system, glucocorticoids have no intrinsic vasoconstrictor action, but exert a "permissive" effect on vascular tone and its response to other endogenous vasopressors such as angiotensin and norepinephrine.[9] Glucocorticoids also enhance myocardial contractility by increasing myocardial ATP and epinephrine synthesis, and have a direct positive inotropic effect.[9,11]

Glucocorticoids derive their name from their essential function in intermediate carbohydrate metabolism: antagonizing the effect of insulin and inhibiting peripheral glucose utilization by cells, and stimulating gluconeogenesis, glycogen synthesis, and lipolysis. Glucocorticoids at physiological levels have countless anti-inflammatory and immunosuppressive actions which are the basis for familiar therapeutic manipulations.

Mineralocorticoid Physiology

Mineralocorticoids derive their name from their principal function: regulating potassium and sodium homeostasis and thereby body fluid volume. Mineralocorticoids have their primary action at the distal collecting tubules of the kidney, where they promote sodium reabsorption and potassium and hydrogen ion excretion.[10]

Etomidate and Its Effect on Adrenocortical Biosynthesis

Etomidate, synthesized by Janssen Pharmaceutica, Belgium in 1971, with human evaluations beginning in 1973, was used clinically for a number of years before its inhibition of adrenal steroidogenesis was reported. As shown in Figure 32-2, etomidate has an imidazole ring, which is probably responsible for the inhibition. Other imidazoles have been shown to have similar effects on steroidogenesis.[12] Etomidate is the most potent of all known inhibitors of corticosteroid biosynthesis

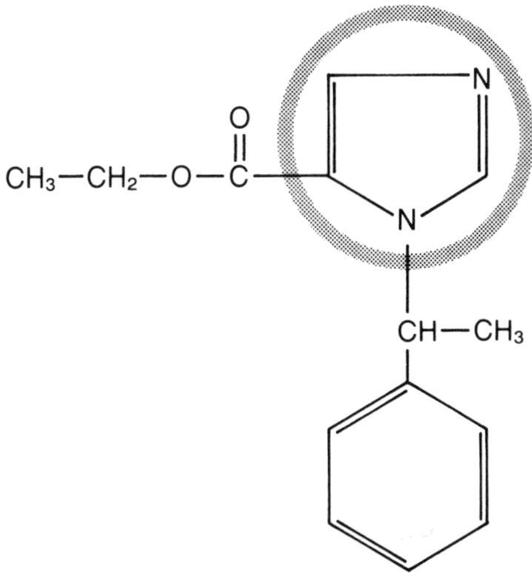

FIGURE 32-2. Structure of etomidate. The imidazole ring (*circled*) is the probable site of interference with steroidogenic enzymes dependent on mitochondrial cytochrome P-450.

and has been used to correct elevated cortisol concentrations of patients with Cushing's syndrome.[13–15]

Etomidate appears to have a selective action on the two mitochondrial-bound cytochrome P450 steroidogenic enzymes. It blocks 11β-hydroxylase ($P450_{11\beta}$) strongly, and cholesterol side chain cleavage enzyme ($P450_{scc}$) more weakly.[14] Both cortisol and aldosterone synthesis require $P450_{11\beta}$, and their production appears to be completely blocked by etomidate, even in subanesthetic concentrations.[2] The block has been well characterized pharmacologically and is dose-dependent and reversible.[16] The duration of action is incompletely characterized and probably varies with clinical conditions, but the effect may last from several hours to several days. The weaker blockade of $P450_{scc}$ may be clinically apparent with larger etomidate doses or in the inhibition of ovarian steroidogenesis discussed below.[18,34]

CLASSICAL ACUTE ADRENOCORTICAL INSUFFICIENCY

Symptoms and Signs

Acute adrenocortical insufficiency can be particularly difficult to diagnose because often the syndrome is precipitated by other coexisting illness or stress. In addition, many of the symptoms are nonspecific. Common symptoms and signs are listed in Table 32-1. Clearly, many of these features can be seen in the postoperative state even with normal adrenocortical function.

Acute bilateral adrenal hemorrhage has been reported in association with meningococcemia (Waterhouse-Friderichsen syndrome), and subsequently following urologic surgery, cardiac surgery, and burns.[19–21] Coagulation disorders and transient hypotension are often cited as possible etiological factors. Two distinct hemodynamic states have been described during acute adrenocortical insufficiency. Classical descriptions have emphasized hypovolemic shock. More recently, a high cardiac output, low systemic vascular resistance state has been defined, perhaps occurring as intravascular volume is repleted.[22–24] Such a picture would be in accord with the known peripheral vasodilation that occurs when the permissive effect of cortisol on vasoconstriction is absent. In both states, there appears to be a direct improvement in myocardial contractility when cortisol is given, independent of the effect of fluid or inotrope therapy. Pulmonary infiltrates may represent a capillary-leak syndrome.[27] The overall picture might well be mistaken for septic shock of unknown etiology. Because the signs are so nonspecific, the diagnosis of acute adrenocortical insufficiency unfortunately is often made post mortem.

Features of chronic adrenocortical insufficiency, which do not have time to manifest themselves in acute cases, include hyperpigmentation, weight loss, anemia, and small heart size. Electrolyte changes may be apparent only to the extent that mineralocorticoid deficiency exists and has had time to affect renal electrolyte clearance.

TABLE 32-1
Symptoms and Signs of Acute Adrenocortical Insufficiency

- Fatigue
- Anorexia
- Nausea and vomiting
- Diffuse abdominal pain
- Listlessness
- Delirium and coma
- Fever
- Dehydration
- Hypovolemic shock
- High output, low resistance shock
- Pulmonary infiltrates

Laboratory Studies

Clinical laboratory testing may be helpful in establishing the diagnosis of adrenocortical insufficiency. Abnormal laboratory findings are summarized in Table 32-2.

Because aldosterone helps regulate sodium retention and potassium excretion, its absence leads to hyponatremia and hyperkalemia.

TABLE 32-2
Laboratory Test Results in Acute Adrenocortical Insufficiency

- Hyponatremia
- Hyperkalemia
- Azotemia
- Metabolic acidosis
- Hypercalcemia
- Hypoglycemia
- Anemia
- Eosinophilia
- Lymphocytosis
- Abnormal ACTH stimulation test

Glucocorticoid deficiency may result in severe hypoglycemia. This deficiency also is apparently responsible for two common abnormal findings in laboratory studies: eosinophilia and lymphocytosis,which probably result from a redistribution of the circulating pools of these cell types in the absence of glucocorticoid activity and may be a valuable aid in diagnosis.[25]

Mineralocorticoid deficiency causes sodium wasting and is followed by dehydration and azotemia. At the same time, potassium and hydrogen ions accumulate. The composite picture is one of hyponatremia, hyperkalemia, azotemia, and acidosis. Few other clinical situations occur in which azotemia coexists with hyponatremia. Hypercalcemia may be present in a minority of cases.

ACTH Stimulation Test

The diagnosis of adrenocortical insufficiency can be confirmed by a standard adrenocorticotropin hormone (ACTH) stimulation test.[26] A baseline measurement of the serum cortisol concentration is obtained. Synthetic ACTH, 250 μg, is given intravenously, and cortisol concentration is measured again from a blood sample taken 30 minutes later. With normal adrenocortical function, basal cortisol concentration usually is greater than 5 μg/dL, and in the sample drawn after ACTH stimulation it should increase by at least 7 μg/dL, to a concentration of 18 μg/dL or higher.

In the stressed patient, ACTH and cortisol secretion may already be maximal, and no increase will be seen when exogenous ACTH is administered. Normal adrenocortical function will be obvious, however, by the very high concentrations of cortisol in both the basal and 30-minute measurements.

Therapy need not be withheld while the test is being performed. Steroid supplementation may begin with dexamethasone, which does not interfere with the cortisol assay. Once the study has been completed, therapy can be changed to hydrocortisone, which has both glucocorticoid and mineralocorticoid properties.

ETOMIDATE-INDUCED ADRENOCORTICAL INSUFFICIENCY

The early clinical reports associated with etomidate describe patients in critical care units with preexisting multisystem failure who received etomidate for days or weeks. These patients appear to have died from overwhelming infection. The role of adrenocortical insufficiency is unclear, but it is particularly notable that the sentinel report of Ledingham and Watt noted a marked increase in ICU mortality to 44% with etomidate as the only identifiable change.[1] Reports also have described patients receiving etomidate on a long-term basis in whom hypotension responsive to corticosteroids developed.[2,3]

A study purporting to show benefits of steroids for cardiopulmonary bypass probably inadvertently revealed etomidate adrenocortical insufficiency.[27,28] The etomidate-anesthetized control group, which received no supplemental steroid, developed hyperthermia to 38°C, hypotension (mean arterial pressure 70 mm Hg), an increased fluid requirement, need for greater inotropic support, and a prolonged stay in the intensive care unit. Three of the 13 control patients, and none of the steroid-supplemented patients, developed hypotension, peripheral vasoconstriction, low urine output, a high volume requirement with a positive fluid balance, a high cardiac output, and signs of interstitial edema in the chest radiograph. These 3 patients improved rapidly (within 3 to 5 hours) after dexamethasone rescue.

A Dutch study that specifically looked for etomidate-induced adrenocortical insufficiency compared an etomidate/fentanyl group with a droperidol/fentanyl group in a nonrandomized study of patients undergoing major vascular surgery.[29] The etomidate patients had a significantly higher fluid requirement, which continued postoperatively, and a higher rate of complications, including need for inotropic and antiarrhythmic therapy and, again, interstitial fluid on chest radiograph. Similarly, a German study of patients receiving etomidate with or without hydrocortisone supplementation for major abdominal surgery showed an increased fluid requirement and decreased serum protein concentration in the group receiving etomidate alone.[30] In another study, patients undergoing abdominal surgery with etomidate had fever and a positive fluid balance as compared with controls, both findings resolving with steroid therapy.[31] The positive fluid balance would be expected in these cases if vasodilation or a capillary-leak syndrome were treated with intravenous fluid therapy to maintain central venous pressures.

Etomidate crosses the placental barrier, causing adrenocortical suppression in the neonates of mothers given etomidate for cesarean section.[32,33]

Even the weaker blockade of cholesterol side chain cleavage enzyme appears to have clinical consequences. Etomidate has now been shown to interfere with ovarian steroidogenesis when given as an anesthetic for laparoscopic oocyte retrieval.[34] This is likely a result of its effect on cholesterol side chain cleavage enzyme in the first step of all steroidogenesis, since the biosynthetic pathway of ovarian steroids differs from that of the adrenocortical steroids beyond this initial step.

Ironically, because one perceived benefit of etomidate is an absence of cardiovascular depression, the drug is most likely to be used in patients with preexisting cardiovascular disease. These patients may be at greater risk for the effects of adrenocortical insufficiency, and any unusual symptoms that appear may be attributed to the preexisting cardiovascular disease or its associated surgery. The correct diagnosis is likely to be made only when it is considered and specifically sought by the alert practitioner.

MANAGEMENT

Awareness of this disorder is paramount. Once adrenocortical insufficiency is considered in the differential diagnosis, both diagnosis and treatment should be straightforward. Management consists of hormone replacement and supportive measures (Table 32-3).

Steroid Replacement

If an ACTH stimulation test is to be performed to confirm the diagnosis, dexamethasone 10 mg may be given initially and

TABLE 32-3
Treatment of Acute Adrenocortical Insufficiency

- Dexamethasone 10 mg IV until rapid ACTH stimulation test performed, then hydrocortisone hemisuccinate 100 mg IV q 6 h until documented return of normal adrenocortical function
- Fluid replacement with an isotonic saline solution
- Intravenous vasopressor and cardiotonic pharmacotherapy. Effective only in conjunction with steroid and fluid replacement therapy
- Hemodynamic monitoring such as central venous catheter, pulmonary artery catheter, or transesophageal echocardiography to guide therapy
- Glucose supplementation as necessary with close monitoring of serum glucose
- Potassium supplementation if indicated after volume status and acidosis are normalized
- Monitoring of urinary volume and electrolytes in conjunction with serum electrolytes

will not interfere with the cortisol assay. Its lack of mineralocorticoid effect is unlikely to be a problem if therapy is subsequently converted to hydrocortisone.

Hydrocortisone hemisuccinate or phosphate (Solu-cortef, Upjohn), 100 mg intravenously every 6 hours, appears to establish adequate glucocorticoid and mineralocorticoid activity, although more frequent administration, perhaps hourly in severe cases, is advocated by some.[25] Replacement therapy should be continued, on a tapering schedule over days to weeks depending on etiology, until normal adrenocortical function is documented by repeat ACTH stimulation testing.

Adjuvant Therapy

The patient with Addison's disease may be markedly hypovolemic as a result of renal fluid losses or vasodilation, in which case fluid replacement with isotonic saline is needed. Vasopressor drugs may be necessary to treat severe hypotension but will almost certainly be ineffective unless fluids, mineralocorticoids, and glucocorticoids also are given.[35] Hypoglycemia must be considered, and if present, appropriately treated with intravenous glucose. Hypercalcemia usually resolves without specific therapy. Although hyperkalemia may be present initially, patients in whom this sign appears may actually have a total body potassium deficit and need potassium replacement as they are rehydrated.

CLINICAL CORRELATES

Importance of the Effect of Etomidate on Adrenocortical Function

Etomidate has been used for induction of anesthesia in more than six million cases in the United States to date. While altered adrenocortical function has been documented, no adverse effects attributed to decreased cortisol levels have been reported.* A recent study suggests the adrenocortical changes are only transient during cardiac surgery.[36]

Several points must be weighed against this benign picture. First, absence of reports is not synonymous with absence of adverse effects. As the previous section illustrates, the effect of etomidate on adrenocortical function may well be masked by unrecognized therapeutic interventions, or mistaken for other clinical entities. Prior to the initial report of high mortality in intensive care patients,[1] similar statements were made about the general safety of etomidate. Adverse effects were not identified until an appropriate search was made. Subsequent to this report, etomidate is no longer used for prolonged sedation in the intensive care unit. However,the state of research has changed little with regard to the effect of etomidate for surgery in other patient groups: appropriate studies have been limited. Moreover, some of the existing studies from Europe do suggest a clinically adverse effect of the known adrenocortical suppression.[27-34] The prudent practitioner should expect and be watchful for adrenocortical insufficiency until appropriate studies are published clearly demonstrating safety in a variety of patient populations and clinical settings.

Etomidate and "Stress-free" Anesthesia

One source of potential confusion for the anesthesiologist is the controversial goal of providing "stress-free" anesthesia, under the assumption that it is more beneficial for the patient.[38] This approach includes avoidance of increased plasma ACTH and cortisol concentrations perioperatively, and has been associated most frequently with high dose opioid techniques or epidural/intrathecal regional anesthesia.

Because etomidate suppresses plasma cortisol concentrations very effectively, it might be thought to meet one goal of stress-free anesthesia. However, there are several unresolved problems:

1. It is unclear when or whether "stress-free" anesthesia is beneficial.
2. Cortisol may have both beneficial and deleterious effects in the perioperative setting.
3. There are multiple other mediators of the stress response besides cortisol.
4. Unlike other "stress-free" anesthetic techniques, which appear to work by suppressing afferent nerve input and thereby all resulting stress responses, etomidate has a specific effect on hormone synthesis by the adrenal cortex. All other stress responses remain unaffected.

Adrenal Cortical Function During Surgery

Conventional clinical wisdom has been that higher serum cortisol production is required for the body to respond adequately to surgery or trauma, perhaps up to 200 mg per day.[39] In fact, this teaching has been the basis for the standard recommendation that "umbrella" steroid coverage is necessary for the patient undergoing trauma or surgery who has previously received chronic steroid therapy. However, while the normal body may respond with this high level of glucocorticoid production, it is less clear that such high levels are necessary or beneficial. This question has been the subject of several studies.[39,40] Moreover, because of the long half-life of cortisol

* Nardini S, Abbott Laboratories, personal communication, 1995

and its slow action at the cellular level, it is probable that adrenocortical hormone production could be diminished or even completely suppressed for some period of time in the perioperative setting without adverse effects.

Future Research

There are at least three areas of incomplete research:

1. Defining the time course of etomidate adrenocortical suppression in various clinical situations
2. Creating a well-defined picture of the onset and time course of acute adrenocortical insufficiency in the perioperative setting, using modern tools such as cardiac output and associated systemic and pulmonary resistance measurements, mixed venous oxygen saturation, transesophageal echocardiography, and renal fluid and electrolyte balance
3. Clarifying whether the stress hormones (including cortisol) are beneficial or detrimental. How much umbrella steroid coverage is necessary for the patient undergoing trauma or surgery who has previously received chronic steroid therapy is a key component.

SUMMARY

Etomidate is a potent inhibitor of adrenocortical steroidogenesis. Etomidate, when used for induction of anesthesia, efficiently performs a pharmacologic adrenalectomy just as surgery begins.

Because of the half-life of existing cortisol, the relatively slow rate at which cortisol influences cellular function and expression, and the fact that a deficiency state may not become apparent until increased cortisol production is called for, there is likely to be a poorly defined and perhaps substantial delay in the appearance of clinical signs of adrenocortical insufficiency after steroidogenesis is suppressed by etomidate. In some cases, adrenocortical synthetic function may return to normal before this lag time has run its course.

Perioperative cortisol requirements remain incompletely characterized despite intense effort over several decades of research.

If signs of adrenocortical insufficiency appear, they are likely to be vague and may mimic other entities, including a typical postoperative course (fever, increased fluid requirement).

Many anesthesiologists are incompletely aware of this clearly documented effect. Medical colleagues outside the field of anesthesia may need to be advised if they are caring for a patient who has received etomidate.

RECOMMENDATIONS

Several leading anesthesiologists have suggested that etomidate should no longer be administered.[41–43] However, the drug does have some advantages, and may be used by the prudent clinician. The following are considerations to keep in mind:

1. Use etomidate when a clinical benefit, such as hemodynamic stability, balances the known adverse effect on adrenocortical function.
2. Assume that complete adrenocortical suppression will be produced for at least several hours and perhaps longer than a day.
3. Consider coverage with hydrocortisone 100 mg intravenously every 8 hours for at least 24 hours after the last dose of etomidate is given. Although good clinical judgment should suffice in most cases, a normal ACTH stimulation test is the only certain documentation that etomidate adrenocortical suppression has resolved.
4. If exogenous glucocorticoid supplementation is not used, watch for subtle signs of early adrenocortical insufficiency such as increasing core temperature and an increased fluid requirement.
5. Ensure that others caring for the patient are aware of both the presentation of acute adrenocortical insufficiency in the perioperative setting and the ability of etomidate to produce this state.

REFERENCES

1. Ledingham M, Watt I: Influence of sedation on mortality in critically ill multiple trauma patients. Lancet 1:1270, 1983
2. Fellows IW, Bastow MD, Byrne AJ, Allison SP: Adrenocortical suppression in multiply injured patients: a complication of etomidate treatment. Br Med J 287:1835, 1983
3. Chee HD, Bronsveld W, Lips PTAM, Thijs LG: Adrenocortical suppression in multiply injured patients: a complication of etomidate treatment. Br Med J 288:485, 1984
4. Diago MC, Amado JA, Otero M, Lopez-Cordovilla JJ: Anti-adrenal action of a sub-anesthetic dose of etomidate. Anaesthesia 43:644, 1988
5. Orth DN, Kovacs WJ, Debold CR: The adrenal cortex. In Wilson JD, Foster DW (eds): Williams textbook of endocrinology, 8th ed. Philadelphia, WB Saunders, 1992:495
6. Simpson ER, Waterman MR: Steroid hormone biosynthesis in the adrenal cortex and its regulation by adrenocorticotropin. In: DeGroot LJ, Cahill GF Jr, Martini L, et al (eds): Endocrinology, 3rd ed. Philadelphia: WB Saunders, 1995:1630
7. Meikle AW: Secretion and metabolism of the corticosteroids and adrenal function and testing. In: DeGroot LJ, Besser GM, Cahill GF Jr (eds): Endocrinology, 2nd ed. Philadelphia: WB Saunders, 1989:1610
8. Feldman D: Mechanism of action of cortisol. In: DeGroot LJ, Besser GM, Cahill GF Jr (eds): Endocrinology, 2nd ed. Philadelphia: WB Saunders, 1989:1557
9. Munck A, Náray-Fejes-Tóth A: Glucocorticoid action-physiology. In: DeGroot LJ, Cahill GF Jr, Martini L, et al (eds): Endocrinology, 3rd ed. Philadelphia: WB Saunders, 1995:1642
10. Mortensen RM, Williams GH: Aldosterone action-physiology. In: DeGroot LJ, Cahill GF Jr, Martini L, et al (eds): Endocrinology, 3rd ed. Philadelphia: WB Saunders, 1995:1642
11. Rovetto MJ, Murphy RA, Lefer AM: Cardiac impairment in adrenal insufficiency in the cat. Reduced adenosinetriphosphate activity of myocardial contractile proteins. Circ Res 26:419, 1970
12. Loose DS, Stover EP, Feldman D: Ketoconazole binds to glucocorticoid receptors and exhibits glucocorticoid antagonist activity in cultured cells. J Clin Invest 72:404, 1983
13. Lambert A, Mitchell R, Frost J, Robertson WR: A simple in vitro approach to the estimation of the biopotency affecting adrenal steroidogenesis. J Steroid Biochem 23:235, 1985
14. Wagner RL, White PF, Kan P, Rosenthal M, Feldman D: Inhibition of adrenal steroidogenesis by the anesthetic etomidate. N Engl J Med 310:1415, 1984
15. Schulte HM, Benker G, Reinwein D, Sippell WG, Allolio B: Infusion of low dose etomidate: correction of hypercortisolemia

in patients with Cushing's syndrome and dose-response relationship in normal subjects. J Clin Endocrinol Metab 70:1426, 1990
16. Crozier TA, Beck D, Wuttke W, Kettler D. In vivo suppression of steroid synthesis by etomidate is concentration-dependent. Anaesthesist 37:337, 1988
17. McKee JI, Finlay WEI: Cortisol replacement in severely stressed patients. Lancet 1:484, 1983
18. Sear JW, Edwards CR, Atherden SM: Dual effect of etomidate on mineralocorticoid biosynthesis. Acta Anaesth Belgica 39(2): 87, 1988
19. Jacobson SA, Blute RD Jr, Green DF, McPhedran P, Weiss RM, Lytton B: Acute adrenal insufficiency as a complication of urologic surgery. J Urol 135:337, 1986
20. Alford WC, Meador CK, Mihalevich J, et al: Acute adrenal insufficiency following cardiac surgical procedures. J Thorac Cardiovasc Surg 78:489, 1979
21. Sheridan RL, Ryan CM, Tompkins RG: Acute adrenal insufficiency in the burn intensive care unit. Burns 19(1):63, 1993
22. Dorin RI, Kearns PJ: High output circulatory failure in acute adrenal insufficiency. Crit Care Med 16:296, 1988
23. Lawton JM: Acute adrenal insufficiency: hemodynamic and echocardiographic characteristics. Wis Med J 91(5):214, 1992
24. Bouachour G, Tirot P, Varache S, Gouello, Harry P, Alquier PH: Hemodynamic changes in acute adrenal insufficiency. Intensive Care Med 20:138, 1994
25. Bondy PK: Disorders of the adrenal cortex. In Wilson JD, Foster DW (eds): Williams' textbook of endocrinology, 5th ed. Philadelphia, WB Saunders, 1985:816
26. Wood JB, Frankland AW, James VHT, et al: A rapid test of adrenocortical function. Lancet 1:243, 1965
27. Jansen NJG, van Oeveren W, vd Broek L, et al: Inhibition by dexamethasone of the reperfusion phenomena in cardiopulmonary bypass. J Thorac Cardiovasc Surg 102:515, 1991
28. Moat NE, MacNaughton PD: Routine dexamethasone therapy for cardiac operations? J Thorac Cardiovasc Surg 107:621, 1994
29. Boidin MP: Can etomidate cause an Addisonlan crisis? Acta Anaesth Belg 37:165, 1986
30. Stuttman R, Allolio B, Becker A, Doehn M, Winkleman W: Etomidate versus etomidate plus hydrocortisone in major abdominal surgery. Anaesthesist 37:576, 1988
31. Boidin MP: Serum levels of cortisol in man during etomidate fentanyl-air anaesthesia compared with neurolept anaesthesia. Acta Anaesthesiol Belg 36:79, 1985
32. Murat I, Estève C, Delleur MM, Bougnères P, Saint-Maurice C: Modifications hormonales induites par l'etomidate chez l'enfant pendant les 24 premieres heures postoperatoires. Ann Fr Anesth Reanim 8:102, 1989
33. Crozier TA, Flamm C, Speer CP, et al: Effects of etomidate on the adrenocortical and metabolic adaptation of the neonate. Br J Anaes 70(1):47, 1993
34. Heytens L, Devroey P, Camu F, Van Steirteghem AC: Effects of etomidate on ovarian steroidogenesis. Human Reproduction 2(2):85, 1987
35. Lefer AM: Corticosteroids and circulatory function. In: Blaschko H, Sayers G, Smith AD (eds): Adrenal gland. In: Greep RO, Astwood EB (eds): Endocrinology, vol 6. In: Geiger SR, ed: Handbook of physiology, section 7. Washington, DC: American Physiological Society, 1975:191
36. Crozier TA, Schlaeger M, Wuttke W, Kettler D: TIVA with etomidate-fentanyl versus midazolam-fentanyl. The perioperative stress of coronary surgery overcomes the inhibition of cortisol synthesis caused by etomidate-fentanyl anesthesia. Anaesthesist 43:605, 1994
37. Wagner RL, White PR: Etomidate inhibits adrenocortical function in surgical patients. Anesthesiology 61:647, 1984
38. Weissman C: The metabolic response to stress: an overview and update. Anesthesiology 73:308, 1990
39. Kehlet H: A rational approach to dosage and preparation of parenteral glucocorticoid substitution therapy during surgical procedures. Acta Anaesthesiol Scand 19:260, 1975
40. Udelsman R, Ramp J, Gallucci WT: Adaptation during surgical stress. A reevaluation of the role of glucocorticoids. J Clin Invest 77:1377, 1986
41. Etomidate. Lancet 2:24, 1983
42. Longnecker DE: Stress free: to be or not to be? Anesthesiology 61:643, 1984
43. Owen H, Spence AA: Etomidate. Br J Anaesth 56:555, 1984

Complications in Anesthesiology, second edition,
edited by Nikolaus Gravenstein and Robert R. Kirby.
Lippincott-Raven Publishers, Philadelphia © 1996.

CHAPTER 33

Fluid and Electrolyte Problems

Richard I. Mazze*
Masahiko Fujinaga
Robert S. Wharton

The successful outcome of major operative procedures on seriously ill patients often requires expert management of fluid and electrolyte therapy and the early recognition and treatment of complications. To accomplish these goals, the physician must have a thorough knowledge of the composition and distribution of fluids and electrolytes within the body; of the normal homeostatic mechanisms for fluid and electrolyte handling; and of the ways in which anesthetic drugs and surgical intervention affect these variables. This knowledge helps to prevent most problems; moreover, complications that do occur can be characterized, so that appropriate treatment can be started. This chapter presents an approach to intraoperative fluid management on the basis of physiologic principles, the nature of the operation, and the type and severity of the patient's illness.

COMPOSITION OF BODY FLUIDS

Volumes and Distribution

In the average healthy young man, total body water accounts for approximately 60% of body weight, and in the young woman, 55%.[1–6] These percentages may vary greatly among individuals, primarily because of differences in the ratio of lean body mass to adipose tissue. The percentage of total body water is inversely proportional to the degree of obesity. Also, with increasing age, a steady decline in total body water as a proportion of body weight occurs; it reaches a low value in geriatric patients of about 52% in men and 46% in women (Table 33-1). In contrast to the large variation in water content from one person to another, the water content of an individual person remains remarkably constant by means of the extremely effective homeostatic mechanisms.

* See Credits on page iv.

Fluid Compartments

Total body water may be divided into two major functional compartments (Fig. 33-1): the intracellular compartment accounts for 55%, and the extracellular compartment 45%. Extracellular water is further divided into a rapidly equilibrating compartment, the functional extracellular fluid volume (FECV) and a very slowly equilibrating space. The former is composed of plasma and interstitial fluid, which together represent approximately 27% of total body water, or 16% of body weight. In a healthy 70-kg man, this value is approximately 12 L. Conservation of the FECV is one of the main priorities of body homeostatic mechanisms.

Slowly equilibrating extracellular water is found in bone, cartilage, connective tissues, and transcellular spaces (cerebrospinal fluid, synovial fluid, and intraluminal fluid of the gastrointestinal tract). In practice, slowly equilibrating extracellular water does not equilibrate with plasma, so it does not enter into problems of fluid and electrolyte balance.

Electrolyte Content

Extracellular Fluid

The predominant cation of extracellular fluid is sodium. Total body stores of sodium are about 4500 mEq (103 g),* of which about 2800 mEq are exchangeable (eg, not incorporated within the crystalline matrix of bone).[3] Normal extracellular sodium concentration is 135 to 145 mEq/L. Other cations present in significant concentrations are potassium, 3.5 to 5.0 mEq/L; magnesium, 1.5 to 2.5 mEq/L; and calcium, 8.5 to 10.5 mg/dL. By comparison, hydrogen ion concentration in

* For conversion of milligrams to milliequivalents:

$$\text{Milliequivalents} = \frac{\text{milligrams}}{\text{molecular weight}} \times \text{valence}$$

TABLE 33-1
Variation in Total Body Water With Age

AGE	SEX	TOTAL BODY WATER (% of Body Weight)
0–1 mo		75.7
1–12 mo		64.5
1–10 y		61.7
10–16 y	Male	58.9
	Female	57.3
17–39 y	Male	60.6
	Female	50.2
40–59 y	Male	54.7
	Female	46.7
≥60 y	Male	51.5
	Female	45.5

Edelman IS, Leibman J: Anatomy of body water and electrolytes. Am J Med 27:256, 1959.

extracellular fluid is only 3.5 to 4.5 × 10^{-5} mEq/L. Major corresponding anions in extracellular fluid are chloride, 95 to 106 mEq/L, and bicarbonate, 22 to 28 mEq/L.

Intracellular Fluid

Potassium and magnesium are the major cations of intracellular fluid and are present in concentrations of approximately 160 and 25 mEq/L, respectively; sodium concentration is only about 10 mEq/L. The predominant intracellular anions are phosphate and sulfate, approximately 100 and 20 mEq/L, respectively; bicarbonate and chloride together contribute about 10 mEq/L. Intracellular proteins exert a net negative charge of 55 mEq/L and make up most of the difference between cation and anion content.[3] An estimated 10% to 15% of intracellular ions are osmotically inactive, presumably bound to intracellular lipids, proteins, or nucleic acids.

Osmotic Pressure, Osmolality, and Tonicity

Extremely important in fluid and electrolyte homeostasis is *osmotic pressure*, the tendency of water to move across a semipermeable membrane from a more dilute to a more concentrated solution. It is measured as the difference in hydrostatic pressure necessary to prevent such movement. Osmotic concentration can be expressed in units of *osmolality* or *osmolarity*. A 1-osmolal solution contains 1 osm of solute per kilogram of water; a 1-osmolar solution contains 1 osm of solute to which sufficient water has been added to result in a final volume of 1 L.

The number of osmoles in a solution is equal to the sum of the number of moles of unionized solute plus the number of equivalents of each ion divided by its valence. Clinical discussions frequently refer to osmolarity, although osmolality is more precise, because laboratory measurements are almost invariably made in milliosmoles per kilogram. In practice, there is little difference between the two measurements.

Determinants of Normal Osmolality

The normal osmolality of extracellular and intracellular fluid is 285 to 295 mOsm/kg. Sodium salts account for 90% to 95% of the osmolality of plasma and interstitial fluid; potassium salts contribute a majority of intracellular osmotic forces. The osmotic concentration of intracellular fluid is subject to very precise homeostatic regulation.

Solutions with the same osmolality are termed *isosmotic*. An isotonic solution is one that is physiologically isosmotic with cell fluid; when it is substituted for extracellular fluid, no net transfer of water into or out of cells occurs. For example, 1.8% urea is isosmotic but is not isotonic, because it diffuses across cell membranes. To be isotonic, a solute must be nondiffusible, as is 0.9% sodium chloride.

Osmolal Differentials

No significant steady-state difference in osmolality can exist across water-permeable cell membranes. If extracellular fluid is made hypotonic or hypertonic, a net movement of water into or out of cells will take place until osmotic concentrations are equal. However, only water, not sodium or potassium ions, is free to move into and out of cells to restore osmotic equilibrium. Thus, when plasma osmolality is low, the intracellular fluid volume will expand at the expense of the FECV whether the latter is low or high; when plasma osmolality is high, intracellular fluid volume will contract, irrespective of extracellular fluid volume. The terms *volume depletion* and *volume overload*, as used clinically, refer only to extracellular fluid volume; changes in intracellular fluid volume may actually be in a direction opposite that of extracellular volume.

Colloid Oncotic Pressure

A slight difference in osmotic pressure exists between the intravascular and interstitial fluid compartments because of

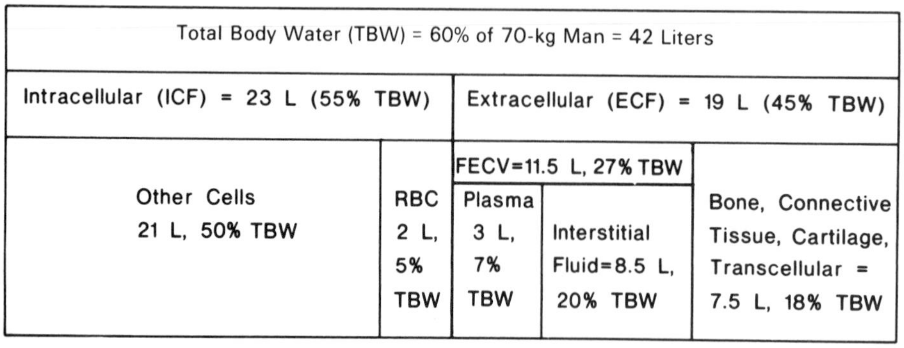

<table>
<tr><td colspan="5">Total Body Water (TBW) = 60% of 70-kg Man = 42 Liters</td></tr>
<tr><td colspan="2">Intracellular (ICF) = 23 L (55% TBW)</td><td colspan="3">Extracellular (ECF) = 19 L (45% TBW)</td></tr>
<tr><td rowspan="2">Other Cells
21 L, 50% TBW</td><td rowspan="2">RBC
2 L,
5%
TBW</td><td colspan="2">FECV=11.5 L, 27% TBW</td><td rowspan="2">Bone, Connective Tissue, Cartilage, Transcellular = 7.5 L, 18% TBW</td></tr>
<tr><td>Plasma
3 L,
7%
TBW</td><td>Interstitial Fluid=8.5 L, 20% TBW</td></tr>
</table>

FIGURE 33-1. Distribution of TBW in a healthy 70-kg man. *ECF*, extracellular fluid compartment; *ICF*, intracellular fluid compartment.

the higher concentration of protein within the intravascular space. This pressure is referred to as the *colloid oncotic pressure* and is about 28 mm Hg. It prevents excessive fluid loss from capillaries. In states of protein deficiency or abnormal capillary permeability to protein, however, the colloid oncotic pressure is decreased and fluid leakage, often significant, can occur.

NORMAL HOMEOSTATIC MECHANISMS

Renal Water and Electrolyte Regulation

Glomerular Filtration

Maintenance of volume and composition of the internal fluid environment is one of the primary functions of the kidneys. Together, the kidneys constitute only 0.4% of total body weight, yet they receive 20% to 25% of cardiac output, or blood at a rate of about 1200 mL/min. Every 24 hours, the 2 million renal glomeruli filter about 160 L of water, containing 24,000 mEq of sodium, 700 mEq of potassium, 5000 mEq of bicarbonate, and 20,000 mEq of chloride.

Proximal Tubular Reabsorption

As glomerular filtrate flows through the proximal convoluted tubules, its volume is reduced by approximately 80% because of the active reabsorption of sodium accompanied by passive reabsorption of chloride and water (Fig. 33-2). Because water diffuses freely across proximal tubular epithelium, tubular fluid remains isosmotic with plasma. About 90% of filtered bicarbonate is absorbed in the proximal tubules. After combining with actively secreted hydrogen ion to form carbonic acid, the latter is rapidly dehydrated to carbon dioxide by carbonic anhydrase present in the brush border of proximal tubular epithelium. Essentially all filtered potassium is actively reabsorbed in the proximal tubules, as are glucose and most amino acids. The fraction of filtered water and electrolytes reabsorbed in the proximal tubules remains relatively constant, despite changes in glomerular filtration rate (GFR). This phenomenon, referred to as *glomerulotubular balance,* prevents fluctuations in the GFR from causing large shifts in sodium balance.

Countercurrent Multiplication and Exchange

As the remaining tubular fluid flows through the loops of Henle, two important events occur that are essential to the ability of the kidneys to concentrate and dilute urine. First, tubular fluid in the ascending limbs of the loops of Henle is rendered hypotonic to plasma by virtue of the active transport of sodium (or perhaps chloride) across the tubular epithelium, which is uniquely impermeable to water. Second, an osmotic gradient is established in the renal medullary and papillary interstitium, as a direct result of the anatomic configuration of the loops of Henle and their associated capillaries. Urea, in large part, contributes to the maintenance of this gradient.

Osmolality of the papillary interstitium in a healthy young person can be as high as 1200 to 1300 mOsm/kg, or four to five times that of plasma. The mechanisms by which this gra-

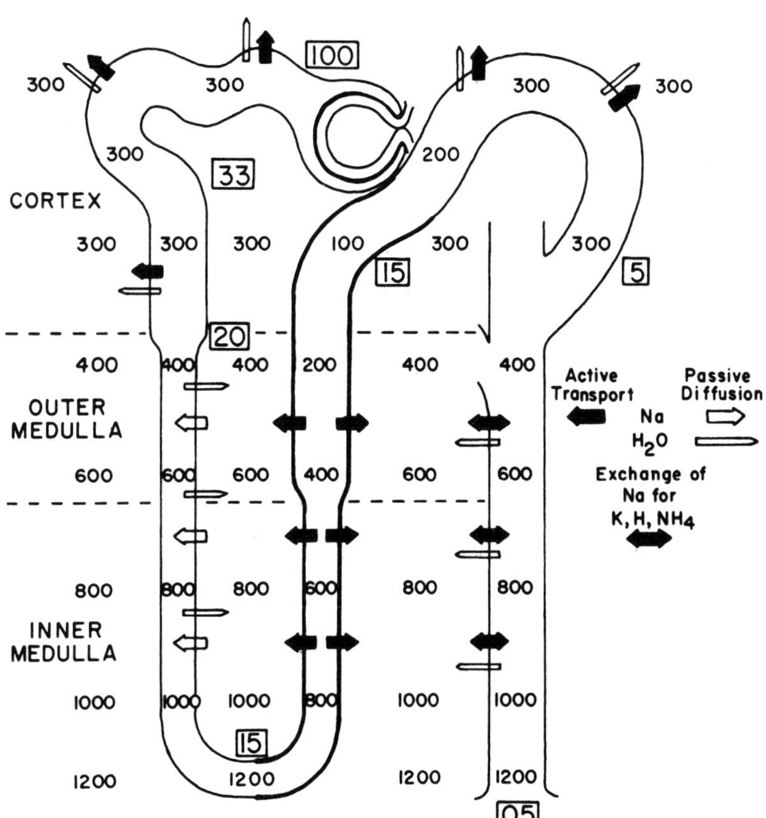

FIGURE 33-2. Passive and active exchanges of water and ions in the nephron in the elaboration of hypertonic urine. Concentrations of tubular urine and peritubular fluid are given in milliosmoles per liter. *Boxed numerals,* the estimated percentage of glomerular filtrate remaining within the tubule at each level. (Adapted from Pitts RF: Physiology of the kidney and body fluids, 3rd ed. Chicago: Year Book Medical Publishers, 1974:134.)

dient is established and maintained are commonly referred to as *countercurrent multiplication* and *countercurrent exchange* (see Chapter 34).

Distal Convoluted Tubular Reabsorption and Excretion

Tubular fluid in the distal convoluted tubules is hypotonic to the surrounding cortical interstitium. Its volume is approximately 15% of that of the initial glomerular filtrate, and its composition is largely unaffected by the patient's volume or osmotic status. From this point on, however, the tubular fluid is subject to numerous regulatory mechanisms. Sodium ions can be reabsorbed or excreted, primarily in exchange for potassium. Hydrogen ions are secreted as required, mostly as titratable acid and ammonium.

Collecting Duct Absorption and Excretion of Water

Nearly all of the water can be passively reabsorbed into the hypertonic medullary interstitium from the collecting ducts, if the latter have been made permeable by the action of antidiuretic hormone (ADH). Conversely, in the absence of ADH, the epithelium of the collecting ducts remains impermeable to water, so that virtually all that reaches the distal tubules is excreted. The net result of these processes is the maintenance of volume, osmolality, and composition of body fluids within very close tolerances, despite highly variable dietary and metabolic loads.

Conservation of Functional Extracellular Fluid Volume: Sodium Regulation

FECV is one of the best defended parameters of fluid and electrolyte physiology; its conservation is accomplished primarily by regulation of sodium excretion. Volume depletion mediated by arterial and possibly left atrial baroreceptors leads to retention of sodium. In all probability, several mechanisms are responsible for sodium excretion; their hierarchy has not been delineated. A brief description of several of these follows.

Aldosterone Release

In the presence of aldosterone, sodium is exchanged for potassium in the distal tubules. The first step in this complex process is the release of renin by the renal juxtaglomerular apparatus, probably as a result of reduced renal perfusion pressure or decreased sodium delivery to the macula densa of the distal tubules. Renin mediates the conversion of circulating angiotensinogen to angiotensin I, which undergoes cleavage in the lungs to form angiotensin II; the latter is a potent stimulator of aldosterone release. In addition, baroreceptors in the carotid sinus, and possibly elsewhere, are thought to mediate aldosterone release in response to depletion of intravascular fluid, extracellular fluid volume, or both.

Until recently, aldosterone was widely believed to be the principal regulator of sodium balance. However, sodium excretion is well regulated in situations in which circulating aldosterone levels are constant and therefore not subject to feedback mechanisms. Hence, factors other than aldosterone release may be equally important in the regulation of sodium excretion.

Alterations in Glomerular Filtration

Changes in GFR might lead to parallel changes in sodium excretion. Although major changes in GFR may affect sodium excretion, this mechanism is unlikely to be precise enough to be a major regulator of sodium balance.

Redistribution of Intrarenal Blood Flow

Redistribution of renal blood flow between cortical and juxtamedullary nephrons experimentally alters sodium excretion.[7] Juxtamedullary nephrons have longer proximal tubules and loops of Henle than do cortical nephrons and therefore are better able to conserve sodium; they appear to be preferentially perfused in states of sodium depletion. When volume is severely depleted, cortical blood flow may be critically impaired.[8] As yet, evidence has been insufficient to establish whether neural, humoral, intrarenal, or a combination of these mechanisms mediate redistribution of intrarenal blood flow.[9]

Peritubular Hydrostatic and Oncotic Pressure

Physical changes in the peritubular environment may significantly affect sodium excretion.[6] Specifically, decreased intracapillary hydrostatic pressure or increased capillary colloid oncotic pressure should facilitate sodium and water reabsorption across tubular epithelium. This theory is supported by the observation that volume replacement with colloid-free solutions results in a greater diuresis than when it is done with plasma substitutes.[10]

Natriuretic Hormone

Atrial natriuretic factor affects sodium excretion directly and also through the inhibition of aldosterone. The factor consists of two low-molecular-weight peptides, atriopeptin I and atriopeptin II, containing 21- and 23-amino acid residues, respectively. Both have potent natriuretic, diuretic, and vasorelaxant properties. Volume expansion, mediated by one or more baroreceptors, is postulated to induce the release of this natriuretic hormone, which inhibits sodium reabsorption at the proximal tubule.[11]

Maintenance of Osmolality: Water Regulation

In contrast to the poorly understood and undoubtedly complex mechanisms for control of the FECV, control of body fluid osmolality is mediated by a single substance, ADH.[1,12] When osmolality is increased by more than 2%, ADH is released from the posterior pituitary gland. ADH acts at the collecting ducts and to a lesser extent at the distal convoluted tubules, rendering them permeable to water, which then passes into the hypertonic medullary interstitium. Vasa rectae carry this water back to the renal venous circulation; in the process, a small volume of concentrated urine is excreted. Secretion of

ADH persists until sufficient water is retained to restore plasma osmolality to normal values.

Conversely, when osmolality decreases, ADH secretion is suppressed. The distal tubules and collecting ducts become impermeable to water, so that tubular fluid reaches the calyceal system with reabsorption of little or no water. The net result is a loss of free water and an increase in plasma osmolality. The mechanism by which increased osmolality triggers ADH secretion is thought to be related to a decrease in intracellular volume of the neurons of the hypothalamic supraoptic nuclei.

Nonosmotic Regulation of Antidiuretic Hormone

Many nonosmotic factors are known to stimulate or inhibit ADH release, and several of these are important to fluid homeostasis of surgical patients.[12,13] The most significant is the release of ADH in response to isosmotic contraction of extracellular water, plasma volume, or both. Secretion in response to volume depletion may be maintained despite significant reductions in plasma osmolality. Although the FECV will be restored toward normal by retention of free water, the resulting hyponatremia has potentially serious consequences. The effector mechanisms responsible for the nonosmotic release of ADH are thought to be located either in the carotid sinus baroreceptors (high-pressure system) or left atrial volume receptors (low-pressure system).

Many drugs used during anesthesia, including narcotics, barbiturates, and inhalation agents, are associated with ADH-like effects.[12,13] Whether these drugs act directly on the pituitary–hypophyseal axis or indirectly through hemodynamic alterations is unknown; the latter mechanism is the most likely explanation. Pain, emotional stress, positive-pressure ventilation, β-adrenergic agents such as isoproterenol, and cholinergic agents such as acetylcholine also are known to stimulate ADH secretion. The importance of nonosmotic stimuli to ADH secretion during the perioperative period should not be underestimated.

Potassium Regulation

Virtually all of the 700 mEq of potassium filtered daily by the glomeruli are actively reabsorbed in the proximal tubules. In the distal tubules potassium appears to be passively secreted into the tubular lumens, in exchange for sodium along a transepithelial electrical gradient. After intake of a potassium load, aldosterone facilitates increased distal tubular secretion of potassium. Tubular secretion of potassium is increased in alkalosis; the mechanism probably involves changes in electrical gradients rather than competition between potassium and hydrogen ions for a single excretory pump.[1] Increased tubular secretion of potassium also may occur when large sodium loads are presented to the distal tubules (eg, when diuretic therapy interferes with sodium reabsorption in the proximal tubules and loops of Henle). An obligatory renal potassium loss of about 20 mEq/day occurs even in states of potassium depletion. In patients with renal disease, potassium balance is usually well maintained until kidney function is severely compromised.[14]

DYNAMICS OF WATER AND SOLUTE BALANCE

Because surgical patients are frequently (though unintentionally) subjected to the stresses of water or sodium deprivation or excess, the dynamics of fluid and electrolyte balance must be examined in normal subjects as well as in patients with renal or cardiac disease.

Normal Fluid and Electrolyte Balance

A healthy 70-kg man eating an unrestricted diet usually consumes 1500 to 2000 mL of water and 50 to 150 mEq each of sodium, potassium, and chloride per day. Intermediary metabolism generates approximately 300 mL of water (mostly from oxidation), 40 to 80 mEq of nonvolatile acids, and 30 g (500 mOsm) of urea.[1,15,16] About 800 mL of water is lost by insensible routes through the lungs and skin, so that each day, the kidneys are required to excrete approximately 1000 to 1500 mL of water, 200 to 400 mEq of electrolytes, 40 to 80 mEq of nonvolatile acid, and 500 mOsm of urea.[5] This total represents an osmotic load of 750 to 1000 mOsm.

Because most people concentrate urine to a maximum osmolality of 750 to 1250 mOsm/kg (the peak value decreases with age), a 24-hour urine volume of 600 to 1000 mL is required to excrete this amount of solute. When insensible water loss and water generated by metabolism are included in these calculations, the daily obligatory water requirement is 1100 to 1500 mL. If less than this amount of water is provided, the total osmotic load cannot be excreted, and solute will be retained.

Water excess is tolerated far better than water restriction by most people. Urine flow can increase to 20 mL/min, accompanied by a decrease in osmolality to as low as 35 mOsm/kg. Thus, a water intake of 20 L/day can be tolerated without the development of significant fluid or electrolyte abnormalities.

Variations in sodium intake within a range of about 1 to 4 g/day (40 to 175 mEq/day) are tolerated with minimal change in extracellular fluid volume. Even a steady sodium load of 10 to 15 g/day may be tolerated, although ultimately, such a diet probably would lead to expansion of extracellular fluid volume by 1 L or more. At the other extreme, a normal person can adapt to a diet almost totally devoid of sodium by reabsorbing essentially all filtered sodium.

Abnormalities of Fluid and Electrolyte Balance

Intrinsic Renal Disease

Patients with renal disease have decreased ability to tolerate extremes of water and sodium intake. Urine-concentrating mechanisms are affected before diluting mechanisms, so that patients with renal disease are less able to tolerate water restriction than are normal patients.[17] Concentration of urine or excretion of a sodium load is decreased roughly in proportion to the decrease in GFR. Some degree of sodium wasting is found in most types of renal disease, and losses of 100 mEq/day or more are not uncommon.[18]

Congestive Heart Failure and Cirrhosis

Certain disease states, notably congestive heart failure (CHF) and hepatic cirrhosis, are associated with an overexpanded extracellular volume and impairment of mechanisms for sodium and water excretion. In CHF, expansion of the FECV is most likely a compensatory mechanism, mediated by carotid sinus baroreceptors.[13] The mechanism for the impairment of sodium and water excretion associated with advanced liver failure is less clear, although a similar baroreceptor mechanism has been postulated.

EFFECTS OF ANESTHESIA ON RENAL FUNCTION

In surgical patients without renal disease, all general anesthetics temporarily depress renal function, including urine flow, GFR, renal blood flow, and electrolyte excretion.[19-21] This consistent and generalized depression of renal function can be attributed to many factors, such as type and duration of the surgical procedure; physical status, especially that of the cardiovascular and renal systems; preoperative and intraoperative blood volume; fluid and electrolyte balance[22,23]; anesthetic agent[19]; and depth of anesthesia.[24] Depression of renal function induced by anesthetic agents is thought to be caused by their indirect effects on the circulatory, sympathetic nervous, and endocrine systems, rather than by their direct effects on the nephrons.

Indirect

Circulatory

During general anesthesia, renal blood flow and glomerular filtration may be depressed as a consequence of cardiovascular depression, renal vasoconstriction, or both. The older agents, cyclopropane and diethyl ether, were associated with marked increases in renal vascular resistance as a result of increased levels of circulating catecholamines.[25,26] Halothane, enflurane, isoflurane, and thiopental, although not evoking a significant catecholamine response, are associated with a moderate increase in renal vascular resistance as blood is shunted away from the kidneys to compensate for hypotension induced by myocardial depression, peripheral vasodilation, or both.[24,27-30] Balanced anesthetic techniques using drugs with α-adrenergic–blocking activity, such as droperidol, have been reported to cause no depression in renal blood flow in well-hydrated patients.[31]

Sympathetic Nervous System

The renal vasculature is richly supplied with sympathetic constrictor fibers but is devoid of sympathetic dilator or parasympathetic innervation. In the resting, unanesthetized, supine patient subjected to no physical or psychic stress, little sympathetic tone is present. A great variety of normal and abnormal physiologic conditions cause mild to moderate increases in sympathetic tone. In patients with these conditions, a relatively greater decrease in renal blood flow than in glomerular filtration occurs; filtration fraction thus increases, and the GFR is maintained.[32]

Conditions causing severe stress, such as fear, pain, hypotension, hemorrhage, and general anesthesia, increase sympathetic tone greatly; renal blood flow is markedly decreased, and GFR is moderately decreased. Sympathetic nervous system involvement in the renal effects of anesthesia is supported by experiments in dogs with one normal and one denervated kidney.[33] Induction of pentobarbital or chloralose anesthesia in these animals is associated with a decrease in renal blood flow and glomerular filtration to the normal kidney, whereas no change is seen on the denervated side.

These findings suggest that spinal or epidural anesthesia will cause only minimal alterations in renal function provided that normal blood pressure can be maintained. The effects of anesthetics on autoregulation of renal blood flow is debated.[34-36] Nonanesthetic drugs that paralyze smooth muscle, such as potassium cyanide and papaverine, also abolish autoregulation, suggesting that autoregulatory resistance changes are of myogenic rather than of sympathetic nervous system origin.

Endocrine

ANTIDIURETIC HORMONE. Antidiuresis associated with anesthesia and surgery is, at least in part, caused by an increase in circulating ADH. The numerous nonosmotic stimuli to ADH secretion that are of importance to surgical patients were discussed earlier.

RENIN–ANGIOTENSIN. The precise role of renin–angiotensin in the renal alterations that occur during anesthesia has not been defined.[37-39] Renin levels do not increase during anesthesia.[39] However, saralasin, the competitive inhibitor of angiotensin II, demonstrates an important role for the maintenance of blood pressure by the renin–angiotensin system during halothane and enflurane anesthesia.

ALDOSTERONE. Whether anesthetic agents act directly on the adrenal gland to cause aldosterone release is unknown. They probably act indirectly through one or several of the following mechanisms: by causing ADH release, which in turn stimulates secretion of aldosterone; by stimulating the sympathetic nervous system, causing renal vasoconstriction; or by inducing peripheral vasodilation. Even though administration of anesthesia leads to aldosterone release, serum sodium concentration often decreases after general anesthesia and surgery. This effect often is related to the fluids administered. Note that Ringer's lactate contains only 130 mEq of sodium per liter.

Direct

Anesthetic agents alter active transport of sodium in in-vitro experimental preparations,[40,41] suggesting that direct effects of anesthetic occur in the renal tubules. However, the direct effects are minor compared with the major indirect effects of anesthesia and operation. Among the anesthetic drugs, only methoxyflurane caused significant nephrotoxicity as a consequence of its biotransformation to fluoride ion.[42-44] Recent work suggests renal biotransformation may be more important than hepatic.[45]

DISORDERS OF FLUIDS AND ELECTROLYTES

Three aspects of body fluid and electrolyte homeostasis are usually discussed: volumes of distribution, osmolality, and electrolyte composition. Disorders of fluid and electrolyte balance are analyzed conveniently in the same terms. Some clinical disorders involve only one of these variables, but many are complex. Treatment of complex disorders is facilitated if the simple underlying disturbances are first identified and then corrected either sequentially or simultaneously, depending on their relative urgency.

Disturbances of Functional Extracellular Fluid Volume

A simple volume disturbance is a deviation from the normal FECV with maintenance of normal osmolality. Because water and electrolytes diffuse freely across capillary endothelium, changes in intravascular volume are reflected throughout the FECV; the usual ratio of 3 to 1 for interstitial fluid volume and plasma volume remains relatively constant in most disturbances. However, in markedly hypoalbuminemic states, decreased plasma colloid oncotic pressure results in a disproportionately high interstitial fluid volume. Isolated disturbances of the FECV do not significantly alter intracellular fluid volume or composition.

Depletion

Contraction of the FECV is the most common fluid disorder in surgical patients.[16,46,47] Nevertheless, mild or moderate degrees of hypovolemia frequently go unrecognized. Two reasons explain this observation. First, major losses of fluid from the extracellular space can occur through internal fluid shifts, without any visible evidence of fluid loss.[46,47] Second, no single set of physical signs or clinical biochemical determinations accurately measures the functional extracellular fluid space.

In the patient undergoing major surgery, the difficulty in assessing FECV is compounded by the effects of preoperative medications, surgical manipulation and the combined cardiovascular, renal, autonomic nervous system, and hormonal effects of the anesthetic agents. Isotope dilution techniques for the determination of FECV have been used as a research tool but are not practical in clinical situations.[48] The complications of severe FECV deficits, such as hypovolemic shock with progressive lactic acidosis, acute renal failure, myocardial infarction, and cerebral ischemia, may be prevented by prompt and adequate volume replacement.

SIGNS. Signs of volume depletion vary with the severity and rapidity of onset of the disturbance. When volume loss is acute, circulatory signs predominate. These may include tachycardia; hypotension; decreased pulse pressure; peripheral vasoconstriction; diminished heart sounds; weak, thready, or undetectable peripheral pulses; collapsed neck veins; low central venous and left atrial pressure; and oliguria.

In the awake patient, neurologic signs, including drowsiness, apathy, lassitude, and stupor, may be seen with increasing degrees of volume depletion. Dryness of mucous membranes and the tongue is observed relatively early, but other tissue signs, such as sunken eyes, furrowed tongue, and decreased skin turgor are usually not apparent until significant deficits have continued for many hours.[15,16]

LABORATORY FINDINGS. Laboratory evidence of volume depletion includes increased hematocrit and, after 24 hours or more, increased blood urea nitrogen; blood urea nitrogen–creatinine ratio greater than 15; increased urine specific gravity (>1.020); and reduced urinary sodium concentration (<20 mEq/L). Calculation of the fractional excretion of sodium is useful to determine whether oliguria is due to volume depletion with normal renal function. A value less than 1% suggests that oliguria is due to a volume deficit.[49]

Fractional excretion of sodium

$$= \text{U/P sodium} \times \text{P/U creatinine}$$

where U = urine concentration and P = plasma concentration. If tissue perfusion is inadequate, metabolic acidosis results from increased lactate production.

ISOSMOTIC DEFICITS. Isosmotic deficits in FECV may occur as a result of external fluid losses (measurable) or internal redistribution of fluid into nonequilibrating compartments (not measurable). Internally sequestered fluid is completely nonfunctional extracellular fluid and should be considered temporarily lost from the body. In addition, effective FECV deficits occur when the capacitance of the vascular system is increased by the vasodilatory action of anesthetic agents and adjuvant drugs, or when myocardial function is depressed to the extent that existing left atrial pressure (preload) is less than that required for optimal cardiac output.

External. Clinically important external losses may be caused by hemorrhage; excessive urine output resulting from intrinsic renal disease, diuretic therapy, inorganic fluoride nephropathy, or osmotic diuresis associated with hyperglycemia or administration of radiographic contrast solutions; or increased gastrointestinal output resulting from vomiting, diarrhea, nasogastric suction, fistula drainage, and preoperative bowel purgation.

Internal. Clinically important internal fluid sequestration is seen in a high percentage of patients undergoing surgery and may result from the primary disease or from the surgery itself. Proper preoperative and intraoperative volume replacement in these patients requires an appreciation of the magnitude of these losses.

Rapid shifts of large volumes of extracellular fluid into a nonfunctional *third space* can result from acute abdominal lesions such as pancreatitis, perforated gastric ulcer with chemical peritonitis, generalized bacterial peritonitis from any cause, volvulus, and intestinal obstruction. Volume deficits greater than 3 L occur frequently and result from accumulation of fluid in the intestinal lumen and free peritoneal cavity, as well as in thickened, inflamed bowel wall, mesentery, and peritoneum. Crush injuries, burns, thrombophlebitis, and fractures, especially of the femur or pelvis, also are associated with major internal fluid sequestration.

In general, intraoperative third-space shifts are related to the degree of tissue dissection and manipulation. Major abdominal surgery, extensive retroperitoneal dissection, and bowel manipulation may result in sequestration of 3 L of fluid.[46,47] Less extensive surgery is associated with lesser fluid shifts.

PREVENTION AND TREATMENT. Preoperatively, the volume status of every patient should be thoroughly assessed. The recent clinical history is likely to indicate possible causes of volume depletion or internal fluid shifts. Records of fluid balance, serial measurements of body weight, and measurements of hematocrit and blood urea nitrogen at intervals yield valuable information. Finally, physical examination may reveal signs of volume deficit, although clinical signs of fluid depletion may not be present until losses exceed 2 L.

Whenever possible, existing deficits should be fully replaced before induction of anesthesia. Significant hypotension during induction usually suggests that this goal has not been accomplished. The best indication of adequate fluid replacement is the reversal of clinical signs of volume deficit and establishment of a urine output of 50 to 100 mL/h.

Monitoring. When significant cardiac or renal impairment is present or large fluid shifts are expected, continuous measurement of urine output with an indwelling catheter is essential. In patients without significant cardiac or pulmonary disease, central venous pressure is usually a good indirect measure of left atrial pressure, or left ventricular preload[50]; as such, it can be used to gauge adequacy of volume replacement, especially when infusions are very rapid.

When marked impairment of myocardial function or severe pulmonary disease is present, central venous pressure may not correlate with left atrial pressure.[51] In this case, if volume status is not known with certainty, or if rapid infusions may be required, left ventricular filling pressure is determined by pulmonary artery occlusion pressure (PAOP), measured by using a balloon-tipped pulmonary artery catheter.[52,53] Alternatively, or as an adjunct to this monitoring, transesophageal echocardiography can be used to monitor left ventricular end diastolic volume and to estimate ejection fraction.

Careful estimation of blood loss and internal fluid shifts, and prompt replacement with appropriate solutions, usually prevent intraoperative hypovolemia. Deterioration of circulatory performance together with diminution of urine output usually means that fluid losses have been underestimated and should be reassessed.

SELECTION OF REPLACEMENT FLUID. Except for insensible losses, virtually all intraoperative losses are isosmotic and should be replaced with isosmotic solutions. The question of which solution to use (eg, normal saline, balanced electrolyte solution, albumin, plasma substitute, whole blood, or packed erythrocytes) is still debated.[54–58] The physiologic approach presented here is that losses should be replaced with fluid of the same composition. Blood loss should be replaced with packed red blood cells (whole blood is seldom available with current blood banking procedures); protein-rich exudates should be replaced with a plasma equivalent; and fluid sequestered as soft-tissue edema should be replaced with balanced salt solution.

Balanced Electrolyte and Saline Solutions. Current practice dictates that, in general, blood loss not expected to result in a hematocrit of less than 21% to 25% should be replaced not with blood but rather with electrolyte solutions, with or without added colloid.[59,60] Aside from eliminating the risk of blood-transmitted disease (eg, acquired immunodeficiency syndrome, hepatitis), oxygen transport to the tissues is well maintained at low hematocrit, assuming that the patient is kept normovolemic. In fact, deliberate hemodilution is commonly used in cardiac surgical and other procedures.[61–63] Decreased oxygen-carrying capacity is compensated by a lowered blood viscosity and a higher cardiac output, without increased myocardial oxygen consumption.[64]

Colloid-free balanced electrolyte or saline solution plus packed erythrocytes are often used for fluid resuscitation after extensive blood loss; this practice is said to result in morbidity that is no higher than that after resuscitation with whole blood and colloid-containing solutions.[10,65] Because colloid-free solutions equilibrate throughout the functional extracellular compartment, the volume of balanced salt solution required to replace a given blood or plasma loss is three or four times greater than the volume lost.[56]

This approach, although well tolerated by most patients, may be associated with perioperative morbidity in patients with decreased cardiopulmonary reserve. In cases of severe hypovolemia, successful treatment is more dependent on the rapidity and adequacy of fluid repletion than on the type of fluid administered.[66]

Hypertonic Solutions. Hypertonic solutions (saline, acetate, or lactate) are also gaining in popularity to reduce the administered water load while maintaining solute delivery.[67] These solutions improve myocardial function, decrease systemic vascular resistance, reduce edema, maintain renal function, and may have a beneficial effect on reduction of cerebral edema in closed head trauma.[68–72] Hypernatremia and increased osmolality are possible side effects. Frequent monitoring of serum sodium is recommended when they are used.

Excess

Isosmotic overload of the functional extracellular compartment is encountered far less frequently in surgical patients than is hypovolemia. In nearly all cases, acute volume overload is iatrogenic and results from the intravenous administration of salt-containing solutions at a rate that exceeds the patient's ability to excrete them. Chronic isosmotic volume expansion is seen in CHF, cirrhosis, and advanced renal insufficiency. All three conditions result from disordered homeostatic mechanisms for sodium excretion.

SIGNS. Clinical signs are related to the degree of overload of the systemic and pulmonary circulation, the rapidity with which overload occurs, and the amount of cardiovascular reserve. Early signs include distention of peripheral veins, increased right and left heart filling pressures, increased pulse pressure, and bounding peripheral pulses. More severe degrees of overload may precipitate heart failure or pulmonary edema,[73-75] heralded by the development of a third-heart sound gallop, decreased pulmonary compliance, pulmonary auscultatory changes, including wheezes or rales, and increasing alveolar–arterial difference in oxygen partial pressure.

PREVENTION. The ability to excrete a large solute load is decreased during anesthesia and operation because of anesthetic-induced depression of renal blood flow and GFR, as well as to the numerous factors that result in ADH release. Still, in patients with normal cardiac and renal reserve, symptomatic volume overload develops only when large excesses of fluid have been administered rapidly. In most patients volume overload may be avoided by monitoring circulatory function and by auscultation of heart and breath sounds. When large volumes of fluid administration are anticipated, monitoring of urine output, central venous pressure, or both is advisable.

MONITORING. Patients with decreased cardiac reserve or renal disease are less able to excrete a volume load during anesthesia than are other patients. Even a mild excess in fluid administration can precipitate CHF or pulmonary edema; therefore, volume replacement must be approached with great caution.

Urine output and central venous pressure should be monitored, but both may be misleading in patients with severely depressed left ventricular function. Oliguria may reflect critically low cardiac output despite administration of the maximum tolerated fluid load. Ideal treatment for patients with extremely poor myocardial reserve undergoing extensive surgical procedures requires direct measurement of arterial pressure perioperatively, as well as measurement of PAOP or monitoring left ventricular systolic function and end diastolic volume via transesophageal echocardiography.

TREATMENT. Treatment of volume overload should vary with the severity of symptoms. Patients with mild overload may require only fluid restriction. Those with pulmonary edema may require diuretics, pharmacologic vasodilation, high inspired fraction of oxygen, and mechanical ventilation, including positive end-expiratory pressure.[76] Inotropic agents are useful if myocardial depression is a factor.

Fluid Shifts Into the Third Space

Fluid sequestered in traumatized tissues does not constitute a part of the FECV. Therefore, a patient should not be considered to be volume overloaded on the basis of fluid shifts into the third space, even when total extracellular fluid volume is expanded by several liters. The return of sequestered fluid into the FECV occurs gradually during the first 5 or 6 postoperative days and usually causes no problems. In fact, reinfusion may occur so gradually that it is undetectable except by serial weight determinations. However, among patients who have a marked tendency to retain sodium, reentry of third-space fluid into the FECV can impose a significant volume overload, so that diuretic administration may become necessary.

DISTURBANCES OF OSMOLALITY

Primary disturbances of serum osmolality are characterized by net total body gains or losses of free water in excess of sodium and may result from either inappropriate perioperative fluid therapy or primary derangements of normal osmoregulatory mechanisms. Associated volume disturbances may be present.

In contrast to isosmotic volume disturbances, which affect only the extracellular fluid compartment, osmotic disorders principally alter the intracellular environment. An excess of extracellular free water results in a rapid redistribution of water into cells, increasing intracellular volume and lowering intracellular osmolality until it again equals that of extracellular fluid. Extracellular free-water deficits have the opposite effects.

Hyperglycemia

Because sodium salts normally account for more than 90% of the osmotic activity of extracellular fluid, alterations in osmolality are usually paralleled by alterations in serum sodium concentration alone. Increased concentrations of other extracellular solutes, most notably glucose, may contribute significantly to plasma osmolality. A plasma glucose concentration of 500 mg/dL, for example, contributes approximately 28 mOsm/kg to plasma osmolality.† Thus, plasma osmolality is increased by 1 mOsm/kg for every 18 mg/dL increase in plasma glucose concentration (molecular weight of glucose, 180). Accordingly, a hyperglycemic patient may have a depressed serum sodium concentration, but a normal or high serum osmolality and a normal or contracted intracellular volume.

Hyperlipidemia and Hyperproteinemia

In states of severe hyperlipidemia or hyperproteinemia, the volume of plasma water is less than usual because of the presence of these substances. Because the serum sodium level is reported as the concentration in milliequivalents per liter of plasma, not of water, the serum sodium concentration will be underestimated. Since proteins and lipids do not contribute to plasma osmolality because of their large molecular size, these states are referred to as *isotonic hyponatremia (pseudohyponatremia)*.[49] Positive diagnosis of osmotic disorders requires that the osmotic contribution of all extracellular particles be estimated or, ideally, that serum osmolality be determined.

---

† For conversion of milligrams per deciliter to milliosmoles per kilogram:

$$\text{Milliosmoles per kilogram} = \frac{\text{(milligrams per deciliter)}}{\text{molecular weight}}$$

TABLE 33-2
Isotonic Hyponatremia

DIAGNOSIS
Decreased serum sodium ion concentration; normal osmolality
CAUSES
Hyperproteinemic states
Hyperlipidemic state
MANAGEMENT
Determine underlying cause
Do not panic
COMPLICATIONS
Related to underlying disease

Layon AJ, Bernards WC, Kirby RR: Fluids and electrolytes in the critically ill. In Civetta JM, Taylor RW, Kirby RR (eds): Critical care, 2nd ed. Philadelphia: JB Lippincott, 1992: 459.

Hyponatremia and Water Intoxication

Variable degrees of hyponatremia commonly occur after surgery, usually as a result of the intravenous administration of sodium-free or hypo-osmotic solutions.[77–79] Less common causes of hypo-osmolar states include diuretic therapy,[80–82] various drug treatments,[83] overhydration during transurethral surgery of the prostate, and the syndrome of inappropriate ADH secretion; the latter two conditions are discussed separately. The terms "hyponatremia" and "hypo-osmolality" are often used synonymously, although the difference between the two should be kept in mind.

Hyponatremia, defined as a serum sodium concentration of less than 135 mEq/L, results when water is retained in excess of sodium; a net positive free-water balance occurs (Tables 33-2 to 33-4). Several factors may predispose the surgical patient to a positive free-water balance.[84] Inappropriately large volumes of sodium-free or hypo-osmotic parenteral fluids may be administered during the perioperative period; pain and emotional stress, administration of narcotics, barbiturates and inhalation anesthetics, and positive-pressure ventilation may result in the secretion of ADH and the retention of free water; reduction of the FECV may occur as a result of third-space sequestration, despite intraoperative volume replacement that is otherwise adequate; depression of renal blood flow and GFR by as much as 70% during anesthesia and surgery, with concomitant decreased ability to excrete a water load; and formation of endogenous free water from oxidation of fats and lysis of lean tissue, which may add water at a rate of 600 mL/day or greater to the free-water load.

Symptoms and Signs

Mild hyponatremia may not be associated with clinically recognizable symptoms or signs. However, when serum sodium decreases to approximately 125 mEq/L or lower, *water intoxication,* characterized by disorientation, confusion, muscle twitching, and hyperactive deep tendon reflexes, may become apparent. *Severe hyponatremia,* serum sodium less than 120 mEq/L may result in convulsions, stupor, coma, or death. These neurologic manifestations reflect a derangement of cerebral function caused by decreased intracellular osmolality and expanded intracellular volume, which lead to cerebral edema and increased intracranial pressure.

For many years postoperative patients were thought to be unable to tolerate water loads. Subsequently, evidence showed that postoperative water intolerance can be ameliorated significantly or even prevented by proper intraoperative volume replacement.[22,84–86] However, when relatively modest deficits of FECV are allowed to persist postoperatively, normal homeostatic mechanisms become operative, resulting in significant retention of free water and marked hyponatremia. The following example may serve to illustrate this important point.

A healthy 70-kg man (total body water 42 L and FECV 12 L) undergoing an uncomplicated cholecystectomy may sustain intraoperative third-space fluid shifts of approximately 2 L. A volume deficit of this magnitude stimulates ADH secretion, resulting in near maximal renal water conservation; thus, urine output might decrease to approximately 500 mL/day. Assuming insensible water losses of 800 mL/day and endogenous water production of 500 mL/day, the daily net obligatory water losses totals approximately 800 mL.

If daily parenteral fluid therapy consists of 3 L of 5% glucose in water, a net positive water balance of more than 4 L results 48 hours after operation. Serum osmolality will drop to approximately 260 to 270 mOsm per kg, and serum sodium concentration to about 125 to 130 mEq/L. Only about one fourth of the net water gain, or about 1 L, will remain in the extracellular compartment; hence, an FECV deficit of approximately 1 L occurs, even though total body water increases by 4 L.

Had the 2-L intraoperative volume deficit been replaced with a corresponding volume of balanced electrolyte solution,

TABLE 33-3
Hypertonic Hyponatremia

DIAGNOSIS
Decreased serum sodium ion concentration; plasma osmolality >290 mOsm/kg water
Hyperglycemia
Mannitol
Glycerol
MANAGEMENT
Correct volume deficit
Insulin to treat hyperglycemia (if present) slowly
Hypotonic saline to correct free-water deficit
Correct underlying cause
Why is patient hyperglycemic?
Why is glycerol or mannitol in use?
COMPLICATIONS
Hypoglycemia
Cerebral edema

Layon AJ, Bernards WC, Kirby RR: Fluids and electrolytes in the critically ill. In Civetta JM, Taylor RW, Kirby RR (eds): Critical care, 2nd ed. Philadelphia: JB Lippincott, 1992: 459.

TABLE 33-4
Hypotonic Hyponatremia

DIAGNOSIS
Decreased serum sodium ion concentration; plasma osmolality <270 mOsm/kg water
Differentiate type by assessment of FECV
CAUSES
Hypovolemic
Extrarenal
Gastrointestinal loss (vomiting, diarrhea)
Burns
Third space (eg, pancreatitis)
Renal
Diuretic agents
Adrenal failure
Renal parenchymal disease
Hypervolemic
Advanced renal disease
Acute renal failure
Chronic renal insufficiency
Edematous states
CHF
Cirrhosis of the liver
Nephrotic syndrome
Severe hypoproteinemia caused by nutritional or gastrointestinal disease
Isovolemic
Stress
Adrenal insufficiency
Hypothyroidism
Drugs
Potassium ion depletion or use of diuretic agents
SIADH
MANAGEMENT
Hypovolemic: isotonic saline
Hypervolemic or isovolemic: restrict free water
Manage underlying disorders
COMPLICATIONS
CNS: seizures, coma, death, pontine myelinolysis, residual effects
Decompensation of underlying disorders

Modified from: Layon AJ, Bernards WC, Kirby RR: Fluids and electrolytes in the critically ill. In Civetta JM, Taylor RW, Kirby RR (eds): Critical care, 2nd ed. Philadelphia: JB Lippincott, 1992: 459.

the volume stimulus to ADH secretion would not have been as great, the patient's ability to handle the postoperative free-water load would have been improved, and a significant osmotic disturbance would not have occurred.

Care must be exercised when infusing large volumes of salt-containing solutions to patients with decreased cardiac reserve; the amount of salt necessary to prevent an osmotic disturbance may be in excess of that which could precipitate CHF. An appropriate balance must be struck in this situation.

Prevention

Most cases of serious hyponatremia and water intoxication can be avoided by adherence to basic principles of fluid therapy. Intraoperative and postoperative administration of electrolyte-free water should be based upon calculated free-water losses; normally, these will not exceed 1000 to 1500 mL/day. Fluid losses and fluid shifts should be fully replaced with isotonic solutions such as normal saline, balanced electrolyte solutions, and blood or plasma substitutes. Finally, parenteral fluid therapy should be guided by determination of serum electrolyte concentrations and, when indicated, serum osmolality.

Treatment

Treatment of hyponatremia and water intoxication will depend on the severity of symptoms and the patient's volume status. If symptoms are mild and the FECV is normal or increased, water restriction alone will be sufficient to correct the problem. When hypovolemia exists as well, correction of the volume deficit with isotonic saline should result in a steady water diuresis and a return of osmolality to normal. Administration of hypertonic saline or 1 M sodium bicarbonate solution is advisable only when hyponatremia is severe and signs of water intoxication are life-threatening (eg, in patients who are in a coma or who have had seizures).

The total sodium deficit can be determined by multiplying estimated total body water (liters) by the deficit in serum sodium (milliequivalents per liter). Total body water, rather than the FECV, is used in this calculation, because the osmotic deficit is distributed throughout intracellular as well as extracellular water. However, only a fraction of the total deficit should be administered to correct signs of severe hyponatremia.

One third of the calculated sodium deficit should be administered as hypertonic saline, at a rate sufficient to increase the serum sodium by only 1 to 2 mEq/L/h to minimize the chance of precipitating central pontine myelinolysis.[87] During this time the patient's condition must be assessed continuously. Complete correction of large sodium deficits using hypertonic saline should not be attempted (ie, only bring the sodium to a level of about 125 mEq/L), and no other fluids should be administered while hypertonic saline is being infused. Rapid intravascular shifts of water in response to the high osmotic load can result in dangerous volume overload, CHF, and pulmonary edema, particularly in patients with reduced cardiac or renal reserve. Furosemide or ethacrynic acid may be of value in treating patients showing signs of fluid overload, but remember that these agents increase sodium loss, particularly at high dosage levels.

Inappropriate Secretion of Antidiuretic Hormone

Causes

The syndrome of inappropriate secretion of ADH (SIADH) is a form of hyponatremia in which a sustained or intermittently increased level of ADH occurs that is inappropriate to the osmotic or volume stimuli that normally cause ADH secretion.[80] The SIADH has been recognized in a wide spectrum of diseases that may be grouped into four broad categories according to their association with malignant tumors, pulmonary infection, disorders of the central nervous system (CNS), and no apparent cause.[89] Occasionally, SIADH occurs postoperatively, especially in the elderly.[90]

A high incidence of SIADH has been reported also in pediatric patients who have undergone posterior spinal fusion.[91]

One or more days after surgery, those affected exhibit a variety of diffuse neurologic signs, including confusion, restlessness, disorientation, and somnolence; in severe cases, profound stupor and seizures may occur. Criteria for diagnosis of SIADH include hyponatremia (serum sodium <130 mEq/L), inappropriately increased urinary osmolality relative to plasma osmolality, normal adrenal and thyroid function, absence of hypovolemia and edema, and correction by strict fluid restriction.

Prevention

In elderly patients undergoing major surgery, stimuli to ADH secretion should be corrected before operation, if possible. Hypovolemia and hypotension during and after surgery should be avoided, volume deficits should be corrected with isotonic solutions. Administration of narcotics should be discontinued when possible as they too have been associated with SIADH, especially morphine sulfate. Urine output must be monitored, and serum electrolytes, checked early in the postoperative period.

Treatment

When hyponatremia is mild, symptoms may not be apparent. In such cases, only water restriction is needed. Restriction of all oral and parenteral water intake will result in a negative water balance, primarily through insensible water losses, with correction of hyponatremia. Infusion of hypertonic saline is not effective, because nearly all administered sodium may be excreted without producing a net negative water balance.

If hyponatremia becomes severe and neurologic symptoms develop, aggressive treatment is indicated. This approach involves establishing a steady diuresis with the intravenous administration of furosemide and measuring and replacing urinary electrolyte losses with appropriate amounts of hypertonic (3%) saline and potassium. Severe hyponatremia can be corrected in several hours in this way, although several more days may be needed to resolve the underlying problem.

Treatment with osmotic agents such as urea, salt supplementation, and water restriction also has been proposed for the severe hyponatremia associated with SIADH.[92,93] Lithium[94] and demeclocycline[95–97] have been used for the treatment of chronic SIADH; however, the onset of action of these agents is slow and they are not recommended for treatment of acute cases in which patients have neurologic symptoms.

Hypo-osmolar Volume Overload During Transurethral Prostatectomy

Pathophysiologic Features

Continuous bladder irrigation during transurethral resection of the prostate frequently results in rapid absorption of large amounts of irrigating solution by venous sinuses opened during surgery.[98–103] The amount of fluid absorbed is related to three factors: the duration of the surgery; the number and size of the venous sinuses opened; and the hydrostatic pressure of the irrigating solution.[104] During prostatectomy, an average of 1200 to 2000 mL of irrigating solution may be absorbed; however, absorption of 4 L has been documented,[105] as has the absorption of large quantities of fluid (3.3 L) in short procedures (20 minutes).[106] Thus, the anesthesiologist must be aware of the potential for volume overload in all cases.

The consequences of absorption of large fluid loads are dependent not only upon the volume that is absorbed, but upon the osmolality of the irrigating fluid and the patient's cardiovascular and renal status. Irrigation solutions are nonelectrolytic so that they inhibit the dispersion of high-voltage electrocautery current.

Irrigating Solutions

In modern practice, the most commonly used solutions are hypo-osmolar, such as 1.5% glycine (212 mOsm/L) or a mixture of 2.7% sorbitol and 0.54% mannitol (Cytal) (195 mOsm/L). In the past, distilled water was used by urologists because it hemolyzed blood in the bladder rapidly and visibility was superior to that with other irrigants. However, in the last 10 to 15 years, water has been abandoned almost completely for transurethral resections, because of the risks of acute volume overload, dilutional hyponatremia, and intravascular hemolysis.

Symptoms and Signs

The symptoms of hypo-osmolar volume overload include restlessness, confusion, nausea, chills, tachypnea, and increased blood pressure, pulse pressure, and central venous pressure. In severe cases, coma, convulsions, cyanosis, pulmonary edema, and cardiovascular collapse may occur.[101,104] The diagnosis is established by determining decreased serum sodium concentration (<125 mEq/L) and serum osmolality (<260 mOsm/kg); intravascular hemolysis may occur at these levels.

Not all patients exhibit the complete constellation of symptoms. In patients with little cardiovascular reserve, for example, CHF and pulmonary edema may develop before body fluid osmolality is sufficiently depressed to cause major signs of water intoxication. To the contrary, in patients who initially are volume depleted, substantial increases in intravascular volume may be tolerated without circulatory overload, and signs only of water intoxication may develop.

Current irrigating solutions are safer than distilled water because their intravascular absorption does not depress plasma osmolality significantly. Thus, intracellular physiologic dysfunction, including the CNS effects of water intoxication, and gross intravascular hemolysis occur less frequently than in the past. However, the risks of hypervolemia, CHF, and pulmonary edema are just as great today as they were when distilled water was used.

Glycine Toxicity

Glycine ($COOHCH_2NH_2$) toxicity is thought to be another cause of CNS complications associated with transurethral prostatectomy.[104,107] Glycine is a nonessential amino acid that, as a 1.5% solution, is used as an irrigant instead of water for such procedures. The distribution of glycine in the body is similar to that of γ-aminobutyric acid, an inhibitory transmitter in the CNS; glycine may act as an inhibitory transmitter in the brain stem and spinal cord.[108,109]

In a report of blindness after transurethral prostatectomy, the serum glycine level was 1029 mg/L (normal value, 13 to 17 mg/L).[107] Vision returned after 12 hours, by which time the glycine level was 143 mg/L. The authors described four similar cases that they attributed to glycine toxicity.

Glycine absorption can also lead to CNS toxicity as a consequence of its metabolism to ammonia. In fact, several cases of delayed awakening after transurethral resection have been attributed to this factor. Peak blood ammonia levels of 500 μM have been reported (normal value, 47 to 65 μM), with 150 μM usually said to be the value at which toxic CNS changes occur.[110] In a prospective evaluation of a 1.5% glycine solution as the irrigant, increased ammonia levels were found in 12 of 26 subjects.[111] However, an inverse correlation was present between blood glycine and ammonia levels, and increases in ammonia levels were not always associated with symptoms of CNS toxicity. At present, the issue of CNS toxicity of glycine and its metabolite, ammonia, during transurethral resection is unsettled.

Prevention and Treatment

Efforts of the surgical team should be directed toward minimizing the absorption of irrigation fluid and early detection of complications. The duration of surgery should be limited; a maximum of 1 hour has been recommended, when possible.[98] Dissection should not be carried into the venous sinuses lying deep in the prostatic capsule, and the hydrostatic pressure of the irrigating fluid should be as low as is compatible with adequate surgical visibility. Distilled water should not be used as an irrigating solution for transurethral prostatectomy. For longer procedures, or resections of prostate glands larger than 45 g, anticipate increased blood loss and fluid absorption. Frequent (eg, every 20 to 30 minutes) determination of serum sodium or osmolality is recommended in such cases.

Anesthetic Management

Early diagnosis is based on observation of the aforementioned signs. Anesthetic techniques that neither alter the patient's sensorium nor significantly interfere with his cardiovascular compensatory mechanisms should be used whenever possible. Spinal anesthesia best meets these requirements; lumbar and caudal epidural anesthesia are acceptable alternative techniques. A sensory block to a level of T10 is optimal.

If general anesthesia is administered, as sometimes it must be, the opportunity to monitor changes in sensorium is lost, and some degree of cardiovascular depression usually occurs. Diagnosis then depends upon demonstration of progressive signs of increasing intravascular volume. If signs of hyponatremia, volume overload, or both develop, surgery should be terminated as rapidly as possible, and corrective therapy should be instituted.

Hypernatremia

Pathophysiologic Features

Hypernatremia is an uncommon but potentially lethal disturbance, characterized by serum sodium concentrations greater than 150 to 155 mEq/L, increased osmolality of body fluids, and decreased intracellular volume.[15,16,112] This fluid and electrolyte disturbance is more common in infants and neonates[113–115]; in many cases, an associated FECV deficit exists. However, hypernatremia rarely causes hypovolemic shock because two thirds of the water that is lost comes from intracellular fluid, with only one third coming from extracellular fluid. Because intravascular volume accounts for only one third to one fourth of extracellular fluid volume, loss from the former compartment is small. Thus, the principal clinical symptoms are attributable to decreased intracellular volume, especially dehydration of CNS cells.[116]

Symptoms and Signs

Symptoms generally do not develop until the serum osmolality approaches 320 to 330 mOsm/kg, at which level serum sodium concentration is about 160 mEq/L.[49] Clinically, hypernatremia due to pure water loss is uncommon because thirst caused by increased plasma osmolality stimulates oral water intake. Typically, water loss causing a hypertonic state occurs only in those who cannot drink water by themselves (eg, infants, very sick adults, anesthetized patients).

Clinical manifestations in the nonanesthetized patient are predominantly neurologic and include restlessness, weakness, irritability, and, in more severe cases, delirium, stupor, fever, and occasional athetoid and choreiform movements. Cardiovascular signs are related to the degree of intravascular volume depletion. Mucous membranes are characteristically dry and sticky.

Causes

Hypernatremia arises whenever free-water loss exceeds water replacement (Tables 33-5 and 33-6). The disorder is most frequently seen in surgical patients who are receiving parenteral or enteric hyperalimentation with high-calorie, high-protein solutions or in infants whose fluid therapy has been mismanaged. The increased solute load results in obligatory urinary excretion of large volumes of water; this loss predisposes to hypernatremia unless sufficient sodium-free water is administered with the alimentation fluid. A similar mechanism is responsible for the hypernatremia seen in association with the osmotic diuresis produced by urea, mannitol, or even excess glucose administration. Hypernatremia can also occur as a result of the administration of hypertonic sodium bicarbonate solution during cardiopulmonary resuscitation.[116]

Excessive nonosmotic renal water loss is characteristic of the ADH-resistant polyuria seen in methoxyflurane nephrotoxicity.[43,44] Diabetes insipidus, high-output renal failure, and the diuretic phase after acute oliguric renal failure all are marked by the inability to conserve free water. Finally, increased insensible water loss, if not replaced, can result in hypernatremia. Increased evaporative water losses occur in patients with fever or abnormal sweating, in patients with extensive burns or large, open granulating wounds, and in patients with tracheotomies breathing unhumidified air. In these situations, evaporative water losses may amount to several liters per day.

TABLE 33-5
Hypernatremia: Pure Water Loss

DIAGNOSIS

Increased serum sodium ion concentration; urine osmolality at least two times plasma osmolality (except in diabetes insipidus); moderate azotemia; decreased urine volume

CAUSES

- Increased insensible loss from skin and lungs
- Increased environmental temperature
- Fever
- Thyrotoxicosis
- Burn injury
- Inadequately humidified ventilator
- Diabetes insipidus

MANAGEMENT

Calculate water deficit:

$$0.6 \times \text{body weight (in kilograms)} \times \frac{\text{Serum sodium ion concentration}}{140} - 1$$

Correct underlying cause if possible
Replace water deficit

COMPLICATIONS

Isotonic water intoxication

Layon AJ, Bernards WC, Kirby RR: Fluids and electrolytes in the critically ill. In Civetta JM, Taylor RW, Kirby RR (eds): Critical care, 2nd ed. Philadelphia: JB Lippincott, 1992: 460.

Prevention and Treatment

An awareness of clinical situations likely to result in abnormal renal and extrarenal water loss is the key to prevention of hypernatremia. Replacement of free-water losses, as indicated by fluid balance records, serial weight measurements, and frequent determination of serum electrolyte concentrations, effectively prevents this complication.

If hypernatremia does occur, treatment consists of correcting the free-water deficit with 5% glucose in water. Assuming total body sodium content is normal, the existing total body water can be calculated as follows:

$$\text{Existing TBW} = \frac{\text{normal sodium concentration}}{\text{existing sodium concentration}} \times \text{normal TBW}$$

The free-water deficit, the difference between existing and normal total body water, should be slowly replaced at rates calculated to reduce serum sodium concentration by no more than 2 mEq/L/h during the first 48 hours.[88] Hyperosmolar disturbances should not be corrected too rapidly. To do so can cause seizures, coma, and death as a result of brain swelling caused, in turn, by a rapid increase in total intracellular fluid.[117] Serum sodium should be determined after partial correction of the disturbance, and therapy should be reevaluated.

TABLE 33-6
Hypotonic Fluid Loss

DIAGNOSIS

Increased serum sodium ion concentration; symptoms of FECV depletion; oliguria (unless due to use of osmotic agents); urinary sodium ion concentration variable

CAUSES

- Gastroenteritis
- Osmotic diuresis
  - Urea from high-protein tube feeding
  - Glucose
  - Mannitol or glycerol
- Peritoneal dialysis

MANAGEMENT

Replace fluid loss with physiologic saline or colloid
Then use hypotonic solutions for slow correction of free-water deficit

COMPLICATIONS

Vascular collapse
Isotonic water intoxication and cerebral edema

Layon AJ, Bernards WC, Kirby RR: Fluids and electrolytes in the critically ill. In Civetta JM, Taylor RW, Kirby RR (eds): Critical care, 2nd ed. Philadelphia: JB Lippincott, 1992: 461.

DISTURBANCES OF POTASSIUM COMPOSITION

Hypokalemia

Symptoms and Signs

Hypokalemia, defined as a serum potassium concentration less than 3.5 mEq per L, is common in surgical patients (Table 33-7). Symptoms are related to physiologic dysfunction in muscle that results from alterations in transmembrane potassium gradients that usually occur when the serum potassium

TABLE 33-7
Hypokalemia

DEFINITION

Serum potassium ion concentration ≤3.5 mEq/L

DIAGNOSIS

Serum potassium ion concentration, spot urinary potassium ion concentration; history; medication list; urinary chloride concentration; arterial pH; carbon dioxide partial pressure; bicarbonate ion concentration

CAUSES

Factitious: White blood cell count (>100,000 at room temperature)
Intracellular shift
  Alkalemia
  Insulin therapy
  β-Adrenergic stimulation
  Anabolism
Gastrointestinal loss
  Diarrhea
  Vomiting
  Enteric or biliary fistula
Renal loss
  Increased urinary flow
  Hypomagnesemia
  Increased mineralocorticoid activity
Drugs

MANAGEMENT

Correct potassium ion abnormality
  Emergency: infusion (peripheral vein) ≤40 mEq/h in a concentration of 40 to 60 mEq/L
  Nonemergency
    Oral: wax matrix potassium chloride 40 to 120 mEq/day
    Intravenous: 10 mEq/h in a concentration of 40 mEq/L
Correct magnesium ion abnormality if present
Determine cause

COMPLICATIONS

Hyperkalemia with rapid or excessive correction because of hypokalemia

Layon AJ, Bernards WC, Kirby RR: Fluids and electrolytes in the critically ill. In Civetta JM, Taylor RW, Kirby RR (eds): Critical care, 2nd ed. Philadelphia: JB Lippincott, 1992:461.

level is less than 2.5 mEq/L. Generalized muscular weakness and muscle cramps are the predominant symptoms of hypokalemia; paralytic ileus frequently occurs. The possibility of a prolonged response to nondepolarizing neuromuscular blocking drugs must be anticipated.[118–120]

Of most concern to anesthesiologists are the cardiac effects of hypokalemia. Myocardial contractility may be depressed. Alterations in resting membrane potential and spontaneous rates of depolarization may result in life-threatening ventricular dysrhythmias. However, the relation between hypokalemia and cardiac dysrhythmias has become controversial.[121–123] Vitez and colleagues suggested that a chronically low potassium concentration (eg, 2.6 to 3.4 mEq/L) is well tolerated by the anesthetized patient, provided that dysrhythmias are not present preoperatively.[123] Additionally, digitalis toxicity is markedly enhanced by hypokalemia.[124] Electrocardiographic (ECG) abnormalities include flattened T waves, sagging ST segments, and the appearance of U waves (Fig. 33-3). Diagnosis is made by measurement of serum potassium but may be suggested by clinical signs and ECG findings.[15,125,126]

Causes

Low serum potassium levels can result either from total body depletion or from factors that promote potassium influx into cells, such as alkalosis[127] or the simultaneous administration of glucose and insulin. Abnormally high gastrointestinal losses of potassium (>40 mEq/day) may result from vomiting, diarrhea, nasogastric drainage, or draining enteric fistulae. Excessive renal potassium losses also are seen after diuretic therapy with furosemide, ethacrynic acid, or the thiazides[128];

TABLE 33-8
Hyperkalemia

DIAGNOSIS

Serum potassium ion concentration

CAUSES

Factitious
  Thrombocytosis
  Leukocytosis
  Hemolysis
  Infectious mononucleosis
Increased intake
  Banked blood (>5 days old)
  Rapid intravenous infusion of potassium ion
Abnormal distribution
  Acidemia (some forms)
  Catabolism
  Extracellular hypertonicity
  Insulin deficiency
  β-Blocking agents
Decreased renal potassium ion secretion
  Acute renal failure
  Decreased mineralocorticoid activity
  Decreased urinary sodium ion
Drugs

MANAGEMENT

Emergency
  10 to 30 mL 10% calcium gluconate
  Saline solution or sodium bicarbonate (50 to 100 mL 7.5% solution)
  Glucose insulin (500 mL 10% dextrose plus 10 U regular insulin, intravenous infusion over 1-hour period)
  Loop diuretic agents
  Sodium or calcium polystyrene sulfonate plus sorbitol, orally (25 g/dose) or by retention enema (50 g/dose)
  Dialysis
  Transvenous pacemaker
Nonemergency
  Potassium ion restriction (40 to 60 mEq/day)
  Correct acidosis or hypovolemia if present
  Treat underlying disease

COMPLICATIONS

Hypokalemia
Dysrhythmias, ventricular fibrillation, asystole

Layon AJ, Bernards WC, Kirby RR: Fluids and electrolytes in the critically ill. In Civetta JM, Taylor RW, Kirby RR (eds): Critical care, 2nd ed. Philadelphia: JB Lippincott, 1992: 462.

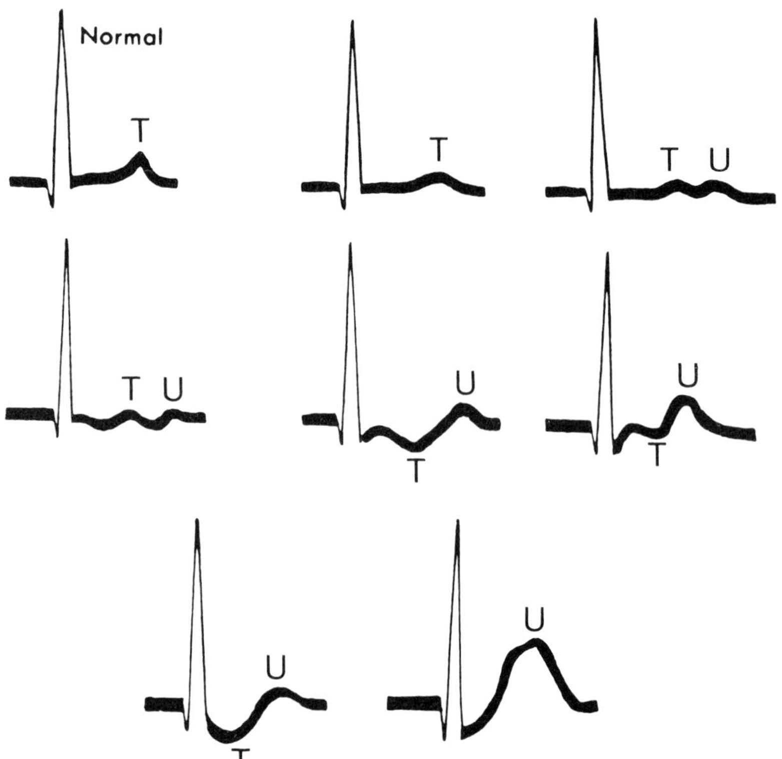

FIGURE 33-3. ECG patterns in hypokalemia. The ECG patterns do not correlate reliably with the severity of hypokalemia. (Goldberger AL, Goldberger E (eds): Clinical electrocardiography, 3rd ed. St. Louis: CV Mosby, 1986: 145.)

during the diuretic phase of acute tubular necrosis; in patients with renal tubular acidosis, hypokalemic periodic paralysis,[129] and hyperaldosteronism; and after glucocorticoid treatment. Severe serum potassium deficits are frequently seen after cardiopulmonary bypass[130]; and after transfusion of large volumes of frozen, thawed, glycerol-preserved, washed, and resuspended red blood cells.[131]

Prevention and Treatment

The risk of potentially fatal dysrhythmias in patients with significant hypokalemia has long made it desirable to postpone elective surgery until deficits can be corrected by oral or intravenous administration of potassium chloride. However, Wong and colleagues have provided an elegant review of the relevant literature in which they conclude that hypokalemia is not an independent risk factor for the development of ventricular dysrhythmias.[132] Furthermore, dangerous complications of oral or intravenous potassium therapy occur in more than 1 of 200 patients so treated.[133] Intravenous replacement of potassium deficits in asymptomatic patients ordinarily should not exceed a rate of 10 mEq/h. Dangerously low serum potassium levels should be treated aggressively, especially when accompanied by cardiac dysrhythmias. In these cases, potassium chloride may be administered at a rate as great as 40 mEq/h, with continuous ECG monitoring. Adequate renal function must be ensured before potassium infusion.

Hyperkalemia

Symptoms and Signs

Hyperkalemia, defined as a serum potassium concentration greater than 5.5 mEq per L, is a much less common problem in surgical patients than hypokalemia (Table 33-8). However, when a significant increased in serum potassium occurs, it may be rapidly fatal; therefore it constitutes a major emergency. Severe disturbances in cardiac rhythm, including heart block, idioventricular rhythm, ventricular fibrillation, and cardiac arrest in asystole, may develop when serum potassium exceeds 7.0 mEq/L (Fig. 33-4).[125]

ECG changes associated with hyperkalemia include tall, peaked T waves, widened QRS complexes, atrioventricular block, and loss of P waves. The definitive diagnosis depends upon laboratory determination of serum potassium concentration. However, a presumptive diagnosis can be made and therapy can be begun on the basis of characteristic ECG changes in a clinical situation in which hyperkalemia is suspected.

Causes

Serum potassium may become increased because of decreased renal potassium excretion, excessively rapid intravenous administration, or abnormal release of intracellular stores.[3,135] Singly or in combination, these factors may result in a fatal increase in serum potassium concentration. Excretion of potassium is decreased in renal failure, hypoaldosteronism, and after administration of aldosterone-inhibiting diuretics, such as spironolactone and triamterene.

High serum potassium levels may follow rapid intravenous administration of potassium supplements or of old, stored blood. Serum potassium concentration increases in stored blood at a rate of about 1 mEq/day, so that 21-day-old blood may have a potassium concentration of 25 to 30 mEq/L.[136] Major trauma, hypoxia, or severe tissue acidosis may result in the release of large amounts of potassium from damaged cells.

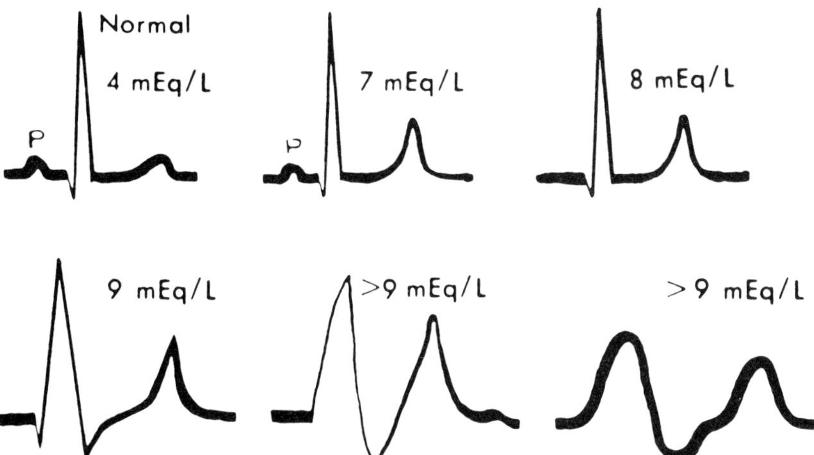

FIGURE 33-4. ECG patterns in hyperkalemia. (Goldberger AL, Goldberger E (eds): Clinical electrocardiography, 3rd ed. St. Louis: CV Mosby, 1986: 142.)

Of unique concern to the anesthesiologist is the marked, sometimes fatal increase in serum potassium that follows the administration of succinylcholine to patients who have sustained major trauma, burns, or spinal cord injuries, or hyperkalemia after succinylcholine administration and who have progressive neuromuscular diseases.[137–142] It is, in part, the concern for children with previously undiagnosed neuromuscular disease that recently has led the Food and Drug Administration and the manufacturers of succinylcholine to revise the indications for succinylcholine use to the difficult or at-risk airway.[143] Subsequently, as a result of intense debate, the revision was downgraded to a warning.[144]

Prevention and Treatment

Patients with hyperkalemia resulting from decreased renal excretion should be dialyzed before elective surgery to reduce serum potassium concentration to normal levels. When massive amounts of blood are transfused, careful attention should be paid to ECG monitoring to detect early signs. Finally, administration of succinylcholine should be avoided for a period beginning several days after, and lasting for 6 months after major trauma, burns, or spinal cord injury to decrease the likelihood of hyperkalemia in these patients.

Emergency treatment of hyperkalemia involves several steps (see Table 33-8)[145,146]: immediate antagonism of the adverse cardiac effects of potassium by intravenous administration of 10% calcium chloride, in 1-mL increments, or 10% calcium gluconate in 1- to 3-mL increments, until the characteristic ECG changes of hyperkalemia have reverted to normal; promotion of the intracellular shift of circulating potassium by intravenous administration of glucose, 50 g, regular insulin, 20 U, and sodium bicarbonate, 100 mEq; and removal of potassium from the body by the rectal administration of a cation exchange resin, such as sodium polystyrene sulfonate (Kayexalate), 25 g, in 200 mL of 10% dextrose; administration of loop diuretics; and, rarely, transvenous pacing. If serum potassium cannot be lowered and controlled effectively by these methods, emergency dialysis is indicated.

REFERENCES

1. Pitts RF: Physiology of the kidney and body fluids, 3rd ed. Chicago: Year Book Medical, 1974
2. Bradbury MWB: Physiology of body fluids and electrolytes. Br J Anaesth 45:937, 1973
3. Hays RM: Dynamics of body water and electrolytes. In Maxwell MH, Kleeman CR (eds): Clinical disorders of fluid and electrolyte metabolism, 3rd ed. New York: McGraw-Hill, 1980: 1
4. Edelman IS, Leibman J: Anatomy of body water and electrolytes. Am J Med 27:256, 1959
5. Atherton JC: Renal physiology. Br J Anaesth 44:236, 1972
6. Bricker NS, Schultze RG, Licht A: Renal function: general concepts. In Maxwell MH, Kleeman CR (eds): Clinical disorders of fluid and electrolyte metabolism, 3rd ed. New York: McGraw-Hill, 1980: 233
7. Barger AC: Renal hemodynamic factors in congestive heart failure. Ann N Y Acad Sci 139:276, 1966
8. Hollenberg NK, Epstein M, Rosen SM, et al: Acute oliguric renal failure in man: evidence for preferential renal cortical ischemia. Medicine (Baltimore) 47:455, 1968
9. Hollenberg NK, Adams DF, Soloman HS, et al: What mediates the renal vascular response to a salt load in normal man? J Appl Physiol 33:491, 1972
10. Siegel DC, Cochin A, Geocaris T, et al: Effects of saline and colloid resuscitation on renal function. Ann Surg 177:51, 1973
11. Atarashi K, Mulrow PJ, Franco-Saenz R, et al: Inhibition of aldosterone production by an atrial extract. Science 224:992, 1984
12. Weitzman R, Kleeman CR: Water metabolism. In Maxwell MH, Kleeman CR (eds): Clinical disorders of fluid and electrolyte metabolism, 3rd ed. New York: McGraw-Hill, 1980: 531
13. Schrier RW, Berl T: Nonosmolar factors affecting renal water excretion. N Engl M Med 292:81, 1975
14. Goldsmith HJ: The chemical pathology of renal failure. Br J Anaesth 44:259, 1972
15. Dougan LR, Finlay WEI: Fluid and electrolyte balance: assessment of the patient. Br J Anaesth 45:945, 1973
16. Shires GT, Canizaro PC, Lowry SF: Fluid, electrolyte, and nutritional management of the surgical patient. In Schwartz ST, Shires GT, Spencer FC, et al (eds): Principles of surgery, 4th ed. New York: McGraw-Hill, 1984: 45
17. Petrie JJB: The clinical features, complications and treatment of chronic renal failure. Br J Anaesth 44:266, 1972
18. Cove-Smith JR, Knapp MS: Sodium handling in analgesic nephropathy. Lancet 2:70, 1973
19. Cousins MJ, Mazze RI: Anaesthesia, surgery, and renal function: immediate and delayed effects. Anaesth Intensive Care 1:355, 1973
20. Larson CP, Mazze RI, Cooperman LH, et al: Effects of anesthetics on cerebral, renal and splanchnic circulations: recent developments. Anesthesiology 41:169, 1974
21. Mazze RI, Barry KG: Prevention of functional renal failure during anesthesia and surgery by sustained hydration and mannitol infusion. Anesth Analg 46:61, 1967
22. Abel RM, Buckley MJ, Austen WG, et al: Etiology, incidence

and prognosis of renal failure following cardiac operations. J Thorac Cardiovasc Surg 71:323, 1976

23. Boba A, Landmesser CM: Renal complications after anesthesia and operation. Anesthesiology 22:781, 1961
24. Mazze RI, Schwartz FD, Slocum HC, et al: Renal function during anesthesia and surgery: I. the effects of halothane anesthesia. Anesthesiology 24:279, 1963
25. Price HL, Linde HW, Jones RE, et al: Sympathoadrenal responses to general anesthesia in man and their relation to hemodynamics. Anesthesiology 20:563, 1959
26. Deutsch S, Pierce EC, Vandam LD: Cyclopropane effects on renal function in normal man. Anesthesiology 28:547, 1967
27. Deutsch S, Bastron RD, Peirce EC Jr: The effects of anaesthesia with thiopentone, nitrous oxide, narcotics, and neuromuscular blocking agents on renal function in normal man. Br J Anaesth 41:807, 1969
28. Cousins MJ, Greenstein LR, Hitt BA, et al: Metabolism and renal effects of enflurane in man. Anesthesiology 44:44, 1976
29. Deutsch S, Goldberg M, Stephen GW, et al: Effects of halothane anesthesia on renal function in normal man. Anesthesiology 27:793, 1966
30. Mazze RI, Cousins MJ, Bar GA: Renal effects and metabolism of isoflurane in man. Anesthesiology 40:536, 1974
31. Gorman HM, Craythorne NWB: The effects of a new neuroleptanalgesic agent (Innovar) on renal function in man. Acta Anaesthesiol Scand Suppl 24:111, 1966
32. Smith HW: Physiology of the renal circulation. Harvey Lect 35:166, 1939
33. Berne RM: hemodynamics and sodium excretion of denervated kidney in anesthetized and unanesthetized dog. Am J Physiol 171:148, 1952
34. Leighton KM, Koth B, Wenkstern BM: Autoregulation of renal blood flow: alteration by methoxyflurane. Can Anaesth Soc J 20:173, 1973
35. Leighton KM, Bruce C: Distribution of kidney blood flow: a comparison of methoxyflurane and halothane effects as measured by heated thermocouple. Can Anaesth Soc J 22:125, 1975
36. Bastron RD, Perkins FM, Pyne JL: Autoregulation of renal blood flow during halothane anesthesia. Anesthesiology 46:142, 1977
37. Pettinger WA: Anesthetics and the renin-angiotensin-aldosterone axis. Anesthesiology 48:393, 1973
38. Miller ED Jr, Bailey D, Kaplan J, et al: the effect of ketamine on the renin–angiotensin system. Anesthesiology 42:503, 1975
39. Miller ED Jr, Longnecker DE, Peach MJ: The regulatory function of the renin–angiotensin system during general anesthesia. Anesthesiology 48:399, 1978
40. Bastron RD, Perkins FM, Kaloyanides GJ: In vitro inhibition of PAH transport by halogenated anesthetics. J Pharmacol Exp Ther 200:75, 1977
41. Andersen NB: Effect of general anesthetics on sodium transport in the isolated toad bladder. Anesthesiology 27:304, 1966
42. Crandell WB, Pappas SG, Macdonald A: Nephrotoxicity associated with methoxyflurane anesthesia. Anesthesiology 27:591, 1966
43. Mazze RI, Shue GL, Jackson SH: Renal dysfunction associated with methoxyflurane anesthesia: a randomized prospective clinical evaluation. JAMA 216:278, 1971
44. Mazze RI, Trudell JR, Cousins MJ: Methoxyflurane metabolism and renal dysfunction: clinical correlation in man. Anesthesiology 35:247, 1971
45. Kharasch ED, Hanki· s DC, Thummel KE: Human kidney methoxyflurane and s· voflurane metabolism: intrarenal fluoride production as a possible mechanism of methoxyflurane nephrotoxicity. Anesthesiology 82:689, 1995
46. Shires T, Williams J, Brown F: Acute change in extracellular fluids associated with major surgical procedures. Ann Surg 154: 803, 1961
47. Hoye RC, Bennett SH, Geelhoed GW, et al: Fluid volume and albumin kinetics occurring with major surgery. JAMA 222: 1255, 1972
48. Blahd WH: Radioisotope techniques. In Maxwell MH, Kleeman CR (eds): Clinical disorders of fluid and electrolyte metabolism, 3rd ed. New York: McGraw-Hill, 1980: 399
49. Jacobson HR: Fluid and electrolyte problems in surgery, trauma and burns. In Kokko JP, Tannen RL (eds): Fluids and electrolytes. Philadelphia: WB Saunders, 1986: 791
50. Weil MH, Shubin H, Rosoff L: Fluid replacement in circulatory shock. JAMA 192:668, 1965
51. Forrester JS, Diamond G, McHugh TJ, et al: Filling pressures in the right and left sides of the heart in acute myocardial infarction. N Engl J Med 285:190, 1971
52. Swan HJC, Ganz W, Forrester J, et al: Catheterization of the heart in man with the use of a flow-directed balloon-tipped catheter. N Engl J Med 283:447, 1970
53. Lappas D, Lell WA, Gabel JC, et al: Indirect measurement of the left-atrial pressure in surgical patients: pulmonary-capillary wedge and pulmonary artery diastolic pressures compared with left atrial pressure. Anesthesiology 38:394, 1973
54. Poole GV, Meredith JW, Pennell T, et al: Comparison of colloids and crystalloids in resuscitation from hemorrhagic shock. Surg Gynecol Obstet 154:577–586, 1982
55. Rackow EC, Falk JL, Fein IA, et al: Fluid resuscitation in circulatory shock: a comparison of the cardiopulmonary effects of albumin, hetastarch, and saline solutions in patients with hypovolemic and septic shock. Crit Care Med 11:839–850, 1983
56. Shoemaker WC: Comparison of the relative effectiveness of whole blood transfusion and various types of fluid therapy in resuscitation. Crit Care Med 4:71, 1976
57. Shoemaker WC, Schluchter M, Hopkins JA, et al: Fluid therapy in emergency resuscitation: clinical evaluation of colloid and crystalloid regimens. Crit Care Med 9:367–368, 1981
58. Tranbaugh RF, Lewis FR: Crystalloid vs colloid in the initial fluid resuscitation of the acutely injured patient. In Askanazi J, Starker PM, Weisman C (eds): Fluid and electrolyte management in critical care. Stoneham, MA: Butterworth, 1986: 189
59. Rush BF, Stewart RA: More liberal use of a plasma expander: impact on a hospital blood bank. N Engl M Med 280:1202, 1969
60. Gollub S, Svigals R, Bailey CP, et al: Electrolyte solution in surgical patients refusing transfusion. JAMA 215:2077, 1971
61. Messmer K: Acute preoperative hemodilution: physiological basis and clinical applications. In: Tuma RF, White JV, Messmer K (eds): The role of hemodilution in optimal patient care. Munich: W Zuckschwerdt Verlag 1989:54
62. Goodnough LT, Grishaber JE, Monk TG, et al: Acute preoperative hemodilution in patients undergoing radical prostatectomy: a case study analysis of efficacy. Anesth Analg 78:932, 1994
63. Feldman JM, Roth JV, Bjoraker DG: Maximum blood savings by acute normovolemic hemodilution. Anesth Analg 80:108, 1995
64. Lasala PA, Chien S, Michelsen CB: Hemorrheology: what is the ideal hematocrit? In Askanazi J, Starker PM, Weisman C (eds): Fluid and electrolyte management in critical care. Stoneham, MA: Butterworth, 1986: 203
65. Moss GS, Siegel DC, Cockin A, et al: Effects of saline and colloid solutions on pulmonary function in hemorrhagic shock. Surg Gynecol Obstet 133:53, 1971
66. Ledingham IMA, Ramsay G: Hypovolaemic shock. Br J Anesth 58:169, 1986
67. McGough EK: Resuscitation in shock, trauma, and burns: hypertonic saline solutions. In Kirby RR (ed): Innovative fluid and electrolyte, nutritional, and transfusion therapy. Problems in Critical Care 346, 1991
68. Maningas PA, Mattox KL, Pepe PE, et al: Hypertonic saline–dextran solutions for the prehospital management of traumatic hypotension. Surgery 157:528, 1989
69. Cross JS, Gruber DP, Burchard KW, et al: Hypertonic saline fluid therapy following surgery: a prospective study. J Trauma 29:817, 1989
70. Hands R, Holcroft JW, Perron PR, et al: Comparison of peripheral and central infusions of 7.5% NaCl/6% dextran 70. Surgery 103:684, 1988
71. Auler AJOC, Pereira MHC, Gomida-Amaral RV, et al: Hemodynamic effects of hypertonic sodium chloride during treatment of aortic aneurysms. Surgery 101:594, 1987

72. Gunnar W, Jonasson O, Merlotti G, et al: Head injury and hemorrhagic shock: studies of the blood brain barrier and intracranial pressure after resuscitation with normal saline solution, 3% saline solution, and dextran 40. Surgery 103:398, 1988
73. Noble WH: Pulmonary edema: a review. Can Anesth Soc J 27: 286, 1980
74. Cooperman LH, Price HL: Pulmonary edema in the operative and postoperative period: a review of 40 cases. Ann Surg 172: 883, 1970
75. Stein L, Beraud JJ, Morissette M, et al: Pulmonary edema during volume infusion. Circulation 52:483, 1975
76. Miles WM, Zipes DP: Circulatory failure. In Andreoli RE, Bennett JC, Carpenter CCJ, Plum F, Smith LH Jr (eds): Cecil essentials of medicine. Philadelphia: WB Saunders, 1993: 34
77. Arieff AI, Schmidt RW: Fluid and electrolyte disorders and the central nervous system. In Maxwell MH, Kleeman CR (eds): Clinical disorders of fluid and electrolyte metabolism, 3rd ed. New York: McGraw-Hill, 1980: 1409
78. Anderson RJ, Chung HM, Kluge R, et al: Hyponatremia: a prospective analysis of its epidemiology and the pathogenetic role of vasopressin. Ann Intern Med 102:164, 1985
79. Kennedy PGE, Mitchell DM, Hoffbrand BI: Severe hyponatraemia in hospital inpatients. Br Med J 2:1251, 1978
80. Fichman MP, Vorherr H, Kleemna CR, et al: Diuretic-induced hyponatremia. Ann Int Med 75:858, 1971
81. Ashraf N, Locksley R, Arieff AI: Thiazide-induced hyponatremia associated with death or neurologic damage in outpatients. Am J Med 70:1163, 1981
82. Abramow M, Cogan E: Clinical aspects and pathophysiology of diuretic-induced hyponatremia. Adv Nephrol Necker Hosp 13:1, 1984
83. Miller M, Moses AM: Drug-induced states of impaired water excretion. Kidney Int 10:96, 1976
84. Bernards WC, Kirby RR: A brief history of fluid and electrolyte therapy: how we got where we are today. In Kirby RR (ed): Innovative fluid and electrolyte, nutritional, and transfusion therapy. Problems in Critical Care 331, 1991
85. Shires T, Jackson DE: Postoperative salt tolerance. Arch Surg 84:703, 1962
86. Crandell WB: Parenteral fluid therapy. Surg Clin North Am 48:707, 1968
87. Ayers JC, Krothapalli RK, Arieff AI: Treatment of symptomatic hyponatremia and its relation to brain damage: a prospective study. N Engl J Med 317:1190, 1987
88. Humes HD: Disorders of water metabolism. In Kakko JP, Tannen RL (eds): Fluids and electrolytes. Philadelphia: WB Saunders, 1986: 118
89. Bartter FC, Schwartz WB: The syndrome of inappropriate secretion of antidiuretic hormone. Am J Med 42:790, 1967
90. Deutsch S, Goldberg M, Dripps RD: Postoperative hyponatremia with the inappropriate release of antidiuretic hormone. Anesthesiology 27:250, 1966
91. Burrows FA, Shutack JG, Crone RK: Inappropriate secretion of antidiuretic hormone in a postsurgical pediatric population. Crit Care Med 11:527, 1983
92. Decaux G, Unger J, Brimioulle S, et al: Hyponatremia in the syndrome of inappropriate secretion of antidiuretic hormone: rapid correction with urea, sodium chloride, and water restriction therapy. JAMA 247:471, 1982
93. Weinberg MS, Donohoe JF: Hyponatremia in the syndrome of inappropriate secretion of antidiuretic hormone: rapid correction with osmotic agents. South Med J 78:348, 1985
94. White MG, Fenter CD: Treatment of the syndrome of inappropriate secretion of antidiuretic hormone with lithium carbonate. N Engl J Med 292:390, 1975
95. Forrest JN, Cox M, Hong C, et al: Superiority of demeclocycline over lithium in the treatment of chronic syndrome of inappropriate secretion of antidiuretic hormone. N Engl J Med 298:173, 1978
96. De Troyer A: Demeclocycline: treatment for the syndrome of inappropriate antidiuretic hormone secretion. JAMA 237:2723, 1977
97. Cherrill DA, Stote RM, Birge JR, et al: Demeclocycline treatment in the syndrome of inappropriate antidiuretic secretion. Ann Intern Med 83:654, 1975
98. Marx GF, Orkin LR: Complications associated with transurethral surgery. Anesthesiology 23:802, 1962
99. Desmond J: Serum osmolality and plasma electrolytes in patients who develop dilutional hyponatremia during transurethral resection. Can J Surg 13:116, 1970
100. Taylor RO, Maxson ES, Carter FH, et al: Volumetric, gravimetric and radioisotopic determination of fluid transfer in transurethral prostatectomy. J Urol 79:490, 1958
101. Still JA, Modell JH: Acute water intoxication during transurethral resection of the prostate, using glycine solution for irrigation. Anesthesiology 38:98, 1973
102. Pennisi SA, Rowland HS, Vinson CE, et al: Hyponatremia as affected by various irrigations used during transurethral electroresection of the prostate. J Urol 86:249, 1961
103. Sunderrajan S, Bauer JH, Vopat RL, et al: Posttransurethral prostatic resection hyponatremic syndrome: case report and review of the literature. Am J Kidney Dis 9:80, 1984
104. Berger JJ: Transurethral resection of the prostate. In Kirby RR (ed): Innovative fluid and electrolyte, nutritional, and transfusion therapy. Problems in Critical Care 376, 1991
105. Maluf NSR, Boren JS, Brandes GE: Absorption of irrigating solution and associated changes upon transurethral electroresection of prostate. J Urol 75:824, 1956
106. Aasheim GM: Hyponatremia during transurethral surgery. Can Anaesth Soc J 230:274, 1973
107. Ovassapian A, Joshi CW, Brunner EA: Visual disturbances: an unusual symptom of transurethral prostatic resection reaction. Anesthesiology 57:332, 1982
108. Aprison MH, Werman R: The distribution of glycine in cat spinal cord and roots. Life Sci 4:2075, 1965
109. Snyder SH, Enna SJ: The role of central glycine receptors in the pharmacologic actions of benzodiazepines. Adv Biochem Psychopharmacol 14:81, 1975
110. Roesch RP, Stoelting RK, Lingeman JE, et al: Ammonia toxicity resulting from glycine absorption during a transurethral resection of the prostate. Anesthesiology 58:577, 1983
111. Hoekstra PT, Kahnoski R, McCamish MA, et al: Transurethral prostatic resection syndrome: a new perspective—encephalopathy with associated hyperammonemia. J Urol 130:704, 1983
112. Orloff MJ, Hutchin P: Fluid and electrolyte response to trauma and surgery. In Maxwell MH, Kleeman CR (eds): Clinical disorders of fluid and electrolyte metabolism, 2nd ed. New York: McGraw-Hill, 1972: 1063
113. Morris-Jones PH, Houston IB, Evans RC: Prognosis of the neurological complications of acute hypernatremia. Lancet 2:1385, 1967
114. Macaulay D, Watson M: Hypernatremia in infants as a cause of brain damage. Arch Dis Child 42:485, 1967
115. Simmons MA, Adcock EW III, Bard H, et al: Hypernatremia and intracranial hemorrhage in neonates. N Engl J Med 291: 6, 1974
116. Feig PU, McCurdy DK: The hypertonic state. N Engl J Med 297:1444, 1977
117. Arieff AI, Guisado R: Effects on the central nervous system of hypernatremic and hyponatremic states. Kidney Int 10:104, 1976
118. Waud BE, Mookerjee A, Waud DR: Chronic potassium depletion and sensitivity to tubocurarine. Anesthesiology 57:111, 1982
119. Miller RD, Roderick LL: Diuretic-induced hypokalemia: pancuronium neuromuscular blockade and its antagonism by neostigmine. Br J Anaesth 50:541, 1978
120. Hill GE, Wong KC, Shaw CL, et al: Acute and chronic changes in intra- and extracellular potassium and responses to neuromuscular blocking agents. Anesth Analg 57:417, 1978
121. McGovern B: Hypokalemia and cardiac arrhythmias. Anesthesiology 63:127, 1985
122. Glaser R: Chronic hypokalemia and intraoperative dysrhythmias. Anesthesiology 64:408, 1986
123. Vitez TS, Soper LE, Wong KC, et al: Chronic hypokalemia

and intraoperative dysrhythmias. Anesthesiology 63:130, 1985
124. Brater DC, Morrelli HF: Digoxin toxicity in patients with normokalemic potassium depletion. Clin Pharmacol Ther 22:21, 1977
125. Vaughan RS, Lunn JN: Potassium and the anaesthetist. Anaesthesia 28:118, 1973
126. Johansson BW, Larsson C: A hypokalemic index ECG as a predictor of hypokalemia. Acta Medica Scandinavica 212:29, 1982
127. Edwards R, Winnie AP, Ramamurthy S: Acute hypocapnic hypokalemia: an iatrogenic anesthetic complication. Anesth Analg 56:786, 1977
128. Harrington JT, Isner JM, Kassirer JP: Our national obsession with potassium. Am J Med 73:155, 1982
129. Melnick B, Chang JL, Larson CE, et al: Hypokalemic familial periodic paralysis. Anesthesiology 58:263, 1983
130. Marcial MB, Vedoya RC, Zerbini EJ, et al: Potassium in cardiac surgery with extracorporeal perfusion. Am J Cardiol 23:400, 1969
131. Rao TLK, Mathru M, Salem MR, et al: Serum potassium levels following transfusion of frozen erythrocytes. Anesthesiology 52:170, 1980
132. Wong KC, Schafer PG, Schultz JR: Hypokalemia and anesthetic implications. Anesth Analg 77:1238, 1993.
133. Lawson BH: Adverse reactions to potassium chloride. Q J Med 43:433, 1974
134. Schultze RG, Nissenson AR: Potassium: Physiology and pathophysiology. In Maxwell MH, Kleeman CR (eds): Clinical disorders of fluid and electrolyte metabolism, 3rd ed. New York: McGraw-Hill, 1980: 113
135. Tanaka K, Pettinger WA: Pharmacokinetics of bolus potassium injections for cardiac arrhythmias. Anesthesiology 38:587, 1973
136. Marshall M: Potassium intoxication from blood and plasma transfusions. Anaesthesia 17:145, 1962
137. Mazze RI, Escue HM, Houston JB: Hyperkalemia and cardiovascular collapse following administration of succinylcholine to the traumatized patient. Anesthesiology 31:540, 1969
138. Gronert GA, Theye RA: Pathophysiology of hyperkalemia induced by succinylcholine. Anesthesiology 43:89, 1975
139. Cooperman LH: Succinylcholine-induced hyperkalemia in neuromuscular disease. JAMA 213:1867, 1970
140. Stone Wa, Beach TP, Hamelberg W: Succinylcholine: danger in the spinal-cord–injured patient. Anesthesiology 32:168, 1970
141. Gronert GA: A possible mechanism of succinylcholine-induced hyperkalemia. Anesthesiology 53:356, 1980
142. Magee DA, Gallagher EG: 'Self-taming' of suxamethonium and serum potassium concentration. Br J Anaesth 56:977, 1984
143. Anectine (succinylcholine chloride) injection, USP and Anectine (succinylcholine chloride) Sterile Powder Flo-Pack (package insert). Research Triangle Park, NC: Burroughs Wellcome, June 1993
144. Morrell RC: FDA group urges sux label wording reduced to "warning." Anesthesia Patient Safety Foundation Newsletter 9(3):25, 1994
145. Tannen RL: Potassium disorders. In Kakko JP, Tannen RL (eds): Fluids and electrolytes. Philadelphia: WB Saunders, 1986: 150
146. Kunis CL, Lowenstein J: The emergency treatment of hyperkalemia. Med Clin North Am 65:165, 1981

FURTHER READING

Layon AJ, Bernards WC, Kirby RR: Fluids and electrolytes in the critically ill. In Civetta JM, Taylor RW, Kirby RR (eds): Critical care, 2nd ed. Philadelphia: JB Lippincott, 1992: 457

Leaf A, Cotran R: Renal pathophysiology, 3rd ed. New York: Oxford University Press, 1980

Mazze RI: Renal physiology and the effects of anesthesia. In Miller RD (ed): Anesthesia, 2nd ed. New York: Churchill Livingstone, 1986: 1223

Schultze RG, Nissenson AR: Potassium: physiology and pathophysiology. In Maxwell MH, Kleeman CR (eds): Clinical disorders of fluid and electrolyte metabolism, 3rd ed. New York: McGraw-Hill, 1980: 113

Complications in Anesthesiology, second edition,
edited by Nikolaus Gravenstein and Robert R. Kirby.
Lippincott-Raven Publishers, Philadelphia © 1996.

CHAPTER 34

Oliguria

James R. Dooley
*Richard I. Mazze**

One of the more ominous signs in clinical practice is the marked reduction or cessation of urinary output in a patient during or after an operation. The decrease can occur suddenly or over a period of several hours or days. It may be the harbinger of the syndrome of acute oliguric renal failure, a disorder that, when well established, is still associated with a mortality rate in excess of 50%.[1] Oliguria in most patients undergoing surgery is readily reversed if promptly treated. Anesthesiologists therefore must be aware that oliguria may occur in many clinical settings, and they must be able to diagnose it correctly and to treat its underlying causes.

CHARACTERISTICS AND DEFINITIONS

Oliguria usually is defined as a urine output of less than 20 mL per hour or less than 400 mL per day in a 70-kg adult. *Renal insufficiency* describes a measurable reduction in renal function with normal serum biochemical values. *Renal failure* is an advanced stage of renal insufficiency in which renal function deteriorates to the extent that homeostatic mechanisms are impaired and serum biochemical parameters are disturbed.

The definition of oliguria implies a state of renal failure, because a urine output of 400 mL per day is usually less than that required to excrete the average daily solute load of 650 to 750 mOsm in maximally concentrated urine (1.2 mOsm/mL). However, renal failure may be present despite a high urine output if water, electrolyte, and acid–base balances are not maintained and if metabolic waste products accumulate.

Thus, the criteria for appropriateness of urine output must include the quality as well as the quantity of urine that is formed. States of renal dysfunction described in terms of the amount of urine voided in a given period (ie, oliguric renal failure, nonoliguric renal failure, and polyuric renal failure) should not be viewed as separate diseases but as part of the continuum of renal failure.

CONCENTRATION AND DILUTION OF URINE

Before a discussion of the clinical presentation and significance of low urine output is presented, a review of the mechanisms for concentration and dilution of urine is appropriate. Two energy-conserving principles are involved in the concentration of urine: countercurrent multiplication and countercurrent exchange.

Countercurrent Multiplication

Countercurrent multiplication was first suggested by Kuhn and Ryffel[2] and is illustrated in Figure 34-1.[3] The principle of countercurrent multiplication of concentration is based on the assumption that at any level along the loop of Henle, a gradient of 200 mOsm/kg can be established between the ascending and descending limbs by active ion transport.

Longitudinal Gradients

In step 1, the loop is filled with fluid containing 300 mOsm/kg of sodium chloride. A gradient of 200 mOsm/kg is established in step 2, the development of the so-called "single effect." Fluid moves down the tubule in step 3 because of the introduction of additional fluid with an osmolality of 200 mOsm/kg. The 200-mOsm gradient is again developed in step 4. The process continues, so that by step 8 a longitudinal gradient of 400 mOsm/kg is present. This value can be as great as 900 to 1200 mOsm/kg in humans and 2500 mOsm/kg in kangaroo rats.

* See Credits on page iv.

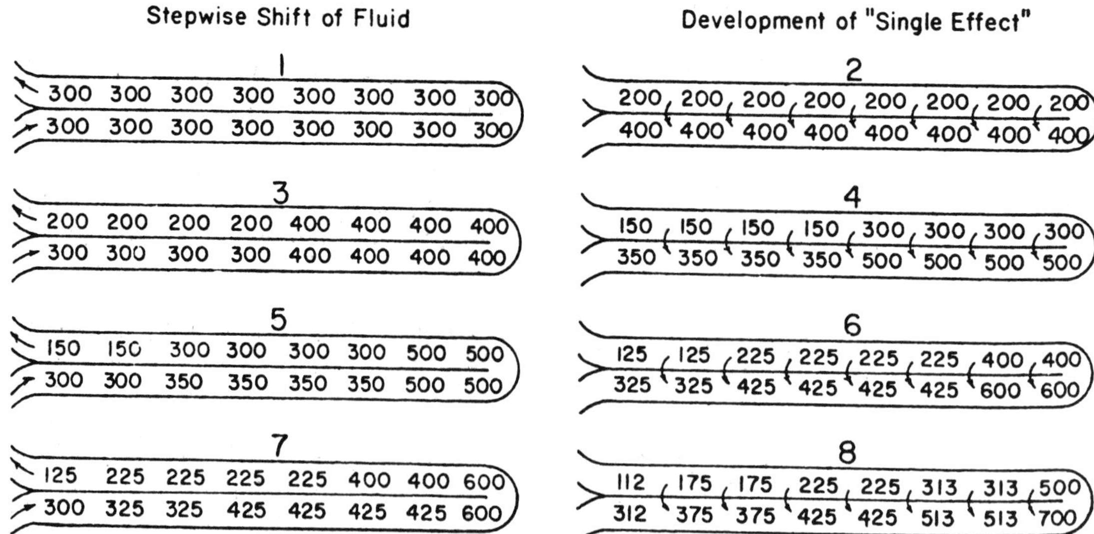

FIGURE 34-1. The principle of countercurrent multiplication of concentration is based on the assumption that at any level along the loop of Henle, a gradient of 200 mOsm/kg can be established between ascending and descending limbs by active transport of ions. (Pitts RF: Physiology of the kidney and body fluids, 3rd ed. Chicago: Year Book Medical Publishers, 1974.)

Longitudinal gradients of this magnitude are possible even though at any given level the system expends only the amount of energy necessary to produce a vertical gradient of 200 mOsm/kg. With development of a gradient, the outgoing fluid is always hypotonic with respect to the inflowing fluid at the same level. In addition, the solute pumped from the ascending limb is progressively concentrated in the interstitial fluid contained in the loop and reaches its greatest concentration at the point of reversal of flow.

The ascending limb of the loop must be impermeable to water. If it is not, the transport of solute between the two ends will be accompanied by the diffusion of an osmotically equivalent amount of water, and a concentration gradient cannot be developed. Finally, the system depicted in Figure 34-1 can do no osmotic work unless an osmotic-equilibrating device is added; the collecting duct plays this role.

Formation of Concentrated Urine

The formation of concentrated urine by countercurrent multiplication is illustrated in Figure 34-2. Isotonic fluid from the proximal tubule enters the descending limb of the loop of Henle. From the corresponding level of the thick, ascending limb, chloride is actively excreted into the interstitium; its concentration is thereby reduced in the ascending limb and increased in the interstitium; sodium follows passively.

Water passively diffuses out of the descending limb into the interstitium, and sodium and chloride passively diffuse into the descending limb. The ascending limb is impermeable to water. The collecting duct serves as an osmotic exchanger, permitting osmotic equilibration of the final urine with the hypertonic interstitium of the medulla and papilla.

In states of dehydration, the concentration of circulating antidiuretic hormone is high, and the permeability of the collecting ducts to water is high. Distal tubular fluid, initially isotonic, enters the collecting ducts and loses water to the hypertonic interstitium. The final urine attains an osmolar concentration equal to that in the interstitium. During antidiuresis, urea, the major end product of protein metabolism, constitutes about 40% of the total medullary and papillary solute concentration; sodium and chloride make up most of the balance.

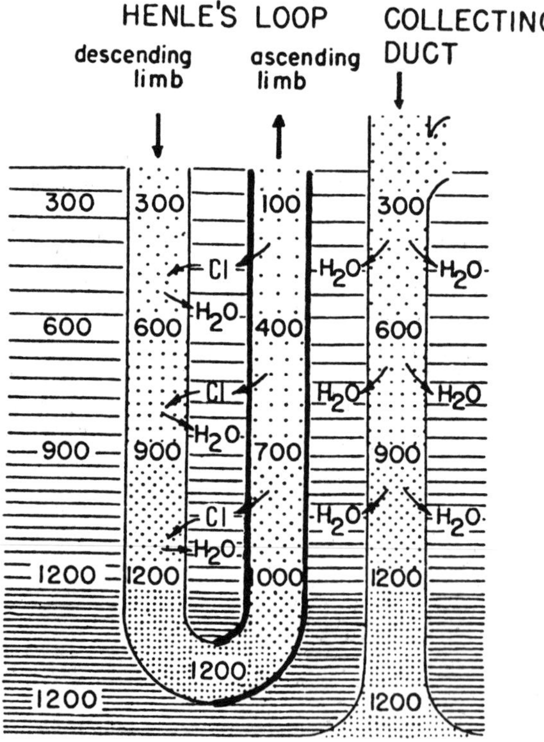

FIGURE 34-2. Countercurrent multiplication of concentration in the formation of hypertonic urine. *Bold lines* (ascending limb), impermeability to water. (Adapted from Pitts RF: Physiology of the kidney and body fluids, 3rd ed. Chicago: Year Book Medical Publishers, 1974. [Adapted from Pitts RF: The physiological basis of diuretic therapy. Springfield: Charles C Thomas, 1959.)

Formation of Dilute Urine

To form dilute urine, the countercurrent multiplication mechanism continues to function qualitatively in the same manner. However, when antidiuretic hormone is absent, the distal tubule[5] and collecting ducts become relatively impermeable to water. Thus, hypo-osmotic urine is excreted, despite the existence of osmotic gradients.

Countercurrent Exchange

Physical Principles

The principle of countercurrent exchange is illustrated in Figure 34-3.[4] Figure 34-3*A* shows a tube through which water flows at the constant rate of 10 mL per minute. A heat source supplies 100 cal/min, so that the fluid entering the system has a temperature of 30°C, and fluid leaving the system has a temperature of 40°C.

In Figure 34-3*B*, the tube is bent upon itself and insulated to prevent heat loss to the outside but is arranged to allow free exchange of heat between the inflowing and outflowing streams. As a countercurrent exchange system, certain aspects of the tube's performance will change. Although the temperature of the outflowing stream remains the same, the temperature at the heat source is much higher than in the straight tube because heat is transferred from the outflowing to the inflowing streams.

If the function of the fluid stream is to cool the heat source, the straight-tube system (see Fig. 34-3*A*) is much more efficient than the bent-tube, countercurrent exchange system (see Fig. 34-3*B*). Conversely, the countercurrent exchange system reduces the effective flow needed to cool the heat source to a small fraction of the true flow.

The Renal Medulla

Figure 34-3*C* illustrates the means by which countercurrent exchange operates in vascular loops to maintain the osmotic gradient in the renal medulla. Blood enters the loop at a concentration of 300 mOsm/kg. As the capillary dips into the medullary and papillary interstitium, water diffuses out from the blood, and osmotically active particles diffuse into the blood. After blood traverses the loop and begins to ascend, the reverse process occurs. Water bypasses the loop and passes directly into the ascending capillary. Because water takes this shortened route, red cells and plasma protein become more concentrated at the tip of the capillary loop. Thus, the loop operates to reduce the effect of blood flow with respect to the dissipation of the interstitial osmotic gradient.

Differences Between the Countercurrent Systems

The two countercurrent systems differ. Countercurrent multiplication of concentration is an active process that requires

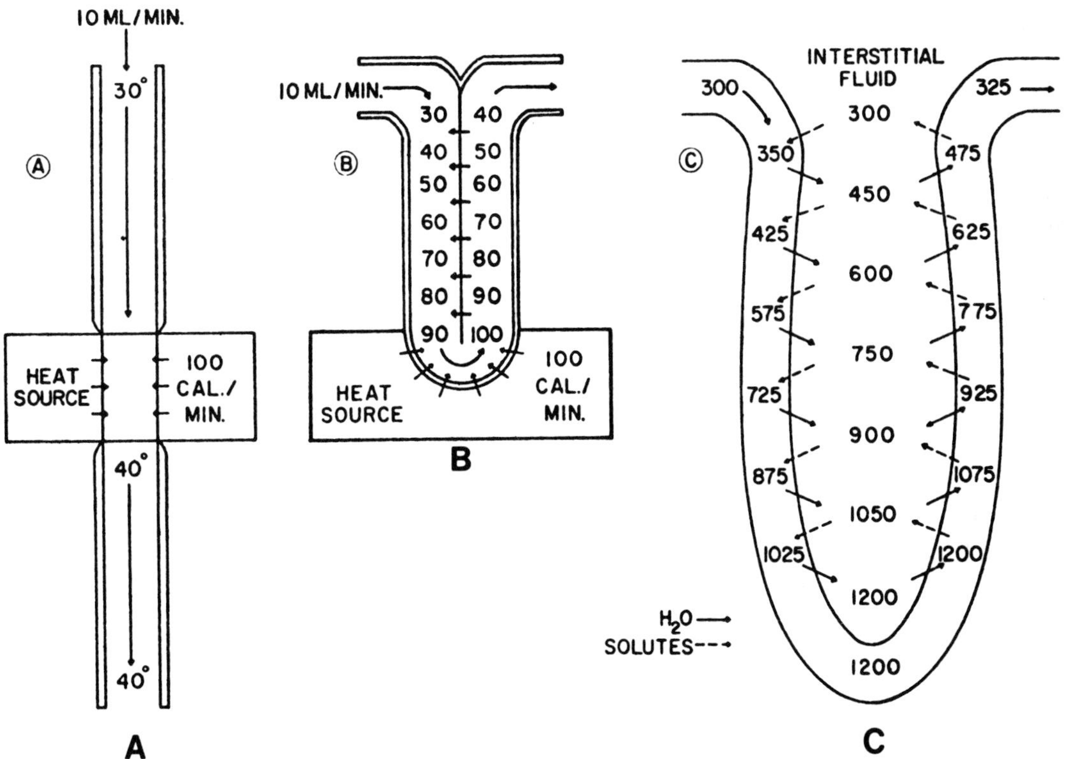

FIGURE 34-3. Countercurrent exchange. (A, B) Thermal models. (C) Operation of countercurrent exchange across the vasa recta reduces the rate of dissipation of the osmolar gradient between cortex and medulla. (Redrawn from Berliner RW, Levinsky NG, Davidson DG, et al: Dilution and concentration of the urine and the action of antidiuretic hormone. Am J Med 24:730, 1958.)

transport of solute from the ascending limb of the loop of Henle into the medullary interstitium; countercurrent exchange is a passive process and depends on the diffusion of solutes and water in both directions across the permeable walls of the vasa recta.

Countercurrent multiplication alone establishes and maintains the gradient of osmolar concentration between the cortex and the tip of the papillae. Countercurrent exchange plays no role in establishing this gradient. However, countercurrent exchange reduces the rate of dissipation of the gradient and hence the rate at which the countercurrent multiplier must pump solute to maintain any given gradient. Together, countercurrent multiplication and countercurrent exchange permit the formation of concentrated urine with a minimum expenditure of energy.

Normal Formation of Urine

Glomerular Filtration

Each day, 160 to 180 L of water are filtered through the glomeruli of a healthy adult. Each liter of filtrate normally contains 300 mOsm of solute, consisting primarily of sodium, chloride, and bicarbonate ions.

Proximal Convoluted Tubules

As the filtrate passes through the proximal convoluted tubules, sodium is actively extruded into the renal cortical interstitium. Chloride follows sodium passively, and water is reabsorbed by osmosis. The ions and water deposited in the interstitium are rapidly removed by the blood that perfuses the cortical capillaries. Although the volume of fluid in the proximal tubule is reduced by approximately 75%, the osmolar concentration remains unchanged at 300 mOsm/kg (see Fig. 34-2).

Descending Limbs of the Loops of Henle

As the tubular fluid flows along the thin, descending limbs of the loops of Henle, water diffuses out into the hypertonic interstitium of the medulla and papilla, and sodium and chloride diffuse in. The volume of tubular fluid decreases, and the osmotic pressure increases progressively, to the point of reversal of flow.

Ascending Limbs of the Loops of Henle

In the thick, ascending limbs of the loops of Henle, chloride is extruded into the interstitium. Because water cannot pass through the ascending limbs, the osmolar concentration of the tubular fluid is reduced. At each level, a gradient of about 200 mOsm/kg is established between the tubular contents and the hypertonic interstitium.

Distal Convoluted Tubules

The fluid that enters the distal convoluted tubules is hypotonic compared with the surrounding cortical interstitial fluid; its volume is reduced to 15% of the original glomerular filtrate. In states of water deprivation, the concentration of circulating antidiuretic hormone is high. Hence, the epithelium of the distal tubules and collecting ducts becomes freely permeable to water; tubular fluid is isotonic with cortical interstitial fluid by the time it reaches the middle of the distal segments. Active extrusion of sodium and passive osmotic diffusion of water are resumed in the distal tubules, thus reducing the volume of tubular fluid that enters the collecting ducts to a small fraction of the original glomerular filtrate.

Collecting Ducts

Collecting duct fluid, initially isosmotic, gives up water and becomes progressively concentrated as it descends through the hypertonic medullary and papillary interstitium. The concentration of the final urine entering the renal pelvis reflects the osmotic milieu of the interstitial tissue at the tips of the papillae.

Vasa Recti

Water, which diffuses out of the descending limbs of the loops of Henle and out of the collecting ducts, is removed by blood that perfuses the vasa recti of the medulla and papilla. These vessels act as countercurrent exchangers, reducing the loss of osmotically active solutes from the medulla and papilla.

Water Diuresis

During water diuresis, the concentration of circulating antidiuretic hormone is so low that the epithelium of the distal tubules and collecting ducts is impermeable to water. Tubular fluid, normally hypotonic as it leaves the loops of Henle, is maintained dilute or is diluted even further throughout the remainder of the nephron by the continued active extrusion of ions. In this manner, the final urine is dilute and its volume great.

CLINICAL ASPECTS

Intraoperative oliguria cannot be diagnosed without a means to monitor urine production. The use of an indwelling bladder catheter is justified in surgical procedures in the following situations: the loss of blood is anticipated to be great; deliberate hypotensive techniques will be used; osmotic diuretic agents will be given; the ureters may be damaged; the operation will be prolonged (>4 hours); the aorta will be cross-clamped; or cardiopulmonary bypass will be used (Table 34-1). In addition, if the patient has extensive tissue damage from trauma or burns, monitoring of urine output during surgery is important.

Presentation

During the operation, urinary output should be noted frequently (at least hourly) and recorded on the anesthesia record. A sudden decrease in urine output is cause for concern. A review of vital signs, blood loss, "third-space" loss (ie, loss from the extravascular, interstitial compartment), surgical manipulation and placement of packs, and intake and output data usually reveal the cause. A mechanical problem with the

TABLE 34-1
Indications for Intraoperative Bladder Catheterization

- Renal insufficiency
- Electrolyte abnormalities
- Lengthy surgical procedure (>4 hours)
- Aortic cross-clamping
- Cardiopulmonary bypass
- Burns
- Anticipation of decreased cardiac output or hypotension
- Large fluid shifts
- Intraoperative administration of diuretic agents
- Surgery that involves or may damage the urogenital system
- Extensive trauma
- Induced hypotension

Modified from: Merrell WJ, Bingham HL: Endocrine/renal system. In Gravenstein N (ed): Manual of complications during anesthesia. Philadelphia: JB Lippincott, 1991: 609.

catheter may account for an apparently low urine volume. Mucus plugs, bladder wall tissue, and blood clots may obstruct drainage holes at the catheter tip. Also, if the patient is placed in a steep head-down position, urine may pool in the bladder dome or kidneys, resulting in scant drainage from the catheter.

If it is believed that urinary output is decreased and there is not a bladder catheter in place, palpation of the bladder may be helpful in the diagnosis. However, a full bladder under these circumstances may reflect urine formed before operation or before the oliguric insult. To make a definitive diagnosis, an indwelling catheter must be placed, and the rate of additional urine formation must be determined.

Postoperatively, patients who have not been catheterized and who have not voided for a prolonged period must be watched carefully, particularly if they had pelvic surgery. In contrast, when a functioning catheter is in place, the clinical presentation of oliguria is obvious. Appropriate treatment, however, necessitates a review of the many possible causes of low urine output.

Classification and Differential Diagnosis

One approach to the differential diagnosis of oliguria is to establish the anatomic location of the initiating disturbance. For convenience, the three categories used to classify acute renal failure may be used to describe oliguria. It should be kept in mind, however, that several types may exist simultaneously (Table 34-2).[5] The categories are postrenal (obstruction or extravasation), prerenal (inadequate renal perfusion), and renal (intrinsic). This classification is important because the specific therapy for prerenal and postrenal disorders is often completely corrective, whereas the therapy for intrinsic renal disease is only 50% effective.[6]

Pattern of Urine Flow

In many cases, the cause of oliguria and azotemia can be determined from the clinical presentation alone. Observation of the pattern of urine flow offers the first clue. Complete anuria is rare; it occurred in only 1 of 85 patients in a series reported by Swann and Merrill.[7] Cortical necrosis, vascular accident, the glomerulitides, and the vasculitides are the likely causes of anuria. Obstruction, at times, may result in anuria, but with this disorder large fluctuations in urine flow may occur as the obstructing body changes position.

Urine Composition

Information about urine composition is helpful in distinguishing oliguria of prerenal origin from that due to established acute tubular necrosis, as shown in Table 34-3.

Urinary Sediment

The urinary sediment also is of diagnostic value. In prerenal oliguria, there is a preponderance of hyaline and finely granular casts, whereas coarse and cellular casts are rare. Oliguria caused by acute tubular necrosis is associated with frequent, dirty-looking, brown cellular casts and numerous epithelial cells, both free and in casts. A paucity of formed elements suggests obstruction. Red blood cells or heme-pigmented casts are rare, except when hemoglobinuria or myoglobinuria is present. Proteinuria is of little diagnostic value because it may be associated with a wide variety of disorders.

Radiography

A supine radiograph of the abdomen helps to determine kidney size and allows visualization of calcified stones. The kidneys are normal or increased in size in acute renal failure, whereas frequently in chronic disease they are small. Urographic studies are used to exclude obstruction and, with modern techniques, are reasonably safe even in cases of acute oliguric renal failure.[8,9]

INTRAVENOUS PYELOGRAPHY. On intravenous pyelography, the appearance of the kidneys is immediate, dense, and persistent in patients with acute tubular necrosis and pyelonephritis but not in those with other forms of oliguria. However, as the serum creatinine concentration increases to more than 1.5 mg/dL, the incidence of acute renal failure increases exponentially. In oliguria of prerenal origin, the findings on the pyelogram are normal. In established oliguric renal failure, no structures appear on the pyelogram, but the pyelogram often is dense enough to allow detection of the calyceal system and observation of filling defects. However, retrograde urography may be necessary in some cases to localize obstructing lesions precisely.

SONOGRAPHY, COMPUTED TOMOGRAPHY, AND RADIONUCLIDES. Sonography and computed tomography have become integral parts of the diagnostic evaluation of oliguria.[10] Radionuclide studies are useful in the diagnosis of renal artery stenosis, chronic pyelonephritis, and lymphomatous infiltration of the kidney. They also may provide functional information for each kidney and obviate the need to resort to invasive measures.[11]

TABLE 34-2
Major Causes of Oliguria

CLASSIFICATION	CAUSE
POSTRENAL	
Obstruction	Calculi, neoplasms of bladder and pelvic organs, prostatitis, surgical accident, urethral instrumentation
Extravasation	Rupture of bladder
PRERENAL	
Hypovolemia	Skin loss (from sweating or burns) Fluid loss (from diuretic agents of osmotic diuresis in diabetes mellitus) Hemorrhage Sequestration (because of burns or peritonitis)
Cardiovascular failure	
Myocardial failure	Infarction, tamponade, dysrhythmias
Vascular pooling	Sepsis, septic abortion, anaphylaxis, extreme acidosis
Vascular obstruction	
Arterial	Thrombosis, embolism, aneurysm
Venous	Thrombosis, vena caval obstruction, diffuse small-vein thrombosis in amyloidosis
RENAL	
Heme pigments	
Intravascular hemolysis	Transfusion reactions, hemolysis (due to toxins or immunologic damage, malaria)
Rhabdomyolysis and myoglobinuria	Trauma, muscle disease, prolonged coma, seizures, heat stroke, severe exercise
Nephrotoxins	
Pregnancy-related	Toxic abortifacents, septic abortion, uterine hemorrhage, eclampsia, postpartum renal failure
Glomerulitis	Post-streptococcal, lupus erythematosus
Vasculitis	Periarteritis, hypersensitivity, angiitis
Malignant nephrosclerosis	
Acute diffuse pyelonephritis or papillary necrosis	
Severe hypercalcemia	
Aminoglycoside antibiotic agents	
Intratubular precipitation	Myeloma, urates after cytotoxic drugs, sulfonamides
Hepatorenal syndrome	

Modified from Levinsky NG, Alexander EA, Venkatachalam MA: Acute renal failure. In Brenner BM, Rector FC (eds): The kidney. Philadelphia: WB Saunders, 1981.

TABLE 34-3
Urine Composition in Prerenal Oliguria, Acute Tubular Necrosis, and Obstruction

PARAMETER	PRERENAL OLIGURIA	ACUTE TUBULAR NECROSIS	OBSTRUCTION
Urinary Sodium (mEq/L)	<10	>25	<30*
Urinary Specific gravity	>1.015	1.010 to 1.015	1.010 to 1.015
Urinary/plasma osmolality ratio	>1.1	≤1.1	≤1.1
Blood urea nitrogen/creatinine ratio	>20/1	10/1	10/1 to 20/1*
Urinary/plasma creatinine ratio	40/1 or more, rarely <10/1	<10/1	<20/1
Fractional excretion of sodium† (%)	<1	>1	<1*

* First 24 hours only.

† Fractional excretion of sodium = $\frac{U_{Na} \times P_{Cr}}{U_{Cr} \times P_{Na}} \times 100$ where Cr = creatinine; Na = sodium; P = plasma; U = urine.

POSTRENAL OLIGURIA

Causes

Postrenal oliguria comprises only a small percentage of oliguric disorders. Obstruction of normal outflow of urine is the most significant disorder in this category (see Table 34-2). Extravasation of urine from a ruptured bladder also is included. Obstruction of urine flow leads to an increase in hydrostatic pressure in the urinary tract proximal to the obstruction; ultimately, a marked decrease in glomerular filtration rate (GFR) ensues. Morphologic damage to the renal parenchyma occurs in proportion to the degree and duration of obstruction and also depends on related factors, such as the virulence of the associated pyelonephritis, which often develops in the presence of urinary stasis.

Extrinsic Obstruction

Passage of urine depends on the patency of compressible structures. Extrinsic obstruction with oliguria may be caused by rapidly growing pelvic tumors or by retroperitoneal fibrosis. This category includes retroperitoneal malignancies, rapidly growing cervical carcinomas, and massive uterine fibromyomata. Complete bilateral ureteral obstruction also may be caused by lymphomatous or leukemic involvement of the lymph nodes.

Iatrogenic oliguria may follow inadvertent ligation or trauma to the ureters. The incidence of these mishaps among patients undergoing gynecologic surgery is reported to be 0.1% to 0.25%.[12] A review of 161 patients with ureteral injuries showed that 72% followed gynecologic surgery; an additional 12% followed obstetric procedures.[13] Approximately 20% to 25% of ureteral injuries are bilateral, resulting in immediate anuria. A common noniatrogenic problem in aged patients is obstructive uropathy and oliguria caused by fecal impaction.

Intrinsic Obstruction

Intrinsic obstruction can be caused by blood clots, calculi, prostatic obstruction, and various neoplasms. Bladder carcinoma accounts for 32% cases of obstructive uremia with oliguria; prostatic carcinoma is half as frequent.[14] Primary ureteral tumors and metastatic tumors of the ureter are rare.[15] Patients with calculi of the genitourinary tract may have sudden oliguria if stones are bilateral or are present in the bladder. Patients with bladder stones often have intermittent anuria or oliguria, as the calculi may act as ball valves.

Intravesical formalin instillation used to control postradiation hemorrhage also has been associated with a high incidence of anuria and oliguria,[16] as has bilateral ureteral obstruction resulting from fungus balls and bilharziasis.[17,18] In one eighth of the kidney transplant recipients in one large series, obstructive uropathy with oliguria developed.[19] Finally, amyloidosis caused a rare case of bilateral ureteral obstruction with resulting anuria.[20]

Benign prostatic enlargement is a frequent cause of impairment of urine flow in older patients after operations around the groin or rectum when pain prevents the relaxation of voluntary sphincters. Overflow incontinence may occur after anesthesia in aged men, with a total urinary output of less than 400 mL/day. This problem may be particularly acute if belladonna alkaloids have been administered as premedication or during the course of the anesthetic. Oliguria also may follow ureteral catheterization if edema obstructs the ureteral orifices.

Urine Extravasation

Extravasation of urine outside of the bladder may occur after trauma to the pelvis and may be associated with oliguria. Damage to the bladder rarely occurs if it is relatively empty at the time of injury; however, pelvic fractures are associated with a 9% to 15% incidence of bladder rupture.[21] Because the ureters are thin, retroperitoneal structures, they are rarely injured, except from direct trauma during surgery.

Treatment

Prompt treatment of postrenal oliguria is essential because prolonged ureteral obstruction may result in irreversible loss of renal function. The degree of renal damage is related to the degree and duration of obstruction and the presence or absence of infection.[22] After obstruction of several weeks' duration, some permanent loss of glomerular function usually occurs, although recovery of normal renal function after 72 days of anuric ureteral obstruction has been reported.[23]

Catheterization of the Bladder

For simple cases of urinary retention after surgery, encouraging the patient to stand may induce urination. If this approach is not possible, if the patient is in severe pain, or if the bladder appears to be overdistended, then a single in-and-out catheterization is the appropriate treatment. If too much time elapses before the first postoperative voiding, the bladder becomes overdistended and atonic; should this problem occur, an indwelling catheter must be inserted for 5 to 7 days.

Surgical

The definitive treatment of more complicated cases of postrenal oliguria is usually surgical. If the obstruction is high in the genitourinary tract, percutaneous nephrostomy may be necessary to provide urinary drainage. If bladder calculi are the cause of obstruction, suprapubic cystostomy or urethral catheterization is the first therapeutic maneuver. Massive diuresis occasionally follows relief of obstruction, so the patient must be observed for signs of hypovolemia and electrolyte imbalance. Hypotension also may occur after rapid decompression of an overdistended bladder. If obstruction is recognized and treated promptly, normal renal function returns rapidly.

PRERENAL OLIGURIA

Causes

Renal Hypoperfusion

Oliguria in patients undergoing surgery is most commonly prerenal; that is, it is caused by inadequate renal perfusion.

Renal hypoperfusion may be caused by cardiac failure or, rarely, by renal artery thrombosis. However, the most likely causes in patients undergoing surgery are inadequate circulating blood volume and intraoperative administration of anesthetic agents. Systemic hypotension may accompany both circumstances along with reflex shunting away from the kidneys to more vital organs occurs.

When renal blood flow is minimally or moderately depressed, a compensatory increase in filtration fraction results; GFR and urine formulation remain relatively unaffected. However, when depression of renal blood flow is marked, GFR, urine formation, and electrolyte excretion also are significantly reduced.

Anesthetic Agents

These changes occur with all anesthetic agents and are due primarily to the direct or indirect effects of the anesthetics on the cardiovascular system. All of the potent volatile anesthetics cause dose-related myocardial depression and peripheral vasodilation, probably by altering calcium flux within myocardial cells and the arteriolar smooth muscle.

Release of catecholamines and other neurohumoral transmitters may also be factors in the reduction of renal blood flow during anesthesia. In the nonanesthetized state, the kidneys maintain perfusion in the presence of hypotension by autoregulating their blood flow. General anesthesia may abolish autoregulation, leading to decreased renal blood flow and GFR during hypotension. In general, anesthetic-induced changes of renal function are readily reversed when administration of the agent is discontinued.[24-28]

Reduction of Circulating Blood Volume

Oliguria resulting from decreased circulating blood volume—whether originally caused by blood loss, sequestration into a surgical third space, dehydration, or gastrointestinal loss—is not as amenable to treatment as is oliguria resulting from anesthetic administration. Treatment is particularly difficult if the hypovolemia is severe and persistent, so that renal ischemia is present as well. In these circumstances, functional lesions develop a renal morphologic component; carried to an extreme, simple prerenal oliguria is converted into oliguric renal failure. The importance of time in the progression of functional renal insufficiency to organic renal failure is illustrated in Figure 34-4.[29]

Drugs

Another cause of prerenal oliguria is massive fibrin thrombosis of the glomerular afferent arterioles as a result of chemotherapy with vinblastine, bleomycin, or cisplatin.[30] Similarly, oliguria and azotemia have occurred after captopril therapy and chronic acetominophen or nonsteroidal antiinflammatory drug use.[31-33] Renal insufficiency may follow treatment with amphotericin B; in this case, renal vasoconstriction is thought to occur concomitantly with nephrotoxicity.

Cardiac Surgery and Cardiopulmonary Bypass

Finally, persistent oliguria and renal failure after open heart surgery may be of prerenal origin. Abel studied 500 consecutive patients who underwent cardiopulmonary bypass and found that in 35, moderate or severe acute renal failure de-

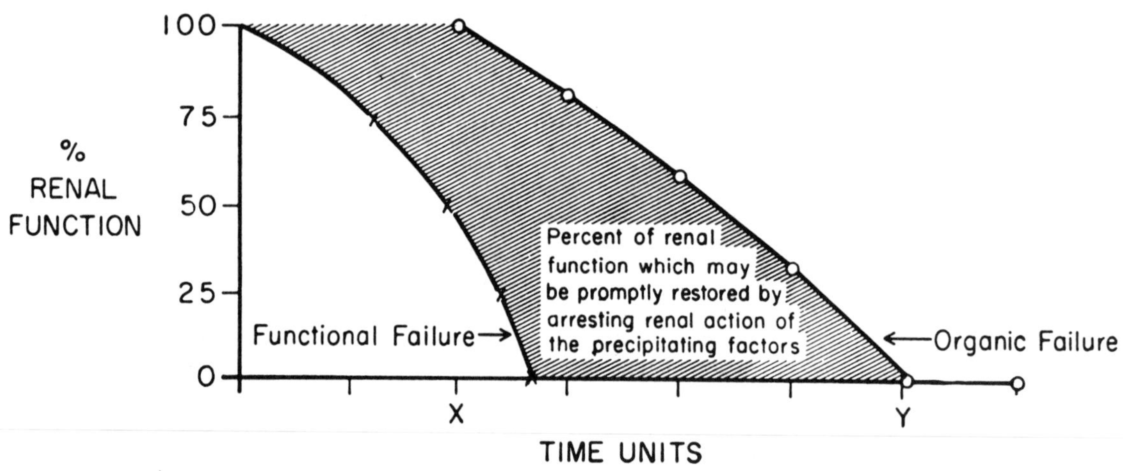

FIGURE 34-4. The importance of time in the progression of functional to organic or parenchymal renal failure. Systemic hypotension may be used as an example of an extrarenal precipitating factor. Reflex spasm of the renal arteries occurs, and renal blood flow is severely reduced. Glomerular filtration rate and urine flow decrease rapidly. Finally, anuria occurs. If renal response to the hypotension is not arrested before time X, renal lesions are initiated. Between times X and Y, therapy will be effective in alleviating the functional component of renal failure and preventing further progression of organic lesions. At time Y, however, organic lesions are of such severity that total organic failure is present, pathologically characterized (in this example) by acute tubular necrosis. At this point, arresting the renal effect of hypotension can have no immediate salutary effect because the patient's condition is one of classic organic renal shutdown. (Barry KG, Malloy JP: Oliguric renal failure. JAMA 179:510, 1962.)

veloped.[34] The mortality rate for this group was 89%; no survivors were reported among patients requiring dialysis. Preoperative renal function and perioperative hemodynamic instability appear to be the factors of greatest importance in postoperative renal dysfunction, particularly when vasopressors, large volume transfusion, and intra-aortic balloon counterpulsation are necessary.[35]

Improvement in renal function has been noted after coronary artery bypass grafting in patients treated with low-dose dopamine infusions. Dopamine, in a dosage of as much as 3 μg/kg/min, results in a marked improvement in creatinine and free water clearance and in a significant increase in the cortical component of renal blood flow, as measured by the xenon isotope washout technique.[36]

Progression to Renal Insufficiency

Renal insufficiency of prerenal origin may develop into classic acute renal failure unless promptly treated. The mechanism by which this progression occurs is reasonably well understood. Renal micropuncture experiments indicate that intratubular obstruction by interstitial edema or intratubular casts may be a contributing factor and that excessive backflow of filtrate across denuded or damaged tubules also may be involved.[37]

The most common factor in the pathogenesis of acute renal failure appears to be suppression of glomerular filtration.[38] Light- and electron-microscopic studies of glomeruli usually fail to reveal structural abnormalities; therefore it is likely that reduced glomerular filtration is caused by vasomotor phenomena.[39]

Alteration of Cortical Perfusion

Hollenberg and colleagues used a krypton isotope washout technique and renal arteriography to measure the intrarenal distribution of blood flow in patients with renal failure.[40] In other studies, they showed similar disproportionate decreases in superficial cortical blood flow in patients with acute renal failure caused by nephrotoxins,[41] in patients undergoing acute renal allograft rejection,[42] and in a patient with irreversible acute renal failure after methoxyflurane anesthesia.[43] They suggested that sustained preglomerular vasoconstriction caused persistent homogeneous reductions in renal cortical perfusion sufficient to induce the cessation of glomerular filtration. They postulated that this chain of events is the pathogenetic final common pathway in acute renal failure.

MECHANISMS. How the reduction in cortical perfusion is induced or sustained is not clear. Evidence suggests that a local intrarenal vasomotor mechanism controlled by a vasoactive mediator, such as the renin–angiotensin system, is the predominant factor. Fifty years ago, hypertrophy of cellular elements of the juxtaglomerular apparatus was observed in the kidney tissue of patients with acute renal failure related to the crush syndrome. A vasopressor substance was postulated to be released from this area, resulting in altered renal blood flow, decreased GFR, and, finally, renal failure.[44]

Increases in plasma renin concentrations have been observed in both clinical[45] and experimental[46] acute renal failure. However, the finding of increased renin concentration has not been consistent, and whether increased renin activity, when it occurs, is a consequence rather than a cause of acute renal failure is unclear.

Experiments with hydralazine and acetylcholine have led to perhaps the most serious defect in the hypothesis of increased renin–angiotensin activity as the common mediator of renal vascular changes in acute renal failure. These drugs block the effects of angiotensin and improve renal blood flow and cortical perfusion, but they do not reverse adverse changes in renal function.[47]

Prevention

Preventing renal ischemia is easier than treating it after it is established. Prevention is advisable particularly in surgical patients with reduced circulating blood volume, in whom the added insult of general anesthesia, with its attendant myocardial depression, decrease in renal blood flow, and peripheral vasodilation, may accelerate the renal ischemic process. The only preoperative renal risk factors that predict postoperative renal dysfunction are shown in Table 34-4, which presents the results of a semiquantitative review of the literature.[48] Consideration of these risk factors should help in the decision to carry out preventive measures.

Preoperative Hydration

Barry and colleagues demonstrated the advantages of preoperative hydration with 15 mL/kg of 0.3% saline and replacement of urine output in six patients anesthetized with light (0.5% to 1.0%) or deep (1.2% to 3.0%) halothane.[49] A control

TABLE 34-4
Preoperative Risk Factors for Postoperative Renal Failure

STRONGLY PREDICTIVE
Poor preoperative renal function (increased blood urea nitrogen or increased creatinine concentration)
Advanced age
Congestive heart failure
POSSIBLY PREDICTIVE
Endocarditis
Hypoalbuminemia
Malignancy
Emergency surgery
Gout
Previous cardiac surgery
Vascular disease
Aneurysm surgery
INCONCLUSIVE
Preoperative use of diuretic agents
Hypotension
Chronic obstructive pulmonary disease
Coronary artery disease
Surgery with coronary artery bypass grafting

Compiled from Novis BK, Roizen MF, Aronson S, et al: Association of preoperative risk factors with postoperative acute renal failure. Anesth Analg 78:143, 1994.

group of six patients were anesthetized with similar halothane concentrations but were not given fluids from the night before operation until the conclusion of anesthesia. Premedication with morphine–scopolamine produced a significant decrease in effective renal blood flow (*p*-aminohippurate clearance), GFR (inulin clearance), and urine flow in the nonhydrated control patients but not in the hydrated patients (Fig. 34-5). Anesthesia with light levels of halothane resulted in greater decreases in these variables in the nonhydrated patients than in the hydrated patients. However, the advantage of hydration was lost with deeper levels of halothane.[49]

In healthy young patients, dehydration plus halothane anesthesia results in moderate changes in renal hemodynamics and function. In older patients, particularly those who might also have marked reductions in circulating blood volume, these changes can be expected to be of greater magnitude and possibly to lead to the development of acute renal failure if not properly treated.

Restoration of Circulating Blood Volume

Restoration of circulating blood volume to values as near normal as possible is a major goal of the preoperative therapy of hypovolemic patients, regardless of the cause of the deficit. During surgery, additional fluid losses may occur from hemorrhage, formation of a surgical third space, pooling of fluids

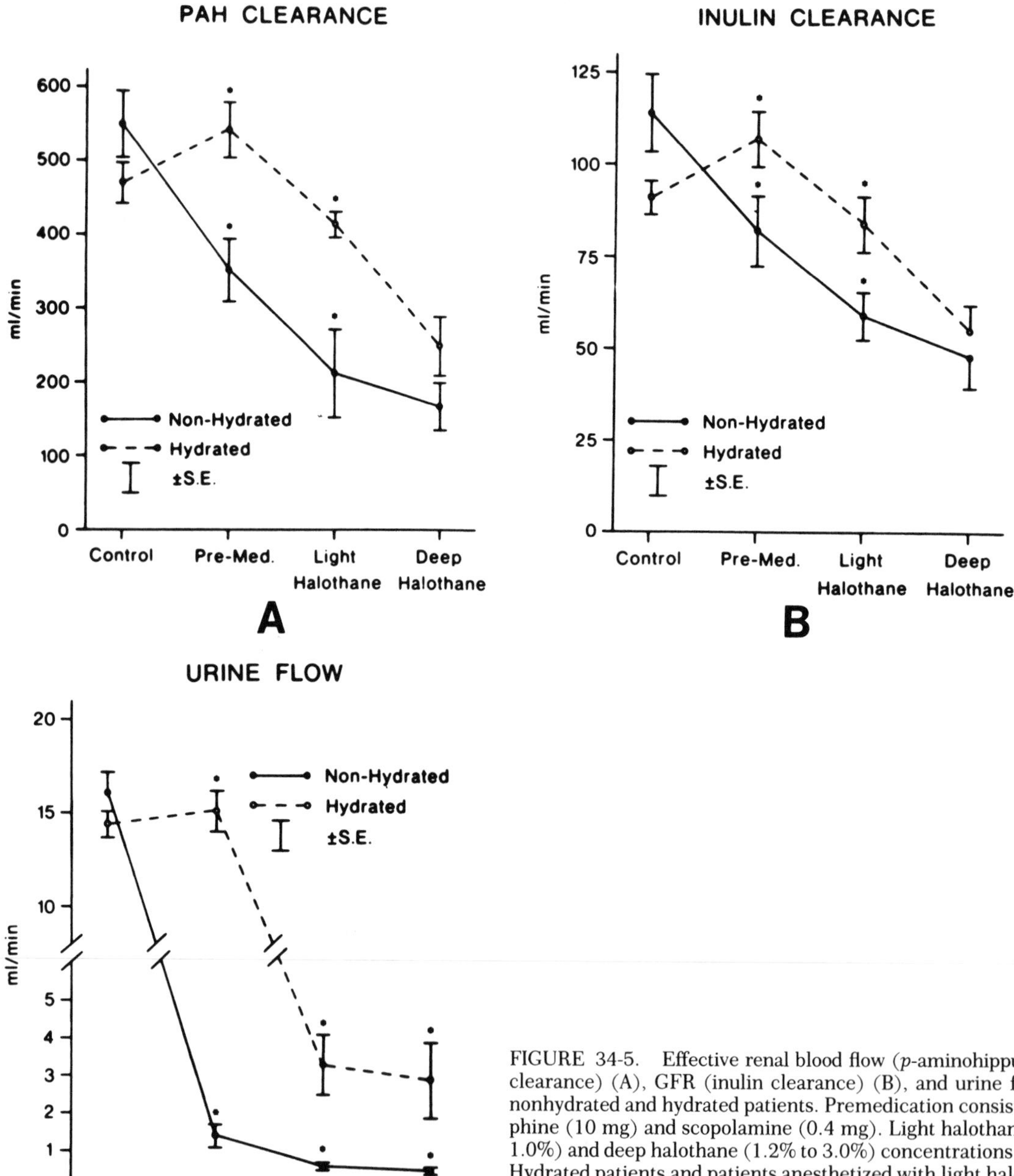

FIGURE 34-5. Effective renal blood flow (*p*-aminohippurate [*PAH*] clearance) (A), GFR (inulin clearance) (B), and urine flow (C) in nonhydrated and hydrated patients. Premedication consisted of morphine (10 mg) and scopolamine (0.4 mg). Light halothane (0.5% to 1.0%) and deep halothane (1.2% to 3.0%) concentrations were used. Hydrated patients and patients anesthetized with light halothane had less depression of renal hemodynamics and function than did nonhydrated and deeply anesthetized patients. *SE*, standard error. (Barry KG, Mazze RI, Schwartz FD: Prevention of surgical oliguria and renal-hemodynamic suppression by sustained hydration. N Engl J Med 270: 1371, 1964.)

in the intestines, or evaporative loss from exposed intestinal surfaces; these conditions must be corrected. Finally, hypovolemia in the postoperative period should be avoided as carefully as in the preoperative and intraoperative periods.

In addition to the obvious causes of hypovolemia, such as hemorrhage and gastrointestinal drainage, more unusual events, such as gram-negative bacterial sepsis, are likely to occur after surgery, particularly in cases of extensive procedures performed in debilitated patients. Release of endotoxins from cell walls of dying bacteria, usually *Escherichia coli*, results in pooling of blood in the microcirculation. Relaxation of precapillary sphincters, combined with intense constriction of postcapillary sphincters, results in stagnation of blood with hypovolemia, hypotension, hypoxemia, and acidosis. Activation of complement by the endotoxin that initiated the process also may lead to intravascular coagulation.

Treatment

Replacement Therapy

In many cases, correction of hypovolemia increases cardiac output, enhances renal perfusion, and prevents parenchymal ischemic changes. A diagnostic and therapeutic maneuver is the rapid infusion of 500 mL of balanced electrolyte solution and the determination of the response of the kidneys to this challenge. An increase in urine flow indicates that additional fluids must be administered, because significant oliguria usually does not occur unless extracellular fluid volume is depleted by 25% or more. In an intensive care unit study, Zaloga and Hughes demonstrated that in hypovolemic oliguric patients, urine output increased from 17 ± 2 mL/hr to more than 0.5 mL/kg/hr following a 500 mL normal saline bolus, while normovolemic oliguric patients remained oliguric following the saline bolus.[50]

In general, replacement fluid should match the type of fluid that has been lost, although organ perfusion may be enhanced by hemodilution. Measurement of central venous pressure can be useful to determine the volume of fluid to be administered. In patients with marked impairment of myocardial function or severe pulmonary disease, however, this parameter may not correlate with left atrial pressure. When volume status is not known with certainty or when rapid infusions are required, left ventricular filling pressure can be estimated by the pulmonary artery occlusion pressure determined with a balloon-tipped, pulmonary artery catheter.[51] Transesophageal echocardiography is as useful or even more so and is less invasive.[52]

Inotropic Support

If replacement of lost fluid does not reverse oliguria, cardiac failure may be present. In that case, administration of inotropic agents, such as dopamine, dobutamine, or epinephrine may be indicated. Digitalis administration in the operating room is uncommon because inotrope administration offers simplicity, control, and fewer hazards.

Diuretic Agents

The efficacy of diuretic agents in the treatment of oliguria is variable. Because these agents are potentially harmful, their mechanisms of action must be understood.

OSMOTIC. Osmotic diuretic agents such as mannitol produce diuresis because they are filtered by the glomeruli but not reabsorbed in the renal tubules; thus, they necessitate the excretion of water. In addition, they increase intravascular volume and may block renin release. Because they increase blood volume, their use is contraindicated in patients with oliguria caused by congestive heart failure.

LOOP. Loop diuretics, such as furosemide and ethacrynic acid, produce diuresis by blocking sodium reabsorption in the loops of Henle and distal convoluted tubules. Furosemide is also a modest vasodilator of the renal vasculature,[53] thus contributing to redistribution of intrarenal blood flow independent of the action of prostaglandin E_2.[54] In addition, furosemide may modulate renin secretion by the macula densa, preventing the harmful effects of vasoconstriction on the glomerular apparatus.

When administered to patients with congestive heart failure, these diuretic agents promote profuse natriuresis with increased urine flow. This effect results in a decrease in intravascular volume and ultimately in improvement in cardiac performance. Loop diuretic agents clearly are beneficial to these patients.[55,56] However, these agents are contraindicated in oliguria of hypovolemic origin, because they may promote diuresis despite a reduced intravascular volume and thereby aggravate renal ischemic changes.

If, after an initial positive response to diuretic treatment, urine flow again decreases to less than 1 mL/kg/h, the treatment should be continued while fluid and electrolyte balance are carefully maintained. When administered in this manner, diuretic agents may prevent functional renal failure from progressing to organic renal disease.[56–58] If these agents are not completely effective, they still may improve the patient's status by converting oliguric renal failure to high-output renal failure, which seems to be more easily managed than the former condition.[56]

CLINICAL APPROACH. Some nephrologists believe that diuretic agents are not indicated except when oliguria is caused by heart failure. They cite the increased salt and water loss and ototoxicity associated with loop diuretic agents and the osmotic nephrosis that may occur after mannitol administration as important disadvantages of this type of therapy.

In general, we believe that diuretic agents are useful in treating oliguria in some patients; their administration should be associated with few complications if basic physiologic principles are followed and the dosage is not excessive. Others advocate the use of diuretic agents in all oliguric patients and suggest the combination of dopamine, 1 to 3 μg/kg/min, and furosemide, 200 to 500 mg, for the treatment of diuretic-resistant, acute oliguric renal insufficiency.[59]

PRIMARY RENAL OLIGURIA

Approximately half of the patients admitted to renal dialysis units have diseases not requiring surgery; oliguria is a part of the complex of symptoms in most of these cases. The causes of oliguria of primary renal origin are indicated in Table 34-2. Few of these patients receive the care of an anesthesiologist, and the differential diagnosis and treatment of their diseases is not discussed extensively here.

Causes

Nephrotoxic Drugs

Worthy of mention are patients treated with potentially nephrotoxic agents. These substances include platinum, a heavy metal used in chemotherapy[60]; ionic and nonionic contrast materials used in digital vascular imaging and selective renal angiography[61]; and nonsteroidal anti-inflammatory agents, such as phenylbutazone, ibuprofen, and indomethacin.[31,32,62,63] Although these agents rarely cause severe oliguria or anuria, when they do, the ability to monitor intraoperative fluid shifts may be critical. Aminoglycoside antibodies account for a significant percentage of all hospital-acquired acute renal failure.[64]

Hemoglobin and Myoglobin

Another example of interest to anesthesiologists is the release of hemoglobin from lysed red blood cells (caused by a blood transfusion reaction or mechanical trauma from intraoperative autologous blood salvage or a roller pump in a cardiopulmonary bypass circuit). Hemoglobin appears in the urine after all binding sites to plasma haptoglobin are occupied and the resorptive capacity of proximal tubular cells is exceeded. In addition, renal tubular cells are sloughed, and heme pigment obstructs the tubular lumens.

Micropuncture studies have shown that obstruction of renal tubules is not the major pathophysiologic event in the development of experimental oliguric renal failure; rather, the primary factor is a reduction in GFR.[37,38] Also, the transfusion of incompatible blood leads to disseminated intravascular coagulation, with deposition of fibrin in renal tubules. Red cell membranes are thought to initiate the coagulation process, ultimately leading to decreases in platelets and in the concentrations of fibrinogen and factors II, V, and VII.[65]

Myoglobinuria after extensive, crushing-type muscle injuries also may lead to oliguric renal failure. The mechanism is probably the same as that after hemoglobin release.[66]

Treatment

Treatment with mannitol, if instituted before hemolysis or shortly thereafter, may ameliorate or prevent renal failure.[29] Hence, 12.5 to 25 g of mannitol frequently is included with the solutions used to prime pump oxygenators for cardiopulmonary bypass. However, when oliguric renal failure is diagnosed, hemodialysis is the treatment of choice.

In most cases, if medical management is meticulous and complications such as infection, hemorrhage, or cardiac dysrhythmias do not supervene, the return of renal function will be complete. However, if oliguria is caused by renal cortical necrosis, and renal function cannot be expected to return, long-term dialysis must be instituted[67] or renal transplantation undertaken.

REFERENCES

1. Brown CB: Established acute renal failure following surgical operations. In Friedman EA, Eliahou HE (eds): Proceedings: Conference on Acute Renal Failure, publication no. (NIH) 74-608. Bethesda, MD: Department of Health, Education, and Welfare, 1973: 187
2. Kuhn W, Ryffel K: Herstellung konzentrierter Lösungen aus verdünnten durch blosse Membranwirkung: Ein Modellversuch zur Funktion der Niere. J Physiol Chem 276:145, 1942
3. Pitts RF: Physiology of the kidney and body fluids, 3rd ed. Chicago: Year Book Medical, 1974
4. Berliner RW, Levinsky NG, Davidson DG, et al: Dilution and concentration of the urine and the action of antidiuretic hormone. Am J Med 24:730, 1958
5. Brezis M, Rosen S, Epstein FH: Acute renal failure. In Brennar BM, Rector FC Jr (eds): The kidney, 3rd ed. Philadelphia: WB Saunders, 1986: 735
6. Harrington JT, Cohen JC: Current concepts: acute oliguria. N Engl J Med 292:89, 1975
7. Swann RC, Merrill JP: The clinical course of acute renal failure. Medicine 32:215, 1953
8. Parfrey PS, Griffiths SM, Barrett BJ, et al: Contrast material-induced renal failure in patients with diabetes mellitus, renal insufficiency, or both. N Engl J Med 320:143, 1989
9. Manske CL, Sprafka JM, Strong JT, et al: Contrast nephropathy in azotemic diabetic patients undergoing coronary angiography. Am J Med 89:615, 1990
10. Balfe DM, McClennon BL: CT of the retroperitoneum in urosurgical disorders. Surg Clin North Am 62:919, 1982
11. Sherman RA, Byan KJ: Nuclear medicine in acute and chronic renal failure. Semin Nucl Med 3:265, 1982
12. Charles AH: Some hazards of pelvic surgery. Proceedings of the Royal Society of Medicine 60:656, 1967
13. Wesolowski S: Ureteral injuries. Int Urol Nephrol 5:39, 1973
14. Chisholm GD, Shackman R: Malignant obstructive uraemia. Br J Urol 40:720, 1968
15. Wanrick S: Carcinoma of pancreas causing ureteral obstruction. J Urol 110:395, 1973
16. Fall M, Petterson S: Ureteral complications after intravenous formalin instillation. J Urol 122:160, 1979
17. Elem B, Sinha SN: Ureterocele in bilharziasis of the urinary tract. Br J Urol 53:428, 1981
18. Biggers R, Edwards J: Anuria secondary to bilateral ureteropelvic fungus balls. Urology 2:161, 1980
19. Mundy AR, Bewick M, Podesto ML, et al: The urological complications of 1000 renal transplants. J Urol 53:397, 1981
20. Mariani AJ, Barrett DM, Kurtz SB, et al: Bilateral localized amyloidosis of the ureter presenting with anuria. J Urol 120:757, 1978
21. Derrick F, Kretkowski R: Trauma to kidney, ureter, bladder and urethra. Postgrad Med 55:183, 1974
22. Taylor PT Jr, Anderson WA: Untreated cervical cancer complicated by obstructive uropathy and oliguric renal failure. Gynecol Oncol 11:162, 1981
23. Hata M, Tachibana M, Deguchi N, et al: Recovery of renal function after 72 days of anuria caused by ureteral obstruction. J Urol 130:37, 1983
24. Burnett CH, Bloomberg EL, Shortz G, et al: A comparison of the effects of ether and cyclopropane anesthesia on renal function of man. J Pharmacol Exp Ther 96:380, 1949
25. Habif DV, Papper EM, Fitzpatrick HF, et al: The renal and hepatic blood flow, glomerular filtration rate, and urinary output of electrolytes during cyclopropane, ether, and thiopental anesthesia, operation, and the immediate postoperative period. Surgery 30:241, 1951
26. Deutsch S, Goldberg M, Stephen GW, et al: Effects of halothane anesthesia on renal function in normal man. Anesthesiology 27: 793, 1966
27. Mazze RI, Cousins MJ, Barr GA: Renal effects and metabolism of isoflurane in man. Anesthesiology 40:536, 1974
28. Cousins MJ, Greenstein LR, Hitt BA, et al: Metabolism and renal effects of enflurane in man. Anesthesiology 44:44, 1976
29. Barry KG, Malloy JP: Oliguric renal failure. JAMA 179:510, 1962
30. Harrel RM, Sibley R, Vogelzang NJ: Renal vascular lesions after chemotherapy with vinblastine, bleomycin, and cisplatin. Am J Med 73:429, 1982
31. Sandler DP, Burr FR, Weinberg CR: Nonsteroidal anti-inflammatory drugs and the risk for chronic renal disease. Ann Intern Med 115: 165, 1991
32. Perneger TV, Whelton PK, Klag MJ: Risk of kidney failure as-

sociated with the use of acetaminophen, aspirin and nonsteroidal antiinflammatory drugs. N Engl J Med 331:1675, 1994
33. Farrow PR, Wilkinsin R: Reversible renal failure during treatment with captopril. Br Med J 1:1680, 1979
34. Abel R: Etiology, incidence, and prognosis of renal failure following cardiac operations. J Thorac Cardiovasc Surg 71:323, 1976
35. Slogoff S, Reul GJ, Keats AS, et al: Role of perfusion pressure and flow in major organ dysfunction after cardiopulmonary bypass. Ann Thorac Surg 50:911, 1990
36. Davis RF, Lappas DM, Kirklin JK, et al: Acute oliguria after cardiopulmonary bypass: renal functional improvement with low dose dopamine infusion. Crit Care Med 10:852, 1982
37. Ruiz-Guinazu A, Coelho JB, Paz RA: Methemoglobin-induced acute renal failure in the rat: in vivo observation, histology and micropuncture measures. Nephron 4:257, 1967
38. Flanigan WJ, Oken DE: Renal micropuncture study of the development of anuria in the rat with mercury-induced renal failure. J Clin Invest 44:449, 1965
39. Olsen TS, Skjolkborg H: The fine structure of the renal glomerulus in acute anuria. Acta Pathologica Microbiologica Scandinavica 70:205, 1967
40. Hollenberg NK, Epstein M, Rosen SM, et al: Acute oliguric renal failure in man: evidence for preferential renal cortical ischemia. Medicine 47:455, 1968
41. Hollenberg NK, Adams DF, Oken DE, et al: Acute renal failure due to nephrotoxins: renal hemodynamic and angiographic studies in man. N Engl J Med 282:1329, 1970
42. Hollenberg NK, Birtch A, Rashid A, et al: Relationships between intrarenal perfusion and function: serial hemodynamic studies in the transplanted human kidney. Medicine 51:95, 1972
43. Hollenberg NK, McDonald FD, Cotran R, et al: Irreversible acute oliguric renal failure: a complication of methoxyflurane anesthesia. N Engl J Med 286:877, 1972
44. Goormaghtigh N: Vascular and circulatory changes in renal cortex in anuric crush syndrome. Proc Soc Exp Biol Med 59:303, 1945
45. Tu WH: Plasma renin activity in acute tubular necrosis and other renal disease associated with hypertension. Circulation 31:686, 1965
46. DiBona GE, Sawin LL: The renin-angiotensin system in acute renal failure in the rat. Lab Invest 25:528, 1971
47. Ladefoged T, Winkler K: Effect of dihydralazine and acetylcholine on renal blood flow, mean circulation time for plasma and renal resistance in acute renal failure. In Gessler U, Schroder K, Weldinger H (eds): Pathogenesis and clinical findings with renal failure. Stuttgart: Georg Thieme, 1971: 7
48. Novis BK, Roizen MF, Aronson S, et al: Association of preoperative risk factors with postoperative acute renal failure. Anesth Analg 78:143, 1994
49. Barry KG, Mazze RI, Schwartz FD: Prevention of surgical oliguria and renal-hemodynamic suppression by sustained hydration. N Engl J Med 270:1371, 1964
50. Zaloga GP, Hughes SS: Oliguria in patients with normal renal function. Anesthesiology 72:598, 1990
51. Lappas D, Lell WA, Gabel JC, et al: Indirect measurement of the left atrial pressure in surgical patients: pulmonary capillary wedge and pulmonary artery diastolic pressures compared with left atrial pressure. Anesthesiology 38:394, 1973
52. Gravenstein N, Good ML: Noninvasive assessment of cardiopulmonary function. In Civetta JM, Taylor RW, Kirby RR (eds): Critical care, 2nd ed. Philadelphia: JB Lippincott, 1992: 291
53. Linder A: Synergism of dopamine and furosemide in diuretic-resistant, oliguric acute renal failure. Nephron 33:121, 1983
54. Kramer HJ, Wasserman C, Dusing R: Prostaglandin-independent protection by furosemide from oliguric ischemic renal failure in conscious rats. Kidney Int 17:455, 1980
55. Cantarovich F, Locatelli A, Fernandez JC, et al: Furosemide in high doses in the treatment of acute renal failure. Postgrad Med J 47(suppl):13, 1971
56. Muth RG: Furosemide in acute renal failure. In Friedman EA, Eliahou HE (eds): Proceedings: Conference on Acute Renal Failure, publication no. (NIH) 74-608. Bethesda, MD: Department of Health, Education, and Welfare, 1973: 245
57. Barry KG, Cohen A, LeBlanc P: Mannitolization: I. the prevention and therapy of oliguria associated with cross-clamping of the abdominal aorta. Surgery 50:335, 1961
58. Stahl WM, Stone AM: Prophylactic diuresis with ethacrynic acid. Ann Surg 172:361, 1970
59. Brun-Brusson C, LeCall JR: Dopamine and furosemide in acute renal failure. Lancet 2:1301, 1980
60. Madias NF, Harrington JT: Platinum nephrotoxicity. Am J Med 65:307, 1978
61. Schwab SJ, Hlatky MA, Pieper KS, et al: Contrast nephrotoxicity: A randomized controlled trial of a nonionic and an ionic radiographic contrast agent. N Engl J Med 320:149, 1989
62. Walshe JJ, Venuto RC: Acute oliguric renal failure induced by indomethacin: possible mechanisms. Ann Intern Med 91:47, 1979
63. Whelton A, Stout RL, Spilman PS, et al: Renal effects of ibuprofen, piroxicam and sulindac in patients with asymptomatic renal failure. Ann Int Med 112:568, 1990
64. Boucher BA, Coffee BC, Kuhl DA, et al: Algorithm for assessing renal dysfunction risk in critically ill trauma patients receiving aminoglycosides. Am J Surg 160:473, 1990
65. Birndor N: DIC and renal failure. J Lab Invest 24:314, 1971
66. Better OS: The crush syndrome revisited (1940-1990). Nephron 55:97, 1990
67. Spurney RF, Fulkerson WJ, Schwab SJ: Acute renal failure in critically ill patients: prognosis for recovery after dialysis support. Crit Care Med 19:8, 1991

FURTHER READING

Kellen M, Aronson S, Roizen M, et al: Predictive and diagnostic tests of renal failure: a review. Anesth Analg 78:134, 1994

Mazze RI: Critical care of the patient with acute renal failure. Anesthesiology 47:138, 1977

Muther RS: Acute renal failure: acute azotemia in the critically ill. In Civetta JM, Taylor RW, Kirby RR (eds): Critical care, 2nd ed. Philadelphia: JB Lippincott, 1992: 1583

Schrier RW, Conger JD: Acute renal failure: pathogenesis, diagnosis, and management. In Schrier RW (ed): Renal and electrolyte disorders, 2nd ed. Boston: Little, Brown, 1980: 375

Complications in Anesthesiology, second edition, edited by Nikolaus Gravenstein and Robert R. Kirby. Lippincott-Raven Publishers, Philadelphia © 1996.

CHAPTER 35

Polyuria

Jeffrey M. Baden
Richard I. Mazze*

Polyuria is defined as daily urinary output greater than 2.5 L in a 70-kg person; the normal 24-hour urinary output ranges from 0.5 to 1.5 L. Any of many physiologic and pathologic processes may result in polyuria. These vary from a transitory excessive intake of fluids to potentially fatal acute renal failure. In addition to conditions that may lead to polyuria but are not associated with surgery, several conditions also occur during anesthesia and operations.

CLINICAL PRESENTATION

The patient may be the first to notice the passage of more than the normal amount of urine. Alternatively, a nurse or physician may notice an increased urinary output. Prolonged and severe polyuria results in dehydration, hypernatremia, and, in some cases, neurologic symptoms such as confusion, apathy, and coma. In the latter circumstances, the symptom of increased urinary output cannot be elicited, and the diagnosis may be obscured. Similarly, when the patient is anesthetized or unconscious because of disease or trauma, the diagnosis is more difficult. In these instances, the only way to assess the rate of urine formation accurately is by using an indwelling bladder catheter.

PATHOPHYSIOLOGIC FEATURES

Inability to Concentrate Urine

Pathologic processes that result in an inability to concentrate urine may be grouped into two broad categories of *diabetes insipidus*: those associated with little or no antidiuretic hormone (ADH) and those in which ADH concentration is normal.[1,2]

Central Diabetes Insipidus

A concentrating defect associated with no ADH or low concentrations of circulating ADH is called *central* diabetes insipidus (Table 35-1). Urine output is high, and urine osmolality typically ranges from 50 to 200 mOsm/kg. Central diabetes insipidus is most frequently acquired as a result of disease or trauma to the pituitary–hypophyseal axis.

Psychogenic polydipsia is the next most common cause of central diabetes insipidus. This condition is often difficult to distinguish from primary, idiopathic central diabetes insipidus. In the latter case, water is drunk because of dehydration secondary to persistent and uncontrollable polyuria. With time, overcompensation tends to occur, resulting in hyponatremia and serum hypo-osmolality. The compulsive water-drinker is overhydrated from the start, manifesting hyponatremia, serum hypo-osmolality, and polyuria secondary to suppression of ADH formation.

DIFFERENTIAL DIAGNOSIS. Deprivation of water for 24 hours or more, with frequent measurements of serum and urine sodium and osmolality, distinguishes these two causes (Table 35-2). Patients with primary, idiopathic central diabetes insipidus cannot increase urinary osmolality to a great extent, despite hypernatremia and serum hyperosmolality, whereas patients with psychogenic polydipsia ultimately can concentrate their urine.

Usually, the underlying cause of central diabetes insipidus cannot be eliminated, even when it can be found. Thus, hormone replacement therapy often is required. Most commonly used these days is desmopressin acetate, which is a synthetic analogue of 8-arginine vasopressin and can be administered intravenously, subcutaneously, or by nasal spray.

In less severe cases, nonhormonal measures may suffice. Reducing the obligatory solute load by dietary restriction occasionally is of value. More success has been achieved by administration of thiazide diuretic agents, which act by contracting the extracellular fluid volume and by reducing delivery

* See Credits, page iv.

TABLE 35-1
Causes of Central Diabetes Insipidus (Absence or Low Concentration of Antidiuretic Hormone)

- Acquired
  - Brain tumor
  - Head trauma
  - Post-neurosurgical
  - Infectious disorders (eg, encephalitis)
  - Vascular disorders (eg, Hand-Schüller-Christian disease or sarcoidosis)
- Psychogenic: polydipsia (compulsive water-drinking)
- Primary, idiopathic
- Familial

of filtrate to the distal nephrons.[3] Chlorpropamide also is effective, in patients who have some residual ADH release from the posterior pituitary gland.

Nephrogenic Diabetes Insipidus

The second major type of diabetes insipidus is *nephrogenic* (Table 35-3).[4] In patients with this condition, renal tubular response to adequate concentrations of ADH is impaired. Nephrogenic diabetes insipidus after administration of methoxyflurane is the most clearly definable, anesthesia-related cause of polyuria.

Because the origin of diabetes insipidus, whether central or nephrogenic, usually is apparent, the following discussion does not distinguish between these major categories. Additional information can be found in Harrington and Cohen's excellent review of clinical disorders of urine concentration and dilution.[5]

PREOPERATIVE POLYURIA

Investigation of the cause of polyuria in patients undergoing surgery should include a determination of the onset of increased urinary output in relation to the time of the operation. In the majority of conditions with which it is associated, polyuria may have been present before the operation.

Causes

In many patients, the cause of polyuria can be readily determined from the history, physical examination, and a few simple laboratory investigations. For example, polyuria, urinary tract infection, weight loss, signs of peripheral vascular disease, neuropathy, and glycosuria are very likely associated with diabetes mellitus, whereas polyuria, headache, and failing vision suggest a hypothalamic tumor.[6,7] However, when chronic renal disease, such as pyelonephritis[8] and nephrocalcinosis,[9] or systemic disease, such as amyloidosis[10] and malnutrition,[11] results in polyuria, the exact cause is more difficult to determine.

In all cases, a careful history of drug intake should be obtained to identify agents that may be directly nephrotoxic, such as lithium carbonate,[12] tetracycline,[13] and gentamicin.[14] Also, treatment with diuretic agents may result in polyuria, either primarily as a therapeutic effect or secondarily as a toxic phenomenon, if potassium replacement has not been adequate.[15]

Every effort should be made to determine and to treat the causes of polyuria. Recognition that a patient is polyuric before surgery is important in the planning of intraoperative and postoperative fluid therapy. Careful preoperative investigation also prevents errors in management that occur when polyuria that is present before operation is first discovered during or after the operation.

INTRAOPERATIVE POLYURIA

Excessive Fluid Administration

A common cause of diuresis is the parenteral administration of excessive amounts of water during the perioperative period. Traumatized patients and patients undergoing extensive operations frequently require large volumes of intravenous fluids to maintain an adequate circulating blood volume. Fluid requirements in these persons are difficult to quantitate because of the shift of large volumes from the intravascular compartment into the extravascular, interstitial compartment, the "third space." The problem is further complicated if large quantities of crystalloids have been administered, because ap-

TABLE 35-2
Water Deprivation Test to Differentiate Causes of Diabetes Insipidus

	MAXIMUM U OSMOLALITY*	MAXIMUM U/P OSMOLALITY	CHANGE AFTER SUBCUTANEOUS VASOPRESSIN (%)	MAXIMUM U/P OSMOLALITY AFTER VASOPRESSIN
Normal	800 to 1200	>1	<9	>1
Diabetes Insipidus				
Central (Psychogenic polydipsia)	400	>1	>9	>1
Central (complete)	100 to 200	<1	>50	Variable
Nephrogenic	<200	<1	<45	<1

P, plasma; *U*, urine.
* In milliosmoles per kilogram water.

TABLE 35-3
Causes of Nephrogenic Diabetes Insipidus (Normal Levels of Antidiuretic Hormone)

CONGENITAL
(with or without hydronephrosis)

ACQUIRED
Hypokalemia (eg, hypokalemia from diuretic therapy)
Hypercalcemia or nephrocalcinosis
Osmotic diuresis (eg, diabetes mellitus)
Nonoliguric acute renal failure
Recovery phase of oliguric acute renal failure
Chronic pyelonephritis or hydronephrosis
Drugs
  Methyoxyflurane
  Demeclocycline
  Gentamicin
  Tetracycline (outdated)
  Lithium carbonate
  Amphotericin B
Period after relief of urinary tract obstruction
Other conditions
  Hypertension
  Cirrhosis
  Malnutrition
  Anorexia nervosa
  Sickle cell disease
  Amyloidosis

proximately three fourths of the amount infused rapidly leaves the intravascular compartment and passes to the interstitium.

Elimination of excess fluid in some cases begins during the operation. If isotonic fluids have been administered, ADH secretion is reduced in response to the expansion of intravascular volume; if hypotonic fluids have been given, decreased serum osmolality is an additional stimulus to reduction of ADH secretion. Most frequently, however, renal excretion of sequestered water begins on the 2nd or 3rd day after surgery.

Osmotic Diuresis

An additional cause of intraoperative polyuria is osmotic diuresis resulting from hyperglycemia. The proximal tubules of the kidney usually reabsorb all filtered glucose provided that a concentration limit, normally 180 to 200 mg/dL glucose in arterial plasma, is not exceeded. During anesthesia and operation, this value may be lower, and glucose intolerance may be present. If the threshold for glucose is exceeded, the transport mechanism becomes saturated; glucose appears in the urine; and excess excretion of water follows. A source of excess glucose during operation may be parenterally administered fluids. Marked inoperative hyperglycemia usually can be prevented by restricting parenteral glucose intake during operation to $\leq$100 g (2 L of intravenous fluids containing 5% glucose).

Administration of Diuretic Agents

Intraoperative polyuria may follow diuretic therapy. Diuretic agents often are administered during surgery to prevent or treat renal failure, to reduce intraocular pressure, or to reduce brain size. Mannitol is the most extensively used osmotic agent, although in the past urea and glucose frequently were administered. The potent loop diuretic agents furosemide and ethacrynic acid also may be administered during the operation. They are of undisputed value in the management of acute fluid overload and have been used instead of or in addition to mannitol for the prevention and treatment of surgically induced renal failure. However, intraoperative urinary output does not predict postoperative renal function if blood volume is maintained, at least in patients undergoing abdominal aortic aneurysmectomy.[16]

Neurosurgical Trauma

Surgical interference with the supraopticohypophyseal axis may lead to an absolute or relative lack of circulating ADH.[17,18] In humans the half-life of endogenous ADH concentrations within the physiologic range is approximately 15 minutes.[19] However, after complete surgical ablation of the pituitary gland, polyuria does not occur for at least 12 hours postoperatively, if it occurs at all. Presumably, sufficient stores of ADH remain in cell bodies and can be released at the pituitary stalk or other sites to prevent the immediate occurrence of polyuria. Nevertheless, urinary output should be carefully monitored whenever surgical procedures are carried out on or near the pituitary gland.

POSTOPERATIVE POLYURIA

Most instances of polyuria in patients undergoing surgery first become manifest postoperatively. Although numerous causes of postoperative polyuria can be cited, the one most clearly related to anesthetic administration is the inorganic fluoride nephropathy characteristic of high-dose methoxyflurane anesthesia.

Methoxyflurane Nephrotoxicity

Crandell and colleagues reported that postoperative polyuria developed in 13 of 41 patients anesthetized with methoxyflurane for abdominal surgical procedures.[20] Inability to concentrate urine despite fluid deprivation and vasopressin administration suggested that the polyuria was of renal origin. In most instances normal urine-concentrating ability was restored in 10 to 20 days, although in 3 patients, abnormalities persisted for more than 1 year.

Mazze and coworkers extended those findings with a controlled, randomized, prospective clinical study, in which renal abnormalities developed in all patients anesthetized with methoxyflurane.[21,22] Patients most affected exhibited ADH-resistant polyuria, marked weight loss, hypernatremia, serum hyperosmolality, increased blood urea nitrogen and serum creatinine concentrations, increased serum uric acid concentration, and decreased uric acid clearance. Renal abnormalities did not develop in any of the control patients anesthetized with halothane.

Subsequent studies in rats[23,24] and in humans[25] demonstrated direct relations among methoxyflurane exposure, serum concentrations of the methoxyflurane metabolite, inorganic fluoride, and the degree of postoperative renal dysfunction. In humans methoxyflurane exposures of 2 minimum alveolar concentration (MAC)–hours or less resulted in peak serum inorganic fluoride concentrations of less than 40 μM and were not associated with nephrotoxicity.[25] Exposures of 2.5 to 5 MAC-hours resulted in peak serum inorganic fluoride concentrations of 50 to 80 μM and were associated with mild biochemical abnormalities and with a delay in the return of maximum preoperative urine-concentrating ability. Longer methoxyflurane exposures resulted in fluoride concentrations greater than 100 μM and in symptoms of marked renal dysfunction.

Patients with methoxyflurane nephrotoxicity also have increased serum and urinary oxalic acid concentrations, and oxalic acid crystals have been found in their renal biopsy specimens.[22,26] However, most evidence suggests that inorganic fluoride, rather than oxalic acid, is the primary nephrotoxic methoxyflurane metabolite.[24,25] An additional factor in the development of methoxyflurane nephropathy is the interaction of the anesthetic with nephrotoxic antibiotic agents. Treatment with tetracycline[27] and gentamicin in humans[14] and animals[28] increases the severity of methoxyflurane-induced renal lesions.

Recently, intrarenal production of fluoride has been suggested to be possibly more important in methoxyflurane-induced nephrotoxicity than is hepatic metabolism.[29] If true, this mechanism might explain why patients with allegedly toxic plasma levels of fluoride ion do not sustain nephrotoxicity with isoflurane[20] or sevoflurane.[31] Nephrotoxicity simply may not be related to plasma fluoride concentrations.[32]

Other Fluorinated Anesthetics

In patients undergoing surgery and exposed to an average of 2.9 MAC-hours of enflurane, serum inorganic fluoride concentrations peaked at 22.2 μM[33]; in volunteers exposed to 9.7 MAC-hours of enflurane, fluoride concentrations peaked at 33.6 μM (Fig. 35-1).[34] Polyuria was not seen in either group of subjects, although the volunteers had a 26% decrease in maximum urinary osmolality, compared with preanesthetic values, in response to vasopressin administration. The concentrations of inorganic fluoride and the functional effects observed in these studies indicate that clinically important nephrotoxicity is unlikely to occur in patients with normal renal function.[35] Again, the relevancy of fluoride plasma concentrations may have to be reassessed in light of the isoflurane and sevoflurane data.[29–32]

Enzyme Induction

The role of enzyme induction in fluoride nephropathy is of great clinical interest. In rats[24] and in humans[25] pretreated with either of the classic enzyme-inducers phenobarbital or pentobarbital, methoxyflurane defluorination was enhanced, and nephrotoxicity was more severe. Another enzyme-inducer, phenytoin, also increased methoxyflurane defluorination in rats.[36] In contrast, phenobarbital pretreatment increases in vitro defluorination of isoflurane only slightly and enflurane defluorination not at all.[37]

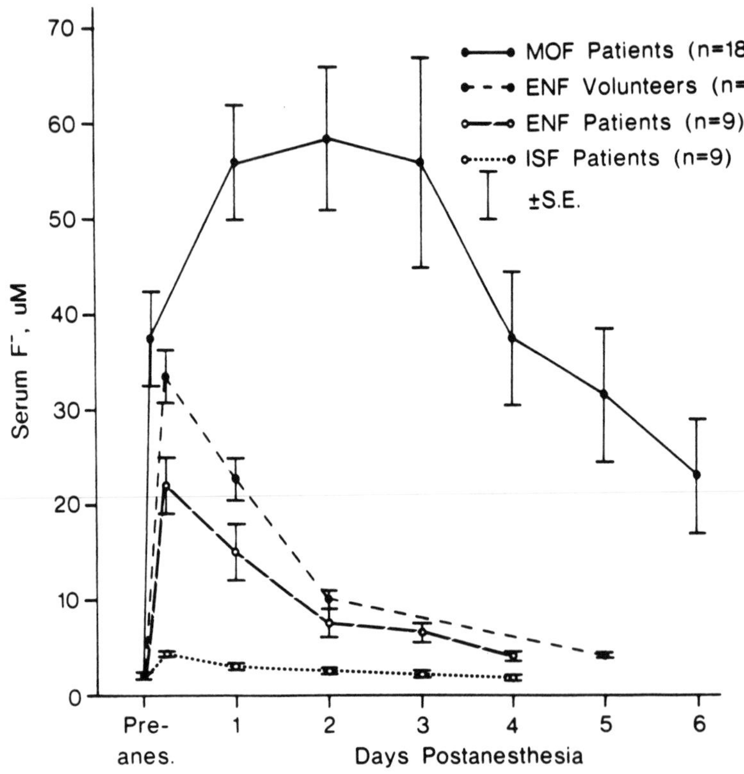

FIGURE 35-1. Serum inorganic fluoride concentrations in patients and volunteers before and after enflurane (*ENF*) anesthesia and in patients before and after isoflurane (*ISF*) and methoxyflurane (*MOF*) anesthesia. A significant increase in serum fluoride concentration immediately followed enflurane anesthesia reached near-peak values of 22.2 ± 2.8 μM in patients and 33.6 ± 2.8 μM in volunteers 4 hours after anesthesia was terminated. After methoxyflurane anesthesia, the mean peak serum fluoride concentration was higher, 61 ± 8 μM, and declined more slowly than after enflurane. After isoflurane, the mean peak serum fluoride concentration was 4.4 ± 0.4 μM. *SE*, standard error.

The result with enflurane is surprising but is consistent with data obtained from a human study in which surgical patients pretreated with a variety of enzyme-inducing drugs showed no increase in serum fluoride concentrations after enflurane anesthesia.[38] However, in several cases isoniazid pretreatment was associated with high serum fluoride concentrations and a transient urine-concentrating defect.[37,38]

A study in rats has confirmed that isoniazid, unlike phenobarbital and phenytoin, significantly increases enflurane defluorination.[39] Furthermore, approximately half of patients undergoing surgery and receiving long-term treatment with isoniazid before enflurane anesthesia have higher serum fluoride concentrations than predicted, but not high enough to produce clinically significant renal impairment.[40]

Renal Failure

Depressed renal function usually returns to normal within a few hours after the operation. Occasionally, however, renal function does not recover rapidly, and acute renal failure may develop.[41] Several factors are responsible for this syndrome, including shock, hypotension, inadequate perioperative fluid replacement, mismatched blood transfusion, and heart failure. The choice of anesthetic is seldom a consideration.

Acute Nonoliguric Renal Failure

Although oliguria is a cardinal sign of acute renal failure, in many patients renal failure is accompanied by normal or even increased urinary output.[42,43] This condition, known as nonoliguric acute renal failure, may be associated with marked biochemical abnormalities. Urinary solute content is relatively low, approximately 300 mOsm/kg, and urinary volume is fixed. This condition has long been recognized as a common form of acute renal failure, making up 50% of cases in two reports.[42,43]

CLINICAL COURSE. Patients with a nonoliguric variety of renal failure spend less time in the hospital and have fewer episodes of sepsis, neurologic abnormalities, and gastrointestinal bleeding; they require less frequent dialysis; and their survival rate is high (74% versus 50% for patients with oliguric renal failure).[43] Presumably, because more nephrons are spared, patients retain some ability to excrete water, electrolytes, and metabolic products.

Diagnosis of nonoliguric acute renal failure is important to prevent serious errors in management of the condition. Death due to overhydration has occurred in patients whose urinary output was fixed in the normal range.[42] In addition, administration of electrolytes, particularly potassium, may be dangerous in patients with nonoliguric renal failure.

Polyuria frequently occurs as the first phase of recovery in patients with oliguric acute renal failure. Daily urinary output doubles for several days, reaching as much as 3 to 6 L/day before returning to normal. Approximately one fourth of the deaths in patients with oliguric renal failure occur during the polyuric phase, so management must be as careful as when urinary output is very low.[43]

Postobstructive Polyuria

Relief of obstruction to urine flow often brings about significant diuresis, the origin of which is incompletely understood.[44] Several factors—including osmotic diuresis from high blood urea nitrogen concentration or excessive salt and water; refractoriness to ADH; or an intrinsic renal tubular insult—may be important. If obstruction is present for less than 2 weeks, prompt return of renal function may occur. After prolonged obstruction, creatinine clearance may not return to normal. Occasionally, a form of nephrogenic diabetes insipidus with obstructive uropathy develops in the kidneys.

REFERENCES

1. Randall RV, Clark EC, Bahn RC: Classification of the causes of diabetes insipidus. Proceedings of the Mayo Clinic 34:299, 1959
2. Chernow B, Willey S, Zaloga GP: Critical care endocrinology. In Shoemaker WC (ed): Textbook of critical care. Philadelphia: WB Saunders, 1989: 736
3. Earley LE, Orloff J: The mechanism of antidiuresis associated with the administration of hydrochlorothiazide to patients with vasopressin resistant diabetes insipidus. J Clin Invest 41:1988, 1962
4. Miller M, Moses AM: Urinary antidiuretic hormone in polyuric disorders and in inappropriate ADH syndrome. Ann Intern Med 77:715, 1972
5. Harrington JT, Cohen JJ: Clinical disorders of urine concentration and dilution. Arch Intern Med 131:810, 1973
6. Blotner H: Primary of idiopathic diabetes insipidus: a systemic disease. Metabolism 7:191, 1958
7. Berliner RW: Outline of renal physiology. In Strauss MB, Welt LG (eds): Diseases of the kidney, 2nd ed. Boston: Little, Brown, 1971: 31
8. Kaye D, Rocha H: Urinary concentrating ability in early experimental pyelonephritis. J Clin Invest 49:1427, 1970
9. Epstein FH: Calcium and the kidney. Am J Med 45:700, 1968
10. Carone FA, Epstein FH: Nephrogenic diabetes insipidus caused by amyloid disease. Am J Med 29:539, 1960
11. Klahr S, Tripathy K, Garcia FT: On the nature of the renal concentrating defect in malnutrition. Am J Med 43:84, 1967
12. Lee RV, Jampol LM, Brown WV: Nephrogenic diabetes insipidus and lithium intoxication: complications of lithium carbonate therapy. N Engl J Med 284:93, 1971
13. Frimpter GW, Timpanelli AE, Eisenmenger WJ, et al: Reversible 'Fanconi syndrome' caused by degraded tetracycline. JAMA 184: 111, 1963
14. Mazze RI, Cousins MJ: Combined nephrotoxicity of gentamicin and methoxyflurane anesthesia in man. Br J Anaesth 45:394, 1973
15. Relman AS, Schwartz WB: The kidney in potassium depletion. Am J Med 24:764, 1958
16. Alpert RA, Roizen MF, Hamilton WK, et al: Intraoperative urinary output does not predict postoperative renal function in patients undergoing abdominal aortic revascularization. Surgery 95:707, 1984
17. Coggins CH, Leaf A: Diabetes insipidus. Am J Med 42:807, 1967
18. Barlow Ed, de Wardener HE: Compulsive water drinking. Q J Med 28:235, 1959
19. Lauson HD: Metabolism of antidiuretic hormones. Am J Med 46:713, 1967
20. Crandell WB, Pappas Sg, Macdonald A: Nephrotoxicity associated with methoxyflurane anesthesia. Anesthesiology 27:591, 1966
21. Mazze RI, Trudell JR, Cousins MJ: Methoxyflurane metabolism and renal dysfunction. Anesthesiology 35:247, 1971
22. Mazze RI, Shue GL, Jackson SH: Renal dysfunction associated with methoxyflurane anesthesia: a randomized, prospective clinical evaluation. JAMA 216:278, 1971

23. Mazze RI, Cousins MJ, Kosek JC: Dose-related methoxyflurane nephrotoxicity in rats: a biochemical and pathologic correlation. Anesthesiology 36:571, 1972
24. Cousins MJ, Mazze RI, Kosek JC: The etiology of methoxyflurane nephrotoxicity. J Pharmacol Exp Ther 190:523, 1974
25. Cousins MJ, Mazze RI: Methoxyflurane nephrotoxicity: a study of dose response in man. JAMA 225:1611, 1973
26. Franscino JA, Vanamee P, Rosen PP: Renal oxalosis and azotemia after methoxyflurane anesthesia. N Engl J Med 283:676, 1970
27. Kuzucu EY: Methoxyflurane, tetracycline, and renal failure. JAMA 211:1162, 1970
28. Barr GA, Mazze RI, Cousins MJ, et al: An animal model for combined methoxyflurane and gentamicin nephrotoxicity. Br J Anaesth 45:306, 1973
29. Kharasch ED, Hankins DC, Thummel KE: Human kidney methoxyflurane and sevoflurane metabolism: intrarenal fluoride production as a possible mechanism of methoxyflurane nephrotoxicity. Anesthesiology 82; 689, 1995
30. Spencer EM, Willatts SM, Prys-Roberts C: Plasma inorganic fluoride concentrations after prolonged (>25 hr) isoflurane sedation: effect on renal function. Anesth Analg 73:731, 1991
31. Kazama T, Ikeda K: The effect of prolonged administration of sevoflurane on serum concentrations of fluoride ion in patients [abstract]. Anesthesiology 75:A346, 1991
32. Brown BB Jr: Shibboleths and jigsaw puzzles: the fluoride nephrotoxicity enigma (editorial). Anesthesiology 82:607, 1995
33. Cousins MJ, Greenstein LR, Hitt BA et al: Metabolism and renal effects of enflurane in man. Anesthesiology 44:44, 1976
34. Mazze RI, Calverley RK, Smith NT: Inorganic fluoride nephrotoxicity. Anesthesiology 46:265, 1977
35. Mazze RI, Sievenpiper TS, Stevenson J: Renal effects of enflurane and halothane in patients with abnormal renal function. Anesthesiology 60:161, 1984
36. Caughey GH, Rice SA, Kosek JC, et al: Effect of phenytoin (DPH) treatment on methoxyflurane metabolism in rats. J Pharmacol Exp Ther 210:180, 1979
37. Hitt BA, Mazze RI: Effect of enzyme induction on nephrotoxicity of halothane related compounds. Environ Health Perspect 21: 179, 1977
38. Dooley JR, Mazze RI, Rice SA, et al: Is enflurane defluorination inducible in man? Anesthesiology 50:213, 1979
39. Rice SA, Sbordone L, Mazze RI: Metabolism by rat microsomes of fluorinated ether anesthetics following isoniazid administration. Anesthesiology 53:489, 1980
40. Mazze RI, Woodruff RE, Heerdt ME: Isoniazid-induced enflurane defluorination in humans. Anesthesiology 57:5, 1982
41. Mazze RI: Critical care of the patient with acute renal failure. Anesthesiology 47:138, 1977
42. Vertel RM, Knochel JP: Nonoliguric acute renal failure. JAMA 200:598, 1967
43. Anderson RJ, Linas SL, Berns AS, et al: Nonoliguric acute renal failure. N Engl J Med 296:1134, 1977
44. Beck C: Disordered renal function: diagnosis. In Civetta JM, Taylor RW, Kirby RR (eds): Critical care, 2nd ed. Philadelphia: JB Lippincott, 1988: 1315

Complications in Anesthesiology, second edition,
edited by Nikolaus Gravenstein and Robert R. Kirby.
Lippincott-Raven Publishers, Philadelphia © 1996.

CHAPTER 36

Urinary Retention

Jeffrey M. Baden
*Richard I. Mazze**

Acute urinary retention is a common complication after surgery and anesthesia. Several mechanisms are involved, including sphincter spasm, bladder neck obstruction, and paralysis of the detrusor muscle. In addition, administration of narcotic and parasympatholytic drugs may result in the inability to void. The serious consequences of unrecognized urinary retention make early diagnosis and correct treatment of this condition mandatory.

NEUROMUSCULAR CONTROL OF THE BLADDER

The smooth muscle of the bladder is arranged in three layers. Only the outer layer, known as the detrusor muscle, is responsible for micturition, the control of which is very complex (Table 36-1). The detrusor muscle is supplied by parasympathetic nerve fibers from the sacral portion of the spinal cord (segments S2 to S4) (Fig. 36-1). Smooth muscle fibers from the detrusor muscle make up the internal sphincter, whereas the external urethral sphincter consists of skeletal muscle. The latter is under conscious control and is supplied by somatic nerve fibers (from the spinal cord in segments S3 and S4) carried in the pudendal nerves.

The bladder also receives sympathetic nerve fibers from the inferior mesenteric ganglion. Sympathetic stimulation inhibits bladder contraction and increases the tone of the internal vesical sphincter. During normal voiding, these nerve fibers are inactive. Sometimes during voiding, however, they may be abnormally stimulated, causing dysergia or inhibiting voiding.

Micturition is an autonomic spinal reflex that is both facilitated and inhibited by higher centers. The urge to void usually occurs when intravesicular pressure reaches 10 cmH_2O, corresponding to a bladder volume of approximately 150 mL. At a volume of 400 mL, a marked sense of fullness usually is present. Micturition involves initial relaxation of the perineal muscles and external urethral sphincters, followed by contraction of the detrusor muscle. Proper function, therefore, requires an intact neuromuscular system and an unobstructed pathway for the flow of urine.[1]

PATHOPHYSIOLOGIC FEATURES OF URINARY RETENTION

Postoperative urinary retention may occur for several reasons. Operations in and around the pelvis and bladder, with subsequent trauma to the detrusor muscle and damage to the pelvic nerves, can inhibit bladder action. Edema around the bladder neck and reflex spasm of the sphincters caused by pain or anxiety may contribute. It is not surprising that the incidence of postoperative urinary retention is highest in operations on the genitourinary tract, rectum, and other pelvic structures.[2,3]

Anesthetics and Adjuvant Drugs

Many of the drugs used in anesthesia are associated with postoperative urinary retention (Table 36-2), especially when there is preexisting obstructive urinary tract disease, such as prostatic enlargement.

Belladonna Alkaloids

Atropine and scopolamine are used as drying agents; in addition, atropine is administered in combination with neostigmine for reversal of paralysis produced by muscle relaxants. The synthetic parasympatholytic agent glycopyrrolate also can predispose to urinary retention. Although contraction of the urinary bladder is inhibited by these drugs only partly, they decrease intravesical pressure, increase bladder capacity, and reduce the frequency of bladder contractions by their para-

* See Credits, page iv.

TABLE 36-1
Control of Micturition

CONTROLLING FACTOR	EFFECT
Parasympathetic nerve fibers (S2 to S4)	Detrusor muscle contraction
Somatic nerve fibers (S3 and S4) (conscious control)	Control of external urethral sphincter
Sympathetic nerve fibers (inferior mesenteric ganglion)	Inhibition of bladder contraction; increase in tone of internal vesical sphincter
Volume of bladder (mL)	
150 (10 cmH_2O intravesicular pressure)	Urge to void
400	Marked sense of fullness

sympatholytic action.[4,5] Their contribution to postoperative urinary retention is unclear, but their potential to affect micturition adversely should be considered, especially when they are administered to patients with lower urinary tract obstructive disease.

General Anesthetics

These drugs differ among themselves in their urodynamic effects but typically predispose to the development of urinary retention.[5] Thiopental, 5 mg/kg, reduces intravesical pressure and increases bladder capacity. Halothane, 1.5% inspired, causes a small, statistically insignificant reduction in intravesical pressure but a marked increase in bladder capacity. Nitrous oxide and neuromuscular blocking agents have very small, inconsistent, and statistically insignificant urodynamic effects.

Regional Anesthetics

Regional anesthesia is commonly believed to cause postoperative urinary retention more frequently than general anesthesia. The mechanism is presumed to be delayed recovery of autonomic and somatic nerve function, with overdistention of the bladder and resultant atony before recovery of bladder innervation.

That spinal anesthesia leads to more difficulty than does general anesthesia has not been supported by experimental data. In a comprehensive study, Scarborough reviewed the records of 65,000 patients having either spinal or general anesthesia and found no difference between the groups in the incidence of postoperative urinary retention.[6] However, Scarborough's study predated the use of the longer-acting local anesthetic agents, such as bupivacaine, which produce motor block of sufficient duration to increase the likelihood of urinary retention.[7]

LONG-ACTING VERSUS SHORT-ACTING LOCAL ANESTHETICS. Among obstetric patients receiving continuous caudal analgesia for vaginal delivery, 63% of patients receiving bupivacaine had urinary retention compared with only 22% of those receiving chloroprocaine.[8] Similarly, among inguinal herniorrhaphy patients receiving regional analgesia with bupivacaine or regional anesthesia with a shorter acting local anesthetic agent plus bupivacaine by local infiltration, 30% of the former group had urinary retention, compared with only 6% of those receiving short-acting drugs.[9] This difference was not related to patient age, dermatome level of anesthesia, or, interestingly, the volume of intravenous fluid received.

Axelsson and colleagues studied the temporal aspects of the urodynamic effects of prolonged spinal analgesia.[10] The intrathecal injection of bupivacaine (22.5 mg in saline or 20

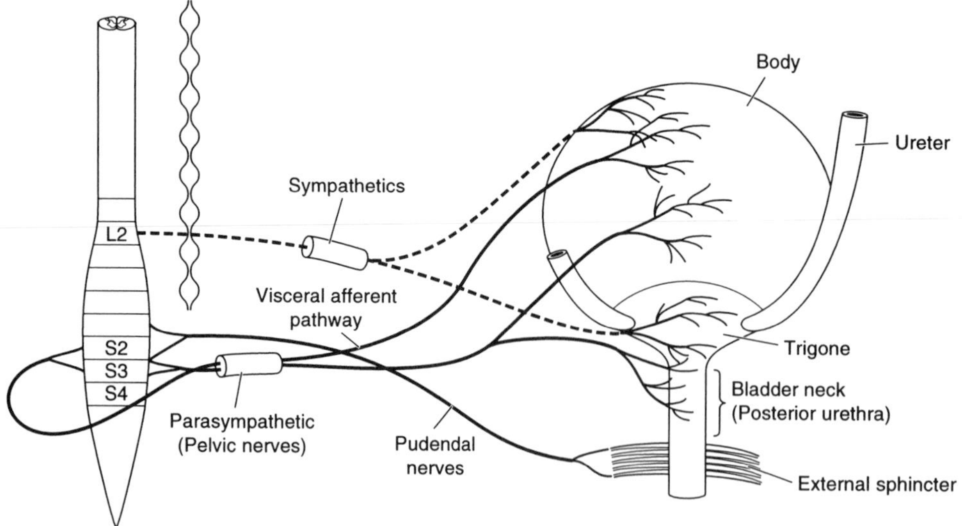

FIGURE 36-1. The innervation of the urinary bladder. (Guyton AG: Renal disease, diuresis and micturition. In: Textbook of medical physiology, 7th ed. Philadelphia: WB Saunders, 1986: 460.)

TABLE 36-2
Anesthetic and Adjuvant Drugs That May Promote Urinary Retention

DRUGS	EFFECT
Belladonna alkaloids	Reduction in intravesicular pressure; increase in bladder capacity; reduction in frequency of bladder contractions
General anesthetics	Variable effects
Regional anesthetics	
Long-acting (eg, bupivacaine)	Significant distention
Short-acting	Insignificant
Spinal and epidural narcotics	As many as 100% of patients affected; greater effect with morphine than with fentanyl
Sedatives and analgesics	Minimal direct effects; possible promotion of retention because of lack of patient awareness

mg in 8% glucose) or of tetracaine (15 mg in 10% glucose) immediately blocked the micturition reflex. When detrusor strength returned, 7 to 8 hours after drug administration, the level of analgesia was L5 or lower. However, patients could not void until full sacral skin sensitivity to pin prick had returned. Considering the duration of bladder denervation and the customary intraoperative hydration rates (300 mL/h or more), they noted that overdistention of the bladder is likely if the patient is not catheterized.

Spinal Narcotics

Spinal narcotics produce urinary retention in as many as 100% of patients; urinary retention is one of the more commonly reported side effects of this mode of postoperative analgesia.[11,12] Doses of morphine of 2, 4, and 10 mg given by epidural injection result in similar degrees of detrusor muscle relaxation and increased bladder capacity.[13] Not unexpectedly, the incidence of urinary retention is the same over the morphine dose range of 0.5 to 8 mg.[14] Thus, the urodynamic effects of spinal narcotics are not dose-related; whether urodynamic effects differ with other narcotics and with the duration of administration is unclear. These effects usually last 14 to 16 hours.[13]

Sedative and Analgesic Agents

Patients who remain heavily sedated and narcotized at the end of an operation are also subject to urinary retention. However, these drugs have minimal, if any, direct urodynamic effects: intramuscular clinical doses of diazepam (10 mg),[5] meperidine (100 mg),[5] and morphine (10 mg)[13] cause very slight if any detrusor relaxation; a 10-mg intravenous dose of morphine causes short-lasting detrusor relaxation, about one-sixth the magnitude of that produced by epidural morphine.[13]

Sedatives and analgesics may result in urinary retention because patients are unaware of bladder distention. Overdistention then leads to atony of the bladder wall and delayed recovery of function when the bladder is emptied.[15] Prolonged treatment, such as indwelling urethral or percutaneous suprapubic catheterization, may be necessary. However, excessive postoperative pain also can make urination impossible. Thus, perioperative administration of narcotic and sedative agents must be accomplished with great skill.

Other Factors

Apart from the use of spinal narcotics, the type and anatomic site of surgery appear to be more important than the type of anesthesia in determining whether urinary retention occurs.[2,3,16] Except for cases of urinary retention relating to spinal narcotics, the overall incidence of this complication is reported to be 1% to 3%. Most cases occur after genitourinary, pelvic, or rectal operations or in the presence of prostatic hyperplasia.[16] In addition, inability to void in the postoperative period is also more likely in the supine position, with peri- and postoperative hypovolemia, and with deep sedation.

CLINICAL PRESENTATION

Physical Findings

Inability to void postoperatively, usually associated with an urgent desire to do so, is the most common clinical presentation. The diagnosis is made by palpating the often tender, distended bladder above the symphysis pubis.

In general, urinary retention may be present in any patient who has not voided within a reasonable period during or after operation. The length of time is variable and depends on the duration of the operation and the amount of fluid administered. A careful examination of any patient who is unable to void must be made if bladder atony and long-term catheterization are to be avoided. However, catheterization may finally be necessary, both to confirm the diagnosis and to institute treatment.

Differential Diagnosis

In addition to impairment of bladder function, several other factors may explain why a patient undergoing surgery is unable to void (Table 36-3). Administration of general anesthesia is associated with a decrease in urine formation, probably because of decreases in renal blood flow and glomerular filtration rate. Inadequate fluid intake before, during, or after surgery also can lead to oliguria and consequent delay in voiding.

TABLE 36-3
Differential Diagnosis of Urinary Retention

Decreased renal blood flow and glomerular filtration rate
Inadequate fluid intake
Acute renal insufficiency or failure
Urinary tract obstruction
Ureteral calculi
Surgical trauma
Blood clots

Patients with acute renal failure usually have oliguria and rarely anuria. Anuria is an important sign of total urinary tract obstruction, such as that due to bilateral ureteral calculi; surgical damage; obstruction of outflow by blood clots; sloughed papillary tissue; compression by pelvic tumors; prostate hypertrophy; urethral strictures; or a neurogenic bladder.

Treatment

Conservative Measures

Lesser degrees of urinary retention are best treated conservatively, by encouraging the patient to urinate (Table 36-4). Most patients are not accustomed to voiding in the horizontal position and can benefit considerably by sitting or standing; early ambulation also is helpful if circumstances permit. Audibly running water, privacy, hot or cold baths, or the suggestion that catheterization may be necessary are techniques that have been successful in inducing patients to void. In general, good nursing care and encouragement give the best results.

Aggressive Measures

PARASYMPATHOMIMETIC DRUGS. When conservative measures fail, other measures are necessary (see Table 36-4). The tone of the detrusor muscle may be increased sufficiently to promote micturition after administration of a parasympathomimetic agent: pilocarpine, as much as 6 to 8 mg orally, or bethanechol, as much as 20 to 50 mg subcutaneously, can be useful. These drugs are administered in small, incremental doses (eg, bethanechol 5 mg subcutaneously hourly) until response is satisfactory or symptoms of excessive cholinergic stimulation, such as biliary or intestinal colic, supervene. They should not be used in cases of obstructive urinary retention, as from prostatic enlargement.

NALOXONE AND PHENOXYBENZAMINE. In cases of urinary retention occurring after administration of a spinal narcotic, a more specific and highly efficacious treatment is use of the narcotic antagonist naloxone. In incremental doses of 100 μg or by infusion at a rate of 10 μg/kg/h, naloxone treats the urinary retention but preserves the analgesia of the epidural or spinal narcotic.[13,17] Phenoxybenzamine reportedly decreases the incidence of urinary retention associated with spinal narcotics when used concurrently; this sympatholytic drug is administered orally, in a dose of 10 mg, 24 hours and 0.5 hour before and 8 and 16 hours after the administration of the spinal narcotic.[18]

Bladder Catheterization

INDICATIONS. When prostatism is likely or when the bladder or surrounding structures have been seriously traumatized, further damage should be prevented, and retention should be alleviated by an indwelling catheter. In patients with vesical neck obstruction undergoing other than prostatic surgery, an indwelling urethral catheter should be inserted at the start of the operation and retained until normal bladder activity resumes. A similar procedure should be followed if surgery is expected to lead to dysfunction or will be prolonged. In other circumstances, catheterization should be performed without delay, as soon as the patient's inability to void becomes apparent.

MAINTENANCE. Great care must be used to insert the catheter by sterile technique and to avoid further trauma to already damaged tissues. Correct management of the catheterized patient is essential. First, the catheter should be kept patent by preventing kinking and obstruction. Most urologists now believe that irrigation of the bladder with normal saline or with a weak acidifying and antiseptic agent, such as mandelamine, is unnecessary because it does not prevent bladder infection if catheterization is protracted.

Routine bacterial culture should be performed and antibiotic therapy should be instituted when necessary. Catheters should be changed at regular intervals to prevent the deposit of urinary salts, which can serve as a nidus for infection and for formation of bladder stones. After catheter removal, the patient should be observed frequently to ensure that urinary retention does not recur. In certain cases, use of suprapubic percutaneous catheters should be considered because they avoid urethral trauma and facilitate a trial of voiding.

Preventive Measures

Assuming that sedatives, parasympatholytic drugs, and intravenous fluids are used with caution, the type of anesthesia

TABLE 36-4
Treatment of Urinary Retention

CONSERVATIVE
Encouragement
Privacy
Sitting or standing
Early ambulation
Audibly running water
Hot or cold baths
Suggestion that catheterization may be necessary
AGGRESSIVE
Parasympathomimetic drugs
Naloxone or phenoxybenzamine
Bladder catheterization

(with the exception of spinal narcotics) appears to have only a small influence on the occurrence and severity of postoperative urinary retention. Care during surgery, with avoidance of injury to the genitourinary tract, is the best form of prophylaxis. The anesthesiologist and surgeon should be constantly alert for this potentially serious but eminently treatable complication.

REFERENCES

1. Karu M: Nervous control of micturition. Physiol Rev 45:425, 1965
2. Bomze EJ: Bladder dysfunction following gynecological surgery. Western Journal of Surgery 62:3225, 1954
3. Egbert LD: Spinal anesthesia for anorectal surgery. Int Anesthesiol Clin 1:811, 1983
4. Brown JH: Atropine, scopolamine and related antimuscarinic drugs. In Gilman AG, Goodman LS, Rall TW (eds): The pharmacological basis of therapeutics, 8th ed. New York: Macmillan, 1990: 150
5. Doyle PT, Briscoe CE: The effects of drugs and anaesthetic agents on the urinary bladder and sphincters. Br J Urol 48:329, 1976
6. Scarborough RA: Spinal anesthesia from the surgeon's standpoint. JAMA 168:1324, 1958
7. Tattersall MP: Isobaric bupivacaine and hyperbaric amethocaine for spinal analgesia. Anaesthesia 38:115, 1983
8. Bridenbaugh LD: Catheterization after long- and short-acting local anesthetics for continuous caudal block for vaginal delivery. Anesthesiology 46:357, 1977
9. Ryan JA Jr, Adye BA, Jolly PC, et al: Outpatient inguinal herniorrhaphy with both regional and local anesthesia. Am J Surg 148:313, 1984
10. Axelsson K, Möllefors K, Olsson JO, et al: Bladder function in spinal anaesthesia. Acta Anaesthesiol Scand 29:315, 1985
11. Cousins MJ, Mather LE: Intrathecal and epidural administration of opioids. Anesthesiology 61:276, 1984
12. Weddel SJ, Ritter RR: Serum levels following epidural administration of morphine and correlation with relief of postsurgical pain. Anesthesiology 54:210, 1981
13. Rawal N, Möllefors K, Axelsson, et al: An experimental study of urodynamic effects of epidural morphine and of naloxone reversal. Anesth Analg 62:641, 1983
14. Martin R, Salbaing J, Blaise G, et al: Epidural morphine for postoperative pain relief: a dose–response curve. Anesthesiology 56:423, 1982
15. Creevy CDP: The care of the urinary bladder after operation. Surgery 7:423, 1940
16. Lund PC: Principles and practice of spinal anesthesia. Springfield: Charles C Thomas, 1971: 631
17. Jones RDM, Jones JG: Intrathecal morphine: naloxone reverses respiratory depression but not analgesia. Br Med J 281:645, 1980
18. Evron S, Samueloff A, Sadovsky E, et al: The effect of phenoxybenzamine on postoperative urinary complications during extradural morphine analgesia. Eur J Anaesthesiol 1:45, 1984

Complications in Anesthesiology, second edition,
edited by Nikolaus Gravenstein and Robert R. Kirby.
Lippincott-Raven Publishers, Philadelphia © 1996.

CHAPTER 37

Disorders of Acid–Base Regulation

Robert R. Kirby
Walter C. Bernards

Disturbances in acid–base homeostasis are common. Currently available techniques, specifically the pH and carbon dioxide partial pressure (P_{CO_2}) electrodes, make the measurement of these disturbances a simple matter. Yet the proper diagnosis and treatment of acid–base disorders remain among the more difficult and poorly performed tasks in the practice of anesthesiology and acute care medicine.

The fault lies in large measure with the frequently changing terminology and the confusing mathematics used to present this subject. Physicians who have little difficulty handling far more difficult problems of various other fluid and electrolyte imbalances are often bewildered when they attempt to understand a subject in which concentrations are expressed as logarithms of inverted fractions. The rote use of derived or artificial parameters such as standard bicarbonate, buffer base, or base excess has done little to increase understanding; when they are applied in the clinical setting without an appreciation of their limitations, serious errors in therapy can result.

This confusion is unnecessary. An understanding of the chemistry of acids and bases sufficient to allow interpretation of the type of acid–base disturbance (ie, respiratory, metabolic, or mixed) and to quantitate the degree of disturbance is within the easy reach of every interested clinician.

CHEMISTRY OF ACIDS AND BASES

It will be helpful to begin with a review of a few fundamentals of chemistry.

Fundamental Concepts

An acid is a molecule or ion with a tendency to dissociate a hydrogen ion or proton (H^+); a base is a molecule or ion with a tendency to bind or associate a H^+. Table 37-1 lists representative acids and their conjugate bases. As can be seen in this table, the charge on a molecule has no direct bearing on its acid property: acids may be cations (positively charged ions), may be anions (negatively charged ions), or may be neutral. The common denominator of an acid then is not its charge but its tendency to dissociate H^+.

Hydrogen Ion Concentration

pH

The concentration of H^+ in most biologic fluids is extremely small. That in blood and extracellular fluid (ECF) is 0.00000004 Mol/L. With severe acidemia, this value might increase to 0.00000016 Mol/L, and with a severe alkalemia, it could decrease to 0.000000016 Mol/L. These are extremely small numbers, are cumbersome to write, and difficult to interpret. Sorenson,[1] in 1909, suggested the expression of H^+ concentration as negative logarithms, for which he introduced the term "potential of hydrogen" (pH). Thus, a H^+ concentration of 0.00000004 Mol/L may be expressed simply as pH 7.4, one of 0.00000016 Mol/L may be expressed simply as pH 6.8, and one of 0.000000016 Mol/L may be expressed as pH 7.8.

Nanoequivalents

Although the pH concept simplified the expression of H^+ concentration and proved to be a help to the chemist, it has been, in some respects, the greatest single reason for the difficulties encountered by clinicians in understanding acid–base chemistry.[2–4] To circumvent this difficulty and return H^+ concentration figures to arithmetic rather than logarithmic expression, Campbell[5,6] in 1962 introduced the term "nanoequivalent" (nanomol), a unit equal to 10^{-9} Mol, or 1 milli-

TABLE 37-1
Examples of Acids and Conjugate Bases

ACID		CONJUGATE BASE
Acetic acid (CH_3COOH)	↔	$CH_3COO^- + H^+$
Dihydrogen phosphate (H_2PO_4)	↔	$HPO_4^- + H^+$
Carbonic acid (H_2CO_3)	↔	$HCO_3^- + H^+$
Ammonium (NH_4^+)	↔	$NH_3 + H^+$
Bicarbonate (HCO_3^-)	↔	$CO_3 + H^+$
Sulfuric acid (H_2SO_4)	↔	$HSO_4^- + H^+$

Bernards WC, Kirby RR: Acid-base chemistry and physiology. In Civetta JM, Taylor RW, Kirby RR (eds): Critical care, 2nd ed. Philadelphia: JB Lippincott, 1992: 344.

TABLE 37-3
Relative Extracellular Concentrations of Physiologically Important Cations and Anions

	CONCENTRATION	
CATION OR ANION	*mMol/L*	*nMol/L*
H^+	0.00004	40
Potassium	4.0	4,000,000
Bicarbonate	24.0	24,000,000
Chloride	100.0	100,000,000
Sodium	140.0	140,000,000

micromol. The normal H^+ concentration of blood and ECF is simply expressed as 40 nMol/L. The range of H^+ concentration compatible with life is approximately 16 to 160 nMol/L (pH 7.8 to 6.8). Table 37-2 lists some comparable values for pH and nanomols per liter.

When the other common ionic constituents of the blood are expressed in nEq/L, as in Table 37-3, one gets a better appreciation of the relatively small number of H^+ present. Why should such a minute amount of H^+ have such a profound effect on body chemistry? The reason lies, in part at least, in the size of the H^+. The atomic radius of a H^+ is only 10^{-13} cm, whereas that of most of the other simple ions in the blood is 10^{-8} cm (ie, the H^+ is only 1/100,000th as large as a sodium or chloride ion). It has access to reaction sites on molecules that are simply not approachable by other larger ions.

pK and the Henderson-Hasselbalch Equation

Some acids, such as hydrochloric acid (HCl) and sulfuric acid (H_2SO_4), are essentially totally dissociated in aqueous solution and are strong acids. Others, such as acetic acid (CH_3COOH) or carbonic acid (H_2CO_3), have a lesser tendency to dissociate an H^+ and are weak acids. In accordance with the law of mass action, the tendency of a weak acid to dissociate a H^+ will depend in part on the total H^+ concentration (ie, acidity) of the solution in which the weak acid exists. The following equilibrium exists:

$$HA \leftrightarrow A^- + H^+ \quad (1)$$

where HA = a weak monobasic acid, and A^- = its conjugate base.

As the concentration of H^+ in the solution increases, the reversible reaction will shift to the left, and the weak acid will become less dissociated. The converse is true as the concentration of H^+ in the solution decreases; the equilibrium will shift to the right, leaving less undissociated acid.

The tendency of any specific weak acid to dissociate is given by its dissociation constant, K:

$$K = \frac{[H^+][A^-]}{[HA]} \quad (2)$$

Just as H^+ concentration commonly is expressed as its negative logarithm and symbolized as pH, so also is the dissociation tendency of weak acids expressed in terms of the negative logarithm of their dissociation constants and symbolized as pK.

From these relations, the very useful Henderson-Hasselbalch equation can be derived. First, Equation 2 is solved for H^+ concentration.

$$[H^+] = K\frac{[HA]}{[A^-]} \quad (3)$$

Both sides are multiplied by −log:

$$-\log [H^+] = -\log K - \log \frac{[HA]}{[A^-]} \quad (4)$$

Substituting pH for $-\log H^+$ and pK for $-\log K$:

$$pH = pK - \log \frac{[HA]}{[A^-]} \quad (5)$$

Finally, inverting the negative log fraction:

$$pH = pK + \log \frac{[A^-]}{[HA]} \quad (6)$$

Equation 6 is the Henderson-Hasselbalch equation.

The log of 1 = 0; the Henderson-Hasselbalch equation thus defines the pK of a weak acid as the pH at which the acid is

TABLE 37-2
pH Values and Corresponding Hydrogen Ion Concentrations

pH	H^+ CONCENTRATION (nMol/L)
6.0	1,000
6.8	160
7.0	100
7.2	63
7.4	40
7.6	25
7.8	16
8.0	10
9.0	1

Bernards WC, Kirby RR: Acid-base chemistry and physiology. In Civetta JM, Taylor RW, Kirby RR (eds): Critical care, 2nd ed. Philadelphia: JB Lippincott, 1992: 344.

50% dissociated—that is, the pH at which equal quantities of acid and its conjugate base are present.

$$\begin{aligned} pH &= pK + \log 1 \\ &= pK + 0 \\ &= pK \end{aligned} \qquad (7)$$

In a solution the pH of which is 1 unit greater than the pK, the ratio of base to acid is 10 to 1; at a pH 2 units greater than the pK, the ratio of base to acid is 100 to 1; and so on.

Over a pH range 2 units greater than and less than its pK, a weak acid is titrated from almost totally in its dissociated or basic form (>99%) to almost totally in its undissociated or acidic form (>99%), respectively. For this reason, the maximum range over which a weak acid can function as a buffer (ie, bind or donate H^+) is 1.5 to 2 pH units on either side of its pK.

NORMAL VALUES AND DEFINITIONS OF TERMS

The blood is in normal acid–base status when pH = 7.4, arterial carbon dioxide partial pressure (Pa_{CO_2}) = 40 mm Hg, and actual bicarbonate concentration = 24 mMol/L (Table 37-4). To decrease the confusion arising from the varying nomenclature in use, the following definitions are commonly used[5]:

Acidemia: H^+ concentration greater than the normal range of 36 to 44 nMol/L (pH less than 7.36)
Alkalemia: H^+ concentration less than the normal range of 36 to 44 nMol/L (pH greater than 7.44)
Acidosis: a physiologic condition that would cause acidemia if it were not compensated
Alkalosis: a physiologic condition that would cause alkalemia if it were not compensated.

Primary and Compensatory Processes

Processes causing acidosis or alkalosis may be conveniently divided into respiratory and metabolic (nonrespiratory) categories. Respiratory acidosis denotes a primary (ie, noncompensatory) increase in Pa_{CO_2} to greater than the normal range of 36 to 44 mm Hg. All other primary processes tending to cause acidemia are, by definition, metabolic. Similarly, respiratory alkalosis denotes a primary decrease in Pa_{CO_2} to less than the normal range of 36 to 44 mm Hg. All other primary processes tending to cause alkalemia are, by definition, metabolic. These definitions of acidosis and alkalosis have been a source of unnecessary confusion. An example helps to clarify their usage.

A patient with chronic obstructive lung disease leading to hypoventilation and a Pa_{CO_2} of 60 mm Hg can achieve a bicarbonate concentration of 34 mMol/L and a normal pH of 7.38 because of renal production and conservation of bicarbonate. To say that acid–base status is "normal" simply because the pH is normal is incorrect. Pulmonary disease is causing a primary increase in Pa_{CO_2}.

The potential semantic dilemma is avoided by using the terms "acidosis" and "alkalosis" to refer to the primary pathologic process and then to describe the degree and type of compensation. In this instance, the patient has chronic respiratory acidosis but has full renal compensation. (In previous years, this renal response was referred to as "compensating renal metabolic alkalosis.")[7]

TABLE 37-4
Normal Acid–Base Values

PARAMETER	VALUE
pH	7.40 ± 0.04
H^+	4.0 ± 4.0 nMol (nEq/L)
Pa_{CO_2}	40.0 ± 4.0 mmHg
Actual bicarbonate	24.0 ± 2.0 mMol/L

Bernards WC, Kirby RR: Acid-base chemistry and physiology. In Civetta JM, Taylor RW, Kirby RR (eds): Critical care, 2nd ed. Philadelphia: JB Lippincott, 1992: 344.

QUANTITATION OF DISTURBANCES

Respiratory

Arterial Carbon Dioxide Partial Pressure

The normal range of Pa_{CO_2} is 36 to 44 mm Hg (see Table 37-4). With the exception of ventilatory compensation for primary metabolic disturbances, an increase of Pa_{CO_2} to greater than 44 mm Hg is a sign of respiratory acidosis, and a decrease to less than 36 mm Hg represents a state of respiratory alkalosis. These diagnoses are among the easiest in medicine, requiring simply a glance at the Pa_{CO_2}.

Alveolar Ventilation

Quantitation also is simple. Assuming a constant rate of carbon dioxide production, an inverse relation exists between the volume of alveolar ventilation and the Pa_{CO_2}. If the former doubles, the Pa_{CO_2} will decrease by 50%; if alveolar ventilation is halved, the Pa_{CO_2} will double. An acute increase in alveolar minute ventilation requires only 5 to 10 minutes for the Pa_{CO_2} to approximate its new level. Conversely, a sudden decrease in ventilation may require 1 hour or more for final equilibrium due to the limited rate of carbon dioxide production.

The presence and quantitation of pure respiratory disturbances then should offer the physician little difficulty and will be discussed no further here.

Metabolic (Nonrespiratory)

A far more difficult problem is to quantitate the metabolic component of an acid–base disturbance, especially if a respiratory disturbance coexists. The reason for this problem is twofold. First, because of the presence of buffers, no direct relation exists between the quantity of H^+ added to or lost from the body and the resultant change in H^+ concentration of the blood; second, changes in ventilation directly affect the parameters used in quantitating metabolic disturbances.

Buffer Capacity of Blood

The H^+ added to the body from any source is to a large degree rapidly removed by buffering. The efficiency of mammalian buffering systems was demonstrated impressively by Pitts.[8] In an investigation in which dogs were given H^+ in a concentration of approximately 14,200,000 nMol/L extracellular fluid (ECF), the H^+ concentration of the blood increased from 36 nMol/L (pH 7.44) to 72 nMol/L (pH 7.14). That is, of the 14,200,000 nMol of H^+ added per liter, only 36 nMol remained as free H^+; the remaining 14,199,964 nMol of H^+ were buffered and appeared as bound hydrogen (HHb, HPr, H_2CO_3, and H_2PO_4). The measurement of the change in free H^+ concentration (ie, pH) clearly is of little direct help in quantitating the total excess acid load.

To quantitate the acid load, an assessment of the total change in blood buffers is necessary. Of course, for every H^+ buffered, a corresponding decrease by one in the total quantity of buffer anions (Hb^-, Pr^-, bicarbonate, and HPO_4^-) and an increase by one in the total quantity of buffer acids (HHb, HPr, H_2CO_3, and H_2PO_4) must occur. If the buffer composition of blood could be measured in the preceding example, the buffer anions would decrease by 14,199,964 nMol/L, and the undissociated buffer acids would increase by a corresponding amount. Measurement of the decrease in buffer anions or of the increase in buffer acids would quantitate the metabolic disturbance.

Bicarbonate and Carbonic Acid

Most of these measurements are not possible in clinical settings. The only buffer pair that can be quantitated is that of bicarbonate–H_2CO_3. This system accounts for 80% or more of the buffer activity of the red cells and ECF against metabolic acids.* In the absence of other causes for variation in the bicarbonate concentration, its concentration change reflects approximately 80% of an acid or alkaline load. In the study by Pitts,[8] 80% of the total acid buffered in the red cells and ECF would have been buffered by bicarbonate, the concentration of which would have decreased by 0.80 × 14,199,964 nMol/L, or approximately 11.4 mMol/L.

Respiratory Effects on Bicarbonate Concentration

The bicarbonate concentration of the blood varies not only with metabolic acid–base status but also with ventilation. An increase in the P_{CO_2} of ECF leads to the hydration of the carbon dioxide to H_2CO_3 and subsequent dissociation to bicarbonate and H^+. Thus, an increase in bicarbonate concentration occurs. A decrease in ECF P_{CO_2} causes the opposite reaction with a subsequent reduction of the bicarbonate concentration. These reactions can be diagrammed as follows:

$$CO_2 + H_2O \leftrightarrow H_2CO_3 \leftrightarrow HCO_3^- + H^+ \qquad (8)$$

DIFFERENTIATION OF RESPIRATORY AND METABOLIC COMPONENTS. If an increase or a decrease in bicarbonate concentration is used to reflect metabolic alkalosis or acidosis, the total change first must be corrected for any alteration due to decreased or increased ventilation. Over the years, several methods have been proposed to make this correction, including determinations of carbon dioxide combining power,[9] standard bicarbonate,[1] buffer base,[2] and base excess.[3] All of these methods are based on in vitro titrations of blood or plasma with carbon dioxide, an approach that varies from the process that occurs in vivo. As a result, unless these methods are well understood, and their limitations appreciated by the clinician using them, a marked hyper- or hypocapnia may be misdiagnosed as representing a primary metabolic disturbance; inappropriate therapy often results.[10–12]

The most direct method for separating the respiratory and metabolic effects on the serum bicarbonate concentration is that provided by Brackett and colleagues[13,14] and Albert and colleagues.[15] They measured the changes in pH and bicarbonate concentration in human volunteers exposed to graded degrees of acute hypo- or hypercapnia, or in patients with uncomplicated chronic hypercapnia. Their results with calculated 95% confidence limits, are combined and summarized in Table 37-5. Bicarbonate changes outside of the ranges shown in Table 37-5 for any given Pa_{CO_2} are due to other than respiratory causes—that is, to a metabolic acid–base derangement.

For example, a patient with an acute respiratory acidosis and a P_{CO_2} of 60 mm Hg would be expected to have a bicarbonate concentration between 25.1 and 27.9 mMol/L. If the bicarbonate concentration was less than 25.1 mMol/L, an associated metabolic acidosis also would be present that could be quantitated by the amount of depression of the bicarbonate concentration. Similarly, a value greater than 27.9 mMol/L would indicate an associated metabolic alkalosis.

ACID–BASE DISTURBANCES

Respiratory Acidosis

When the elimination of carbon dioxide is less than its production, the Pa_{CO_2} increases. In surgical patients, the most common causes are respiratory center depression by anesthetic agents or narcotics, persistent neuromuscular blockade; or failure of the anesthesiologist to provide adequate alveolar ventilation. These changes may be exacerbated by pulmonary disease or instability of the rib cage.

Compensation

The change in pH in response to an increase in Pa_{CO_2} can be predicted (see Table 37-5). Renal and hepatic compensation is slow and not complete for 48 to 72 hours. An increase in extracellular H^+ is associated with H^+–potassium ion exchange

* Hemoglobin accounts for 90% of the buffering of carbon dioxide in its transport from the tissues to the lungs, but plays only a minor role in the buffering of the nonrespiratory acids. The percentage of metabolic acids buffered by HCO_3^- increases to greater than 80% with increasing degrees of respiratory compensation.

TABLE 37-5
Acute and Chronic Changes in Arterial Carbon Dioxide Partial Pressure, Arterial pH, and Bicarbonate Concentration

	ARTERIAL pH		BICARBONATE CONCENTRATION (mMol/L)	
Pa_{CO_2} (mmHg)	*Acute*	*Chronic*	*Acute*	*Chronic*
15	7.61–7.74	—	15–21	—
20	7.55–7.66	—	18–23	10–14
25	7.49–7.59	0	20–24	13–16
30	7.45–7.53	7.38–7.51	21–26	17–23
35	7.40–7.48	—	22–27	—
40	7.37–7.44	7.37–7.51	23–27	22–31
45	7.33–7.39	—	24–28	—
50	7.31–7.36	7.35–7.47	24–28	27–35
60	7.24–7.29	7.33–7.44	25–28	31–40
70	7.19–7.23	7.30–7.42	26–29	33–44
80	7.14–7.18	7.28–7.39	26–29	—
90	7.09–7.13	—	27–29	—
100	—	7.24–7.35	—	42–54

Bernards WC, Kirby RR: Acid-base chemistry and physiology. In Civetta JM, Taylor RW, Kirby RR (eds): Critical care, 2nd ed. Philadelphia: JB Lippincott, 1992: 347.

across cell membranes so that hypercapnia is commonly associated with hyperkalemia.

Treatment

Correction of respiratory acidosis should be achieved slowly and, primarily, by correcting the underlying cause, particularly when the persistent effects of respiratory depressant or neuromuscular blocking drugs are responsible. Chronic carbon dioxide retention is associated with decreased central drive to ventilation, which then becomes dependent on peripheral chemoreceptors. If the P_{CO_2} is reduced rapidly in these patients, the sudden increase in CSF pH may produce convulsions and unconsciousness.[16] Thus, P_{CO_2} should be reduced slowly over a period of several hours to a day or more. In general, the lower level should be no less than that "normally" maintained by the patient with spontaneous respiration.

Respiratory Alkalosis

Hypocapnia occurs when effective ventilation is increased. The most common cause is manual or mechanical alveolar hyperventilation. However, the condition occurs frequently when the respiratory center is stimulated by pain, anxiety, fear, pregnancy, or a primary metabolic acidosis (eg, salicylate intoxication) (Table 37-6). Peripheral hypoxic chemoreceptor stimulation occurs at high altitude and also probably accounts for the hypocapnia of sepsis, anemia, and heart failure. Although carbon dioxide depletion is common in hepatic failure, decreased lactate and urea metabolism cause more important metabolic than respiratory disturbances of acid–base status. Potentially deleterious effects of respiratory alkalosis are listed in Table 37-7.

TABLE 37-6
Clinical States in Which Respiratory Alkalosis May Occur

THERAPY
Salicylates
Analeptic drugs
Doxapram

HORMONE THERAPY
Progesterone
Epinephrine

HYPERMETABOLIC STATES
Fever
Exercise
Thyrotoxicosis

ANOXIA

CNS LESIONS
Meningitis
Encephalitis
Hemorrhage
Trauma

HEPATIC FAILURE

SHOCK

GRAM-NEGATIVE BACTEREMIA
(without fever or shock)

INTERSTITIAL PULMONARY DISEASE

IATROGENIC HYPERVENTILATION

Bernards WC, Kirby RR: Acid-base chemistry and physiology. In: Civetta JM, Taylor RW, Kirby RR (eds): Critical care, 2nd ed. Philadelphia: JB Lippincott, 1992: 350.

TABLE 37-7
Effects of Acute Respiratory Alkalosis

- Decreased cardiac output
- Increased difference between alveolar and arterial oxygen partial pressures
- Leftward shift of the hemoglobin dissociation curve
- Bronchoconstriction with increased ventilation–perfusion imbalance
- Hypotension
- Hypokalemia
- Decreased cerebral blood flow
- Decreased cerebral spinal fluid pressure
- Posthyperventilation hypoxia
- Resetting of central chemoreceptors

Bernards WC, Kirby RR: Acid-base chemistry and physiology. In Civetta JM, Taylor RW, Kirby RR (eds): Critical care, 2nd ed. Philadelphia: JB Lippincott, 1992: 351.

Compensation

The initial change in H^+ and bicarbonate can be predicted from Table 37-5. Within hours, renal and hepatic mechanisms counteract the change in pH so completely that the hypocapnia of altitude is accompanied by a near normal or normal pH. Respiratory alkalosis appears to be the only acid–base disturbance in which compensation restores pH to normal.

Treatment

Respiratory alkalosis is better prevented than treated. In particular, mechanical ventilation should be guided by monitoring of end-tidal carbon dioxide partial pressure or Pa_{CO_2}. Maintenance of arterial oxygen partial pressure may be difficult when ventilation is reduced to correct profound hypocapnia, because the depletion in carbon dioxide stores causes an apparent reduction in the respiratory quotient, R. Consequently, as is predicted from the alveolar air equation,

$$PA_{O_2} = FI_{CO_2}(P_B - P_{H_2O}) - Pa_{CO_2}\left(FI_{O_2} + \frac{1 - FI_{O_2}}{R}\right) \quad (9)$$

where PA_{O_2} = alveolar oxygen partial pressure, P_B = barometric pressure, P_{H_2O} = water vapor pressure, and FI_{O_2} = fraction of inspired oxygen, alveolar oxygen partial pressure and hence arterial oxygen partial pressure decrease as Pa_{CO_2} increases. Additional oxygen should be provided during weaning.

Metabolic Acidosis

Metabolic acidosis (Table 37-8) is commonly classified according to the anion gap (AG), which is defined as:

$$AG = Na^+ - (Cl^- + HCO_3^-) \quad (10)$$

A normal AG is 12 to 15 mMol/L. Those conditions associated with an increased AG may be further divided according to the presence or absence of hypoxia, a distinction that may have important therapeutic implications. Most of the conditions listed are the result of the addition of organic acids or substances (paraldehyde, ethylene glycol, methanol, or fructose) that produce acid by their metabolism.

Some conditions may result from an increased alkaline loss (diarrhea or biliary or pancreatic fistulae) (see Table 37-8). Administration of large volumes of stored blood, particularly when acid–citrate–dextrose was used as an anticoagulant, produced an acute metabolic acidosis that subsequently converted to metabolic alkalosis over the next 2- to 3-day period as the citrate was metabolized.

Infusion of several liters of normal saline or smaller volumes of hypertonic saline during resuscitation may result in a slight hyperchloremic metabolic acidosis from dilution of extracellular bicarbonate. Although the pH of saline is decreased compared with the normal blood value, the titrable acidity (actual acid load) is minuscule. The pH is low because no buffers are present in saline; thus a very small amount of acid causes a significant reduction of pH.

Lactic Acidosis

TYPE A. Lactic acidosis is commonly associated with hypoxia. In the early stages of shock, hypovolemia, sepsis, and overall oxygen consumption may not be altered because of an offsetting increase of oxygen extraction. However, the distribution of oxygen uptake is modified: consumption by the liver, muscle, kidneys, and gut decreases, while that of the heart and brain increases.[18] Decreased oxygen availability in the affected tissues leads to anaerobic glycolysis and the accumulation of lactic acid.

After cardiac arrest, the increase in myocardial H^+ is the result of carbon dioxide accumulation and failure of sufficient generation of adenosine triphosphate to drive sodium ion–H^+ exchange. If sodium bicarbonate is given to correct the acidosis, it will result in the liberation of carbon dioxide that causes further increase in intracellular H^+ and acidosis.[19–24]

TYPE B. The lactic acid in type B lactic acidosis originates from metabolic causes such as congenital pyruvate dehydrogenase deficiency. It is not associated with hypoxia. Severe

TABLE 37-8
Types of Metabolic Acidosis

INCREASED ANION GAP
Renal failure
Diabetic ketoacidosis
Salicylism
Lactic acidosis (and starvation)
Toxins: methanol, paraldehyde, ethylene glycol

HYPERCHLOREMIC
Renal tubular acidosis
Acetazolamide therapy
Diarrhea
Ureteral diversions
Addition of hydrochloric acid (ammonium chloride, hydrochloric acid, arginine, lysine)
Early renal failure

Bernards WC, Kirby RR: Acid-base chemistry and physiology. In Civetta JM, Taylor RW, Kirby RR (eds): Critical care, 2nd ed. Philadelphia: JB Lippincott, 1992: 345.

renal and hepatic disease play a role. Rapid lactic acidosis may occur in uremia; hepatic gluconeogenesis is decreased, but renal gluconeogenesis, which increases lactic acid production, is increased.

Fructose, sorbitol, and xylitol are used in parenteral nutrition as a source of carbohydrate because they are metabolized in the absence of insulin and produce less venous irritation. However, all lead to an increase in lactate production; 30% to 40% of a fructose load is converted to lactate.

Compensation

Metabolic acidosis stimulates ventilation, producing hypocapnia that limits the decrease in pH. The P_{CO_2} decreases slowly to reach its nadir at 12 to 24 hours. A useful rule is that the anticipated P_{CO_2} is approximately equal to the last two numbers of the pH; for example, at pH 7.20, the anticipated P_{CO_2} is 20 mm Hg.

Treatment

Metabolic acidosis long has been treated by sodium bicarbonate. The quantity required can be estimated from the numerical expression of the Henderson-Hasselbalch equation, assuming that the bicarbonate is distributed throughout the ECF volume (20% body weight). Half the estimated deficit was given slowly over a 10-minute period and subsequent therapy was dictated by frequent acid–base assessment.

Although such therapy may be appropriate for some causes of metabolic acidosis (uremia, diarrhea and fistulae, renal tubular acidosis), in the presence of hypoxia it neither corrects the acidosis nor improves the cardiovascular status. Kette and colleagues showed that 10 minutes of ventricular fibrillation in pigs (sustained by external chest compression and mechanical ventilation) resulted in an average increase of intramyocardial P_{CO_2} from 54 to 346 mm Hg and of H^+ from 65 to 441 nMol/L.[25] These increases were correlated inversely with coronary perfusion pressure and survivability. The P_{CO_2} elaborated by the bicarbonate neutralization of ECF H^+ may contribute to a worsening of intramyocardial acidosis.[26,27] In experimental metabolic acidosis, sodium bicarbonate leads to an increase in intracellular H^+ in the heart, liver, muscle, and red blood cells.[20,24] In addition, it promotes cerebrospinal fluid acidosis, hypoxia, circulatory depression, hyperosmolality, and hypernatremia.

Sodium bicarbonate has no place in the treatment of diabetic ketoacidosis. It does not decrease ketone body concentration, increase pH, or improve patient survival. This condition should be managed with fluid and insulin to restore glucose metabolism, an approach that has the additional advantage of improving hepatic metabolism of accumulated lactate, itself a store of bicarbonate.

Several alternatives to bicarbonate have been tried experimentally, including sodium dichloroacetate; equimolar mixture of sodium bicarbonate and sodium carbonate[28,29]; and tromethamine (THAM) buffer. These agents do not increase intracellular H^+; however, improved outcome has yet to be demonstrated. The safest treatment of hypoxic metabolic acidosis is removal of the cause and aggressive cardiorespiratory support. Survival depends on the ability of the individual to increase cardiac output and oxygen delivery in the face of tissue hypoxia and anaerobic metabolism.

Metabolic Alkalosis

Severe metabolic alkalosis has a mortality as high as 65% when the pH is 7.65 or greater.[30] Causes include loss of gastrointestinal fluid, adrenal hyperplasia, loop diuretics, and cortisol (Table 37-9). In addition, a significant amount of alkali is administered to surgical patients, often without the physician's recognition. Organic anions, such as lactate, acetate, pyruvate, gluconate and citrate are metabolized with the formation of bicarbonate. One liter of lactated Ringer's solution contains 25 mMol of bicarbonate precursor, and Normosol contains bicarbonate precursor in a concentration of 50 mMol/L.

A surgical patient often receives 10 L or more of solution during surgery and the first 2 postoperative days and thus accumulates a significant alkaline load in intravenous fluids if they consist of balanced electrolyte solution. Add to this the several hundred milliequivalents of bicarbonate precursor as citrate in bank blood (1 mol citrate = 3 mol bicarbonate) plus the acid and chloride loss caused by nasogastric suction, and the reason why significant alkalosis develops postoperatively in so many of these patients becomes clear.

Compensation

Respiratory compensation occurs but is variable. The Pa_{CO_2} is seldom greater than 50 mm Hg and can be predicted:

$$Pa_{CO_2} = 0.9 \times HCO_3^- + 9 \qquad (11)$$

Treatment

Most cases of metabolic alkalosis are iatrogenic and preventable. Acidic gastric losses should be replaced with a high concentration chloride solution (half- or full-strength saline). Patients already alkalotic and in need of continuing replacement of ongoing ECF losses should be given saline solution and not balanced electrolyte solution with its hidden alkali load. This simple step, the administration of chloride-rich saline solution, will prevent or correct nearly all cases of metabolic alkalosis.

TABLE 37-9
Causes of Metabolic Alkalosis

- Loss of acidic gastrointestinal fluid
- Volume depletion, especially associated with low concentration of potassium ion or chloride ion
- Diuretic therapy
- Excess adrenal cortical hormone
- Hepatic coma
- Administration of exogenous base
  - Lactate or acetate (intravenous fluids)
  - Citrate (bank blood)
  - Bicarbonate

Bernards WC, Kirby RR: Acid-base chemistry and physiology. In Civetta JM, Taylor RW, Kirby RR (eds): Critical care, 2nd ed. Philadelphia: JB Lippincott, 1992: 349.

Hypokalemia

Hypokalemia almost invariably accompanies alkalosis, and can reach staggering levels. Body potassium deficits of 1000 mEq have been reported; 300 to 500 mEq deficits are common. Although metabolic alkalosis, with potassium deficits as high as 500 mMol, can be corrected with chloride alone, the accompanying hypokalemia can be life-threatening and requires correction. The usual practice of administering 40 mEq of potassium ion in 1 L of 5% dextrose can actually lead to an acute decrease of the serum concentration of potassium ion as the glucose causes an intracellular movement of potassium. With significant hypokalemia, potassium should be administered at a rate of 10 to 40 mMol/h, with frequent serum level determinations.

Salt-wasting Nephropathy

Not every case of metabolic alkalosis is correctable with chloride alone. A syndrome of saline-resistant metabolic alkalosis or "chloride-wasting nephropathy" is characterized by persistent urinary excretion of chloride in the presence of metabolic alkalosis. This situation may occur when body potassium depletion becomes severe, in excess of 500 mMol. Severe potassium depletion of this magnitude may alter the renal tubular handling of chloride, leading to chloride wasting and metabolic alkalosis. This syndrome is reversible with potassium replacement.

EFFECTS OF ACID–BASE DISTURBANCES

Circulation

For respiratory disturbances, the direct depressant actions of P_{CO_2} may be offset by the associated sympathetic stimulation. Carbon dioxide acts as a peripheral vasodilator and a pulmonary vasoconstrictor. However, its secondary sympathetic stimulation leads to vasoconstriction in organs such as the kidneys. Thus, hypoventilation induces renal vasoconstriction and cerebral vasodilation. Sympathetic activation also leads to increases in stroke volume, heart rate, and cardiac output.

When P_{CO_2} is maintained constant, the cardiovascular effect of pH depends on the source and distribution of H^+. In general, a decrease in pH leads to myocardial depression with decreased stroke volume and cardiac output. However, in the presence of myocardial ischemia, intracellular H^+ decreases from hydrolysis of adenosine triphosphate and the local production of carbon dioxide.[18,25] In this situation, the heart is particularly vulnerable to attempts at correcting the acidosis with bicarbonate. The resulting increase in P_{CO_2} leads to further increase in intracellular H^+, myocardial depression, and impaired tissue oxygenation.[19–24]

Ventilation

Hypercapnia stimulates central and peripheral chemoreceptors maximally at a Pa_{CO_2} of about 80 mm Hg; at greater values of Pa_{CO_2}, ventilation is depressed. An increase of Pa_{CO_2} induces a rapid increase in ventilation by stimulation of aortic and carotid bodies. The accompanying decrease in pH produces a slower but additional central stimulus to ventilation. Carbon dioxide and H^+ cause separate and additive rightward shifts of the oxyhemoglobin dissociation curve. The P_{50} is increased by about 2 mm Hg per 0.1 pH unit reduction.

Tissue oxygen delivery is the product of cardiac output and arterial oxygen content. To some extent, the shift in the oxygen dissociation curve induced by hypercapnia and acidosis compensates for the hemodynamic depression. Consequently, in metabolic acidosis, a slight undercorrection rather than overcorrection is preferable, because metabolic alkalosis has a detrimental effect both on cardiac output and on the hemoglobin–oxygen dissociation curve.

Central Nervous System

In general, carbon dioxide and H^+ have no direct effect on cerebral metabolism except as a consequence of altered cerebral perfusion. Hypocapnia has been shown to have some effect on increasing pain threshold. Tetany, in alkalotic states, is caused by a decrease in the ionized calcium concentration. However, in cardiac arrest, with reduced to absent perfusion (depending on the efficacy of resuscitative efforts), lactic acid accumulation increases the destruction of neural elements. Hyperglycemia aggravates this situation by providing additional substrate for anaerobic glycolysis and lactic acid production.

REFERENCES

1. Jorgenson K, Astrup P: Standard bicarbonate: its clinical significance and a new method for its determination. Scand J Clin Lab Invest 2:122, 1957
2. Singer RB, Hastings AB: An improved clinical method for the estimation of disturbances of the acid-base balance of human blood. Medicine 27:223, 1948
3. Astrup P, Siggaard-Andersen O, Jorgensen K, et al: The acid-base metabolism: a new approach. Lancet 1:1035, 1960
4. Henderson vs. Hasselbalch (Editor's Choice). Anesth Analg 45: 491, 1966
5. Campbell EJM: RI pH. Lancet 1:681, 1962
6. Campbell EJM: RI pH. Lancet 2:154, 1962
7. Winters RW: Terminology of acid-base disorders. Ann N Y Acad Sci 133:211, 1965
8. Pitts RF: Mechanisms for stabilizing the alkaline reserves of the body. Harvey Lect 48:172, 1952-53
9. Van Slyke DD, Cullen GD: Studies of acidosis: I. the bicarbonate concentration of the blood plasma—its significance and its determination as a measure of acidosis. J Biol Chem 30:289, 1917
10. Roos A, Thomas IJ: The *in vivo* and *in vitro* carbon dioxide dissociation curves of true plasma. Anesthesiology 28:1048, 1967
11. Bunker J: The great transatlantic acid–base debate. Anesthesiology 26:591, 1965
12. Arbus G, Hebert L, Levesque P, et al: Application of 'significant band' for acute respiratory alkalosis. N Engl J Med 280:117, 1969
13. Brackett NC, Cohen JJ, Schwartz WB: Carbon dioxide titration curve of normal man: effect of increasing degrees of acute hypercapnia on acid-base equilibrium. N Engl J Med 272:6, 1965
14. Brackett NC, Wingo CF, Muren O, et al: Acid-base response to chronic hypercapnia in man. N Engl J Med 280:124, 1969
15. Albert M, Dell R, Winters R: Quantitative displacement of acid-base equilibrium in metabolic acidosis. Ann Intern Med 66:312, 1967
16. Cotev S, Severinghaus JW: Role of cerebrospinal fluid pH in management of respiratory problems. Anesth Analg 1969; 48: 42
17. Narins RG, Emmett M: Simple and mixed acid-base disorders: a practical approach. Medicine (Baltimore) 56:161, 1987

18. Arieff AI: Indications for use of bicarbonate in patients with metabolic acidosis. Br J Anaesth 67:165, 1991
19. Guidelines for advanced cardiac life support and emergency cardiac care. JAMA 268:2210, 1992
20. Graf H, Leach W, Arief A: Evidence for a detrimental effect of bicarbonate therapy in hypoxic lactic acidosis. Science 227:754, 1986
21. Weil MH, Rackow EC, Trevino R, et al: Differences in acid-base state between venous and arterial blood during cardiopulmonary resuscitation. N Engl J Med 315:153, 1986
22. Grundler W, Weil MH, Rackow EC: Arteriovenous carbon dioxide and pH gradients during cardiac arrest. Circulation 74:1071, 1986
23. Young GP: Reservations and recommendations regarding sodium bicarbonate administered during cardiac arrest. J Emerg Med 6:321, 1988
24. von Planta M, Weil MH, Gazmuri RJ, et al: Myocardial acidosis associated with CO_2 production during cardiac arrest and resuscitation. Circulation 80:684, 1989
25. Kette F, Weil MH, Gazmuri RJ, et al: Intramyocardial hypercarbic acidosis during cardiac arrest and resuscitation. Crit Care Med 21:901, 1993
26. Ostrea EM, Odell GB: The influence of bicarbonate administration on blood pH in a 'closed system': clinical implications. J Pediatr 80:671, 1972
27. Poole-Wilson PA: Is early decline of cardiac function due to carbon dioxide retention? Lancet 2:1285, 1975
28. Sun JH, Filley GF, Hord K, et al: Carbicarb: an effective substitute for $NaHCO_3$ for the treatment of acidosis. Surgery 102:835, 1987
29. Bersin RM, Arieff AI: Improved hemodynamic function during hypoxia with Carbicarb, a new agent for the management of acidosis. Circulation 77:227, 1988
30. Schwartz W, Van Yipserle de Strihau IC, Kassirer J: Role of anions in metabolic alkalosis and potassium deficiency. N Engl J Med 279:630, 1968

FURTHER READING

Bernards WC, Kirby RR: Acid-base chemistry and physiology. In Civetta JM, Taylor RW, Kirby RR (eds): Critical care, 2nd ed. Philadelphia: JB Lippincott, 1992: 343

Bevan DR: Acid base. In Kirby RR, Gravenstein N (eds): Clinical anesthesia practice. Philadelphia: WB Saunders, 1994, 732

Gravenstein JS: Fluid electrolytes and acid base balance. In Gravenstein N (ed): Manual of complications in anesthesia. Philadelphia: JB Lippincott, 1991: 353

Complications in Anesthesiology, second edition,
edited by Nikolaus Gravenstein and Robert R. Kirby.
Lippincott-Raven Publishers, Philadelphia © 1996.

CHAPTER 38

Transfusion Problems

Neil S. Yeston
Richard C. Dennis

RED BLOOD CELL FUNCTION

The primary indication for transfusing red blood cells is to maintain or restore the blood's oxygen-carrying capacity. Oxygen delivery to the tissues depends directly on cardiac output and the arterial oxygen content of the blood. Most oxygen is bound to hemoglobin, but a small portion is dissolved in the plasma. The most important functional feature of hemoglobin is its ability to bind reversibly with oxygen. The hemoglobin molecule releases oxygen to the tissues more easily when it is fully saturated; a marked increase in oxygen affinity occurs when it is only partially saturated.

The P_{50}, or partial pressure of oxygen at which the hemoglobin is 50% saturated, is a measure of oxygen affinity. The normal adult value is 26 mm Hg. Fever, acidosis, and increased levels of 2,3-diphosphoglycerate (2,3-DPG) diminish oxygen-hemoglobin affinity, facilitating oxygen release when tissue oxygen requirements are increased. Tissue oxygen consumption ($\dot{V}O_2$) is calculated from the product of the cardiac output CO and the difference between the arterial oxygen concentration (CaO_2) and the mixed venous oxygen concentration ($C\bar{v}O_2$).

$$\dot{V}O_2 = CO \times (CaO_2 - C\bar{v}O_2) \quad [1]$$

Oxygen Delivery Variables

The normal oxygen transport system has a large reserve capacity that responds to physiologic stress and provides a margin of safety if any portion of the system becomes impaired. This feature is best demonstrated by the relation between normal oxygen consumption in a 70-kg person (250 mL/minute) and oxygen delivery ($\dot{D}O_2$) (1000 mL/minute). The amount of available oxygen is four times the amount that is normally consumed.

The supply side of the equation, $\dot{D}O$, is defined as the product of CaO_2 and CO (equation 2). Content is defined as the amount of oxygen that is carried by hemoglobin (Hb) plus that dissolved in plasma (Equation 3):

$$\dot{D}O_2 = CaO_2 \times CO \quad [2]$$

$$CaO_2 = (Hb \times 1.34 \times SaO_2) + (.0031 \times PaO_2) \quad [3]$$

in which 1.34 is the amount of oxygen (mL) per gram of hemoglobin; SaO_2 is the hemoglobin saturation (%) with oxygen; and 0.0031 is the solubility of oxygen in plasma (mL/dL).

The solubility coefficient of oxygen in plasma is so low that the contribution of the oxygen partial pressure relative to total oxygen delivery is almost insignificant. For example, if a patient has a hemoglobin concentration of 14 g/dL, SaO_2 of 100%, a PaO_2 of 100 mm Hg, and a cardiac output of 5 L/minute, the amount of delivered oxygen is 988 mL/minute of oxygen. If the PaO_2 were to increase by 100% (eg, from 100 to 200 mm Hg), maintaining the same hemoglobin concentration and CO, $\dot{D}O_2$ would increase only 1.6% to 1004 mL/minute.

Conversely, alterations in the hemoglobin concentration may impact significantly on oxygen delivery. For example, a 20% increase in hemoglobin concentration from 15 to 18 g/dL, assuming the negligible effect of PaO_2 and given a constant cardiac output of 5 L/minute, yields a 20% increase in $\dot{D}O_2$ (from 973 to 1167 mL/minute). A similar magnitude of influence can be found for cardiac output.

Hemoglobin Concentration and Blood Volume

The relation between hemoglobin concentration and blood volume is also of critical importance. A normal hemoglobin concentration and a reduced blood volume is much more deleterious than a reduced hemoglobin concentration and normal blood volume. Using the $\dot{D}O_2$ formula (see Equation 38-2), if a hemoglobin concentration of 15 g/dL is reduced to a concentration of 10 g/dL (assuming a PaO_2 of 60 mm Hg and a SaO_2 of 90%), $\dot{D}O_2$ would fall from 990 to 612 mL/minute.

Examples such as this are used to justify the concept that a hemoglobin concentration of 10 g/dL, assuming an arterial saturation of 90% or greater, is optimal for oxygen delivery. However, if the hemoglobin concentration of 10 g/dL was associated with a cardiac output of only 3 L/minute as a result of a reduction in blood volume (SaO_2 = 90% and PaO_2 = 60 mm Hg), $\dot{D}O_2$ would fall from 610 to 366 mL/minute, clearly an example of only marginal or inadequate oxygen delivery despite an acceptable hemoglobin concentration. Conversely, even if the hemoglobin concentration was reduced further to 8 g/dL, as long as it was compensated for by an increase in CO (eg, 6 L/minute), $\dot{D}O_2$ could be sustained at 600 mL/minute.

A normal or minimally acceptable hemoglobin concentration associated with a reduced blood volume may not be adequate to meet cellular demands, but a reduced hemoglobin concentration associated with a normal blood volume and an appropriately compensated CO often meets the challenge of $\dot{D}O_2$.

The importance of the association between hemoglobin concentration and blood volume was illustrated by Spence and colleagues,[1] who, while caring for a group of Jehovah's Witnesses, failed to identify a difference in outcome for patients undergoing major surgical procedures whose preoperative hemoglobin concentration exceeded 10 g/dL compared with those whose values were less than 10 g/dL but greater than 6 g/dL of hemoglobin. If blood volume was reduced intraoperatively (>500 mL of blood loss), the mortality rate rose from 0% to 7.4%.

Optimal Hemoglobin Concentration

Most clinicians have supported a "transfusion trigger" of 10 g/dL despite experimental and clinical data that support the efficacy of support at lower hemoglobin levels. In an attempt to identify the limits of cardiac compensation in acute anemia, Wilkerson and colleagues,[2] using a paralyzed, anesthetized, normovolemic, anemic primate model, identified a net positive increase in myocardial lactate production when hematocrit fell below 10%. They further observed that compensatory mechanisms in the animals for low hemoglobin concentration—increase in CO, decrease in systemic vascular resistance, increase in left ventricular blood flow, and decrease in left ventricular resistance—did not occur until the hemoglobin concentration fell below 7 g/dL (hematocrit of 21%).

The animals used by Wilkerson were healthy primates that were anesthetized, paralyzed, and euthanized within 6 hours, and correlation with the clinical setting was unclear. Accordingly, Levine and colleagues[3] selected a normovolemic, anemic, primate model, but they attempted to recreate surgical stress and anemia by performing laparotomy on 19 adult baboons, followed by an exchange transfusion of 6% hetastarch, yielding a final hematocrit of 15%. The animals were then observed for 2 months. The results indicated no morbidity or mortality, with all hematocrit values approaching baseline at the conclusion of the study.

It could be hypothesized that these animals were able to survive extremely low hemoglobin concentrations as a result of their presumably normal coronary arteries' ability to increase myocardial oxygen delivery in compensation for maximal oxygen extraction. Case and associates[4] showed that coronary artery stenosis and anemia produced a far greater depression in myocardial performance than anemia alone or the combination of coronary artery stenosis and normal hemoglobin concentration. In a retrospective review, Nelson and coworkers suggested that postoperative myocardial ischemia increased significantly in a high-risk group of vascular surgical patients when the hematocrit fell below 28%.[5]

These study results demonstrate that there is no universal or optimal hemoglobin concentration. The transfusion trigger instead must be individualized in response to the variability in co-morbidity associated with most critically ill patients. For example, the young, healthy trauma victim, who in most instances can be assumed to have normal coronary artery anatomy, may safely sustain hemoglobin concentrations far below 10 g/dL, if a normal blood volume and cardiac output exist. However, persons with coronary artery disease, who usually cannot augment coronary artery blood flow and may not be able to appropriately increase CO in compensation for acute anemia, may require higher hemoglobin concentrations and should be transfused.

This conclusion has been supported by the National Institutes of Health Consensus Development Conference.[6] The group concluded that:

> . . . the decision to transfuse a specific patient should take into consideration the duration of anemia, the intravascular volume, the extent of the operation, the probability for massive blood loss, and the presence of coexisting conditions such as pulmonary function, inadequate cardiac output, myocardial ischemia, and cerebral vascular or peripheral circulatory output, myocardial ischemia, and cerebral vascular or peripheral circulatory disease. These factors are representative of the universe of considerations that compromise clinical judgment. No single measure can replace good clinical judgment for decisions regarding perioperative transfusion. However, current experience would suggest that otherwise healthy patients with hemoglobin values of 10 g/dL or greater rarely required perioperative transfusion. Whereas those with acute anemia with resulting hemoglobin values of less than 7 mg/dL frequently require red blood cell transfusion, it appears that some patients with chronic anemia, such as those with chronic renal failure, tolerate hemoglobin values of less than 7 g/dL. The decision to transfuse red blood cells depends on clinical assessment that is aided by laboratory data such as arterial oxygenation, mixed venous oxygen tension, cardiac output, the oxygen extraction ratio, and blood volume when indicated.

2,3-Diphosphoglycerate

Reduced levels of red cell 2,3-DPG increase hemoglobin-oxygen affinity and diminish oxygen release to tissue. Levels of 2,3-DPG rapidly decrease in red blood cells stored in the liquid state to less than 10% after 2 weeks.[7] Transfusion of 2,3-DPG–depleted red cells has potentially adverse clinical implications.[8] Restoration of 2,3-DPG in circulating transfused red cells may take 24 to 48 hours in healthy persons and considerably longer in metabolically deranged patients.[9] Proponents of infusion of 2,3-DPG–enriched red blood cells suggest that near-normal oxygen release is critical during the acute phase of resuscitation, when oxygen delivery is impaired because of decreased red cell mass and diminished CO.[10] Fresh blood, citrate-phosphate-dextrose-adenine (CPDA) blood less than 14 days old, and cryopreserved red cells provide enough

2,3-DPG for near-normal oxygen release when it is most needed.

COLLECTION, STORAGE, AND USE OF BLOOD PRODUCTS

Red Cells

Fresh, warm whole blood most effectively restores red cell mass, plasma volume, platelets, and clotting factors. However, it is unrealistic to expect the blood bank to have donors of each blood type available at a moment's notice. In addition, the requirement for testing blood for hepatitis and acquired immunodeficiency syndrome (AIDS) necessitates storage, during which time platelets and clotting factors rapidly deteriorate. Fresh whole blood is therefore only rarely available, and component therapy is the mainstay of blood banking practice (Table 38-1).

Whole blood is collected from a donor into a closed system of plastic bags containing an anticoagulant. Packed red blood cells (hematocrit = 70% to 80%) are prepared by removing approximately 200 mL of plasma by centrifugation or gravity sedimentation. The cells are stored in a liquid state at 4°C or frozen at −80°C. Most blood banks use the former method.

Clinicians have difficulty assessing the therapeutic effectiveness of blood product transfusions because of biologic variability, the diverse disease processes treated, and the lack of standardization of blood product units. A unit of whole blood is defined as 450 mL (±10%) plus 63 mL of anticoagulant. If one donor has a borderline low but acceptable hemoglobin of 12.5 g/dL and a "short draw" of 405 mL and another donor has a hemoglobin of 17 g/dL and a "large draw" of 495 mL, the amount of hemoglobin in the acceptable unit can vary from 50.6 to 84.1 g. Using this definition, 8 small-volume, low-hemoglobin units are equivalent to 5 large-volume, high-hemoglobin units.

To confuse matters more, not all transfused red cells survive. Taking all these variables into account, it is possible to devise a clinical scenario in which 6.7 small, 50.6-g hemoglobin units transfused near the end of their storage period are required to provide the same number of red cells as 3 large units transfused after a brief storage period. It is little wonder that the incremental rise in hemoglobin after transfusion often differs from the predicted norm.

Characteristics of Storage Solutions

Citrate-Phosphate-Dextrose

Citrate-phosphate-dextrose (CPD) is an anticoagulant preservative in which blood is stored at 1°C to 6°C. The acceptable duration of storage has been set by United States regulations that require that at least 70% of the transfused red blood cells remain in circulation for 24 hours after infusion. Red cells preserved in CPD for 1, 2, or 3 weeks yield 90%, 80%, and 70% 24-hour posttransfusion survival rates, respectively.[11] As a result, blood stored in CPD solution is outdated after 21 days of storage. The changes in CPD blood that occur with storage are listed in Table 38-2.

Citrate-Phosphate-Dextrose With Adenine

The addition of a small amount of adenine (0.25 to 0.5 mM) to CPD-stored blood creates the preservative CPDA, which can prolong storage from 21 to 35 days.

Adenine-Glucose-Mannitol-Sodium Chloride

Adenine-glucose-mannitol-sodium chloride (Adsol) preservative has been approved for the storage of packed red blood

TABLE 38-1
Characteristics of Component Therapies

BLOOD COMPONENT	CONTENT	VOLUME (mL)	HEMATOCRIT (%)	PLATELETS	PLASMA (mL)	SHELF-LIFE
Whole blood	450 mL blood; RBC, plasma, WBC platelets; 63 mL CPD, 60 g hemoglobin	500	40–45	Nonviable	180–305	42 days in Adsol 35 days in CPDA 21 days in CPD 4°C
Red blood cells	RBC, WBC, platelets; 60 g hemoglobin	250–350	70	Nonviable	40–115	42 days in Adsol 35 days in CPDA 21 days in CPD
Frozen RBC	RBC, minimal WBC and platelets, no plasma; 54 g hemoglobin	170–190	90	None	0	24 years at −80°C 72 hours at 4°C
Platelets, single donor	Platelets; some WBC, plasma, and RBC	300	0	$3–8 \times 10^{11}$	250	24 hours at 22°, open
Platelets, random	Platelets; some WBC, plasma, and RBC	50	0	5.5×10^{10}	50	5 days at 22°C, closed
Fresh frozen plasma	Plasma; 200 units of all coagulation factors, complement, 400 mg fibrinogen	220	0	0	200–275	1 year at −18°C 24 hours at 4°C

RBC, red blood cell; *WBC,* white blood cell; *CPD,* citrate-phosphate-dextrose; *CPDA,* CPD + adenine.

Yeston NS, Niehoff JM, Dennis RC: Transfusion therapy. In Civetta JM, Taylor RW, Kirby RR (eds): Critical Care, 2nd ed. Philadelphia: JB Lippincott, 1992:433

TABLE 38-2
Changes in Citrate-Phosphate-Dextrose Blood With Storage

TEST	NORMAL	STORAGE (days) 1	21
pH	7.4	7.1	6.9
$PaCO_2$ (mm Hg)	40.0	48.0	140.0
Plasma bicarbonate (mEq/L)	26.0	18.0	11.0
Plasma potassium (mEq/L)	4.0	3.9	21.0
2,3-DPG (μM/mL)	18.0	4.8	<1.0
Platelets (%)	100.00	10.0	0
Factors V and VIII (%)	100.0	70.0	20.0

cells for 49 days. This 14-day increase in storage time over that approved for CPD with adenine adds tremendous flexibility to blood banking. The 24-hour posttransfusion survival of red blood cells stored in Adsol for 49 days is only 65%.

Biochemical Changes

Independent of the medium in which blood is stored, the biochemical changes associated with storage (see Table 38-2) are similar, as are the complications. All three preservatives significantly deplete the blood of 2,3-DPG. Because the storage medium that allows the greatest flexibility should be used, additional research is needed to find a medium in which blood can be easily stored and retrieved for a period longer than 49 days. Despite the advantages offered by CPDA and Adsol, coagulation, pulmonary, and metabolic problems and transfusion reactions occur when blood is stored in either solution.

Cryopreservation

If any technique has the potential to provide the optimally stored red cell product, it is cryopreservation. Red cells stored at −80°C in 40% glycerol for as long as 21 years demonstrate acceptable in vitro storage criteria and clinical efficacy. The 24-hour posttransfusion survival rates of cryopreserved red cells ranges from 80% to 90%.[11] Oxygen release is similar to that of fresh whole blood because the 2,3-DPG level is normal. Antigenic immune reactions are minimized by the near elimination of platelets and leukocytes. Large quantities of red blood cells, including rare blood types, can be stockpiled. Recognizing these distinct advantages, the Department of Defense approved cryopreserved red cells for routine preservation.

Oxyhemoglobin Dissociation Curve

In 1954, Valtis and Kennedy described an in vitro leftward shift of the oxyhemoglobin dissociation curve. The magnitude of this shift is related directly to the time blood has been stored.[12] After transfusion of CPD blood stored 7 days or longer, all patients' dissociation curves also shift to the left. The magnitude of the leftward shift is related to volume and storage time of the infused blood. In some cases, the curve remains shifted to the left for as long as 24 hours after transfusion. Because of the leftward shift in the dissociation curve, tissue hypoxia may develop after infusion of stored blood.

CHARACTERISTICS. The oxyhemoglobin dissociation curve (Fig. 38-1) is obtained by plotting the partial pressure of oxygen (PO_2) in blood against the percentage of hemoglobin saturated with oxygen. As hemoglobin becomes more saturated, its affinity for oxygen also increases. This relation is reflected by the sigmoid shape of the curve, which indicates that a decrease in arterial PO_2 makes considerably more oxygen available to the tissues than if the curve were linear. Greater efficiency of blood transport of oxygen to the tissues results.

Shifts in the dissociation curve are quantitated as the PaO_2 at which, at 37°C and pH 7.4, hemoglobin is 50% saturated (P_{50}; Fig. 38-1). A low P_{50} indicates a leftward shift in the oxygen dissociation curve and an increased affinity of hemoglobin for oxygen. With this shift, a lower than normal PaO_2 saturates hemoglobin in the lungs; subsequent release of oxygen to the tissues occurs at a capillary PO_2 that is lower than normal. Increased affinity may be sufficient to ensure that oxygen is not released to the tissues, unless the tissue PO_2 is in the hypoxic range.

DECREASED DELIVERY OF OXYGEN TO TISSUE FROM STORED BLOOD. A close relation between oxygen affinity of stored blood and intraerythrocytic 2,3-DPG has been established.[13] The 2,3-DPG concentrations decrease with storage in CPD or acid-citrate-dextrose (ACD), although the decrease is less in CPD-stored blood (Fig. 38-2). Although ACD blood is no longer used, most of the work on 2,3-DPG was performed with this preservative. The problems are the same with all types of stored blood. Alkalosis and hypothermia shift the curve leftward even more (see Fig. 38-1).

Autotransfusion

Autotransfusion is the process of collecting and reinfusing the patient's own blood for intravascular volume replacement. Advantages in the event of acute hemorrhage include immediate availability of blood without the need to type and crossmatch and elimination of the risks of alloimmunization and transmission of infectious diseases. The patient receives blood containing higher levels of 2,3-DPG than those in banked units.

Candidates for emergency autotransfusion include patients injured by blunt or penetrating chest trauma with an acute chest tube blood loss of 1500 mL or more; those suffering an acute recoverable (eg, intraoperative) blood loss who desire to avoid homologous transfusion or when there is no available homologous blood; and those who have massive blood loss when homologous blood is available but is insufficient for resuscitation.

The Sorenson system consists of a soft inner collection bag contained in a rigid outer canister.[14] Anticoagulant is added by drip to the suction tubing or contained in the collection bag. The system must be monitored closely because insufficient or excessive amounts of anticoagulopathy can be administered inadvertently. The Sorenson system is relatively

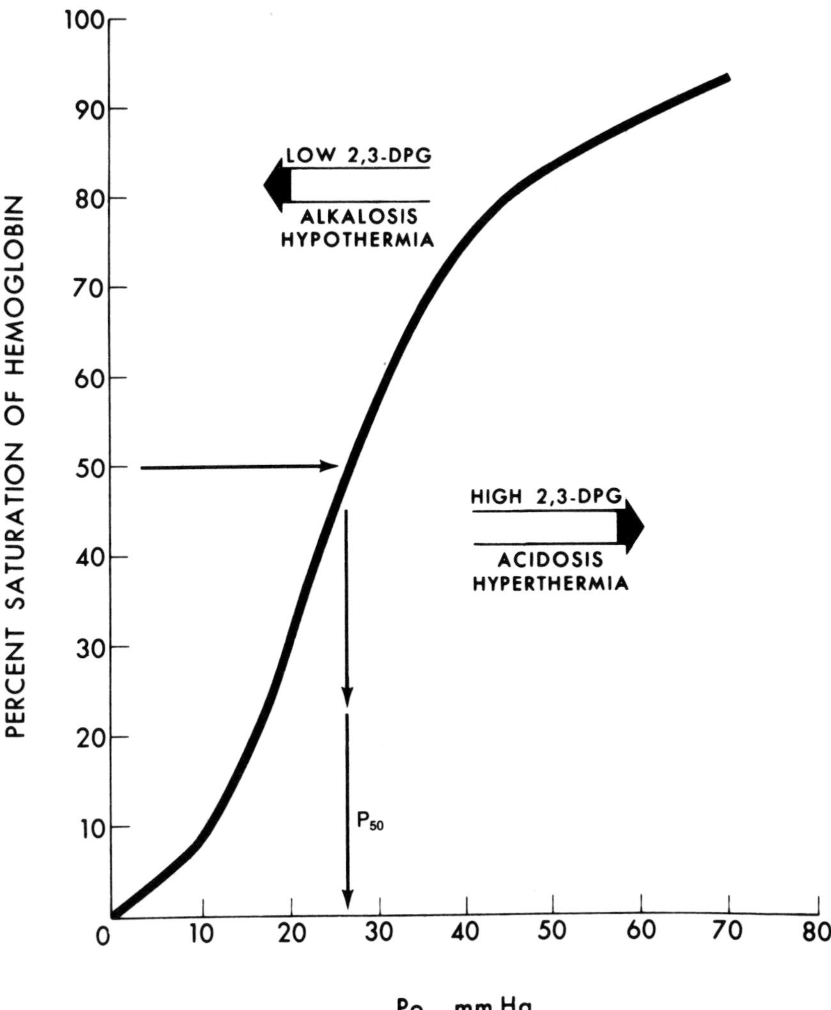

FIGURE 38-1. Factors that shift the oxyhemoglobin dissociation curve.

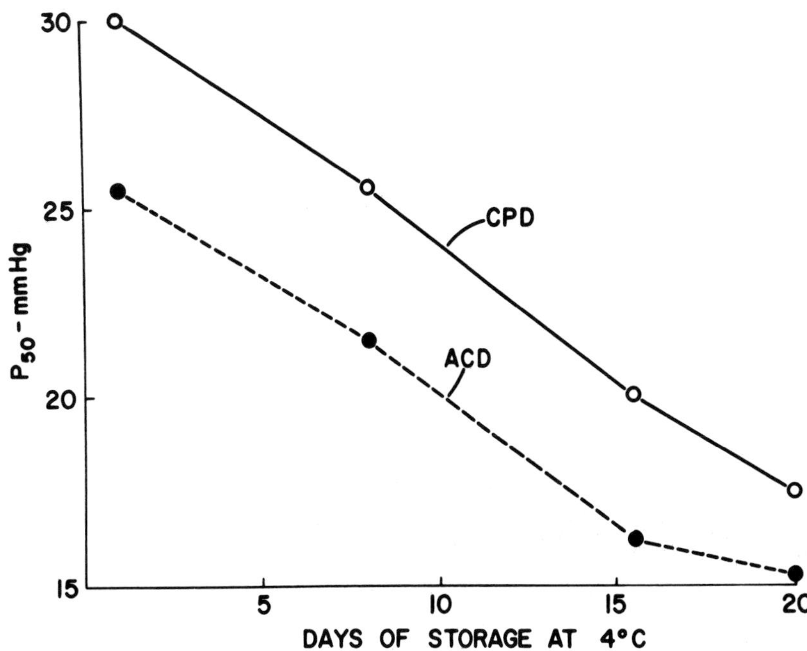

FIGURE 38-2. Relation between P_{50} and days of storage of ACD- and CPD-stored blood. (Dawson RB Jr, Ellis TJ: Hemoglobin function of blood stored at 4°C in ACD and CPD with adenine and inosine. Transfusion 10:113, 1970.)

inexpensive, can be employed in a variety of clinical situations, and is easy to use.

The IBM blood cell processor centrifuges and washes blood collected by the Sorenson or other salvage systems. As much as 500 mL of blood can be washed in each cycle; depending on the amount of debris, more than one cycle may be required. A cycle takes approximately 15 minutes. The final product is washed red blood cells suspended in saline. This system is expensive, but it does not require constant operator attention, and the processor can be used for other blood banking purposes.

The Haemonetics Cell Saver is a dedicated cell-washing unit that provides a product similar to the IBM system. Shed blood is anticoagulated and aspirated directly into the apparatus. It is then washed, concentrated, and stored in a transfer pack. As much as 3 units of blood can be processed for retransfusion in 9 minutes. The device is expensive, as is the disposable plastic ware. Excluding the risk of infection from homologous transfusion, the Cell Saver break-even cost is approximately 2 units of autologous transfused blood. Both the IBM and the Haemonetics units yield red cells with virtually no plasma, clotting factors, or oncotic properties.

Complications

HEMATOLOGIC. The most reproducible hematologic complication of autotransfusion is thrombocytopenia.[15] Platelet counts approach 50,000μL when patients receive more than 400 mL of autologous processed blood.[16,17] Platelets collected from the Sorenson autotransfusion system function abnormally in vitro but aggregate normally in vivo after transfusion. Hypofibrinogenemia is the most reproducible coagulation factor abnormality.[17] Platelet counts and fibrinogen levels, however, return to normal by 48 to 72 hours.[14] In an evaluation of autotransfusion patients with traumatic hemothoraces, Symbas found that no patient demonstrated evidence of a coagulopathy if the autotransfused volume was less than 50% of the patient's total blood volume (5 units).[18]

Although good data are lacking, it is reasonable to speculate that devices (eg, Sorenson) returning partially activated, filtered whole blood are more likely to produce disseminated intravascular coagulation (DIC) and less likely to produce dilutional coagulopathy than systems (eg, IBM, Haemonetics) returning washed red cells. In addition, dilutional thrombocytopenia may occur earlier in systems that wash red cells in saline. Some researchers recommend administering fresh frozen plasma (FFP) after 4 to 6 units of autologous washed red cells are transfused.[19] Platelets also may be given after a 6- to 8-unit replacement (see Table 38-1). When in doubt, a blood sample should be assessed for platelet count, prothrombin time (PT), and partial thromboplastin time (PTT).

NONHEMATOLOGIC. Nonhematologic complications of autotransfusion include sepsis, air embolization, tumor embolization, and particulate microemboli.[14,19] The risk of sepsis due to autotransfusion appears to be minimal following an isolated thoracic injury. Although blood has been transfused without incident after contamination, this practice is not advisable.[20]

Platelet or fat microemboli can be eliminated by the use of a micropore filter.[21] Air embolism has been reported in systems using automated roller pumps when the aspirate reservoir was allowed to run dry and when the bag containing red cells to be reinfused is pressurized. Air emboli are rare with standard gravity-assisted reinfusion techniques.

Predonation

Predonation or predeposit autologous transfusion requires blood donation before surgery. The blood may be stored in the liquid phase for as long as 49 days (Adsol) or cryopreserved and then made available at the time blood loss is anticipated. This process is suitable only for elective surgery. The increased public awareness of disease transmission by blood products (eg, AIDS; hepatitis B; non-A, non-B hepatitis; cytomegalovirus) has renewed interest in the concept of autologous blood banking.

The requirements for predonation are similar to those of routine homologous donation at most centers. A patient is a candidate for predonation if the hemoglobin concentration is 11 g/dL or greater (hematocrit of 34%). Numerous predonation schedules are available. They can be as short as blood donations every fourth day[22] (if the previous hemoglobin and hematocrit criteria are met) or, more commonly, 1 unit per week.[23] In general, the final phlebotomy is performed 3 days before the surgical event.

Human recombinant erythropoietin was administered to patients scheduled for elective orthopedic surgery in the preoperative period.[24,25] The mean number of autologous units collected per patient and the mean red cell volume were clinically and statistically greater in the erythropoietin group than those in the control group. The role of erythropoietin in the predonation schema needs further clarification, although early evidence suggests questionable benefit.[26]

Few complications have arisen as a result of predonated blood, and most donors are acceptable. Although some centers have reported success in patients with coronary artery disease, pregnancy, and the extremes of age as being free from complications,[27] others find predonation in these groups to be relatively contraindicated. Errors in identification of blood can occur during phlebotomy, processing, or transfusion, and a transfusion reaction remains a possibility. The true cost of autologous transfusion probably exceeds that of homologous transfusion, because donor recruitment is only a small percentage of the cost of transfusion therapy. Red cells stored by cryopreservation are estimated to be three to four times more costly than liquid-preserved red cells. Routine type and crossmatch and disease testing should still be done, even with predonated units in case improper identification has occurred.

Although predonation of autologous blood generally is safe and effective, the practice is grossly underused throughout the country. Despite the growth of autologous blood donation from 30,000 units in 1982 to 397,000 units in 1987,[28] Toy and associates[29] found that only 5% of patients who were scheduled for major elective surgery and who were potential candidates for predonation actually received autologous blood. If those same patients had donated autologous blood preoperatively and received their blood when indicated, the incidence of homologous blood transfusions would have been reduced by 68%.

TABLE 38-3
Hemorrhagic Diathesis

SIGNS	CAUSES
Venipuncture site bleeding	Dilutional thrombocytopenia
Oozing in surgical field	Low concentrations of factors V and VIII
Hematuria	Disseminated intravascular coagulation and fibrinolysis
Gingival bleeding	Hemolytic transfusion reaction
Ecchymoses	
Petechiae	
Suture line bleeding	

COAGULATION DEFECTS

The major clinical signs and causes of a hemorrhagic diathesis are listed in Table 38-3.

Blood Transfusion Coagulopathies

Blood transfusion–induced coagulopathies often present a vicious cycle. The bleeding is usually caused by blood that lacks certain coagulation factors. To replace a continuing blood loss, more stored blood must be given, but this is the blood that initially caused the coagulopathy. A bleeding tendency may be exacerbated by infusion of the required amount of stored blood. This practice establishes the vicious cycle, which must be interrupted by appropriate therapy.

Thrombocytopenia

Dilutional thrombocytopenia is the most important cause of a hemorrhagic diathesis from transfusion.[30] Although primarily quantitative, the platelet defect is also qualitative, and a storage temperature of 4°C accounts for most of the damage to platelets.[31] Taking into account viability and survival time, platelets retain only 60% of their hemostatic function after 3 hours of storage. After 24 hours, only 12% of the original platelet function is still present. When blood stored for more than 24 hours is infused, especially in patients who have lost large amounts of blood, the available platelet pool is diluted (Fig. 38-3). When the platelet count decreases to less than 20,000/mm^3, a bleeding problem is likely to develop.[30,31]

A closer examination of Figure 38-3 indicates that the observed platelet counts are slightly higher than what would be expected from a pure dilutional thrombocytopenia. This finding is consistent with a study that implies that platelets are being released into the circulation, countering the effects of dilution. If so, the most likely source of such platelet reserve is the spleen, which normally pools about one third of the circulating platelets. An alternative explanation may be the circulation of nonfunctional platelets (transfused in the blood units) and release of immature platelets from bone marrow.

Use of the absolute platelet count alone can be criticized. Patients with leukemia may have platelet counts of less than 10,000/μL but do not bleed. These patients have chronic thrombocytopenias but no large surgical wounds. In patients without chronic thrombocytopenia, spontaneous bleeding may begin when the platelet count is less than about 65,000/μL.

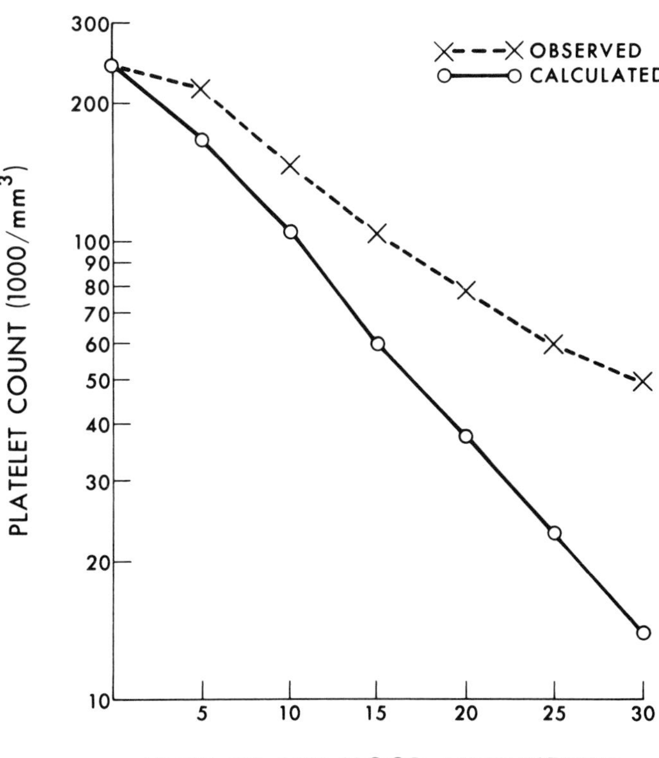

FIGURE 38-3. Comparison between mean observed platelet counts in 21 patients receiving more than 15 U of ACD-stored blood and platelet count (predicted) in a person receiving platelet-free blood. The moderately close approximation of these two curves suggests that the thrombocytopenia is dilutional, resulting from infusion of platelet-free solutions (ACD blood stored for >24 hours). (Miller RD, Robbins TO, Tong MJ: Coagulation defects associated with massive blood transfusions. Ann Surg 174:794, 1971.)

Factors V and VIII

Although concentrations of factors V and VIII gradually decline by 20% to 50% of normal after 21 days of storage, these values usually are not low enough to be the primary cause of a bleeding diathesis.[30] The practice of giving FFP containing all the clotting factors except platelets, prophylactically or therapeutically, for bleeding from blood transfusion is questionable.[32] A National Institutes of Health consensus development conference concluded that FFP specifically was not indicated prophylactically in massively transfused patients.[33] FFP should not be given unless the PT, PTT, or both are at least 1.5 times the normal value.

Disseminated Intravascular Coagulation and Fibrinolysis

DIC and fibrinolysis have occurred in patients given bank-stored blood and in patients undergoing certain operative procedures, such as removal of abruptio placenta,[34] prostatic surgery,[35] portacaval shunt, and neurosurgery resulting in brain injury.[36] Although the precise causes are unknown, some hormone or toxic material releases tissue thromboplastin as a result. Thromboplastin triggers the coagulation system, resulting in consumption and decreased blood concentrations of factors I, II, V, VIII, and platelets. Thrombi and fibrin are deposited in the microcirculation of vital tissues, possibly interrupting their blood flow.

In response to this hypercoaguable state, the fibrinolytic system is activated, lysing some of the excess fibrin. This process is called secondary fibrinolysis (Fig. 38-4); primary fibrinolysis refers to activation of the fibrinolytic system without concomitant DIC. Heparin sometimes is used for the treatment of DIC with secondary fibrinolysis, and ε-aminocaproic acid is used to treat primary fibrinolysis.

Fresh Frozen Plasma

FFP is removed from a unit of whole blood within 6 hours of collection and frozen at −18°C. Freezing protects factors V and VIII; the remainder of the coagulation factors are stable during liquid storage. All the components of the coagulation, fibrinolytic, and complement systems and the proteins that maintain oncotic pressure and modulate immunity are present in FFP. Fats, carbohydrates, and minerals are present in concentrations similar to those in the circulation.

Treatment with FFP is indicated for deficiencies of factors II, V, VIII, IX, and XI. Treatment can also be given to reverse the effects of warfarin, for antithrombin III deficiency, to treat thrombotic thrombocytopenic purpura, and to treat humoral immunodeficiencies. Fresh frozen plasma is not indicated as a volume expander or as a nutritional source.

It has been suggested that FFP be administered in response to abnormal clotting parameters (PT >16 seconds or PTT >60 seconds) in patients about to undergo major surgical procedures.[37] However, the sensitivity and specificity of the PT and PTT laboratory determinations are 40% to 63% and 47% to 67%, respectively, when used preoperatively in predicting perioperative bleeding.[38] Other researchers, however, have confirmed a strong correlation between postoperative bleeding and preoperative abnormal clotting tests if the PT and PTT were more than 1.5 times normal; these values are associated with factor V and VIII levels of less than 20% of normal and fibrinogen levels in the range of 75 mg/dL.[39] However, patients who had abnormalities in PT and PTT preoperatively that were not in excess of 1.5 times normal failed to show

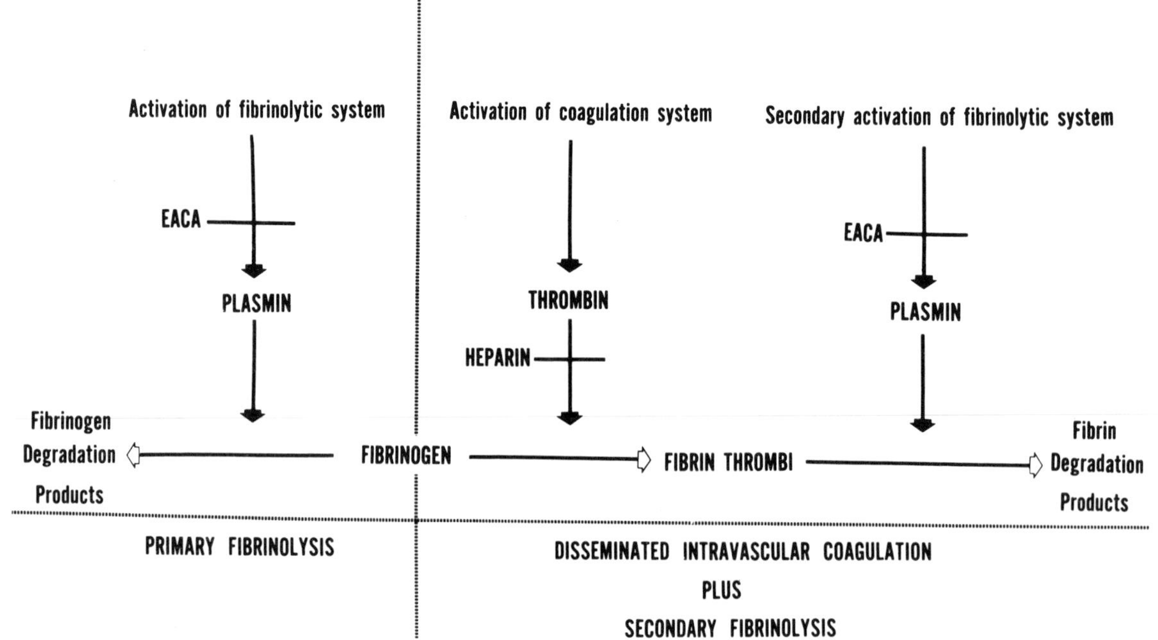

FIGURE 38-4. Primary fibrinolysis and secondary fibrinolysis with DIC. Although ε-aminocaproic acid (*EACA*) inhibits primary fibrinolysis, it also inhibits secondary fibrinolysis, one of the main defenses against DIC. (Miller RD: Complications of massive blood transfusion. Anesthesiology 39: 82, 1973.)

evidence of significant bleeding in the postoperative period. (See Appendix).

Cryoprecipitate

Cryoprecipitate is a plasma concentrate consisting primarily of factor VIII and fibrinogen in approximately 10 mL of plasma. A single unit of cryoprecipitate contains approximately 100 clotting units of factor VIII and 250 mg of fibrinogen. A clotting unit of factor VIII is the amount of factor VIII in 1 mL of fresh normal plasma. Cryoprecipitate is stored frozen and can be prepared for infusion at 37°C (ie, complete thawing) in 10 minutes. Temperatures greater than 37°C diminish the factor VIII activity.

Cryoprecipitate is recommended for the replenishment of factor VIII or fibrinogen. An average adult dose is 8 to 10 units, which results in an increase of 2% per unit in the factor VIII level. The most satisfactory way to judge the amount required is to measure the patient's circulating factor VIII level. Cryoprecipitate carries a greater risk of disease transmission because it is pooled from multiple donors.

Platelets

Platelets initiate vasoconstriction and platelet aggregation at sites of damaged vascular endothelium. A platelet has a life span of 10 days. One third of the platelets released from the marrow into the vascular space are stored in the spleen. When additional platelets are required to maintain hemostasis, splenic platelets are released. Marrow production increases if platelet mobilization is inadequate.

General Considerations

Platelets are removed from a unit of fresh whole blood, first by differential centrifugation into platelet-rich plasma and then by repeat centrifugation, at which time most of the plasma is removed. The platelet pellet is resuspended in 50 mL of residual plasma and stored at 22°C. Platelets also can be collected by single-donor platelet pheresis. Heparinized, citrated donor blood flows into a continuous centrifuge that separates the blood into its components. The platelets are harvested, and the plasma and remaining cells are reinfused into the donor. Platelets so collected must be used within 24 hours of collection or be frozen. An advantage of this system is that 6 to 8 units of platelets can be collected from a single donor, reducing the danger of disease transmission compared with the collection of platelet transfusions from six or eight different donors.

The number of platelets present in a unit to be transfused is variable. A unit of platelets should contain 5.5×10^{10} platelets. A normal platelet count ranges between 15 and 44 $\times 10^{10}$/L. A small unit from a donor with a low normal platelet count may contain only 6×10^{10} platelets, but a large unit from a donor with a high normal count may contain 22 $\times 10^{10}$ platelets. Platelet units contain only 70% of the platelets in the original unit of whole blood; a fresh unit of platelets can be as small as 4×10^{10} or as large as 15×10^{10}. Because donor platelet counts are not routinely measured, the variation can be even greater. Because platelet units are stored for as long as 5 days in the blood bank, their therapeutic effectiveness deteriorates. A fresh, large unit can have many times the number of functional platelets available as a stored, smaller unit.

As a result of the release of thromboxane A_2, a prostanoid instrumental in the initiation of the vasoconstriction phase of the clotting mechanism,[40] and the aggregation resulting in a platelet plug, platelets effectively initiate clotting. When available in adequate numbers (>100,000 thrombocytes/mm^3) and free from thrombocytopathy, platelets reduce the bleeding time to normal (5 to 8 minutes). Platelet counts below 50,000/μL correlate with increased bleeding time.[41] Levels below 20,000/μL render the person at risk for microvascular bleeding and usually signal the need for prophylactic platelet transfusion.[42] Patients scheduled for surgery or those who are about to receive large-bore hemodynamic monitoring catheters and who have platelet counts less than 50,000 platelets/μL deserve prophylactic platelet transfusions. In general, transfusion of platelets to achieve a posttransfusion platelet count of 50,000/μL or greater is the accepted standard.[43] On average, 1 unit of administered platelets results in a net gain of 5,000–10,000 or more platelets/μL after the transfusion. (See Appendix I).

Platelet Mass

The concept of platelet mass is critically important to the understanding of platelet function. Large platelets contain a greater number of platelet granules than smaller platelets. Because platelet granules are partly responsible for platelet function, large platelets are more hemostatically effective than smaller ones. Consequently, a low platelet count of predominantly large platelets can be as hemostatically effective as a higher platelet count comprising primarily small platelets. The platelet mass and number merit consideration.

Desmopressin

1-Desamino-8-D-arginine-vasopressin (desmopressin, DDAVP) has been shown to reduce significantly the bleeding time in patients with von Willebrand's disease,[44] uremia,[45] primary or acquired platelet disorders, and aspirin ingestion.[46] DDAVP administration also has decreased intraoperative and postoperative blood loss in patients undergoing Harrington rod insertion[47] or cardiac bypass surgical procedures.[48] The mechanism of efficacy is probably related to an overall increase in the von Willebrand factor released from endogenous storage pools as a result of DDAVP stimulation.[49] It may be effective in patients who take aspirin before surgery.[50]

Too few studies are available for wholesale recommendations. In most cases, tachyphylaxis occurs with prolonged therapy. DDAVP has been shown to be associated with significant hypotension[51] secondary to vasodilation and with hyponatremia because of its antidiuretic properties.[46] When DDAVP is used, it should be administered over at least a 15-minute period with careful blood pressure monitoring.

TRANSFUSION COMPLICATIONS

The transfusion of blood and blood products is associated with serious and even fatal complications.

Hemolytic Reactions

Most hemolytic reactions are the result of clerical errors. A small percentage of reactions results from laboratory "failures." Clinical manifestations of hemolysis are immediate symptoms that start after 50 mL or less of blood have been given and include fever and chills. More severe manifestations are headache, severe back pain, substernal tightness, dyspnea, and shock. Few symptoms may be present in anesthetized or obtunded patients. Objective findings include facial flushing, cyanosis, distended neck veins, tachycardia, and profound shock, usually occurring within 1 hour of transfusion. DIC may follow. Hemoglobinuria, hemoglobinemia, jaundice, oliguria, anuria, and acute renal failure may supervene. The severity of the reaction depends on the antibody titer, the affinity (ie, strength of binding) of the antibody, and the dose of offending red cells that has been administered. Hemolytic reactions caused by interdonor incompatibility involve mostly the ABO and Kell blood groups.

The renal failure associated with hemolysis is thought to be caused by the stroma-antibody complexes released into the circulation, rather than hemoglobin precipitation in the tubular lumina. Damage probably results from a combination of hypotension and vasoconstriction, leading to a reduction in renal blood flow and the deposition of fibrin thrombi. The severity of renal dysfunction ranges from mild (ie, quickly resolving diminution of urine output with little alteration in the clearance of metabolites) to acute tubular necrosis and bilateral renal cortical necrosis.

Management depends on the prompt recognition of symptoms and immediate discontinuation of the transfusion (Table 38-4). The blood should be quickly checked against the patient's identification and then returned to the blood bank along with another sample of the patient's blood for repeat typing and crossmatch. Blood bank personnel then test for a hemolytic antibody, and blood and urine are checked for free hemoglobin. Often, the urine test is positive for free hemoglobin because of the presence of red blood cells related to a Foley catheter or surgical trauma. The simple technique of centrifuging a tube of urine and identifying pink discoloration of the supernatant aids in differentiating hemoglobinuria (ie, pink supernatant) from hematuria (ie, pink sediment).

Some authorities recommend infusion of 25 g of mannitol over 5 minutes as soon as a hemolytic reaction is suspected. Others suggest the use of furosemide or ethacrynic acid, because these drugs may be more effective in maintaining renal blood flow. Intravenous fluids should be increased to maintain urine output of more than 100 mL/hour. Hypotension should be corrected with crystalloids or plasma expanders. Vasoactive drugs may be necessary. Additional blood transfusions should be avoided until the blood bank evaluation is complete. If renal failure develops, dialysis or hemofiltration may be required.

TABLE 38-4
Steps in the Treatment of Hemolytic Reaction

1. Stop the transfusion.
2. Maintain a urine output of at least 75 to 100 mL/h by generous administration of intravenous fluids:
   Mannitol, *12.5 to 50* g, given slowly, intravenously
   If intravenous fluids and mannitol are insufficient, furosemide, *40* mg, intravenously
3. Alkalinize the urine. Because bicarbonate is preferentially excreted in the urine, usually only 40 to 70 mEq of sodium bicarbonate per 70 kg body weight is required to increase the urine pH to 8, whereupon repeated urine pH determinations indicate the need for additional bicarbonate.
4. Assay plasma and urinary hemoglobin concentrations.
5. Determine platelet count, partial thromboplastin time, and serum fibrinolysis level.
6. Return unused blood to blood bank for repeated crossmatching.
7. Prevent hypotension to ensure adequate renal blood flow.

Minor Reactions

Minor reactions to blood transfusions usually are not serious and are febrile or allergic in origin. A febrile reaction is characterized by chills, fever, and urticaria and probably is caused by antigens to which the recipient has leukocytes and perhaps platelet antibodies.[52] Allergic reactions are similar and are characterized by urticaria or, in more severe cases, by chills and fever as well.

Although the cause of these reactions is rarely determined, they occur more frequently in patients who have had a previous transfusion reaction or who have a history of allergies. Supportive therapy that includes antihistamines or aspirin may be needed. If the reaction begins with chills and fever with no urticaria, the plasma and urine should be examined for free hemoglobin to exclude a hemolytic transfusion reaction. Chills and fever may signal bacterial contamination, but this problem is exceedingly rare.

Febrile reactions due to antileukocyte antibodies represent the majority of untoward reactions and are seen in almost 7% of all blood product recipients. Prior transfusions contribute to the development of the responsible antibodies. The incidence of developing antileukocyte antibodies is high and increases with repeated exposure.

Transfusion-Mediated Transfer of Allergy

The recipient of a blood transfusion may demonstrate an allergic reaction to medication or food ingested by the donor. The reaction may vary in severity from urticaria to frank anaphylaxis. Alternatively, allergic transfusion reactions develop as a result of the passive transfer of sensitizing antibodies. The recipient subsequently encounters the allergen to which he now has antibody, and an allergic reaction ensues. Ramirez reported the first case of such a phenomenon in 1919, when a patient who had been recently transfused from a donor known to be allergic to animal dander developed wheezing during a carriage ride. Several months later, no sensitivity was present.[53]

Pulmonary Reactions

Pulmonary insufficiency is often attributed to microaggregates in stored, transfused blood. Canine models show increased shunt and diminished pulmonary diffusing capacity after transfusion, which can be prevented with a micropore filter.[54,55] However, primates resuscitated with stored blood administered without a micropore filter do not develop pulmonary insufficiency.[56] A retrospective analysis of combat injuries concluded that the volume of blood transfused was less closely related to the development of pulmonary dysfunction than to the magnitude and location of injuries incurred.[57] The exact role of blood transfusions in the development of pulmonary dysfunction remains unsolved.

Graft-Versus-Host Disease

Graft-versus-host disease (GVHD) follows infusion of immunocompetent cells into an immunoincompetent recipient who is incapable of rejecting the foreign cells. Consequently, the infused immunocompetent cells initiate rejection of the host's normal tissues. Blood product transfusions into patients with cell-mediated immune deficiency may cause GVHD. Acute GVHD also occurs in recipients of allogeneic bone marrow transplants and in persons with primary immunodeficiencies who receive viable allogeneic lymphocytes. Blood products at risk for inducing GVHD are whole blood, red packed blood cells, buffy coats, granulocytes, fresh plasma, and platelets. In animal studies, the number of lymphocytes transfused appears to be a critical determinant. GVHD is not seen after transfusion of frozen blood, FFP, cryoprecipitate, or washed red cells. Irradiated blood products also may be given safely.[58]

The clinical presentation of GVHD involves many organ systems, including the skin, liver, gastrointestinal tract, and bone marrow. Fever occurs first, with a rash developing 24 to 48 hours after that. The rash is a generalized erythroderma starting on the face (frequently behind the ears) and then spreading to the trunk and extremities. Bullae can form. Skin biopsies show extensive lymphocytic infiltration. Anorexia, nausea, vomiting, diarrhea, hepatocellular dysfunction manifested by elevated liver enzymes, and pancytopenia also occur.

Infections

Hepatitis

The incidence of posttransfusion hepatitis is 5% to 10% nationwide, with great regional variation.[59,60] Fifty percent of patients developing posttransfusion hepatitis progress to chronic active hepatitis, with 20% of those patients developing cirrhosis. Of the latter group, 15% die.[61] Given the 20 million units of red blood cells and fresh frozen plasma and platelets transfused in this country in 1 year, the morbidity and mortality rates are significant.[28] Mandatory screening for hepatitis B virus has reduced successfully the risk of viral transmission, although zero incidence has not been achieved. Most cases of posttransfusion hepatitis are a consequence of the transmission of non-A, non-B hepatitis virus.[61]

Although evidence for the hepatitis virus was poorly detected in the blood banking industry, later data suggest that much non-A, non-B hepatitis may be hepatitis C virus, for which an anti–hepatitis C monoclonal antibody has been developed.[62–64] Mandatory screening for hepatitis C has reduced the incidence of infection per unit of red blood cells transfused to 0.3 per 1000 units.

Although there is the potential for the transmission of hepatitis A virus through blood transfusions, the incidence is extremely low.

Acquired Immunodeficiency Syndrome

AIDS involves the development of a life-threatening opportunistic infection or Kaposi's sarcoma in a person with no underlying immunosuppressive disease who has not received any immunosuppressive therapy. AIDS is associated with abnormal cell-mediated immunity. Transmission of the virus through blood transfusion accounts for approximately 1% of all reported cases in the United States.[65]

All blood banks eliminate donors with known risk factors and screen blood products for human immunodeficiency virus (HIV). The ELISA and the Western blot tests are available. The ELISA is 99% sensitive and has a specificity of 93% to 97%. It has been estimated that approximately 1000 patients per year may be potentially infected with blood contaminated with the HIV virus. The risk of acquiring HIV virus through blood transfusion despite HIV antibody testing is approximately 1 in 225,000.[66] Because testing requires antibody detection to determine the potential for disease transmission, the fact that viremia can occur for a significant interval without antibody production in certain persons helps to explain why screening is not 100% effective. The risk of disease transmission must be balanced by sound indications and clinical judgment when transfusion is being contemplated.

Other Viral Infections

Cytomegalovirus (CMV) and Epstein-Barr virus (EBV) are associated with posttransfusion infection and are transmitted by lymphocytes. Transmission and clinical symptoms occur primarily in compromised recipients, such as premature infants, immunosuppressed transplant patients, and patients undergoing open-heart surgery. The "postperfusion syndrome," occurring 3 to 6 weeks after thoracotomy, consists of fever, lymphocytosis with atypical cells, a negative heterophile test, splenomegaly, and mild abnormalities in liver function. Cytomegalovirus infection in immunocompromised patients ranges from a mild, self-limited febrile illness to extensive disseminated disease resulting in death.

In addition to a mononucleosis-like syndrome, CMV also causes retinitis, pneumonia, hepatitis, gastrointestinal ulcerations, pericarditis, and encephalitis. Between 51% and 72% of donors have anti-CMV antibodies, but only 5% are capable of transmitting the infection. However, the potentially devastating complications of CMV disease in the postoperative transplant recipient suggest that seronegative blood be given when transfusion is required in the seronegative recipient who has received a seronegative organ donation. There are those who believe that seronegative blood should be administered to all transplant recipients regardless of the status of their antibodies, because prior CMV disease does not protect against new infection (Hull D: personal communication).

Acid-Base Alterations

The pH of CPD solution is approximately 6.6. When this solution is added to 1 unit of freshly drawn blood, the pH of the blood immediately decreases to approximately 7.0 to 7.1. The pH of bank blood continues to decrease to about pH 6.6 after 21 days of storage. Much of the progressive acidosis can be explained by the increasing carbon dioxide partial pressure (PCO_2; see Table 38-1). The PCO_2 is high because the plastic blood container does not permit escape of carbon dioxide; however, with adequate pulmonary ventilation in the transfusion recipient, the high PCO_2 should be of little consequence.

Bicarbonate Therapy

Even when P_{CO_2} is returned to 40 mm Hg, acidosis continues to affect stored blood (see Table 38-1). In 1965, Howland and Schweizer recommended intravenous administration of sodium bicarbonate (44.6 mEq for every 5 units of bank blood infused), particularly in patients who have abnormal respiratory or renal compensatory mechanisms.[67] Since 1986, considerable controversy has surrounded bicarbonate therapy, and it is specifically not recommended in conditions of significant lactic acidosis nor as routine treatment in cardiac arrest.[68]

Excessive bicarbonate administration also may result in a hyperosmolal state, causing intracellular dehydration. Administration of 0.5 to 1.0 mEq/kg of sodium bicarbonate increases the plasma osmolality to 349 mOsm/kg in dogs experimentally and in humans during treatment of cardiac arrest.[69,70] Although plasma osmolality has not been measured when bicarbonate has been given empirically, the amount recommended is in the range described above. A hyperosmolal state seems possible. The evolution of carbon dioxide from bicarbonate (>1 L/50 mEq) may worsen myocardial cellular acidosis, because it is freely diffusible across all cell membranes.[71]

Citrate Intoxication

Citrate intoxication is not caused by the citrate ion but is the result of the binding of citrate to calcium. The signs of citrate intoxication are those of hypocalcemia: hypotension, narrow pulse pressure, increased intraventricular end-diastolic pressure and central venous pressures, and a prolonged QT interval on the electrocardiogram.[72] At one time, most investigators felt that citrate intoxication occurred only when at least 1 unit of blood was infused every 3 to 4 minutes in a 70-kg patient.

In a later study of patients receiving a mean of 5.8 L of CPD blood at a rate of 0.6 mL/kg/minute, ionized calcium decreased from a mean of 1.1 to 0.5 mM, a value that could cause minor circulatory changes.[73] The investigators concluded that calcium administration should be considered when evidence of myocardial depression is present with a blood infusion rate greater than 0.4 mL/kg/minute. However, even without calcium therapy, ionized calcium concentrations returned to normal shortly after cessation of blood administration.

The rapid return of these concentrations to normal can be explained by the metabolism of citrate by the liver and mobilization of calcium from endogenous stores. Hypothermia, liver disease, and hyperventilation may increase the possibility that citrate intoxication can occur. Excluding these conditions, ionized calcium concentrations begin to decrease only when 1 unit of blood is infused every 10 minutes, and therefore, citrate intoxication is rare.

REFERENCES

1. Spence RK Carson JA, Poses R, et al: Elective surgery without transfusion: influence of preoperative hemoglobin level and blood loss on mortality. Am J Surg 159:320, 1990
2. Wilkerson DK, Rosen AL, Seagal LR, et al: Limits of cardiac compensation in anemic baboons. Surgery 103:665, 1988
3. Levine E, Rosen A, Seagal L, et al: Physiologic effects of acute anemia: implications for a reduced transfusion trigger. Transfusion 30:11, 1990
4. Case RB, Berglund E, Sarnoff SJ: Ventricular function: changes in coronary resistance and ventricular function resulting from acutely induced anemia and the effect thereon of coronary stenosis. Am J Med 55:397, 1955
5. Nelson AH, Fleisher LA, Rosenbaum SH: Relationship between postoperative anemia and cardiac morbidity in high risk vascular patients in the intensive care unit. Crit Care Med 21:860, 1993
6. National Institutes of Health Consensus Development Conference Statement: Perioperative Red Cell Transfusion. U.S. Department of Health and Human Services. Bethesda, MD: Public Health Service. 1988: 7:1.
7. Beutler E, Meul A, Wood LA: Depletion and regeneration of 2,3-diphosphoglyceric acid in stored red blood cells. Transfusion 9: 109, 1969
8. Weisel RD, Dennis RC, Manny J, et al: Adverse effects of transfusion therapy during abdominal aortic aneurysmectomy. Surgery 83:682, 1978
9. Valeri CR, Hirsch NM: Restoration of in vivo erythrocyte adenosine triphosphate, 2,3-diphosphoglycerate, potassium ion, and sodium ion concentration following transfusion of acid-citrate-dextrose stored human red blood cells. J Lab Clin Med 73:722, 1969
10. Dennis RC, Hechtman HB, Berger RL, et al: Transfusion of 2,3-DPG–enriched red blood cells to improve cardiac function. Ann Thorac Surg 26:17, 1978
11. Valeri CR: Blood banking and the use of frozen blood products. Boca Raton, FL: CRC Press, 1976
12. Valtis DJ, Kennedy AC: Defective gas-transport function of stored red blood cells. Lancet 1:119, 1954
13. Bunn HF, May MH, Koholaty WF, et al: Hemoglobin function in stored blood. J Clin Invest 48:311, 1969
14. Noon GP, Solis RT, Natelson EA: A simple method of intraoperative autotransfusion. Surg Gynecol Obstet 143:65, 1976
15. Bell W: The hematology of autotransfusion. Surgery 84:695, 1978
16. Davidson SJ: Emergency unit autotransfusion. Surgery 84:703, 1978
17. Klebanaoff G, Watkins D: A disposable autotransfusion unit. Am J Surg 116:475, 1968
18. Symbas PN: Extraoperative autotransfusion from hemothorax. Surgery 84:722, 1978
19. Dowling J: Autotransfusion: its use in the severely injured patient. In the Proceedings of the First Annual Bentley autotransfusion seminar. San Francisco, 1972: 11
20. Glover JL, Smith R, Yaw PB, et al: Autotransfusion of blood contaminated by intestinal contents. JACEP 7:142, 1978
21. Raines S, Buth J, Brewster DC, et al: Intraoperative autotransfusion: equipment, protocol and guidelines. J Trauma 16:616, 1976
22. Autologous Blood Transfusions Council on Scientific Affairs: . JAMA 256:2378, 1986
23. Lonser RE, Taber B: Autologous transfusion in a community hospital. In the Proceedings of the Haemonetics Research Institute advanced component seminar. Boston, MA, 1980
24. Goodnough LT, Rudnick S, Price TH, et al: Increased preoperative collection of autologous blood with recombinant human erythropoietin therapy. N Engl J Med 321:1163, 1989
25. Goodnough LT, Price TH, Rudnick S, et al: Preoperative red cell volume production in patients undergoing aggressive autologous blood phlebotomy with and without erythropoietin therapy. Transfusion 32:441, 1992
26. Goodnough TH, Freidman KD, Johnston M, et al: A phase III trial of recombinant human erythropoietin in therapy in non-anemic orthopedic patients subjected to aggressive removal of blood for autologous use: dose, response, toxicity, and efficacy. Transfusion 34:66, 1994
27. Pendyck J, Avorn J, Kuriyan N, et al: Blood donation in the elderly. JAMA 257:1186, 1987
28. Surgenor DM, Wallace EL, Hao SHS, et al: Collection and transfusion of blood in the United States 1982–1988. N Engl J Med 322:1646, 1990

29. Toy PTCY, Strauss RG, Stehling LC, et al: Predeposited autologous blood for elective surgery: a national multicenter study. N Engl J Med 316:517, 1987
30. Miller RD, Robbin TO, Tong MJ: Coagulation defects associated with massive blood transfusions. Ann Surg 174:794, 1971
31. Lim RC Jr, Olcott C IV, Robinson AJ, et al: Platelet response and coagulation changes following massive blood replacement. J Trauma 13:577, 1973
32. Counts RB, Halsch C, Simon TL, et al: Hemostasis in massively transfused patients. Ann Surg 190:91, 1979
33. National Institutes of Health: Fresh-frozen plasma: indications and risks (NIH consensus development summary). Conn Med 49:295, 1985
34. Himansu KB: Fibrinolysis and abruptio placenta. Br J Obstet Gynaecol 76:481, 1969
35. Friedman NJ, Hoag MS, Robinson AJ: Hemorrhagic syndrome following transurethral prostatic resection for benign adenoma. Arch Intern Med 124:341, 1969
36. Goodnight SH, Kenoyer G Rapaport SI, et al: Defibrination after brain-tissue destruction. N Engl J Med 290:1043, 1974
37. Coffin CM: Current issues in transfusion therapy. Postgrad Med 8:343, 1987
38. Braunstein AH, Oberman HA: Transfusion of plasma components. Transfusion 249:281, 1984
39. Murray DJ, Olson J, Strauss R, et al: Coagulation changes during packed red cell replacement of major blood loss. Anesthesiology 69:839, 1988
40. Giorgio A, Finegold H, Ragno G, et al: Effect of autologous fresh- and liquid-preserved platelets on an aspirin-induced thrombocytopathy in the baboon. Presented at the American Association of Blood Banks Joint Congress. Los Angeles, November 10–15, 1990: S-164
41. Harker LA, Schlicter SJ: The bleeding time as a screening test for evaluation of platelet function. N Engl J Med 287:155, 1972
42. Daly PA: Platelet transfusion—clinical applications in the oncology setting. Am J Med Sci 280:130, 1980
43. Handin RI, Valeri CR: Hemostatic effectiveness of platelets stored at 22°C. N Engl J Med 285:538, 1971
44. Mannucci PM, Ruggeri ZM, Pareti FI, et al: 1-Desamino-8-D-arginine vasopressin: a new pharmacological approach to the management of haemophilia and von Willebrand's disease. Lancet 1:869, 1977
45. Mannucci PM, Remuzzi G, Pusinieri F, et al: Desamino-8-D-arginine vasopressin shortens the bleeding time in uremia. N Engl J Med 308:8, 1983
46. Kobrinsky NL, Israels ED, Gerrard JM, et al: Shortening of bleeding time by 1-desamino-8-D-arginine vasopressin in various bleeding disorders. Lancet 1:1185, 1984
47. Kobrinsky NL, Letts RM, Patel LR, et al: 1-Desamino-8-D-arginine vasopressin (desmopressin) decreases operative blood loss in patients having Harrington rod spinal fusion surgery. Ann Intern Med 107:446, 1987
48. Saltzman EW, Weinstein MJ, Weintraub RM, et al: Treatment with desmopressin acetate to reduce blood loss after cardiac surgery. A double-blind randomized trial. N Engl J Med 314: 1402, 1986
49. Mannucci PM: Desmopressin (DDAVP) for treatment of disorders of hemostasis. Prog Hemost Thromb 8:19, 1986
50. Grotz I, Koehler J, Olsen D, et al: The effect of desmopressin acetate on postoperative hemorrhage in patients receiving aspirin therapy before coronary bypass operations. J Thorac Cardiovasc Surg 104:1417, 1992
51. D'Alauro FS, Johns RA: Hypotension related to desmopressin administration following cardiopulmonary bypass. Anesthesiology 69:962, 1988
52. De Rie MA, van der Plas-van Dalen CM, Engelfriet CP, et al: The serology of febrile transfusion reactions. Vox Sang 49:126, 1985
53. Ramirez MA: Horse asthma following blood transfusion: report of a case. JAMA 73:984, 1919
54. Snyder EL, Underwood PA, Spivack M, et al: An in vivo evaluation of microaggregate blood filtration during total hip replacement. Ann Surg 190:75, 1979
55. Rosario MD, Rumsey EW, Arakaki G, et al: Blood microaggregates and ultrafilters. J Trauma 18:498, 1978
56. Ketai LH, Grum CM: C3a and adult respiratory distress syndrome after massive transfusion. Crit Care Med 14:1101, 1986
57. Collings JA, James PM, Bredenberg CE: The relationship between transfusion and hypoxemia in combat casualties. Ann Surg 188:513, 1978
58. Brubaker DB: Human posttransfusion graft-versus-host disease. Vox Sang 45:401, 1983
59. Rutledge R, Sheldon GF, Collins ML: Massive transfusion. Crit Care Clin 4:791, 1986
60. Stevens CE, Aach RD, Hollinger FB, et al: Hepatitis B virus antibody in blood donors and the occurrence of non-A non-B hepatitis in transfusion recipients. Ann Intern Med 101:733, 1984
61. Alter HJ, Purcell RH, Shih JW, et al: Detection of antibody to hepatitis C virus and prospectively followed transfusion recipients with acute and chronic non-A non-B hepatitis. N Engl J Med 321:1494, 1989
62. Choo QL, Ku OG, Weiner AJ, et al: Isolation of a cDNA clone-derived from blood-borne non-A non-B viral hepatitis genome. Science 244:359, 1989
63. Ku OG, Choo QL, Alter HL, et al: An assay for circulating antibodies to a major etiologic virus of human non-A non-B hepatitis. Science 244:362, 1989
64. Stevens CE, Taylor PE, Pindyck J, et al: Epidemiology of hepatic C virus: a preliminary study in volunteer blood donors. JAMA 263:49, 1990
65. Curran JW, Lawrence DW, Jaffe H, et al: Acquired immunodeficiency syndrome (AIDS) associated with transfusions. N Engl J Med 310:69, 1984
66. Dodd RY: The risk of transfusion transmitted infection. N Engl J Med 327:369, 1992
67. Howland WS, Schweizer O: Physiologic compensation for storage lesion of bank blood. Anesth Analg 44:8, 1965
68. American Heart Association: Guidelines for cardiopulmonary resuscitation and emergency cardiac care. JAMA 268:2210, 1992
69. Mattor JA, Weil MH, Shubin H, et al: Cardiac arrest in the critically ill: II. Hyperosmolal states following cardiac arrest. Am J Med 56:162, 1974
70. Bishop RL, Wiesfeldt ML: Sodium bicarbonate administration during cardiac arrest. JAMA 235:507, 1976
71. Von Planta M, Weil MH, Gazmuri RJ, et al: Myocardial acidosis associated with CO_2 production during cardiac arrest and resuscitation. Circulation 80:684, 1989
72. Bunker JP, Bendixen HH, Murphy JA: Hemodynamic effects of intravenously administered sodium citrate. N Engl J Med 266: 372, 1962
73. Linko K, Sapelin I: Electrolyte and acid-base disturbances caused by blood transfusions. Acta Anaesthesiol Scand 30:139, 1986

APPENDIX
Clinical Recommendations for Transfusion

In 1994, the National Institutes of Health National Heart Lung and Blood Institute published their recommendations for the use of red blood cells (RBCs), platelets, and fresh frozen plasma (FFP).[1] The indications are summarized here.

I. Rationale for component use

Blood transfusion can be lifesaving therapy for patients with a variety of medical and surgical conditions. Advances in the use of blood components have made whole blood transfusions rarely necessary. Blood component therapy provides better treatment for the patient by giving only the specific component needed. Such therapy helps to conserve blood resources, because components from 1 unit of blood can be used to treat several patients.

II. Red blood cell transfusion[2]

RBC transfusions increase oxygen-carrying capacity in anemic patients. Transfusing 1 unit of RBCs usually increases the hemoglobin by about 1 g/dL and the hematocrit by 2% to 3% in the average 70-kg adult.

In deciding whether to transfuse a specific patient, the physician should consider the age of the person; the cause, degree, and time course of the anemia; hemodynamic stability; and the presence of coexisting cardiac, pulmonary, or vascular conditions. There is no across-the-board threshold or "trigger." Undertransfusion and overtransfusion should be avoided.

A. Transfuse red blood cells

Transfuse red blood cells only to increase oxygen-carrying capacity in anemic patients. When a treatable cause of anemia can be identified and time permits, specific therapy (eg, vitamin B_{12}, iron, folate) should be used in preference to transfusion. If volume expanders are indicated, fluids such as crystalloid or nonblood colloid solutions should be administered.

B. Do not transfuse red blood cells

1. For volume expansion only
2. In place of a hematinic
3. To enhance wound healing
4. To improve general well-being

III. Platelet transfusion[3]

Platelet transfusions are administered to control or prevent bleeding associated with deficiencies in platelet number or function. One unit of platelet concentrate should increase the platelet count in the average adult recipient by at least 5000 platelets/μL.

Prophylactic platelet transfusion may be indicated to prevent bleeding in patients with severe thrombocytopenia. For the clinically stable patient with an intact vascular system and normal platelet function, prophylactic platelet transfusions may be indicated for platelet counts of less than 10,000 to 20,000/μL.

A. Transfuse platelets

Transfuse platelets to control or prevent bleeding associated with deficiencies in platelet number or function.

B. Do not transfuse platelets

1. To patients with immune or thrombotic thrombocytopenic purpura, unless there is clinically significant bleeding
2. Prophylactically with massive blood transfusion
3. Prophylactically after cardiopulmonary bypass

A patient undergoing an operation or other invasive procedure is unlikely to benefit from prophylactic platelet transfusions if the platelet count is 50,000/μL or more and thrombocytopenia is the sole abnormality. Platelet transfusions at higher platelet counts may be required for patients with systemic bleeding and for patients at higher risk of bleeding because of additional coagulation defects, sepsis, or platelet dysfunction related to medication or disease.

IV. Fresh frozen plasma transfusion[4]

FFP transfusions should be administered only to increase the level of clotting factors in patients with a demonstrated deficiency. Laboratory tests should be used to monitor the patient with a suspected clotting disorder. If prothrombin time (PT) and partial thromboplastin time (PTT) are less than 1.5 times normal, FFP transfusion is rarely indicated.

A. Transfuse fresh frozen plasma

Transfuse fresh frozen plasma to increase the level of clotting factors in patients with a demonstrated deficiency. Patients who have been given the anticoagulant warfarin sodium become deficient in vitamin K–dependent coagulation factors II, VII, IX, and X. If these patients are bleeding or require emergency surgery, they may be candidates for FFP transfusion to achieve immediate hemostasis when time does not permit warfarin reversal by stopping the drug and, when necessary, administering vitamin K. Patients with thrombotic thrombocytopenic purpura or hemolytic uremic syndrome may benefit from FFP transfusion.

B. Do not transfuse fresh frozen plasma

1. For volume expansion
2. As a nutritional supplement
3. Prophylactically for less than one blood volume hemorrhage and replacement
4. Prophylactically after cardiopulmonary bypass

V. Risks common to all blood components

Infection and alloimmunization are the major complications associated with transfusion of blood components. Risk is associated with the number of donor exposures.

The risk of infection is geographically variable. Risks listed below are per unit transfused.[5-8]

A. Hepatitis C virus (HCV) can be transmitted by blood transfusion. With the introduction of a screening test to detect anti-HCV in donated blood and the discarding of positive units, the estimated risk of transfusion-related hepatitis C has been decreased to approximately 1 in 3300 transfusions.
B. Human immunodeficiency viruses pose a relatively small transfusion hazard. The wide range of estimated risk (1 in 40,000 to 225,000) reflects geographic variance.
C. Other infectious diseases or agents, such as hepatitis B (1 in 200,000), human T-cell lymphotropic virus types I and II (1 in 50,000), cytomegalovirus, malaria, and rare diseases (<1 in 1 million) may be transmitted through transfusion.
D. Fatal hemolytic transfusion reactions can occur (approximately 1 in 600,000). They are caused by an ABO incompatibility, primarily due to errors in patient identification at the bedside.
E. Recipients of any blood component may produce antibodies against donor antigens (ie, alloimmunization). This condition can result in an inadequate response to transfusion.
F. Allergic reactions, febrile reactions, and circulatory overload may also occur.

REFERENCES

1. National Blood Resource Education Program Expert Panel on the Indications for the Use of Red Blood Cells, Platelets, and Fresh Frozen Plasma: National Blood Resource Education Program, Office of Prevention, Education, and Control. NIH Publication No. 93-2974a. Bethesda, MD: National Heart, Lung, and Blood institute, Revised August 1993
2. Office of Medical Applications of Research. National Institutes of Health: Perioperative red cell transfusion. JAMA 260:2700, 1988
3. Office of Medical Applications of Research. National Institutes of Health: Platelet transfusion therapy. JAMA 257:1777, 1987
4. Office of Medical Applications of Research. National Institutes of Health: Fresh frozen plasma: indications and risks. JAMA 253:551, 1985
5. Donahue JG, Munoz A, Ness P, et al: The declining risk of post-transfusion hepatitis C virus infection. N Engl J Med 327: 369, 1992
6. Petersen LR, Satten G, Dodd RY, et al: Current estimates of the infectious window period and risk of HIV infection from seronegative blood donations. In the program abstracts of the Fifth National Forum on AIDS, Hepatitis, and Other Blood-Borne Diseases, in Atlanta, 1992 March 29–April 1. Princeton: Symedco, 1992: 37
7. Dodd RY: The risk of transfusion-transmitted infection. N Engl J Med 327:419, 1992
8. Linden J, Paul B, Dressler KP: A report of 104 transfusion errors in New York state. Transfusion 32:601, 1992

Complications in Anesthesiology, second edition,
edited by Nikolaus Gravenstein and Robert R. Kirby.
Lippincott-Raven Publishers, Philadelphia © 1996.

CHAPTER 39

Difficulties in Sickle Cell States

Orah S. Platt
Fredrick K. Orkin

Sickle cell anemia is a common chronic hemolytic anemia among black Americans. Most patients with this and other sickling disorders are otherwise healthy and are able to function effectively at school, in the workplace, and at home. However, prolonged periods of well-being are often punctuated by unexpected, acute episodes of clinical deterioration that tip the delicate balance and make the patient vulnerable to serious and even fatal complications. Surgery is one of the situations that can destabilize the condition of an otherwise well patient, making the anesthetic treatment of these patients a challenge. This chapter reviews the physical basis and pathophysiologic features of sickling disorders and provides a framework for anesthetic treatment of affected patients.

PATHOPHYSIOLOGIC FEATURES

In 1910, Herrick described hemolytic anemia in a black Jamaican medical student whose peripheral blood contained "peculiar, elongated and sickle-shaped red blood corpuscles."[1] During the ensuing decades, others noted the reversibility of sickling with oxygenation.[2] Demonstrating that this phenomenon occurs only in erythrocytes containing a genetically determined abnormal hemoglobin (hemoglobin S), Pauling termed the sickle cell disorder a "molecular disease" in 1949.[3] Subsequently, others extended this medical paradigm. A single amino acid substitution, valine for glutamic acid, was identified as the basis for hemoglobin polymerization with deoxygenation, followed by sickling of erythrocytes, hemolysis, and vascular occlusion.

Molecular Basis of Sickling

The normal hemoglobin molecule (hemoglobin A) is composed of four globin polypeptide chains, each of which is folded such that it provides a pocket for an oxygen-binding heme. Specific amino acid composition influences hemoglobin's function: hydrophilic amino acids on the molecule's surface help keep it in solution, whereas other amino acids are important in forming linkages among the four globin chains as the molecule becomes oxygenated. As one oxygen molecule binds to each heme in a sequential, *cooperative* process, the affinity of the remaining hemes for oxygen increases. The oxyhemoglobin dissociation curve rises first slowly and then steeply; when an oxygen molecule has combined with each of the four hemes, it flattens again.

Hemoglobin S

Hemoglobin S differs from normal hemoglobin A by a single amino acid substitution: normally, the sixth amino acid of the β-globin chain is a hydrophilic glutamic acid, a charged amino acid that is exposed on the surface of the deoxygenated hemoglobin A molecule and helps to keep this bulky protein in solution. In contrast, in hemoglobin S, the hydrophilic glutamic acid is replaced by hydrophobic, uncharged valine. This amino acid, when exposed on the surface of the deoxygenated hemoglobin S molecule, results in decreased solubility that begins gel formation. Subsequently, deoxyhemoglobin S can polymerize into a complex, filamentous, crystal-like structure.[4]

Polymerization

The kinetics of this polymerization reaction have been studied in detail. There are two thermodynamically measurable steps: a rate-limiting lag phase (the *delay time*); and a thermodynamically favorable polymerization phase. The shorter the delay, the faster the polymerization. Factors favoring a short delay include increased hemoglobin concentration, decreased pH, increased 2,3-diphosphoglycerate concentrations, decreased temperature, increased ionic strength, and decreased oxygen saturation.

Clinical Implications

Erythrocytes with the highest mean corpuscular hemoglobin concentrations are especially susceptible to polymerization, providing the rationale for clinical management that includes ensuring optimal hydration to reduce the intraerythrocytic hemoglobin concentration. Even at 100% oxygen saturation, some erythrocytes irreversibly sickle in persons who are homozygous for the abnormal gene (SS); the process accelerates as the oxygen saturation decreases to less than 85% (Table 39-1). The relatively weak forces holding deoxyhemoglobin S molecules together are easily reversed by increasing temperature, improving hydration, and adding ligands (eg, oxygen).

Effects of Other Hemoglobins

A decreased tendency to polymerize occurs when other hemoglobins coexist with hemoglobin S in a variety of heterozygous states and when fetal hemoglobin (hemoglobin F) persists in the circulation: hemoglobin F is more protective against sickling than is normal hemoglobin A which, in turn, is more protective than hemoglobin C (see Table 39-1). Thus, the persistence of hemoglobin F accounts for the mildness or asymptomatic nature of the SS state in the first 6 months of life, despite the presence of up to 80% hemoglobin S. This protection exists because hemoglobin F contains λ rather than β-globin chains. Similarly, persons heterozygous for hemoglobins S and A (AS) (sickle cell trait) rarely have symptoms (see Table 39-1), and even then only under the most extraordinary physiologic circumstances. Hemoglobin A_2 represents a normal variant comprising less than 3% of hemoglobin in the adult and about 0.5% of hemoglobin in the newborn.

Vascular Occlusion

When SS red cells become deoxygenated, there is a delay before the deoxyhemoglobin S inside the cell begins to polymerize. If this process takes place in a very narrow vessel, the now rigid red cells, full of polymerized deoxyhemoglobin S, can occlude the vessel and cause tissue ischemia. This situation is called a *crisis* in the ischemic tissue.

Most often, however, the delay is longer than the transit time through the capillary bed, and no occlusion takes place. Likewise, factors that shorten the delay increase the chance that occlusion will occur. For this reason, hypoxic, acidotic, dehydrated patients are vulnerable to occlusion, and certain tissues such as the hypoxic, low-flow spleen and bone marrow, and the hypoxic, hyperosmolar renal papillae are especially susceptible.

Red Cell Survival

Besides causing vascular occlusion, the sickling process results in markedly shortened red cell survival, as low as 15% of normal.[5] The bone marrow of affected persons is unable to compensate through erythropoietin stimulation because of the decreased affinity of hemoglobin S for oxygen.[6] Thus, the accelerated red cell destruction manifests itself as a chronic hemolytic anemia.

Oxygen Transport

Sickle cell blood has a decreased affinity for oxygen principally because intraerythrocytic polymerization impairs oxygen binding.[7] In addition, in compensation for anemia, intraerythrocytic 2,3-diphosphoglycerate concentrations are higher than those in normal red cells, resulting in a shift of the oxyhemoglobin dissociation curve far to the right. This change, in turn, facilitates oxygen delivery to the tissues. The partial pressure of oxygen at which hemoglobin S is 50% saturated is 49.7 mm Hg for whole SS blood, compared with the normal value of 30 to 32 mm Hg at pH 7.13 and 37°C.[8]

Although the considerable shift in the oxyhemoglobin dissociation curve compensates for the otherwise markedly reduced delivery of oxygen, it also promotes the formation of deoxyhemoglobin, with further polymerization.[9] In addition, a marked increase in cardiac index also helps to offset the oxygen flux deficit.[10]

Rheologic Features

Symptoms in sickle cell disease are related not to anemia but to rheologic changes—alterations in blood viscosity and the

TABLE 39-1
Features of the Common Sickling Disorders

DISORDER	SYMPTOMS	SPLENOMEGALY	CONCENTRATION OF CIRCULATING HEMOGLOBIN (g/dL)	BLOOD CELLS		HEMOGLOBINS (%) PRESENT ON ELECTROPHORESIS
				Sickled	*Target*	
SS disease	++++	0	6 to 8	Many	Many	90 to 100 S; remainder F
S–β-thalassemia	++ to +++	++	7 to 8	Few	Many	65 to 85 S; remainder A, A_2, and F
SC disease	+ to ++	++ to +++	9 to 11	Few	Very many	40 to 60 each S and C
S with hereditary persistence of Hb F	0 to +	0	Normal	0	±	70 to 80 S; 20 to 30 F
AS disease (sickle cell trait)	0	0	Normal	0	0	20 to 40 S; remainder normal A

resultant impairment in flow.[11] The increase in viscosity is directly related to the number and degree of sickled cells.[12] With deoxygenation, it is greatest for SS blood, followed in order by SC, SF, and AS, an observation consistent with the differential influence that these other hemoglobins have on hemoglobin S polymerization and severity of symptoms (see Table 39-1).[13] Whereas SS-containing red cells become less filterable within 0.12 second of deoxygenation, AS-containing red cells (ie, those from persons with sickle cell trait) undergo no change in 5 seconds,[14] emphasizing the importance of transit time in the hypoxic microcirculation. Even with complete deoxygenation, AS blood sickles after about 70 seconds compared with 2 seconds for SS blood.[15]

A variety of other factors also influence the viscosity of sickle cell blood. Admixture of normal cells with sickle cells attenuates the increase in viscosity associated with deoxygenation,[16] providing the rationale for transfusion as both therapy and prophylaxis. Not unexpectedly, a decrease in temperature is associated with an increase in the viscosity of sickle cell blood,[17] consistent with the observation that exposure to cold may precipitate a sickling crisis. Equilibration of deoxygenated sickle cell blood with clinical concentrations of halothane is also associated with increased viscosity.[18]

The Vicious Cycle

An understanding of the foregoing altered rheologic properties of SS blood and the factors that precipitate sickling provides a ready appreciation of the "vicious cycle of erythrostasis" that has been recognized clinically for more than half a century.[19] In persons with SS blood, sickling normally occurs during deoxygenation as the erythrocytes migrate slowly through the capillary microcirculation. Sickling increases blood viscosity, further slowing the circulation and leading, in turn, to further deoxygenation, acidosis, and enhanced sickling.

Beyond the microcirculation, oxygenation of those erythrocytes not irreversibly sickled enables them to assume the normal discoid shape. However, under physiologically stressful circumstances characterized by hypoxemia, hypotension, acidosis, cooling, and circulatory stasis, the cycle accelerates, eventually yielding static masses of sickled erythrocytes that occlude the circulation. Although most closely associated with sickle cell anemia (SS blood), this process also occurs, but with less severity, in heterozygous states (hemoglobins SC, S–β-thalassemia, and S with persistence of F) and, under extraordinary physiologic conditions, the heterozygous AS state (sickle cell trait). The interrelated factors that may precipitate the vicious cycle and produce vaso-occlusion in sickling disorders are shown schematically in Figure 39-1.

CLINICAL ASPECTS

Epidemiologic Features

Worldwide in its distribution, the sickle cell gene is especially prevalent in central Africa, Mediterranean areas (eg, Greece, Italy, Turkey, and Saudi Arabia), and India. The migration of black West Africans is believed to have introduced the gene

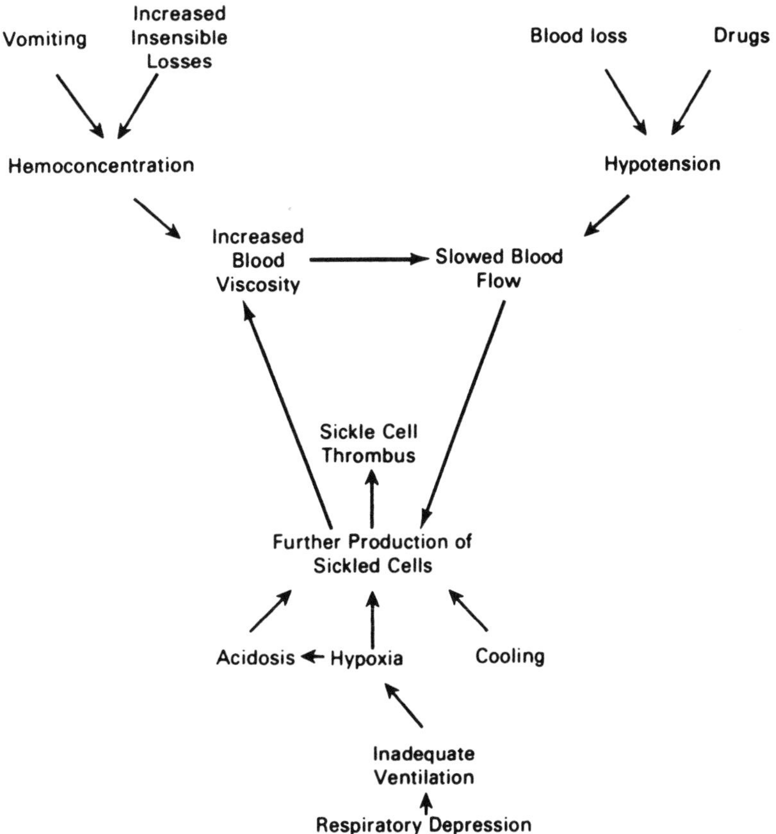

FIGURE 39-1. The vicious cycle of sickle cell disease and the interrelation of factors precipitating crisis in the patient undergoing anesthesia and surgery.

to the United States. Thus, sickle cell disorders in the United States are largely associated with, but not necessarily restricted to, black persons.[20]

Inheritance

Inheritance of the abnormal gene is generally in accordance with Mendelian laws. However, both the normal and abnormal hemoglobin genes are codominant, with each retaining the ability to produce hemoglobin when present. Thus, the SS anemia produces symptoms, whereas AS anemia (sickle cell trait) is rarely symptomatic; the other heterozygous states are characterized by symptoms of intermediate severity (see Table 39-1).

Incidence

The SS state is present in 1 in 625 black Americans at birth; heterozygous states are less frequently encountered: SC, 1 in 833 black persons; S–β-thalassemia, 1 in 1667; and S with persistence of F, 1 in 25,000. The prevalence of AS anemia (sickle cell trait) is estimated at about 8% among black Americans, and perhaps 0.8% for other races.[21]

Features of Sickle Cell Disorders

Table 39-1 presents a summary of the salient clinical characteristics of sickle cell disorders. Given the differing propensities of the genotypes to give rise to sickling under similar physiologic conditions, these disorders present a very wide spectrum of unpredictable symptoms. Children less than 6 months old have few, if any, clinical manifestations because of the protective effect of residual fetal hemoglobin; however, overwhelming sepsis is a special risk in their attacks.[22,23]

Hemoglobin SS Disease

Sickle cell anemia is a severe disorder characterized by chronic hemolytic anemia and repeated episodes of vaso-occlusive crises, producing widespread tissue infarction and organ dysfunction. Manifestations are protean, but commonly include painful crises of the abdomen, back, and extremities; jaundice; renal insufficiency; bone deformities; leg ulcers; and major neurologic deficits (eg, hemiplegia, blindness). Congestive heart failure and severe infections such as osteomyelitis and pneumonia may occur.[24]

Heterozygous Disorders

HEMOGLOBIN SC DISEASE AND S–β-THALASSEMIA. Hemoglobin SC and S–β-thalassemia produce symptoms similar to that noted in SS disease but generally are less severe and less frequent. Patients with hemoglobin SC usually have palpable spleens and appear particularly prone to retinopathy, aseptic necrosis of the femoral heads, and renal papillary necrosis. Some cases of S–β-thalassemia are as severe as SS disease, whereas other heterozygous diseases may be asymptomatic. Family studies, as well as laboratory studies, are usually necessary to differentiate them. Hemoglobin S in association with hereditary persistence of hemoglobin F is rare; affected persons usually are asymptomatic.

HEMOGLOBIN AS DISEASE. Patients with AS blood (sickle cell trait) are rarely symptomatic. Although this disorder is generally benign, AS blood can sickle under extraordinary physiologic circumstances characterized by severe hypoxemia,[15,25] dehydration and stasis, or both. Severe crises have occurred during high-altitude flying in an unpressurized aircraft and with very strenuous physical exercise.[25–31]

Diagnosis

The diagnosis of sickle cell disorders generally is not difficult but requires a complete history and physical examination, complete blood count, examination of the peripheral blood smear, and a test designed to detect hemoglobin S (see Table 39-1).

An evolving variety of laboratory methods are available to screen for or detect hemoglobin S. Currently, the standard method for mass screening is hemoglobin electrophoresis on cellulose acetate; positive results are confirmed with electrophoresis on citrate agar, which differentiates the abnormal hemoglobins. A simpler screening method is the tube solubility (dithionite) test, which is based on the insolubility of reduced hemoglobin S in a solution of slightly acidic phosphate buffer, producing turbidity. This test can be performed with a drop of blood in only 5 minutes.[32]

The sodium metabisulfite test ("sickle prep"), an older method, involves microscopic examination of a wet mount of blood for sickling.[32] At the other end of the spectrum are methods developed for prenatal testing of minute quantities of blood to identify DNA fragments associated with specific hemoglobinopathies.[33,34]

SS Disease in the Newborn

The early diagnosis of sickle cell anemia, before symptoms occur, is the first critical step in preventing the major cause of death, pneumococcal sepsis, in children with this disease. As a result, mass screening of all newborns, when possible, has been recommended.[35] Because the sickle mutation affects the β-globin chain of hemoglobin, a chain that is not prominent *in utero*, newborns with sickling disorders are neither anemic nor symptomatic.

The diagnosis is made at birth by hemoglobin electrophoresis. Normal newborns have mostly hemoglobin F with a small but measurable amount of hemoglobin A; those with hemoglobin AS have mostly hemoglobin F and a mixture of hemoglobins A and S; newborns with sickle cell SS disease have only hemoglobins F and S.

SS Disease in Older Children and Adults

After the first few months of life, as the production of hemoglobin S increases and the production of hemoglobin F decreases, the clinical syndrome of sickle cell anemia emerges. The typical patient is moderately anemic, with hematocrit and reticulocyte counts in the 20s. The peripheral smear is quite bizarre, full of long, slender sickle forms, target cells, nucleated red cells, and red cell fragments. Numerous Howell-Jolly bodies are evidence of splenic dysfunction, even though the spleen is frequently enlarged in the first few years of life. Jaundice, increased lactate dehydrogenase, and increased bilirubin reflect the chronic hemolytic nature of the anemia.

These laboratory findings compose the chronic picture of the disease both when the patient is well and when he or she is in crisis. As in the newborn period, the definitive diagnosis is made by hemoglobin electrophoresis; the pattern reveals predominantly hemoglobin S, with varying amounts of hemoglobin F and no hemoglobin A. The various screening tests that are used for detection of asymptomatic sickle cell trait are also abnormal in SS anemia.

Sickle Cell Trait

Persons with sickle cell trait are neither anemic nor symptomatic; the peripheral smear is entirely normal. This trait can be diagnosed with a positive sodium metabisulfite "sickle prep" or positive dithionate precipitation screening test. Hemoglobin electrophoresis confirms the diagnosis, revealing a pattern with hemoglobins A and S.

Other Sickle Cell Syndromes

Hemoglobin SC disease is associated with mild anemia (hematocrit in the low 30s) and a reticulocyte count of 5% to 10%. The peripheral smear shows numerous target cells, and only rare, if any, sickle forms. The sickle screening tests are positive, and the hemoglobin electrophoresis reveals hemoglobins S and C. The combination of sickle cell trait with β-thalassemia results in clinical severity that varies with the degree of output of normal hemoglobin A from the β-thalassemia gene. In the S–β-thalassemia syndromes, the red cells are microcytic, and splenomegaly can be prominent.

TREATMENT

Although the treatment of a group of chronic diseases is beyond the scope of this chapter, the anesthesiologist must understand the therapeutic setting on which anesthetic management is superimposed. For simplicity, the discussion relates to the patients most severely affected, typically those with sickle cell anemia.

Supportive Measures

Given the chronic nature of these disorders, and especially the episodic severe complications, affected persons require close medical supervision, counseling, and education. In particular, they must understand the importance of maintaining good hydration and in seeking medical attention early when fever or other signs of illness develop. Splenic infarction renders these persons more susceptible to infection, especially in the case of infants and young children; care often includes chronic penicillin therapy and periodic vaccination against *Streptococcus pneumoniae* and *Haemophilus influenzae.*

Maintenance Therapy

In the absence of specific therapy for the hemolytic anemia, these patients require daily folic acid supplementation. Although diluting the patient's concentration of abnormal hemoglobin (to <50% of circulating hemoglobin) by periodic blood transfusion and exchange transfusion can reduce sickling and, thus, blood viscosity, the problems of isoimmunization, iron overload, disease transmission (eg, hepatitis or acquired immunodeficiency syndrome), and high cost preclude its routine use. Transfusion therapy has become part of obstetric care in many centers, however.[36] Such therapy corrects the mother's anemia and reduces the number of sickling crises, but fetal outcome is apparently unchanged.[37]

Enhancement of Endogenous Hemoglobin F Production

This approach has been the focus of recent research with a variety of approaches, including cytotoxic and cytostatic agents,[38–40] erythropoietin,[41] or hydroxyurea.[39,42,43] Further evaluation is underway. Bone marrow transplantation has been used in a few especially severe cases in which a co-existing hematologic malignancy is present. Immunologic problems are much more common in these patients, already alloimmunized from frequent transfusions, rendering this treatment largely of theoretic interest, even in such rare circumstances.[44] Genetic engineering promises to repair or replace the abnormal hemoglobin *in vivo.*

Therapy for Sickle Cell Crises

Although these disorders have no cure, much can be done to ameliorate and even abort them. Often crises are characterized by the symptoms associated with the involved organs: musculoskeletal (pain, tenderness, and erythema); chest (pleuritic pain, fever, and cough); splenic sequestration (enlarged spleen, severe anemia, and possible severe hypotension); abdominal (much like an acute abdomen); and neurologic (altered mental status, motor deficits, sensory deficits, or both).

Given the cyclical nature of the underlying disorder, treatment should be prompt and directed toward specific problems: analgesics for painful crises, oxygen for hypoxemia, and bicarbonate for acidosis. Oxygen therapy also reduces hemoglobin production by decreasing erythropoietin concentrations. Thus, it should be intermittent to avoid the rebound increase in abnormal hemoglobin that follows discontinuation of continuous oxygen administration.[45]

Blood Transfusion

Transfusion decreases the fraction of abnormal hemoglobin in the patient's circulation, in turn decreasing the amount of sickling and improving microvascular perfusion. However, the role of transfusion is limited due to the need for more than half of the patient's red cells to be of donor origin, the related possibility of intravascular volume overload, and the previously mentioned problems associated with frequent transfusions. When blood is given, packed red cells are infused as part of a partial exchange transfusion.[46] Typically, this therapy is reserved for the more severe and life-threatening crises, such as cerebrovascular accident, splenic or hepatic sequestration, acute chest syndrome,[47] and priapism.

ANESTHETIC MANAGEMENT

Preoperative Assessment

As in other clinical settings, the goal of preoperative assessment is the identification of treatable risk factors associated with adverse patient outcome. Thus, the focus is on those factors that may precipitate sickling, infection, and hypoxia. An especially careful review of systems is necessary, given that repeated vaso-occlusive crises over a lifetime lead to compromised organ function (Table 39-2). Again, to facilitate discussion, we assume that the patient has sickle cell anemia.

Heart

Most sickle cell anemia patients have abnormal cardiac examinations, including cardiomegaly, a hyperdynamic circulation, and systolic ejection murmurs.[48–50] These findings primarily are the result of the compensation for chronic anemia.[51] Electrocardiographic evidence of both left and right ventricular hypertrophy is common.[50] Interestingly, myocardial infarction is an extremely rare event, presumably because of the short transit time through the coronary circulation. However, subtle myocardial injury and myocardial dysfunction may be relatively common.

In one study, one third of affected children had decreased left ventricular contractility, and 15% had ischemic electrocardiographic changes and decreased ejection fractions during exercise.[52] From a practical, clinical point of view, the more severely affected patients may have rapidly developing congestive heart failure under stress, such as a volume load (hydration or transfusion). The patient must be examined carefully and observed for signs of mild congestive failure when intravenous fluids are administered.

TABLE 39-2
Complications of Sickle Cell Disorders

- Painful (vaso-occlusive) crisis
- Cardiac irregularities
- Hepatic crisis
- Cholelithiasis
- Aseptic necrosis of bone
- Bone marrow necrosis and fat embolism
- Cerebral vascular occlusion
- Hematuria
- Priapism
- Splenic infarction and sequestration
- Postsplenectomy sepsis

Sears DA: Hematologic diseases requiring critical care. In Civetta JM, Taylor RW, Kirby RR (eds): Critical care, 2nd ed. Philadelphia: JB Lippincott, 1992: 1729.

Lungs

Repeated episodes of occlusion in the lungs result in progressive obliteration of the pulmonary vascular bed, pulmonary hypertension, and chronic lung disease. In one study, the arterial partial pressure of oxygen in asymptomatic children at rest was between 65 and 85 mm Hg, with alveolar–arterial oxygen partial pressure differences of 27 to 42 mm Hg while they breathed room air, and 186 to 246 mm Hg with breathing of 100% oxygen. These values were consistent with a 12% to 16% pulmonary shunt, due to undefined anatomic pathways and abnormal heterogeneity of ventilation–perfusion ratios.[53] The mean membrane-diffusing and pulmonary-diffusing capacities are less than normal.[54] Pulmonary function tests often document reduced vital and total lung capacities.[55]

Kidneys

Most affected patients have lost the ability to concentrate urine (hyposthenuria) and have a fixed water loss.[56] They should not be left for long periods perioperatively without adequate intravenous fluid replacement. Baseline urine specific gravity, serum electrolytes, and body weight are important in determining the optimum fluid and electrolyte replacement strategy. In addition, chronic renal failure occurs. Blood urea nitrogen and creatinine measurements facilitate drug dosage adjustments for renal failure.

Liver

The most common liver complication of this disease is bilirubin gallstone formation. Cholecystectomy is the most common surgical procedure. Mild hepatic dysfunction can result from gallbladder disease, hepatic infarction, and transfusion-related hepatitis. Baseline liver function studies are helpful to evaluate subsequent hepatic decompensation. Production of pseudocholinesterase is often mildly impaired.[57] Drugs with predominantly hepatic clearance should be used with particular care.

Skin

Chronic leg ulcers can be a serious problem for older patients. If these are present, care must be taken to protect them from further trauma during long operative procedures.

Blood

All patients with sickle cell disease have a chronic hemolytic anemia. In general, because of cardiovascular compensatory mechanisms, this anemia is tolerated well, and transfusion is not indicated. The distribution of red cell antigens varies among racial groups. Black persons are commonly negative for part of the Rh complex, Duffy, and Kell antigens. Because Caucasian donors are largely positive for these antigens, black patients, not surprisingly, become sensitized to them and can have serious crossmatching and transfusion reaction problems. Therefore, be sure to determine if patients have been previously transfused. For elective transfusions, the patient should have minor group antigen testing, and minor group compatible red cells should be used.

Preoperative Management

Because of the substantial amount of co-existing disease in these patients, and the difficulty in treating many of their perioperative complications satisfactorily, prevention of problems must receive special emphasis. Even elective surgery should be avoided or performed only when the patient is truly in optimum general medical condition. The need for enhanced postoperative care and supervision makes outpatient care generally unwise.

Given the importance of avoiding circulatory stasis, hypovolemia must be treated preoperatively and assiduously avoided through the rest of the perioperative period. Depending on the surgical procedure, prophylactic antibiotics may be indicated. Preanesthetic sedatives and narcotics should be avoided, if possible, lest cardiorespiratory depression aggravate the sickling process.

Prophylactic Transfusion

Prophylactic transfusion is a controversial therapy. Patients likely to benefit from it are those who are hypoxic, unstable, and undergoing procedures that are likely to cause considerable blood loss, or who face long postoperative recovery periods with prolonged bedrest. A healthy, steady-state patient does not require preoperative transfusion to undergo general anesthesia for short procedures, such as myringotomy. In contrast, a patient having a hip replacement for aseptic necrosis of the femoral head is likely to experience reduced postoperative morbidity and enhanced healing with transfusion therapy.

OUTCOME. Difference in patient populations (eg, disease severity, complexity of surgery), as well as the general trend of improved patient outcome after anesthesia, make comparison of reports of clinical experience with transfusion difficult. In fact, the incidence of death and severe morbidity is rather similar in some reports of conservative transfusion (eg, replacement of surgical blood loss)[58–60] and more aggressive prophylactic transfusion.[61,62] Nonetheless, prophylactic transfusion therapy remains a common procedure for more severely affected patients having complex surgery.

TECHNIQUES. Patients can tolerate simple transfusion of packed red cells if they are carefully monitored for signs of cardiovascular overload. In most cases, a partial or complete exchange transfusion is preferable to remove part or all of the patient's abnormal red cells while replacing, isovolemically, normal red cells. The goal is less than 30% hemoglobin S. Although venous access may be a problem, adults usually can undergo phlebotomy from one arm while being transfused in the other. Automated blood exchanges can be efficiently and safely done in many blood banks equipped with apheresis machines.

A simple alternative method to reduce the patient's circulating hemoglobin S to less than 30% can be achieved by transfusing about 5 mL/kg of packed cells every 2 weeks while simultaneously following serial hemoglobin electrophoresis. This procedure may take a few months to complete. Details of various transfusion regimens are outlined in a helpful monograph available upon request from the National Institutes of Health.[63]

RECOMMENDATIONS. The multicenter national preoperative transfusion study group findings[64] compared the perioperative complication rates of 551 sickle cell patients, randomized to either aggressive transfusion, wherein the Hb S was decreased to <30% and the Hb was increased to 10.0 g/dL, or conservative transfusion in which the goal was a Hb of 10.0 g/dL independent of Hb S concentrate. The investigators observed a generally similar serious complication rate in both groups. The only significant complication difference related to a 14% transfusion complication in the aggressively transfused group as compared to a 7% rate in the conservatively transfused group. The immediate preoperative Hb S levels averaged 34% in the aggressively transfused group as compared to 58% in the conservatively transfused one. A preoperative HbS of <60% and a Hb level no greater than 11 g/dL in high risk sickle cell patients appear to be appropriate goals.

Intraoperative Management

The key to successful intraoperative management is the maintenance of normal tissue oxygenation and perfusion, acid–base regulation, body temperature, and hydration.[58,65–69] Thus, the operating room should be warmer than is customary, and the patient should be treated, if necessary, with heating blankets, or, even better, forced heated air blankets, airway humidification, and warmed intravenous fluids. In the postanesthetic care unit, heating lamps are among additional approaches to maintain normothermia, especially if shivering is present. Special care must also be taken with boards used to stabilize intravenous access sites in extremities, casts, and dressing to maintain good circulation.

Monitoring

Meticulous assessment of oxygenation, blood pressure, urine output, and pH is essential throughout the perioperative period, with prompt correction of underlying derangements. Although preoxygenation occasionally is not undertaken in healthy patients immediately before induction, it is mandatory in patients with sickle cell disease. During the anesthetic, the inspired oxygen concentration should be adjusted so that the patient maintains an arterial partial pressure of oxygen of at least 80 to 100 mm Hg. Even mild degrees of hypoxemia present an especially serious risk for these patients and are difficult to assess clinically (because of the anemia); thus, oxygenation must be monitored closely throughout the entire perioperative period. Fortunately, with pulse oximetry, continuous monitoring largely has supplanted frequent, inconvenient, and costly periodic blood gas determinations.

Anesthetic Agents and Techniques

As is true in other clinical settings, the choice of anesthetic agent and technique is not as critical as the care with which the anesthetic is administered.[58,64] Searle notes, "a fit patient will tolerate considerable physiologic insults during anaesthesia, but the patient with sickle cell anemia will not."[58]

TECHNIQUES. Although general anesthesia is usually chosen, regional techniques and conduction anesthesia are not contraindicated for surgery or postoperative pain therapy. A recent case report describes the use of epidural analgesia for management of obstetric labor pain occurring during sickle cell crisis.[70] If a conduction anesthetic technique is chosen, the patient should receive substantial intravenous hydration (eg, Ringer's lactate 1.5 L) before the block is administered, to reduce the likelihood and magnitude of sympathectomy-induced hypotension; hydration should be used rather than vasoconstrictors to treat hypotension whenever possible. Although limb tourniquets, for intravenous regional anesthesia, as well as for extremity surgery, may seem ill-advised, they are not contraindicated; however, optimal limb exsanguination and minimal ischemia time are important objectives.

OUTCOME. As noted earlier in the discussion of prophylactic transfusion therapy, the incidence of death and serious complications after surgery in patients with sickle cell disease is highly variable in studies that span more than three decades. During this period, many aspects of anesthesia care have changed, making comparisons of study results very difficult. In particular, the true incidence of additional complications of anesthesia and surgery attributable to sickle cell disease is difficult to estimate. Very likely, the medical literature is heavily biased, because death and severe complications are more likely to be reported than lesser problems. Nonetheless, several studies are mentioned here so that the reader may appreciate the spectrum of anesthetic-related complications.

COMPLICATIONS. A frequently cited review describes the clinical outcome of general anesthesia administered on 284 occasions to 200 patients with a variety of sickle cell disorders in one Jamaican hospital during the period 1958 to 1978.[60] Of the 211 anesthetics delivered to sickle cell anemia patients, only nine were associated with significant intraoperative complications, including airway obstruction (1), hypotension (4), cardiac dysrhythmia (2), asystole (1, with death) and apnea (1). In contrast, postoperative complications occurred in 32 of these sickle cell patients, including pulmonary complications (10), wound infections (8), prolonged febrile courses (3), and episodes of jaundice and bone pain attributable to sickle cell disease (4).

Transfusion

In the previously mentioned review,[60] most patients (79%) were anesthetized without preoperative transfusion and had a mean hemoglobin of 8.2 g/dL. Intraoperatively, 31 patients, 16 of whom had not received any transfusions before surgery, required transfusions. Postoperatively, 15 patients, eight of whom had not received previous transfusions, required transfusions. No relation was apparent between complication rate and choice of anesthetic agent or type of surgery. The complication rate in the patients who were transfused was slightly higher than the complication rate in patients who were not. This observation probably reflected the severity of the underlying condition, which was related to both the prevalence of postoperative complications and the need for transfusion.

A rather similar clinical experience with conservative use of transfusion during the period 1956 to 1967 was reported from an American hospital.[59] These studies are often cited to support the notion that selective use of transfusion (eg, to replace operative blood loss or treat crisis), rather than prophylactic transfusion, is associated with a low rate of adverse outcomes.

A review of pediatric cases describes the outcomes experienced by 27 children with sickling disorders (25 SS) who received 34 general anesthetics during the period 1967 to 1978.[69] These patients were treated preoperatively with a simple transfusion regimen including administration of 15 to 20 mL/kg of packed red cells; the goal was to reach a hematocrit of 36% (with hemoglobin A hematocrit of 15%). No operative or postoperative morbidity or mortality occurred.

Such a favorable experience was not reported in another series of 12 children with sickling disorders having 29 anesthetics during the period 1962 to 1971.[62] Among this group, seven simple and four exchange transfusions were administered preoperatively, two transfusions intraoperatively, and five postoperatively. Postoperative complications occurred in seven children, including wound infections, bacteremia, and pneumonia. Thus, more liberal use of transfusion therapy is not necessarily associated with optimum clinical outcome.[64]

Postoperative Care

Complications in these patients occur more commonly postoperatively than intraoperatively. Thus, vigilance must not wane after surgery. Among the supportive maneuvers that may be needed beyond the customary immediate postoperative period, sometimes for several days, are supplemental oxygen, intravenous hydration (and transfusions), and chest physiotherapy. Particular attention must be directed to respiratory care, because atelectasis and pneumonia occur more frequently,[59,62,71] and the complications may initiate the vicious cycle of sickling.

Considerations for Sickle Cell Trait

No evidence shows in general that patients with sickle cell trait are at any increased risk of complications during general anesthesia.[25,71–73] Yet, as was noted earlier, extraordinarily stressful physiologic conditions, typically involving extreme physical exertion or high-altitude flying, have been associated with severe sickling manifestations.[26–31] A particularly well-documented case report describes sudden death during cesarean section in a patient with sickle cell trait.[74]

Similar catastrophe might occur when patients with sickle cell trait undergo cardiopulmonary bypass or cerebral aneurysm clipping. However, reports from these surgical settings are characterized by poor documentation of the sickling disorder or are confounded by co-existing problems. Nonetheless, patients with sickle cell trait can have intravascular occlusion if they become severely hypoxic or acidotic. This observation emphasizes the importance of identifying a susceptibility of patients who are undergoing surgery to any degree of sickling before anesthesia, by using one of the previously described procedures. The status of these patients should be monitored carefully and supervised closely to avoid any complicating hypoxia or acidosis.

REFERENCES

1. Herrick JB: Peculiar elongated and sickled-shaped red blood corpuscles in a case of severe anemia. Arch Intern Med 6:517, 1910
2. Scriver JB, Waugh TR: Studies on a case of sickle-cell anemia. Can Med Assoc J 23:375, 1930
3. Pauling L, Itano HA, Singer SJ, et al: Sickle cell anemia, a molecular disease. Science 110:543, 1949
4. Murayama M: Molecular mechanism of red cell 'sickling.' Science 153:145, 1966
5. McCurdy PR, Sherman AS: Irreversibly sickled cells and red cell survival in sickle cell anemia: a study with both DF ^{32}P and ^{51}Cr. Am J Med 64:253, 1978
6. Sherwood JB, Goldwasser E, Chilcote R, et al: Sickle cell anemia patients have low erythropoietin levels for their degree of anemia. Blood 67:46, 1986
7. Seakins M, Gibbs WN, Milner PF, et al: Erythrocyte HbS concentration: an important factor in the low oxygen affinity of blood in sickle cell anemia. J Clin Invest 52:422, 1973
8. Charache S, Grisolia S, Fiedler AJ, et al: Effect of 2,3-diphosphoglycerate on oxygen affinity of blood in sickle cell anemia. J Clin Invest 49:806, 1970
9. Milner P: Oxygen transport in sickle cell anemia. Arch Intern Med 133:565, 1974
10. Leight L, Snider TH, Clifford GO, et al: Hemodynamic studies in sickle cell anemia. Circulation 10:653, 1954
11. Klug P, Lessin L, Radice P: Rheologic aspects of sickle cell disease. Arch Intern Med 133:577, 1974
12. Harris JW, Brewster HH, Ham TH, et al: Studies on the destruction of blood cells: X. the biophysics and biology of sickle cell disease. Arch Intern Med 97:145, 1956
13. Charache S, Conley CL: Rate of sickling of red cells during deoxygenation of blood from persons with various sickling disorders. Blood 24:25, 1964
14. Messner MJ, Harris JW: Filtration characteristics of sickle cells: rates of alteration of filterability after deoxygenation and reoxygenation, and correlations with sickling and unsickling. J Lab Clin Med 76:537, 1970
15. Zarkowsky HS, Hochmuth RM: Sickling times of individual erythrocytes at zero pO_2. J Clin Invest 56:1023, 1975
16. Anderson R, Cassell M, Mullinax GL, et al: Effect of normal cells on viscosity of sickle-cell blood. Arch Intern Med 111:286, 1963
17. Rubenstein E: Studies on the relationship of temperature to sickle cell anemia. Am J Med 111:286, 1963
18. Laasberg LH, Hedley-Whyte J: Viscosity of sickle cell disease and trait blood: changes with anesthesia. J Appl Physiol 35:837, 1973
19. Ham TH, Castle WB: Relation of increased hypotonic fragility and of erythrostasis to the mechanism of hemolysis in certain anemias. Trans Assoc Am Physicians 55:127, 1940
20. Serjeant GR: Sickle cell disease. New York: Oxford University Press, 1985: 14
21. Motulsky AG: Frequency of sickling disorders in US blacks. N Engl J Med 288:31, 1973
22. O'Brien RT, McIntosh S, Aspnes GT, et al: Prospective study of sickle cell anemia in infancy. J Pediatr 89:205, 1976
23. Karayalcin G: Sickle cell anemia in the neonatal period. South Med J 72:492, 1979
24. Karayalcin G, Rosner F, Chandra P, et al: Sickle cell anemia: clinical manifestations in 100 patients and review of literature. Am J Med Sci 51:51, 1976
25. Sears DA: The morbidity of sickle cell trait: a review of the literature. Am J Med 64:1021, 1978
26. Conn HO: Sickle-cell trait and splenic infarction associated with high-altitude flying. N Engl J Med 251:417, 1954
27. Oker WB, Bruno MS, Weinberg SB, et al: Fatal intravascular sickling in a patient with sickle cell trait. N Engl J Med 263: 947, 1960
28. Jones SR, Binder RA, Donowho EM: Sudden death in sickle cell trait. N Engl J Med 282:323, 1970
29. Koppes GM, Daly JJ, Coltman CA Jr, et al: Exertion-induced rhabdomyolysis with acute renal failure and disseminated intravascular coagulation in sickle cell trait. Mil Med 139:313, 1974
30. Helzlsouer KJ, Hayden FG, Rogol AD: Severe metabolic complications in a cross-country runner with sickle cell trait. JAMA 249:777, 1983
31. Kark JA, Posey DM, Schumacher HR, et al: Sickle cell trait as a risk factor for sudden death in physical training. N Engl J Med 317:781, 1988
32. Diggs LW: Screening tests for sickle cell disease. Postgrad Med 51:267, 1972
33. Orkin SH: Prenatal diagnosis of hemoglobin disorders by DNA analysis. Blood 63:249, 1984
34. Saili RK, Chang C-A, Levenson CH, et al: Diagnosis of sickle cell anemia and $S\beta$-thalassemia with enzymatically amplified DNA and nonradioactive allele-specific oligonucleotide probes. N Engl J Med 319:537, 1988
35. Newborn screening for sickle cell disease and other hemoglobinopathies. JAMA 258:1205, 1987
36. Morrison JC, Blake PG, Reed CD: Therapy for the pregnant patient with sickle hemoglobinopathies: a national focus. Am J Obstet Gynecol 144:268, 1982
37. Koshy M, Burd L, Wallace D, et al: Prophylactic red-cell transfusions in pregnant patients with sickle cell disease: a randomized cooperative study. N Engl J Med 319:1447, 1988
38. Ley TJ, DeSimone J, Anagnou NP, et al: 5-Azacytidine selectively increases β-globin synthesis in a patient with β+-thalassemia. N Engl J Med 307:1469, 1982
39. Veith R, Galanello R, Papayannopoulou, et al: Stimulation of F-cell production in patients with sickle cell anemia treated with cytarabine or hydroxyurea. N Engl J Med 313:1571, 1985
40. Platt OS: Chemotherapy to increase fetal hemoglobin in patients with sickle cell anemia. Am J Pediatr Hematol Oncol 7:258, 1985
41. Al-Khatti A, Veith RW, Papayannopoulou, T, et al: Stimulation of fetal hemoglobin synthesis by erythropoietin in baboons. N Engl J Med 317:415, 1987
42. Charache S, Dover GJ, Moyer MA, et al: Hydroxyurea-induced augmentation of fetal hemoglobin production in patients with sickle cell anemia. Blood 69:109, 1987
43. Rodgers GP, Dover DJ, Noguchi CT, et al: Hematologic responses of patients with sickle cell disease to treatment with hydroxyurea. N Engl J Med 322:1037, 1990
44. Johnson FL, Look AT, Gockerman J, et al: Bone-marrow transplantation in a patient with sickle cell anemia. N Engl J Med 311:780, 1984
45. Embury SH, Garcia JF, Mohandas N, et al: Effects of oxygen inhalation on endogenous erythropoietin kinetics, erythropoiesis and properties of blood cells in sickle cell anemia. N Engl J Med 311:291, 1984
46. Lanzkowsky P, Shende A, Karayalcin G, et al: Partial exchange transfusion in sickle cell anemia. Am J Dis Child 132:1206, 1978
47. Mallouh AA, Asha M: Beneficial effect of blood transfusion in children with sickle cell chest syndrome. Am J Dis Child 142: 178, 1988
48. Ng ML, Liebman J, et al: Cardiovascular findings in children with sickle cell anemia. Dis Chest 52:748, 1967
49. Sproule BJ, Halden ER, et al: A study of cardiopulmonary alterations in patients with sickle cell disease and its variants. J Clin Invest 37:486, 1957
50. Lindsay J Jr, Meshel JC, Patterson RH: The cardiovascular manifestations of sickle cell disease. Arch Intern Med 133:643, 1974
51. Finch CA: Pathophysiologic aspects of sickle cell anemia. Am J Med 53:1, 1972
52. Alpert BS, Gilman PA, et al: Hemodynamic and ECG responses to exercise in children with sickle cell anaemia. Br Heart J 40: 690, 1978
53. Wall MA, Platt OS, et al: Lung function in children with sickle cell anemia. Am Rev Respir Dis 120:210, 1979
54. Femi-Pearse D, Gazioglu KM, Yu PN: Pulmonary function studies in sickle cell disease. J Appl Physiol 28:574, 1970

55. Miller GJ, Serjeant GR: An assessment of lung volumes and gas transfer in sickle cell anemia. Thorax 26:309, 1974
56. Buckalew VM, Someren A: Renal manifestations of sickle cell disease. Arch Intern Med 133:660, 1974
57. Shelley TW: The liver in sickle cell disease: a clinicopathologic study of 70 patients. Am J Med 69:833, 1980
58. Searle JF: Anaesthesia in sickle cell states: a review. Anaesthesia 28:48, 1973
59. Holzmann L, Finn H, Lichtman HC, et al: Anesthesia in patients with sickle cell disease: a review of 112 cases. Anesth Analg 48: 566, 1969
60. Homi J, Reynolds J, Skinner A, et al: General anaesthesia in sickle cell disease. Br Med J 1:1599, 1979
61. Rutledge R, Croom RD, Davis JW, et al: Cholelithiasis in sickle cell anemia: surgical considerations. South Med J 79:28, 1986
62. Spigelman A, Warden MJ: Surgery in patients with sickle cell disease. Arch Surg 104:761, 1972
63. Charache S, Lubin B, Reid CD: Therapy of sickle cell disease. In: Management and therapy of sickle cell disease. NIH Publication 84:2117, 1984
64. Vichinsky EP, Haberkern C, Neumeyr L, et al. Randomized prospective study of conservative versus aggressive transfusion in the perioperative management of sickle cell disease. N Engl J Med (in press)
65. Bentley PG, Howard ER: Surgery in children with homozygous sickle cell anaemia. Ann R Coll Surg Engl 61:55, 1979
66. Esseltine DW, Baxter MRN, Bevan JC: Sickle cell states and the anaesthetist. Can J Anaesth 35:385, 1988
67. Howells TH, Huntsman RG: Anaesthesia in sickle cell states. Br Med J 1:174, 1973
68. Burrington JD, Smith MD: Elective and emergency surgery in children with sickle cell disease. Surg Clin North Am 56:55, 1976
69. Janik JS, Seeler RA: Surgical procedures in children with sickle hemoglobinopathy. J Pediatr 91:505, 1977
70. Finer P, Blair J, Rowe P: Epidural analgesia in the management of labor pain and sickle cell crises: a case report. Anesthesiology 68:799, 1988
71. Gilbertson AA: Anaesthesia in West African patients with sickle cell anaemia, haemoglobin SC disease, and sickle cell trait. Br J Anaesth 37:614, 1965
72. Murphy SB: Difficulties in sickle cell states. In Orkin FK, Cooperman LH (eds): Complications in anesthesiology. Philadelphia: JB Lippincott, 1983: 476
73. Diggs LW: The sickle cell trait in relation to the training and assignment of duties in the Armed Forces: III. hyposthenuria, hematuria, sudden death, rhabdomyolysis and acute tubular necrosis. Aviat Space Environ Med 55:358, 1984
74. Dunn A, Davies A, Eckert G, et al: Intraoperative death during caesarian section in a patient with sickle cell trait. Can J Anaesth 34:67, 1987

FURTHER READING

Schechter AN, Noguchi CT, Rodgers GP: Sickle cell disease. In Stamatoyannopoulos G, Nienhuis AW, Leder P (eds): The molecular basis of blood diseases. Philadelphia: WB Saunders, 1987: 179

Complications in Anesthesiology, second edition,
edited by Nikolaus Gravenstein and Robert R. Kirby.
Lippincott-Raven Publishers, Philadelphia © 1996.

CHAPTER 40

Immediate Reactions to Local Anesthetics

Benjamin G. Covino
Robert R. Kirby

Local anesthetic agents are relatively free of side effects if administered in an appropriate dose and in an appropriate anatomic location. However, systemic and localized toxic reactions can occur after their use, usually because of an accidental intravascular or intrathecal injection or the administration of an excessive dose. In addition, specific adverse effects are associated with the use of certain agents, such as allergic reactions to the aminoester or the procaine family of drugs, and methemoglobinemia after the use of prilocaine. Finally, regional anesthetic procedures, such as epidural and spinal anesthesia, may cause significant hemodynamic alterations by means of inhibition of sympathetic pathways.

SYSTEMIC TOXICITY

Most systemic reactions to local anesthetics involve the central nervous system (CNS) and the cardiovascular system. In general, the CNS is more susceptible to the systemic actions of local anesthetic agents than the cardiovascular system. Studies in dogs and sheep demonstrate that a substantially smaller dose and lower concentration in blood of local anesthetic is required to produce CNS toxicity compared with the dose and blood concentrations needed to achieve cardiovascular collapse (CC). In addition, the majority of toxic reactions to local anesthetics in humans involve the CNS. On the other hand, although local anesthetic–induced cardiovascular depression occurs less frequently, adverse effects involving the cardiovascular system tend to be more serious and more difficult to manage.

Central Nervous System Toxicity

Symptoms and Signs

The symptoms of local anesthetic induced CNS toxicity are summarized in Table 40-1. Human volunteers receiving intravenous infusions of local anesthetics describe feelings of lightheadedness and dizziness, followed frequently by visual and auditory disturbances such as difficulty in focusing, and tinnitus. Other subjective CNS symptoms include disorientation and occasionally feelings of drowsiness.

Objective signs of CNS toxicity are usually excitatory in nature and include shivering, muscular twitching, and tremors initially involving muscles of the face and distal parts of the extremities. Ultimately, generalized convulsions of a tonic-clonic nature occur. If a sufficiently large dose of a local anesthetic agent is administered systemically, the initial signs of CNS excitation are rapidly followed by a state of generalized CNS depression. Seizure activity ceases and respiratory depression and ultimately respiratory arrest occur. In some patients, CNS depression occasionally may occur without a preceding excitatory phase, particularly if other CNS depressant drugs have been used concomitantly.

Excitation and Inhibition

The excitatory effect of local anesthetics in the brain involves the selective blockade of inhibitory pathways in the cerebral cortex.[1,2] The specific sites of action may involve either inhibitory cortical synapses or inhibitory cortical neurons. The CNS effect of local anesthetics is not believed to be related to inhibitory neurohumoral agents such as γ-aminobutyric acid, because lidocaine does not block the inhibitory effects of γ-aminobutyric acid, nor the release of this agent in cortical neurons obtained from the brain of cats.[3]

The initial inhibition of inhibitory pathways by local anesthetic agents allows facilatory neurons to function unopposed, which results in an increase in excitatory activity leading to convulsions. After an increase in the dose of local anesthetics administered, these agents then tend to inhibit both inhibitory

TABLE 40-1
Symptoms of Local Anesthetic–Induced Central Nervous System Toxicity

INITIAL EVENTS
Tinnitus
Lightheadedness
Confusion
Circumoral numbness
EXCITATION PHASE
Tonic–clonic convulsions
DEPRESSION PHASE
Unconsciousness
Generalized CNS depression
Respiratory arrest

and facilatory pathways resulting in a generalized state of CNS depression.

Potential Toxicity of Various Agents

Differences exist with regard to the potential CNS toxicity of various local anesthetic agents. For example, in cats, a dose of approximately 35 mg/kg of procaine is required to cause convulsions.[4] Bupivacaine induces convulsions at a mean dose of 5 mg/kg. Lidocaine, mepivacaine, and prilocaine are agents of intermediate potency with regard to the dose required to produce convulsions.

A correlation exists between the anesthetic potency of the various agents and their potential CNS toxicity (Fig. 40-1). Bupivacaine is approximately eight times more potent than procaine in regional anesthesia and approximately seven times more toxic with respect to the production of seizures. In dogs approximately 20 mg/kg of lidocaine is required to produce seizures compared with 8 mg/kg for etidocaine and 5 mg/kg for bupivacaine.[5] Thus the relative CNS toxicity of bupivacaine, etidocaine, and lidocaine is approximately 4:2:1, which is similar to the relative potency of these agents for the production of regional anesthesia in humans. Intravenous infusion studies in volunteers also have demonstrated a relation between the intrinsic anesthetic potency of various local anesthetics and the dose required to induce signs of CNS toxicity.[6–8]

CONCENTRATIONS IN BLOOD. A comparison of the blood concentration of various local anesthetic agents associated with CNS excitation and convulsions and the relative anesthetic potency of the various compounds again reveals that a correlation exists between CNS toxicity and local anesthetic activity. In monkeys, bupivacaine produces convulsions at a blood concentration of approximately 4.5 μg/mL whereas lidocaine-induced convulsions occur at a mean blood concentration of 25 μg/mL.[9]

Studies in which blood concentrations of local anesthetics have been determined at the time of convulsions after the accidental intravenous injection of local anesthetics in patients also have shown that a correlation exists between the activity of these agents and their effect on the CNS. For example, convulsions occur at venous blood concentrations of approximately 2 to 4 μg/mL of the more potent agents such as bupivacaine and etidocaine, whereas venous blood concentrations in excess of 10 μg/mL are usually required for convulsive activity with a less potent agent such as lidocaine.

RATES OF INJECTION AND INFUSION. Although a general relation exists between anesthetic potency and CNS toxicity, the rate of injection and rapidity with which a particular blood concentration is achieved also will influence toxicity. Volunteers could tolerate an average dose of 236 mg of eti-

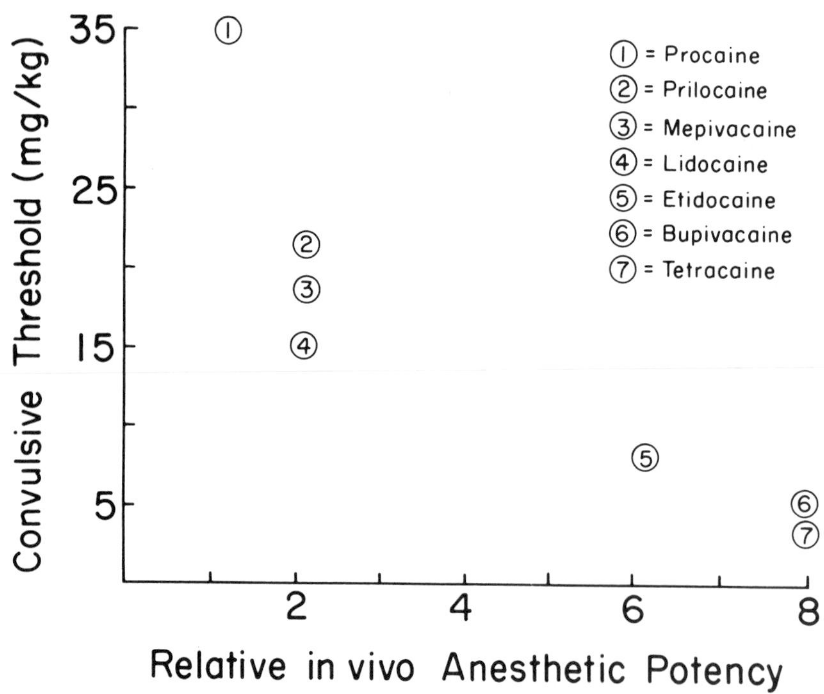

FIGURE 40-1. Relation in cats and dogs between the convulsive threshold and the relative in vivo potency of various local anesthetic agents.

docaine given intravenously and a venous blood concentration of 3.0 μg/mL before the onset of CNS symptoms when etidocaine was infused at the rate of 10 mg per minute.[10] When etidocaine was infused at 20 mg per minute, it required only 161 mg to achieve a similar serum concentration.

Intra-arterial injection (eg, into a cervical artery), with either antegrade (eg, carotid) or retrograde (eg, thyrocervical trunk) infusion into the CNS obviously results immediately in a very high regional brain local anesthetic concentration even though the peripheral venous concentration would be quite low.

ACID–BASE STATUS. The acid–base status can markedly affect the CNS activity of local anesthetic agents.[4] In cats, the convulsive threshold of various local anesthetics is inversely related to the arterial carbon dioxide partial pressure (Pa_{CO_2}) (Fig. 40-2). The convulsive threshold dose of procaine was decreased from approximately 35 to 17 mg/kg when the Pa_{CO_2} was increased from 25 to 40 mm Hg to 65 to 81 mm Hg. Similarly, the convulsive threshold of mepivacaine, prilocaine, lidocaine, and bupivacaine were decreased when the Pa_{CO_2} was increased.

A decrease in arterial pH is associated with a decrease in the convulsive threshold. The relation between Pa_{CO_2}, pH and the CNS activity of local anesthetic agents has been evaluated by Englesson.[11] Respiratory acidosis, with a resultant increase in Pa_{CO_2} and a decrease in arterial pH, consistently decreases the convulsive threshold of local anesthetic agents. However, an increase in Pa_{CO_2} in response to an increased arterial pH, as may occur during metabolic alkalosis, exerts less of a potentiating effect on the CNS activity of local anesthetic agents.

The relation between Pa_{CO_2} and the effect of local anesthetics on the CNS may be due to several factors. An increase in Pa_{CO_2} enhances cerebral blood flow so that more anesthetic agent is delivered to the brain. Hypercapnia increases diffusion of carbon dioxide across the nerve membrane with a resultant decrease in intracellular pH. Local anesthetic agents that diffuse across the nerve membrane then encounter an area of decreased pH, which tends to favor the conversion of the base form to the cationic form, increasing the intraneuronal concentration of the cationic form. Because the cationic form of local anesthetics does not diffuse well across the nerve membrane, ionic trapping occurs, which tends to potentiate the CNS effects of local anesthetic agents.

PLASMA PROTEIN BINDING. Hypercapnia, acidosis, or both decrease the plasma protein binding of local anesthetic agents.[12,13] Therefore, an increase in Pa_{CO_2} or decrease in pH increases the proportion of free drug available for diffusion into the brain. On the other hand, acidosis increases the cationic form of the local anesthetic, which will decrease the rate of diffusion.

CARDIOVASCULAR SYSTEM TOXICITY

Local anesthetic agents can produce profound effects on the cardiovascular system (Table 40-2). The systemic administration of these agents can exert a direct action both on cardiac muscle and on peripheral vascular smooth muscle. In addition, sympathetic blockade after epidural or spinal anesthesia may also result in profound cardiovascular depression.

Direct Cardiac Effects

Electric Activity

Detailed electrophysiologic studies on cardiac muscle show that local anesthetics such as lidocaine do not alter the resting cardiac cell membrane potential.[14] The primary effect is a

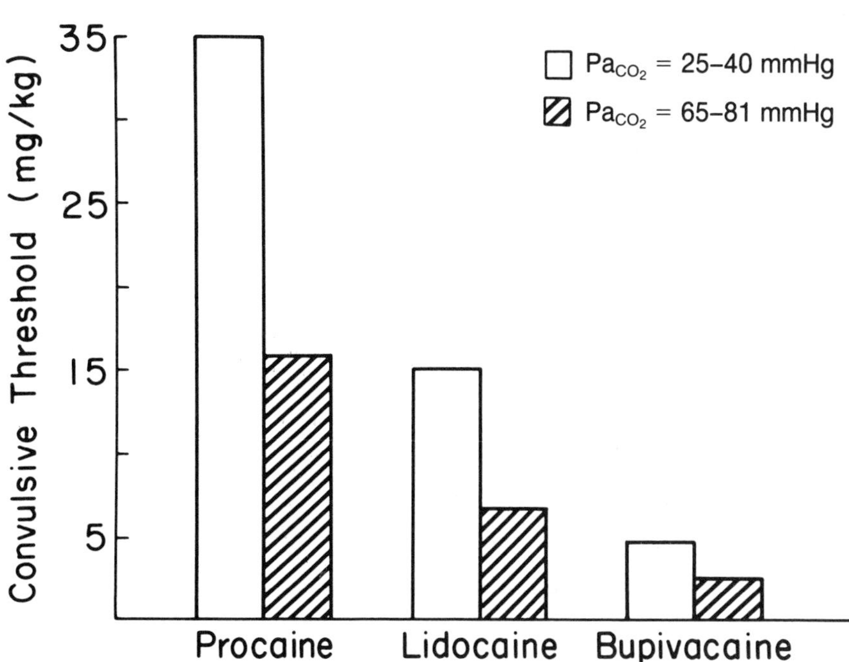

FIGURE 40-2. Effect of Pa_{CO_2} on the convulsive threshold of various local anesthetics in cats.

TABLE 40-2
Symptoms of Local Anesthetic–Induced Cardiovascular Toxicity

INITIAL EVENTS
Hypertension and tachycardia during CNS-excitation phase
INTERMEDIATE PHASE
Myocardial depression
Decreased cardiac output
Mild to moderate hypotension
TERMINAL PHASE
Peripheral vasodilatation
Profound hypotension
Sinus bradycardia
Conduction defects
Ventricular dysrhythmias
Cardiovascular collapse

decrease in the maximum rate of depolarization, similar to their effects on the nerve membrane. Lidocaine is believed to decrease the maximum rate of depolarization by an interaction with the fast sodium channels. This decrease in sodium conductance results in a decreased rate of depolarization. Action potential duration and the effective refractory period are decreased by lidocaine. However, the ratio of effective refractory period to action potential duration is increased both in Purkinje fibers and in ventricular muscle.

The considerable interest in the cardiac electrophysiologic effects of bupivacaine arises from the observation that this agent may precipitate cardiac dysrhythmias in various animal species, including humans. Bupivacaine markedly depresses the rapid phase of depolarization ($\dot{V}$max) in isolated guinea pig papillary muscle preparations.[15] In addition, the recovery from a steady-state block is much slower in bupivacaine-treated papillary muscles than in those treated with lidocaine. This slow recovery results in an incomplete restoration of $\dot{V}$max between action potentials when heart rate exceeds 10 beats/min. In contrast, recovery from lidocaine is complete, even at rapid heart rates. A decrease in rate of depolarization and action potential duration leading to conduction block and electric inexcitability also is observed in canine Purkinje fibers.[16] These results suggest that bupivacaine may be capable of producing unidirectional block and a reentrant type of cardiac dysrhythmia.

Electrophysiologic studies in intact dogs and in humans essentially reflect the findings observed in isolated cardiac tissue.[17,18] As the dose and blood concentrations of lidocaine are increased, a prolongation of conduction time through various parts of the heart occurs. These are reflected in the electrocardiogram as an increase in the PR interval and QRS duration. Extremely high concentrations of local anesthetics depress spontaneous pacemaker activity in the sinus node, resulting in sinus bradycardia and sinus arrest. A similar depression at the atrioventricular node also occurs, resulting in prolonged PR intervals and partial and complete atrioventricular dissociation.

Mechanical Activity

Local anesthetic agents also exert profound effects on the mechanical activity of cardiac muscle. Studies on isolated atria from guinea pigs show that all local anesthetics exert a dose-dependent negative inotropic action.[19] The ability of local anesthetic agents to depress the contractility of cardiac muscle is proportional to their ability to suppress conduction in peripheral nerves. Thus, the more potent local anesthetic agents tend to depress cardiac contractility in smaller doses and lower concentrations than the less potent local anesthetic agents (Table 40-3).

In general, local anesthetics can be divided into three groups in terms of their myocardial depressant effect. The more potent agents, bupivacaine, tetracaine, and etidocaine, depress cardiac contractility at the lowest concentrations. The agents of moderate anesthetic potency, lidocaine, mepivacaine, prilocaine, chloroprocaine, and cocaine, form an intermediate group of compounds in terms of their potency as myocardial

TABLE 40-3
Comparative Effects of Local Anesthetic Agents on Cardiac Contractility and Cardiac Output

AGENT	RELATIVE POTENCY	CONCENTRATION (μg/mL) FOR 50% DECREASE IN CONTRACTILITY*	DOSE FOR 50% DECREASE IN CARDIAC OUTPUT†
Procaine	1	277	100
Chloroprocaine	1	102	30
Cocaine	2	56	—
Lidocaine	2	67	30
Prilocaine	2	42	40
Mepivacaine	2	55	40
Etidocaine	6	—	20
Bupivacaine	8	6	10
Tetracaine	8	6	

* Data from isolated guinea pig atria.[19]
† Data from dogs.[22,23]

depressants. Finally, procaine, which is the least potent of the local anesthetics, is also the least depressant in terms of decreasing contractility of atrial tissue.

Studies on the isolated whole rabbit heart confirm the results observed on isolated atria.[20] Again, the more potent local anesthetics, bupivacaine, tetracaine, and etidocaine, depress ventricular contractility by 25% at concentrations of approximately 1 to 1.5 μg/mL. Lidocaine, mepivacaine, and prilocaine require concentrations of approximately 10 to 15 μg/mL to cause a similar decrease of 25% in the maximum rate of tension development.

Studies in dogs in which a strain gauge arch was sutured to the right ventricle revealed that all local anesthetic agents evaluated are capable of exerting a negative inotropic action.[21] As in the isolated atrial and ventricular muscle studies, a relation appears to exist between the local anesthetic potency of various agents and their ability to decrease myocardial contractility in intact animals. For example, tetracaine is approximately eight to 10 times more potent than procaine in humans as a local anesthetic. Similarly, it is approximately eight times more potent as a depressant of myocardial contractility.

Additional investigations have been conducted in closed-chest anesthetized dogs in which cardiac output has been measured by means of a thermodilution technique. The hemodynamic effect of the various clinically useful ester and amide local anesthetics were compared.[22,23] Statistically significant decreases in cardiac output were observed at doses of approximately 20 mg/kg of tetracaine, 40 mg/kg of chloroprocaine, and 100 mg/kg of procaine. A similar study involving the amide local anesthetics revealed that the more potent amino-amides, bupivacaine and etidocaine, caused a marked decrease in cardiac output at doses of approximately 5 to 10 mg/kg, whereas the less potent local anesthetics, mepivacaine, prilocaine and lidocaine, required doses of 10 to 30 mg/kg to cause significant depression of cardiac output.

Mechanisms

The mechanism by which local anesthetics depress myocardial contractility is not precisely known. Procaine and tetracaine increase the release of calcium from isolated skeletal muscle preparations.[24] The relative potency of tetracaine and procaine in terms of their ability to increase the rate of calcium efflux from sartorius muscle is also proportional to their local anesthetic activity. A similar displacement of calcium from cardiac muscle would result in a decrease in myocardial contractility. However, studies in the isolated guinea pig heart have shown that an increase in the extracellular concentration of calcium fails to reverse the negative inotropic action of bupivacaine or lidocaine.[25]

Direct Peripheral Vascular Effects

Biphasic Action

Local anesthetic agents exert significant effects on peripheral vascular smooth muscle. Both in vitro and in vivo studies demonstrate that these agents have a biphasic action on smooth muscle of peripheral blood vessels. Johns, DiFazio, and Longnecker directly measured the diameter of arterioles in the cremaster muscle of rats before and after the topical application of lidocaine.[26] Concentrations of lidocaine varying from 1 to 10^3 μg/mL produced a dose-related state of vasoconstriction varying from 88% to 60% of the control vascular diameter (Fig. 40-3). An increase in the concentration of lidocaine to 10^4 μg/mL produced approximately a 27% increase in arteriolar diameter indicative of a significant degree of vasodilation.

Other studies using an isolated rat portal vein preparation also demonstrated that local anesthetic drugs stimulate spontaneous myogenic contractions and augment basal tone at low concentrations.[27] As the concentration of local anesthetic increases, inhibition of myogenic activity occurs. No correlation was found between the anesthetic potency of various agents and their effect on vascular smooth muscle. For example, prilocaine produced the greatest enhancement of myogenic activity, whereas etidocaine was least effective. Prilocaine, mepivacaine, and procaine also caused the greatest increase in basal tone, whereas minimal changes were seen with lidocaine, tetracaine, bupivacaine, and etidocaine.

In vivo studies confirm the biphasic affect of local anesthetic on the peripheral vasculature. For example, the intra-arterial administration of mepivacaine in volunteers results in a decrease in forearm blood flow without any change in arterial pressure, suggesting that mepivacaine causes vasoconstriction that increases peripheral vascular resistance.[28] Similar studies with lidocaine also show an increased tone in capacitance vessels with less consistent effect on resistance vessels. Animal studies in which vascular tone is reduced by α-adrenergic receptor blockade or by spinal cord section show that hind limb vascular resistance increases after administration of mepivacaine and procaine.

Dose

As the dose of local anesthetic agent administered and the concentration of the agent to which the vascular smooth mus-

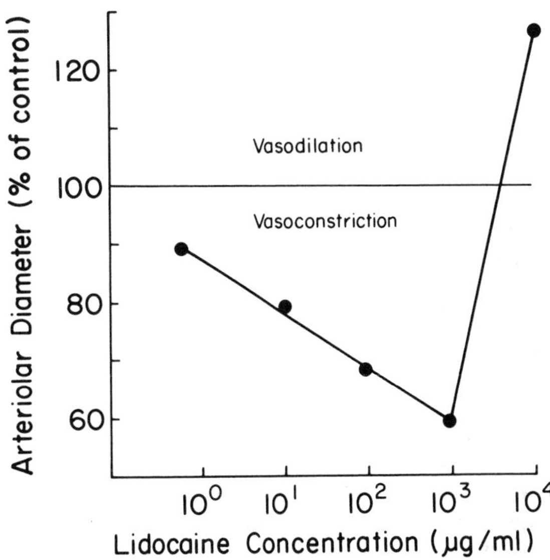

FIGURE 40-3. Biphasic effect of lidocaine on arteriolar diameter.

cle is exposed increase, the stimulatory or vasoconstrictor action of these agents changes to one of inhibition and vasodilation. Femoral blood flow in dogs after intra-arterial administration of mepivacaine increases as the dose of the agent is increased.[29] A comparison of the peripheral vascular effects of local anesthetic agents fails to demonstrate a good correlation between the relative anesthetic potency of these agents and their ability to cause peripheral vasodilation. However, a correlation does appear to exist between the duration of action as local anesthetics and their duration of vasodilation. Thus, lidocaine, mepivacaine, and prilocaine cause a duration of peripheral vasodilation of approximately 5 minutes after intraarterial injection into the femoral artery of dogs. Agents such as bupivacaine, etidocaine, and tetracaine, which are long-acting, produce a prolonged period of vasodilation.

Contractility

An increase in contractility of vascular smooth muscle after the administration of local anesthetics is most apparent in the pulmonary vascular system. Wollenberger and Krayer originally reported that procaine markedly increased pulmonary vascular resistance (PVR) in their Starling heart-lung preparation.[30] Studies in intact dogs with pulmonary artery catheters also showed that both the ester and amide agents can cause marked increases in pulmonary artery pressure and PVR.[22,23] Increases in pulmonary artery pressure achieved statistical significance at doses of approximately 10 to 15 mg/kg of procaine, chloroprocaine, and tetracaine. Peak increases in PVR of approximately 300% were observed after administration of these three ester agents.

Similar studies with amides also revealed significant increases in pulmonary artery pressure at doses varying from 3 to 10 mg/kg of bupivacaine, etidocaine, mepivacaine, lidocaine, and prilocaine. Increases of 100% to 200% in PVR were observed after the administration of 3 mg/kg of bupivacaine and etidocaine. Mepivacaine, lidocaine, and procaine in doses of 10-mg/kg resulted in increases of 50% to 100%. The pulmonary vascular tree also changes from a state of vasoconstriction to one of vasodilation as the dose of local anesthetics markedly increases. Thus, at doses of local anesthetics that approach lethal concentrations, decreases in pulmonary artery pressure and PVR occur with both the ester and amide type local anesthetic agents.

Mechanisms

The biphasic peripheral vascular effect of local anesthetic agents may be related to changes in smooth muscle calcium concentrations. A competitive antagonism exists between local anesthetic drugs and calcium ions in smooth muscle.[31] Local anesthetic compounds may displace calcium from membrane binding sites resulting in diffusion of this ion into the smooth muscle cytoplasm. Such an increase in cytoplasmic calcium concentration should stimulate the interaction between contractile proteins leading to an increase in myogenic tone, which would produce a state of vasoconstriction. However, as the concentration of local anesthetic agent at the smooth muscle membrane is increased, the displacement of calcium by these agents will ultimately decrease both the cytoplasmic calcium concentration and the interaction between the contractile protein elements of smooth muscle. A state of muscle relaxation leading to vasodilation will result.

COCAINE. All local anesthetic agents studied to date, with the exception of cocaine, appear to exert this biphasic effect on vascular smooth muscle. Cocaine produces a state of vasoconstriction at most doses. Although direct blood flow studies in dogs show that the initial effect of cocaine is one of vasodilation, a long period of vasoconstriction follows, regardless of the dose administered.[32]

This unique property of cocaine is not related to a direct effect on vascular smooth muscle, but to inhibition of the uptake of norepinephrine. Thus, after the release of norepinephrine from postganglionic sympathetic fibers, the decrease in the reuptake of norepinephrine by tissue binding sites results in an excess amount of free norepinephrine that leads to a prolonged and profound state of vasoconstriction. This property of cocaine does not occur with other local anesthetics.

COMPARATIVE CARDIOVASCULAR EFFECTS

The more potent local anesthetic agents are more cardiotoxic than the less potent, local anesthetics. Bupivacaine and etidocaine are associated with rapid and profound cardiovascular depression.[33-35] This differs from the usual cardiovascular depression seen with local anesthetics. The onset of cardiovascular depression occurs relatively early and, in some cases, severe cardiac dysrhythmias are observed. In addition, the cardiac depression appears resistant to various therapeutic modalities.

Cardiotoxicity of Potent Agents

Cardiotoxicity of the more potent agents such as bupivacaine appears to differ from that of lidocaine (Table 40-4, Fig. 40-4).

Ratio of Cardiovascular Collapse to Convulsion

The dose and blood concentration of lidocaine, bupivacaine, and etidocaine associated with the development of convulsive activity and CC has been determined in adult sheep in which continuous intravenous infusions of these various local anesthetics was administered.[36,37] A CC/CNS dose ratio of 7.1 ± 1.1 existed for lidocaine, indicating that seven times as much drug was required to induce irreversible CC as was needed for the production of convulsions (see Fig. 40-4). In comparison, the CC/CNS ratio for bupivacaine was 3.7 ± 0.5 and for etidocaine 4.4 ± 0.9. Thus, although the CNS was more sensitive to the toxic effects of the potent local anesthetics, a smaller difference existed between the dose causing convulsions and that leading to irreversible CC compared with lidocaine.

deJong and Bonin indicated that a narrow margin of safety exists in mice between the dose of bupivacaine to cause CNS toxicity and the dose to cause cardiovascular toxicity compared with lidocaine.[38] Studies in sheep in which the blood concentrations of various local anesthetics were determined and re-

TABLE 40-4
Ventricular Dysrhythmias After Lidocaine and Bupivacaine in Animals

STUDY (reference)	ANIMAL	VENTRICULAR DYSRHYTHMIAS (% incidence)	
		Lidocaine	*Bupivacaine*
39	Nonanesthetized, paralyzed cat	6 PVC	100 PVC
23	Anesthetized dog	0	0
41	Nonanesthetized dog	0	40 VT and VF
40	Nonanesthetized sheep	0	80 to 100 PVC and VT
47	Hypoxic, acidotic sheep	0	17 to 50 VT and VF
25	Isolated guinea pig heart	0	33 to 50 PVC, bigeminy, and trigeminy

PVC, premature ventricular contractions; *VF*, ventricular fibrillation; *VT*, ventricular tachycardia.

lated to the onset of CNS and cardiovascular toxicity also reveal a narrower CC/CNS ratio for the more potent local anesthetics.[36,37] For example, lidocaine was found to possess a CC/CNS blood concentration ratio of 3.6 ± 0.3, compared with values of 1.6 to 1.7 for bupivacaine and etidocaine (see Fig. 40-4). Tissue concentrations of the various local anesthetics that were determined at the time of CC indicate a greater uptake of bupivacaine and etidocaine by the myocardium compared with lidocaine. Thus, the enhanced sensitivity of the myocardium to these more potent agents appears to be due to a greater myocardial uptake.

Ventricular Dysrhythmias

Several groups of investigators have reported the development of ventricular dysrhythmias in animals exposed to toxic doses of bupivacaine. deJong and colleagues were the first to show that bupivacaine caused cardiac dysrhythmias in awake but paralyzed cats, whereas such changes were not observed with lidocaine.[39] Studies in unanesthetized sheep also demonstrated that severe cardiac dysrhythmias occur after the rapid intravenous administration of bupivacaine, whereas no cardiac irregularities were observed when lidocaine was injected intravenously (Table 40-5).[40] Although no cardiac dysrhythmias were observed in the canine toxicity studies conducted by Liu and associates, these dogs were anesthetized with pentobarbital.[22,23] Subsequent studies in unanesthetized dogs demonstrated the occurrence of ventricular tachycardia and ventricular fibrillation in some of the animals receiving intravenous bupivacaine.[41] No dysrhythmias occurred when the same dogs were given intravenous lidocaine.

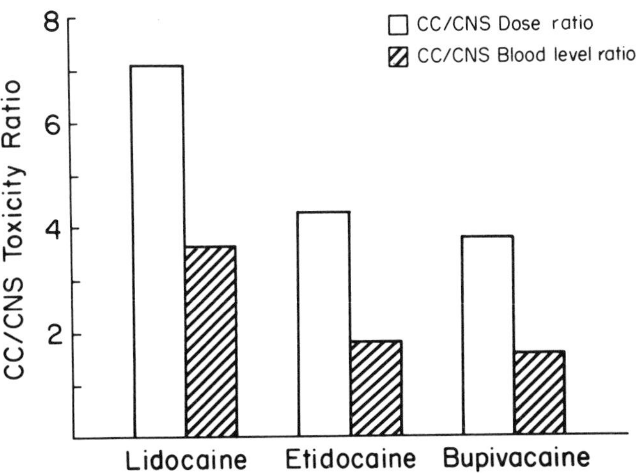

FIGURE 40-4. Cardiovascular collapse/central nervous system toxicity ratio of lidocaine, etidocaine, and bupivacaine in sheep.

MECHANISMS. Whether the occurrence of ventricular dysrhythmias is a toxic effect related to bupivacaine alone or may be produced by other local anesthetics is unknown. The incidence of ventricular fibrillation has been determined in preliminary studies in awake dogs in which convulsant and supraconvulsant doses of lidocaine, mepivacaine, bupivacaine, and etidocaine were administered intravenously.[42] Ventricular fibrillation was observed in approximately 50% of dogs after the rapid intravenous injection of a convulsant or supraconvulsant dose of bupivacaine. Ventricular fibrillation did not occur in lidocaine-, mepivacaine-, or etidocaine-treated dogs. However, in a previous study, ventricular fibrillation developed in one of four dogs that received 10 mg/kg of etidocaine.[43] In addition, ventricular dysrhythmias were observed in awake paralyzed cats after the administration of etidocaine, although the frequency was less than that associated with the use of bupivacaine.[39]

The results suggest that the occurrence of ventricular fibrillation is not related to the basic piperidine ring structure of bupivacaine, because mepivacaine, which contains the piperidine moiety, failed to cause these abnormalities. In addition, a precise correlation does not appear to exist between the frequency of ventricular arrhythmias and the lipid solubility and protein binding of local anesthetics. Large doses of etidocaine, which is more lipid soluble than bupivacaine and equally protein bound, may cause ventricular dysrhythmias and fibrillation, but the incidence appears to be lower than that observed with bupivacaine.

The possibility that the cardiac dysrhythmias observed in bupivacaine-treated animals may be related to the intensity of convulsive activity has also been investigated, particularly

TABLE 40-5
Electrocardiographic Changes or Dysrhythmias After Intravenous Lidocaine or Bupivacaine in Sheep

	INCIDENCE (%)			
	Lidocaine		*Bupivacaine*	
ELECTROCARDIOGRAPHIC CHANGES	5.7 mg/kg	11.4 mg/kg	2.1 mg/kg	4.2 mg/kg
Sinus tachycardia	100	100	0	0
Supraventricular tachycardia	0	0	44	60
Atrioventricular blocks	0	0	56	60
Ventricular tachycardia	0	0	11	80
Multiforme premature ventricular contractions	0	0	44	100
Wide QRS complexes	0	0	100	100
ST-T wave change	14	40	44	60

Adapted from Kotelko DM, Shnider SM, Dailey PA, et al: Bupivacaine-induced cardiac arrhythmias in sheep. Anesthesiology 60:15, 1984.

because dogs that received pentobarbital that did not convulse did not demonstrate these electrocardiographic abnormalities. Isolated guinea pig hearts perfused with a bupivacaine solution revealed evidence of conduction block, bigeminy, and trigeminy; those perfused with lidocaine did not.[25] In addition, Reiz and associates observed ventricular fibrillation in intact pigs in which bupivacaine was injected directly into the left anterior descending coronary artery.[44] Thus, these ventricular dysrhythmias apparently are not related to the occurrence of convulsive activity.

ELECTROPHYSIOLOGIC STUDIES. Various electrophysiologic studies have been conducted to determine the cause of bupivacaine-associated ventricular dysrhythmias. Bupivacaine decreases maximum diastolic potential, action potential amplitude, the maximum rate of depolarization, and conduction velocity in isolated cardiac tissue preparations.[15,16,45,46] In particular, the rate of recovery between beats is extremely slow in the presence of bupivacaine, which can result in conduction block of a unidirectional type leading to a reentrant type of dysrhythmia.[15] Intact dog studies have shown that bupivacaine lowers the ventricular tachycardia threshold and significantly increases the Q-TU intervals, resulting in an undulating type of ventricular tachycardia, similar to that seen in torsades de pointes.[47]

Enhanced Cardiotoxicity in Pregnancy

Several of the cardiotoxic reactions reported after the use of bupivacaine have occurred in pregnant patients. As a result, the 0.75% solution is no longer recommended for use in obstetric anesthesia. Whether the pregnant patient is more susceptible to the toxic effects of local anesthetics is uncertain.

Studies have been conducted in pregnant and nonpregnant sheep in an effort to determine their relative sensitivity to toxic doses of bupivacaine.[48] The CC/CNS dose ratio decreased from 3.7 ± 0.5 in nonpregnant sheep to 2.7 ± 0.4 in pregnant animals. However, little difference was observed in the CC/CNS blood concentration ratio, which varied from 1.6 ± 0.1 in nonpregnant animals to 1.4 ± 0.1 in pregnant ewes. However, the blood concentration of bupivacaine at which CC occurred was lower in pregnant animals.

Measurements of cardiac tissue concentrations have failed to demonstrate a greater myocardial uptake of bupivacaine in pregnant sheep at the time of CC. Thus, if the pregnant patient is more susceptible to the cardiotoxic effects of bupivacaine, the effect apparently is not related to a greater myocardial uptake of drug. It may result from increased circulating concentrations of progesterone and a resulting depression of the maximum rate of Purkinje fiber depolarization.[49]

Cardiac Resuscitation

Cardiopulmonary resuscitation is extremely difficult in patients in whom cardiotoxicity has occurred after the administration of a toxic dose of bupivacaine. Studies in acidotic and hypoxic sheep also have indicated that cardiac resuscitation after bupivacaine-induced toxicity is difficult.[48] Resuscitation of hypoxic dogs rendered toxic with bupivacaine is possible if massive doses of epinephrine and atropine are administered.[50] In addition, Kasten and Martin reported that bretylium, but not lidocaine, could reverse the cardiodepressant effects of bupivacaine in dogs and also raise the ventricular tachycardia threshold.[47] Ropivacaine, which is almost as potent as bupivacaine, appears to be far more amenable to vigorous cardiac resuscitation than bupivacaine.

Acidosis and Hypoxia

Changes in acid–base status alter the potential cardiovascular toxicity of local anesthetic agents. Hypercapnia, acidosis, and hypoxia tend to potentiate the negative chronotropic and inotropic action of lidocaine and bupivacaine. In particular, the combination of hypoxia and acidosis appears to markedly potentiate the cardiodepressant effects of bupivacaine.

Studies in intact sheep also have demonstrated that hypoxia and acidosis markedly increase the frequency of cardiac dysrhythmias after the intravenous administration of bupivacaine and also increase the mortality rate.[48] Enhanced toxicity in the presence of acidosis does not appear related to a greater myocardial tissue uptake of local anesthetic, because investigations in sheep[52] demonstrated a *decreased* cardiac concentration of bupivacaine in the presence of acidosis.

Marked hypercapnia, acidosis, and hypoxia occur very rapidly in some patients after seizure activity due to the rapid accidental intravascular injection of local anesthetic agents.[53] Thus, the cardiovascular depression observed with the more potent agents, such as bupivacaine, may be related in part to the severe acid–base changes that occur after the administration of toxic doses of these agents.

INDIRECT CARDIOVASCULAR EFFECTS

Certain regional anesthetic techniques such as epidural or spinal anesthesia are associated with sympathetic blockade that may result in profound hypotension. In general, the degree of hypotension is related to the extent of the sympathetic blockade.

Epidural Anesthesia

Cardiovascular alterations after epidural blockade are related to (1) the level of blockade, (2) the dose administered, (3) the specific local anesthetic agent chosen, (4) the addition of vasoconstrictors, and (5) blood volume status.

Level of Blockade

Epidural anesthesia to the level of the T5 dermatome or below usually is not accompanied by significant cardiovascular alterations. As the level of anesthesia extends from T5 to T1, a 20% decrease in blood pressure has been observed.[54] This hypotensive state is related almost exclusively to sympathetic inhibition and peripheral vasodilation below the level of block, which results in a significant decrease in systemic vascular resistance (SVR). At T1 and above, a decrease in heart rate and cardiac output may occur as a result of the blockade of sympathetic fibers terminating in the heart. A decrease in cardiac output may be related in part to the inhibition of myocardial sympathetic fibers, resulting in decreased cardiac contractility, and also to a decrease in venous return due to venodilation and expansion of capacitance vessels.

Dose

Relatively large amounts of local anesthetic drug are required to achieve a satisfactory degree of epidural blockade. These local anesthetic agents are absorbed rather rapidly and substantial blood concentrations may be achieved. The absorbed local anesthetic agent may produce systemic effects involving the cardiovascular system as discussed above.

Bonica and coworkers showed that blood concentrations of lidocaine of less than 4 μg/mL after epidural blockade resulted in a slight increase in blood pressure due mainly to an increased cardiac output.[54] Doses of epidural lidocaine that produced blood concentrations in excess of 4 μg/mL caused hypotension in part as a result of the negative inotropic and peripheral vasodilator actions of the drug.

Choice of Local Anesthetic Drug

Differences in the onset of epidural anesthesia occur as a function of the specific agent administered. For example, chloroprocaine, lidocaine, and etidocaine produce a fairly rapid onset of anesthesia, whereas bupivacaine exerts a significantly slower onset of action. The more rapidly acting agents produce a more profound degree of hypotension because of the more rapid blockade or sympathetic fibers.[55] In addition, certain agents such as etidocaine penetrate nerve fibers more readily and may be associated with a more profound degree of sympathetic blockade and hypotension.

Addition of Vasoconstrictor Agents

Epinephrine is frequently added to local anesthetics intended for epidural use to decrease the rate of vascular absorption and prolong the duration of anesthesia. Absorbed epinephrine may produce transient cardiovascular alterations. An exaggerated decrease in arterial blood pressure has been reported after the use of epinephrine containing local anesthetics for epidural blockade.[56] The absorbed epinephrine is believed to stimulate β_1-adrenergic receptors, resulting in an increase in heart rate and cardiac output that counteracts the peripheral vasodilator state to some extent. Although absorbed epinephrine may be responsible for the early cardiovascular changes observed after epidural blockade, the more prolonged hypotension seen after epidural anesthesia with epinephrine containing local anesthetics is probably related to a more profound degree of sympathetic blockade.

Blood Volume

Cardiovascular depression is more severe and more dangerous after the production of epidural anesthesia in hypovolemic patients. Bonica and co-workers demonstrated that epidural anesthesia in hypovolemic volunteers was associated with profound hypotension due to peripheral vasodilation and a decrease in cardiac output and heart rate.[57] The addition of epinephrine to the anesthetic solution resulted in a less profound degree of hypotension in these subjects but was unable to prevent a significant decrease in blood pressure. The failure of epinephrine to increase cardiac output sufficiently in these subjects to prevent a marked decrease in blood pressure is obviously due to the diminished circulating blood volume.

Regional Blood Flow

The effect of epidural blockade on regional blood flow to various organs has been studied in monkeys.[58] Epidural blockade to the midthoracic level is associated with marked increase in hind limb blood flow. Studies in humans also show that blood flow increases in the legs after epidural blockade, while a decrease in blood flow in the arms occurs, suggesting a compensatory vasoconstrictor action above the level of the block. An extensive spread of epidural anesthesia will cause vasodilation in both upper and lower levels.

Epidural blockade to the level of the T10 dermatome does not cause a significant change in coronary, cerebral, renal or hepatic blood flow. However, extension of the block to T1 causes a marked decrease in blood flow to all of these areas. Coronary flow decreased 52% at the time when arterial pressure fell by 47%. Thus, the reduction in coronary flow appears to be related directly to the decrease in blood pressure.

Cerebral blood flow decreased by approximately 35% when epidural anesthesia to the level of the T1 dermatome was achieved. Normally, cerebral blood flow remains constant at arterial mean pressures between 50 and 150 mm Hg. Although a mean decrease of approximately 50% in mean blood pressure occurred in these monkeys, the results suggest that high epidural anesthesia may interfere with normal autoregulation of cerebral blood flow.

Renal blood flow is also affected by epidural blockade that extends to the midthoracic level or higher. A 14% decrease was observed in humans in whom a T5 level of epidural anesthesia was produced. In monkeys, a decrease in renal blood flow of approximately 30% to 40% occurred when a T1 level of block was achieved. The reduction in renal blood flow in the absence of significant changes in blood pressure also indicates that epidural anesthesia may alter normal renal autoregulation.

Changes in hepatic blood flow appear to parallel alterations in blood pressure after epidural blockade. Decreases in blood pressure of 14% to 47% resulted in reductions in hepatic flow of 20% to 40%. Pulmonary blood flow increased markedly in monkeys when low and high thoracic levels of epidural block were achieved. This was believed to be related to the opening of pulmonary arteriovenous shunts after sympathetic blockade.

Spinal Anesthesia

Sympathetic Blockade

In general, a decrease in blood pressure occurs after the induction of spinal anesthesia because of the blockade of sympathetic fibers. The degree of hypotension appears to be related almost exclusively to the extent of sensory and sympathetic blockade. Studies in humans have shown that subarachnoid anesthesia to the level of the T5 dermatome caused a decrease in stroke volume, cardiac output, and SVR.[59]

The decrease in cardiac output and stroke volume after spinal anesthesia that extends to the midthoracic level is not believed related to a decrease in myocardial contractility but rather to a decrease in venous return. Placement of patients in a slightly head-down position or the infusion of crystalloid solutions are usually sufficient to reverse the hypotensive state.

Studies have been carried out in monkeys in which the level of sensory anesthesia after the intrathecal administration of tetracaine has been correlated with the degree of hypotension.[60] Anesthesia to the level of the T10 dermatome resulted in a decrease in blood pressure of approximately 15%, due almost exclusively to a decrease in SVR with little change in cardiac output. However, extension of the level of sympathetic and sensory block to T1 was associated with a 35% decrease in blood pressure. This exaggerated state of hypotension was caused in part by a decrease in SVR but also by a significant reduction in cardiac output.

Regional blood flow was also studied.[60] Spinal anesthesia to the level of the T10 dermatome was associated with a decrease in coronary, cerebral, hepatic, and renal blood flow and an increase in pulmonary blood flow. Extension of sympathetic blockade to T1 caused a further decrease in coronary, cerebral, hepatic and renal blood flow and an even greater increase in pulmonary blood flow.

Direct Versus Indirect Effects

The direct cardiovascular effect of local anesthetic agents and the circulatory alteration due to the regional anesthetic procedure can be compared. For example, the blood concentration of lidocaine after the administration of 400 mg of this agent into the lumbar epidural space is similar to that produced by the intravenous injection of 1 mg/kg of lidocaine. Little or no change in blood pressure, SVR, cardiac output and heart rate is usually observed after the intravenous administration of 1 mg/kg of lidocaine. However, the epidural administration of 400 mg of lidocaine results in a significant decrease in arterial blood pressure due primarily to a decrease in SVR with little or no change in cardiac output or heart rate. These results clearly indicate that the cardiovascular effects after epidural or spinal anesthesia are due to sympathetic blockade and the subsequent reduction in peripheral vascular tone rather than to a direct action of the local anesthetic agent on the cardiovascular system.

PHARMACOKINETIC DETERMINANTS

The most common cause of local anesthetic induced toxic reactions is an accidental rapid intravascular injection. Although intravenous toxicity is related primarily to intrinsic anesthetic potency, the duration of a toxic reaction is related primarily to the distribution and elimination kinetics of the various drugs. The toxicity of extravascularly administered local anesthetic is related in part to their local anesthetic potency, but more importantly to their rate of vascular absorption, tissue redistribution, and elimination.

Both CNS and cardiovascular toxic reactions to local anesthetics are dependent on the blood concentration of these agents and the concentrations achieved in the brain and heart. Any factors that tend to increase the rate of absorption, alter the rate of tissue redistribution, and decrease the rate of elimination augment the blood and tissue concentration of these drugs, thereby enhancing their potential toxicity.

Differences exist between the various agents with regard to their basic pharmacokinetic properties that will directly influence their potential for toxic reactions.

Absorption Phase

The absorption of local anesthetic agents is related to the site of injection, dose administered, addition of vasoconstrictor agents to the local anesthetic solution, and the pharmacologic profile of the specific agent used.

Site of Injection

The rate of absorption of local anesthetic agents from various anatomic sites varies markedly (Fig. 40-5).[61–67] In general,

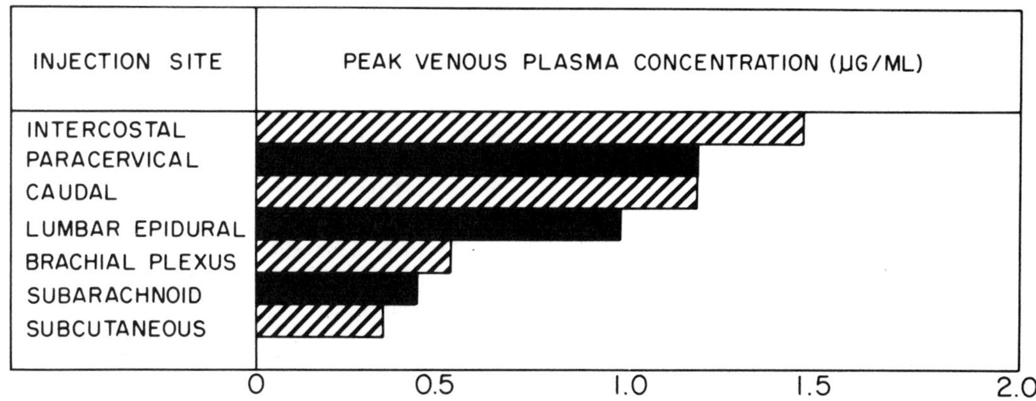

FIGURE 40-5. Relative rates of absorption of lidocaine (100 mg) from various injection sites.

intercostal nerve blockade is associated with the most rapid rate of absorption and the highest blood concentrations regardless of which agent is used.[61] The paracervical area and the caudal canal also represent sites of relatively rapid absorption.[62,63] Higher anesthetic blood concentrations are seen after caudal and paracervical blocks as compared with lumbar epidural injections. Peripheral nerve blocks such as brachial plexus blockade and sciatic-femoral blockade result in slower absorption and lower blood concentrations than occur after intercostal or epidural blocks. The slowest rate of absorption and the lowest blood concentrations occur after subcutaneous and subarachnoid administration of local anesthetics.[66,67] For every 100 mg of lidocaine injected, a peak venous plasma concentration of approximately 1.5 μg/mL is attained after intercostal nerve blocks; 1.2 μg/mL after paracervical and caudal blocks; 1.0 μg/mL after injection into the lumbar epidural space; 0.6 μg/mL after brachial plexus blocks; and approximately 0.3 to 0.4 μg/mL after subcutaneous and subarachnoid administration.

This relation of administration site to rate of drug absorption has obvious clinical implications, because the same dose of a local anesthetic agent may be potentially toxic in one injection area but not in others. For example, average peak blood concentrations in excess of 6 μg/mL have been reported with 300 to 500 mg of lidocaine and mepivacaine administered for paracervical and intercostal nerve blockade compared with average peak blood concentrations of 3 to 5 μg/mL when the same dose of these two agents was administered for lumbar epidural anesthesia.

Because adverse events become manifest when the blood concentration of lidocaine and mepivacaine exceeds 5 μg/mL, the potential for systemic toxicity is significantly greater after paracervical and intercostal nerve blockade compared with lumbar epidural anesthesia despite the use of the same total dose of local anesthesia agent for both procedures.

Dose

In general, a linear relation exists between the dose of local anesthetic agent administered, the rate of absorption, and the subsequent peak blood concentration. For most local anesthetics, the peak blood concentration achieved after regional anesthesia is a function of the total dose of drug administered (Fig. 40-6).[68] Alterations in volume and concentration within the clinical range do not markedly influence the rate of absorption and subsequent peak venous blood concentration provided the total dose remains the same (Fig. 40-7).

Addition of Vasoconstrictor Agents

Vasoconstrictor agents are frequently added to local anesthetic solutions to decrease the rate of vascular absorption or identify intravascular injection and thus reduce the potential toxicity of these agents. For peripheral nerve blocks all of the currently available local anesthetic agents appear to benefit from the addition of epinephrine (Fig. 40-8). After interscalene blockade a difference of approximately 50% in the peak venous plasma concentrations of lidocaine, prilocaine, etidocaine, and bupivacaine exists when these agents are administered with and without epinephrine.[69] However, blood concentrations of the newer local anesthetic agent, ropivacaine, are not significantly altered by the addition of epinephrine.[70]

Differences exist with regard to the effect of epinephrine in reducing the rate of vascular absorption after central neural blocks. The addition of epinephrine to lidocaine and mepivacaine is associated with a significant decrease in the rate of vascular absorption from the epidural space. However, epi-

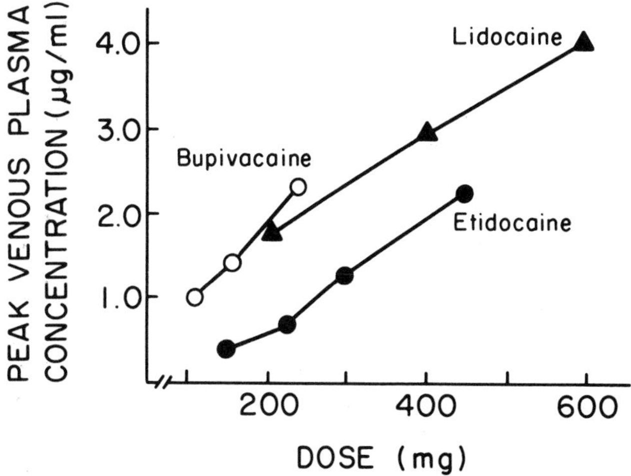

FIGURE 40-6. Relation between peak concentrations in venous plasma and epidural dose of lidocaine, etidocaine, or bupivacaine.

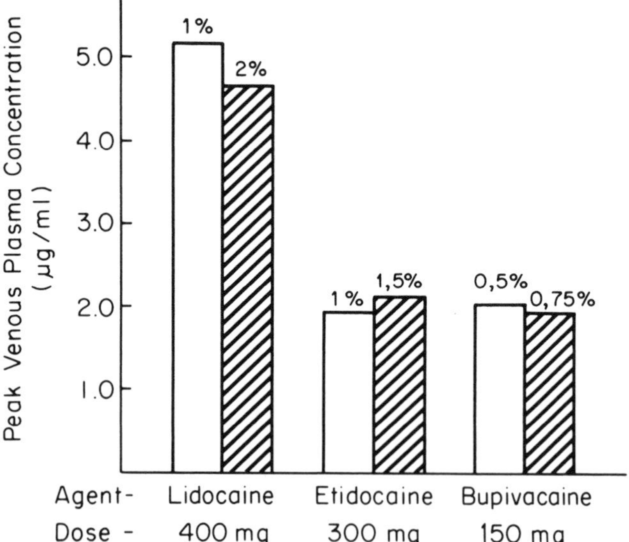

FIGURE 40-7. Relation between peak concentrations in venous plasma and concentrations of various local anesthetics administered epidurally.

nephrine appears to exert minimal influence on the peak venous plasma concentrations of prilocaine, bupivacaine and etidocaine after administration into the lumbar epidural space (Fig. 40-9).[61] In addition, the absorption of lidocaine and bupivacaine from the subarachnoid space does not appear to be influenced by the addition of epinephrine.[71]

Pharmacologic Characteristics

The rate of absorption of local anesthetic agents is also determined by the pharmacologic properties of the specific drugs. Lidocaine and mepivacaine show similar peak venous blood concentrations after lumbar epidural administration (see Fig. 40-9). However, the concentration of prilocaine in blood is significantly less than that of lidocaine after administration of identical doses of these agents for epidural anesthesia or interscalene blockade (see Figs. 40-8 and 40-9).[61,69]

Distribution Phase

The blood concentration of local anesthetic agents after absorption from the site of injection is a function of the rate of distribution from vascular to tissue compartments and of elimination through metabolic and excretory pathways.

The disposition kinetics of local anesthetic agents can be calculated best after intravenous administration. The shape of the curve relating anesthetic concentration in blood to time after intravenous injection is similar for all agents (Fig. 40-10). The initial, or α, phase represents the fast disappearance from blood into rapidly equilibrating tissues (ie, tissues with a high vascular perfusion). A second, slower β phase of disappearance is a function of distribution to slowly equilibrating tissues and metabolism.

The initial distribution phase is related to the rate of uptake of local anesthetic agents by vessel rich tissues, such as lung, brain, heart, liver and kidney. The lungs, in particular, appear to play an important role in the removal of local anesthetics from the circulation during the very early phase of tissue redistribution. Studies in pigs and in humans showed that 25% of lidocaine was taken up by the lungs within seconds after intravenous administration.[72]

The percentage of local anesthetic extracted by the lungs is dose-related.[73] Forty percent of lidocaine was taken up by lung tissue immediately after intravenous injection of 0.5 mg/kg in pigs. At a dose of 2 mg/kg the maximum uptake fell to 25%, indicating that the ability of the lungs to absorb local anesthetics is limited. Human studies have shown that 80% to 90% of the injected dose of lidocaine is extracted during the first passage through the lungs.[74] Differences exist regarding the degree of uptake of various local anesthetic agents by the lungs.[75] Measurements of prilocaine, lidocaine, and etidocaine in lung tissue 10 minutes after subcutaneous injection in guinea pigs revealed significantly higher concentrations of prilocaine compared with the other agents. The concentration of lidocaine, in turn, was greater than that of etidocaine. The results suggest that protein binding may be the most important determinant of lung uptake because prilocaine, which is least protein-bound, was concentrated to the greatest extent in the lung, whereas etidocaine, which is highly protein-bound, showed the lowest concentrations.

Local anesthetic agents are distributed throughout all body tissues, but the relative concentration in different tissues varies as a function of time after injection.[76] One minute after the intravenous injection of lidocaine, approximately 70% of the injected dose was found in vessel rich tissues. Within 4 minutes approximately 30% of the total injected dose of lidocaine was present in skeletal muscle. Although the concentration of local anesthetic agent per gram of muscle tissue was not large, skeletal muscle is the largest mass of tissue in the body and serves as the greatest reservoir for local anesthetic agents.

Elimination Phase

The second, slow-disappearance phase primarily represents elimination of the injected local anesthetic from the body. The rate of elimination is a function of drug metabolism and

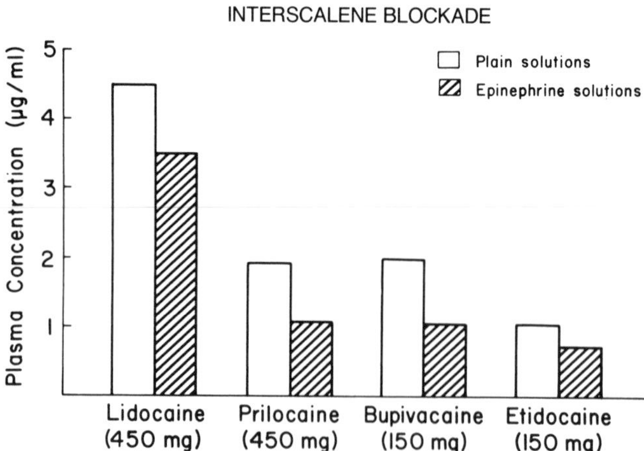

FIGURE 40-8. Effect of epinephrine on peak concentrations in venous plasma of various local anesthetics after interscalene administration.

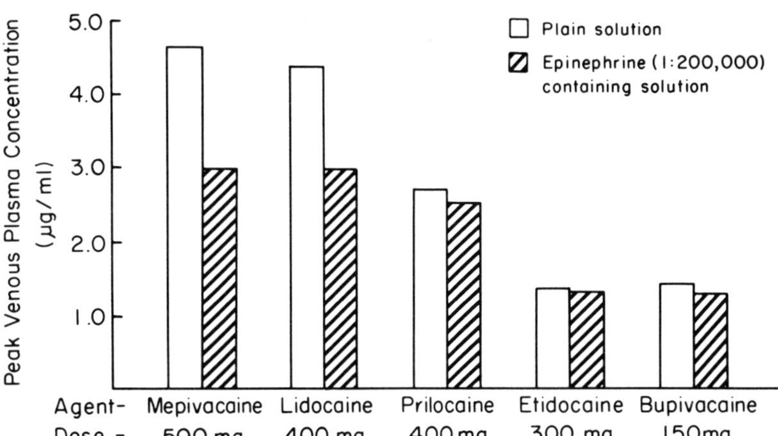

FIGURE 40-9. Effect of epinephrine on peak concentrations of various local anesthetics in venous plasma after lumbar epidural administration.

excretion. Metabolism of local anesthetic agents is dependent on the chemical structure of the various drugs. The amino-esters (eg, procaine) are hydrolyzed in plasma by cholinesterase enzymes. The amino-amides such as lidocaine are metabolized primarily in the liver by microsomal enzymes.

The rate of hydrolysis of amino-ester agents varies markedly. In vitro studies show that chloroprocaine has the most rapid rate of hydrolysis (4.7 µmol/mL/hour); a rate of 1.1 µmol/mL/hour was observed for procaine, and 0.3 µmol/mL/hour for tetracaine.[6] The rapid degradation of chloroprocaine is responsible for the low systemic toxicity of the agent. On the other hand, tetracaine is potentially the most toxic ester agent because of its intrinsic potency and relatively slow rate of hydrolysis.

The elimination pharmacokinetics of the amido-amides have been studied extensively (Table 40-6).[65] Prilocaine, which is a secondary amine, has the shortest half-life. The remaining amino-amides are tertiary amines whose elimination half-lives vary from 1.6 hours for lidocaine to 3.5 hours for bupivacaine. A correlation exists between the clearance rate of the various amide drugs and their potential systemic toxicity. Prilocaine is cleared most rapidly and is least toxic of the amino-amides. Conversely, bupivacaine is cleared most slowly and is potentially the most toxic amide agent.

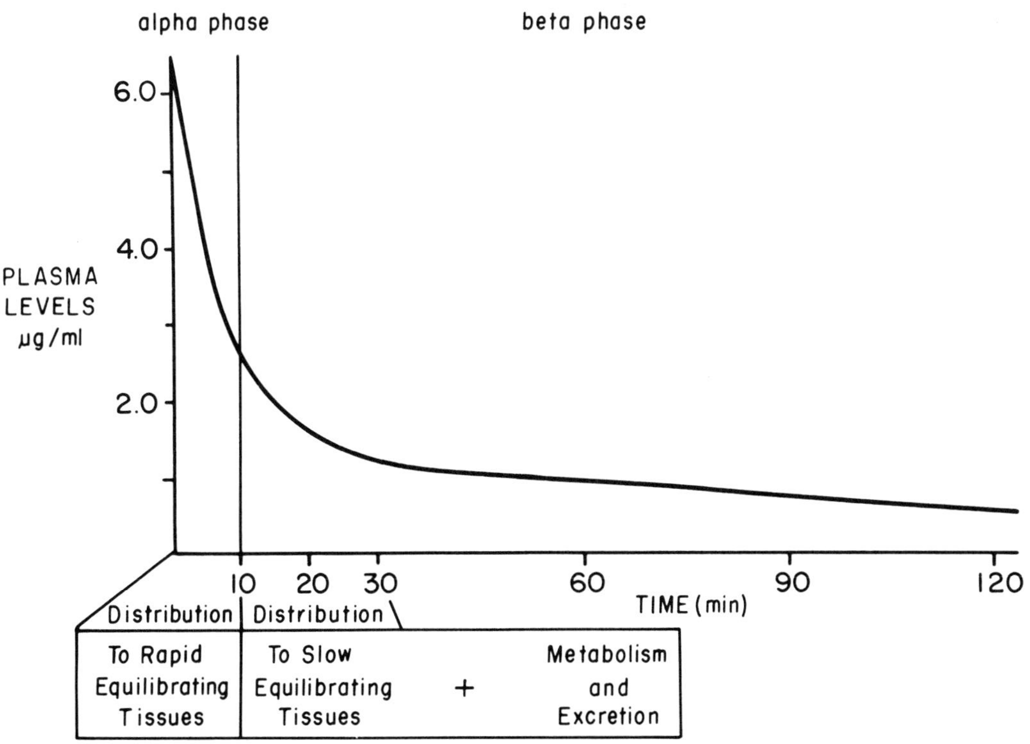

FIGURE 40-10. Typical plasma concentration curve of a local anesthetic after intravenous administration.

TABLE 40-6
Pharmacokinetic Properties of Amide Local Anesthetics

AGENT	HALF-LIFE (min) α	HALF-LIFE (min) β	VOLUME OF DISTRIBUTION AT STEADY STATE (L)	ELIMINATION HALF-LIFE γ (h)	CLEARANCE (L/min)
Prilocaine	0.5	5.0	261	1.5	2.8
Lidocaine	1.0	9.6	91	1.6	0.9
Mepivacaine	0.7	7.2	84	1.9	0.8
Bupivacaine	2.7	28.0	72	3.5	0.5
Etidocaine	2.2	19.0	133	2.6	1.2

Hepatic Metabolism

The liver is the primary site of metabolism for amide local anesthetic agents. Prilocaine undergoes the most rapid rate of hepatic degradation. The rate of metabolism of lidocaine and mepivacaine appear to be similar. Studies in humans have shown that approximately 70% of injected lidocaine is taken up by the liver and presumably metabolized in subjects with normal hepatic function.[77] Similar studies with etidocaine and bupivacaine revealed a 70% to 80% hepatic uptake of etidocaine.[78] However, the hepatic extraction and presumably metabolism of bupivacaine averaged 50% of the injected dose after an initial extraction ratio of 70% to 80%.

Renal Clearance

The kidneys are the main excretory organ for local anesthetic agents and their metabolites. Among ester local anesthetic drugs, procaine is hydrolyzed almost completely in plasma and less than 2% of unchanged drug is excreted by the kidney. Similarly, only small amounts of unchanged chloroprocaine and tetracaine are found in urine.

Small amounts of the amide-type local anesthetic agents are excreted unchanged by way of the kidneys.[65] Less than 10% of intravenously administered lidocaine was found in the urine of human volunteers. Approximately 80% of administered lidocaine could be recovered in human urine in the form of various metabolites. From 1% to 16% of administered mepivacaine appears unchanged in human urine, whereas 25% to 40% is excreted as degradation products. Only 16% of unchanged bupivacaine has been recovered from human urine. Less than 1% of etidocaine has been found in urine as the unchanged drug.

FACTORS INFLUENCING PHARMACOKINETICS AND TOXICITY

Pregnancy

Local anesthetic drugs easily cross the placenta by passive diffusion. Excessive doses in obstetrical patients can result in high fetal blood concentrations and fetal depression. The rate and degree of diffusion appear to be inversely correlated with the degree of plasma protein binding (Fig. 40-11).[79] Prilocaine shows the highest umbilical vein/maternal blood ratio and lowest plasma protein binding capacity. On the other hand, the umbilical vein/maternal blood ratio of bupivacaine and etidocaine is very low and these agents are approximately 95% protein-bound. Lidocaine and mepivacaine occupy an intermediate position in terms of both placental transmission and protein binding.

Placental transmission is influenced mainly by the degree of maternal plasma protein binding of the various agents and the rate of fetal tissue uptake. Fetal plasma binding is approximately 50% less than binding in maternal plasma so that more unbound drug is present in the fetus. Those drugs that demonstrate the highest degree of protein binding also tend to be more lipid soluble, such that the rate of tissue uptake of the unbound drug is enhanced.

Thus, maternal/fetal blood anesthetic concentrations may differ markedly among agents, but the total amount of drug transferred across the placenta can be similar for agents of

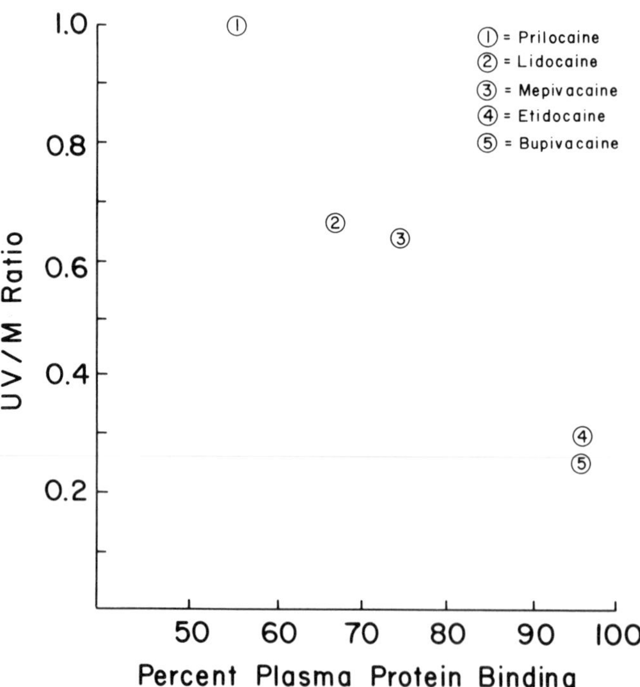

FIGURE 40-11. Relation between the ratio of concentration in umbilical vein to that in maternal vein plasma and the plasma protein binding of various local anesthetics.

high and low protein binding capacity. Those agents that possess a high protein binding capacity originally were postulated to be potentially less toxic for the fetus. However, if the rate of fetal tissue uptake is greater for drugs of high protein binding and high lipid solubility, the potential fetal toxicity will be similar for all the local anesthetic compounds.

Age

Studies of the kinetics of lidocaine and mepivacaine in human neonates showed a significant prolongation of the elimination half-life of both drugs.[80,81] The elimination half-life of lidocaine averaged 2.3 hours in the neonate compared with a value of approximately 1.6 hours in adults. Mepivacaine showed an elimination half-life of 8.7 hours in neonates compared with average half-lives of 1.9 to 2.3 hours in adults. This prolonged elimination half-life is related in part to the greater tissue accumulation of lidocaine and mepivacaine in neonates, and also immaturity of neonatal hepatic enzyme systems.

A pharmacokinetic study comparing lidocaine between adults whose mean age was approximately 65 years and those whose mean age was approximately 25 years revealed a significant prolongation of the elimination half-life in the older population.[82] This difference probably resulted from a significantly greater volume of distribution in the older group. No other pharmacokinetic difference was observed. The greater percentage of adipose tissue in older adults may account for the larger volume of distribution of lidocaine, which, in turn, would result in a decreased rate of drug elimination.

Acid–Base Status

Hypercapnia and acidosis, as discussed previously, increase the toxicity of local anesthetic agents. Changes in the pharmacokinetics of local anesthetics in the presence of hypercapnia and acidosis may account in part for the enhanced toxicity. An inverse correlation has been reported between hydrogen ion concentration and the degree of plasma protein binding of lidocaine. Thus, acidosis results in a greater fraction in blood of free drug that is available for diffusion to tissues. Indeed, higher tissue concentrations of lidocaine have been observed in acidotic animals compared with nonacidotic animals.[83]

Pseudocholinesterase

Any change in the physiologic status that influences drug distribution and elimination will alter the pharmacokinetic properties of local anesthetics and their potential toxicity. For example, among the amino-ester agents, the rate of elimination is related to the rate of hydrolysis by plasma pseudocholinesterase. Patients with atypical plasma cholinesterase or decreased concentrations of plasma cholinesterase tend to hydrolyze amino-esters more slowly, resulting in a decreased rate of elimination of these compounds.[65] In addition, patients with hepatic disease show decreased concentrations of plasma cholinesterases, because these enzymes are produced in the liver. The in vitro plasma half-life of procaine has been reported to increase from approximately 39 to 138 seconds in patients with liver disease.

Hepatic Blood Flow

Alterations in hepatic blood flow or hepatic metabolism markedly influence the rate of degradation and the elimination half-life of the amino-amide compounds. A direct relation between hepatic blood flow and extraction of lidocaine by the liver has been demonstrated.[77] Patients with decreased myocardial contractility resulting in passive congestion of the liver and decreased hepatic blood flow show a significant prolongation in the elimination half-life of lidocaine.[84]

Studies performed in patients during and after recovery from acute hepatitis have revealed marked differences in the half-life of lidocaine.[85] During the active phase, the half-life of lidocaine was approximately 160 minutes. Several months after recovery, a normal lidocaine half-life of 80 minutes was observed in the same subjects.

Renal Failure

The pharmacokinetics of lidocaine also have been studied in patients with renal failure.[86] Although the elimination half-life of lidocaine was found to be unchanged, the rate of disappearance from blood of glycinexylidide, a secondary metabolite of lidocaine was markedly decreased. No change in the elimination half-life of monoethylglycinexylidine was found in these patients, because this primary metabolite of lidocaine is dependent on hepatic metabolism for its elimination.

OTHER SYSTEMIC EFFECTS AND TOXICITY

A variety of miscellaneous systemic actions have been ascribed to local anesthetic drugs, most of which are related to the generalized membrane stabilizing property of this class of drugs. Local anesthetics have been reported to possess neuromuscular blocking, ganglionic blocking, and anticholinergic activity. Little evidence suggests that any of these miscellaneous effects are clinically important under normal conditions.

Methemoglobinemia

A unique systemic side effect is the formation of methemoglobinemia after the administration of large doses of prilocaine.[87,88] A dose–response relation exists between the amount of epidural prilocaine administered and the incidence of methemoglobinemia (Fig. 40-12). In general, prilocaine doses of 600 mg are required for the development of clinically significant concentrations of methemoglobinemia. The formation of methemoglobinemia is believed to be related to the chemical structure of prilocaine.[89] This agent lacks a methyl group in the benzene ring. The metabolism of prilocaine in the liver results in the formation of *o*-toluidine, which is actually responsible for the oxidation of hemoglobin to methemoglobin. The methemoglobinemia associated with prilocaine is spontaneously reversible or may be treated by the intravenous administration of methylene blue.

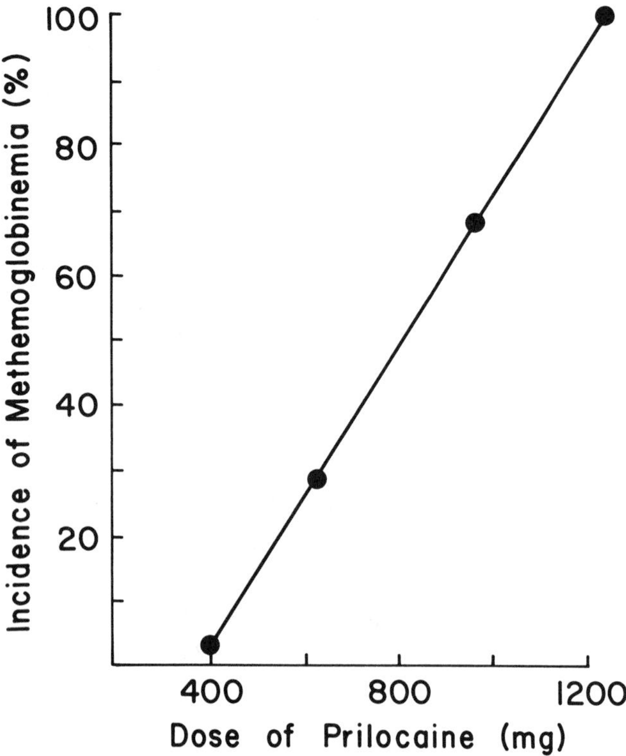

FIGURE 40-12. Relation between epidural dose of prilocaine and incidence of methemoglobinemia.

Allergic Reaction

Reports of allergic reactions, hypersensitivity, or anaphylactic responses to local anesthetic agents appear periodically. Unfortunately, systemic toxic reactions are frequently misdiagnosed as representing allergic or hypersensitivity type reactions. The amino-ester agents such as procaine can produce allergic type reactions. These agents are derivatives of paraminobenzoic acid, which is known to be allergenic. The amino-amide local anesthetics are not derivatives of paraminobenzoic acid and allergic reactions to the amino-amides are extremely rare. However, several cases have been reported that suggest this class of agents can, on rare occasions, produce an allergic type phenomenon.[90]

Aldrete and colleagues used a technique of intradermal injections to study the frequency of allergic type responses to both amino-ester and amino-amide local anesthetics in patients with and without a presumptive history of local anesthetic allergy.[91,92] Positive skin reactions were observed in 25 of 60 patients who did not describe any previous allergic symptoms. In all cases the cutaneous reactions occurred after the injection of an amino-ester type of agent such as procaine, tetracaine, and chloroprocaine. No cutaneous reactions occurred after the use of the amino-amide agents, namely lidocaine, mepivacaine, or prilocaine.

Eleven patients were studied who had a history of alleged local anesthetic allergy. Eight of these patients showed a positive skin reaction to procaine, tetracaine, or chloroprocaine. However, no positive cutaneous response was seen after the administration of lidocaine, mepivacaine, or prilocaine. No signs of systemic anaphylaxis occurred in any of the subjects.

Remember that although the amino-amide agents appear to be relatively free from allergic type reactions, solutions of these agents may contain a preservative, methylparaben, whose chemical structure is similar to that of paraminobenzoic acid. Patients to whom methylparaben was administered intradermally demonstrated a positive skin reaction.[92]

Local Tissue Toxicity

Local anesthetic agents that are used clinically rarely produce localized nerve damage. Studies on isolated frog sciatic nerve revealed that concentrations of procaine, cocaine, tetracaine, and dibucaine required to produce irreversible conduction blockade are far in excess of the concentration of these agents used clinically.[93] A comparison of lidocaine, tetracaine, or etidocaine administered subdurally in rabbits revealed histopathologic spinal cord changes after the use of 2% tetracaine, which is considerably greater than the maximum concentration of 1% used for spinal anesthesia in humans.[94] In recent years, prolonged sensory motor deficits have been reported in some patients, usually after the epidural or subarachnoid injection of large doses of this particular drug and after use of spinal microcatheters. The latter scenario is thought to be related to very high anesthetic concentrations in the area of the cauda as a result of repeated dosing and poor mixing.[95–97]

Chloroprocaine

NEUROTOXICITY. Studies in animals have proven contradictory regarding the potential neurotoxicity of chloroprocaine. Barsa and associates, using an isolated rabbit vagus nerve preparation, reported that chloroprocaine was associated with signs of neural irritation, whereas the use of lidocaine under similar conditions failed to cause local toxic effects.[98] However, histologic examination of rabbit sciatic nerves exposed to chloroprocaine for 6 hours did not reveal any signs of nerve damage.[99] When doses sufficient to cause total spinal anesthesia in dogs were administered, chloroprocaine produced total paralysis in approximately 30%, whereas none of the bupivacaine-treated dogs showed evidence of permanent neurologic sequelae.[100] Studies of a similar nature in sheep and monkeys failed to show any difference in neurotoxicity between chloroprocaine and other local anesthetics or control solutions.[101]

Paralysis has also been observed in rabbits in whom chloroprocaine solutions were administered intrathecally.[102] However, the paralysis was believed to be related to the sodium bisulfite that is used as an antioxidant in chloroprocaine solutions. Pure solutions of chloroprocaine without sodium bisulfite did not cause paralysis, whereas sodium bisulfite alone was associated with paralysis.

A detailed series of studies has been conducted on the isolated rabbit vagus nerve to investigate the neurotoxicity of the various components of commercial chloroprocaine solutions.[103] Commercial solutions of 3% chloroprocaine contain the local anesthetic agent, 0.2% sodium bisulfite, and hydrogen ions yielding a pH of approximately 3.0. Application of commercial 3% chloroprocaine to isolated vagus nerves for 30 minutes resulted in irreversible conduction blockade. A 3% chloroprocaine solution with sodium bisulfite buffered to a pH of 7.0 caused reversible conduction block. A 3% chloroprocaine solution with a pH of 3.0, but without sodium bisulfite, also resulted in reversible blockade. Application of a 0.2% sodium bisulfite solution at a pH of 3.0 resulted in irreversible conduction block, whereas the use of an 0.2% sodium bisulfite solution with a pH of 7.0 caused no conduction block.

The results of these studies suggest that the combination of a low pH and sodium bisulfite are responsible for the neurotoxic reactions observed after the use of large amounts of chloroprocaine solution. Chloroprocaine does not appear to be neurotoxic, and current preparation of chloroprocaine contain either only very small concentrations of sodium bisulfite (those with epinephrine) or none at all.

BACK PAIN. Currently, available chloroprocaine avoids the combination of sodium bisulfite and low pH. However, the newer solution, Nesacaine MPF (without preservatives) (Astra Pharmaceutical Products, Westboro, MA) has been associated with severe, dull, deep lumbar ache, sometimes associated with erector spinae spasm, after epidural anesthesia.[104-106] The cause may be related to the antioxidant ethylenediamine tetraacetic acid or the large volumes of chloroprocaine used and infiltration of the interspinous ligaments before needle insertion.

Skeletal Muscle

Skeletal muscle appears to be more sensitive to the local irritant properties of local anesthetic agents than other tissues. Changes have been observed with most of the clinically used local anesthetic agents such as lidocaine, mepivacaine, prilocaine, bupivacaine, and etidocaine.[107,108] In general, the more potent longer-acting agents such as bupivacaine and etidocaine appear to cause a greater degree of localized skeletal muscle damage than the less potent, shorter-acting agents such as lidocaine and prilocaine. This effect is reversible; muscle regeneration occurs rapidly and is complete within 2 weeks after injection. These changes in skeletal muscle have not been correlated with any overt clinical signs of local irritation.

DIAGNOSIS

The cause of an adverse response to local anesthetic administration is usually readily apparent to knowledgeable observers. Yet often the anesthesiologist is confronted by a vague history or merely a statement of "allergy to local anesthetic" provided by the patient. Establishing the correct diagnosis requires a comprehensive description of the reaction, which, in turn, may require obtaining medical records and contacting the health care personnel who administered the local anesthetic. The differential diagnosis of local anesthetic reactions is presented in Table 40-7.

TREATMENT

Apart from discontinuing the injection of the local anesthetic, the minor symptoms of toxicity seldom must be treated, provided that adequate respiration and cardiovascular function are maintained (Table 40-8). Nevertheless, the early symp-

TABLE 40-7
Differential Diagnosis of Local Anesthetic Reactions

CAUSE	CLINICAL FEATURES	COMMENTS
Local anesthetic toxicity Intravascular injection	Immediate convulsion or cardiac dysrhythmias	Injection into vertebral or carotid artery may cause convulsion after administration of small dose
Relative overdose	Onset in 5 to 15 minutes of irritability, progressing to convulsions	
Reaction to vasoconstrictor	Tachycardia, hypertension, headache, apprehension	Possible variation with vasopressor used
Vasovagal reaction	Rapid onset; bradycardia, hypotension, pallor, faintness	Rapidly reversible with elevation of legs
Allergy Immediate	Anaphylaxis (decreased blood pressure, bronchospasm, edema)	Allergy to amides extremely rare
Delayed	Urticaria	Cross-allergy possible (eg, with preservatives in local anesthetics and food)
High spinal or epidural block	Gradual onset; bradycardia,* hypotension, possible respiratory arrest	Possible loss of consciousness with total spinal block; onset of cardiorespiratory effects more rapid than with high epidural or with subdural block
Concurrent medical episode (eg, asthma attack or myocardial infarction)	Possible mimicking of local anesthetic reaction	Medical history important

* Sympathetic block above T4 adds cardioaccelerator nerve blockade to the vasodilatation seen with blockade below T4; total spinal block may have rapid onset.

Covino BG: Clinical pharmacology of local anesthetic agents. In Cousins MJ, Bridenbaugh PO (eds): Neural blockade in clinical anesthesia and management of pain, 2nd ed. Philadelphia: JB Lippincott, 1988:135.

TABLE 40-8
Treatment of Acute Local Anesthetic Toxicity

AIRWAY
Establishment of clear airway; suction, if required

BREATHING
Oxygen with face mask
Encouragement of adequate ventilation (prevent cycle of acidosis, increased uptake of local anesthetic into CNS, and lowered seizure threshold)
Artificial ventilation, if required

CIRCULATION
Elevation of legs
Increase in IV fluids if blood pressure decreases
Cardiovascular support drug if decrease in blood pressure persists (see below) or if heart rate decreases
Cardioversion if ventricular arrhythmias occur

DRUGS
CNS depressant
Midazolam 1 to 2 mg IV or Diazepam, 5 to 10 mg IV *or*
Thiopental, 50 mg IV, incremental doses until seizures cease
Muscle relaxant: succinylcholine, 1 mg/kg, if control of ventilation with above measures inadequate (requires artificial ventilation and may necessitate intubation)

CARDIOVASCULAR SUPPORT
Atropine, 0.5–1.0 mg IV, if heart rate decreases
Ephedrine, 10–25 mg IV, to restore adequate blood pressure
Epinephrine for cardiovascular collapse

IV, intravenous.
Modified from Covino BG: Clinical pharmacology of local anesthetic agents. In Cousins MJ, Bridenbaugh PO (eds): Neural blockade in clinical anesthesia and management of pain, 2nd ed. Philadelphia: JB Lippincott, 1988:135.

toms of toxicity (eg, lightheadedness and dysarthria) warrant close attention, lest they progress unnoticed to greater severity. Even minimal evidence of toxicity warrants constant verbal contact, administration of oxygen, cardiovascular monitoring, and encouragement to breathe with a normal minute volume.

Convulsions

Should convulsions occur, the immediate goal is their cessation before cerebral hypoxia supervenes. Currently, three pharmacologic approaches are recommended. However, simple nonpharmacologic measures, such as maintaining a patent airway and administering oxygen, should be instituted before any drug treatment is begun. The cornerstone of therapy is the prevention of hypoxia and acidosis.

Barbiturates

Thiopental (50 to 100 mg intravenously), rapidly terminates a convulsion. The small dose required adds minimal respiratory and cardiovascular depression; nonetheless, respiration must be observed closely and augmented, if necessary. Similarly, tracheal intubation should be performed, if necessary, to provide a patent airway.

Benzodiazepines

Midazolam, 1 to 2 mg, or diazepam, 5 to 10 mg intravenously, are also effective in terminating convulsion, although onset is slower than that of thiopental and duration of action is longer. The same concerns about respiratory adequacy pertain, and, regardless which drug is chosen, the possibility of respiratory and cardiovascular depression still exists.

Succinylcholine

Succinylcholine, 30 to 50 mg intravenously, will also terminate a convulsion but poses additional considerations: because the drug produces muscular paralysis, pulmonary ventilation ceases, and the patient is thus totally dependent on the airway management skills of those in attendance. Thus, it should be administered only by persons skilled in airway maintenance and tracheal intubation. Also, muscular activity is abolished, which is the external manifestation of the cerebral excitation underlying the convulsion. Without terminating the convulsive process in the brain, high cerebral oxygen utilization continues and threatens cerebral hypoxia. If ventilation is maintained with oxygen, and cardiovascular function is adequate to maintain oxygen delivery to the tissues, no deleterious CNS sequelae are likely.

Cardiovascular Depression

Because CNS toxicity is apparent before cardiovascular toxicity, cardiovascular depression all too likely will go unnoticed. As soon as treatment of the convulsion is begun, the patient's blood pressure and pulse should be determined, if they are not already known. Hypotension, if present, should be treated by correction of hypoxemia, elevation of the legs, increase of the rate of intravenous fluid administration, and, if necessary, intravenous administration of a vasopressor. Because hypotension is usually due to both myocardial depression and peripheral vasodilation, the preferred agent is one that stimulates both α- and β-adrenergic receptors, such as ephedrine, 10 to 25 mg intravenously, incrementally. If bradycardia is present, atropine, 0.5 to 1.0 mg, should be administered intravenously. Do not hesitate to use more potent agents, such as epinephrine, if necessary, to prevent irreversible brain damage or death.[109,110]

Typically, cardiovascular depression is minimal, if present at all. However, when profound cardiovascular depression occurs, it requires immediate institution of standard cardiopulmonary resuscitation. The possibility that catastrophe can occur unexpectedly requires the immediate availability of proper monitoring and resuscitative equipment, as well as experienced personnel, wherever regional anesthesia is administered.

PREVENTION

Because most toxic reactions are due to accidental intravascular injection, careful technique will avoid potential reactions in most situations (Table 40-9). For example, when aspirating

TABLE 40-9
Prevention of Toxicity From Neural Blockade

EXAMINATION OF PATIENT

Identify significant systemic disease, age, and other factors to permit individualization of local anesthetic dose

PREMEDICATION

Benzodiazepine or other appropriate CNS depressant in moderate dosage

PREPARATION

Ensure adequate intravenous fluid available
Equipment
Oxygen administration and suction equipment
Airway (oropharyngeal airway, laryngoscope, endotracheal tube)
Resuscitative drugs: benzodiazepine or thiopental; succinylcholine; atropine; vasopressor
Discard any cloudy solutions or those containing crystals
Separation of neural blockade tray from any other drugs

PREVENTION

Personally check dose of local anesthetic and vasoconstrictor
Use test dose, 5% to 10% of total dose
Aspirate frequently and discard solution colored by blood
Monitor cardiovascular signs (rapid increase in heart rate if epinephrine injected intravenously)
Speak constantly with patient after peak plasma concentration

* Local anesthetic toxicity may result in convulsions; however, with rapid and appropriate treatment, these should never be fatal. See also discussion of cardiac effects of bupivacaine in text.

Covino BG: Clinical pharmacology of local anesthetic agents. In Cousins MJ, Bridenbaugh PO (eds): Neural blockade in clinical anesthesia and management of pain, 2nd ed. Philadelphia: JB Lippincott, 1988:135.

before injecting local anesthetic solution, sufficient time should be allowed for blood to appear in the needle or catheter; similarly, use of a short-bevel needle with a clear plastic hub facilitates recognition of vascular entry.

Test Dose

Use of a test dose is frequently helpful in detecting accidental intravascular or intrathecal injection. Typically, 3 to 5 mL of anesthetic solution is used. If no medical contraindication exists, epinephrine should be added to produce a 1:200,000 solution, which will cause a sudden increase in heart rate and blood pressure if injected intravascularly unless the patient has been taking β-adrenergic blocking agents. A period of 3 to 4 minutes is usually required after an epidural test dose to elicit signs of subarachnoid block. Subsequent injections should be made slowly and incrementally, with periodic aspiration. The patient should be questioned throughout the injection of the local anesthetic to ascertain whether any early symptoms of toxicity (eg, circumoral numbness or tinnitus) are developing.

Benzodiazepines

An additional safeguard is the administration of a benzodiazepine (eg, diazepam or midazolam) intravenously, before administration of the local anesthetic. Such premedication raises the convulsive threshold and provides anxiolysis. In a swine model, in which benzodiazepine-sedated animals received infusions of bupivacaine, premedication decreased the incidence of convulsions and delayed the onset of ventricular dysrhythmias.[111] However, premedication did not alter the dose of bupivacaine or the blood concentration associated with cardiovascular collapse. Most animals progressed directly to collapse without first manifesting convulsions.

REFERENCES

1. Tanaka K, Yamasaki M: Blocking of cortical inhibitory synapses by intravenous lidocaine. Nature 209:207, 1966
2. DeJong RH, Robles R, Corbin RW: Central actions of lidocaine: synaptic transmission. Anesthesiology 30:19, 1969
3. Warnick JE, Kee RD, Yim GKW: The effects of lidocaine on inhibition in the cerebral cortex. Anesthesiology 34:327, 1971
4. Englesson S: The influence of acid-base changes on central nervous system toxicity of local anesthetic agents: I. an experimental study in cats. Acta Anaesthesiol Scand 18:79, 1974
5. Liu PL, Feldman HS, Giasi R, et al: Comparative CNS toxicity of lidocaine, etidocaine, bupivacaine and tetracaine in awake dogs following rapid IV administration. Anesth Analg 62:375, 1983
6. Foldes FF, Davidson GM, Duncalf D, et al: The intravenous toxicity of local anesthetic agents in man. Clin Pharmacol Ther 6:328, 1965
7. Scott DB: Evaluation of the toxicity of local anesthetic agents in man. Br J Anaesth 47:56,61, 1975
8. Scott DB: Evaluation of the toxicity of local anesthetic drugs. Br J Anaesth 53:553, 1981
9. Munson ES, Tucker WK, Ausinsch B, et al: Etidocaine, bupivacaine, and lidocaine seizure thresholds in monkey. Anesthesiology 42:471, 1975
10. Scott DB: Evaluation of clinical tolerance of local anesthetic agents. Br J Anaesth 47:328, 1975
11. Englesson S, Grevsten S: The influence of acid-base changes on central nervous system toxicity of local anaesthetic agents. Acta Anaesthesiol Scand 18:88, 1974
12. Burney RG, DiFazio CA, Foster JA: Effects of pH on protein binding of lidocaine. Anesth Analg 57:478, 1978
13. Apfelbaum JL, Gross JB, Shaw LM, et al: Changes in lidocaine protein binding may explain its increased CNS toxicity at elevated CO_2 tensions (abstract). Anesthesiology 61:A213, 1984
14. Gettes LS: Physiology and pharmacology of antiarrhythmic drugs. Hosp Pract 16:89, 1981
15. Clarkson CW, Hohdeghem LM: Mechanism for bupivacaine depression of cardiac conduction: fast block of sodium channels during the action potential with slow recovery from block during diastole. Anesthesiology 62:396, 1985
16. Wojtczak JA, Pratilas V, Griffin RM, et al: Cellular mechanisms of cardiac arrhythmias induced by bupivacaine (abstract). Anesthesiology 61:A37, 1984
17. Lieberman NA, Harris RS, Katz RI, et al: The effects of lidocaine on the electrical and mechanical activity of the heart. Am J Cardiol 22:375, 1968
18. Sugimoto T, Schaal SF, Dunn NM, et al: Electrophysiological effects of lidocaine in awake dogs. J Pharmacol Exp Ther 166:146, 1969
19. Feldman HS, Covino BM, Sage DJ: Direct chronotropic and inotropic effects of local anesthetic agents in isolated guinea pig atria. Reg Anesth 7:149, 1982
20. Block A, Covino BG: Effect of local anesthetic agents on cardiac conduction and contractility. Reg Anesth 6:55, 1981
21. Stewart DM, Rogers WP, Mahaffrey JE, et al: Effect of local anesthetics on the cardiovascular system in the dog. Anesthesiology 24:620, 1963
22. Liu PL, Feldman HS, Covino BM, et al: Acute cardiovascular toxicity of procaine, chloroprocaine and tetracaine in anesthetized ventilated dogs. Reg Anesth 7:14, 1982
23. Liu PL, Feldman HS, Covino BM, et al: Acute cardiovascular

toxicity of intravenous amide local anesthetics in anesthetized ventilated dogs. Anesth Analg 61:317, 1982
24. Kuperman AS, Altura BT, Chezar JA: Action of procaine on calcium efflux from frog nerve and muscle. Nature 217:673, 1968
25. Tanz RD, Heskett T, Loehning RW, et al: Comparative cardiotoxicity of bupivacaine and lidocaine in the isolated perfused mammalian heart. Anesth Analg 63:549, 1984
26. Johns RA, DiFazio CA, Longnecker DE: Lidocaine constricts or dilates rat arterioles in a dose-dependent manner (abstract). Anesthesiology 61:A204, 1984
27. Blair MR: Cardiovascular pharmacology of local anesthetics. Br J Anaesth 47:247, 1975
28. Jorfeldt L, Lofstrom B, Pernow B, et al: The effect of mepivacaine and lidocaine on forearm resistance and capacitance vessels in man. Acta Anaesthesiol Scand 14:183, 1970
29. Aberg G, Dhuner K-G: Effects of mepivacaine (Carbocaine) on femoral blood flow in the dog. Acta Pharmacol Toxicol 31: 267, 1972
30. Wollenberger A, Krayer O: Experimental heart failure caused by central nervous system depressants and local anesthetics. J Pharmacol Exp Ther 94:439, 1948
31. Aberg G, Anderson R: Studies on mechanical actions of mepivacaine (Carbocaine) and its optically active isomers on isolated smooth muscle: role of Ca^{++} and cyclic AMP. Acta Pharmacol Toxicol 31:321, 1972
32. Nishimura N, Morioka T, Sato S, et al: Effects of local anesthetic agents on the peripheral vascular system. Anesth Analg 44: 135, 1965
33. Edde RR, Deutsch S: Cardiac arrest after interscalene brachial plexus block. Anesth Analg 55:446, 1977
34. Prentiss JE: Cardiac arrest following caudal anesthesia. Anesthesiology 50:51, 1979
35. Albright GA: Cardiac arrest following regional anesthesia with etidocaine or bupivacaine. Anesthesiology 51:285, 1979
36. Morishima HO, Pedersen H, Finster M, et al: Etidocaine toxicity in the adult, newborn and fetal sheep. Anesthesiology 58:342, 1983
37. Morishima HO, Pedersen H, Finster M, et al: Bupivacaine toxicity in pregnant and nonpregnant ewes. Anesthesiology 63: 134, 1985
38. deJong JA, Bonin JD: Deaths from local anesthetic-induced convulsions in mice. Anesth Analg 59:401, 1980
39. deJong RH, Ronfeld RA, DeRosa RA: Cardiovascular effects of convulsant and supraconvulsant doses of amide local anesthetics. Anesth Analg 61:3, 1982
40. Kotelko DM, Shnider SM, Dailey PA, et al: Bupivacaine-induced cardiac arrhythmias in sheep. Anesthesiology 60:10, 1984
41. Sage D, Feldman H, Arthur GR, et al: The cardiovascular effects of convulsant doses of lidocaine and bupivacaine in the conscious dog. Reg Anesth 10:175, 1985
42. Feldman HS, Arthur GR, Norway SB, et al: Cardiovascular effects of mepivacaine and etidocaine in the awake dog (abstract). Anesthesiology 61:A229, 1984
43. Eicholzer AW, Feldman HS: Acute toxicity of etidocaine following various routes of administration in the dog. Toxicol Appl Pharmacol 37:13, 1976
44. Nath S, Haggmark S, Johansson G, et al: Differential depressant and electrophysiologic cardiotoxicity of local anesthetics: an experimental study with special reference to lidocaine and bupivacaine. Anesth Analg 65:1263, 1986
45. Wojtczak JA, Griffen RM, Pratilas V, et al: Is it possible to resuscitate a bupivacaine-intoxicated heart? (abstract). Anesthesiology 61:A207, 1984
46. Moller RA, Covino BG: Toxic cardiac electrophysiologic effects of bupivacaine and lidocaine at high concentrations (abstract). Anesthesiology 63:A223, 1985
47. Kasten GW, Martin ST: Bupivacaine cardiovascular toxicity: comparison of treatment with bretylium and lidocaine. Anesth Analg 64:911, 1985
48. Thigpen JW, Kotelko DM, Shnider SM, et al: Bupivacaine cardiotoxicity in hypoxic-acidotic sheep (abstract). Anesthesiology 59:A-24, 1983
49. Moller RA, Datta S, Fox J, et al: Effects of progesterone on the cardiac electrophysiologic action of bupivacaine and lidocaine. Anesthesiology 76:604, 1992
50. Kasten GW, Martin ST: Successful resuscitation after massive intravenous bupivacaine overdose in the hypoxic dog (abstract). Anesthesiology 61:A206, 1984
51. Feldman HS, Arthur GR, Pitkanan M, et al: Treatment of acute systemic toxicity after the rapid intravenous injection of ropivacaine and bupivacaine in the conscious dog. Anesth Analy 73:373, 1991
52. Nancarrow C, Runciman WB, Mather LE, et al: The influence of acidosis on the distribution of lidocaine and bupivacaine into the myocardium and brain of the sheep. Anesth Analg 66: 925, 1987
53. Moore DC, Crawford RD, Scurlock JE: Severe hypoxia and acidosis following local anesthetic-induced convulsions. Anesthesiology 53:259, 1980
54. Bonica JJ, Berges PV, Morikawa K: Circulatory effects of peridural block: I. effects of level of analgesia and dose of lidocaine. Anesthesiology 33:619, 1970
55. Stanton-Hicks M, Murphy TM, Bonica JJ, et al: Circulatory effects of peridural block: V. properties of circulatory effects, and blood levels of etidocaine and lidocaine. Anesthesiology 42:398, 1975
56. Bonica JJ, Akamatsu TS, Berges PV, et al: Circulatory effects of peridural block: II. effects of epinephrine. Anesthesiology 34:514, 1971
57. Bonica JJ, Kennedy WF, Akamatsu TJ, et al: Circulatory effects of peridural block: III. effects of acute blood loss. Anesthesiology 36:219, 1972
58. Sivarajan M, Amory DW, Lindbloom LE: Systemic and regional blood flow during epidural anesthesia without epinephrine in the rhesus monkey. Anesthesiology 45:300, 1976
59. Ward RJ, Bonica JJ, Freund FG, et al: Epidural and subarachnoid anesthesia: cardiovascular and respiratory effects. JAMA 191:275, 1965
60. Sivarajan M, Amory DW, Lindbloom LE, et al: Systemic and regional blood flow changes during spinal anesthesia in the Rhesus monkey. Anesthesiology 43:78, 1975
61. Braid DP, Scott DB: The systemic absorption of local analgesic drugs. Br J Anaesth 37:394, 1965
62. Evans JA, Chastain GM, Phillips JM: The use of local anesthetic agents in obstetrics. South Med J 62:519, 1969
63. DiGiovanni AJ: Inadvertent intraosseous injection: a hazard of caudal anesthesia. Anesthesiology 34:92, 1971
64. Lund PC, Bush DF, Covino BG: Determinants of etidocaine concentration in the blood. Anesthesiology 42:497, 1975
65. Tucker GT, Mather LE: Clinical pharmacokinetics of local anesthetics. Clin Pharmacokinet 4:241, 1979
66. Schwartz ML, Meyer MB, Covino BG, et al: Antiarrhythmic effectiveness of intramuscular lidocaine: influence of different injection sites. J Clin Pharmacol 14:77, 1974
67. Giasi RM, D'Agostino E, Covino BG: Absorption of lidocaine following subarachnoid and epidural administration. Anesth Analg 58:360, 1979
68. Scott DB, Cousins MJ: Clinical pharmacology of local anesthetic agents. In Cousins MJ, Bridenbaugh PO (eds): Neural blockade. Philadelphia: JB Lippincott, 1972: 86
69. Wildsmith JA, Tucker GT, Cooper S, et al: Plasma concentrations of local anaesthetics after interscalene brachial plexus block. Br J Anaesth 49:461, 1977
70. Hickey R, Blanchard J, Hoffman J, et al: Plasma concentrations of ropivacaine given with or without epinephrine for brachial plexus block. Can J Anaesth 37:878, 1990
71. Feldman HS, Arthur GS, Covino BG: Cardiovascular effects of total spinal anesthesia following intrathecal administration of bupivacaine with and without epinephrine in the dog. Reg Anesth 9:22, 1984
72. Post C: Studies on the pharmacokinetic function of the lung with special reference to lidocaine. Acta Pharmacol Toxicol 44:1, 1979
73. Lofstrom JB, Alm B-E, Bertler A, et al: Lung uptake of lidocaine. Acta Anaesthesiol Scand Suppl 70:80, 1978

74. Lofstrom JB: Tissue distribution of local anesthetics with special reference to the lung. Int Anesthesiol Clin 16:53, 1978
75. Covino BG, Vassallo HG: Local anesthetics: mechanism of action and clinical use. New York: Grune & Stratton, 1976
76. Benowitz NL: Clinical applications of the pharmacokinetics of lidocaine. Cardiovascular Clinics 6:77, 1974
77. Stenson RE, Constantino RT, Harrison RC: Interrelationships of hepatic blood flow, cardiac output and blood levels of lidocaine in man. Circulation 43:205, 1971
78. Wiklund L, Berlin-Wahlin A: Splanchnic elimination and systemic toxicity of bupivacaine and etidocaine in man. Acta Anaesthesiol Scand 21:521, 1977
79. Covino BG: Pharmacokinetics of local anesthetic agents. In Prys-Roberts C (ed): Pharmacokinetics of anesthesia. Oxford: Blackwell Scientific, 1985: 270
80. Meffin P, Long GJ, Thomas J: Clearance and metabolism of mepivacaine in the human neonate. Clin Pharmacol Ther 14: 218, 1973
81. Mihaly GW, Moore RG, Thomas J, et al: The pharmacokinetics and metabolism of the anilide local anesthetics in neonates: I. lignocaine. Eur J Pharmacol 13:143, 1978
82. Nation RL, Triggs EJ, Selig M: Lignocaine kinetics in cardiac patients and aged subjects. Br J Clin Pharmacol 44:1, 1977
83. Morishima HO, Pedersen H, Finster M, et al: Toxicity of lidocaine in adult, newborn, and fetal sheep. Anesthesiology 55: 57, 1981
84. Thomson PD, Melmon KL, Richardson JA, et al: Lidocaine pharmacokinetics in advanced heart failure, liver disease and renal failure in humans. Ann Intern Med 78:499, 1973
85. Williams RL, Blaschke TF, Meffin PJ, et al: Influence of viral hepatitis on the disposition of two compounds with high hepatic clearance: lidocaine and indocyanine green. Clin Pharmacol Ther 20:290, 1976
86. Collinsworth KA, Strong JM, Atkinson AF Jr, et al: Pharmacokinetics and metabolism of lidocaine in patients with renal failure. Clin Pharmacol Ther 18:59, 1975
87. Scott DB, Owen JA, Richmond J: Methemoglobinemia due to prilocaine. Lancet 2:728, 1964
88. Lund PC, Cwik JC: Propitocaine (Citanest) and methemoglobinemia. Anesthesiology 26:569, 571, 1965
89. Hjelm M, Holmdahl MH: Biochemical effects of aromatic amines: II. cyanosis, methemoglobinemia and Heinz-body formation induced by a local anesthetic agent (prilocaine). Acta Anaesthesiol Scand 2:99, 1965
90. Brown DT, Beamish D, Wildsmith JAW: Allergic reaction to an amide local anesthetic. Br J Anaesth 53:435, 1981
91. Aldrete JA, Johnson DA: Evaluation of intracutaneous testing for investigation of allergy to local anesthetic agents. Anesth Analg 49:173, 1970
92. Aldrete JA, O'Higgins JW: Evaluation of patients with history of allergy to local anesthetic drugs. South Med J 64:1118, 1971
93. Skou JC: Local anesthetics: II. the toxic potencies of some local anesthetics and of butyl alcohol, determined on peripheral nerve. Acta Pharmacol Toxicol 10:292, 1954
94. Adams HJ, Mastri AR, Eicholzer A, et al: Morphologic effects of intrathecal etidocaine and tetracaine on the rabbit spinal cord. Anesth Analg 53:904, 1974
95. Moore DC, Spierdijk J, vanKleef JD, et al: Chloroprocaine neurotoxicity: four additional cases. Anesth Analg 61:155, 1982
96. Rigler ML, Drasner K: Distribution of catheter-injected local anesthetic in a model of the subarachnoid space. Anesthesiology 75:684, 1991
97. FDA Safety Alert: Cauda equina syndrome associated with use of small-bore catheters in continuous spinal anesthesia. Rockville, MD: Food and Drug Administration, 1992
98. Barsa JE, Batra M, Fink BR, et al: Prolonged neural blockade following regional analgesia with 2-chloroprocaine. Anesth Analg 61:961, 1982
99. Pizzalato D, Renegar OJ: Histopathologic effects of long exposure to local anesthetics on peripheral nerves. Anesth Analg 38:138, 1959
100. Ranindran RS, Turner MS, Muller J: Neurologic effects of subarachnoid administration of 2-chloroprocaine-CE, bupivacaine, and low pH normal saline in dogs. Anesth Analg 61:279, 1982
101. Rosen MA, Baysinger CL, Shnider SM, et al: Evaluation of neurotoxicity after subarachnoid injection of large volumes of local anesthetic solutions. Anesth Analg 62:802, 1983
102. Wang BC, Hillman DE, Spiedholz NI, et al: Chronic neurological deficits and Nesacaine-CE: an effect of the anesthetic, 2-chloroprocaine, or the antioxidant, sodium bisulfite? Anesth Analg 63:445, 1984
103. Gissen AJ, Datta S, Lambert D: The chloroprocaine controversy: II. is chloroprocaine neurotoxic? Reg Anesth 9:135, 1984
104. Fillbuck EF, Opper SE: Back pain following epidurally administered Nesacaine MPF. Anesth Analg 69:113, 1989
105. Levy L, Randall GI, Pandit SK: Does chloroprocaine (Nesacaine NPF) for epidural anesthesia increase the incidence of backache? Anesthesiology 71:476, 1989
106. Stevens RA, Chester WL, Artusio JD, et al: Back pain after epidural anesthesia with chloroprocaine in volunteers: preliminary report. Reg Anesth 16:199, 1991
107. Benoit PW, Belt WD: Some effects of local anesthetic agents on skeletal muscle. Exp Neurol 34:264, 1972
108. Libelius R, Sonesson B, Stamenovic BA, et al: Denervation-like changes in skeletal muscle after treatment with a local anesthetic (Marcaine). J Anat 106:297, 1970
109. Kaplan RA, Ward RJ, Posner K, et al: Unexpected cardiac arrest during spinal anesthesia: a closed claims analysis of predisposing factors. Anesthesiology 68:5, 1988
110. Keats AS: Anesthesia mortality: a new mechanism. Anesthesiology 68:2, 1988
111. Bernards CM, Carpenter RL, Rupp SM, et al: Effect of midazolam and diazepam premedication on central nervous system and cardiovascular toxicity of bupivacaine in pigs. Anesthesiology 70:318, 1989

FURTHER READING

Covino BG: Clinical pharmacology of local anesthetic agents. In Cousins MJ, Bridenbaugh PO (eds): Neural blockade in clinical anesthesia and management of pain, 2nd ed. Philadelphia: JB Lippincott, 1988: 111

Reiz S, Nath S: Cardiotoxicity of local anaesthetic agents. Br J Anaesth 58:736, 1986

Scott DB: Toxic effects of local anaesthetic agents on the central nervous system. Br J Anaesth 58:732, 1986

Complications in Anesthesiology, second edition,
edited by Nikolaus Gravenstein and Robert R. Kirby.
Lippincott-Raven Publishers, Philadelphia © 1996.

CHAPTER 41

Complications of Spinal and Epidural Anesthesia

Leroy D. Vandam

The practice of anesthesiology reflects the art as well as the knowledge of the times, and the same may be said of the complications that ensue. With experience and study, the results of a technique should improve; if not, the technique should be abandoned in favor of methods offering more acceptable morbidity and mortality. In this context, the popularity of spinal and epidural anesthesia has waxed and waned over the years, but their widespread use today is an indication of better understanding and progressive improvement in their administration.

HISTORY OF SPINAL AND EPIDURAL ANESTHESIA

Before a presentation of the complications resulting from these kinds of regional anesthesia, a brief history may provide insight into the problems that concern us.

Within a year of the demonstration of the local anesthetic properties of cocaine in 1884, Corning, a New York neurologist, attempted to relieve the symptoms of a patient with urologic complaints by injecting a solution of cocaine into the vicinity of the spinal cord. Numbness in the lower half of the body was apparent after 20 minutes. We shall never know whether Corning succeeded in giving a spinal or epidural anesthetic because the needle was capped with a syringe and Corning did not comment on the escape of cerebrospinal fluid (CSF).

Quincke, in 1891, performed subarachnoid puncture for the first time in an effort to relieve hydrocephalus. It was but a step further to inject cocaine into the subarachnoid space, and this Bier attempted in 1898. After several administrations to patients, he, as the subject, became the first to have the common complication of postural headache. Copious quantities of CSF escaped because the syringe did not fit the needle.

Others—Matas in America and Tuffier in France—followed suit. Subsequent reports contained more than a few references to headache, nausea and vomiting (because of the practice of barbotage), and meningitis. Moreover, because the sterility of cocaine solutions could not be ensured, residual neurologic deficit occurred. Furthermore, the immediate onset of arterial hypotension was noted. Thus patients given spinal anesthesia customarily were placed for operation in the head-down position.

In 1901 Cathelin succeeded in producing epidural anesthesia by injection through the sacrococcygeal ligament into the caudal canal. In the 1st decade of the 20th century, many of the details of spinal anesthesia as we know them today were introduced: the use of dextrose to weight the anesthetic solution, thereby permitting hyperbaric control; substitution for cocaine of the more easily sterilized procaine (Novocain); and addition of epinephrine to prolong the effect of nerve block. As early as 1921, Antoni advocated the use of a small-gauge lumbar puncture needle to minimize CSF leakage and development of headache. At the same time, Pages achieved more uniform success with lumbar epidural anesthesia, perfected and popularized a decade later by the Italian surgeon Dogliotti.

Ultimately, the clamor over the neurologic sequelae of spinal anesthesia reached a crescendo in the 1940s, culminating in Thorsen's monograph on the subject.[1] Both he and a group working with Kennedy,[2] an eminent neurologist, proclaimed that neurologic disease and paralysis were too high a price to pay for the fine muscle relaxation achieved with spinal anesthesia. Several other studies illuminated the causes and suggested preventive measures to eliminate neurologic complications. The problem of hypotension was more or less solved by prophylactic administration of sympathomimetic amines and intravenous fluid administration to correct the disproportion between blood volume and the dilatated vascular space. Finally, new local anesthetics, knowledge of their mode of action and metabolism, and detailed technical studies led to a resurgence of epidural anesthesia in the 1950s and 1960s.

In this chapter, the complications of spinal and epidural anesthesia are presented together because the techniques are almost identical. The complications may be immediate, largely because of the physiologic effects of nerve block, or delayed, owing to pathophysiologic changes that result from the techniques and drugs used.

FUNCTIONAL ANATOMY

The anatomic basis of these techniques provides clues to development of complications.

Subarachnoid and Epidural Puncture

For prevention of neurologic sequelae, knowledge of the anatomy of the spinal column and its contents is essential in the performance of subarachnoid and epidural puncture. Subarachnoid puncture should be performed preferably below the L2–L3 interspace to avoid direct injury to the spinal cord, which usually terminates at that level. This rule is less important in epidural anesthesia, in which entry is made at any level of the spinal column, depending on the segmental area to be anesthetized.

Needle Entry

For lumbar puncture, vertebral spines are identified by their rectangular surfaces; usually the L4–L5 space is chosen, as approximated by a line drawn between the highest points of the iliac crests. Entry by way of the lumbosacral space, the largest of all, is not easy because of the overhanging L5 spine: the approach, from below upward, starts at the level of the S2 foramen with the needle angled upward and medially (the Taylor approach). Because repeated attempts at lumbar puncture may result in back pain and neurologic damage, the back should be maximally flexed to open the interspaces. For obese patients, in whom landmarks are not obvious, and for patients with arthritis, the sitting position helps to straighten and to flex the spine.

Pertinent Structures

Progressing inward, the needle passes through several structures easily recognized by sense of touch and resistance (Fig. 41-1). Disinfection of the skin must be meticulous, and attention should be paid to epidermal abnormalities (eg, pigmentation, alopecia, or dimpling) that might suggest spinal dysraphism or low termination of the cord. A needle, regardless of the type of point, with a close-fitting stylet is essential to limit the introduction of bits of epidermis, subcutaneous tissue, or periosteum into the epidural or subarachnoid space and thus to help avoid infection or transplantation of epidermal cells to the meninges.[3,4]

The longitudinal furrow of the back results from fixation of the skin by connective tissue to the supraspinous ligament, but it does not necessarily represent the midline, unless the spine is erect and flexed. The supraspinous ligament spans

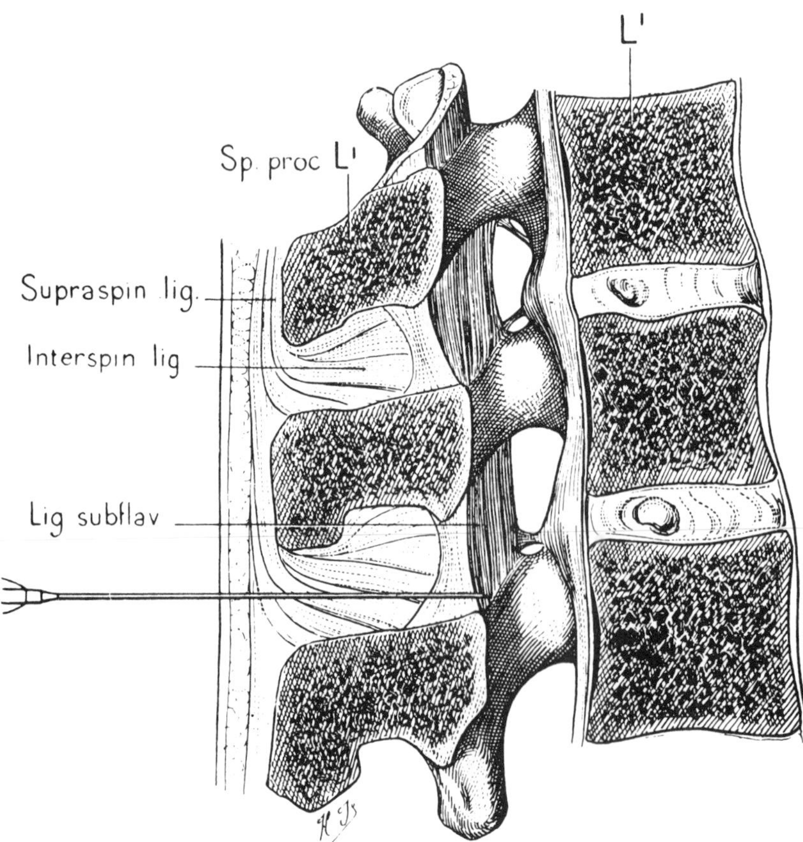

FIGURE 41-1. Sagittal section of the lumbar spine shows the direction of the needle perpendicular to the surface of the skin and the anatomic structures through which it passes. *Interspin lig,* interspinous ligament; *Lig subflav,* ligamentum subflavum; *Sp proc,* spinous process; *Supraspin lig,* supraspinous ligament. (Labat G: Regional anesthesia. Philadelphia: WB Saunders, 1923)

the apices of the spinous processes and, similar to other ligaments, contains relatively few pain receptors; thus midline puncture can be pain-free. Any pain is felt deep in the back or segmentally and rarely is referred to the buttocks or thighs.

Paresthesias

A paresthesia, the sensation of electric shock referred to a dermatome of the lumbosacral plexus, suggests that a nerve has been touched. Repeated paresthesias call for abandonment of the procedure. Once the needle is in the subarachnoid space, the local anesthetic should not be injected if a paresthesia is present, because permanent damage could occur. Introduction of a catheter into the epidural or subarachnoid space results in a higher incidence of paresthesias than does introduction of the needle alone.[5]

Loss of Resistance

The interspinous ligament, a dense collagenous structure and a good guide to the midline, offers resistance to injection and provides the anatomic basis for the loss-of-resistance test for entry into the epidural space. Deep to the junction of the vertebral arches is the paired ligamentum flavum, consisting of yellow elastic tissue confluent in the midline and offering less resistance as the needle is advanced beyond it. This change in resistance is often mistaken as entry into the subarachnoid space but more likely indicates entry into the epidural or subdural space.

Epidural Space

Contents

The epidural space, within the spinal column surrounding the dural sac, extends from the foramen magnum above to the sacrococcygeal ligament below. It varies in capacity according to the cross-sectional area of the canal and diameter of the spinal cord, which is largest in the cervical, upper thoracic, and lumbar regions. This space contains nerve roots partly ensheathed in meninges, semiliquid fat, areolar tissue, and radicals of the peridural plexus of veins. The space may be partially occluded by fibrous tissue adhesions between dura mater and vertebrae, particularly in aged patients.

Paravertebral Venous Plexus

The paravertebral plexus of veins, a valveless, large-capacity system that is subject to changes in pressure transmitted from the abdomen, drains the structures of the back. The veins act as accessory pathways for the caval system in returning blood from the periphery. The plexus is ladder-like, lacking venous radicals in the midline where lumbar puncture ordinarily is done. Perforation of one of these veins is the usual cause of a bloody spinal tap and the source of epidural hematoma in persons with clotting abnormalities. Occasionally, the tip of a catheter placed in the epidural space may enter one of the veins. If this error is not recognized, injection of anesthetic solution may result in a toxic reaction as well as failure to obtain anesthesia.

Changing pressures in this venous system affect pressures within the dural sac. Dilation of the veins, both inside and outside of the dura, increases CSF pressure. The resulting change in pressure can be seen during myelography when the patient coughs or strains and the contrast medium rises several segments. It is the basis of Queckenstedt's test and the reason why straining or coughing after injection of a local anesthetic may result in high levels of anesthesia. In the relief of spinal headache caused by CSF hypotension, application of a tight abdominal binder may be effective by increasing intra-abdominal venous pressure, raising pressure in the epidural plexus, and secondarily increasing CSF pressure.

Negative Pressure

Pressure in the lumbar epidural space becomes negative (subambient) just after the needle perforates the ligamentum flavum; this change is a useful sign in identifying the space during administration of epidural anesthesia. The negative pressure has been ascribed to one or more of several factors: tenting of the dura as the needle is inserted, with creation of a partial vacuum; spinal flexion, which increases the capacity of the epidural space through an accordion-like effect; and transmission of negative intrathoracic pressure to the lumbar epidural space.

Dura Mater

The dura mater is an avascular collagenous membrane with predominantly vertically directed fibers, recognizable by a characteristic loss of resistance as the membrane is tented and perforated by a needle. The poor vascularity of the dura leads to slow healing, with the result that the perforation may persist and allow leakage of CSF. It has been recommended that the dura be entered with the bevel of the needle parallel to the long axis of the fibers to limit the size of the opening. This approach has been shown to be effective in decreasing the incidence of post–dural puncture headache.[6,7]

Subdural Space

The subdural space is a virtual space between the dura and the arachnoid that can be seen during laminectomy, when the dura is incised and the underlying arachnoid prevents escape of CSF. The importance of this space in spinal anesthesia lies in the possibility that the local anesthetic may be injected here rather than into the subarachnoid space, thus causing failure of the block.[8]

Arachnoid

The arachnoid is a webbed membrane that contains the CSF and acts as a framework for blood vessels supplying the spinal cord. It is not sensed as a distinct structure when lumbar puncture is performed. CSF and local anesthetics are absorbed by the spinal arachnoidal granulations through perineural lymphatic vessels and in epidural anesthesia after exit through the intervertebral perineural spaces.

Subarachnoid Space and Spinal Cord

In the lumbar area, the important structures in the subarachnoid space comprise the anterior and posterior nerve roots forming the cauda equina, which pass through the intervertebral foramina, where the dorsal root ganglia are found. Each dorsal and ventral nerve root comprises many rootlets, arising in a continuous line from the lateral spinal sulcus. The individual fibers, rather than a conglomeration in bundles as in peripheral nerves, permit easy penetration and rapid onset of anesthesia. Some fibers are myelinated and others nonmyelinated; the latter contain nodes of Ranvier, where local anesthetic penetration takes place.

In the lumbar area, the nerve roots may be traumatized during puncture, as indicated by paresthesias. However, because they are not under tension, the roots usually are not transfixed by the needle and therefore are deflected. Injury may occur more frequently than is realized, particularly in the motor roots, where contact does not result in paresthesia. Injection of a local anesthetic into a nerve root, as suggested by intensification of paresthesia, severe pain, and occasionally loss of consciousness, results in permanent neurologic damage, probably because the anesthetic diffuses along the nerve into the spinal cord, where pressure ischemia occurs.[9]

Anterior and Posterior Compartments

Above the cauda equina, the subarachnoid space is incompletely divided into anterior and posterior compartments by the dentate ligament, which arises from the cord in a continuous line between anterior and posterior nerve roots, to attach by a series of digitations between the dura and arachnoid (Fig. 41-2). As such, the dentate ligament acts as a baffle, a feature possibly important in localizing anesthesia when an attempt is made to produce unilateral block.

Blood Supply

The blood supply to the spinal cord is segmentally derived from cervical, thoracic, lumbar, and sacral arteries by their passage along the nerve roots to anastomose on the surface with the anterior and posterior spinal arteries (Fig. 41-3). Higher in the cord, the anterior and posterior spinal arteries originate from the vertebral, basilar, and branches of the thyrocervical arteries. The cord is thus vascularized by an anastomosing network with penetration of the vessels from the periphery.

The blood supply of the cord is controlled by the same physiologic mechanisms as is the brain. These vessels usually are not injured during lumbar puncture; blood-stained CSF originates in the peridural venous plexus. However, subarachnoid apoplexy may follow rupture of a sclerotic vessel, and ischemia of the cord may result from arteriosclerotic occlusion of one of these vessels, producing characteristic neurologic syndromes. Some believe that the progressive development of neurologic disease caused by arachnoiditis results from occlusion of the blood vessels by an organizing inflammatory process at the periphery of the cord. Finally, because of sys-

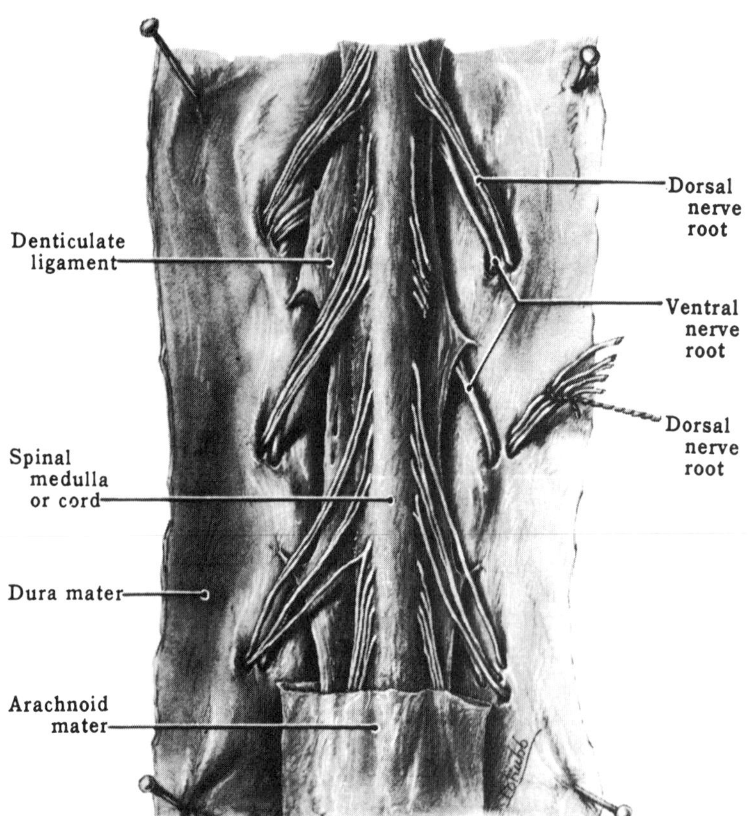

FIGURE 41-2. A portion of the spinal cord and its membranes, shown from behind. The dura mater is unopened below; the arachnoid is removed above. The multiple radicles of the spinal nerve roots and the dentate ligament can be seen. (Grant JCB: Atlas of anatomy, 7th ed. Baltimore: Williams & Wilkins, 1978)

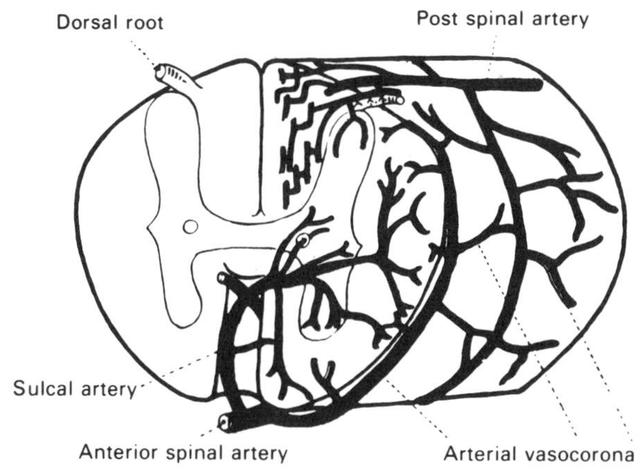

FIGURE 41-3. The blood supply of the spinal cord: the anterior and posterior spinal arteries, the anastomoses on the surface, and the penetration of the cord. (Vandam LD: Spinal anesthesia. In Hale DE (ed): Anesthesiology. Philadelphia: FA Davis, 1963)

temic hypotension or because of the pressure of large volumes of local anesthetic in the epidural space, ischemia of the cord may precipitate residual damage.

PHYSIOLOGIC EFFECTS

When an anesthetic is injected into the epidural or subarachnoid space, anesthesia develops at the point of injection. Spinal nerve roots, dorsal root ganglia, and the periphery of the cord are the sites of action. In epidural anesthesia, the local anesthetic affects these structures by diffusion across the meninges and passage through the intervertebral foramina, where the spinal nerves are reached. The major effects ultimately result from the anesthetization of anterior and posterior spinal nerve roots.

Because of the initial high concentration gradient and lipid solubility of the local anesthetics, absorption takes place rapidly, according to the diameter of the nerve fiber. As in many forms of regional anesthesia, fibers of smallest diameter are often affected first. A lesser concentration is needed, and the surface area for penetration is larger. However, structure also is important, because sympathetic B fibers are most susceptible. Because of their varying effects on receptors, the amide local anesthetics may not follow these general rules.

Thus, in general, neurologic function disappears in the following order: autonomic activity; sensation to pinprick; sensation of heat and cold; vibratory sense and sense of position; motor power; and touch. From this sequence of action, one can deduce that differential block is possible, depending on the concentration of anesthetic injected.

Respiratory Insufficiency

Spinal

The excellent muscle relaxation obtained with spinal anesthesia is unrivaled by any other anesthetic technique, perhaps including the use of neuromuscular blocking agents, which act only at the neuromuscular junction. The muscle paralysis of spinal anesthesia results from interference with conduction in motor nerves and is aided by blockade on the sensory side of the spinal reflex arc. Skeletal muscle relaxation requires the use of high concentrations of anesthetic or anesthetics with a special affinity to block motor fibers.

CLINICAL PRESENTATION. Paralysis of the lower intercostal muscles is the price paid for good operating conditions in the upper abdomen. If, in addition, abdominal packs and retractors interfere with diaphragmatic action, respiration may be seriously compromised. If this dysfunction is significant, ventilation should be assisted. Many patients complain of difficulty in breathing, probably because proprioceptive sense from intercostal and abdominal muscles is lost. High paralysis is accompanied by a feeling of suffocation and signs of motor and sensory paralysis in the arms. If phrenic nerve roots are blocked, the accessory muscles of respiration may be called into action, although these too may be affected. The patient is unable to talk because of an inability to move air, and consciousness may be lost. Paralysis of respiration is treated with positive-pressure oxygen by mask or tracheal intubation until the level of anesthesia recedes.

Epidural

Respiratory paralysis is not as common during epidural anesthesia because the anesthetic does not diffuse as easily in the epidural space as in CSF. In a survey of complications of epidural anesthesia involving 30,088 administrations, Dawkins reported the onset of massive anesthesia in approximately 0.1% (Table 41-1).[10] After apparently uneventful administration and a lapse of approximately 20 minutes, respiration ceased and the pupils dilated, with no decrease in blood pressure. With respiratory support, recovery took place in about 1.75 hours. To account for this reaction, either subdural injection or massive transudation into CSF must have occurred. Usubiaga noted similar cases in a review of the world literature.[11]

Circulatory Depression

Spinal

Marked arterial hypotension after administration of spinal anesthesia was an early concern and still is a controversial aspect of this technique, despite prophylactic and therapeutic use of vasopressor drugs. Even if temporary, a major decrease in blood pressure may so decrease cerebral or coronary blood flow in patients with arteriosclerosis that an ischemic accident may occur.

MECHANISMS. The arterial hypotension of spinal anesthesia results from interruption of sympathetic innervation to systemic veins and arteries and interference with baroreceptor reflexes that control pressure. The consistency and magnitude of the decrease in pressure are directly proportional to, and the chance for compensatory vasoconstriction in nonanesthetized areas of the body is inversely proportional to, the height of the sympathetic blockade. Blood pressure tends

TABLE 41-1
Complications After Lumbar and Thoracic Epidural Block

	NO. CASES	NO. COMPLICATIONS (%)
Dural puncture	43,152	1,090 (2.5)
Accidental total spinal anesthesia	48,297	102 (0.2)
Blood vessel puncture	6578	189 (2.8)
Toxic reaction	66,366	144 (0.2)
Massive subdural anesthesia	16,644	28 (0.1)
Severe hypotension	42,900	797 (1.8)
Backache	9107	185 (2.0)
Transient paralysis	32,718	48 (0.1)
Permanent paralysis	32,718	7 (0.02)

Dawkins CJM: Analysis of the complications of extradural and caudal block. Anaesthesia 24:554, 1969.

to decrease more if the initial pressure is high. Postural effects are marked, as in any kind of neurogenic hypotension. Hypotension is aggravated by reduced blood volume. In a study of spinal anesthetics given without prophylactic vasopressors, Dripps and Deming found that 90% of patients sustained a decrease in systolic pressure that was 35% of control pressure.[12]

A study of the circulation indicates that a decrease in total systemic vascular resistance accounts for the hypotension in some patients, whereas in others a decrease in cardiac output is found.[13] The latter probably results from systemic venous dilatation and pooling of blood, with decreased venous return to the heart. Accessory factors include bradycardia resulting from the block of accelerator impulses to the heart and, possibly, a decrease in the release of catecholamines from sympathetic nerve endings, also an effect that decreases myocardial contractility.

Skeletal muscle relaxation and decrease in amplitude of respiration, with consequent diminution in negative intrathoracic pressure and venous return to the thorax, seem not to be essential to the development of hypotension. Vasoconstriction in nonanesthetized areas of the body may compensate partially for the decrease in pressure. With total autonomic blockade, the reflex response to hypotension initiated by the baroreceptors, vasoconstriction, and acceleration of the pulse is inactivated.

Epidural

Hypotension during epidural anesthesia occurs for the same reasons as it does during spinal anesthesia. At the same levels of anesthesia, the circulatory response to epidural block is qualitatively similar with the two techniques. A difference, however, is that absorption of local anesthetic from the epidural space into the circulation can depress systemic vascular and myocardial function. All of the local anesthetics exert a quinidine-like effect on the myocardium, reducing contractility, diminishing irritability, and slowing conduction time; in addition, peripheral vasodilatation occurs.

In comparisons of spinal and epidural anesthesia of equal extent, the hypotension observed with the latter technique tends to be less profound. One possible reason for this difference is that in epidural anesthesia little or no differential occurs between sensory and sympathetic blockade: that is, sympathetic block does not ascend as high as in spinal anesthesia. The concomitant use of epinephrine in epidural anesthesia does not entirely prevent development of hypotension. Despite an increase in heart rate and stroke volume, peripheral resistance is diminished.

Pressor drugs are seldom given prophylactically before epidural anesthesia; their use in spinal anesthesia is less common now than it was in the past. As in spinal anesthesia, many accessory factors are involved in the circulatory depression observed with epidural anesthesia: adequacy of blood volume; height of sympathetic blockade; the amount of local anesthetic and epinephrine absorbed into the systemic circulation; and a tendency in aged patients for the level of anesthesia to ascend.

Cerebral and Coronary Arterial Blood Flow

Cerebral and coronary blood flow may remain unchanged during the hypotension of spinal and epidural anesthesia because of vasodilatation and decrease in resistance, the means by which circulation ordinarily is maintained in these vascular beds. However, if arteriosclerosis, which would preclude vasodilatation, is present, or if the mean arterial blood pressure decreases to less than 60 to 70 mm Hg, vasodilatation may be insufficient to compensate, and ischemia may result. Thus, the hypotension tolerated depends on the pressure to which the patient is accustomed and the presence of vascular disease.

Because little decrease in cerebral metabolic rate occurs during spinal anesthesia, hypotension may threaten the brain more than it does the heart. Measurements of cerebral blood flow indicate that vasodilatation compensates for the hypotension, but signs of cerebral ischemia, such as yawning, syncope, and nausea, are seen frequently in normal patients in the supine position when systolic blood pressure decreases to less than 70 to 80 mm Hg.

Hepatic and Renal Blood Flow

Hepatic and renal blood flow are maintained to a point during spinal and epidural anesthesia because the decrease in mean arterial pressure is accompanied by vasodilatation. Urinary output usually ceases at systolic pressures of less than 60 or

70 mm Hg, but the renal parenchyma may still be well perfused. Changes in hepatic function after spinal anesthesia differ little from those observed after general anesthesia.

The operation performed is a more important influence. During spinal anesthesia with hypotension, estimated hepatic blood flow is markedly decreased, and postoperative hepatic dysfunction is greater than after anesthesia with normotension. In animal models, vasodilatation in the liver and kidneys has been found helpful in the prevention of ischemia and avoidance of irreversible shock.

Prophylactic Vasopressor Administration

In the 1930s, prophylactic injection of vasopressor drugs was used to counteract the decrease in blood pressure encountered during spinal anesthesia. The rationale was to maintain tissue perfusion in the heart and brain, despite vasoconstriction in the kidneys and liver. This practice is far less common today. In a study of the actions of several vasopressor drugs, Dripps and Deming found methamphetamine to be useful, but little statistical difference was noted among the drugs studied.[12]

In view of the circulatory alterations, a drug with both myocardial and peripheral stimulating properties seems a logical choice so that cardiac output and peripheral vascular resistance are maintained. Most clinicians prefer ephedrine because of its predominantly central actions; a few select phenylephrine, for its peripheral actions. If pressure decreases to threatening levels or cardiac arrest occurs after anesthesia has taken effect, epinephrine should be injected intravenously to increase pressure quickly and prevent permanent neurologic damage.[13,14] If more than one or two subsequent injections are required, a continuous infusion of vasopressor may be started to titrate blood pressure to an appropriate level.

Attempts to lessen the degree of hypotension often include intravenous infusion of fluids before spinal anesthesia is administered. This approach helps to some degree, especially in obstetric cases. The incidence of postanesthetic catheterization increases, however, because of diuresis and overdistention of the urinary bladder.

Bowel and Urinary Dysfunction

Hyperactive Peristalsis

Interruption of sympathetic innervation to the bowel leaves parasympathetic nerve action unopposed, with resultant smooth muscle contraction, hyperactive peristalsis, and sphincter relaxation. In addition to muscle paralysis, contraction of the bowel is one of the reasons that abdominal relaxation is excellent during spinal anesthesia; this effect accounts for the scaphoid appearance of the abdomen.

Excessive peristalsis should alert the surgeon to anticipate intestinal spillage during intestinal anastomoses. Hyperactive peristalsis leading to perforation is one reason that spinal anesthesia is deemed dangerous in the presence of intestinal obstruction, a fear that is more theoretical than real. Defecation and colostomy movements often occur because of sphincter relaxation. Preanesthetic use of morphine, with its depressant effect on intestinal smooth muscle, may counteract parasympathetic stimulatory effects.

Urinary Retention

Spinal and caudal anesthesia have always been associated with a high incidence of postoperative inability to void and a consequent need for catheterization. In the sacral region, sympathetic and parasympathetic nerves are blocked, with resulting detrusor and sphincter paralysis. These autonomic effects considerably outlast motor and sensory blockade. Inability to empty the bladder is exaggerated by overdistention when intravenous fluid therapy is excessive.

Nausea and Vomiting

Incidence

In 1923, Labat, commenting on spinal anesthesia, stated, "Under the best conditions nausea frequently occurs in the Trendelenburg position and in the case of operations on the organs of the upper abdominal cavity, especially the stomach. This is increased by rough manipulation and heavy packing of the bowels against the diaphragm."[15] Babcock, one of the pioneers of spinal anesthesia, found that vomiting occurred in 13% and nausea in 18% of his patients. He believed that nausea was a premonitory sign of hypotension, cyanosis, or respiratory depression.[16] Among other reasons suggested for the onset of nausea during spinal anesthesia are cerebral ischemia, psychologic factors, the presence of bile in the stomach because of relaxation of the sphincters, increased peristalsis, a specific action of the drug on the spinal medulla, the effect of preanesthetic medication and bodily motion, and use of a vasoconstrictor drug. Nausea and vomiting occur in at least 13% and perhaps as many as 42% of spinal anesthetics.[17]

Mechanisms

Vomiting is a complex coordinated motor reflex. The neural network lies in the lateral gray reticular formation of the medulla, which coordinates the several components of the process. Vomiting may be incited directly or reflexively by stimulation of the chemoreceptive trigger zone in the floor of the fourth ventricle, which is sensitive to drugs with central actions such as morphine or apomorphine. Vagal and sympathetic afferent nerve fibers transmit the effects of emetic agents acting locally on the bowel and carry other kinds of reflexes from the thorax and abdomen. Thus, the medulla is the integrative area, but vomiting may be initiated from almost any site in the body. Davis and Pollock stated that "the persistence of vomiting after blocking of the pain fibers (cerebrospinal) indicates that strong visceral afferent impulses continue to reach the higher centers through the sympathetic and vagal chains."[18]

According to these concepts, many instances of nausea and vomiting during spinal anesthesia are initiated reflexively from the operative field, as supported by the data presented in Table 41-2.[17] Among patients with a sensory level to pinprick at the T4 segment or higher, the incidence of nausea and vomiting was increased, even though pain did not occur. Because few of the operations performed necessitated such high levels, probably the local anesthetic had spread in the subarachnoid space without providing complete anesthesia.

Table 41-3 shows that intrathecal use of epinephrine was

TABLE 41-2
Incidence of Nausea and Vomiting During Spinal Anesthesia in Relation to Position, Sensory Level, and Need for Supplementation

	NAUSEA AND VOMITING (176 cases)	NO NAUSEA OR VOMITING (763 cases)	
	No. (%)	*No. (%)*	AVERAGE *P*
POSITION			
Supine	82 (47)	400 (53)	
Lithotomy	29 (16)	139 (18)	
Lateral	25 (14)	69 (9)	
Trendelenburg	27 (15)	58 (8)	<0.30
Prone	8 (5)	69 (9)	
Fowler	3 (2)	10 (1)	
Other	2 (1)	18 (2)	
SENSORY LEVEL OF ANESTHESIA			
T10 & below	37 (21)	205 (27)	
T4–T9	111 (63)	439 (57)	
Above T4	26 (15)	45 (6)	
Not recorded	2 (1)	74 (10)	
SUPPLEMENTATION WITH GENERAL ANESTHESIA			
Intravenous	58 (33)	265 (35)	
Inhalation	11 (6)	18 (2)	
Intravenous-inhalation	80 (46)	180 (24)	
None	27 (15)	300 (39)	

Crocker JS, Vandam LD: Concerning nausea and vomiting during spinal anesthesia. Anesthesiology 20:587, 1959.

associated with a higher incidence of vomiting. Epinephrine not only prolongs anesthesia but also delays onset and the time for full attainment of a satisfactory sensory level. For these reasons, the level of anesthesia is difficult to control, and often the dose of anesthetic is reduced when epinephrine is added. In these circumstances, sensory blockade may be inadequate.

NEUROLOGIC SEQUELAE OF SPINAL AND EPIDURAL ANESTHESIA

Because of the neurologic sequelae, criticism of spinal anesthesia reached a peak in the late 1940s. To this day, people fear the method because they believe that neurologic sequelae are common. Some anesthesiologists avoid the technique because of the possibility of a lawsuit, should postanesthetic complications develop. Yet carefully observed series of anesthetics have demonstrated that major neurologic consequences are rare and that the frequency of minor neurologic sequelae is minimal.[19,20] Analysis of postanesthetic deaths places spinal anesthesia in a favorable position with regard to mortality.[21] With few exceptions, however, central neuraxis blocks have not been documented to possess clear advantages compared with general anesthesia.[22] If clinical impressions overrule careful observation, patients may be denied a valuable anesthetic technique.

Spinal anesthesia, believed to be the method of choice for certain operations, was studied prospectively during the period

TABLE 41-3
Incidence of Pain, Hypotension, Need for Supplementary Vasopressor, and the Use of Epinephrine in Relation to Nausea and Vomiting During Spinal Anesthesia

	CASES (no.)	NAUSEA AND VOMITING No. (%)	NO NAUSEA OR VOMITING No. (%)	AVERAGE *P*
Pain	176	72 (41)	80 (10)	<0.01
Hypotension	176	79 (45)	172 (23)	<0.01
Supplementary vasopressor drugs	176	79 (45)	194 (26)	<0.01
Intrathecal epinephrine	97	48 (50)	136 (33)	<0.01

Crocker JS, Vandam LD: Concerning nausea and vomiting during spinal anesthesia. Anesthesiology 20:587, 1959.

from 1948 to 1951 at the University of Pennsylvania.[9] Data from a total of 8460 patients given 10,098 spinal anesthetics were available for review. During the hospital stay, patients were seen daily by an anesthesiologist or by a trained nurse. Before leaving the hospital, they were requested to reply to a questionnaire that would be mailed within 6 months. The advantage of the immediate phase of the study was that all of the details of anesthesia, the operation, and immediate postoperative effects could be gathered in one institution. This search for complications probably exaggerated the reporting of symptoms, but only by these means could neurologic problems that might otherwise have passed undetected be discovered. A parallel study was conducted in a group of 1000 persons given general anesthesia for the same kinds of operation performed during spinal anesthesia to uncover the symptoms that might be common to the patient or to the operation. In a smaller series, 100 patients were given spinal anesthesia only after induction of general anesthesia to exclude symptoms that could arise purely on a psychologic basis.

Data were obtained for 89% of the anesthetics, for periods ranging from 6 months to 10 years.[9] No instance of adhesive arachnoiditis, transverse myelitis, or cauda equina syndrome was found. Minor neurologic deficits were noted; none was progressive, and most were of little consequence. Eleven patients had exacerbation of preexisting neurologic disease after anesthesia. Neurologic complications of spinal anesthesia resulted from lumbar puncture per se or injection of the local anesthetic.

In lumbar puncture, several factors are involved. Best known are those attributable to leakage of CSF, causing the syndrome of decreased intracranial pressure: headache and ocular and auditory symptoms. Another group of complications involves trauma of lumbar puncture. Backache and infection have been reported many times as sequelae of lumbar puncture, but neurologic deficit resulting from trauma has not been emphasized.

The complications of spinal anesthesia, followed by those resulting from epidural anesthesia, are presented here in detail. Although these data were gathered many years ago, the results are applicable today.

Cerebral Complications

As with any kind of anesthesia, cerebral hypoxia can result from arterial hypotension or respiratory inadequacy; the resultant ischemia may produce transient neurologic symptoms or may produce irreversible changes if hypoxia is severe or cardiac arrest occurs. Cerebrovascular accidents have been reported after transient hypotension during spinal anesthesia and after excessive hypertensive responses to the injection of a vasopressor drug. In the majority of cases, CNS symptoms such as coma, loss of memory, mental deterioration, confusion, and psychoses can be attributed to unrecognized or untreated episodes of hypoxia. It is important, however, that other causes of neurologic disease be sought before any neurologic changes are ascribed to the spinal anesthetic.

Decreased Intracranial Pressure

The overall incidences of headache, ocular, and auditory complications are shown in Table 41-4.[23] In this study, headaches were postural, with onset on assumption of the erect position, and usually were relieved by recumbency; their location was frontal, occipital, vertex, nuchal, or a combination, probably depending on the intracranial pain-sensitive structures involved. Severity, duration, and time of onset varied. Patients described in subjective terms (such as constricting band, heaviness, vacuum-like, dead weight, or worse on moving) how or what they felt.

TABLE 41-4
Syndrome of Decreased Intracranial Pressure

COMPLICATION	CASES No. (%)
"Spinal" headache	1011 (11.0)
Ocular difficulties	34 (0.4)
Auditory difficulties	35 (0.4)

Vandam LD, Dripps RD: Long-term follow-up of patients who received 10,098 spinal anesthetics: III. syndrome of decreased intracranial pressure (headache and ocular and auditory difficulties). JAMA 161:586, 1956.

Occipital headache, nuchal pain, and stiffness of the neck were not signs of meningitis, because fever and CSF pleocytosis was not found. Rather, spasm and pain in the cervical muscles were interpreted as reactions to pain similar to those that occur in other areas of the body. Stiffness of the neck and tender spots in cervical muscles are common accompaniments of headache, regardless of the cause. A similar incidence of headache was found in a control series of 1000 patients given general anesthesia, but headaches were nonspecific in nature.

Ocular difficulties included diplopia, blurring, difficulty in focusing, spots before the eyes, photophobia, and scintillation. Auditory complaints included decreased hearing, obstruction, and tinnitus. Few of these symptoms were found in patients receiving general anesthesia. The symptoms enumerated were related to lumbar puncture rather than to introduction of the spinal anesthetic. Controlled series of lumbar puncture in our experience[23] and in that of others[1] have revealed the same kinds of symptoms.

When a second lumbar puncture for diagnostic or therapeutic reasons was performed in a patient after the onset of a spinal headache, CSF pressure was observed to be very low.[23] Although not an invariable finding, this observation suggested that headache and the associated symptoms result from leakage of CSF through a dural opening left by the lumbar puncture needle. When CSF pressure is lowered, intracranial vasodilatation, aggravated by assumption of the erect position, results in traction on pain-sensitive dilatated blood vessels, giving rise to a vascular type of headache.[23–25] No increase in CSF pressure after spinal anesthesia was found in these studies.

"Spinal" Headache

Incidence. An incidence of 18% was found by Thorsen in 50,000 cases collected from various sources,[1] whereas an overall incidence of headache in the cited series was 11%.[23] Occurrence of headache according to age in this series is shown in Table 41-5. The incidence decreased after the 5th decade; the highest frequency occurred in the 3rd and 4th decades. In part, this difference among age groups may be attributed to an elevation of pain threshold in the aged, perhaps because of a progressive decrease in neural elements. Vibratory sensibility decreases with advancing age, as does the elasticity of the cerebral vessels. The differences among age groups were not attributable to factors that might affect CSF pressure, such as earlier ambulation in young patients or more adequate parenteral fluid replacement in one group than in another.

In women, the incidence of headache was almost twice that in men (Table 41-6).[23] The main reason for this difference is the inclusion of obstetric cases in the group of women studied; headache after vaginal delivery occurred in 22% of patients, twice the overall figure. This finding may relate to changes in intra-abdominal pressure during labor, which influence CSF pressure and lumbar puncture leakage; to changes in blood volume; and to the lesser attention paid to parenteral fluid replacement after delivery. Even when obstetric cases are not included, headache still occurs more frequently in women (see Table 41-6).

Although other investigators may disagree,[26] the role of the psyche in the development of headache seems negligible. To prove this point, spinal anesthesia was given to 100 patients during general anesthesia.[23] Although none of these people knew that spinal anesthesia had been administered, the percentage of postural headache was the same as in the series at large.

Needle Diameter. The most conclusive data on development of lumbar puncture headache[23] are shown in Table 41-7, which relates the diameter of the needle to headache. The incidence, severity, and duration of headache decreased progressively with smaller needle diameters. Use of a 26-G needle resulted in a low incidence. When a 16-G needle was used for continuous spinal anesthesia, the number and severity of headaches and ocular complaints were so prohibitive that this technique was later reserved for older patients or for patients with conditions for which safety and better control were major considerations. At the time, for routine use and minimization of technical difficulty, a 22-G needle proved best. The overall incidence of headache with this needle was nearly 9%, but the headaches usually were mild. Today, use of a 27-G needle seems prudent, with a reported incidence of headache of less than 2%.[27] However, other investigators suggest that needle bevel orientation and patient age are factors more significant than a needle size less than 22-G.[28]

Early Ambulation. After surgery patients were encouraged to ambulate early, and thus onset of headache took place soon thereafter. In some cases, headache appeared when the patient lifted his or her head or arose from bed for the first time. In cases of severe headache, patients soon learned the value of recumbency to relieve symptoms. The first onset of headache after several days or even weeks explains why, in some series, the reported incidence was exceptionally low (Table 41-8): patients simply were not observed postoperatively over a sufficient time. In the University of Pennsylvania series, onset of headache rarely was reported long after the patient had

TABLE 41-6
Gender in Relation to Incidence of "Spinal" Headache

SEX	SPINAL ANESTHETICS No.	"SPINAL" HEADACHES No. (%)
Male	4063	302 (7)
Female	5214	709 (14)
Vaginal delivery	938	220 (22)
Other procedures	4276	489 (12)
Total	9277	1011 (21)

Vandam LD, Dripps RD: Long-term follow-up of patients who received 10,098 spinal anesthetics: III. syndrome of decreased intracranial pressure (headache and ocular and auditory difficulties). JAMA 161:586, 1956.

TABLE 41-5
Age in Relation to Incidence of "Spinal" Headache

AGE (yr)	SPINAL ANESTHETICS No.	"SPINAL" HEADACHES No. (%)
10–19	537	41 (10)
20–29	1994	321 (16)
30–39	1833	261 (14)
40–49	1759	192 (11)
50–59	1736	133 (8)
60–69	1094	45 (4)
70–79	297	7 (2)
80–89	27	1 (3)
Total	9277	1011 (11)

Vandam LD, Dripps RD: Long-term follow-up of patients who received 10,098 spinal anesthetics: III. syndrome of decreased intracranial pressure (headache and ocular and auditory difficulties). JAMA 161:586, 1956.

TABLE 41-7
Gauge of Needle for Lumbar Puncture in Relation to Incidence of "Spinal" Headache

NEEDLE GAUGE	SPINAL ANESTHETICS No.	"SPINAL" HEADACHES No. (%)
16	839	151 (18)
19	154	16 (10)
20	2698	377 (14)
22	4952	430 (9)
24	634	37 (6)

Vandam LD, Dripps RD: Long-term follow-up of patients who received 10,098 spinal anesthetics: III. syndrome of decreased intracranial pressure (headache and ocular and auditory difficulties). JAMA 161:586, 1956.

TABLE 41-8
Time of Onset of "Spinal" Headache in Postoperative Period

TIME OF ONSET AFTER OPERATION	"SPINAL" HEADACHES No. (%)
Day of operation	89 (9)
1 day	302 (29)
2 days	216 (21)
3 days	123 (13)
4–6 days	115 (11)
7–12 days	12 (1)
1 month	2 (0.2)
5 months	2 (0.2)
No data	150 (15)

Vandam LD, Dripps RD: Long-term follow-up of patients who received 10,098 spinal anesthetics: III. syndrome of decreased intracranial pressure (headache and ocular and auditory difficulties). JAMA 161:586, 1956.

left the hospital.[23] Such a delay in headache is not easily explained. It is possible that slow leakage of CSF continues without causing symptoms until loss overbalances production or until a certain pain threshold is reached.

Patients commonly are required to remain recumbent in bed after spinal anesthesia in an attempt to prevent headache, but neither we nor others have evidence that this technique is effective.[28] Leakage of CSF probably takes place during operation and afterward, even if the patient is recumbent.[29,30]

Duration. The duration of headache from lumbar puncture may be extraordinarily long, from 1 day to 12 months; 53% of headaches ended within 4 days[23] (Table 41-9). Because of poor blood supply, the dura does not heal readily. Leakage from a needle opening has been seen at laminectomy and at postmortem examination as long as 14 days after lumbar puncture.

Prevention. If headache does not follow lumbar puncture, the arachnoid may have prolapsed through the dural opening, thereby preventing leakage; this finding has been observed at laminectomy. To prevent leakage, a variety of lumbar puncture techniques and special needles have been devised. Oblique needle insertion to puncture the dura and arachnoid at different levels is unlikely to prolapse the arachnoid consistently.[31] Insertion of the needle bevel parallel to the longitudinal fibers of the dura so that fibers are spread rather than sectioned has been recommended.[28] In our series of 100 spinal anesthetics,[23] in which the bevel of the needle was inserted parallel to the fibers, headaches were slightly fewer but not significantly different from those occurring in the larger series. The issue of the influence of the needle bevel is easily circumvented by using a pencil-point needle, which eliminates cutting of the longitudinally or horizontally oriented fibers and which has been suggested to reduce the incidence of post–dural puncture headache.[32]

Treatment. Headache can be relieved with analgesic agents or by attempts to increase CSF pressure. Hydration with saline-containing fluids and application of a tight abdominal binder may relieve a milder headache. The mechanism of relief of headache by way of epidural fluid injection is not clear; perhaps the dura is buttressed, or epidural fluid passing through the opening increases CSF pressure directly. During the past 25 years, success in relieving headache has been achieved in about 90% of cases by means of a "blood patch"[33,34]: ten to 20 mL of the patient's venous blood is collected aseptically and injected into the epidural space at the leakage site. The clot thus formed stems escape of CSF, increases CSF pressure, and almost immediately relieves the symptoms.

Ocular Symptoms

In the study of spinal anesthesia,[23] 34 patients had difficulty with vision (see Table 41-4). The diverse complaints included diplopia, sensitivity to light, and spots before the eyes. In all but 8 cases, visual complaints were associated with typical postural headache. In 3 cases lateral rectus muscle palsy was proven, and in 3 others prolonged diplopia suggested that palsy might have been present. These cases followed use of a 16-G needle for continuous spinal anesthesia. Five of the headaches were severe, and 3 were localized to the occiput. Thus, the palsies and the other ocular complaints seemed related to CSF leakage.

Ocular nerve palsies appeared suddenly, about 1 week after anesthesia, and persisted from a few weeks to 6 months, with eventual restitution of functional vision. Many reports of cranial nerve palsy after spinal anesthesia have appeared; the abducens nerve usually is involved.[35] One theory contends that with brain displacement and traction on supporting structures, a motor nerve such as the abducens, with its long intracranial course, can be compressed against bone; alternatively, as the nerve passes through the cavernous sinus, venous dilatation might cause pressure.

Auditory Difficulties

Thirty-five patients in the series had difficulty in hearing (see Table 41-4).[23] In many dizziness was associated, and nausea was common. Dizziness, nausea, and difficulty in hearing were

TABLE 41-9
Duration of "Spinal" Headache

DURATION	"SPINAL" HEADACHES (1011 Cases) No. (%)
1–2 d	245 (24)
3–4 d	296 (29)
5–7 d	193 (19)
8–14 d	79 (8)
3–6 wk	49 (5)
3–6 mo	19 (2)
7–12 mo	38 (4)
No data	92 (9)

Vandam LD, Dripps RD: Long-term follow-up of patients who received 10,098 spinal anesthetics: III. syndrome of decreased intracranial pressure (headache and ocular and auditory difficulties). JAMA 161:586, 1956.

found in the control series receiving general anesthetics but usually could be ascribed to underlying medical disease. After spinal anesthesia, patients noted buzzing, loss of hearing, and a roaring sound. With few exceptions, these complaints also were associated with postural headache, and hence a decrease in CSF pressure was implicated. Anatomic communication exists between the subarachnoid space and cochlea. Hughson demonstrated that a decrease in CSF pressure is associated with a decrease of intralabyrinthine pressure followed by inability of the ear to transmit high tones.[23] In several patients, an audiogram was restored to normal values when CSF pressure was artificially increased.

INJURIES LOCALIZED TO THE SPINAL CORD AND ITS COVERINGS

Traumatic Lumbar Puncture

Major Sequelae

Another group of complications is related to traumatic lumbar puncture. In a comparison of single-dose and continuous spinal anesthesia, Dripps found a much higher incidence of technical difficulties, paresthesias, and bloody taps with continuous spinal anesthesia.[5] Although backache and infection have been emphasized as sequelae of lumbar puncture, neurologic deficit has not been. The following is a case in point.

CASE 1. A 23-year-old man was to undergo excision of an anal fistula. Spinal anesthesia was selected, although the skin of the back was scarred, the result of burns sustained in childhood. Many attempts at lumbar puncture with a 22-G needle were made at two interspaces, with the patient in the sitting position. Paresthesias occurred in both legs. Although the subarachnoid space was entered and clear CSF obtained, anesthesia was abandoned because paresthesias were induced every time an attempt was made to withdraw fluid.

On the 1st postoperative day, severe postural headache developed, beginning in the nuchal region and radiating around the side of the face to the eyes. Tenderness and pain at the lumbar puncture site were present, with radiation to the low back. Neither numbness nor difficulty in voiding or walking was noted.

One week later, the patient still had postural headache and severe back pain. He walked with the aid of a cane in a semi-stooped position and complained of pain in the left calf, without paresthesias or numbness. After urination, he sensed that the bladder was incompletely emptied, and his sexual drive was considerably diminished. Neurologic examination was normal, except for tenderness over the L3–L5 spines.

Subsequently, his condition improved, and he resumed work as a machinist. However, 8 months after the operation, after exacerbation of back and leg pain, findings were suggestive of a protruded disc at L3–L4 or L4–L5.

Little doubt was cast on the relation between traumatic puncture and development of back and leg pain. Because the anesthetic was not injected, an intraneural or intraspinal injection was not the cause. The decision to abandon spinal anesthesia was based on inability to avoid paresthesias with repositioning of the needle.[37]

CASE 2. A 32-year-old woman was scheduled for cesarean section. She had had spinal anesthesia for a previous cesarean section without complication. With the patient in lateral decubitus position, numerous attempts at lumbar puncture with a 22-G needle were made, producing multiple paresthesias in the legs, thighs, and feet that were more severe on the left side. Blood-tinged CSF was recovered. Ultimately, subarachnoid tap produced a scant quantity of clear CSF. The anesthetic was injected without additional paresthesias, but supplementary general anesthesia was required.

Postoperatively, sensation returned more slowly in the left than in the right leg. Backache at the puncture sites and a feeling of weakness in the left leg were present. At first, the patient was unable to lift the left leg because of motor weakness and loss of position sense. On standing she tended to lose balance, and she bore weight on the right leg. She also complained of spasmodic pain with voiding. Symptoms gradually abated, and on the 8th postoperative day, neurologic signs (hypalgesia over the anterior left thigh and slight motor weakness in the entire limb but with normal reflexes) were minimal. Three months later, the patient showed marked improvement but complained of occasional loss of balance, a sensation of flexion in the third and fourth toes, and several episodes of involuntary defecation. Neurologic examination was normal. After 5 years of observation, residual complaints were pain and numbness in the heels and toes during fatigue.

This patient had undergone spinal anesthesia previously and had no antecedent neurologic disease. Inexperience on the part of a novice anesthesiologist, failure to flex the spine adequately in a pregnant woman, and faulty selection of landmarks were probably responsible for lumbar puncture difficulty. Surely related to trauma were back pain at the puncture site; multiple paresthesias, particularly in the left leg, in which subsequently involvement was severe; and recovery of blood-stained CSF.

Minor Sequelae

The remainder of the patients (Table 41-10) had no antecedent neurologic disease; a solution of tetracaine and dextrose solution was used in 13 of the 17 cases. The common denominator in all cases was multiple insertion of a lumbar puncture needle, with production of paresthesias in lumbar and sacral dermatomes; blood-stained fluid was seen only once. In all patients, subsequent complaints of pain, paresthesia, or numbness, could be related to paresthesia occurring at lumbar puncture. The duration of complaints ranged from 1 day to many months, but the symptoms were never incapacitating or progressive.

Symptoms in patients 7, 10, and 14 resembled those of meralgia paresthetica.[38] Those in patient 10 were unusual in that pain and paresthesias at puncture were felt in the shoulder girdle, a symptom known as Lhermitte's sign, ascribed to reduction in CSF pressure with traction on adhesions or other mechanical effects on the spinal cord.[39] An intraneural injection was doubtful in these cases, because this event usually results in excruciating paresthesia with injection, loss of consciousness, and onset of permanent sensory and motor deficit immediately postoperatively.

Trauma to ligaments, fascia, or bone can give rise to low

TABLE 41-10
Minor Sequelae of Lumbar Puncture in 17 Patients

PATIENTS				ATTEMPTS			
No.	*Age (years)*	*Sex*	OPERATION	*No.*	SITE OF PARESTHESIA	SEQUELAE	DURATION OF SEQUELAE
1	24	M	Coccygeal sinus	3	R leg	Shooting pain, R leg	1 day
2*	28	F	Coccygeal sinus	1	L leg	Shooting pain and numbness, L leg	2 days
3	34	M	Appendectomy	1	L buttock, penis	Paresthesia, L buttock and penis	2 days
4	43	F	Hemorrhoidectomy	4	L thigh, buttock	Pain, L thigh to knee	1 day
5	47	F	Hysterectomy	2	R buttock, groin	Weakness and pain, R leg	8 days
6	29	F	Cesarean section	2	R leg	Paralysis and pain, R leg	2 weeks
7†	36	M	Appendectomy	2	R thigh	Numbness and tingling, R thigh	3 weeks
8†	41	M	Varicose veins (ligation and stripping)	1	R leg	Numb area, R foot	2 weeks
9	54	F	Cholecystectomy	1	L leg	Sharp pain, L leg	Few weeks
10	30	F	Laparotomy	2	R leg and shoulder	Pain, R shoulder and thigh; numbness, R thigh; paresthesias	1 month
11	31	F	Vaginal plastic	4	None	Pain, L calf and foot; numbness	1 month
12	35	F	Hysterectomy	1	L Leg	Pain, L leg	Months
13	38	M	Appendectomy	Many	R toes, both heels	Burning pain, heels	Months
14	29	F	Delivery	2	R leg	Numbness, R thigh	6 months
15	39	M	Incision and drainage of rectal abscess	2	L leg	Pain, L leg	1 year, intermittent
16	40	M	Cholecystectomy	5	R leg	Shooting pain, R foot	6 months
17	55	M	Cholecystectomy	1	L leg	Pain, L leg	Intermittent

F, female; *L,* left; *M,* male; *R,* right.

* Cerebrospinal fluid was bloody in this patient only.

† A 22-gauge needle was used in all but these patients, in whom a 20-gauge needle was used.

Vandam LD, Dripps RD: Long-term follow-up of patients who received 10,098 spinal anesthetics: IV. neurological disease incident to traumatic lumbar puncture during spinal anesthesia. JAMA 172:1483, 1960.

back pain and sciatic radiation, a syndrome produced experimentally on injection of hypertonic saline into the back.[40] Disc infection as a sequela of traumatic puncture also has been reported.[41] Injury to the cauda equina may have caused a radiculitis not sufficient to be associated with sensory deficit. Still another possibility is a sterile inflammatory reaction resulting from introduction of blood into the subarachnoid space.[42]

Not all traumatic lumbar punctures are followed by neurologic complaints, and paresthesias occur in cases handled by even the most skillful anesthesiologists. In a large series, they were encountered during lumbar puncture in 13% of single-dose spinal anesthetics and in 30% of continuous spinal catheter anesthetics. Few patients had subsequent disability.[5]

Perhaps patients with marked obesity, spinal curvature, or arthritis should be offered another form of anesthesia. In any situation a position and technique that will make lumbar puncture easier should be used. When difficulty is encountered with midline insertion, a lateral approach should be tried. Blood-stained CSF should be allowed to clear before injection of anesthetic. Injection should never be made in the presence of a paresthesia, to avoid injection into a nerve root or spinal cord. When paresthesia is produced, the needle should be repositioned or inserted at another interspace. Finally, the question of when to abandon lumbar puncture arises. If a technique other than spinal anesthesia can be used safely (as usually it can), a patient should be spared further discomfort and possible complications.

INFECTIOUS SEQUELAE

Meningitis

Meningitis may occur after diagnostic lumbar puncture or the administration of spinal or epidural anesthesia. In the latter situation, the dural sac may have been entered. The presence of an epidural abscess after a catheter or needle insertion can spread infection to the subarachnoid space. Soon after introduction of subarachnoid block meningism (stiffness of the neck and headache) and meningitis were frequent. Meningism may indicate spinal headache.

Bacterial meningitis also may occur. Diagnostic puncture to identify the organism and appropriate antibiotic treatment are essential. Repeated lumbar puncture after spinal anesthesia occasionally yields CSF with increased protein and pleocytosis. At one time, these findings were interpreted as indicators of meningitis.[43] However, the increased protein content is thought merely to reflect increased protein concentrations in the circulation after operation.[44] In addition, the numbers of cells usually are increased after lumbar puncture with production of paresthesias.[44]

Chemical

From time to time epidemics of chemical meningitis have occurred.[45,46] This complication, which may also occur after paravertebral nerve block, epidural anesthesia, and caudal anesthesia, is characterized by fever, headache, cervical rigidity, nausea and vomiting, transient neurologic signs, prostration, and coma. The CSF is opalescent, though sterile, and contains a variety of white cells. The syndrome lasts for several days and has been attributed to pyrogens in the apparatus and solutions used. Treatment is directed entirely toward symptoms; antibiotic agents are not required. The possibility of disease caused by coxsackievirus also must be considered.

Bacterial

Meningitis has ceased to be a problem in spinal anesthesia because of increased attention to asepsis. The following report of coincident, acute, purulent otitis media gives rise to interesting speculation.[47]

CASE 3. A 12-year-old mentally retarded boy had incapacitating bilateral pes planus. A diagnostic spinal anesthetic was done to exclude spasm from the orthopedic problem. A tetracaine spinal anesthetic to the level of T12 was given with a 22-G needle inserted at the L3–L4 interspace after recovery of clear CSF. Mild headache was present 2 days afterward. Twelve days later, abrupt onset of frontal headache, stiffness of the neck, and fever to 39.1°C occurred. Purulent secretion was seen in the right auditory canal, and the ear drum was injected. Marked spasm of the anterior and posterior cervical muscle groups was elicited, with referred pain to forehead and low back. Tests for Brudzinski's and Kernig's signs were positive.

The white blood cell count was 8100 cells/mL. Lumbar puncture yielded grossly clear CSF, with 20 red blood cells and 150 white blood cells, of which 60% were neutrophils and 40% lymphocytes. The protein content was 58 mg/dL, glucose 56 mg/dL, and chloride 118 mEq/dL. The initial pressure was 20 mm Hg. Bacterial culture was negative. Within 24 hours of antibiotic treatment, symptoms disappeared.

The 12-day interval between anesthesia and the onset of meningitis tended to exclude anesthesia as the cause. Meningism and meningitis are not uncommon in association with acute otitis media. The early disappearance of symptoms and the paucity of CSF changes suggested meningism rather than frank bacterial meningitis.

Spinal anesthesia should not be administered in the presence of infection, especially if bacteremia is a possibility. Weed and colleagues were able to produce meningitis in several animal species by performing occipital or lumbar puncture within 5 hours of intravenous injection of pathogenic bacteria.[48] Meningitis began not at the puncture site but intracranially, and bacteria were recovered from the subarachnoid space. Thus, the hypothesis that resistance to infection may be reduced by spinal puncture was suggested. Others have reported meningitis and epidural abscess in humans when spinal anesthesia was given in the presence of acute infectious disease.[49,50]

COMPLICATIONS RELATED TO INJECTION OF LOCAL ANESTHETICS

Two major complications of spinal anesthesia deserve special mention because of the resulting disabling illness: cauda equina syndrome and chronic adhesive arachnoiditis.

Cauda Equina Syndrome

The cauda equina syndrome involves symptoms localized to areas innervated by the lumbar and sacral nerves. In chemical, neural injury, the small fibers are affected first, just as they may be the first to be affected by local anesthetics. Thus, the syndrome presents with autonomic disability, problems in the evacuation of bladder and bowel, and disturbance of sweating and temperature control in lumbar and sacral dermatomes. In addition, sensation to pinprick, temperature, and position may be altered.

A form of cauda equina syndrome can follow traumatic lumbar puncture when injection of local anesthetic is intraneural. The solution travels along the nerve root to origins in the spinal cord, possibly causing ischemia of cells.

In the past, when neither traumatic tap nor intraneural injection could be implicated and the cauda equina syndrome developed, a toxic substance, possibly a detergent used in cleaning apparatus or a contaminant of the local anesthetic, was assumed to have been introduced into the subarachnoid space. At one time, when ampules were soaked in phenol for sterilization, the substance could seep through inapparent cracks into ampules. This problem was implicated in a major lawsuit in Great Britain.[51] Apparatus and ampules are sterilized today by autoclaving or ethylene oxide. Suspicious-looking ampules that have discolored solutions or seem to have less than the volume of solution expected should be discarded. In the United States, use of disposable spinal trays, for practical purposes, has eliminated this problem.

Another possible explanation for the cauda equina syndrome is the development of vascular insufficiency. Arterial hypotension and hypoxemia may damage the spinal cord as well as the brain, particularly in the patient with hypertension. Similarly, vascular accidents involving the cord have been reported. In addition, an increase in pressure with injection of large volumes of solution may decrease blood flow in the superficial vessels of the cord. Vasoconstrictor drugs combined with the local anesthetic also may enhance this effect.

Recently, the syndrome was reported as a complication of continuous spinal anesthesia when 26-G or smaller microcatheters were used.[52] Very high local anesthetic concentration and exposure to larger doses with this technique are thought to be contributory. The United States Food and Drug Administration ordered these microcatheters removed from the market in 1992.[53]

Adhesive Arachnoiditis

Adhesive arachnoiditis, a stereotypical pathologic reaction of the central nervous system, occurred long before spinal anesthesia was used.[54] Appearing diffusely or in patches, this sterile, organizing, inflammatory process may be idiopathic or may occur in response to trauma, chemical irritation, or infection. The subarachnoid space becomes obliterated by adhesions, with dense attachment of the arachnoid to dura. At laminectomy, the dura can hardly be peeled away from the underlying arachnoidal membrane. Blood vessels are entrapped in the organizing inflammatory process, with resultant ischemia and destruction of cells and tracts within the spinal cord, producing a variety of neurologic deficits. On pathologic examination, the blood vessels are obliterated by an organizing endarteritis.

Relation to Spinal Anesthesia

Adhesive arachnoiditis occurring after spinal anesthesia presents the additional features of variable location and progressive involvement of the spinal cord and brain; hence, it is called chronic progressive adhesive arachnoiditis. Hydrocephalus, syringomyelia, and varieties of paraplegia and tetraplegia typify the end stage of this process. The cause is unknown, but it has been attributed to contamination of the local anesthetic with a chemical preservative (methylparaben) or to an allergic response. The latter is suggested by the vasculitis that sometimes is concomitant. This finding may be the explanation for the development of neurologic sequelae after unintended injection of chloroprocaine into the subarachnoid space during the administration of epidural anesthesia. The lesion has been reproduced experimentally by injection of a variety of chemical irritants, including detergents, into the subarachnoid space.[55] Figure 41-4 shows a normal-looking spinal cord at laminectomy and a cord in a case of adhesive arachnoiditis.

Arachnoiditis does not seem to occur today, although without continued surveillance of spinal and epidural techniques we cannot be certain that it has been eliminated. If improvement has occurred, credit should go to meticulous preparation of equipment and solutions, which are sterilized and continuously surveyed in pharmaceutical houses and hospital pharmacies. Storage times, lot numbers, and date of expiration must be known.

Arachnoiditis presents typical manifestations at myelography, although many radiologists prefer not to inject an additional chemical irritant for diagnosis. To exclude other lesions, laminectomy is necessary. The best treatment for adhesive arachnoiditis is to attempt to decompress the cord and reestablish CSF circulation.

MINOR NEUROLOGIC SEQUELAE

Incidence

In one study of 10,098 cases, 71 cases were found in which subjective or both subjective and objective evidence of neurologic disease was present after spinal anesthesia.[56] Subjective complaints comprised numbness, tingling, heaviness, or burning; some were associated with neurologic deficit. Symptoms usually were present in the immediate postoperative period and lasted from a few days to more than 6 months without progression. Of note is that the majority of complaints were confined to the lumbar and sacral areas. In 85 others (1% of the total number of patients), reported symptoms were called "irritative," for want of a better term. Cramps and twisting, pulling, or drawing sensations in the lower extremities arose and subsided in the first few days after operation. Because 0.9% of patients given general anesthesia had iden-

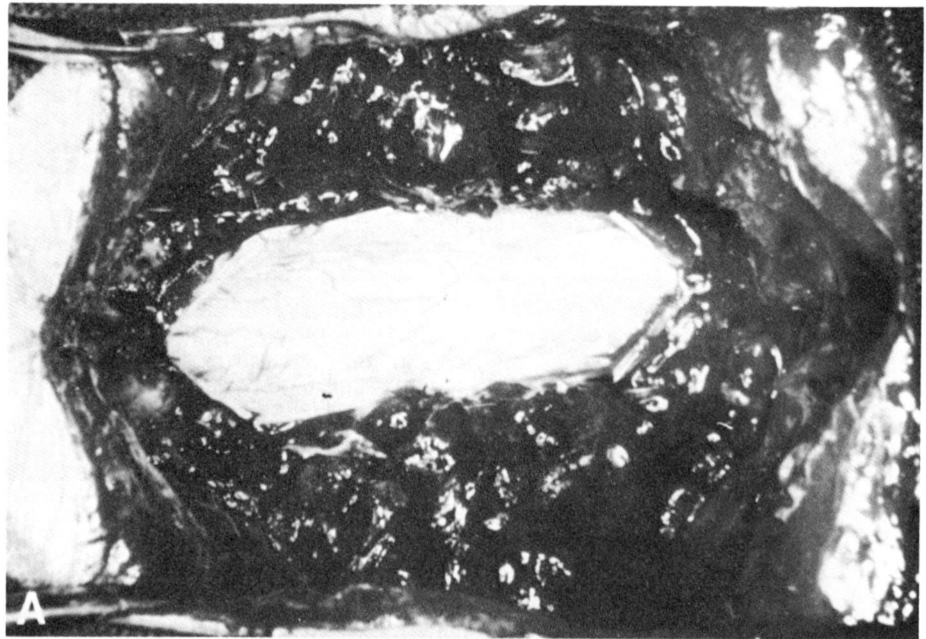

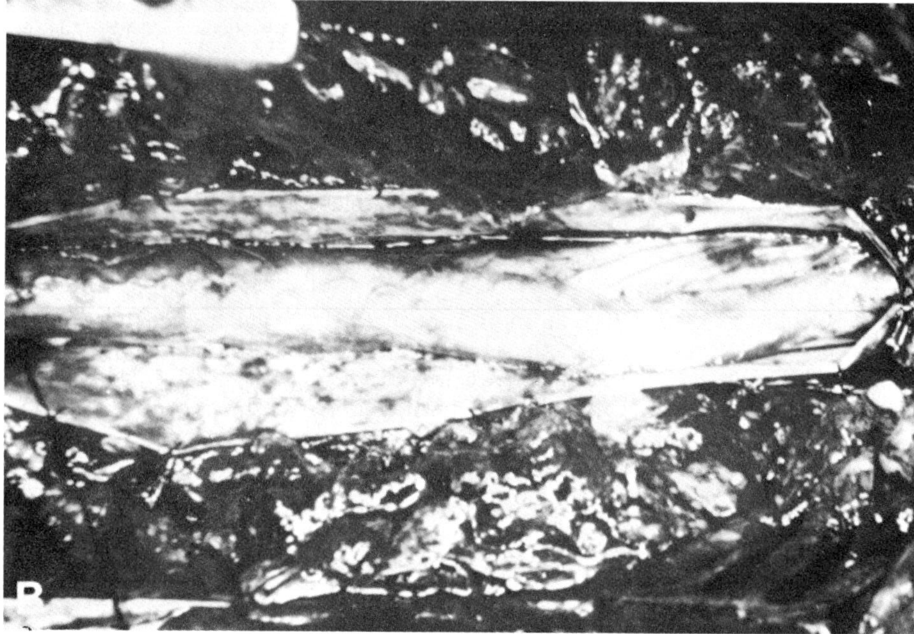

FIGURE 41-4. (**A**) Normal spinal cord at laminectomy. The dura has been opened, and the arachnoid is still intact. The arachnoid is transparent. The delicate anastomosing network of blood vessels on the surface of the cord can be seen. (**B**) Adhesive arachnoiditis at laminectomy. In contrast to **A,** the dura has been opened and stripped, only with difficulty, from the underlying arachnoidal membrane. The latter is opaque, thickened, vascularized, and adherent to the underlying spinal cord, which cannot be seen. The subarachnoid space is obliterated. (Vandam LD: Spinal anesthesia. In Hale DE (ed): Anesthesiology. Philadelphia: FA Davis, 1963)

tical symptoms, these symptoms were not believed to be specific for spinal anesthesia.

Bias

Many of these people were apparently symptom-free postoperatively, yet 6 months later some said that neurologic symptoms had appeared from the time of operation.[56] No doubt the investigation sensitized patients to the possibility of development of disease, and they were, therefore, prone to associate minor complaints with the anesthetic. Nevertheless, similar findings were not encountered in a control group of patients given general anesthesia.

Trauma

Numbness usually is not found as a sequela of lumbar puncture, and few of the 71 patients had headache.[56] Comparatively few instances of traumatic puncture occurred, and on only a few occasions was blood-stained CSF obtained. When paresthesias were produced at the time of lumbar puncture, no obvious relation to the subsequent site of neurologic involvement could be found. One might conclude, then, that the trauma of lumbar puncture played little role.

Was trauma of another kind responsible? Can the operation performed or mechanical factors associated with operation be implicated? In some instances, the complaints may be related to positioning of legs in stirrups. There may have been a direct cause in patients for whom varicose veins were ligated, hemorrhoidectomy was performed, or herniorrhaphy carried out in proximity to the area of numbness. These operations did not comprise a large share of those reported. The influence of position on the operating table, application of restraining straps, or subsequent intramuscular injection into the thigh could not be established.

Local Anesthetic

Consideration must be given to the part played by the local anesthetic. Complaints were confined almost entirely to the lumbar and sacral areas,[56] the general level of the spine at which lumbar puncture is done and, consequently, where the concentration of anesthetic is highest. No relation between a specific anesthetic injected and the number of complications was found. Weighting the anesthetic with dextrose and position at the time of injection could not be related to the side on which the subsequent difficulty occurred.

In all likelihood, these neurologic complaints were related nonspecifically to the anesthetic agent. The majority of injectable spinal anesthetic solutions are hypertonic, with mean values for osmolality outside the CSF range, which is 257 to 305 mOsm/L; the damage caused by these anesthetics is related directly to the variation from isotonicity of the solution used.[57] Moreover, vasoconstrictor drugs injected into the subarachnoid space may cause neurologic sequelae, as has been found in the rhesus monkey,[58] though at concentrations far greater than those used in clinical practice; one study failed to implicate these drugs in the development of disease. Neurologic sequelae have followed injection of various foreign substances into the subarachnoid space.[59] The delicacy of spinal structures and their peculiar vascularity invite complications.

Finally, the neurologic complaints described[56] and the syndrome of meralgia paresthetica are similar, as noted earlier. The latter is characterized by numbness and paresthesias in the area of distribution of the lateral femoral cutaneous nerve, not an uncommon ailment.[60] The cause is unknown and has been attributed to arthritis of the spine, spinal trauma, excessive smoking of tobacco, or lower abdominal stresses such as pregnancy or the wearing of a truss, tight undergarments, or a cartridge belt. The course of the lateral femoral cutaneous nerve in the retroperitoneal space and lower abdomen, its proximity to the anterior superior spine of the ilium, and its final penetration of the fascia lata suggest that the nerve may be susceptible to trauma. Approximately half of the patients described numbness coinciding with the distribution of the lateral femoral cutaneous nerve.[56] That nerve fibers constituting the lateral femoral cutaneous nerve can be selectively affected by a substance injected into the subarachnoid space hardly seems possible.

ANTECEDENT NEUROLOGIC DISEASE AND POSTANESTHETIC SEQUELAE

An important means of preventing neurologic disease after spinal anesthesia involves proper preoperative examination of the patient. A basic tenet, hitherto undocumented, was that afflictions of the CNS and spinal column contraindicate use of spinal anesthesia.

Spinal Cord Tumor

CASE 4. A 42-year-old woman underwent repair of a diaphragmatic hernia. Lumbar puncture was performed with a 22-G needle at the L4–L5 interspace. A transient paresthesia was produced in the left leg, but CSF was clear and flowed freely. Spinal anesthesia to the level of T5 was obtained. Postoperatively, the patient complained of backache. Before leaving the hospital, she experienced heaviness in the legs and tingling sensations in the toes. Six months later, she gradually had become incapacitated with backache, falling episodes, spreading numbness, loss of strength, and paresthesias in the legs.

Neurologic findings included ataxia, positive Romberg's and Babinski's signs on the left, absence of abdominal reflexes, diminution or loss of sense of position in the legs, hypesthesia to pinprick to the level of T10, partial loss of motor power in the left leg, and spasm of the back muscles. Red and white blood cell counts were normal; the result of blood serologic testing was negative; and free hydrochloric acid was present in gastric juice. CSF pressure and dynamics were normal. The protein concentration in the CSF was 47 mg/dL; Kolmer's test was negative; and cells were not present. A cystometrogram disclosed a hypotonic bladder. Radiographic examination of the back showed degenerative and hypertrophic changes in the thoracic spine. Myelography was avoided because of the possibility that arachnoiditis was present. Physical therapy was prescribed. One year after spinal anesthesia, a meningioma was found at laminectomy. Postoperatively, rapid improvement occurred, and 6 months later the patient had recovered completely.

Early onset of symptoms of spinal cord compression by tumor after lumbar puncture can be attributed to displacement of the mass or to vascular engorgement. Michelsen[61] and Nicholson and Eversole[62] reported similar experiences with spinal cord tumors and administration of spinal anesthesia. Michelsen suggested that CSF dynamics and the protein content be tested routinely in spinal anesthesia. A spinal anesthetic should not be injected, however, if lumbar puncture yields a suspicious-appearing fluid (cloudy, discolored) or if flow is not free.

Central Nervous System Viral Disease

Herpes Zoster

CASE 5. A 25-year-old woman with right-lower-quadrant abdominal pain underwent operation for appendicitis. Spinal anesthesia to T6 was obtained with tetracaine and glucose, injected through a 22-G needle at the L3–L4 intervertebral space. One tap was made without paresthesia, and CSF was clear. At operation, the appendix was not inflamed. On the 2nd postoperative day, herpetic lesions appeared on the left in the distribution of dermatomes T6 and T4. These lesions persisted for 4 weeks. Three weeks after operation, sensations of pins and needles arose in both thighs, with radiation down the backs of the legs. At the same time, severe backache with difficulty in straightening of the trunk occurred. The sensory disturbances lasted 12 days and the backache 2 weeks. One month after anesthesia, appreciation of pinprick was diminished over the outer surface of the right foot and the anterior surface of the tibia. One week later these signs disappeared. The only complaint after 1 year was a subjective difference in the temperature of the legs.

Herpes zoster is a viral disease that affects the posterior root ganglia, posterior nerve roots, and dorsal horns. Persistent sensory and motor paralysis often results. However, a clear relation between the neurologic deficit of spinal anesthesia and herpes zoster has not been established. Trophic lesions of a herpetiform type may, in rare instances, be induced by spinal anesthesia, one of the explanations offered by Carter for an eruption arising after lumbar puncture.[63]

Trauma may be the cause if the lumbar puncture needle injures a ganglion, because herpetiform eruptions can be produced by manipulation of a nerve root. Arnold found these eruptions in three cases among 640 spinal anesthetics.[64] He found no relation to lumbar puncture site and assumed that a toxic injury had occurred. Spinal anesthesia probably should be avoided if a diagnosis of CNS viral disease is made preoperatively. This admonition is borne out by the report of Nicholson and Eversole on a spinal anesthetic followed by neurologic deficit, in a patient with varicella.[62]

Mumps Encephalitis

CASE 6. A 36-year-old woman was scheduled for cholecystectomy. She was in the 3rd month of pregnancy and reported a history of eclampsia, hypertension, and jaundice. Lumbar puncture was performed, without paresthesia, with a 22-G needle inserted at the L3–L4 interspace. CSF was clear and flowed freely. Spinal anesthesia to T5 was achieved with tetracaine, glucose, and epinephrine.

Immediately postoperatively, the patient had weakness of the right leg and diffuse impairment of pinprick sensation. A mild, transient postural headache lasted for 2 days. Within several days, the leg seemed stronger, but buckled on the 10th postoperative day when she attempted to stand. At this time, the patient volunteered that she had had mumps followed by convulsions and encephalitis 10 years previously. Both legs were affected at that time, especially the right, which weakened with exercise. When she was seen 3 years later her right leg, though much stronger, continued to have intermittent pain.

In this patient, spinal anesthesia seemed to precipitate symptoms that had been dormant for years. A history of encephalitis was not elicited on the preoperative visit, despite specific inquiry for antecedent disease. For one reason or another, many patients forget important events in describing their medical history. Reasons for the recrudescence of a disease usually are speculative. In this case, it may be of significance that the maximum concentration of anesthetic in the subarachnoid space came in contact with the lumbar nerve roots on the previously affected, right side.

Backache and Sciatic Pain

Backache is a common complaint after spinal and general anesthesia. When followed by sciatic pain, backache becomes a neurologic problem because protrusion of an intervertebral disc and compression of a spinal nerve root may be present. In the University of Pennsylvania study,[23] several cases with a common pattern were seen: recurrence of backache and sciatica after spinal anesthesia, with symptoms strongly suggesting disc protrusion. Though questioned before anesthesia, none of the patients mentioned having had back pain.

CASE 8. A 59-year-old man was given spinal anesthesia with tetracaine and glucose for suprapubic prostatectomy. Lumbar puncture was performed after two insertions of a 22-G needle. No pain or paresthesia occurred, and CSF was clear. On standing 2 days postoperatively, he had severe low back pain with radiation to the left foot. At this time, he said that he had had shooting pains in the left leg before anesthesia. One week after anesthesia, examination disclosed right sacroiliac tenderness, and straight leg raising was limited to 70°. Radiographs of the back showed increased density of bone, extensive osseous degenerative disease in the lower lumbar and sacral regions, marginal lipping of the vertebrae, and narrowing of the L4–L5 space. His symptoms improved with traction to the affected leg, and recovery was complete 10 months later.

Many reasons can be offered as to why spinal anesthesia might be inadvisable in the presence of backache, although backache is just as common after general anesthesia. Traumatic lumbar puncture may injure a disc or a vertebra. Hemorrhage into a ligament can act as a focus of pain, with radiation in a sciatic distribution. Some physicians believe that muscle relaxation while the patient lies on an operating table causes back strain. Other positions on the table (eg, lithotomy) also certainly can produce strain.

The situation is even more complex when disc disease is already present. Rarely, spinal anesthesia is selected for laminectomy. However, the incidence of persistent pain and neurologic deficit after operation for protruded disc is sufficiently high that spinal anesthesia probably should be avoided. If diagnostic myelography has been done, arachnoiditis from that source is not uncommon. Finally, arachnoiditis has been found at a second laminectomy performed because of persistent backache. In some cases the arachnoiditis probably developed as a result of trauma during the first disc operation.[65]

Metastatic Malignancy of the Spine

CASE 9. A 77-year-old man was given continuous spinal anesthesia with tetracaine and glucose for abdominoperineal resection of the rectum. Lumbar puncture was performed with a 16-G needle after two insertions, without pain or paresthesia. The CSF was clear, and a sensory level to T4 was obtained. Six months later, shooting pains in the left hip and anterior thigh developed, with radiation to the knee. The possibility of arachnoiditis was raised by a consulting neurologist, but radiographs of the back showed destruction of the L1–L3 vertebrae by metastatic tumor.

Nicholson and Eversole also reported a case of spinal cord compression after anesthesia, caused by metastatic tumor.[62] Aside from the possibility that lumbar puncture may accentuate symptoms, the most important aspect of the relation between anesthesia and spinal column disease is the likelihood that the patient may attribute the disease to the anesthetic. The patient may be encouraged in this belief by physicians; the prospect of death from metastatic disease is not an easy matter to discuss. Usually the possibility of spinal anesthetic complications dominates the thinking of consultants, and the more likely causes for disease are relegated to a secondary role.

Diabetes Mellitus and Peripheral Neuropathy

Operations on patients with diabetes often are performed with the use of spinal anesthesia, a method that does little to upset metabolic balance. However, the patient with diabetes often has complicating ailments. Vascular disease and peripheral neuropathy are accompanied by neurologic symptoms that may be confused with complications of spinal anesthesia.[66]

CASE 10. A 68-year-old man with severe diabetes mellitus and prostatic obstruction underwent prostatectomy. Spinal anesthesia with tetracaine and glucose was administered by means of a 22-G needle at the L3–L4 interspace. Three insertions of the needle were made; CSF was clear; and a sensory level to T10 was obtained. Postoperative bleeding and a transfusion reaction left the patient anemic; the postoperative course was marked by fever, confusion, phlebitis, and wound sepsis. Two months later, he complained of weakness and lack of control of his legs dating from the hospital stay. Although subjective improvement had occurred, examination disclosed an equivocal Romberg's sign, hyperactivity of the reflexes, and a shuffling gait. One month later, weakness of the muscles of the left leg and a stocking type of hypesthesia were found. Thereafter, symptoms improved.

Details are lacking to make this picture more interpretable. The extent of diabetic control, adequacy of circulation to the legs, and blood and spinal fluid serologic parameters were unknown. Nonetheless, the symptoms may have resulted from spinal anesthesia. These improved, however, and may be attributable to several factors: anemia, vascular disease, poor diabetic control and nutrition, and probably peripheral neuropathy.

Case 10 illustrates that spinal anesthesia may be held responsible for the first appearance or exacerbation of any concurrent neurologic disease. Marinacci and Courville emphasized this possibility in a study of 482 patients whose complaints were attributed to spinal anesthesia.[67] Of this group, 478 were shown to have an entirely unrelated neurologic condition, either an infectious neuritis or peripheral neuropathy. The electromyogram played an important role in evaluating the complaints and differentiating among them. Differentiation was based on the following criteria: distribution of denervation, that is, the electromyographic changes, and the time at which denervation activity was first detected by electromyography. Samaha has reviewed the value of electrodiagnostic studies in the identification of neuromuscular disease.[68]

EPIDURAL AND CAUDAL ANESTHESIA

Because the only major difference between spinal and epidural anesthesia is the injection site, complications of both are qualitatively the same. However, a thorough prospective study of neurologic sequelae has not been performed. The complications must be rare indeed. If so, a lack of such problems may be ascribed to the lessons learned from administration of spinal anesthesia and to the availability of more reliable anesthetics and equipment. In general, the types of complications that might occur (eg, technical, physiologic, and pathologic) are suggested by Dawkins' retrospective survey of approximately 350 articles on epidural and caudal block, including records of 4000 anesthetics done by that author over a period of 25 years (see Table 41-1).[10] A discrepancy exists in the total numbers of cases quoted for any one complication, because complete figures were lacking. Usubiaga's survey of the world literature revealed the same kinds of complications.[11]

Bleeding

Blood vessel puncture is the most common complication. No mention is made of epidural hematoma,[69] a problem that can also occur spontaneously,[70] particularly after needle puncture in the presence of blood clotting abnormalities iatrogenically or pathologically induced. Onset of severe backache after anesthesia, with progressive signs of spinal cord compression, strongly suggests hematoma formation. CT or MRI scanning reveals the site of blockage, and immediate evacuation of the clot is necessary to avoid permanent deficit. Epidural abscess formation after spinal and epidural anesthesia is more delayed in onset but presents systemic signs of infection and a similar neurologic picture. Treatment consists of surgical drainage and antibiotic therapy.

Inadvertent Subarachnoid Puncture

A second common complication entails inadvertent subarachnoid puncture. Usually the needle is withdrawn, and epidural injection is made at another spinal interspace. Total spinal anesthesia still may arise, however, if the anesthetic injected epidurally enters the dural puncture opening. With accidental puncture, severe and prolonged postural headache is common because of the large-gauge needle used. Treatment, including use of an epidural blood patch, is the same as that suggested for post–lumbar puncture headache.

Dawkins gives no details on reported cases of paralysis, but relates two incidents of his own.[10] In one, gross destruction of the posterolateral portion of the spinal cord from T6 to T12 was found at necropsy after anesthesia in a 70-year-old man with inoperable carcinoma of the pancreas. In the second instance, transient sensory and motor paralysis of the lower extremities followed epidural block given for deliberate hypotension during resection of a parotid tumor. It is probable,

TABLE 41-11
Complications After Caudal Block

	CASES	COMPLICATION
	No.	No. (%)
Dural puncture	13,639	171 (1.2)
Accidental total spinal anesthesia	6,334	9 (0.1)
Blood vessel puncture	639	4 (0.6)
Failure to find sacral hiatus	2,803	87 (3.1)
Toxic reaction	3,332	6 (0.2)
Sepsis	3,767	8 (0.2)
Breakage of needle	850	12 (1.4)
Breakage of catheter	5,379	6 (0.1)
Severe hypotension	3,189	201 (6.3)
Transient paralysis	22,968	5 (0.02)
Permanent paralysis	22,968	1 (0.005)

Dawkins CJM: Analysis of the complications of extradural and caudal block. Anaesthesia 24:554, 1969.

therefore, that neurologic complications may follow epidural anesthesia for the same reasons that they may follow spinal anesthesia. Finally, Dawkins notes that the sequelae of caudal block usually are those associated with the technical aspects of that approach to the epidural space (Table 41-11).[10]

REFERENCES

1. Thorsen G: Neurological complications after spinal anesthesia. Acta Chirurgica Scandinavica 95(suppl):121, 1947
2. Kennedy F, Effron AS, Perry G: The grave spinal cord paralyses caused by spinal anesthesia. Surg Gynecol Obstet 91:385, 1950
3. Dickson WEC: Cerebrospinal fluids in meningitis. Postgrad Med J 20:69, 1944
4. Lumbar puncture and epidermoid tumors. Lancet 1:635, 1977
5. Dripps RD: A comparison of the malleable needle and catheter technics for continuous spinal anesthesia. New York State Journal of Medicine 50:1595, 1950
6. Mihic DN: Post-spinal headache and relationship of needle bevel to longitudinal dural fibers. Reg Anesth 10:76, 1985
7. Norris MC, Leighton BL, Desimone CA: Needle bevel direction and headache after inadvertent dural puncture. Anesthesiology 70:729, 1989
8. Sechzer PH: Subdural space in spinal anesthesia. Anesthesiology 24:896, 1963
9. Dripps RD, Vandam LD: Long-term follow-up of patients who received 10,098 spinal anesthetics: I. Failure to discover major neurological sequelae. JAMA 156:1486, 1954
10. Dawkins CJM: Analysis of the complications of extradural and caudal block. Anaesthesia 24:554, 1969
11. Usubiaga JE: Neurological complications following epidural anesthesia. Int Anesthesiol Clin 13:1, 1975
12. Dripps RD, Deming MVN: An evaluation of certain drugs used to maintain blood pressure during spinal anesthesia: comparison of ephedrine, paredrine, pitressin-ephedrine and methedrine in 2,500 cases. Surg Gynecol Obstet 83:312, 1946
13. Greene NM: Physiology of spinal anesthesia, 3rd ed. Baltimore: Williams & Wilkins, 1981: 63
14. Caplan RA, Ward RJ, Pasner KL, et al: Unexpected cardiac arrest during spinal anesthesia: a closed claims analysis of predisposing factors. Anesthesiology 68:5, 1988
15. Labat G: Regional anesthesia. Philadelphia: WB Saunders, 1923: 449
16. Babcock WW: Spinal anesthesia. Am J Surg 5:571, 1928
17. Crocker JS, Vandam LD: Concerning nausea and vomiting during spinal anesthesia. Anesthesiology 20:587, 1959
18. Davis L, Pollock LJ: Role of autonomic nervous system in production of pain. JAMA 106:350, 1936
19. Phillips OC, Ebner H, Nelson AT, et al: Neurologic complications following spinal anesthesia with lidocaine. Anesthesiology 30: 284, 1969
20. Kane RE: Neurologic deficits following epidural or spinal anesthesia. Anesth Analg 60:150, 1981
21. Beecher HK, Todd D: A study of the deaths associated with anesthesia and surgery. Ann Surg 140:2, 1954
22. Brown DL: Anesthetic choice. In Brown DL (ed): Risk and outcome in anesthesia. Philadelphia: JB Lippincott, 1992: 193
23. Vandam LD, Dripps RD: Long-term follow-up of patients who received 10,098 spinal anesthetics: III. syndrome of decreased intracranial pressure (headache and ocular and auditory difficulties). JAMA 161:586, 1956
24. Marshall J: Lumbar puncture headache. J Neurol Neurosurg Psychiatry 13:71, 1950
25. Page F: Intracranial hypotension. Lancet 1:1, 1953
26. Redlich FC, Moore BD, Kimbell I: Lumbar puncture reactions: relative importance of physiological and psychological factors. Psychosom Med 8:836, 1946
27. Kang SB, Goodnough DE, Lee YK, et al: Comparison of 26- and 27-G needles for spinal anesthesia for ambulatory surgery patients. Anesthesiology 76:734, 1992
28. Lybecker H, Moller JT, May O: Incidence and prediction of postdural puncture headache: a prospective study of 1021 spinal anesthetics. Anesth Analg 70:389, 1990
29. Jones RJ: The role of recumbency in the prevention and treatment of spinal headache. Anesth Analg 53:788, 1974
30. Carbaat PAT, van Cravel H: Lumbar puncture headache: controlled study on the preventive effect of 24 hours bed rest. Lancet 2:1133, 1981
31. Ready LB, Woodland RV, Haschke RH: Spinal needle angle affects rate of fluid leak across human dura (abstract). Anesthesiology 63:A241, 1985
32. Dixon CL: The Sprotte, Whitacre and Quincke spinal needles. Anesthesiology Reviews 5:42, 1991
33. DiGiovanni AJ, Dunbar BS: Epidural injections of autologous blood for post-lumbar puncture headache. Anesth Analg 49:268, 1970
34. Szeinfeld M, Shmeidan IH, Moser MM, et al: Epidural blood patch: evaluation of the volume and spread of blood injected into the epidural space. Anesthesiology 64:820, 1986
35. Bryce-Smith RM, Macintosh RR: Sixth-nerve palsy after lumbar puncture and spinal analgesia. Br Med J 1:275, 1971
36. Hughson W: A note on the relationship of cerebrospinal and intralabyrinthine pressures. Am J Physiol 101:396, 1932
37. Selander D, Dhuner KG, Lundborg G. Peripheral nerve injury due to injection needles used for regional anaesthesia: an experimental study of the acute effects of needle point trauma. Acta Anaesthesiol Scand 21:182, 1977
38. Musser JA, Sailer J: Meralgia paresthetica of Roth. J Nerv Ment Dis 27:16, 1900
39. Hogeman O: Lhermitte's sign due to cervical exostosis. Acta Soc Med Upsal 17:192, 1952
40. Kellgren JH: On the distribution of pain arising from deep somatic structures with charts of segmental pain areas. Clin Sci 4:35, 1939
41. Bromley LL, Craig JD, Kessel AWL: Infected intervertebral disc after lumbar puncture. Br Med J 1:132, 1949
42. Jackson IJ: Aseptic hemogenic meningitis: experimental production of aseptic meningeal reactions due to blood and its breakdown products. Archives of Neurology and Psychiatry 62: 572, 1949
43. Black MG: Spinal fluid findings in spinal anesthesia. Anesthesiology 8:382, 1947
44. Marx GF, Saifer A, Orkin LR: Cerebrospinal fluid cells and proteins following spinal anesthesia. Anesthesiology 24:305, 1963
45. Goldman WW, Sanford JP: An 'epidemic' of chemical meningitis. Am J Med 29:94, 1960
46. DiGiovanni AJ: 'Chemical meningitis' tied to cleaning fluid bacteria. JAMA 214:2129, 1970

47. Vandam LD, Dripps RD: Exacerbation of pre-existing neurologic disease after spinal anesthesia. N Engl J Med 255:843, 1956
48. Weed LH, Wegefarth P, Auer JB, et al: The production of meningitis by release of cerebrospinal fluid during an experimental septicemia: preliminary note. JAMA 72:190, 1919
49. Berman RS, Eisele JH: Bacteremia, spinal anesthesia, and development of meningitis. Anesthesiology 48:376, 1978
50. Loarie DJ, Fairley HB: Epidural abscess following spinal anesthesia. Anesth Analg 57:351, 1978
51. Foreign letters (London). JAMA 154:532, 1954
52. Hurley RJ, Lambert D: Cauda equina syndrome after continuous spinal anesthesia. Anesth Analg 72:817, 1991
53. FDA Safety Alert (special edition). ASRA News (special edition) July 1992, 1
54. Mackay RP: Chronic adhesive arachnoiditis: a clinical and pathological study. JAMA 112:802, 1939
55. Hurst EW: Adhesive arachnoiditis and vascular blockage caused by detergents and other chemical irritants: an experimental study. Journal of Pathology and Bacteriology 70:167, 1955
56. Vandam LD, Dripps RD: Long-term follow-up of patients who received 10,098 spinal anesthetics: II. Incidence and analyses of minor sensory neurological defects. Surgery 38:463, 1955
57. Sawinski VJ, Goldberg AF, Goldberg NB: Osmolality of spinal anesthetic agents. Anesthesiology 27:86, 1966
58. Brizzee KR, Wu JJ: Studies on the effects of intrathecal injections of ephedrine sulphate on the spinal cord. Journal of Neuropathology and Clinical Neurology 1:234, 1951
59. Wilson G, Rupp C, Wilson WW: The dangers of intrathecal medication. JAMA 140:1076, 1949
60. Schneck JM: Meralgia paresthesia. J Nerv Ment Dis 105:77, 1947
61. Michelsen JJ: Neurologic manifestations following spinal anesthesia. Neurology 2:255, 1952
62. Nicholson MJ, Eversole UH: Neurologic complications of spinal anesthesia. JAMA 132:679, 1946
63. Carter HR: Herpes zoster: a case following lumbar puncture. Am J Psychiatry 94:373, 1938
64. Arnold DG: Herpes zoster as a sequel of spinal anesthesia. Int Coll Surg 4:66, 1941
65. Smolik EA, Nash FP: Lumbar spinal arachnoiditis: a complication of the intervertebral disc operation. Ann Surg 133:490, 1951
66. Jordan WR: Neuritic manifestations in diabetes mellitus. Arch Intern Med 57:301, 1936
67. Marinacci AA, Courville CB: Electromyogram in evaluation of neurological complications of spinal anesthesia. JAMA 168: 1337, 1958
68. Samaha FJ: Current concepts: electrodiagnostic studies in neuromuscular disease. N Engl J Med 285:1244, 1971
69. Janis KM: Epidural hematoma following postoperative epidural anesthesia. Anesth Analg 51:689, 1972
70. Spurny OM, Rubin S, Wolf JW, et al: Spinal epidural hematoma during anticoagulant therapy. Arch Intern Med 114:103, 1964

FURTHER READING

Bromage PR: Epidural analgesia. Philadelphia: WB Saunders, 1978

Brown DL: An atlas of regional anesthesia. Philadelphia: WB Saunders, 1992

Cousins MJ, Bridenbaugh PO (eds): Neural blockade, 2nd ed. Philadelphia, JB Lippincott, 1988

Greene NM: Physiology of spinal anesthesia, 3rd ed. Baltimore: Williams & Wilkins, 1981

Kane RE: Neurologic deficits following epidural or spinal anesthesia. Anesth Analg 60:150, 1981

Mulroy MF: Spinal headaches: management and avoidance. In Brown DL (ed): Regional anesthesia at the Virginia Mason Medical Center: a clinical perspective. Problems in Anesthesia 602, 1987

Complications in Anesthesiology, second edition,
edited by Nikolaus Gravenstein and Robert R. Kirby.
Lippincott-Raven Publishers, Philadelphia © 1996.

CHAPTER 42

Complications of Diagnostic and Therapeutic Nerve Blocks

Terence M. Murphy

Murphy's law states, "If things can go wrong, they will."[1] Risk is identified with virtually everything done in medicine. These considerations are equally true for nerve blocks and all other forms of anesthesia. Sequelae of nerve blocks are identified characteristically by damage to the nerve, subsequent palsies, and pain. Nerve blocks can produce damage to or have effects on other structures, adjacent to and remote from the nerve being blocked (Table 42-1). Problems can result from the needle or the injected drug and may include local toxicity or systemic central nervous system effects. In this text, other chapters deal with systemic effects of local anesthetics and with the complications of spinal and epidural anesthesia. This chapter concerns primarily the complications arising from peripheral nerve blocks.

BASIC CONSIDERATIONS

The success of diagnostic and therapeutic blocks depends on several critical factors (Table 42-2).

Anatomic Concerns

A knowledge of anatomy is a prerequisite for successful performance of regional anesthesia and helps in the anticipation, interpretation, and prevention or correction of possible complications from any block. Performing nerve blocks without thorough anatomic knowledge is like sailing an uncharted sea. Reliance placed on surface landmarks learned by rote not only is accompanied by a high incidence of failure (as much as 80% in one series[2]) but also is associated with inability to recognize the potential for involvement of adjacent structures other than the intended nerves. For practitioners inexperienced in applied anatomy, frequent recourse to standard regional anesthesia texts is necessary. In the following discussion, reference is made to anatomic features as they relate to the individual blocks.

Pharmacologic Characteristics of Local Anesthetics

Knowledge of the pharmacologic characteristics of local anesthetics also is essential, especially with regard to systemic and local toxicity. Because the concentration of the drug injected appears to be associated with the incidence of neuritis, it frequently is limited when applied to peripheral nerves.[3,4] Systemic toxic responses can be minimized by the prophylactic administration of a benzodiazepine (eg, midazolam) before performance of the block.[5] This class of drugs raises the threshold for convulsion, and if patient alertness is not a priority, is a useful premedicant.

Technique

Correct positioning of the needle is important. A block is produced more efficiently if the small muscles of the hand are used to hold the needle as a pen would be held; the anesthesiologist should use delicate movements of the fingers and wrist, instead of locking the needle in the hand and directing it with motion at the elbow and shoulder joints. The fingers and hand are considerably more sensitive and capable of meticulous, fine movement because they have much greater cortical representation than do the large muscles of the upper arm and shoulder.

Needle Position

Needle position may be determined in various ways. In some instances, the point is rested adjacent to a bony landmark, such as a vertebral transverse process in a patient undergoing

TABLE 42-1
Relative Risk of Complications of Common Peripheral Nerve Blocks

	RETROBULBAR	STELLATE GANGLION	PARAVERTEBRAL		CELIAC PLEXUS	INTRAVENOUS REGIONAL ANESTHESIA
			Lumbar	*Thoracic*		
Systemic toxicity	+	+	+	+	++	++++
Intramuscular injection	+	++	+	+	++	+
Pneumothorax	–	+	+++	+	+	–
Subarachnoid or epidural injection	+	++	++	++	+	–
Inadvertent nerve block (eg, phrenic or recurrent laryngeal)	+	+	++	++	++	–

+, risk; –, no risk.

Modified from James CF: Local and regional anesthesia. In Gravenstein N (ed): Manual of complications during anesthesia. Philadelphia: JB Lippincott, 1991: 432.

a stellate ganglion block. In other cases, detection of loss of resistance follows when the needle tip pops through fascial planes (eg, in the posterior triangle of the neck or in the axillary sheath for brachial plexus block). Frequently, when the needle actually touches the nerve, the patient experiences a paresthesia over the dermatomal distribution. Placement of the needle also can be controlled with radiography, a nerve stimulator, or even two-dimensional ultrasound imaging. Sometimes a combination of these methods is used for precise placement.

Once a quantity of local anesthetic has been injected at the intended site, a search for additional sites of paresthesia is potentially dangerous in an area that might already be partially anesthetized; accidental trauma to the nerve may occur repeatedly without awareness by the patient or anesthetist.

TABLE 42-2
Elements of Successful Diagnostic and Therapeutic Block

KNOWLEDGE OF ANATOMY

- Refer to standard texts when necessary; do not grope blindly!

KNOWLEDGE OF PHARMACOLOGY OF LOCAL ANESTHETICS AND OPIOIDS

- Dose and concentration
- Duration
- Toxic effects

TECHNIQUE

- Fine, hand-controlled movement
- Intermittent aspiration tests
- Correct needle positioning (eg, by bony landmarks or fascial "pop")

EQUIPMENT

- Stainless steel reusable needles with markers
- Glass syringes
- Nerve stimulator when appropriate
- Resuscitation devices

Precautions

Blocks always should be performed with means for resuscitation immediately available. An oxygen source, a means to administer positive-pressure ventilation, an established intravenous route for resuscitative fluids and drugs, suction apparatus to clear the airway, and an assistant to help or summon aid are essential. The postanesthesia care unit is an optimal location in which to perform these blocks if space, time, and personnel are sufficient.

Equipment

Needles

In regional anesthesia, equipment of good quality repays the capital investment. Attempting some of the more technically difficult blocks with poor-quality, disposable syringes and needles only decreases the chances of success and probably increases the risk of complications. Stainless steel needles with shallow bevels reduce the incidence of nerve trauma, because they tend to displace structures rather than to cut through them[6] (Fig. 42-1).

Because of the possibility (albeit remote) of needle breakage during the performance of nerve blocks and the sometimes great difficulty that results in recovering the embedded portion, needles with security beads are advantageous. These beads permit ready recovery if the needle separates from the hub. Use of a marker is advised for blocks in which the depth of needle insertion is critical. The marker can be set on the needle at the appropriate length. Although special markers are available, the rubber stopper from the local anesthetic bottle is one that is usually readily available, and it serves admirably.

Nerve Stimulators

To reduce the possibility of nerve damage even further, use of a nerve stimulator to elicit paresthesias or motor responses is a distinct advantage; this technique allows the patient to be sedated more adequately. Nerve stimulation just before con-

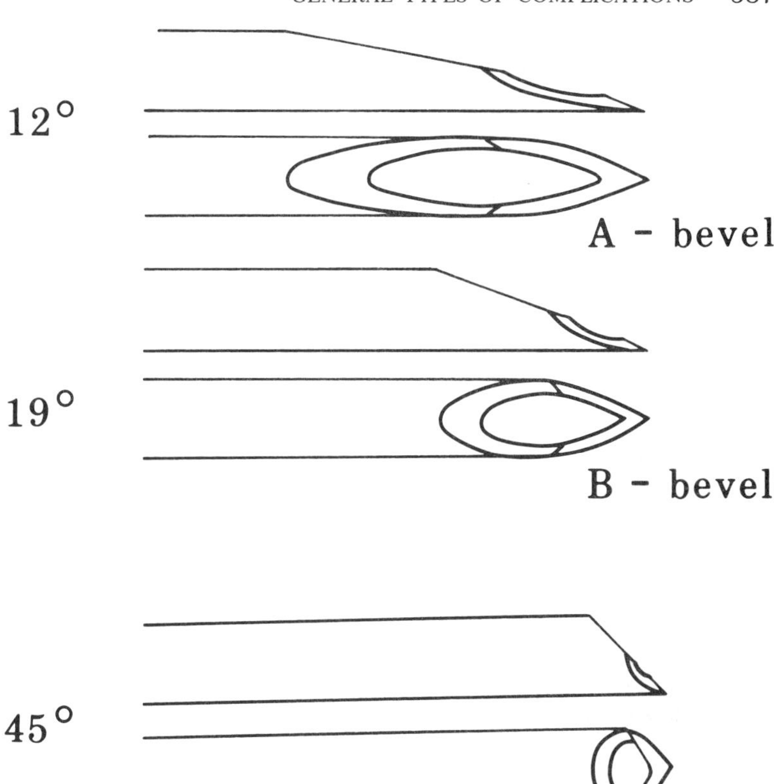

FIGURE 42-1. Regional block needles: 12° (A-bevel), 19° (B-bevel), and 45°-bevel needles. (Winnie AP: Perivascular techniques of brachial plexus block. In Plexus anesthesia, vol 1. Philadelphia: WB Saunders, 1983: 213)

tact with the needle point should reduce the incidence of needle-induced nerve trauma and improve the chance that the block will be successful.[7]

Syringes and Jet Injectors

A freely sliding glass control syringe allows the anesthesiologist to work with much greater dexterity during the injection of the anesthetic and especially during aspiration for cerebrospinal fluid and blood. Occasionally, jet injector devices have been used instead of syringes for superficial nerve blocks, such as injection of myofascial trigger points or oral blocks in dental practice. Although jet injectors appear to be quite safe, hematomas have resulted.[8]

GENERAL TYPES OF COMPLICATIONS

A variety of complications can and will occur from time to time (Table 42-3).

Inadequate Anesthesia

With diagnostic blocks, problems seldom result from repeating the block until the desired effect is achieved. The failed block can always be considered a placebo within a diagnostic series of blocks!

Extensive Anesthesia

Total Spinal or High Epidural Blockade

Any block performed near the neuraxis (eg, paravertebral, stellate ganglion, retrobulbar, or interscalene block) can involve spread of the anesthetic into the epidural or subarachnoid compartment. Worse, this spread may lead to total spinal anesthesia. These complications, though serious, do not necessarily pose any great difficulty to a vigilant anesthesiologist who is accustomed to caring for patients with epidural and spinal anesthesia.

Paravertebral Spread

If, of course, the specific block was intended as a diagnostic maneuver, its spread to other neurologic structures invalidates its purpose, and the procedure must be repeated at a later time. The continuity of the paravertebral space permits free flow of local anesthetic between adjacent segmental nerves. This effect is seen particularly in the cervical and thoracic areas, where injection at one paravertebral site often results in the extension of anesthesia over several dermatomes if large volumes are used. (An alternative explanation is, of course, peridural spread.)

When surgery is planned, adjacent dermatomal involvement (eg, spread to the cervical plexus during interscalene brachial plexus block) usually is of no great importance. However, the diagnostic value of segmental paravertebral diagnostic blocks

TABLE 42-3
Generalized and Local Complications of Nerve Blocks

- Inadequate anesthesia
- Excessive anesthesia (total spinal or high epidural)
- Prolonged blockade
- Tissue toxicity (rare and reversible)
- Infection
- Neuritis
- Nerve injury
- Pneumothorax
- Bleeding

can be invalidated if spread occurs. In this case, therefore, use of very small amounts (1 to 2 mL) of drug, accurately placed on the desired segmental nerve, is optimal.

Prolonged Block

The treatment of prolonged block usually consists of observation until sensation returns. The anesthetized area must be protected with slings, splints, and padding to prevent trauma to the insensitive part by pressure, heat, or other stimuli. After undue prolongation of block, the advice and assistance of colleagues in other specialties, such as neurology and physical medicine, can be of a great help, both to document the extent of the block and to follow its temporal progress by means of electromyography.[9,10]

Irreversibility of block with long-acting agents such as bupivacaine and etidocaine has not been reported. However, the duration of action of these agents can vary considerably and occasionally can be as great as 20 hours.[11] I recall a 0.5% bupivacaine axillary block used for hand surgery; when the patient required another operation the next day, the anesthetic was still effective, and thus two operations 24 hours apart were performed with the same anesthetic.

LOCAL COMPLICATIONS

Tissue Toxicity

Local Anesthetics

When used in conventional clinical concentrations, local anesthetics do not produce nerve damage. In the experimental laboratory, concentrations far in excess of those used clinically produce irreversible nerve block.[12] Local anesthetic agents can cause histologic alterations in muscle, although this change appears to be reversible; recovery is complete within a matter of weeks.[13]

Epinephrine

Epinephrine frequently is added to local anesthetic solutions for prolongation of the block and β-adrenergic stimulation of the cardiovascular system. Provided a solution of appropriate strength is used (1:200,000 appears optimal[4]), epinephrine is not associated with undue complications or toxic effects.[14] However, most investigators advise against the use of epinephrine in digital blocks because of possible ischemic sequelae such as gangrene[3]; similar precautions also pertain to ring blocks of the penis.

Infection

In the laboratory, infection has been potentiated by topical anesthetic agents applied to the wound.[15] Although infection has occurred subsequent to nerve block, occasionally with disastrous results,[16,17] it is rarely seen if correct techniques of sterilization and asepsis are followed. One explanation for its infrequency is that local anesthetics appear to have antimicrobial activity, inhibiting the growth of pathogenic bacteria and some fungal organisms. Gram-negative bacteria are especially sensitive to these agents, as is the tubercle bacillus. Both lidocaine and procaine appear to interfere with protein production in the cell wall or cytoplasmic membrane of these organisms.[18]

Rare severe infections have been reported and attributed to the sequelae of peripheral nerve blocks. Pudendal block at the time of delivery has been implicated in infection with bowel organisms, especially *Escherichia coli* in deep structures; this organism produces dramatic and occasionally fatal infection, with peritonitis, in the subgluteal, retropsoas, and retroperitoneal areas.[16] Even atlanto-occipital subluxation has been blamed on infection resulting from local anesthetic infiltration of the tonsillar bed.[19]

DIFFERENTIAL DIAGNOSIS OF NERVE DAMAGE

Positioning

Nerve damage (neuritis) can result from factors other than the regional anesthetic technique.[20-22] Brachial plexus injury follows stretching and/or compression. Pressure on, or trauma to many nerves in the body has been described during positioning. For example, the lateral popliteal nerve may be compressed between the head of the fibula and a lithotomy stirrup, resulting in footdrop. If this complication occurs in a patient who has undergone regional anesthesia, it is quite likely that the footdrop may be attributed to the nerve block, unless the risk of pressure against the stirrup had been considered.

Similarly, if the leg is suspended lateral to the stirrup, the saphenous nerve can be damaged, resulting in sensory loss along the medial aspect of the calf and dorsum of the foot. The sciatic nerve can be traumatized by intramuscular injections into the buttock pre- or postoperatively. During a hip-pinning operation, paralysis of all muscles below the knee and the hamstrings may occur in a thin patient lying on a hard table.

Other Causes

The pudendal nerve is vulnerable in orthopedic operations involving a traction post, in which the nerve lying in Alcock's canal is compressed against the ischial tuberosity. The femoral nerve can be damaged by a self-retaining retractor during lower abdominal explorations. Nerve damage also can follow the use of a tourniquet.[23]

The aforementioned causes must be eliminated as possibilities before untoward sequelae are ascribed to the anesthetic technique. Similarly, it should be determined whether complications are dermatomal, and therefore segmental, or peripheral in distribution; this distinction permits a diagnostic impression of the defect's origin. Many positional injuries are difficult and sometimes impossible to ascribe to any substandard or negligent act by the anesthetist.[24]

NEEDLE INSERTION

Nerve Injury

In many cases paresthesias are elicited to locate a nerve before the anesthetic agent is injected. However, contact between a needle and a nerve risks nerve injury. With supraclavicular and axillary block techniques in which paresthesia are sought, the incidence of neurologic sequelae ranges from 0% to slightly more than 5%. These sequelae vary from mild paresthesias to severe sensory disturbances, pain, and paralysis and last from a few days to more than 1 year.[25,26]

That transient nerve injury is related, at least in part, to needle trauma is suggested by a study that noted an incidence of 2.8% when paresthesias were actively sought compared with 0.8% when the axillary artery was used as the landmark in axillary block.[25] In addition, nerve injury occurs less frequently with short-beveled needles.[6,26] Paresthesias, when necessary, should be elicited gently and with a short-beveled needle to minimize injury.

Pneumothorax

Incidence

Pneumothorax is a risk associated with any block that involves insertion of a needle in the region of the thoracic cage (see Table 42-1). The incidence varies indirectly with experience. Thoracic paravertebral blocks, somatic and especially sympathetic, are associated with the greatest incidence, 4% to 8%, even among skilled anesthetists.[3] With a brachial plexus block, pneumothorax occurs most frequently when the classic supraclavicular approach is used. With experienced practitioners the incidence is about 1%.[3,4] The incidence probably is lower with intercostal and stellate ganglion blocks, especially when the latter is performed from the anterior rather than posterior approach. The overall incidence may be greater than is reported because some cases are relatively asymptomatic.

Treatment

The treatment of pneumothorax is well established.[3,27] If it is less than 20%, treatment of symptoms and observation are usually all that is required until spontaneous recovery occurs. For pneumothoraces greater than 25%, closer observation is required, and preparations must be made to proceed with more active therapy should the lung fail to reexpand in the first 24 hours. This therapy involves active decompression, usually by thoracostomy tube insertion in the midclavicular line of the second intercostal space, or the midaxillary line of the fifth intercostal space, followed by attachment to an underwater seal.[27] However, not all chest pain that follows nerve blocks is caused by pneumothorax, and careful physical examination and chest radiograph are mandatory before diagnosis.

Prevention

Prevention of pneumothorax during regional anesthesia is best achieved by meticulous adherence to technique and by patient cooperation to avoid sudden movements in response to any discomfort or paresthesia. If the anesthesiologist believes that the needle has broached the integrity of the pleura or a lung, the patient should remain at quiet bed rest for the next 12 to 24 hours. A latent period may exist between needle insertion into the pleura and development of pneumothorax, which conceivably may be precipitated by exertion.[3] In patients who require a chest tube, further in-hospital observation is necessary once the chest tube has been withdrawn, because collapse can occur again.

Bleeding

Bleeding can occur any time a blood vessel is damaged during needle insertion. It is usually of greater significance within rather than outside of the central neuraxis. Of course, it is a greater risk in patients who are taking anticoagulant agents. Permanent nerve damage has been attributed to the effect of hematoma on the brachial plexus nerves[28] and the spinal cord. To prevent this complication, nerve blocks should be avoided in patients who have bleeding disorders and in those who are taking anticoagulant agents, if the results of coagulation studies are abnormal.

SPECIFIC NERVE BLOCKS

Head and Neck

Before the advent of routine tracheal intubation and general anesthesia, much head and neck surgery was performed with regional blocks. Subsequently, the need for specific blocks about the head and neck diminished, as did their routine use for surgical practice. However, on occasion, optimal anesthesia is achieved with some of these blocks, either alone or in conjunction with general anesthesia. They are especially useful in the diagnostic and therapeutic management of painful conditions. However, several potential complications, some serious and even life-threatening, must be recognized (Table 42-4).

As compact and complicated anatomic structures, the head and the neck pose a challenge to the regional anesthetist. Meticulous placement of the needle and use of small doses of local anesthetic are required for accurate and discrete results. However, landmarks in this region tend to be constant and predictable; for the practitioner who acquires the requisite skills, it can be a most useful and satisfactory method for surgical anesthesia and especially for diagnostic anesthesia.

Eye

Anesthesiologists increasingly provide service for ophthalmic surgery, and occasionally for diagnostic blocks in and around

TABLE 42-4
Complications of Nerve Block of the Head and Neck

OPHTHALMIC REGION
- Central nervous system toxic reactions
- Puncture or transfixation of globe

TRIGEMINAL NERVE
- Subarachnoid injection
- Perforation of middle meningeal artery
- Damage to cavernous sinus
- Puncture of oral cavity

MANDIBULAR NERVE
- Infection
- Intrathecal injection

MAXILLARY NERVE
- Infratemporal and orbital hematoma
- Local tissue damage

FRONTAL NERVE
- Orbital hematoma from block within orbit

FACIAL NERVE
- Facial weakness during performance of mandibular or maxillary blocks

GLOSSOPHARYNGEAL NERVE
- Block of cranial nerves X and XI
  - Weakness of trapezius and sternocleidomastoid muscles
  - Hoarseness
  - Ipsilateral gag reflex loss
- Puncture of carotid artery or internal jugular vein

VAGUS NERVE
- Local damage when branches blocked

PHRENIC NERVES
- Inadvertent spread of agent after deep cervical plexus, interscalene, or stellate ganglion block
- Respiratory embarrassment in patients with severe lung disease

STELLATE GANGLION
- Pneumothorax
- Subarachnoid spread
- Regional spread
  - Recurrent laryngeal nerve
  - Somatic nerves of brachial plexus
  - Phrenic nerve
- Horner's syndrome

the orbit. Although these blocks usually are safe,[29] profound central nervous system toxic reactions can occur as a result of spread through vascular or other conduits (perhaps the optic nerve sheath) to the brain.[30] Direct injection within the orbit can transfix the globe with the needle. Reports suggest that recovery typically occurs but that particular notice should be taken of an early warning sign, clouding of the anterior chamber on injection; of course, injections should cease immediately.

Trigeminal Nerve

INTRATHECAL INJECTION. Gasserian ganglion block is performed less frequently now that thermal gangliolysis is used to treat tic douloureux.[31] The complications of gasserian block stem primarily from the entrance of the needle and subsequent injection of drug into the subarachnoid space by way of invagination of dura that surrounds the gasserian ganglion (Meckel's cavity). A very small quantity of local anesthetic injected into this space can produce profound anesthesia of the ipsilateral cranial nerves. A patient in my clinic was given a test injection of 0.25 mL of 1% lidocaine, which produced anesthesia of all of the ipsilateral cranial nerves and was associated with brief loss of consciousness. Thus, it is of paramount importance to ensure that no backflow of cerebrospinal fluid occurs before the injection of local anesthetics, and especially neurolytic agents.

DAMAGE TO INTRACRANIAL STRUCTURES. Ideally, this block is performed with radiographic control; advancement of the needle too far can result in damage to intracranial structures, particularly the cavernous sinus and its contents (cranial nerves II and VI) and the brain itself. Also, if the needle is directed too far posteriorly and misses the foramen ovale, it may enter the middle meningeal artery at the foramen spinosum or even the carotid artery in the foramen lacerum. To prevent the needle from entering the oral cavity en route, a finger can be placed in the patient's mouth during insertion to guide its path.

Mandibular Nerve

PHARYNGEAL PENETRATION. In "walking" the needle posteriorly off the lateral pterygoid plate, the nerve can be missed completely, and the needle can enter the pharynx. On injection into the pharynx, the patient may complain of a bitter taste and may even spit the local anesthetic out! Although injection into the pharynx is of no great consequence, the needle now has been inserted into an unsterile area; withdrawal through the infratemporal fossa may lead to infection. However, in dentistry numerous intraoral injections are made into branches of the cranial nerves by way of the oral cavity without great morbidity.

INTRATHECAL INJECTION. Unintended intrathecal injection can occur during attempted block of the main branches of the mandibular nerve, resulting in anesthesia of the brain stem.[32] The dental literature describes puzzling central nervous system symptoms after attempted injection of branches of the trigeminal system at peripheral sites in the jaw. The hypothesis has been advanced that retrovascular transmission of local anesthetic agent centrally may produce central nervous system toxicity and ocular complications.[33] Similar phenomena have been reported after injection of the scalp[34] and tonsils.[35] Aspiration tests before injection of head and neck blocks are equally if not more important than they are for blocks performed in other body sites.

Maxillary Nerve

INFRATEMPORAL HEMATOMA. The approach to the maxillary nerve traverses the infratemporal fossa as the needle passes through the coronoid notch or anterior to the ramus of the mandible. The goal is to place the needle in the pterygopalatine fossa. Complications are primarily those of damage to or injection into the very rich vascular plexus lying in this fossa. The five terminal branches of the maxillary artery and the veins draining the orbit by way of the inferior orbital fissure are contained therein. Hematoma formation is common after this particular block. Because of the venous communications through the inferior orbital fissure with this fossa, fairly extensive orbital hematoma ("black eye") can result.[3]

LOCAL TISSUE DAMAGE. The needle may be advanced through the inferior orbital fissure into the back of the orbit and produce local tissue damage. Therefore, the depth of needle insertion is important, and a marker should be used. This complication is less likely to happen with an approach through the coronoid notch with the jaw closed. In this case, the path of the needle impinges on the back of the maxilla. The higher elevation necessary to enter the orbit by way of the inferior orbital fissure is unlikely to occur. The maxillary nerve also can be approached along the inferolateral aspect of the orbital floor.[36] Damage to the orbital contents can result if strict adherence to technique is not followed.

Frontal Nerve

Nerve blocks of the supratrochlear and supraorbital branches of the first division of the trigeminal nerve are best performed at or above the eyebrow. Attempts to block the nerve from within the orbit, below the eyebrow, are likely to produce a black eye because of injury to the loose vascular connective tissue in the orbit, which permits hematoma should a blood vessel be punctured.[3]

Facial Nerve

Block of the facial nerve results in ipsilateral facial weakness and occurs occasionally during the performance of a mandibular or maxillary nerve block by the extraoral route. It is caused by infiltration of the superficial and deep subcutaneous tissues over the ramus of the mandible, producing anesthesia of the pes anserinus, the branches of the facial nerve that lie in the parotid gland. Block of the facial nerve also can occur as a complication of glossopharyngeal block performed at the styloid process, where the facial nerve trunk emerges from the stylomastoid foramen.

Glossopharyngeal Nerve

The glossopharyngeal nerve may be blocked from an intraoral or extraoral approach.[37] With the latter, the usual route is by way of a site halfway between the angle of the mandible and the mastoid process, with the styloid process used as an end point. Invariably, block of the glossopharyngeal nerve produces a block of cranial nerves X and XI also, resulting in weakness of the trapezius and the sternomastoid muscles as well as hoarseness on occasion. A glossopharyngeal block interferes with the gag reflex on the ipsilateral side. The proximity of the carotid arterial system and internal jugular vein calls for mandatory aspiration tests. In general, blocks from within the oral cavity have very few complications and a high success rate.[37]

Vagus Nerve

The main trunk of the vagus nerve is rarely, if ever, blocked as a primary therapeutic maneuver. The branches to the larynx, however, are often blocked when tracheal intubation is attempted without use of muscle relaxants or deep general anesthesia. To render the laryngeal inlet analgesic, the superior laryngeal nerves (primarily the internal branches) are blocked as they pass beneath the greater cornu of the hyoid. This is a relatively simple block and is associated with a low morbidity, which is restricted to damage at the point of needle insertion. The recurrent laryngeal nerves are intentionally blocked only in rare cases but frequently as a complication of stellate ganglion block. However, the distribution of these nerves is blocked with a transtracheal spray of the region in which the needle is inserted, between the thyroid and cricoid cartilages in the sagittal plane. This technique is effective for anesthetizing this area and is associated with low morbidity.

Phrenic Nerve

Block of the phrenic nerves also is seldom the primary goal in regional anesthesia, although attempts are occasionally made to block them to abort persistent attacks of singultus (hiccups). The phrenic nerve is adherent to the anterior surface of the anterior scalene muscle. Thus, it is probably blocked more often than is realized as a complication of other local anesthetic procedures in and around the base of the neck, particularly in deep cervical plexus, interscalene, and stellate ganglion blocks. For example, during interscalene block, the nerve is predictably anesthetized by direct involvement or by the paravertebral spread of the anesthetic to the cervical plexus.

Investigators have speculated on the inadvisability of performing bilateral interscalene blocks because of the risk of bilateral phrenic nerve block and respiratory embarrassment.[38] However, unless the patient's respiratory function is severely compromised, blocking one or even two phrenic nerves is unlikely to produce any detectable effects and probably can be demonstrated only by fluoroscopy. The phrenic nerves supply only the central part of the diaphragm; the remainder is supplied by intercostal nerves. For the otherwise healthy patient at rest, phrenic nerve block appears to pose no risk of respiratory embarrassment. In the "respiratory cripple," or thoracic level paraplegic, however, phrenic nerve block may be followed by significant respiratory dysfunction.

CERVICOTHORACIC SYMPATHETIC BLOCK

Stellate Ganglion

For the diagnosis and therapy of upper-extremity pain, a stellate ganglion block often is performed. The stellate ganglion is the group of autonomic fibers believed to be the confluence of the upper thoracic and inferior cervical ganglion on the sympathetic chain. Through this ganglion pass most, though not necessarily all, of the sympathetic efferent fibers to the upper extremity.[39]

Many approaches have been described for this block, which have been reviewed extensively.[40] However, the anterior approach is used most frequently; local anesthetic is usually deposited at the level of C7 or C6 so that caudal spread of the solution in the prevertebral plane will block the fibers that pass from the upper thoracic sympathetic chain to the extremity. Depending on the technique chosen, the needle is introduced in the paratracheal region at the base of the neck at C7 or C6 and passes in close proximity to several important structures. The most serious and not infrequent complications are unintended intravascular injection into a vertebral or even carotid artery, and pneumothorax.

Anterior Approach

The anterior approach, like that of other blocks, depends on location of a bony landmark, such as the transverse process of C6 (Chassaignac's tubercle) or C7. The needle is then withdrawn anteriorly until the point clears the prevertebral muscle mass and, more importantly, the prevertebral fascia.

Complications

VERTEBRAL ARTERY INJECTION. If the needle is advanced in error between the transverse processes into the paravertebral space such that it locates the posterior tubercle, which may be erroneously interpreted as the anterior tubercle, withdrawal can leave the needle point in the lumen of the vertebral artery. Injection of very small quantities of local anesthetic drug into this artery result in profound effects, such as convulsions,[41] aphasia, hemiparesis,[42] and reversible blindness.[43]

I have had experience with three such cases, in which injection of less than 0.25 mL of 1% lidocaine resulted in unconsciousness and convulsions. Although an aspiration test should prevent these complications, in the these three instances the test results were negative. Therefore, a small test dose, perhaps as little as 0.125 mL, injected slowly, is advisable. Treatment of the convulsions involves airway support, oxygen administration, and intravenous benzodiazepine or thiopental.

PNEUMOTHORAX. Pneumothorax after stellate ganglion block is attributable to direct puncture of the parietal pleura of the cupola in the thoracic inlet; its likelihood varies with the vertical extent of the apical lobe of the lung. Thus, it occurs more frequently in patients in whom the apical pleura is higher, such as tall, thin persons rather than those who are short and fat. The incidence of pneumothorax also is greater with blocks done at the lower level (C7) than with blocks performed at C6.

REGIONAL SPREAD. Other less serious complications of stellate ganglion block result from spread to the somatic nerves of the brachial plexus and the recurrent laryngeal nerve. Involvement of the latter is quite common because it lies in the same fascial compartment, anterior to the prevertebral fascia, as the sympathetic chain. However, if the needle is advanced too far posteriorly and not withdrawn to the prevertebral fascia, block of the cephalic components of the brachial plexus (dermatomes and myotomes of C5 and C6 and perhaps of C7 and C8) may result. This problem usually is transient with reversible agents.

Spread to the recurrent laryngeal nerve is often distressing to the patient, who should be warned about this possibility. It usually results in hoarseness, cough, and a diminution of the voice to a whisper for the duration of the block. Block of the right stellate ganglion, but not the left, results in a significant decrease in heart rate. The functional significance of this phenomenon is unknown.[44]

OTHER COMPLICATIONS. Subarachnoid spread from incorrect needle positioning or by way of dural sleeves is possible but infrequent. When it occurs, the patient may need urgent resuscitative and supportive treatment for the resulting total spinal anesthesia. Horner's syndrome of ptosis, miosis, enophthalmos, and anhydrosis is not really a complication but rather a result of the sympathetic block produced; although occasionally bothersome, it is tolerated well by most patients. Thoracic duct trauma also has been reported with this block.[45]

NERVE BLOCKS OF THE TRUNK

Potential complications are numerous because of the proximity of vital structures and organs (Table 42-5).

Lumbar Sympathetic Block

Lumbar sympathetic block frequently is performed for diagnosis and treatment of reflex sympathetic dystrophy. It also has been used for intermittent claudication[46] and relief of pain in the first stage of labor.

TABLE 42-5
Complications of Blocks of the Trunk

LUMBAR SYMPATHETIC BLOCK

- Paravertebral sensory, somatic block
- Puncture of aorta or inferior vena cava
- Puncture of kidney or ureter (L2 approach)
- Peridural or subarachnoid spread
- Peritoneal injection

THORACIC PARAVERTEBRAL BLOCK

- Pneumothorax
- Peridural or subarachnoid spread

CELIAC PLEXUS BLOCK

- Postural hypotension
- Puncture of aorta or vena cava (retroperitoneal hematoma)
- Pneumothorax

Posterior Approach

The lumbar sympathetic chain is situated on the anterolateral border of the lumbar vertebrae. Invariably it is approached posteriorly. In the preferred approach, a needle is inserted 10 cm from the midline, usually at the level of L2 or L3, advanced at a 45° angle, and walked along the vertebral body until it just slips off, at which time it should be adjacent to the lumbar sympathetic chain.[47,48] It then will have advanced beyond the psoas sheath, and injected local anesthetic will be distributed in the retroperitoneal fascial plane wherein lies the lumbar sympathetic chain.

If the needle is not advanced far enough anteriorly, the injected drug will be confined within the limits of the psoas sheath, involve the lumbar plexus, and produce a somatic rather than a sympathetic block. Even if the needle is placed correctly, the drug still can diffuse back between the origins of the psoas major muscle, following the path of the lumbar arteries into the paravertebral space and then to the paravertebral nerves, especially if the patient is turned supine.[49]

If the needle is advanced too far anteriorly, it may enter the aorta or the inferior vena cava from the left or right side, respectively, or their tributaries. Another complication of the more lateral approach is puncture of the lower pole of the kidney or ureters.[50] I have demonstrated this problem in two of six cadavers tested with the needle at the level of L2 but not at L3. The clinical significance of this finding is not mentioned in the literature, but probably the needle should be inserted at L3. This complication is easily avoidable if the block is performed with fluoroscopic guidance.

Pain is encountered at the skin, the lumbar fascia, and the periosteum of the vertebral body. With the classic paravertebral approach, in addition to these sites, the sensitive periosteum of the transverse process is encountered, and frequently paresthesia occurs on contact with the paravertebral nerve.

As with all blocks around the neuraxis, the complication of peridural and subarachnoid spread is ever present.[51] Unintentionally, the needle may be inserted through the paravertebral foramen. This problem can result from faulty technique or from indistinct landmarks, as in an extremely obese patient. Local anesthetic can spread up the perineural sheaths that have been described to accompany the segmental nerves beyond the paravertebral foramina.[52]

Complications

Careful aspiration and the use of a test dose markedly reduce the risk of intravascular and intradural complications.

SOMATIC SPREAD. The most frequent complication of lumbar sympathetic block is that of somatic spread. This problem occurs despite good technique in about 5% to 15% of patients. Depending on the agent used, the sequelae of somatic spread can have relatively little or no significance. That is, when the block is done for reflex sympathetic dystrophies, the sequela may be just a band of temporary numbness over the L2 or L3 dermatomes. However, if the concentration of local anesthetic is sufficient to produce motor blockade, spread can seriously compromise the patient's ability to walk for some time, depending on the local anesthetic agent used (eg, several hours with bupivicaine). Therefore, an agent such as 0.225% bupivacaine, which will give prolonged sympathetic blockade, should be used. If it spills into the lumbar plexus, it is hoped that only somatic analgesia, not motor block, will result.

To prevent spread to somatic nerves, the anesthesiologist must abstain from infiltrating the whole track with local anesthetic. Instead, a skin wheal should be raised and a small amount (1 to 2 mL) of local anesthetic injected at the sensitive lumbar fascia. Excessive infiltration, including the intrapsoas path of the needle, may result in anesthetization of components of the lumbar plexus and produce weakness of hip flexion.

PERITONEAL OR VISCERAL INJECTION. Theoretically, complications may arise from positioning of the needle point too anteriorly, resulting in the injection of drugs into the peritoneal cavity or viscera. However, I am unaware of its occurrence in practice. Retroperitoneal hemorrhage also may occur.[53]

Thoracic Paravertebral Block

Somatic and sympathetic paravertebral nerve blocks performed in the thoracic region are associated with a higher risk of pneumothorax than are brachial plexus and intercostal blocks. This observation probably is related to the increased depth of needle insertion, which leads to some loss of control, and to the proximity of the pleura to the target nerves. As with other paravertebral blocks, peridural spread or subarachnoid spread results from misplacement of needles or movement of anesthetic by way of dural sheaths that accompany the nerves. This complication can occur even after intercostal blocks.[54]

Celiac Plexus Block

Celiac plexus block, in combination with intercostal blockade, is used with success by skilled practitioners for anesthesia in patients undergoing surgery. However, it is more frequently used as a diagnostic maneuver during attempts to clarify causes of obscure abdominal pain. It is often used successfully as therapy in patients whose source of pain is an intra-abdominal malignancy. Because blockade of the celiac plexus leads to sympathetic denervation of a large area of the splanchnic bed, the patient's ability to maintain adequate blood pressure is compromised; postural hypotension is a frequent complication.

Another possible complication is the puncture of large vessels, such as the aorta or inferior vena cava. Although this complication could lead to a retroperitoneal hematoma, that problem does not seem to occur frequently. Unless meticulous attention to needle direction is maintained, a pneumothorax also may result.

INTRAVENOUS REGIONAL BLOCK

Used since the turn of the century, the intravenous regional block has a long and proven safety record. Although very careful monitoring reveals sinus bradycardia after release of

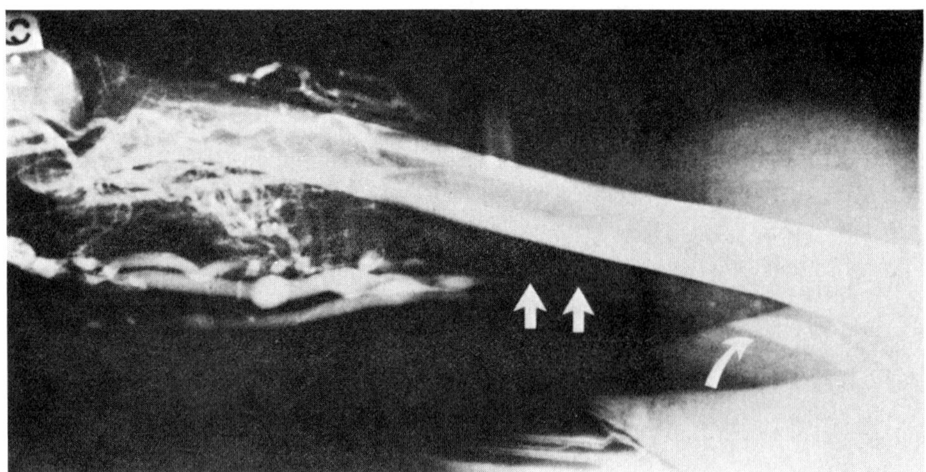

FIGURE 42-2. Phlebograph of the arm after injection of contrast material into a peripheral vein of the exsanguinated arm. Pressure of tourniquet cuff (*double arrow*) was 300 mmHg. The filled axillary vein at the proximal side of the cuff area (*curved arrow*) and a continuous narrow streak of contrast under the cuff on the medial side of the humerus can be seen. (Rosenberg PH, Kalso EA, Tuominen MK, et al: Acute bupivacaine cardiotoxicity as a result of venous leakage under the tourniquet during a Bier block. Anesthesiology 58: 96, 1983)

the tourniquet in 65% of these blocks, this bradycardia usually is limited to a reduction of only about 10 beats/min.[55]

Isolated cases in which resuscitation was required after use of this technique have been reported.[56] These cardiovascular complications, related presumably to the high circulating blood levels of local anesthetic agent after release of the cuff, appear to be self-limiting in most cases and, were it not for close monitoring, probably would go undetected. However, deaths after the use of bupivacaine[57] and acute systemic toxicity have been associated with venous leakage of this agent under the tourniquet during these procedures (Fig. 42-2).[58] Even with the tourniquet appropriately inflated, local anesthetic enters the systemic circulation.[59] This appears to be a consequence of the high pressure created in the venous system, especially when the injection cannula is in the forearm rather than the hand and/or when the tourniquet is too small and fails to occlude all vascular channels. Bupivacaine is no longer used for intravenous regional anesthesia because the central nervous system–cardiac toxicity ratio is so much lower than that for prilocaine or lidocaine. Chronic neurologic deficits after this technique require careful assessment of possible causes because prolonged application of a tourniquet can lead to neural impairment.[23]

Guanethidine instead of a local anesthetic agent has been administered into the vascular system of the isolated limb as a therapy for reflex sympathetic dystrophy.[60] This technique appears to be safe. However, because guanethidine is not available in North America, reserpine has been used as a substitute; in some patients, this drug produces postural hypotension after the release of the tourniquet.[61]

EPIDURAL AND SPINAL NARCOTICS

The demonstration that profound analgesia can be produced by the administration of narcotics directly to the neuraxis has led to an explosion of experimental and clinical effort to outline the mechanisms involved and to realize its full therapeutic potential. This particular form of therapy has proven effective in controlling postoperative, obstetric, and posttraumatic pain, and especially in controlling the chronic pain of patients with cancer.[62,63]

Respiratory depression as a side effect has been shown to occur less frequently than previously feared. Nevertheless, some factors increase the risk of this problem (Table 42-6).[62] Low-dosage naloxone infusion (5 μg/kg/h) prevents morphine-induced respiratory depression without affecting its analgesia.[64] Use of this technique varies widely; in some centers the method is used extensively for postoperative pain relief, whereas in others a more selective and cautious approach with intensive monitoring has been adopted.

Central neuraxis narcotic treatment of cancer pain is most gratifying. These patients do not seem to be as prone to the side effects that have been described when the technique is used in patients who have not been treated previously with narcotic agents. The patient with cancer for whom oral narcotic analgesia has ceased to be effective or for whom the side effects interfere with the quality of life can often obtain much improved pain control through long-term administration of epidural opiates, usually morphine. By means of indwelling epidural catheter systems, these patients enjoy excellent, safe, long-term pain control at home.[65] Respiratory depression has not proven to be an important problem because tolerance to oral narcotics already has developed. The other side effects of epidural narcotic administration, itching and urinary re-

TABLE 42-6
Factors Increasing the Risk of Respiratory Depression With Epidural Narcotics

- Intrathecal administration
- Age >70 years
- Dose of morphine >10 mg
- Residual parenteral narcotics
- Other central nervous system–depressant drugs
- Lack of tolerance to opioids
- Preexisting respiratory disease

Cousins MJ, Mather LE: Intrathecal and epidural administration of opioids. Anesthesiology 61:42, 1984.

tention, also seem to be tolerated better during long-term use by the cancer patient than after the administration of narcotics for postoperative pain control.

Because neuraxial narcotics do not produce motor or sympathetic blockade, they may have important potential for replacing some conventional diagnostic block techniques, especially so because this application permits functional and subjective testing of the pain. Some of the shorter-acting synthetic narcotics are more useful and safer in selected applications.[66,67]

REFERENCES

1. Murphy E: 'Murphy's law.' Quoted by Frank E, Winelhake W, Van deStadt J, et al: Formulations of natural law. Journal of Irreproducible Results 21:4, 1974
2. Brechner T, Brechner V: Accuracy of needle placement during diagnostic and therapeutic nerve block. In Bonica JJ, Albe-Fessard (eds): Advances in pain research and therapy, vol 1. New York: Raven Press, 1976: 679
3. Moore DC: Complications of regional anesthesia. Clinical Anesthesiology 7:217, 1969
4. Bonica JJ, Buckley FP: Regional anesthesia with local anesthetics in the management of pain. In Bonica JJ (ed): The management of pain. Philadelphia: Lea & Febiger, 1990, 1883
5. de Jong RH, Heavner JE: Diazepam prevents local anesthetic seizures. Anesthesiology 34:523, 1971
6. Selander D, Dhuner KG, Lundborg G: Peripheral nerve injury due to injection needles used for regional anesthesia. Acta Anaesthesiol Scand 21:182, 1977
7. Magora F: Obturator nerve block: evaluation of technique. Br J Anaesth 41:695, 1969
8. Tabita PV: Side effects of the jet injector for the production of local anesthesia. Anesthesia Progress 26:102, 1979
9. Jebsen RH: Electrodiagnosis in the nerve root syndrome. N Z Med J 65:107, 1966
10. Logstrom B, Wennberg A, Widen L: Late disturbances in nerve function after block with local anesthetics: an electroneurographic study. Acta Anaesthesiol Scand 10:111, 1966
11. Bromage PR, O'Brien P, Dunford LA: Etidocaine: a clinical evaluation for regional analgesia in surgery. Can Anaesth Soc J 21:523, 1974
12. Skou JC: Toxicity of local anesthetics. Acta Pharmacol Toxicol 10:292, 1954
13. Benoit PW, Belt WD: Destruction and regeneration of skeletal muscle after treatment with a local anesthetic, bupivacaine (Marcaine). J Anat 107:547, 1970
14. Dhuner KG: Frequency of general side reactions after regional anaesthesia with mepivacaine with and without vasoconstrictors. Acta Anaesthesiol Scand Suppl 48:23, 1972
15. Barker M, Rodeheaver GI, Edgerton MT, et al: Damage to tissue defenses by a topical anesthetic agent. Ann Emerg Med 11:307, 1982
16. Hibbard LT, Snyder EN, McVann RM: Subgluteal and retropsoal infection in obstetric practice. Obstet Gynecol 39:137, 1972
17. Wenger DR, Gitchell RG: Severe infections following pudendal block in anesthesia: need for orthopaedic awareness. J Bone Joint Surg [Am] 55:202, 1973
18. Schmidt RM, Rosenkranz HS: Anti-microbial activity of local anesthetics: lidocaine and procaine. J Infect Dis 121:597, 1970
19. Sipila P, Plava A, Soril M, et al: Atlantoaxial subluxation: an unusual complication after local anesthesia for tonsillectomy. Arch Otolaryngol 107:181, 1981
20. Stoelting R: Nerve injury during anesthesia. American Society of Anesthesiologists Newsletter 58:6, 1994
21. Dawson DM, Krarup C: Perioperative nerve lesions. Archives of Neurology 46:1355, 1989
22. Britt BA, Gordon RA: Peripheral nerve injuries associated with anesthesia. Can Anaesth Soc J 11:514, 1964
23. Moldaver J: Tourniquet paralysis syndrome. Arch Surg 68:136, 1954
24. Kroll DA, Caplan RA, Posner K, et al: Nerve injury associated with anesthesia. Anesthesiology 73:202, 1990
25. Selander D, Dhuner K-G, Lundborg G: Peripheral nerve injury due to injection needles used for regional anesthesia: an experimental study of the acute effects of needle point trauma. Acta Anaesthesiol Scand 21:182, 1977
26. Selander D, Edshage S, Wolff T: Paresthesiae or no paresthesiae? nerve lesions after axillary blocks. Acta Anaesthesiol Scand 23: 27, 1979
27. Brown DL, Kirby RR: Pulmonary barotrauma. In Civetta JM, Taylor RW, Kirby RR (eds): Critical care, 2nd ed. Philadelphia: JB Lippincott, 1992: 1437
28. Wooley EJ, Vandam LD: Neurological sequelae of brachial plexus nerve block. Ann Surg 149:53, 1959
29. Backer CL, Tinker JH, Robertson DM, et al: Myocardial reinfarction following local anesthesia for ophthalmic surgery. Anesth Analg 59:257, 1980
30. Smith JL: Retrobulbar bupivacaine can cause respiratory arrest. Ann Ophthalmol 14:1005, 1982
31. Loeser JD: What to do about tic douloureux. JAMA 239:1153, 1978
32. Nique TA, Bennett CR: Inadvertent brainstem anesthesia following extraoral trigeminal V_2-V_3 blocks. Oral Surg 51:468, 1981
33. Cooley RL, Cottingham AJ Jr: Ocular complications from local anesthetic injections. General Dentistry 27:40, 1979
34. Von Bahr G: Multiple embolisms in the fundus of an eye after an injection in the scalp. Acta Ophthalmol (Copenh) 41:85, 1963
35. Ellis PP: Visual loss following tonsillectomy. Arch Otolaryngol 87:128, 1968
36. Adriani J: Labat's regional anesthesia: techniques and clinical applications, 3rd ed. Philadelphia: WB Saunders, 1967, 94
37. DeMeester TR: Glossopharyngeal nerve block for endoscopy. Clin Trends Anesthesiol 6:2, 1976
38. Kumar A, Battit GE, Froese AD, et al: Bilateral cervical and thoracic epidural blockade complicating interscalene block: reports of two cases. Anesthesiology 35:650, 1971
39. Kuntz A: Autonomic nervous system, 3rd ed. Philadelphia, Lea & Febiger, 1945, 136
40. Moore DC: Stellate ganglion blocks. Springfield: Charles C Thomas, 1954
41. Korevaar WC, Burney RG, Moore PA: Convulsions during stellate ganglion block: a case report. Anesth Analg 58:329, 1979
42. Scott DL, Ghia JM, Teeple E: Aphasia and hemiparesis following stellate ganglion block. Anesth Analg 62:1038, 1983
43. Szeinfeld M, Laurencio M, Pallares VS: Total reversible blindness following attempted stellate ganglion block. Anesth Analg 60: 689, 1981
44. Rogers MC, Battit GE, McPeek B, et al: The lateralization of sympathetic control of the human sinus node. Anesthesiology 48:139, 1978
45. Thompson KJ, Melding P, Hatangdi VS: Pneumochylothorax: a rare complication of stellate ganglion block. Anesthesiology 55: 589, 1981
46. Hatangdi VS, Boas RA: Lumbar sympathectomy: a single needle technique. Br J Anaesth 57:285, 1985
47. Parks FW, Chalmers JA: Paravertebral sympathetic block in treatment of superficial and deep thrombosis of leg veins. Journal of Obstetrics and Gynaecology of the British Commonwealth 64:419, 1957
48. Reid W, Watt JK, Gray TC: Phenol injection of the sympathetic chain. Br J Surg 57:45, 1970
49. Bryce-Smith R: Injection of the lumbar sympathetic chain. Anaesthesia 6:150, 1951
50. Kuzmarof IM, MacIsaac SG, Sioufi J, et al: Iatrogenic ureteral injury secondary to lumbar sympathetic ganglion blockade. Urology 16:617, 1980
51. Evans JA, Dobben GD, Gay GR: Peridural infusion of drugs in sympathetic blockade. JAMA 200:573, 1967
52. Gay GR, Evans JA: Total spinal anesthesia following lumbar

paravertebral block: a potentially lethal complication. Anesth Analg 50:344, 1971

53. Learned LO, Calhoun RF: Retroperitoneal hemorrhage as a complication of lumbar paravertebral injections: report of three cases. Anesthesiology 12:391, 1951
54. Maddaugh RE, Menk EJ, Reynolds WJ, et al: Epidural block using large volumes of local anesthetic solution for intercostal nerve block. Anesthesiology 63:214, 1985
55. Kew MC, Lowe JP: The cardiovascular complications of intravenous regional anaesthesia. Br J Surg 58:179, 1971
56. Thorn-Alquist AM: Intravenous regional anaesthesia: a seven year survey. Acta Anaesthesiol Scand 15:23, 1971
57. Heath ML: Deaths after intravenous regional anaesthesia. Br Med J 9:3, 1982
58. Reynolds F. Bupivicaine and intravenous regional anesthesia (editorial). Anesthesia 39:105, 1984
59. Rosenberg PH, Kalso EA, Tuominen MK, et al: Acute bupivacaine cardiotoxicity as a result of venous leakage under the tourniquet during Bier block. Anesthesiology 58:95, 1983
60. Hannington-Kiff JG: Intravenous regional sympathetic block with guanethidine. Lancet 1:1019, 1974
61. Benzon HT, Chomker CM, Brunner EA: Treatment of reflex sympathetic dystrophy with regional intravenous reserpine. Anesth Analg 59:500, 1980
62. Cousins MJ, Mather LE: Intrathecal and epidural administration of opioids. Anesthesiology 61:42, 1984
63. Twycross RG, Lack SA: Symptom control in far advanced cancer: pain relief. London: Pitman, 1983
64. Rawal N, Schott U, Dahlstrom B, et al: Influence of naloxone infusion on analgesia and respiratory depression following epidural morphine. Anesthesiology 64:194, 1986
65. Cherry DA, Gourley GK, Cousins MJ, et al: A technique for the insertion of an implantable portal system for the long-term epidural administration of opioids in the treatment of cancer pain. Anaesth Intensive Care 13:145, 1985
66. Cherry DA, Gourley GK, McLachlan M, et al: Diagnostic epidural opioid blockade and chronic pain: preliminary report. Pain 21: 143, 1985
67. Ready LB: Acute peridural narcotic therapy. Problems in Anesthsia 2:327, 1988

FURTHER READING

Bridenbaugh PO. Complications of local anesthetic neural blockade. In Cousins MJ, Bridenbaugh PO (eds): Neural blockade in clinical anesthesia and management of pain, 2nd ed. Philadelphia: JB Lippincott, 1988: 695

Brown DL, Flynn JF, Owens BD: Pain control. In Civetta JM, Taylor RW, Kirby RR (eds): Critical care, 2nd ed. Philadelphia: JB Lippincott, 1992: 219

James CF: Local and regional anesthesia. In: Gravenstein N (ed): Manual of complications during anesthesia. Philadelphia: JB Lippincott, 1991: 421

Murphy TM: Chronic pain. In Miller RD (ed): Anesthesia, 4th ed. New York: Churchill Livingstone, 1994: 2345

Complications in Anesthesiology, second edition,
edited by Nikolaus Gravenstein and Robert R. Kirby.
Lippincott-Raven Publishers, Philadelphia © 1996.

CHAPTER 43

Complications of Neurolytic Blocks

Terence M. Murphy

Neurolytic blocks have been used since the advent of nerve block technology for the control of chronic pain and spasticity. However, increased use of epidural narcotics and improved delivery systems for long-term maintenance have lessened the need for neurodestruction as a means of controlling chronic pain. As a result, neurolytic blockade is little used in contemporary medical practice. However, it still is indicated in selected conditions and forms a small but important part of the practice of anesthesiologists concerned with control of chronic pain.

Neurolytic blocks are used primarily for the treatment of pain in patients with cancer. They also are useful for the relief of persistent spasticity in patients with spinal cord injuries or progressive neurologic diseases such as multiple sclerosis. The main hazard of these agents is possible spread to other adjacent and vital structures.

The incidence of complications has been reported by several investigators. Swerdlow reported a rate of 50% but included intrathecal chlorocresol, a particularly toxic agent.[1] Nathan and Scott described a 10% incidence of complications with intrathecal phenol.[2] Kuzucu and colleagues, in a large series of 300 neurolytic subarachnoid blocks with alcohol, reported a 7% incidence of complications in the period immediately after the block but a long-term incidence of only 1%.[3] In a series of 1000 patients receiving phenol lumbar sympathetic blocks, the most common complication was neuralgia, which occurred in approximately 10% of patients, but usually was mild, responded well to simple analgesics, and was self-limiting, lasting only a few weeks.[4]

Complications arise because of the impossibility of guaranteeing that the agent, when it is injected by a percutaneous needle technique, will be deposited at and produce an effect only on the intended target. Even when performed by experienced clinicians and with meticulous attention to technique, tissues other than the intended target sometimes become involved.

NEUROLYTIC AGENTS AND TECHNIQUES

A variety of agents have been used with varying degrees of success (Table 43-1).

Absolute Alcohol

Absolute alcohol is used to effect somatic nerve block, peripherally or within the subarachnoid space. For sympathetic blockade, 50% alcohol suffices. Alcohol is very irritating to tissues and therefore very painful on injection. However, this discomfort is short-lived; analgesia rapidly follows the burning sensation, and the temporary discomfort is tolerated well by most patients. Supplemental analgesia can reduce this discomfort on injection but is not advisable, because preservation of the patient's ability to respond is important for following more closely the extent of analgesia.

Technical Aspects

If an extensive block is required, additional injections at various levels are usually advisable, rather than attempts to inject larger volumes at one site. Because it is less dense than cerebrospinal fluid, alcohol floats and forms a layer on the surface. Thus, during subarachnoid alcohol blocks it is important to ensure that the desired nerve is uppermost. If alcohol is accidentally injected intravascularly, it is rapidly diluted, with little or no undesirable effects.

Duration of Effect

Analgesia lasts as long as several months; when pain returns, injection can be repeated. In contrast to the effect of phenol, the analgesia is immediate. Thus any deficiencies noted in the extent of the blockade at the time of the procedure can be rectified promptly. When the alcohol is injected into the subarachnoid space, neurolytic concentrations tend to be limited to the site of injection.[5]

TABLE 43-1
Neurolytic Agents for Central or Peripheral Blockade

- Alcohol
- Phenol
- Chlorocresol
- Silver nitrate
- Ammonium compounds
- Tetracaine
- Hypertonic saline (normo- or hypothermic)

Phenol

Technical Aspects

Phenol is used for peripheral somatic and subarachnoid nerve blocks as well as sympathetic blocks. Concentrations of 1% to 10% are recommended. Usually, at least 5% phenol is needed; often 10% is necessary. When used in the subarachnoid space, phenol commonly is mixed with glycerine, which effects a hyperbaric solution but delays its release into the tissues. As a result, the final extent of the block may not be evident until the following day. What may appear to be an adequate block at the time of the procedure often diminishes significantly. Diminution occurs because phenol probably has a dual effect, acting both as a local anesthetic in weaker concentrations at the periphery of the injected bolus and as a neurolytic agent in stronger concentrations at the injection site.[6] Therefore, a more extensive block than is required usually is advisable.

Phenol, though its effects are less predictable than those of alcohol, is less painful on injection.

Duration

Like other neurolytic agents, the duration of analgesia of phenol is variable and may last from several weeks to 12 months. Systemic side effects are mild and nonspecific, because commonly only small doses, of less than 500 to 1000 mg maximum, are administered at a single time—much less than the toxic dose of 8 to 15 g.[7]

Chlorocresol

Used as a 2% solution in glycerine, chlorocresol is very effective, but because of its greater diffusion and penetration has a greater incidence of toxic side effects than does phenol.[1] Though more efficacious in pain relief than phenol, this agent also produces almost twice the number of instances of urinary and bowel sphincter paralysis, persistent numbness, and paresthesia (Table 43-2).[1] Pain relief is sometimes delayed for as long as 24 hours.

Silver Nitrate

Silver nitrate should be avoided because its use has been associated with meningitis.[6,8]

Ammonium Compounds

Ammonium compounds have been used in various concentrations (5% to 20%) in an attempt to damage pain fibers selectively while preserving the function of other fibers.[9,10] However, this selectivity does not appear to be possible. These compounds do not prevent the postneurolytic neuralgia seen with destructive blocks. The role of ammonium compounds in neurolytic block techniques is undecided at this time.

Tetracaine

Tetracaine in concentrations greater than those used for clinical anesthesia (eg, 1%, with the total dose restricted to 50 mg) has been used to effect prolonged block.[11]

Osmotic Neurolysis

The instillation of normothermic or hypothermic hypertonic saline solution into the subarachnoid space frequently is very uncomfortable for the patient and is associated with severe but transient pain, vertigo, weakness, and vomiting.[12–14] Among the complications of this procedure are severe hypertension, sinus tachycardia or bradycardia, ventricular ectopic beats, and pulmonary edema.[15,16] Some of these untoward effects are avoided by performing the procedure during general anesthesia.[12,13] The use of osmotic neurolysis in therapy is controversial.

Barbotage

The analgesic effect of barbotage is speculated to result from a partial demyelinization of the spinal cord, resulting from the alteration in local pressure.[16] The principal complication, occurring in 80% of patients In Lloyd and coworkers' series, is severe headache.[17] In that series, one death was attributed to thrombosis of the basilar vessels.[17]

GENERAL COMPLICATIONS

Complications may be categorized as in Table 43-3.

Failure of Neurolytic Block

Failure of nerve block is perhaps one of the most frustrating complications associated with neurolytic blocks. Often, after what appears to be meticulous placement of drugs in the appropriate anatomic site with confirmatory testing, the subsequent neurolytic block is short-lived, incomplete, or even absent. Knowledge of the action of these agents is incomplete and does not always permit full explanation of such enigmatic results. However, an incomplete block can always be repeated, if necessary.

Sometimes when working in vital areas in which precision is paramount, the anesthetist should risk the possibility of an incomplete block, use a conservative approach, and be prepared to return later, rather than proceed with an overly generous initial dose and as a result involve an adjacent vital structure. The possibility of failure can be minimized by meticulous adherence to technique and by the use of ancillary aids, such as biplane fluoroscopy (in addition to contrast media) or a nerve stimulator, in an effort to position the needle more accurately at the target.

TABLE 43-2
Complications of Intrathecal Neurolytic Blocks

DURATION OF COMPLICATIONS	DRUGS ADMINISTERED	CASES (no.)	BLADDER PARESIS	BOWEL PARESIS	MUSCLE PARESIS	HEADACHE	PARESTHESIA	NUMBNESS	HYPERESTHESIA	OTHERS
BRIEF										
≤72 hours	Phenol*	145	7			5		7		Nausea
	Chlorocresol†	138	4		7	4	1	13	2	Backache and nausea (2)
	Phenol and chlorocresol	17	2	2			1	2		Involuntary movements of contralateral leg
	Total	300	13	2	7	9	2	22	2	6
LONGLASTING										
>7 days	Phenol*	145	8	1	3		1	4		
	Chlorocresol†	138	11	1	7	1	1	5		
	Phenol and chlorocresol	17	3	1		1		1		
	Total	300	22	3	10	2	2	10		

* 5% or 7% in glycerin.

† 1:50 or 1:40 in glycerin.

Adapted from Swerdlow M: Complications of neurolytic blockade. In Cousins MJ, Bridenbaugh PO (eds): Neural blockade, 2nd ed. Philadelphia: JB Lippincott, 1988, 723.

TABLE 43-3
Complications of Neurolytic Blocks

- Failure of block
- Spread to other, nontarget structures
- Sphincter disturbances (bladder and/or bowel)
- Denervation
  - Trophic changes
  - Neuritis
  - Anesthesia dolorosa
  - Corneal damage

Often, the pain felt by many patients with cancer is attributable not as much to the noxious afferent input as it is to other less specific but still very real causes, such as anxiety and depression. In those cases, although it interrupts afferent input, a neurolytic block will not put an end to complaints that are generated psychologically. Therefore, the block may be deemed to have failed. Hence, diagnostic evaluation should be carried out before a neurolytic block is considered, and only if pain relief is obtained by repeated diagnostic procedures is a neurolytic block performed.

Spread to Other Structures

Like conventional local anesthetics, neurolytic substances can spread to involve structures other than their intended target when they are injected percutaneously. The result ranges from a relatively mild focal necrosis of musculoskeletal tissue, causing some self-limiting discomfort for a day or so, to effects on vital structures such as the optic nerve or spinal cord, with consequences of blindness and myelitis.[18]

To prevent spread of hyperbaric or hypobaric neurolytic solutions with segmental neurolytic subarachnoid blocks, the patient should not be moved from the blocking position too soon, to prevent involvement of other nerves or the spinal cord. However, concentrations of alcohol[5] and phenol[19] decrease so rapidly that within 10 to 15 minutes the patient may adopt a more comfortable position without risk of gravitational or turbulent spread of the agent in the cerebrospinal fluid.

A test dose of local anesthetic often can confirm needle position or detect placement of the needle in a dural sleeve or other site that might lead to accidental intrathecal injection.[20]

Sphincter Disturbance

With neurolytic blocks involving the sacral roots or the cauda equina, control of the bladder and bowel sphincters often may be disturbed. Temporary disturbance of bladder or bowel function may occur with use of segmental thoracic or lumbar neurolytic blocks. This risk should be explained to the patient beforehand. This complication usually is of a limited duration, resolving within several days to about 4 weeks.

If neurolytic block of the cauda equina or sacral roots is undertaken, the possibility of long-term sphincter disturbance must be appreciated by both the patient and the anesthesiologist before performance of the block. Thus, the patient's pelvic or lower-extremity pain must be so severe that he or she is willing to accept the possibility of bladder or bowel incontinence. Neurolytic blocks involving sphincter control are usually reserved until these functions are already compromised by the neoplastic disease causing the pain.

Bladder Dysfunction

In patients with bladder dysfunction, the most common presentation is retention of urine with overflow incontinence. This problem usually is caused by spillage of neurolytic agent onto sacral roots of the cauda equina, anywhere between their origins at the T12–L1 level to their emergence by way of the sacral foramina. In lumbar neurolytic blocks, therefore, the neurolytic substance should be deposited in the most peripheral location possible in the subarachnoid space—that is, just within the theca rather than in a central position within the cauda equina.

If anesthetic effects are noted at a remote site (eg, sacral dermatomes) and not at the intended target, the injection should be stopped immediately. This complication often can be avoided by initial use of a diagnostic dose of local anesthetic to ascertain the position of the needle. The likelihood of incontinence also can be reduced by tilting the table in the appropriate direction for hyperbaric and hypobaric solutions so that the neurolytic agent tends to flow away from the sacral roots.

Most bladder dysfunction difficulties are temporary, and an indwelling catheter and continuous drainage prevent urinary retention and minimize infection that could result in permanent damage. As recovery occurs and the patient no longer needs the catheter, micturition is performed on a time-contingent basis. The anesthesiologist facing any of these complications should not hesitate to seek the assistance of a urologist.

DENERVATION

Trophic Changes: Sloughing

Sloughing of areas of skin and subcutaneous tissues after alcohol injections and neurolytic procedures on branches of the trigeminal nerve has been described.[18] The mechanism of this process is not entirely clear. Because the nerves are in close proximity to the corresponding arteries, injection of a neurolytic solution may involve destruction of an artery. However, in general, the collateral circulation should be more than adequate to compensate for this vascular interruption, particularly in the head and the neck. Perhaps local conditions compromise collateral perfusion. Also, denervated tissues undergo trophic changes and become subject to undetected trauma that progresses to infection and tissue destruction.

Neuralgia

The discomfort that follows a neurolytic block of a peripheral nerve often is referred to as "postneurolytic neuralgia." This problem most frequently is seen when neurolytic blocks are performed on nerves distal to the foramina through which they emerge, in the skull or spinal cord. It can be so severe that, in general, peripheral neurolytic block is not advised for use in any patient with a long life expectancy and is reserved instead for terminally ill patients. An exception is neurolytic block of the peripheral branches of the trigeminal system; this technique appears to be relatively free from the occurrence of such complications.[21] However, the success of thermogangliolysis in the treatment of tic douloureux[22] has markedly decreased the need for neurolytic blocks of the trigeminal nerve. For the most part, then, neurolysis should be produced centrally, at a subarachnoid level, so that the neurolytic block involves the dorsal root selectively.[21]

The time after which postneurolytic neuralgia appears is variable, but 6 months is a figure often quoted.[21] A second neurolytic block at this stage, performed proximal to the site of the original procedure, can afford a few more months of pain relief and is justified in a terminally ill patient but not in a person with a long life expectancy.

New pain after a neurolytic block is often described by the patient as a sequela of the block procedure. However, it may have other causes. After the cessation of the primary pain, discomfort that previously had not troubled the patient often becomes more evident.

Painful paresthesia is the only reported toxic effect of phenol injection of peripheral nerves for spasticity; it occurs in less than 10% of cases.[23]

Anesthesia Dolorosa

Another complication of neurolytic procedures is anesthesia dolorosa, the patient's distress at the numbness produced. The denervated area can become painful, much as an amputated extremity can be a source of phantom limb pain. Why this phenomenon occurs is poorly understood. It may involve imbalances in the afferent neuronal input to the central nervous system, at the spinal cord or at higher levels.[24]

The patient should be permitted to experience the sequelae of a neurolytic block by initial use of temporary agents, especially long-acting local anesthetic agents, such as bupivacaine and etidocaine. Some patients prefer to have pain rather than numbness! However, even if numbness is well tolerated for the duration of a temporary diagnostic block, it may be more disturbing if present for a considerable period after neurolysis. Treatment for anesthesia dolorosa is unsatisfactory, but some patients may respond to carbamazapine, in dosages of as much as 1400 mg/day, or to combinations of amitriptyline, 75 to 150 mg/day, with or without fluphenazine, 3 to 6 mg/day. This long-term deafferentation is one reason that the procedure is best reserved for the terminally ill. Patients whose pain is of a nonmalignant origin are not candidates for neurolytic procedures.

Corneal Damage

The sequela to neurolytic block of the gasserian ganglion—corneal damage—is often the most distressing aspect of this procedure. The cornea is rendered insensitive; therefore, the accumulation of foreign objects (eg, dust or dirt) produces a chronic conjunctivitis that can lead to ulceration and infection.

Several suggestions have been made to cope with this problem. A lateral tarsal fusion can reduce the conjunctival surface area at risk without impairing vision. Also, meticulous cleansing of the conjunctival sac with appropriate lubricants and antibiotic agents and the wearing of special spectacles with side screens can reduce the incidence of complications.

Hemifacial numbness after gasserian ganglion block also results in analgesia of the ipsilateral half of the oral cavity and spillage of accumulated saliva from that side of the mouth. For many patients this problem is distressing. It is perhaps best treated with an antisialagogue such as diphenhydramine or even glycopyrrolate to reduce saliva production.

NEUROLYTIC EPIDURAL BLOCK

The injection of neurolytic agents into the epidural space has been used in the past. This procedure involves a relatively large volume of neurolytic agent; therefore, accidental subarachnoid injection, a potential complication of all epidural injections, must be avoided. However, relatively few other complications appear to occur, except temporary sphincter impairment interfering with bladder control.[25]

Epidurally injected alcohol is very painful unless preceded by a local anesthetic block. Epidurally injected phenol is less painful and has been used in concentrations of 5% to 10%.[26,27] Theoretically, epidurally administered neurolytic agents offer advantages. Spread to the cranial cavity is unlikely, and meningeal irritation can be avoided. The potential problems are listed in Table 43-4.

NEUROLYTIC LUMBAR SYMPATHETIC BLOCK

Chemical sympathectomy with neurolytic agents administered by a percutaneous technique into the lumbar sympathetic chain is used quite extensively and safely to improve blood supply to the lower extremities in elderly patients with peripheral vascular disease.[28,29] These techniques, usually performed with fluoroscopic control, appear to be safe, with relatively few complications (see Table 43-4). Somatic neuralgia, usually in the genitofemoral nerve distribution, occurs in fewer than 10% of patients.

Ejaculatory failure has been reported in a younger patient subjected to bilateral chemical sympathectomy in connection

TABLE 43-4
Complications of Neurolytic Epidural and Lumbar Sympathetic Blocks

EPIDURAL

- Accidental subarachnoid injection
- Temporary interference with bladder control
- Pain with alcohol injection (prevented by local anesthetic)
- Spread to cranial vault (very rare)

LUMBAR SYMPATHETIC

- Somatic neuralgia (primarily genitofemoral nerve)
- Ejaculatory failure (usually short-lived)

with Buerger's disease. The complication, however, was short-lived, and spontaneous recovery occurred at 2 weeks.[30] It seems to have been associated with bilateral interruption of sympathetic chains and also has been reported in about 2% of patients after neurolytic celiac plexus block.[31]

NEUROLYTIC CELIAC PLEXUS BLOCK

The most frequent indication for neurolytic celiac plexus block is the relief of intra-abdominal cancer pain, primarily from the stomach and pancreas. Because the celiac plexus provides innervation to most of the gut from the lower esophagus to the splenic flexure of the colon, its application is potentially widespread.[31] Various agents have been used to achieve neurolysis. Brown recommends 50% alcohol, formulated from absolute alcohol, and 0.25% bupivacaine to a total dose of 50 mL.[32] I prefer to use the alcohol *without* any added local anesthetic—the burning discomfort is very short-lived (less than 30 to 60 seconds). It is then possible to assess if the block is complete. If the local anesthetic is used with the alcohol, it is not possible to assess if any relief is the action of the local anesthetic or the alcohol until several hours have elapsed. Patients are "warned" ahead of time about the anticipated burning pain, and they cope well.

Potential complications are listed in Table 43-5.[33] Epidural or spinal spread can occur because of the proximity of the celiac ganglion to the central neuraxis.[33] Aortic puncture occurs frequently (in approximately one third of cases) but rarely is problematic. The neurolytic solution also can involve the lumbar nerve roots, an apparently infrequent complication. An increase in bowel motility and bowel movements can be expected for a few days. Hypotension is a common problem but usually for only the first 24 hours after the block. It usually responds to administration of fluids, and a vasopressor such as ephedrine may be needed in the immediate post-block recovery period (1–3 hours). Partial to complete pain relief is present in over 70% of patients for at least 3 months after the block.[33]

TABLE 43-5
Complications of Celiac Plexus Block

- Spread to central neuraxis
- Aortic puncture
- Kidney puncture
- Increased bowel motility and bowel movements
- Hypotension
- Spread to lumbar roots: neuritis
- Failure of ejaculation
- Intravascular injection
- Pneumothorax
- Spinal or paraspinal pain
- Loss of anal and bladder sphincter control

Swerdlow M: Complications of neurolytic neural blockade. In Cousins MJ, Bridenbaugh PO (eds): Neural blockade. Philadelphia: JB Lippincott, 1988: 719.

TABLE 43-6
Prevention of Complications of Neurolytic Blocks

- Always perform diagnostic blocks before neurolytic blocks. These usually include a short-acting agent (eg, lidocaine), a long-acting agent (eg, bupivacaine), and a placebo; ideally, these are administered on separate occasions before neurolytic blockade.
- Always warn the patient beforehand regarding complications, and allow the patient to play an active part in the decision to proceed with neurolysis, once he or she is aware of the risks and complications. "Permanent blocks" are rarely permanent and often must be repeated within several months. Obtain a signed informed consent.
- When contemplating nerve block for a patient with preexisting neurologic deficits or disease of the nervous system (eg, poliomyelitis or multiple sclerosis), it is necessary to document fully the nerve deficits before the block procedure, so that any preexisting defect will not be ascribed retrospectively to the anesthetic technique or agent.
- Do not perform neurolytic blocks in a patient with a long life expectancy.
- Avoid neurolytic blocks on peripheral nerves (with the exception of the branches of the trigeminal and glossopharyngeal), except in the terminally ill patient.
- Segmental subarachnoid block, unilateral or bilateral (as required), is the preferred neurolytic block for treatment of pain in the trunk.
- Neurolytic blocks are best used for treatment of pain in the head, thorax, or abdomen; block of nerves of the brachial or lumbosacral plexus can compromise the function of the extremities. If neurolysis involves the cauda equina, sphincter incontinence may result.
- Do not administer premedication to a patient undergoing neurolytic block.
- Use a test dose.
- Neurolytic agents should be used only by physicians experienced in performing regional nerve block procedures.
- Neurolytic block rarely solves a patient's pain problem by itself. Other modalities of supportive therapy (eg, medications, psychotherapy, or support) frequently are required, even if noxious input has been totally eliminated.

RECOMMENDATIONS

Selective neurolytic blocks have a definite role in the treatment of chronic pain and the relief of spasticity. Because of the meticulous technique required and the potential for complications, they probably should be undertaken only by experienced practitioners. Like the pain relief, which in many cases is temporary, most complications are not permanent and resolve with time. Many of the reported impairments of sphincter dysfunction last only a few days to 1 week.[2,9,35] Even when motor weakness complicates neurolytic block, it can resolve in a short time.[9,36,37]

Because the pain relief resulting from neurolytic nerve blocks is relatively finite, these techniques are eminently suitable for patients with finite pain, such as that of terminal cancer. However, they are rarely indicated for the management of pain of nonmalignant causes, in which the pain may persist for years.

Prevention of the complications associated with neurolytic blocks can be enhanced by adherence to the principles summarized in Table 43-6.

REFERENCES

1. Swerdlow M: Intrathecal chlorocresol. Anaesthesia 28:297, 1973
2. Nathan PW, Scott TG: Intrathecal phenol for intractable pain: the safety and dangers of the method. Lancet 1:76, 1958
3. Kuzucu EY, Derrick WS, Wilbur SA: Control of intractable pain with subarachnoid alcohol block. JAMA 195:541, 1966
4. Reid W, Watt JK, Gray TG: Phenol injection of the sympathetic chain. Br J Surg 57:45, 1970
5. Matsuki M, Kato Y, Ichiyanagi K: Progressive changes in the concentration of ethyl alcohol in human and canine subarachnoid spaces. Anesthesiology 36:617, 1972
6. Nathan PW, Sears RA: Effect of phenol on nervous conduction. J Physiol 150:565, 1960
7. Esplin DW: Antiseptics and disinfectants; fungicides; ectoparasiticides. In Goodman LS, Gilman A (eds): The pharmaceutical basis of therapeutics, 4th ed. New York: Macmillan, 1970: 1036
8. Maher RM: Intrathecal chlorocresol (parachlormetacresol) in treatment of pain of cancer. Lancet 1:965, 1963
9. Swerdlow M: Intrathecal and extradural block. In: Relief of intractable pain, 3rd ed. Amsterdam: Excerpta Medica, 1983
10. Wright BD: Treatment of intractable coccygodynia by transsacral ammonium chloride injection. Anesth Analg 50:519, 1971
11. Khalili AA, Ditzler JW: Neurolytic substances in relief of pain. Med Clin North Am 52:163, 1968
12. Hitchcock E: Hypothermic subarachnoid irrigation for intractable pain. Lancet 1:1133, 1967
13. Hitchcock E: Osmolytic neurolysis for intractable facial pain. Lancet 1:434, 1969
14. Robbie DS: General management of intractable pain in advanced cancer of the rectum. Proc R Soc Lond 62:1225, 1969
15. Thompson GE: Pulmonary edema complicating intrathecal hypertonic saline injection of intractable pain. Anesthesiology 35: 425, 1971
16. O'Higgins JW, Padfield A, Clapp H: Possible complications of hypothermic-saline subarachnoid injection. Lancet 1:567, 1970
17. Lloyd JW, Hughes JT, Davies-Jones GAB: Relief of severe intractable pain by barbotage of cerebral spinal fluid. Lancet 1: 354, 1972
18. Moore DC: Complications of regional anesthesia. Springfield, IL: Charles C Thomas, 1965:119–140
19. Ichyanagi K, Matsuki M, Kinefuchi S, et al: Progressive changes in concentrations of phenol and glycerine in human subarachnoid space. Anesthesiology 42:622, 1975
20. Galizia EJ, Lahiri SK: Paraplegia following coeliac plexus block. Br J Anaesth 46:539, 1974
21. Bonica JJ, Buckley FP, Moricca G, Murphy TM: Neurolytic Blockade and Pituitary Hypophysectomy. In Bonica JJ (ed): The management of pain, 2nd ed. Philadelphia: Lea & Febiger, 1990: 1980
22. Sweet WH, Wepsic JG: Controlled thermocoagulation of trigeminal ganglion and rootlets for differential destruction of pain fibers: I. trigeminal Neuralgia. J Neurosurg 40:143, 1974
23. Moritz U: Phenol block of peripheral nerves. Scand J Rehabil Med 5:160, 1973
24. Melzack R: Phantom limb pain: implications for treatment of pathological pain. Anesthesiology 35:409, 1971
25. De Beule F, Schottee A: Nouvelle étapes dans la lutte contre la douleur. Alcoholisation paravertébrale et épidural. Alcoholisation de plexus solaire. Rev Belge Sci Med 67:357, 1934
26. Laurie H, Vanasupa R: Comments on the use of intraspinal phenol pantopaque for relief of pain and spasticity. J Neurosurg 20: 60, 1963
27. Finer B: Epidural injection of carbolic acid in incurable cancer. Lancet 2:1179, 1958
28. Cousins MJ, Reest TS, Glynn CJ, et al: Neurolytic lumbar sympathetic blockade: duration of denervation and relief of rest pain. Anaesth Intensive Care 7:121, 1979
29. Hatangdi VS, Boas RA: Lumbar sympathectomy: a single needle technic. Br J Anaesth 57:285, 1985
30. Baxter AD, O'Kafo BA: Ejaculatory failure after chemical sympathectomy. Anesth Analg 63:770, 1984
31. Black A, Dwyer B: Coeliac plexus block. Anaesth Intensive Care 1:315, 1973
32. Brown DL: Atlas of regional anesthesia. Philadelphia: WB Saunders, 1992: 245
33. Eisenberg E, Carr DB, Chalmers TC: Neurolytic celiac plexus block for treatment of cancer pain: a meta-analysis. Anesth Analg 80:290, 1995
34. Moore DC: Celiac (splanchnic) plexus block with alcohol. Adv Pain Res Ther 2:357, 1979
35. Stovner J, Endresen R: Intrathecal phenol for cancer pain. Acta Anaesthesiol Scand 16:17, 1972
36. Hughes JT: Thrombosis of posterior spinal arteries. Neurology 20:659, 1970
37. Wilkinson HA, Mark VH, White JC: Further experiences with intrathecal phenol for relief of pain. Journal of Chronic Disease 17:1055, 1964

FURTHER READING

Dixon C: Pain management consultation in adult patients. In Kirby RR, Gravenstein N (eds): Clinical anesthesia practice. 1994

Murphy TM: Chronic pain. In Miller RD (ed): Anesthesia, vol 4. New York: Churchill Livingstone, 1994: 2345

Swerdlow M: Complications of neurolytic neural blockade. In Cousins MJ, Bridenbaugh PO (eds): Neural blockade. Philadelphia: JB Lippincott, 1988: 719

Complications in Anesthesiology, second edition,
edited by Nikolaus Gravenstein and Robert R. Kirby.
Lippincott-Raven Publishers, Philadelphia © 1996.

CHAPTER 44

The Allergic Response and Anesthesia

Marc Goldberg

The incidence of allergic reactions in hospitalized patients is 1% to 4%.[1] Allergy can be considered a set of undesirable physiologic changes that occur in response to ingestion of a foreign substance.[2] True allergy requires an immune mediator and thus previous exposure to a foreign material for recognition. Many foreign substances, though, elicit a noxious response on first exposure, by nonimmunologic mechanisms. Most adverse reactions to drugs are called "allergy," even though evidence of a true allergic reaction is difficult to obtain.

Antigens are foreign substances, usually complex organic molecules, which because of structural similarity to lymphocyte-bound recognition sites can stimulate antibody production. Because most drug molecules are relatively small, they must bind to a protein to become antigenic.[3] Small protein-bound immunogenic compounds are called "haptens."

Anaphylaxis is defined as an "explosive, untoward physiologic reaction" to foreign proteins or other substances.[4] Not all allergic reactions are anaphylactic; allergic reactions may be very mild or may take the form of delayed or cytotoxic reactions.

DETERMINANTS OF SUSCEPTIBILITY

Some patients are more likely than others to have drug allergies. Those who have any food or pollen allergy have a two- to tenfold greater likelihood of having allergies to certain drugs such as radiographic contrast media.[5,6] However, given the low incidence, a history of allergy in a patient is an unreliable predictor of the risk of an allergic reaction.[7] Patients with cardiac disease or asthma have a higher incidence of allergy.[6] Cross reactions to drugs similar in structure (eg, penicillin and the cephalosporins,[8] thiopental and amylbarbital[9]) may occur in some patients. An atopic history, though, may not be of predictive value when considering reactions to anesthetic drugs.[10] The risk of anaphylaxis is not related to gender, age, or season but is increased with intermittent exposure to the antigen and with parenteral antigen administration. Whether atopy increases the risk of anaphylaxis is controversial; some evidence deemphasizes the link.[11]

Genetic Factors

Various factors indicate a genetic basis for allergic susceptibility. Patients with higher immunoglobulin E (IgE) concentrations tend to have more allergies than other patients. Marsh and colleagues, using inheritance analysis, determined that the trait of high IgE concentrations is inherited in an autosomal recessive pattern, whereas low concentrations of IgE are inherited in an autosomal dominant fashion.[12] These findings are consistent with the incidence in the general population of high IgE concentrations and the familial tendency toward atopy. High IgE production, perhaps resulting from a defect in the normal control of the IgE-producing system, increases the number of allergic determinants recognized and thus the likelihood of reaction.

Genetic Markers

The human leukocyte antigen (HLA) system has been identified as a marker of allergic responsiveness. HLA antigens appear on the surface of all cells in the body; each person has a specific combination of parental antigens. The presence or absence of a certain antigen type has been correlated positively with certain diseases. HLA-B7, a specific HLA type, is found commonly in patients who react to ragweed pollen but rarely in nonreactive persons.[13] Furthermore, patients with generalized allergic hyperresponsiveness frequently have HLA-A1, HLA-B8 or HLA-B8, HLA-Dw3 phenotypes, whereas among patients who have hyporesponsiveness the HLA-A1 and HLA-B8 phenotypes are less common.[12]

Adrenergic and Cholinergic Receptors

The cellular "defect" that produces allergic reactions in susceptible patients is not completely known. In vitro studies have shown decreased β-adrenergic receptors on the lymphocytes of allergic patients compared with nonallergic patients.[14,15] β-Adrenergic antagonists such as propranolol not only increase symptoms of asthma but also have been reported to potentiate anaphylaxis.[16,17] The link between decreased β-receptor activity and allergy is that activation of β-receptors stimulates a prolonged increase in intracellular cyclic adenosine monophosphate concentrations. This reaction in turn inhibits cell degranulation and release of vasoactive mediators. Allergic and asthmatic patients may have defective or decreased numbers of β-adrenergic receptors.[16]

Allergic and asthmatic patients also have increased cholinergic sensitivity and may have increased α-adrenergic sensitivity.[15] The resulting adrenergic imbalance causes some of the manifestations of anaphylactic reaction. The clinical relevance of this receptor theory is that α-adrenergic agents (eg, phenylephrine) and cholinergic stimuli possibly should be avoided during anaphylactic reactions.

Antibody–Antigen Interaction

"Immune surveillance"[18] is the lymphocyte-based system by which organisms differentiate their own cellular characteristics from those of foreign substances. During fetal development, every lymphocyte develops a unique pattern of surface markers, composed of IgD and IgM, by genetic recombination. As a result, the number of different foreign antigens that can be recognized is almost infinite. Foreign substances ingested later react with the lymphocyte whose surface markers most closely match their own.

B Lymphocytes

The interaction of antigen with lymphocyte membrane-bound antibody activates the lymphocyte. The cell then clones itself and produces and secretes immunoactive substances. Lymphocytes originating in the bursa of Fabricus (B lymphocytes), which mature primarily in the bone marrow, secrete immunoglobulins. These secreted proteins have the same recognition areas as those that were fixed to the original lymphocyte membrane. Serum antibody proteins act primarily by adhering to antigen to enhance antigen recognition and elimination; by activating complement; and by fixing to mast cells and basophils, thus initiating the inflammatory process.

T Lymphocytes

Lymphocytes activated in the thymus (T lymphocytes) recognize both foreign antigens and the cell membrane–based HLA system. T cells, like B cells, undergo proliferation and secrete immunoactive lymphokines, which are short-lived hormone-like messengers capable of causing other blood elements to become active, to aggregate, to secrete vasoactive mediators, and to lyse, thus promoting inflammation or anaphylaxis. The subsets of T cells include helper cells, delayed hypersensitivity cells, killer cells, and suppressor cells. T cells are involved in allergic reactions primarily because they facilitate or suppress the activation of B cells and the formation of antibodies.

Immunoglobulins

The antibody immunoglobulin fraction of serum protein is significant[19]: 9 to 20 mg of protein per mL of serum is immunoglobulin, that is, as much as 33% of total serum protein. An immunoglobulin is a large (150,000 to 900,000 Da) polypeptide made up of three fragments: two identical, called the Fab fragments, and a third, called the Fc fragment. The Fab fragments function together as the antibody recognition–antigen binding sites, and the Fc portion is required for complement fixation. A typical immunoglobulin molecule is shown in Figure 44-1.

Five immunoglobulin types are distinguished by the types of heavy polypeptide chains that form the molecule. The five heavy chains (α, δ, ε, γ, and μ) form IgA, IgD, IgE, IgG, and IgM, respectively. By far the most common immunoglobulin is IgG, composing about 80% of the total, followed by IgA (10%), IgM (5%), and IgD and IgE (<1% each).[19]

IgM. IgM is found on nonactivated lymphocytes in monomeric form and when secreted into serum, in a pentameric structure, with ten Fab sites per molecule. IgM is very efficient in causing complement activation. Increased serum IgM is usually the first immune response to a new antigen.

IgG. The IgG molecule is the second immunoglobulin generated in response to exposure to a new antigen. In addition to causing activation of other cellular elements, it contains multiple binding sites for complement. It is the only immunoglobulin capable of crossing the placenta. Transplacental passage of anti-D, the maternal IgG antibody formed in response to Rh-positive fetal red blood cells, causes Rh hemolytic disease ("erythroblastosis fetalis") in subsequent Rh-positive fetuses.

IgD and IgA. IgD functions principally as a primary receptor on lymphocyte membranes, as does IgM. Serum IgA has no known unique defense functions, although mucosal IgA plays a role in combatting enteral infective agents.

IgE. IgE is unique among the immunoglobulins in that it has a high avidity for tissues, mast cells, and basophils.[20] Production of IgE requires introduction of small amounts of antigen into the organism; ingestion of larger amounts of antigen stimulates production of IgG or IgM.

In contrast to IgG and IgM, as much as 50% of serum IgE is specific for a certain antigen. The serum IgE response to antigen ingestion is short-lived, with a half-life of 2.7 days,[21] but IgE persists much longer on the cell membranes of mast cells and basophils. Interaction of IgE with its antigen triggers the anaphylactic response, stimulating basophils and mast cells to release histamine, slow-reacting substance of anaphylaxis (a combination of leukotrienes C_4, D_4, and E_4), and other mediators. Relatively small amounts of antigen are capable of causing an IgE-mediated anaphylactic response because of a cascade effect in which mediator release causes further mediator release.

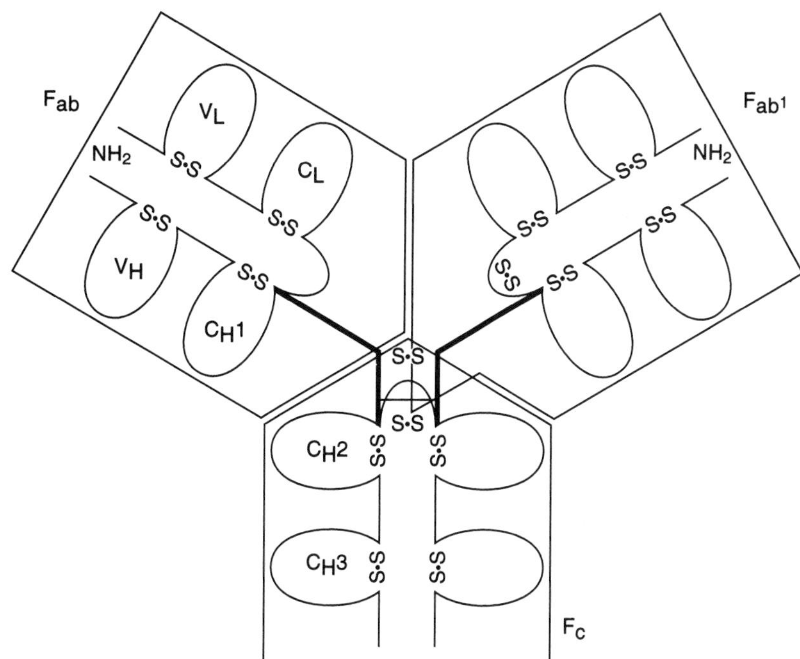

FIGURE 44-1. The five types of immunoglobulin share the same light (*L*) chain structure; they are differentiated by the type of heavy (*H*) chain: α, δ, ϵ, γ, or μ. The chains are covalently linked by disulfide bonds. The ability to recognize different antigens is provided by the variable (*V*) parts of the heavy and light chains. The Fab and Fab[1] sections of the molecule, which can be separated from the entire molecule by pepsin, are the portions that control antigen recognition. The Fc fragment is the area at which immunoglobulin molecules adhere to cell membranes. C, constant region. (Redrawn after Austyn JM, Wood KJ. Principles of cellular and molecular immunology. New York: Oxford University Press, 1993, 335.)

IgE is responsible for immediate hypersensitivity reactions (type I allergic reactions).[22] Mast cells and basophils carry IgE receptor molecules with extreme specificity for circulating IgE. When two or more molecules of IgE are bound and when an allergen contacts two or more IgE-based receptor sites, "bridging" or linkage between the receptor sites occurs. This reaction prompts activation of cell membrane–associated enzymes that temporarily increase the concentration of intracellular cyclic adenosine monophosphate and increase membrane phospholipid methylation; a cellular influx of calcium ions follows.[20] Calcium and cAMP are the intracellular messengers that cause release of the mediators of anaphylaxis.

MECHANISMS

Type I Reactions

A variety of mechanisms may cause anaphylaxis. Type I hypersensitivity is mediated by IgE, formed by the patient's B lymphocytes after previous exposure to the allergen. Agents that produce anaphylaxis mediated by IgE include antibiotics,[23,24] foreign proteins,[25,26] drugs,[26–31] latex,[32] and foods.[33] Exposure to minute quantities of allergens can produce IgE antibodies; subsequent exposure to equally small quantities can produce anaphylaxis.[20] Cross reaction to closely related foreign substances (eg, to penicillin and the cephalosporins in approximately 5% of patients allergic to penicillin)[8] may occur. Distinct sensitization to different parts of a drug may occur; some patients have anti-insulin[34] and anti-protamine[35] antibodies as a consequence of treatment with neutral protamine Hagedorn NPH insulin.

Anaphylactoid Reactions

Anaphylactoid reactions differ from anaphylactic reactions in that neither immunoglobin nor past exposure to the "allergen" is required. Thus, the instigators of anaphylactoid reactions are not truly allergens. These substances usually have basic, positively charged components that cause direct displacement of histamine from mast cells and basophils.[36] Patients with a history of atopy, multiple allergies, or drug reactions are more likely to have anaphylactoid reactions than are other patients.[37] However, if enough drug of this type is injected fast enough, in almost all patients an anaphylactoid reaction with hypotension and cutaneous manifestations develops. Examples of anesthetic-related drugs that act in this manner are curare,[38–40] morphine,[41] atracurium,[42–45] thiopental,[41,46,47] and dextran.[48]

Inhibition of Cyclo-oxygenase

Aspirin and nonsteroidal anti-inflammatory agents may cause anaphylactic reactions by inhibiting the enzyme cyclo-oxygenase.[49] This enzyme is required for synthesis of prostaglandins from arachidonic acid. The drugs thus decrease the availability of prostaglandins that mediate bronchodilatation, predisposing the patient to the effects of other bronchoconstricting agents. Aspirin-induced anaphylaxis is more common in asthmatic patients.

Complement Activation

A final immune-related cause of anaphylaxis is complement activation (Fig. 44-2).[50,51] Circulating immune complexes (such as IgA–anti-IgA) and some drugs cause activation of the classic complement cascade, a chain reaction of serum proteins that eventually causes destruction of foreign substances. Ingested substances or immune complexes interact with preformed but not completely specific IgG or IgM; thus previous exposure to the "antigen" is not necessary. Immune complexes and drug–antibody reactions activate complement protein C1, which initiates the classic complement cascade.

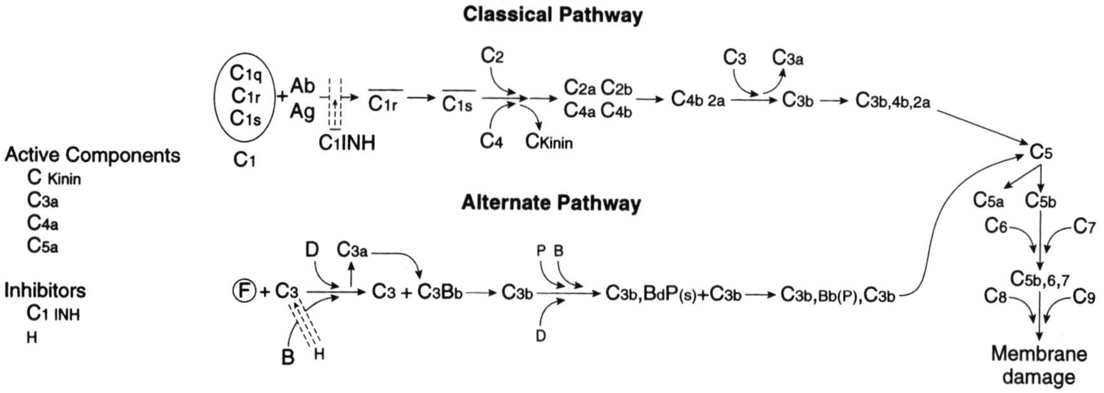

FIGURE 44-2. The classic complement pathway is activated when the C1 complex attaches to an antibody–antigen (*Ab–Ag*) complex. The alternate pathway is activated when a foreign substance (*F*) activates C3. Both pathways produce by-products that are cytotoxic or chemotactic. The pathways converge to a final end point, the C6-C9 complex, which is cytotoxic. Complement is involved in all anaphylactic reactions, whether through direct activation or through activation by the by-products of the reaction. (Redrawn after Bernier GM: Antibody and immunoglobins: structure and function. In Bellanti JA (ed): Immunology. Philadelphia: WB Saunders, 1971, 95)

In some anaphylactic reactions, however, changes in complement concentrations may result from intravascular volume redistribution rather than from complement activation.[52] Certain drugs cause activation of the alternate complement cascade by the direct interaction of the inciting substance and the C3 protein, which then activates the remainder of the complement cascade (see Fig. 44-2).[53]

Other Reactions

Two other anaphylactic syndromes that have been described are exercise-induced[54] and idiopathic[55] anaphylaxis. Extensive immunologic studies in these patients rarely disclose the source of the allergic stimulus, although occasionally a cause, such as endogenous progesterone,[56] is found.

In addition, not all drug reactions described by the patient as "allergic" are immunologic or anaphylactoid reactions. They may be toxic effects of the drug itself. The unintended intravascular injection of lidocaine with epinephrine and the intravascular administration of radiographic contrast media are two common examples of adverse reactions not necessarily caused by allergy.

MANIFESTATIONS

Anaphylactic reactions most often begin within 5 minutes of ingestion of the allergen, although rarely reactions may develop as long as 24 hours later. Pruritus, urticaria, and angioedema are often the initial symptoms. Nausea, abdominal pain, and diarrhea, sometimes bloody, occur in 20% to 50% of patients. Anaphylactic reactions during anesthesia are listed in Table 44-1.

Airway

Upper-airway manifestations include sneezing, dyspnea, and airway obstruction caused by pharyngeal edema. Wheezing

TABLE 44-1
Anaphylactic Reactions in Anesthesia and Intensive Care

SYSTEM	SIGNS
RESPIRATORY	• Cyanosis, wheezing, or increased peak airway pressure (23%) • Acute pulmonary edema • Bronchospasm (23%)
CARDIOVASCULAR	• Tachycardia • Dysrhythmia • Pulmonary hypertension • Decreased systemic vascular resistance • Cardiovascular collapse >68% • Cardiac arrest (11%)
CUTANEOUS	• Urticaria • Flushing (55%) • Perioral edema • Periorbital edema

Modified from Levy JH: Anaphylactic reactions in anethesia and intensive care. Boston: Butterworth, 1986: 19.

and bronchospasm may follow shortly. Intraoperative signs of anaphylaxis include decreased lung compliance, increased airway pressures, a prolonged exhalation phase, and pulmonary edema.

Cardiovascular System

Cardiac dysrhythmias and cardiovascular collapse may occur. Myocardial ischemia, caused by coronary artery vasoconstriction produced by histamine and leukotriene D_4, may cause decreased myocardial contractility.[57] The peripheral vasodilating effects of histamine may lead to severe decreases in preload and afterload and thereby to severe hypotension.

Beaupre and colleagues described a patient whose unexpected anaphylactic reaction to the cephalosporin antibiotic cefazolin was monitored by transesophageal echocardiography.[58] The patient's mean arterial blood pressure decreased by 51% and the pulmonary artery occlusion pressure by 47%; systemic and pulmonary artery occlusion also decreased. Left ventricular systolic and diastolic volumes decreased 60% to 70%. However, in part because of a compensatory increase in heart rate, the cardiac index increased 89%. No electrocardiographic or echocardiographic evidence of myocardial ischemia was seen. Myocardial contractility actually improved during this episode. Because the patient had severe coronary artery stenosis, the hypotension was treated with fluid infusion rather than with epinephrine, and hemodynamics returned to prereaction levels within 15 minutes.

Only one fourth of deaths during anaphylaxis are caused by cardiovascular collapse; two thirds are caused by respiratory insufficiency. Intense bronchospasm may be the presenting sign. Hypoxemia can occur rapidly,[59] and death can ensue within several minutes.

In fatal cases of anaphylaxis, severe lung hyperinflation with scattered atelectasis, pulmonary edema,[60] hemorrhages, bronchorrhea, and eosinophilic bronchiolar infiltration is seen. Edema of the hypopharynx, epiglottis, and larynx are prominent.

MEDIATORS

Anaphylaxis, as a syndrome, appears the same whether it is mediated by IgE, immune complexes, or nonantigenic drugs. Mast cell degranulation, histamine release, complement activation, and prostaglandin synthesis potentiate the release and activation of the anaphylactic process by positive-feedback pathways. The mediators of allergic and anaphylactic responses are listed in Table 44-2.

Allergy Testing

In vivo and in vitro allergy tests are used. The ideal test would be an inexpensive, prospective, in vitro assay.

Intradermal Skin Test

In this type of test, small quantities of allergen, in 1:1000 weight-to-volume dilutions, are injected 0.3 mm into the dermis.[61] Reactivity is graded on a scale of 0 to 4+, depending on the area of erythema and wheal produced. Most people have sufficient IgE antibody to raise small wheals to common antigens. However, the testing procedure is very time-consuming, requiring 20 minutes between injections.

Prick or Scratch Test

Much higher concentrations of antigen are required for this test than for the intradermal test. The allergen is placed on the skin, and a small lancet introduces it into the epidermis.

TABLE 44-2
Mediators of Allergic and Anaphylactic Reactions

Histamine	Histamine H_1 receptors mediate bronchospasm, increase vascular permeability, decrease atrioventricular conduction, decrease coronary artery blood flow, and cause chemotaxis
Slow reacting substance of anaphylaxis (leukotrienes C_4, D_4, and E_4)	Decreases pulmonary compliance and increases vascular permeability
Eosinophil chemotactic factor of anaphylaxis	Attracts eosinophils to aid elimination of antigen–antibody complexes
Platelet-activating factor	Releases lysozomes, prostaglandins, and platelet factor 4; contracts smooth muscle
Serotonin	Causes bronchoconstriction
Prostaglandin (D_2)	Increases cyclic adenosine monophosphate concentration and contracts airway smooth muscle
Neutrophil chemotactic factor	Releases lysozyme and accelerates complement-aided neutrophil killing of parasites
Bradykinin	Increases vascular permeability and causes pain
Coagulation cascade	Activated during anaphylaxis, resulting in decreased fibrin and thrombin levels and production of fibrin split products
Heparin	Released during anaphylaxis; function unknown

The prick test is faster and easier to perform, allows testing of several antigens in one session, and is more comfortable than intradermal testing. In addition, its results correlate well with those of intradermal testing.[62] Intradermal tests are more sensitive and have better reproducibility, but both types of test correlate well with clinical signs of allergy and with in vitro tests for presence of IgE.

Several factors affect the usefulness of skin testing. The maximum response to histamine and allergen occurs in the evening and the minimum in the morning.[61] Some areas of the body react more than others. In infants and persons older than 60 years, reaction is less pronounced than in young adults. Reactions are suppressed by a variety of medications.

Both the allergen and its diluent must be tested to ensure that a reaction is not caused by the diluent. In approximately 2% to 8% of patients without clinical allergy, the test reaction is positive, and variations in the quantity of test allergen may cause an unknown percentage of false-negative results. With intradermal testing, anaphylactic reactions may occur; immediate treatment must be available.

Prausnitz-Kustner Test

This test requires injection of the serum from a sensitive person into the dermis of a nonsensitive person and introduction of allergen near the site of serum injection. Appearance of a dermal reaction is proof of transference of a sensitizing antibody. Prausnitz-Kustner testing carries the risk of transmission of serum-borne diseases.

In Vitro Test

This type of test determines the presence of specific IgE, affinity of antibody for antigen, and the ability of antigen to cause cell activation.[63] Equilibrium dialysis determines the affinity of antibody for haptens. Complement activity can be used to assay antigen–antibody affinity. A variety of radioimmunoassay techniques have been developed.

RADIOALLERGOSORBENT TEST. The most clinically useful in vitro technique is the radioallergosorbent test (RAST). Initially, the allergen in question is bound to a polysaccharide and exposed to serum from a potentially allergic patient. IgE antibodies from the patient react with the antigen. After washing, the polysaccharide is is subjected to reaction with radiolabeled anti-human IgE, and the residual radioactivity is quantified.

RAST has several advantages: there is no risk to the patient; quantitative results are not changed by concomitant drug administration; and there is good correlation with clinical signs of allergy. However, the test is expensive, and some allergens are not yet available for use in RAST.

LYMPHOCYTE HISTAMINE RELEASE TEST. Another method of demonstrating antibody–antigen interaction is to expose target cells, such as lymphocytes, to serum antibodies with antigen and determine the degree of cell activation or mediator release. The lymphocyte histamine release test has been used, but it does not differentiate immunologically mediated histamine reactions from direct drug-mediated release. This method is expensive and has less clinical utility than does RAST.

TEST FOR DECREASE IN COMPLEMENT AND IMMUNOGLOBULIN E. During an allergic reaction, immediate decreases in complement alone or in both complement and IgE may indicate anaphylactoid or immune sensitivity. The results are correlative, however, and not absolute proof of the cause of a reaction.

ANESTHETIC DRUGS THAT MAY CAUSE REACTIONS

Induction Agents

Thiopental

Thiopental was first reported to be responsible for a hypersensitivity reaction in 1952,[64] and since then a variety of anaphylactic reactions in different circumstances have been reported.[41,42–47,65–68] The incidence of anaphylaxis to thiopental is 1 in 29,000 to 1 in 36,000 patients, with a 10% to 15% mortality rate.[65–67] Relatively few patients who have thiopental anaphylaxis are patients considered at high risk (those with atopy, with other drug or food allergies, or with asthma).

IMMUNOGLOBULIN E–MEDIATED REACTIONS. Until the advent of IgE assays, little evidence was available that IgE actually mediated thiopental reactions. Lilly and Hoy described a patient with asthma in whom anaphylaxis developed during his seventh exposure to thiopental.[65] Shortly after the episode, the patient's serum concentration of IgE decreased markedly, suggesting that the reaction was of IgE origin. Fisher performed Prausnitz-Kustner and passive cutaneous anaphylaxis tests on serum from patients with clinical thiopental-related anaphylaxis; one patient who had received thiopental five times was found to have an anti-thiopental IgE antibody.[27]

DIRECT RELEASE OF HISTAMINE. Direct drug-mediated release of histamine is a prominent cause of anaphylactoid reaction to thiopental. Hirshman described a patient with asthma in whom severe bronchospasm and hypotension developed after thiopental administration.[69] Serum IgE concentrations did not change, but leukocyte histamine release testing demonstrated substantial histamine release on exposure to thiopental and morphine.

Other Barbiturates

Other barbiturates have been reported to cause anaphylaxis. Thiamylal anaphylaxis has been reported rarely, and methohexital sensitivity was noted in 1 in 7000 patients.[70,71] Oral administration of amylbarbital has been implicated as a cause of subsequent thiopental anaphylaxis.[9]

Ketamine

A macular rash developed in a 3-year-old child 6 minutes after his fifth exposure to ketamine.[72] Prausnitz-Kustner testing was negative, making an immunologic mechanism of reaction unlikely. Doenicke administered ketamine along with other anesthetics to volunteers, and found no evidence of histamine release or immunoglobulin development.

Althesin

A steroidal hypnotic agent used in Europe, althesin (alphaxalone–alphadolone) is associated with a high incidence, approximately 1 in 1000 patients, of allergic reactions.[66,73] Anaphylaxis has been reported to develop within 2 weeks of initial exposure to althesin.[74] Although the fatality rate associated with the drug is very low, the high incidence of reactions has made althesin unpopular. Repeated exposure to althesin or to drugs dissolved in the same vehicle, cremophor EL, has been cited as contributory to althesin reactions.[75]

Propanidid

Like althesin, propanidid is associated with far higher incidence of allergic or anaphylactic reactions, 1 in 750 administrations, than is thiopental or ketamine.[66] Cremophor EL is used as a vehicle for propanidid. Although this substance is not antigenic by itself, it seems to promote reactions and cross reactions to drug formulations that contain it. The dose-related cardiac depression caused by propanidid must be differentiated from true anaphylaxis.

Etomidate

Etomidate has been called an "immunologically safe" induction agent; no anaphylactic reactions were reported in more than 3,000,000 administrations.[76] Several cases of urticaria or flushing have occurred, but two patients in whom hypotension developed had also been given muscle relaxants.[76] Although etomidate has minimal histamine-releasing or cardiovascular effects when used as an induction agent, it has been shown to interfere with adrenal cortisol production.[77] Use of etomidate for long-term sedation was associated with an increased surgical mortality in a small series of patients.[77]

Propofol

Clinical features of anaphylaxis are relatively rare after propofol administration. However, numerous case reports have begun to appear. The relation of the drug to bronchospasm and hypotension is difficult to establish because of concomitant administration of other drugs. Anaphylaxis may occur in response to the vehicle (10% soybean oil, 2.25% glycerol, and 1.2% purified egg phosphatide) or to the propofol itself.[78,79] In Laxenaire and colleagues' series, 9 of 14 patients with life-threatening reactions to propofol had a history of allergy (atopy or allergy to antibiotics, muscle relaxants, colloids, or lidocaine) preoperatively.[80] The authors recommended that propofol not be used in an anesthetic regimen that includes a histamine-releasing drug such as atracurium for patients at risk for releasing excessive histamine.[80] Patients allergic to soybean oil, egg phosphatide, or glycerol may have anaphylactic reactions to propofol.

Muscle Relaxants

All of the muscle relaxants used currently, with the possible exception of vecuronium, have been associated with histamine release or anaphylaxis. The frequency of anaphylaxis attributable to relaxants probably has been underestimated; some relaxant-caused reactions have been attributed to induction agents.[68] Patients who have hypersensitivity reactions to relaxants tend to have other drug allergies, asthma, or atopy.[80,81,82] Adverse reactions are seen five to eight times more often in women than in men.[81] Eighty-five percent of patients who react to relaxants have not been exposed previously, suggesting cross sensitivity to other relaxants, other drugs such as penicillin, or even substances such as cosmetics.[81] Succinylcholine and gallamine cause a disproportionately high proportion of reactions relative to their frequency of use,[68] whereas reactions to pancuronium and vecuronium are less common. The benzylisquinolone structure appears to be responsible for histamine release.[82]

Whether reactions are caused by direct histamine release or are mediated by antibody–antigen mechanisms can be distinguished only by the Prausnitz-Kustner test, a passive cutaneous serum transfer test, or an assay for specific anti-relaxant IgE.[10] Skin testing with low concentrations of muscle relaxants does not differentiate immune-mediated sensitivity from direct histamine release by mast cells and may not be predictive of anaphylaxis. For example, pancuronium, which causes sensitivity infrequently, often causes skin wheals in nonatopic patients.[83] A positive result on skin testing to succinylcholine has been considered a contraindication to its use.[27]

Succinylcholine

Erythema, macular rashes,[84] upper-airway edema,[85] bronchospasm,[84] and hypotension[84,86] have been reported after succinylcholine injection. The frequency of succinylcholine anaphylaxis is approximately 1 in 5000 administrations, and the female-to-male ratio for its occurrence is 8:1.[81] Inadequate anesthesia for tracheal intubation and the use of other drugs (ie, induction agents) must be considered before bronchospasm is attributed to succinylcholine.

Harle and colleagues demonstrated the presence of IgE antibodies reactive against choline in sera from nine of ten patients who had anaphylaxis when given succinylcholine and thereby proved an immunologic basis for hypersensitivity to succinylcholine in some patients.[28] However, Fisher and Roffe failed to find any predictive value in IgE concentrations after anaphylactoid reactions to relaxants.[10]

d-Tubocurarine

This drug, and to a lesser extent dimethylcurarine, cause dose-related histamine release.[40] This effect is enhanced by rapid administration of larger doses of curare, such as a 0.6-mg/kg bolus. Anaphylactoid reactions and the effects of histamine release seem more pronounced in asthmatic and atopic patients than in others. Whether histamine or other vasoactive mediators, such as the slow-reacting substance of anaphylaxis, is more important in the promotion of bronchospasm by curare is uncertain.[87] Reports of anaphylactoid reactions to curare in patients at low risk are rare. In one patient, cross sensitivity appears to have developed between curare and alcuronium, a pancuronium analogue.[81]

Gallamine

Approximately 20 reports of anaphylaxis in response to gallamine have been published since its introduction in 1949. Evans and McKinnon described a patient with no risk factors who, on exposure to gallamine, had severe erythema, angioedema, and hypotension without bronchospasm.[88] The result of a subsequent skin test to gallamine was strongly positive. All reported cases of gallamine hypersensitivity have occurred in women, but this disproportion may reflect the small number of case reports and the overall greater incidence of relaxant-related anaphylaxis in women.

Pancuronium

Pancuronium has been noted to cause histamine release[83] and anaphylaxis,[89] but the incidence of patient sensitivity to pancuronium is extremely low.

Vecuronium

Vecuronium has not been reported to cause anaphylaxis, and it does not alter serum histamine concentrations in doses as large as 3.5 times the dose effective in 95% of subjects (ED_{95}), which is much larger than the clinical dose range.[90] Vecuronium and pancuronium appear to be the safest and least likely to cause cross reactions. Vecuronium, with only one quaternary ammonium group, may pose particularly little risk of sensitizing patients to other muscle relaxants.

Atracurium

Atracurium causes histamine release but to a much smaller degree than does curare and only at multiples of the usual intubating dose. Mercer reported a severe anaphylactic reaction to atracurium in an asthmatic woman who had not been exposed to the drug previously.[42]

Mivacurium

Mivacurium causes histamine to be released in an amount that is related to the dose and rate of administration, particularly in some patients when twice the ED_{95} is given over only 10 to 15 seconds. Savarese and associates determined that the changes in blood pressure and other histamine-related events can be described by the dose ratio (ED_{50} for histamine-related events divided by the ED_{95} for neuromuscular blockade, where ED_{50} = the dose effective in 50% of subjects).[91] Others have shown that oral premedication with histamine H_1 and H_2 antagonists substantially reduce histamine release after the administration of 0.21 mg/kg, which is three times the ED_{95}.[92]

Narcotics

Although morphine, dihydromorphone, and meperidine are known to cause histamine release, only one report of an IgE-mediated anaphylactic reaction to a narcotic, meperidine, has been published.[93] Fahmy documented an anaphylactic response to morphine, noting marked increases in plasma histamine concentrations and a decrease in systolic blood pressure and systemic vascular resistance (Fig. 44-3).[94] Philbin and colleagues demonstrated that previous administration of the histamine blocking agents diphenhydramine and cimetidine can attenuate the decrease in blood pressure and systemic vascular resistance caused by 1 mg/kg morphine.[95]

Local Anesthetics

Allergy to local anesthetic compounds is uncommon. The vast majority of "reactions" reported by patients are caused by rapid intravascular injection, rapid systemic uptake of the an-

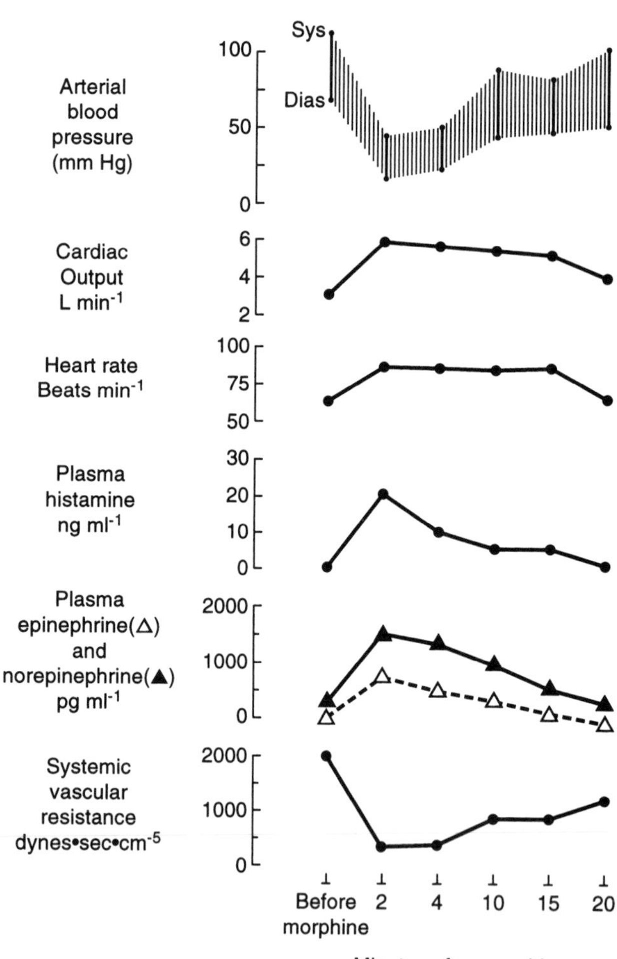

FIGURE 44-3. Hemodynamic, histamine and catecholamine changes during an anaphylactoid reaction to 0.3 mg/kg intravenous morphine. *Sys*, systolic; *Dias*, diastolic. (Redrawn after Fahmy NR: Hemodynamics, plasma histamine, and catecholamine concentrations during an anaphylactoid reaction to morphine. Anesthesiology 55: 330, 1981)

esthetic, or the effects of epinephrine injected with the anesthetic. Probably fewer than 1% of adverse reactions to local anesthetics are allergic in origin.

Esters

Ester-containing compounds (tetracaine and procaine) are especially likely to cause true allergic reactions because they are metabolized to and resemble *p*-aminobenzoic acid. *p*-Aminobenzoic acid is a common environmental chemical irritant and is found in many sunscreens, the use of which may be the first exposure before exposure during anesthesia. Furthermore, the methylparaben preservative used in many preparations of local anesthetics, rather than the anesthetic itself, may be the actual source of allergy.

Amides

Brown described a patient who gave a history of a severe reaction to lidocaine.[96] Skin testing with prilocaine produced a transient local flare and no systemic effects. Intradermal injection of 0.2 mL 0.5% bupivacaine produced urticaria, visual difficulties, and a feeling of "tightness" in the throat. A marked reduction of complement C4 and small reduction of C3 suggested an allergic reaction, but no antibodies to lidocaine or bupivacaine were identified.

This case appears to be the sole documented allergic reaction to an amide-type local anesthetic. The strong reaction to skin testing and the reaction, however mild, to a similar agent suggest that skin testing may be dangerous or of little value in the evaluation of local anesthetic allergy. More useful is avoidance of agents of the class alleged to have caused a reaction in the past and, particularly, use of preservative-free preparations of the drugs.

BLOOD TRANSFUSION

Blood transfusion causes a typically mild allergic reaction during approximately 3% of administrations.[97] Major transfusion reactions involving hemolysis and renal failure are caused by administration of incorrectly ABO–cross-matched blood; however, these reactions are rare.

Most (75%) immunologic reactions are manifested by fever; about 10% are anaphylactic.[98] Donor serum contains elements such as leukocytes, platelets, and plasma proteins to which the recipient either has antibodies or to which antibodies develop. Centrifugation and filtration to remove platelets, fibrin, and leukocytes can reduce the incidence of fever by 77% to 98%.[98]

Natural deficiency of IgA occurs in 1 in 700 patients; repeated transfusions of donor serum containing IgA causes production of recipient anti-IgA antibodies. Washing red blood cells to remove leukocytes and plasma reduces by half the incidence of transfusion reactions.[97] Antibodies also may be formed against clotting factors and against the antigens composing the various minor blood group systems (Lewis, P, MNSs, Kell, Duffy, and Rh). An uncommon allergic reaction to blood is the development of pulmonary edema and arterial hypoxemia without other manifestations of anaphylaxis.

Transfusion reactions may be avoided by seeking a history of past transfusion or reaction; taking care in the matching of blood and rejecting non–cross-matched blood; maintaining sterile administration conditions; screening for unusual antibodies in patients who receive multiple transfusions; and, in the patient at high risk, use of prophylactic antihistamines. Most blood transfusion reactions are the result of a clerical error rather than a cross-matching error.

OTHER DRUGS

Plasma Expanders

Dextran

Dextran causes allergic reactions infrequently. Studying a series of 1.3 million administrations, Ljungstrom and coworkers reported a 0.013% incidence of reaction to dextran 40 and a 0.025% incidence of reaction to dextran 70.[48] Allergic tendencies did not predispose to anaphylaxis, but increasing age, diabetes, cardiovascular and pulmonary disease, and chronic infection were prominent among patients with severe reactions. The male-to-female ratio for all dextran reactions was 1.5:1. Administration of 20 mL of dextran 1 (Promit) markedly reduces the incidence of severe reactions. This low–molecular-weight dextran, serving as an antigen, creates an environment of antigen excess in which it occupies all antibody binding sites, which therefore are not available for dextran 40 or 70.[99]

Symptoms typically begin rapidly after infusion is begun, with pruritus, chills, and mild respiratory distress after a small-volume infusion of dextran. Rapid fluid administration is vital to success during resuscitation. Because several fatal dextran reactions have occurred after administration of only 0.5 mL, Ljungstrom and coworkers advise against in vivo skin testing.[99]

Hydroxyethyl Starch and Plasma Fractions

This plasma expander is associated with allergic reactions in 0.006% of administrations. Commercial preparations of heat-treated albumin or plasma protein fractions may cause non-allergic vasodilatation if infused rapidly, perhaps by production of a kallikrein factor during the heating process.[100]

Protamine

Mechanisms

ALLERGIC. Protamine sulfate is used to reverse the anticoagulant effects of heparin. It is capable of causing a decrease in systemic vascular resistance and hypotension in almost all patients if given quickly.[101] Protamine is a protein derived from salmon sperm cells and is thus immunogenic.[102] Patients who have allergies to fish, who have had vasectomies (and perhaps have autoantibodies to sperm cells), who have taken neutral protamine Hagedorn insulin on a long-term basis, and who have been exposed repeatedly to protamine have been reported to have anaphylactic reactions. IgG antibodies to protamine have been demonstrated.[102]

Protamine is a basic compound that can cause direct release of histamine. Administration into the left atrium or aorta rather than into a vein has been claimed to decrease the amount of histamine released, probably by bypassing the histamine-rich pulmonary parenchyma.[103]

A marked decrease in systemic vascular resistance is the principal manifestation of protamine reactions. In several patients noncardiogenic pulmonary edema has developed.[104] A rare syndrome of pulmonary vasoconstriction has been described in patients who have mitral insufficiency or pulmonary artery hypertension.[105]

NONALLERGIC. Other proposed nonallergic causes of hypotension from protamine include calcium chelation, a direct negative inotropic effect, and an unspecified adverse effect caused by the heparin–protamine complex.[101]

Treatment

If allergy to protamine is known or possible, protamine should be avoided and heparin allowed to metabolize. Alternately, slow intravenous infusion of small test doses (eg, 5 to 10 mg) of protamine may be attempted, or left atrial or aortic administration may be used. Pretreatment with antihistamines and steroids before exposure to protamine may prevent reactions. Other agents capable of reversing the anticoagulant effect of heparin, such as hexadimethrine, and platelet factor 4 (Pf4)[106] are still under investigation.

Chymopapain

Chymopapain was first used in 1964 for chemonucleolysis of herniated lumbar intervertebral discs. Thousands of patients were treated, and approximately 80% reported relief of symptoms. However, because of the incidence and severity of allergic reactions to this substance, it is no longer available in the United States.

Because chymopapain is an enzyme, patients may have anti-IgE antibodies to it.[107] These antibodies are derived from exposure to papaya or meat tenderizers. The incidence of anaphylactic reactions to chymopapain ranges from 0.35% to 5%.[108] Patients may lack the usual predisposing factors noted in other types of allergy, except for a 2:1 female-to-male ratio in the incidence of reaction. Kapsalis and associates prospectively used a RAST-like test for the presence of anti-chymopapain IgE in 1263 patients; in 67 the test result was positive, but only 7 had anaphylaxis.[108] Five patients had anaphylaxis and a negative IgE test.

The use of prednisone and histamine-blocking drugs as prophylaxis against reaction is controversial. Hall and colleagues suggested that pretreatment would not decrease the incidence of anaphylaxis to less than the 0.35% they reported and would result in 99% of patients receiving unnecessary treatment.[107]

Administration of intervertebral chymopapain was most often performed during local anesthesia with sedation. Subjective symptoms are thus easily identified. Bruno and coworkers reported severe hypotension after a test dose of chymopapain.[109] Thus, full preparation for the treatment of anaphylaxis was required during and after chymopapain instillation. Because the drug is not available, the discussion, although interesting, is moot.

Radiographic Contrast Media

Clinical Manifestations

The incidence of severe and fatal allergic reactions to contrast media is 0.08%.[37] A true immunologic basis for these reactions, with antibody formation, is unusual. However, the common contrast media are hyperosmolar; are capable of chelating calcium, releasing histamine, activating complement; and may cause electrocardiographic signs of ischemia and dysrhythmias. Adverse reactions include nausea, sensations of "warmth," pruritus, and urticaria. Serious reactions include rapid development of upper-airway edema, bronchospasm, hypotension, and ventricular dysrhythmias.

Risk Factors and Prophylaxis

Risk factors for more serious reactions include a history of any allergy, atopy, or allergy to contrast media or to seafood; the iodine content (>20 g) of the dose of contrast media used; and cardiac disease. Recommended prophylaxis for the patient at high risk consists of cancellation of proposed studies unless absolutely indicated and administration of prednisone and diphenhydramine for 24 hours before the study.[110] Steroid administration has been shown to increase the concentration of an inhibitor of complement activity, C1 esterase inhibitor, and to decrease the likelihood of an anaphylactoid reaction.[111]

A multi-institutional, randomized study demonstrated that two orally administered doses of corticosteroid (32 mg methylprednisolone) 12 and 2 hours before challenge with contrast media is very effective in reducing the incidence of allergic reactions.[112] The author noted that this regimen reduced the incidence of reactions with conventional ionic media to that approximating the rate associated with newer, nonionic contrast media without steroid pretreatment. Although the newer contrast media appear preferable, their cost is about 15 times that of the conventional media. Thus, they should be reserved for special indications.

Latex

In the past decade, latex has been identified as another source of intraoperative anaphylaxis. Latex is virtually ubiquitous in the operating room (Table 44-3) and may be the source of as many as 10% of the anaphylactic events in the operating room.[113] Patients who have myelodysplasia or congenital genitourinary abnormalities, who have undergone multiple procedures, and who wear a latex appliance are especially at risk. In addition, all health care workers are at potentially increased risk for latex allergy because of their frequent exposure to latex. Latex allergy may be either a contact dermatitis or a type I, IgE-mediated acute hypersensitivity. Latex allergy among occupationally exposed physicians results in an overall latex allergy incidence of 10%, with a slightly higher incidence of 5 of 43 (12%) among anesthesiologists.[114] Hospital physicians who are atopic (those who have allergic rhinitis or

TABLE 44-3
Latex-Containing Medical Equipment

ANESTHESIA-RELATED	ACCESSORY EQUIPMENT
Endotracheal tubes	Surgical gloves
Face masks	Adhesive tape
Pharyngeal airways	Elastic bandages
Bite blocks	Rubber pads
Teeth protectors	Protective sheets
Ventilator hoses	Urinary catheters
Ventilator bellows	Drains
Blood pressure cuffs	Electrode pads
	Intestinal tubes
	Stomach tubes
	Condom urinals
	Rubber dams (dentistry)

Gerber AC, Jörg W, Zbinden S, et al: Severe intraoperative anaphylaxis to surgical gloves: latex allergy, an unfamiliar condition. Anesthesiology 71:801, 1989.

conjunctivitis, asthma, or eczema) have a 24% incidence of latex allergy.[114] If latex allergy is possible, skin-prick testing is sensitive and specific in indicating IgE latex antibody.[115]

POSTANESTHETIC HEPATITIS

Possible Allergic Basis

Inhalational anesthetics have not been implicated in immediate hypersensitivity reactions, but one of the purported mechanisms of "halothane hepatitis" is immunologic damage by cell-mediated immunity. In vitro, halothane decreases chemotaxis and transiently depresses lymphocyte activation.[116,117] Halothane and other anesthetics cause bone marrow depression after long exposures.[118]

Postanesthetic hepatitis has been described as a syndrome characterized by skin rash; fever; bronchospasm; eosinophilia; presence of autoantibodies to thyroglobulin and to liver and kidney microsomes; and positive results on skin challenge tests to halothane.[119] These symptoms resemble the clinical course of disease known to be caused by cell-mediated immunity. Mathieu and colleagues demonstrated in guinea pigs the production of anaphylactic and hemolytic antibodies to trifluoroacetate, which is a metabolite of halothane, enflurane, and fluroxene.[120] On reexposure to the metabolite, antibody concentrations decreased, suggesting that antibody–antigen complexes were formed (see Chap. 51).

Autoimmune Mechanisms

Vergani and colleagues hypothesized that halothane alters hepatocyte membrane antigenicity and produces an autoimmune response in susceptible patients.[119] Serum from patients who had fulminant, halothane-associated hepatitis was capable of reacting immunologically with the hepatocytes of rabbits exposed to halothane within the same 12-hour period. Neuberger and associates isolated an IgG antibody from patients who had fulminant anesthetic-related hepatitis and showed its specificity to liver cell membranes altered by halothane.[121] The antibody was absent from patients who had hepatitis not associated with halothane. Halothane presumably altered a membrane determinant of hepatocytes, making them susceptible to autoantibody production and cytotoxic lymphocytes.

PROPHYLAXIS

Drug Therapy

The most effective prophylaxis against repeated drug allergy is avoidance of the agent in question. This approach usually is possible in anesthetic practice. Yet certain drugs known to be allergens (eg, intravascular contrast media and protamine) must be used occasionally despite the potential for anaphylaxis. Prophylactic use of histamine H_1– and H_2–blocking drugs has been shown to decrease the anaphylactoid properties of 1 mg/kg morphine as an anesthetic.[95]

Diphenhydramine and Prednisone

Administration of diphenhydramine, 50 mg orally in two doses before and two doses after contrast media, and prednisone, 20 mg every 6 hours from 18 hours before to 12 hours after contrast media, decrease the expected 21% to 37% incidence of severe reactions to 0% to 4% per administration; mild reactions occur in 5%.

Cromolyn Sodium

Prophylactic use of cromolyn sodium has been suggested but not documented to decrease allergic sensitivity. Cromolyn sodium acts by preventing the release of vasoactive mediators from basophils and mast cells.[122] It inhibits mediator release stimulated by cell-bound IgE–antigen interaction, by exercise-induced asthma, and by non-IgE mechanisms. The mediator inhibition can be overcome if the antigen is present in large amounts. Tachyphylaxis to cromolyn sodium has been reported in vitro and in vivo.[122]

Cromolyn sodium has a biphasic effect; acutely it stabilizes mast cells, decreases activity of irritant receptors, and has an α-adrenergic blocking effect. Chronic administration gradually decreases airway responsiveness to histamine and causes increased bronchodilatation in response to atropine. The mechanism of mast cell stabilization is controversial, but theories include phosphodiesterase inhibition; phosphorylation of proteins and binding of calcium required for histamine secretion; and inhibition of oxygen-free radical formation.

Cromolyn sodium has a short serum half-life and must be administered as an inhalant four times daily. A 4- to 8-week trial period in allergic patients with asthma may be required before clinical benefit is seen. Longer-lasting, faster-acting, orally administered analogues of cromoglycate are being investigated.

TREATMENT

Despite careful history-taking, pretesting, and prophylaxis, some patients still have allergic reactions during anesthesia. Prompt recognition and early treatment are the keys to moderating morbidity and mortality. Immediate steps should include increase in the inspired oxygen concentration, increase in the rate of infusion of intravenous fluids, and discontinuation of anesthesia. Infusions of potential allergens such as blood or antibiotic agents also should be stopped.

Drug Therapy

Pharmacologic treatment is summarized in Table 44-4. Adrenergic agonists act by supporting cardiac output and blood pressure and biochemically slow the anaphylactic process by decreasing mediator release. If hypotension is the predominant sign of reaction, epinephrine is the preferred drug. It should not be given intravenously in the absence of hypotension.[123] If bronchospasm is more prominent, aminophylline or isoproterenol (β_1-selective agents) are useful. Bronchodilators (eg, albuterol) can be given with a metered dose inhaler placed in the anesthetic circuit.[124] Antihistamines are not particularly useful once an allergic reaction is underway but are not harmful.

Steroids have several anti-inflammatory actions that are potentially useful in the treatment of or prophylaxis against allergic reactions.[125,126] In the intravascular space, they cause vasoconstriction and decreased vascular permeability; lymphopenia, including a decrease in B lymphocytes; a decrease in the tissue histamine concentration; a decrease in chemotactic activity; and an increase in the catabolism of immunoglobulins.[125] At the intracellular level, they decrease the release of vasoactive mediators from lysosomes; increase intracellular concentrations of cyclic adenosine monophosphate by adenyl cyclase activation; decrease macrophage activation and phagocytosis; increase the sensitivity of β-adrenergic receptors; and inhibit sensitivity to prostaglandins.

TABLE 44-4
Treatment of Anaphylactic Reactions Occurring During Anesthesia

PRIMARY MEASURES

1. Stop administration of antigen
2. Maintain airway; administer 100% oxygen
3. Discontinue anesthesia
4. Institute rapid intravascular volume expansion: crystalloid 2–4 L to help maintain blood pressure
5. Epinephrine 3–8 μg/kg, intravenous bolus, with dose adjusted to degree of hypotension

ADDITIONAL CONSIDERATIONS FOR INTRAVENOUS MEDICATION (depending on signs and symptoms)

1. Aminophylline 5–6 mg/kg over 20-minute period (loading dose); then 0.5–0.9 mg/kg/h infusion (maintenance dose), with dosage reduced 50% in patients with cardiac or renal failure
2. Epinephrine 1–4 μg/min, norepinephrine 2–4 μg/min, or isoproterenol 0.5–1.0 μg/min, adjusted to degree of hypotension
3. Hydrocortisone 0.25–1.0 g, methylprednisolone 0.1–1.0 g, or dexamethasone 4–20 mg, all intravenously
4. Diphenydramine 25–50 mg intravenously
5. Atropine 0.5–2.0 mg intravenously

REFERENCES

1. Girsh LS, Perelmutter LL:. The diagnosis of drug allergies utilizing in vitro mast cell test and IgE inhibition test. Allergologia et Immunopathologia 10:229, 1982
2. Middleton E, Reed CE, Ellis EF: Introduction. In Middleton E, Reed CE, Ellis EF (eds): Allergy: principles and practice. St. Louis: CV Mosby, 1983: xxi
3. Levine BB, Redmond AP: The nature of the antigen-antibody complexes initiating the specific wheal and flare reaction in sensitized man. J Clin Invest 47:556, 1968
4. Wasserman SI: Anaphylaxis. In Middleton E, Reed CE, Ellis EF (eds): Allergy: principles and practice. St. Louis: CV Mosby, 1983: 689
5. Ansell G, Tweedie MCK, West ER, et al: The current status of reaction to intravascular contrast media. Invest Radiol 15:532, 1980
6. Ansell G: Adverse reaction to contrast media: scope of problem. Invest Radiol 5:374, 1970
7. Fisher MM, Outhred A, Bowey CJ: Can clinical anaphylaxis to anaesthetic drugs be predicted from allergic history? Br J Anaesth 59:690, 1987
8. Girard JP: Common antigenic determinants of penicillin G, ampicillin and the cephalosporins demonstrated in men. Int Arch Allergy Appl Immunol 33:428, 1968
9. Davis J: Thiopentone anaphylaxis. Br J Anaesth 50:1159, 1971
10. Fisher MM, Roffe DJ: Allergy, atopy and IgE: the predictive value of total IgE and allergic history in anaphylactic reactions during anaesthesia. Anaesthesia 39:213, 1984
11. Horowitz L: Atopy as factor in penicillin reactions. N Engl J Med 292:1243, 1975
12. Marsh DG, Hsu SH, Hussain R, et al: Genetics of human response to allergens. J Allergy Clin Immunol 65:322, 1980
13. Steensgaard J, Johansen AS: Biochemical aspects of immune complex formation and immune complex disease. Allergy 35: 457, 1980
14. Conolly ME, Greenacre JK: The lymphocyte β-receptor in normal subjects and patients with bronchial asthma: the effect of different forms of treatment on receptor function. J Clin Invest 58:1307, 1976
15. Casale TB: The role of the autonomic nervous system in allergic disease. Ann Allergy 51:423, 1983
16. Shelhamer JH, Marom Z, Kalineer M: Abnormal β-adrenergic responsiveness in allergic subjects: II. the role of selective $beta_2$-adrenergic hyporeactivity. J Allergy Clin Immunol 70:57, 1983
17. Jacobs RL, Rake GW, Fournier DC, et al: Potentiated anaphylaxis in patients with drug-induced β-adrenergic blockade. J Allergy Clin Immunol 68:125, 1981
18. Burnet FM: Immunological surveillance. Sydney: Pergammon, 1970
19. Plojak RJ: Immunoglobulin structure and function. In Middleton E, Reed CE, Ellis EF (eds): Allergy: principles and practice. St. Louis: CV Mosby, 1983: 19
20. Sullivan TJ, Kulczycki A: Immediate hypersensitivity responses. In Parker CW (ed): Clinical immunology. Philadelphia: WB Saunders, 1980: 115
21. Waldmann TA, Iio A, Ogawa M, et al: The metabolism of IgE: studies in normal individuals and in a patient with IgE myeloma. J Immunol 177:1139, 1976
22. Wasserman SI. Mediators of immediate hypersensitivity. J Allergy Clin Immunol 72:101, 1983
23. Levine BB: Immunological mechanisms of penicillin allergy: a haptenic model system for the study of allergic diseases of man. N Engl J Med 275:1115, 1966
24. Pollen RH: Anaphylactoid reaction to orally administered demethylchlortetracycline. N Engl J Med 271:673, 1964
25. Hilgard P: Immunological reactions to blood and blood products. Br J Anesth 51:45, 1979
26. Kapalis AA, Stern IJ, Bornstein I: Correlation between hypersensitivity to parenteral chymopapain and the presence of IgE anti-chymopapain and the presence of IgE anti-chymopapain antibody. Clin Exp Immunol 33:150, 1978

27. Fisher MM: Reaginic antibodies to drugs used in anesthesia. Anesthesiology 52:318, 1980
28. Harle DG, Baldo BA, Fisher MM: Detection of IgE antibodies to suxamethonium after anaphylactoid reactions during anesthesia. Lancet 1(8383):930, 1984
29. Moudgil GC: Anaesthesia and allergic drug reactions. Can Anaesth Soc J 33:400, 1986
30. Bird AG: Severe drug reactions during anaesthesia. Adverse Drug Reactions and Acute Poisoning Reviews 6:117, 1987
31. Levy JH: Allergic reactions during anesthesia. J Clin Anesth 1:39, 1988
32. Holzman RS: Latex allergy: an emerging operating room problem. Anesth Analg 76:635, 1993
33. Yunginger JW, Sweeney KG, Sturner WQ, et al: Fatal food-induced anaphylaxis. JAMA 260:1450, 1988
34. Mattson JR, Patterson R, Roberts M: Insulin therapy in patients with systemic insulin allergy. Arch Intern Med 135:818, 1975
35. Lakin JD, Blocker TJ, Strong DM, et al: Anaphylaxis to protamine sulfate by a complement-dependent IgG antibody. J Allergy Clin Immunol 61:102, 1978
36. Sheffer AL, Wasserman SI: Anaphylaxis. In Cohen AS (ed): Rheumatology and immunology, vol 4. The science and practice of clinical medicine. New York: Grune and Stratton, 1979: 468
37. Goldberg M: Systemic reactions to intravascular contrast media: a guide for the anesthesiologist. Anesthesiology 60:46, 1984
38. Basta SJ, Savarese JJ, Ali HH, et al: Histamine-releasing potencies of atracurium, dimethyl tubocurarine, and tubocurarine. Br J Anaesth 55:1055, 1981
39. Baldo BA, Fisher MM: Detection of serum IgE antibodies that react with alcuronium and tubocurarine after life-threatening reactions to muscle-relaxant drugs. Anaesth Intensive Care 11: 194, 1983
40. Comroe JH, Dripps RD: The histamine-like action of curare and tubocurarine injected intracutaneously and intra-arterially in man. Anesthesiology 7:260, 1946
41. Fisher MM: Severe histamine mediated reactions to intravenous drugs used in anaesthesia. Anaesth Intensive Care 3:180, 1975
42. Mercer JD: A severe anaphylactic reaction to atracurium. Anaesth Intensive Care 12:262, 1984
43. Aldrete JA: Allergic reaction after atracurium. Br J Anaesth 57:929, 1985
44. Tettzlaff JE, Gellman MD: Anaphylactoid reaction to atracurium. Can Anaesth Soc J 33:647, 1986
45. Rowlands DE: Harmless cutaneous reactions associated with the use of atracurium: a report of 1200 anaesthetics. Br J Anaesth 59:693, 1987
46. Westacott P, Ramachandran PR, Jancekwicz Z: Anaphylactic reaction to thiopentone: a case report. Can Anaesth Soc J 31: 434, 1984
47. Wright PJ, Shortland JR, Stevens JD, et al: Fatal haemopathological consequences of general anaesthesia. Br J Anaesth 62: 104, 1989
48. Ljungstrom KG, Renck H, Strindberg K, et al: Adverse reactions to dextran in Sweden 1970-1979. Acta Chirurgica Scandinavica 149:253, 1983
49. Flower RJ, Vane JR: Inhibition of prostaglandin biosynthesis. Biochem Pharmacol 23:1439, 1974
50. Fearon DT: Complement. J Allergy Clin Immunol 71:520, 1983
51. Hasselbacher P, Hahn J: In vitro effects of radiocontrast media on the complement system. J Allergy Clin Immunol 66:217, 1980
52. Fisher MM, Teisnner B, Charlesworth J: Significance of sequential changes in serum complement levels during acute anaphylactoid reactions. Crit Care Med 12:351, 1984
53. Fearon DT, Austen KF: The alternate pathway of complement: a system for host resistance to microbial infection. N Engl J Med 303:259, 1980
54. Sheffer AL, Austen KF: Exercise-induced anaphylaxis. J Allergy Clin Immunol 66:106, 1980
55. Lieberman P, Taylor WW: Recurrent idiopathic anaphylaxis. Arch Intern Med 139:1032, 1979
56. Meggs WJ, Pescovitz OH, Metcalfe D, et al: Progesterone sensitivity as a cause of recurrent anaphylaxis. N Engl J Med 311: 1236, 1984
57. Bristow MR, Ginsberg R, Harrison DL: Histamine and the human heart: the other receptor system. Am J Cardiol 49:249, 1982
58. Beaupre PN, Roizen MF, Cahalan MK, et al: Hemodynamic and two-dimensional transesophageal echocardiographic analysis of an anaphylactic reaction in a human. Anesthesiology 60:482, 1984
59. Velasquez JL, Gold MI: Anaphylactic reaction to cephalothin during anesthesia. Anesthesiology 43:476, 1975
60. Borish L, Matloff SM, Findley SR: Radiographic contrast media-induced noncardiogenic pulmonary edema: case report and review of the literature. J Allergy Clin Immunol 74:104, 1984
61. Wilson HS: Diagnostic procedures in allergy: I. allergy skin testing. Ann Allergy 51:411, 1983
62. Leynadier F, Sansarricq M, Didier JM, et al: Prick tests in the diagnosis of anaphylaxis to general anaesthetics. Br J Anaesth 59:83, 1987
63. Gleich GJ, Yunginger JW, Stobo JD: Laboratory methods for studies of allergy. In Middleton E, Reed CE, Ellis EF (eds): Allergy: principles and practice. St. Louis: CV Mosby, 1983: 271
64. Evans F, Gould J: Relation between sensitivity to thiopentone, sulphonamides, and sunlight. Br Med J 7:417, 1952
65. Lilly JK, Hoy RH: Thiopental anaphylaxis and reagin involvement. Anesthesiology 53:335, 1980
66. Stoelting RK: Allergic reactions during anesthesia. Anesth Analg 62:341, 1983
67. Chung DCW: Anaphylaxis to thiopentone: a case report. Can Anaesth Soc J 23:319, 1976
68. Dundee JW: Hypersensitivity to intravenous anaesthetic agents. Br J Anaesth 48:57, 1976
69. Hirshman CA, Peters J, Cartwright-Lee I: Leukocyte histamine release to thiopental. Anesthesiology 56:64, 1982
70. Reichert EF, Bassett PA: A rare allergic reaction to sodium methohexital. Journal of Oral Surgery 30:910, 1972
71. Driggs RL, O'Day RA: Acute allergic reaction associated with methohexital anesthesia: report of six cases. Journal of Oral Surgery 30:906, 1972
72. Mathieu A, Goudsouzian N, Snide MT: Reaction to ketamine: anaphylactoid or anaphylactic? Br J Anaesth 47:624, 1975
73. Watkins J, Clark A, Appleyard TN, et al: Immune-mediated reactions to althesin (alphaxalone). Br J Anaesth 48:881, 1976
74. Brown TCK, Doolan LA: Althesin reaction in a child. Anaesth Intensive Care 11:390, 1983
75. Beamish D, Brown DT: Adverse response to IV anaesthetics. Br J Anaesth 53:55, 1981
76. Watkins J: Etomidate: an 'immunologically safe' anaesthetic agent. Anaesthesia 38S:34, 1983
77. Wagner RL, White PF, Kan PB, et al: Inhibition of adrenal steroidogenesis by the anesthetic etomidate. N Engl J Med 310:1415, 1984
78. Laxenaire MC, Guéant JL, Barmejo E, et al: Anaphylactic shock due to propofol. Lancet 2:739, 1988
79. Jamieson V, Mackenzie J: Allergy to propofol? Anaesthesia 43: 70, 1988
80. Laxenaire M-C, Mata-Barmejo, Monet-Vautrin DA, et al: Life-threatening anaphylactoid reactions to propofol (Diprivan®). Anesthesiology 77:275, 1992
81. Fisher MM, Munro I: Life threatening anaphylactoid reactions to muscle relaxants. Anesth Analg 62:559, 1983
82. Levy JH, Adelson DM, Walker BF: Wheal and flare responses to muscle relaxants in humans. Agents Actions 34:302, 1991
83. Bodman RI: Pancuronium and histamine release. Can Anaesth Soc J 25:40, 1978
84. Matthews MD, Ceglaraski JZ, Pabari M: Anaphylaxis to suxamethonium: a case report. Anaesth Intensive Care 5:235, 1977
85. Cohen S, Lia KH, Marx GF: Upper airway edema: an anaphylactoid reaction to succinylcholine? Anesthesiology 56:467, 1982
86. Ravindran RS, Klemm JE: Anaphylaxis to succinylcholine in a patient allergic to penicillin. Anesth Analg 59:944, 1980

87. Hirshman CA: Airway reactivity in humans: anesthetic implications. Anesthesiology 58:170, 1983
88. Evans PJD, McKinnon I: Anaphylactoid reaction to gallamine triethodide. Anaesth Intensive Care 5:239, 1977
89. Brauer FS, Ananthaqnarayan CR: Histamine release by pancuronium. Anesthesiology 49:434, 1978
90. Tullock WC, Diana P, Cook DR, et al.: Neuromuscular and cardiovascular effects of high-dose vecuronium. Anesthesia and Analgesia 70:86, 1990
91. Savarese JJ, Ali HH, Basta SJ, et al: The cardiovascular effects of mivacurium chloride (BW B109OU) in patients receiving nitrous oxide–opiate–barbiturate anesthesia. Anesthesiology 70:386, 1989
92. Doenicke A, Mayer M, Nebauer AE: Mivacurium and histamine levels: oral premedication with H_1/H_2 antagonists prevents side effects. Anesthesiology 79:A931, 1993
93. Levy JH, Rockoff MA: Anaphylaxis to meperidine. Anesth Analg 61:301, 1982
94. Fahmy NR: Hemodynamics, plasma histamine, and catecholamine concentrations during an anaphylactoid reaction to morphine. Anesthesiology 55:329, 1981
95. Philbin DM, Moss J, Akins CW, et al: The use of H_1 and H_2 histamine antagonists with morphine anesthesia: a double-blind study. Anesthesiology 55:292, 1981
96. Brown DT, Beamish D, Wildsmith JAW: Allergic reaction to an amide local anaesthetic. Br J Anaesth 53:435, 1981
97. Goldfinger D, Lowe C: Prevention of adverse reactions to blood transfusion by the administration of saline-washed red blood cells. Transfusion 21:277, 1981
98. Wenz B: Microaggregate blood filtration and the febrile transfusion reaction: a comparative study. Transfusion 23:95, 1983
99. Ljungstrom KG, Renck H, Hedin H, et al: Prevention of dextran-induced anaphylactic reactions by hapten inhibition. Acta Chirurgica Scandinavica 149:341, 1983
100. Alving BM, Hojima Y, Pisano TJ, et al: Hypotension associated with prekallikrein activator (Hageman-factor fragments) in plasma protein fraction. N Engl J Med 299:66, 1978
101. Horrow JC: Protamine allergy. J Thorac Cardiovasc Anesth 2: 225, 1988
102. Lakin JD, Blocker TJ, Strong DM, et al: Anaphylaxis to protamine sulfate by a complement-dependent IgG antibody. J Allergy Clin Immunol 61:102, 1978
103. Frater RW, Oka Y, Hong Y, et al.: Protamine-induced circulatory changes. Journal of Thoracic and Cardiovascular Surgery 87:687, 1984
104. Olinger GN, Becker RM, Bonchek LI: Noncardiogenic pulmonary edema and peripheral vascular collapse following cardio-pulmonary bypass: rare protamine reaction? Ann Thorac Surg 29:20, 1980
105. Lowenstein E, Johnston WE, Lappas DG, et al: Catastrophic pulmonary vasoconstriction associated with protamine reversal of heparin. Anesthesiology 59:470, 1983
106. Kurrek MM, Winkler M, Robinson DR, Zapol WM: Platelet factor 4 injection produces acute pulmonary hypertension in the awake lamb. Anesthesiology 82:183, 1995
107. Hall BB, McCulloch JA: Anaphylactic reactions following the intradiscal injection of chymopapain under local anesthesia. J Bone Joint Surg [Am] 65:1215, 1983
108. Kapsalis AA, Stern IJ, Bornstein I: Correlation between hypersensitivity to parenteral chymopapain and the presence of IgE anti-chymopapain antibody. Clin Exp Immunol 33:150, 1978
109. Bruno LA, Smith DS, Bloom MJ, et al: Sudden hypotension with a test dose of chymopapain. Anesth Analg 63:533, 1984
110. Greenberger PA, Patterson R, Simon R, et al: Pretreatment of high risk patients requiring radiographic contrast media studies. J Allergy Clin Immunol 67:185, 1981
111. Lasser EC, Long JH, Hamblin AE, et al: Activation systems in contrast idiosyncrasy. Invest Radiol 15:52, 1980
112. Lasser EC: Pretreatment with corticosteroids to alleviate reactions to intravenous contrast material. N Engl J Med 317: 845, 1987
113. Slatter JE: Rubber anaphylaxis. N Engl J Med 320:1126, 1989
114. Arellano R, Bradley J, Sussman G: Prevalence of latex sensitization among hospital physicians occupationally exposed to latex gloves. Anesthesiology 77:905, 1992
115. Wrangso K, Wahlberg JE, Axelsson IGK: IgE-mediated allergy to natural rubber in 30 patients with contact urticaria. Contact Dermatitis 19:264, 1988
116. Vosw BM, Kimber I: The effects of halothane on antibody-dependent cellular cytotoxicity in rats. Immunology 32:609, 1977
117. Salo M, Lassila O, Viljanen M, et al: Effect of halothane anaesthesia on secondary antibody response and mitogen-induced lymphocyte transformation in the chicken. Acta Pathologica et Microbiolica Scandinavica 86:105, 1978
118. Cullen BF, Van Belle G: Lymphocyte transformation and changes in leukocyte count: effects of anesthesia and operation. Anesthesiology 43:563, 1975
119. Vergani D, Miele-Vergani G, Alberti A, et al: Antibodies to the surface of halothane-altered rabbit hepatocytes in patients with severe halothane-associated hepatitis. N Engl J Med 303:66, 1980
120. Mathieu A, Padua D, Kahan BD, et al: Humoral immunity to a metabolite of halothane, fluroxene, and enflurane. Anesthesiology 42:612, 1975
121. Neuberger J, Gimson AES, Davis M, et al: Specific serological markers in the diagnosis of fulminant hepatic failure associated with halothane anaesthesia. Br J Anaesth 55:15, 1983
122. Johnson HG: Cromoglycate and other inhibitors of mediator release. In Middleton E, Reed CE, Ellis EF (eds): Allergy: principles and practice. St Louis: CV Mosby, 1983: 613
123. Levy JH: Cardiovascular changes during anaphylactic/anaphylactoid reactions. J Clin Anesth 1:426, 1989
124. Gold MI, Marcial E: An anesthetic adapter for all metered dose inhalers. Anesthesiology 68:964, 1988
125. Claman HN: How corticosteroids work. J Allergy Clin Immunol 55:145, 1975
126. Morris HG: Factors that influence clinical responses to administered corticosteroids. J Allergy Clin Immunol 66:343, 1980

FURTHER READING

Austyn JM, Wood KJ. Principles of cellular and molecular immunology. New York, Oxford University Press, 1993

Goodwin SR: Drugs and drug reactions. In Gravenstein N (ed): Manual of complications during anesthesia. Philadelphia: JB Lippincott, 1991: 479

Levy JH (ed): Anaphylactic reactions in anesthesia and intensive care. Boston: Butterworth-Heinemann, 1992

Stoelting RK: Allergic reactions during anesthesia. Anesth Analg 62: 341, 1983

Complications in Anesthesiology, second edition,
edited by Nikolaus Gravenstein and Robert R. Kirby.
Lippincott-Raven Publishers, Philadelphia © 1996.

CHAPTER 45

Complications of Prior Drug Therapy

Margaret Wood

The typical hospitalized patient in the United States receives from 8 to 10 medications during an admission; adverse responses occur in about 5% of patients. For patients receiving 10 to 20 drugs, the incidence of adverse reactions may increase to more than 40%.[1-3] Hence, the probability of a drug interaction varies directly with the number of drugs to which a patient is exposed. Most patients undergoing surgery receive several drugs during their hospitalization, and the patient who, during preoperative evaluation, denies taking any drugs is rare.

Current anesthetic practice relies on a wide variety of drugs, each chosen for a specific purpose, such as loss of consciousness, muscle relaxation, analgesia, sedation, and in some cases amnesia. The effects of these drugs may be modified by previous administration of other drugs, with resultant adverse drug reactions or complications.

Adverse drug reactions are classified into two main groups. *Type A reactions* are the result of an exaggerated but predictable pharmacologic effect and are usually dose-dependent. *Type B reactions* are adverse reactions that are unpredictable and unrelated to the expected pharmacologic effect.[4] Most drug reactions encountered by anesthesiologists are of type A.

MECHANISMS AND SITES OF DRUG INTERACTION

Whenever more then one drug is administered, the potential for an adverse drug interaction arises. Pharmacologic effect may be exaggerated or diminished by *pharmacokinetic interactions*, in which the administration of one drug alters the disposition (absorption, distribution, metabolism, or elimination) of another drug, or by *pharmacodynamic interactions*, in which one drug alters the response or *sensitivity* to another drug.

Type A Pharmacokinetic Interactions

Direct Physical or Chemical Incompatibility

Pharmaceutical incompatibility can occur when drugs are physically mixed, because many drugs are incompatible in the same solution. For example, if thiopental (pH 10.8) mixes in the intravenous tubing with succinylcholine (pH 3.0 to 4.5) or meperidine (pH 3.5), a dense white precipitate results from the change in hydrogen ion concentration. Figure 45-1 shows the compatibility of many drugs that are administered by anesthesiologists.

Interference at Absorption Sites

Delayed absorption leads to unpredictable clinical effects. The rate of absorption of drugs administered orally depends principally on the rate of gastric emptying. Acetaminophen absorption has been used as a model to study the effect of drugs on gastric absorption and the rate of gastric emptying. The administration of narcotic analgesic agents during labor slows gastric emptying, delaying the absorption of acetaminophen.[5] Probably the absorption of other drugs also is delayed by the administration of narcotics during labor.

Preanesthetic medication also can affect gastric emptying and absorption: diazepam has no effect, but opioids such as morphine markedly reduce acetaminophen absorption.[6] In addition, the anticholinergic agent glycopyrrolate reduces gastric absorption of acetaminophen, whereas atropine has no effect.[7]

Local blood flow determines the absorption, or uptake, of drugs that are administered subcutaneously or intramuscularly. The addition of epinephrine to a local anesthetic produces vasoconstriction and thereby retards absorption into the blood, with consequent decrease in toxicity and increased

	Aminophylline	Atracurium	Atropine	Calcium Chloride	Cefazolin	Cimetidine	Curare	Diazepam	Dopamine	Droperidol	Epinephrine	Erythromycin	Fentanyl	Furosemide	Gentamicin	Heparin	Lidocaine	Mannitol	Metoclopramide	Midazolam	Morphine	Nafcillin	Nitroprusside	Pancuronium	Phenytoin	Ranitidine	Succinylcholine	Thiopental	Trimethophan	Vancomycin	Vecuronium
Aminophylline			C		C	I		C	C		I	C		C	C	C	C		C		I	C			I			C	I	I	
Atracurium																												I			
Atropine	C			C		C				C	C		C			C	C		C	C	C	C				C					
Calcium Chloride	I		C		I				C		I						C	I													
Cefazolin	C			I		I		C							I		I		I		C					C					
Cimetidine	I		C					C			C	C	C	C	C	C	C	C	C		C	C	C		I	C				C	
Curare																												C			
Diazepam	C					C					I			I			Δ			I		C		C		I					
Dopamine	C			C													C	C													
Droperidol			C										C						C	C	C	I									
Epinephrine	I		C	I		C		I						I			C									C					
Erythromycin	C					C										I	C		Δ		C					C					
Fentanyl			C			C				C						C			C	C	C					C		I			
Furosemide	C					C		I			I				I		C									C					
Gentamicin	C				I	C			C					I		I	C				C	I				C					
Heparin	C		C		C	C		I	Δ	C	C	I	C	C	I		C		C		C	C	C	C	I		C		C		
Lidocaine	C			C	I	C		C	C		C	C			C	C			C						I	C					
Mannitol				I	C	C			C										C												
Metoclopramide	C		C		I	C				C		Δ	C			C	C	C		C	C										
Midazolam			C					I		C			C						C		C							I			
Morphine	I		C		C	C				C		C	C		C	C			C	C		C			I	C	C	I		C	
Nafcillin	Δ		C			C		C		I					I	C					C										
Nitroprusside						C										C															
Pancuronium							C									C					C						C	I			
Phenytoin	I					I										I	I				I									I	
Ranitidine			C		C	C		I			C	C	C	C	C		C				C		C					I		C	
Succinylcholine												-				C					C							I			
Thiopental	C	I					C						I							I	I					I	I				I
Trimethophan	I															C															
Vancomycin	I			C	I	C										I					C				C						
Vecuronium																												I			

FIGURE 45-1. Drug compatibility chart. C, compatible; *I*, incompatible; Δ, concentration dependent. (Goodwin SR: Drugs and drug reactions. In Gravenstein N (ed): Manual of complications during anesthesia. Philadelphia: JB Lippincott, 1991: 484)

duration of effect. Furthermore, 85% to 95% of intragluteal drug injections given with a 22-G needle and intended to be intramuscular actually are administered subcutaneously.[8] Uptake from the relatively nonvascular fatty tissue is unpredictable and differs considerably from uptake in blood-rich muscle.

Alteration in Drug Distribution by Protein Binding

Numerous drugs are bound to plasma proteins; only the free (unbound) fraction readily diffuses across biologic membranes to reach the receptor site and exert its pharmacologic effect. Because many drugs share common binding sites on plasma proteins, drug–drug displacement interactions occur, with consequent increases in the free fractions of the displaced drugs. Pharmacologic activity is intensified and toxicity is more likely in these circumstances. For example, 84% of thiopental is bound to plasma proteins. Other drugs administered before thiopental can compete for its binding sites and produce a displacement interaction. The administration of sulfafurazole may enhance thiopental anesthesia by competitive displacement of thiopental from binding sites on plasma proteins.[9] Prolongation of anesthesia has been demonstrated in rats after injection of radiographic contrast media that displaces barbiturates.[10]

Alteration in Drug Metabolism

Many drugs are metabolized by cytochrome P450 enzymes in the liver. Microsomal drug activity can be increased (enzyme induction) or reduced (enzyme inhibition) by previously administered agents. Increase in the activity of drug-metabolizing enzymes results in more rapid metabolism of the drugs and a resultant decrease in drug concentrations.

Patients receiving an enzyme-inducing agent (such as phenobarbital, isoniazid, or ethanol) on a long-term basis may be better able to metabolize inhalation anesthetic agents to produce a greater quantity of metabolites than would otherwise occur. Some investigators have speculated that enzyme induction plays a role in halothane hepatotoxicity, by production of increased amounts of toxic metabolites that covalently bind to liver macromolecules.[11]

One of the metabolites of the fluorinated ethers, methoxyflurane and enflurane, is inorganic fluoride ion. Inorganic fluoride has been shown to be responsible for the acute polyuric renal failure that occurs after methoxyflurane administration.[12] Enzyme induction with isoniazid that increases P450 2E1 activity (a specific P450 enzyme responsible for volatile anesthetic defluorination) enhances the metabolism of methoxyflurane. The liberation of increased amounts of the nephrotoxic fluoride ion causes a parallel increase in toxicity.[13]

Although enflurane also is metabolized to produce free fluoride ion by cytochrome P450 2E1, the previous administration of enzyme-inducing drugs is unlikely to increase the risk of nephrotoxicity with this agent in patients with normal renal function, because the fluoride does not normally attain a sufficient concentration.[14]

ENZYME INHIBITION. Inhibition of drug metabolism results in increased drug concentrations and enhanced pharmacologic activity. Examples of drugs causing enzyme inhibition include sulfaphenazole, monoamine oxidase (MAO) inhibitors, allopurinol, and perhaps the best known, cimetidine.

The histamine H_2–receptor antagonist cimetidine, through binding of its imidazole group to cytochrome P-450, can inhibit the metabolism of a wide variety of drugs that are metabolized by the mixed-function oxidase systems of the liver. These include diazepam, propranolol, meperidine, lidocaine, and chlordiazepoxide.[15–17] Cimetidine is prescribed for many surgical patients for anesthetic and non–anesthetic-related indications. In the perioperative period it may interact with central nervous system depressants and cause postoperative somnolence or confusion.[18] By contrast, ranitidine, also a histamine H_2–receptor agonist, is relatively devoid of many of cimetidine's interactions.[19] Disulfram inhibits cytochrome P450 2E1 isozyme activity, and therefore inhibits enflurane defluorination.

The inhalation anesthetics inhibit drug metabolism and hence increase the concentration of many previously or concomitantly administered drugs. Included among the latter are propranolol, fentanyl, lidocaine, and verapamil, all of which may undergo increases in their therapeutic effects and toxicity.[20–23]

Drugs that inhibit plasma cholinesterase activity prolong the duration of effect of succinylcholine.[24,25] Patients undergoing eye surgery may have been receiving the anticholinesterase echothiophate, which is used in the treatment of glaucoma.

MAO inhibitors reduce the metabolism of many sympathomimetic agents. The administration of indirectly acting sympathomimetic amines during anesthesia for treated patients leads to increased pharmacologic effect and may promote a hypertensive crisis.[26]

Alteration in Excretion

Previous administration of one drug also can alter the excretion of another. For example, forced alkaline diuresis has been used therapeutically to hasten the elimination of phenobarbital taken in overdose. Drugs that are ventilatory depressant agents, such as narcotic analgesics given as part of a preanesthetic regimen, can delay the pulmonary excretion of the inhalation anesthetics.

An important interaction occurs between digoxin and quinidine: when quinidine is administered to patients receiving digoxin, an increase in digoxin concentration occurs.[27] This effect is attributable in part to a reduction in the renal clearance of digoxin and in part to a reduction in digoxin's volume of distribution. Anesthesiologists should be cautious in the perioperative use of quinidine when patients are receiving digoxin.

Type A Pharmacodynamic Interactions

Pharmacodynamic interactions are mediated by changes at the receptor site. Drugs with similar pharmacologic actions can interact to produce additive or synergistic effects. Two drugs with central nervous system–depressant activity (eg, alcohol, benzodiazepines, narcotics, propofol, and thiopental) produce greater sedation than would be anticipated for either drug alone. As shown in Figure 45-2, the combination of fentanyl and midazolam results in a synergistic effect, whereby a dose of fentanyl that is only 25% of the dose effective in 50% of subjects (ED_{50}), given with 23% of the ED_{50} for midazolam, results in the ED_{50} for the combination.[28] If the drugs were additive in effect, the requirement would fall on the diagonal line of the ED_{50} isobologram.

Many drugs have pharmacologic effects other than those for which they are prescribed. The potentiation of the nondepolarizing muscle relaxants by the aminoglycoside and polymyxin antibiotic agents, which themselves possess weak relaxant properties, is a well-recognized example.[29]

Previous drug therapy may depress physiologic homeostatic reflex responses. β-Adrenergic receptor blocking agents, such as propranolol, predispose patients to heart failure by decreasing reflex sympathetic stimulation of the heart. They also may potentiate the cardiovascular depressant effects of inhalation anesthetic agents and reduce the sympathetic response to stress and hypovolemia. However, this blockade of cardiac stimulation can be beneficial in patients with myocardial ischemia.

Type B Interactions

Type B interactions, which are idiosyncratic and unrelated to a drug's primary pharmacologic activity, are uncommon in clinical anesthetic practice. MAO inhibitors interact with me-

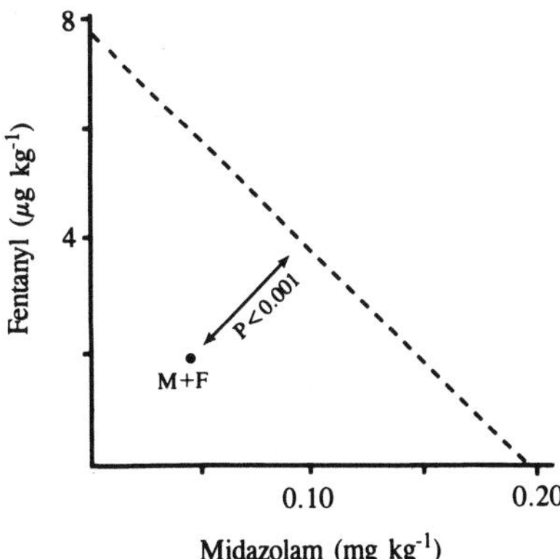

FIGURE 45-2. ED_{50} isobologram for the anesthetic interaction of midazolam (*M*) and fentanyl (*F*). *Dashed line* connects the ED_{50} values of each drug for inability to open eyes on command and represents the relative doses required if the drug effects were additive. (Ben-Shlomo I, Abd-El-Khalim H, Ezry J, et al: Midazolam acts synergistically with fentanyl for induction of anaesthesia. Br J Anaesth 64: 45, 1990)

peridine to produce a syndrome of excitation, rigidity, coma, hypo- or hypertension, and hyperpyrexia.[30] The mechanism of this interaction is not known, but it is thought not to be related to inhibition of drug metabolism.[31,32]

SELECTED DRUG REACTIONS

The Boston Collaborative Drug Surveillance Study indicated that patients receive an average of nine drugs during a hospitalization.[3] Thus, each patient is subjected to considerable risk for drug interactions and adverse drug effects. Although most adverse responses to drugs are transient and of minor consequence, about 3% of patients have life-threatening reactions.[3] As many as 90% of all adverse reactions are caused by a defined group of drugs, including aspirin, digoxin, anticoagulant agents, diuretic agents, antimicrobial agents, steroids, and hypoglycemic agents.[2] Among the most common untoward responses are dysrhythmia, central nervous system depression, fluid overload, and hemorrhage.

Selected interactions associated with many of the drugs administered to or taken by patients who undergo surgery are grouped in the following discussion by major pharmacologic classes. These drugs may elicit a broad range of adverse responses, from those of doubtful clinical significance to those causing life-threatening reactions. Several potentially serious drug interactions that may result in anesthetic complications are discussed in more detail.

Adrenocorticosteroids

The first postoperative death caused by adrenocortical suppression after adrenocorticosteroid therapy was reported in 1952[33]; other reports followed.[34,35] Long-term steroid administration results in suppression of the hypothalamic–pituitary–adrenal axis so that stress, including that produced by surgery or anesthesia, does not elicit the normal increase in adrenocortical hormone output. After this type of therapy, the stress response is suppressed for as long as 9 months. Thus, preoperative and intraoperative steroid supplementation is commonly advocated for patients who have received oral corticosteroids during the year before surgery (Table 45-1).

Side Effects

It may be undesirable to administer exogenous steroids to patients who have the ability to respond to stress with an increase in plasma cortisol. Corticosteroid treatment has many deleterious side effects: increased susceptibility to infection, delayed wound-healing, increased risk of gastrointestinal hemorrhage, electrolyte imbalance, hypertension, and venous thrombosis.[36,37]

Perioperative Supplementation

Many patients come to surgery while receiving steroids or having received them in the recent past. The selection of patients for steroid supplementation in the perioperative period is controversial.

PRO. The recommendation that some form of steroid supplementation ("cover") be given to all patients receiving steroids at the time of operation is followed widely.[38] However, in the majority of patients, adrenal stress responsiveness to surgery returns to normal very rapidly after treatment is stopped. Therefore, routine coverage after more than 2 months of cessation of therapy is probably unnecessary.

One common regimen suggests that for patients currently receiving steroid treatment, 100 mg hydrocortisone should be given every 6 hours for 72 hours after major surgery, whereas 24 hours' therapy is adequate for minor surgery.[39] For very short procedures, a single intramuscular injection of hydrocortisone as part of the preanesthetic medication regimen is sufficient. Other studies have advocated lower dosages of hydrocortisone supplementation: 25 mg intravenously at the start of the procedure, followed by 100 mg intravenously over the next 24-hour period.[40] A lower dosage may be associated with a decreased incidence of side effects.[41]

CON. Some anesthesiologists believe that steroid-treated patients who are undergoing surgery do not need routine supplemental cortisol as part of their preanesthetic medication and that the current policy of supplemental steroid coverage is based not on data but on tradition. Kehlet and Binder studied 104 glucocorticoid-treated patients who underwent surgery without supplementary steroid coverage[42]: of 8 patients in whom unexplained hypotension developed during anesthesia, only 1 had concomitantly low plasma cortisol concentrations. Other patients had minimal adrenal cortical activity preoperatively and yet no signs of adrenal insufficiency during anesthesia. The investigators concluded that acute stress-induced adrenal insufficiency during surgery in steroid-treated patients is infrequent.[42] Furthermore, when hypotension did occur during anesthesia, blood pressure returned to normal spontaneously or with volume correction. Other data describe such a minimal cortisol response to minor surgical procedures using local anesthesia and lasting less than 1 hour that replacement beyond the usual daily dose seems unnecessary and possibly detrimental.[40,43]

Clinical Recommendations

It cannot be determined, on clinical grounds alone, which patients receiving chronic steroid therapy have adrenocortical insufficiency and therefore truly require perioperative steroid coverage. In one study[40] of renal transplant recipients chronically receiving 5 to 10 mg prednisone per day, although 63% had normal ACTH stimulation tests 97% had normal or increased urinary cortisol concentrations as evidence of adequate circulating cortisol to meet requirements during stress.[44] The insulin hypoglycemia and ACTH stimulation tests allow selection of patients whose hypothalamic–pituitary–adrenal axis has lost the ability to respond to stress with increased endogenous output. A positive test result indicates that steroid coverage is unnecessary and can be withheld. However, it is rarely performed in the perioperative setting and thus of little clinical use.

Despite these conflicting points of view, the majority of

TABLE 45-1
Endocrine Drug Interactions

PREVIOUS DRUG THERAPY	COMPLICATIONS	PREVENTION, TREATMENT, OR SIGNIFICANCE	REFERENCES
Adrenocortical steroids	• Chronic steroid therapy causes suppression of the pituitary adrenal axis and adrenocortical insufficiency • Predisposes patient to hypotension and respiratory insufficiency if steroid coverage not provided • Sudden increase in steroid therapy may lead to delayed wound healing, infection, exacerbation of hypertension, and venous thrombosis	• No steroid "coverage" required if steroid therapy terminated 2 months before surgery • If patient currently receiving steroids suggested premedication consists of hydrocortisone 100 mg parenterally, 1 hour before anesthesia and every 6 hours thereafter for ≥12–24 hours • Monitor cardiovascular system and fluid volume status; be prepared to treat intraoperative hypotension with hydrocortisone, judicious fluid administration, and anesthesia dose reduction	33–44
Drugs for diabetes: insulin	• Anesthetic risk relates to pathophysiologic processes associated with diabetes • Intraoperative hypoglycemia and hyperglycemia are serious complications • Central nervous system manifestations of hypoglycemia are masked by general anesthesia • β-Adrenergic blockers mask signs and may prolong hypoglycemia • Antidiabetogenic effects of insulin antagonized by corticosteroids, oral contraceptives, thiazide, and loop diuretics	• Monitor blood glucose frequently	48
Oral hypoglycemic drugs: sulfonylureas (eg., chlorpropamide, and tolbutamide)	• Hypoglycemia may occur as long as 60 hours after last dose • Interact with aspirin, phenylbutazone, and sulfonamide to cause enhanced hypoglycemic effect by displacement from binding sites • Interact with chloramphenicol, dicoumarol, and anticoagulants to cause enhanced hypoglycemic effect by inhibition of metabolism	• Monitor blood glucose	

authorities advocate the doctrine, "When in doubt, give steroid coverage." They advise further that all patients currently receiving glucocorticoid therapy should be assumed to have hypothalamic–pituitary–adrenocortical suppression until it is proven otherwise. Therefore, these patients should be treated with some form of replacement therapy. It is appropriate to consider the amount of glucocorticoid treatment, and the extent and duration of surgery in choosing a replacement regimen.[40]

Hypoglycemic Drugs

Diabetes mellitus is discussed elsewhere. Important drug interactions involving insulin and oral hypoglycemic agents are summarized in Table 45-1.[45–48]

Calcium Channel–Blocking Drugs

Indications

The range of indications for the use of the calcium channel–blocking drugs has increased greatly since their introduction. They are used in the management of supraventricular dysrhythmias, angina pectoris, coronary vasospasm, hypertension, myocardial protection during cardiac surgery, and cerebral arterial spasm.[49,50] Most commonly used are verapamil, nifedipine, diltiazem, and the newer dihydropyridine calcium channel blockers such as nicardipine. Drug interactions have been reported between these drugs and the volatile inhalation anesthetics and muscle relaxants. In addition, complications during anesthesia may result from their physiologic effects (Table 45-2).

TABLE 45-2
Antihypertensive Drug Interactions

PREVIOUS DRUG THERAPY	COMPLICATIONS	PREVENTION, TREATMENT, OR SIGNIFICANCE	REFERENCES
Antihypertensive drugs (in general)	• Interact with anesthetics and drugs that produce vasodilation to cause intraoperative hypotension • Labile cardiovascular responses, and both hypo- and hypertension may occur	• Continue therapy to time of surgery • Careful monitoring of cardiovascular system and fluid volume status essential • Treat hypotension with judicious fluid administration and suitable inotrope • Treat hypertension vigorously with nitroprusside or nitroglycerin • Titrate anesthetic requirements cautiously	
CENTRAL α-ADRENERGIC RECEPTOR AGONISTS			
Clonidine	• Decreases sympathetic outflow from central nervous system • Clonidine withdrawal syndrome with rebound hypertension. • Halothane MAC decreased	• Continue clonidine to time of surgery • Treat postoperative hypertension with nitroprusside	101
Methyldopa through metabolite α-methylnorepinephrine	• Halothane MAC decreased		
PERIPHERAL α-ADRENERGIC RECEPTOR ANTAGONISTS			
Prazosin	• Peripheral vasodilation unaccompanied by tachycardia • Higher doses of pressors required to produce same increase in blood pressure		102
α_1- AND α_2-ADRENERGIC RECEPTOR ANTAGONISTS			
Phenoxybenzamine, phentolamine, others	• α-Adrenergic receptor blockade results, causing a decrease in peripheral resistance and tachycardia • Used in pheochromocytoma	• Tachycardia may be treated by β-adrenergic receptor antagonist	
ADRENERGIC NEURON BLOCKING AGENTS			
Guanethidine	• No effect on halothane MAC		103, 143
Reserpine	• Prevents norepinephrine reuptake at nerve terminal • Intraoperative hypotension reported; antagonizes indirect pressors and potentiates direct pressors • Depression and possible suicide • Halothane MAC decreased	• Use direct sympathomimetic agents cautiously	104–106 143
DIURETIC AGENTS			
Hydrochlorothiazide, furosemide, others	• Interact with anesthetics and drugs that produce vasodilation to cause hypotension • May cause hypovolemia with hypokalemia and may cause dysrhythmias • May enhance nondepolarizing neuromuscular blockade	• Continue administration of drug • Monitor volume status and serum potassium	140
VASODILATORS			
Hydralazine	• Reflex tachycardia that may precipitate angina	• Combine hydralazine with β-adrenergic receptor blocking agent (eg, propranolol)	107

Minoxidil	• Profound reflex sympathetic activity and sodium retention • Should be given with diuretic agent and β-adrenergic receptor blocking agent	• Monitor cardiovascular system and fluid volume status	108
Diazoxide	• Profound reflex sympathetic activity • May precipitate myocardial ischemia	• For hydralazine and minoxidil, watch for hypoglycemia	109
Nitroglycerin	• Potentiates pancuronium-induced neuromuscular blockade	• Use peripheral nerve stimulator	138
Nitropruisside	• Cyanide toxicity and metabolic acidosis	• Monitor dose and acid–base status • Hydroxocabalamin combines with cyanide ions to yield vitamin B_{12} and decreases cyanide concentrations	
GANGLIONIC BLOCKING AGENTS			
Trimethaphan	• Inhibits plasma cholinesterase • Prolonged apnea with succinylcholine	• Avoid succinylcholine • Use nerve stimulator to monitor neuromuscular function	139
ANGIOTENSIN-CONVERTING ENZYME INHIBITORS			
Captopril, enalapril, lisinopril	• Inhibit generation of angiotensin II. • Enhance hypotensive response to nitroprusside • Intraoperative hypotension	• Titrate nitroprusside dose cautiously	110
β-ADRENERGIC RECEPTOR BLOCKING AGENTS			
Propranolol, nadolol, timolol, metoprolol, esmolol	• Blunt sympathetic response to anesthesia and surgery • Interact with inhalational anesthetics to potentiate depression of cardiovascular system • Bradycardia, bronchospasm, and worsening of congestive heart failure may occur	• Continue adminstration to day of surgery, and do not discontinue abruptly • Treat hypotension with calcium and inotrope such as dopamine • Treat bradycardia with atropine, isoproterenol or pacing • Use more cardioselective β-adrenergic blocking agent (esmolol) if respiratory disease present	79–98
β-ADRENERGIC RECEPTOR AGONISTS			
Ritodrine (β_2-adrenergic agonist), others	• Pulmonary edema, hypokalemia, dysrhythmias, and hypotension	• Monitor serum potassium and fluid volume status	
PHOSPHODIESTERASE INHIBITORS			
Aminophylline, others	• Inhibit phosphodiesterase, leading to increased concentrations of cyclic adenosine monophosphate • Dysrhythmias during halothane anesthesia • Toxic effects include seizures, dysrhythmias, cardiorespiratory arrest, and coma	• Monitor for cardiac dysrhythmias • Avoid halothane or reduce infusion rate of aminophylline • Isoflurane is volatile anesthetic of choice • Monitor serum theophylline concentration (therapeutic range is 10–20 μg/mL)	
CALCIUM CHANNEL–BLOCKING AGENTS			
Verapamil, nifedipine, diltiazem, others	• Bradycardia, heart block, and hypotension	• Continue therapy • Carefully titrate anesthetics	55–58
	• Potentiate cardiovascular depressant effects of inhalational anesthetics • Halothane MAC decreased		62
	• Interact with β-adrenergic blocking agents • Potentiate neuromuscular relaxants	• Use nerve stimulator	65

MAC, minimum alveolar concentration.

Effects

These drugs produce systemic and coronary artery vasodilatation to varying degrees and depress heart rate, atrioventricular conduction, and myocardial contractility (Table 45-3).[51,52] How an individual anesthetic agent affects the pharmacologic activity of a particular calcium channel–blocking drug is sometimes difficult to predict, because each exerts a different hemodynamic effect; physiologic reflexes also modify the initial effect. For example, reflex sympathetic stimulation in response to calcium channel blocker–induced vasodilatation modifies heart rate changes.

Anesthetic Interactions

Inhalational anesthetic agents inhibit baroreceptor reflex activity and sympathetic nervous system function, may depress myocardial function, and produce vasodilatation. Thus, the potential exists for additive negative inotropic and vasodilatory effects from the interaction of a calcium channel–blocking drug and an inhalation anesthetic. Studies in animals indicate that verapamil and nifedipine enhance the hemodynamic effects of halothane, enflurane, and isoflurane in a dose-related manner.[53–57] Although the qualitative effects of verapamil administration during isoflurane and enflurane are similar to those during halothane anesthesia, verapamil appears to produce less hemodynamic depression during isoflurane anesthesia than during the administration of equipotent concentrations of enflurane.[55]

IN VITRO VERSUS IN VIVO RESPONSES. Although verapamil, nifedipine, and diltiazem have dose-dependent vasodilatory as well as negative chronotropic, dromotropic, and inotropic effects in isolated tissue preparations, studies in awake animals with intact physiologic reflexes show very different effects.[58] Nifedipine, which is a potent vasodilator, reduces blood pressure. The consequent reflex stimulation of the sympathetic nervous system results in an increase in heart rate and cardiac output. Therefore, in a halothane anesthesia swine model, equihypotensive doses of verapamil and diltiazem have more pronounced effects on cardiac conduction and myocardial contractility than does nifedipine, which predominantly reduces systemic vascular resistance.[58]

Animal studies indicate that caution should be exercised when these agents are administered during inhalation anesthesia in humans. Verapamil has been used to treat cardiac dysrhythmias during light halothane anesthesia without serious ill effects, although blood pressure decreased and the PR interval increased.[59]

One study of patients undergoing coronary artery bypass graft surgery showed that halothane anesthesia produces a marked reduction in mean arterial pressure, cardiac index, and left ventricular contractility (as measured by the rate of change in left ventricular pressure) and that verapamil, 0.15 mg/kg administered over a 10-minute period, causes further depression of left ventricular contractility and a small increase in left ventricular end-diastolic pressure.[60] Systemic vasodilatation increases; mean arterial pressure decreases; and heart rate does not change.

Another study showed that verapamil 0.075 mg/kg causes a rapid reduction in systemic vascular resistance and arterial blood pressure but no change in heart rate or cardiac index during narcotic anesthesia in patients with good ventricular function about to undergo coronary artery bypass graft surgery.[61] No patients experienced any untoward complications. Apparently, verapamil can be administered safely to these patients during narcotic anesthesia.

PHARMACOKINETIC AND PHARMACODYNAMIC INTERACTIONS. Before it is assumed that these changes are totally pharmacodynamic, it should be remembered that the inhalation anesthetic agents inhibit drug metabolism. During halothane, isoflurane, or enflurane anesthesia in dogs, verapamil concentrations are increased because of a reduction in clearance.[23] Therefore, the interaction between the calcium antagonists and volatile anesthetics probably is both pharmacodynamic and pharmacokinetic in origin. Verapamil also decreases MAC for halothane in dogs.[62]

Other Interactions

Animal data suggest that the calcium channel–blocking agents also have important effects at the neuromuscular junction, such as a progressive dose-dependent reduction in twitch height (see Table 45-2).[63,64] The effects of the depolarizing and nondepolarizing relaxants are augmented by verapamil.[65] Although human studies are few, they suggest that verapamil can prolong the duration of neuromuscular blockade.[66] Calcium antagonists also interact with other drugs that may be administered perioperatively, such as digoxin,[67] β-adrenergic receptor antagonists,[68] quinidine,[69] and theophylline.[70]

TABLE 45-3
Hemodynamic Effects of Calcium Channel–Blocking Agents

	NEGATIVE CHRONOTROPIC	NEGATIVE DROMOTROPIC	NEGATIVE INOTROPIC	VASODILATATION	
				Systemic	*Coronary*
Verapamil	+++	++	++	++	++
Nifedipine	+/0	+/0	+/0	+++	+++
Diltiazem	+	+	++	++	++

+, effect; ++, greater effect; +++, greatest effect; 0, little or no effect

Clinical Recommendations

Although calcium channel–blocking agents interact with a wide variety of drugs and may produce complications during anesthesia, they should not be discontinued before anesthesia and surgery. Clinical experience suggests they are beneficial. If potential problems are recognized and the anesthetic regimen modified, patients can be anesthetized safely while continuing to receive these drugs. Moreover, several case reports suggest that a cardiovascular withdrawal syndrome may be associated with the calcium antagonists; thus, they should be continued to the time of surgery.[71,72]

Varying degrees of hypotension, bradycardia, and heart block may be more likely during surgery and general anesthesia in patients receiving calcium channel blocking agents on a long-term basis. Careful titration of anesthesia and attention to intravascular volume is important. Adverse effects can be managed by administration of calcium, β-adrenergic receptor agonists, or an appropriate inotrope.

Cardiac Glycosides

The proportion of elderly people in the population is constantly increasing, and therefore so too is the prevalence of atherosclerotic heart disease. Many patients who undergo surgery take cardiac glycosides (digitalis) for the management of atrial tachydysrhythmias or congestive heart failure. Patients frequently also take diuretic agents that produce potassium loss and hypokalemia (Table 45-4).[73,74] This depletion may make them more susceptible to digitalis toxicity, manifested by cardiac dysrhythmias. Patients receiving digitalis therapy appear to be more prone to dysrhythmias, independent of diuretic therapy or sodium potassium concentration. Although the relation between hypokalemia and the effect of digitalis therapy on ventricular ectopy has been questioned, most clinicians treating a patient who is receiving digitalis prefer to correct hypokalemia preoperatively.

Amrinone

Amrinone is a bipyridine that is neither a glycoside nor a catecholamine and that functions as an inotrope and a vasodilator.[75] It augments myocardial contractility and is popular in the treatment of congestive heart failure and after cardiac surgery, particularly in the setting of pulmonary hypertension. Cardiac output increases, but blood pressure and pulse usually change very little. However, in the presence of any of the volatile anesthetics, blood pressure can decrease significantly. Milrinone, a bipyridine derivative, has also been shown to be effective in cardiac failure, by increasing cardiac contractility and reducing systemic vascular resistance.

β-Adrenergic Receptor Antagonists

Propranolol, one of the most commonly administered β-adrenergic receptor antagonists in the United States, is used to treat a wide variety of diseases and syndromes, including ischemic heart disease, hypertension, cardiac dysrhythmias, thyrotoxicosis, pheochromocytoma, obstructive cardiomyopathy, and simple anxiety. Other β-adrenergic receptor blocking agents that have been introduced differ in selectivity; intrinsic sympathomimetic activity; and membrane-stabilizing, local anesthetic or "quinidine-like" effect.

Actions

All β-adrenergic receptor antagonists competitively block the effects of endogenous and exogenous catecholamines. Therapy results in decreased heart rate and myocardial contractility by antagonism at the β_1-adrenergic receptor. Bronchoconstriction and peripheral vasoconstriction produced by antagonism of β_2-adrenergic receptors occur with propranolol but less so with esmolol. Thus, in patients with bronchial asthma and obstructive airway disease, propranolol can precipitate bronchospasm. Esmolol is much less likely to do so. One complication of preoperative β-receptor blocking therapy is the development of intraoperative bronchoconstriction.

Adverse Effects

Adverse effects of β-adrenergic receptor blockade are predictable on the basis of pharmacologic principles and include bronchospasm; cardiac failure; peripheral vasoconstriction and precipitation of Raynaud's phenomenon; masking of hypoglycemia in diabetic patients; and severe bradycardia accompanied by inadequate cardiac output. In the past, these adverse effects made anesthesiologists apprehensive when patients taking β-adrenergic receptor antagonists required surgery.

Anesthetic Interactions

Because inhalation anesthetic agents depress myocardial contractility in a dose-dependent fashion, concern has been

TABLE 45-4
Digoxin and Amrinone Interactions

PREVIOUS DRUG THERAPY	COMPLICATIONS	PREVENTION, TREATMENT, OR SIGNIFICANCE	REFERENCES
Digoxin	Interacts with diuretics to produce hypokalemia and may enhance digitalis toxicity, manifested by cardiac dysrhythmias; may interact with succinylcholine to enhance digitalis toxicity	Discontinue on day of surgery; monitor serum potassium and correct hypokalemia preoperatively if time permits	73, 74
Amrinone	Cardiotonic drug that is not a cathecholamine or cardiac glycoside; hypotension may occur		75

expressed that β-adrenergic receptor blockade may impair the ability of the patient receiving general anesthesia to compensate for hypovolemia, blood loss, and hypoxia, and that anesthetic-induced hypotension will be potentiated.[77,78]

The hemodynamic changes produced by the interaction of propranolol and enflurane have been shown in dogs to be greater than those produced by equipotent concentrations of halothane.[79-81] Cardiac function is well maintained in the presence of β-blockade with propranolol during isoflurane anesthesia in dogs. Induced hemorrhage is better tolerated than during enflurane anesthesia.[82] A narcotic muscle relaxant technique is also compatible with β-adrenergic blockade; enflurane probably should be avoided in this situation, although halothane and isoflurane may be used with caution.[83,84]

Withdrawal

Despite the possible complications with long-term β-adrenergic receptor blockade, withdrawal of therapy also may have adverse effects; a withdrawal syndrome after discontinuation of therapy has been described.[85] Several case reports describe angina, ventricular tachycardia, myocardial infarction, and even death after abrupt withdrawal,[86,87] although the significance of this problem has been disputed.[88] Clinical features suggest a hyperadrenergic state, and changes in adrenergic sensitivity have been noted.

Because of an adaptive decrease in the number of β-adrenergic receptors in response to physiologic concentrations of catecholamines, blockade of this *down-regulation* by propranolol results in increased β-adrenergic receptor density. This effect has been demonstrated and implies that the increased sensitivity to β-adrenergic agonists after propranolol withdrawal may be a valid mechanism to account for the syndrome.[86] The existence of the withdrawal syndrome contraindicates withdrawal of propranolol before surgery.

Angina Pectoris and Myocardial Infarction

Despite these potential adverse effects, many clinical studies have documented the beneficial effect of β-adrenergic receptor blockade in angina pectoris and myocardial infarction. Blockade reduces the oxygen requirement of the left ventricle by effecting a reduction in heart rate and myocardial contractility and an inhibition of the pressor response to exercise, all of which are changes in determinants of myocardial oxygen consumption. Propranolol and other β-adrenergic receptor blocking agents reduce myocardial infarct size and protect against dysrhythmias.[89-91] β-adrenergic receptor blockade reduces mortality after myocardial infarction. These effects clearly are beneficial perioperatively.

If a suitable anesthetic regimen is selected, these patients can be anesthetized safely.[92,93] β-Adrenergic receptor blockade reportedly provides excellent myocardial protection from the sympathetic stimulation induced by fear and anxiety.[94] This protective effect also occurs when sympathetic stimulation is elicited by anesthesia induction, tracheal intubation, surgical manipulation, and postoperative pain.[95-98] Sudden discontinuation of antihypertensive drugs may lead to serious postoperative rebound hypertension.

Clinical Recommendations

In current anesthetic practice, therapy with β-adrenergic receptor blocking agents is continued to the time of surgery and through the postoperative period. Because propranolol is a competitive antagonist, isoproterenol or other β-receptor agonists will reverse its effect, if necessary. Bradycardia can be treated initially with 0.1 mg atropine given intravenously every 5 minutes to a maximum dose of 3.0 mg. Calcium chloride can be used to treat any accompanying hypotension. If atropine and calcium are ineffective, cardiac pacing is useful; in rare instances, an isoproterenol infusion may be required.

Antihypertensive and Vasodilator Drugs

The treatment of hypertension has advanced considerably in recent years through better understanding of the mechanisms and sites of drug action. Many patients receiving antihypertensive medication undergo anesthesia and surgery. Hypertension affects 15% to 20% of the North American population.

Perioperative Continuation of Medication

It was once common practice to recommend discontinuation of antihypertensive agents before elective anesthesia and surgery. However, Foex and Prys-Roberts demonstrated that patients with untreated or inadequately treated hypertension were at greater risk for lability of blood pressure during anesthesia.[99] Therefore, in patients with untreated hypertension, blood pressure should be controlled before elective surgery. Goldman and Caldera later found that if intraoperative and immediate postoperative blood pressures were monitored closely and treated effectively to prevent hypertensive or hypotensive episodes, patients with mild to moderate hypertension (diastolic pressure not >100 mm Hg) were at no greater risk than were normotensive patients.[100]

Effective intra- and postoperative management of hypertension is as important as preoperative management and control. Ideally, the quality of patients' antihypertensive therapy should be evaluated as part of their preoperative assessment. The majority of patients who have diastolic pressures of less than 110 mm Hg can be treated safely intraoperatively, provided that their status is monitored carefully and that hyper- and hypotension are treated rigorously. Patients with severe hypertension must be treated adequately before anesthesia is induced. Antihypertensive medication should be continued until and on the day of surgery to prevent rebound hypertension.

Adverse Responses

Adverse responses to antihypertensive agents are listed in Table 45-2. Most potential anesthetic complications are caused by interference with cardiovascular homeostatic mechanisms or by direct interactions produced by the antihypertensive agents themselves. Over the last few years, many new agents with different mechanisms have been introduced for the management of hypertension, such as calcium channel blockers, angiotensin converting enzyme inhibitors, and new sympatholytic drugs (guanabenz, guanfacine, prazosin, and mixed antagonists such as labetalol). Vasodilators such as minoxidil are also used.

CLONIDINE. Clonidine, an α_2-adrenergic receptor agonist, should not be discontinued abruptly before anesthesia because a clonidine withdrawal syndrome may ensue.[101] This syndrome resembles a hyperadrenergic state, similar to that noted with abrupt cessation of β-adrenergic blocking drugs. Hypertension, tachycardia, and an increase in catecholamine concentrations occur. Clonidine should be continued until the day of surgery; if it is discontinued, the dose should be tapered slowly and another antihypertensive agent substituted. Alternatively, a transcutaneous patch can be substituted for the oral preparation; a parenteral form of the drug is unavailable in the United States.

THIAZIDE DIURETIC AGENTS. Intraoperative hypotension may occur in patients receiving thiazide diuretic agents when inhalation anesthetics and vasodilators are administered, because plasma volume may be low. Volume status should be assessed carefully and the serum potassium concentration monitored. Hypokalemia may increase the risk of dysrhythmia and the toxicity of digitalis, and it enhances the action of nondepolarizing muscle relaxants.

Clinical Recommendations

HYPERTENSION. The treatment of intraoperative hypertension is sometimes difficult. Many antihypertensive agents are not available in parenteral form, and the choice of antihypertensive therapy is limited and controversial.[101–110]

Parenteral hydralazine, a potent peripheral vasodilator, is popular for treatment of pregnancy-induced hypertension. Reflex tachycardia often accompanies its use and can precipitate myocardial ischemia; it is prevented by concurrent use of a β-adrenergic blocking agent.

Many anesthesiologists use labetalol or sodium nitroprusside to attenuate intraoperative hypertension. Labetalol is a mixed α- and β-adrenergic receptor antagonist that during general anesthesia appears to exert both effects to a similar degree, whereas in the ambulatory setting, it is predominantly a β-receptor antagonist. Sodium nitroprusside is a potent, rapidly acting agent the effect of which is readily reversed after discontinuation. Nitroglycerin, which produces smooth muscle relaxation with predominant venodilatation, is also popular. Esmolol, an ultrashort-acting β-adrenergic receptor antagonist, is also used by many anesthesiologists to treat acute increases in heart rate and blood pressure. Equally important is that postoperative hypertension is aggressively controlled with parenteral agents to prevent myocardial ischemia, pulmonary edema, and cerebrovascular accidents. Continuation of antihypertensive therapy to the time of surgery minimizes the likelihood of postoperative hypertension.

HYPOTENSION. Intraoperative hypotension can occur in patients taking antihypertensive medications. Intravascular volume must be carefully maintained and a decrease in blood pressure treated by the judicious administration of fluids and a vasopressor, if required. The antihypertensive medications act in many ways. Knowledge of their mechanism of action allows prediction of the effect of a pressor amine's coadministration.

In general, drugs that inhibit the reuptake of norepinephrine diminish the effects of sympathomimetic agents that rely in part on an indirect effect (ie, release of endogenous catecholamines, such as ephedrine and methamphetamine) but potentiate the response to directly acting sympathomimetics (such as phenylephrine, methoxamine, and epinephrine). When an indirectly acting pressor is administered in this situation, decreased amounts of norepinephrine are available to act as neurotransmitter; thus, the beneficial effects are diminished.

Vasodilators that directly relax smooth muscle and drugs that block α-adrenergic receptors in blood vessels decrease the efficacy of both directly and indirectly acting vasopressors.[104–106] Thus, the action of vasopressors in patients receiving antihypertensive medication is unpredictable, and these agents should be cautiously titrated to achieve the desired response.

Antidepressant Drugs

Monoamine Oxidase Inhibitors

MAO inhibitors interfere with the action of an enzyme responsible for the metabolic breakdown of sympathomimetic amines, including norepinephrine. Examples include pargyline, nialamide, tranylcypromine, and isocarboxazid (Table 45-5). These drugs are used infrequently today but still are prescribed for the management of depression unresponsive to other therapy.

Of vital importance are the life-threatening reactions that occur when certain drugs are given to patients taking these drugs. MAO plays only a minor role in terminating the action of norepinephrine released at sympathetic nerve terminals or of exogenously administered directly acting sympathomimetic amines. The reuptake of norepinephrine into the sympathetic nerve terminal is the primary mechanism by which its action is terminated. Hence, MAO inhibitors do not potentiate the effects of exogenously administered directly acting vasopressors. The administration of indirectly acting sympathomimetic agents to a patient receiving a MAO inhibitor, however, leads to increased pharmacologic effect and possibly a hypertensive crisis. Hypertensive crises also have been reported in these patients when they eat foods containing tyramine (eg, certain cheeses or wine).

Atypical reactions occur rarely in patients who are taking MAO inhibitors and who have received narcotic analgesics, especially meperidine.[111,112] A syndrome or hyperpyrexia, muscle rigidity, coma, and hypo- or hypertension has been described.[30,31] MAO inhibitors also inhibit drug metabolism in the liver; the action of the barbiturates and alcohol may be prolonged.[111,112]

CLINICAL RECOMMENDATIONS. Given the wide variety of drug interactions that may occur, MAO inhibitors should be discontinued before surgery if possible and another anti-

TABLE 45-5
Central Nervous System Drug Interactions

PREVIOUS DRUG THERAPY	COMPLICATIONS	PREVENTION, TREATMENT, OR SIGNIFICANCE
SEDATIVE-HYPNOTIC AGENTS		
In general	• May interact with general anesthesia to produce postoperative somnolence • Reduce anesthetic requirements	• Titrate anesthetics
Benzodiazepines (eg, diazepam)	• Withdrawal syndrome after abuse or chronic use if discontinued for surgery • Halothane minimum alveolar concentration decreased by diazepam and midazolam	• Lower halothane dose
Barbiturates	• Chronic therapy causes enzyme induction • Increased incidence of drug interactions	• Careful preoperative assessment of other drug therapy
ANTIDEPRESSANT AGENTS		
Tricyclic (eg, amitriptyline, imipramine, and nortriptyline)	• Tricyclics block reuptake of norepinephrine • Cardiovascular instability • Intraoperative dysrhythmias • Increased sensitivity to sympathomimetic pressor agents, tachycardia and hypotension • Interact with pancuronium and halothane to produce tachydysrhythmias	• Monitor for dysrhythmias • Avoid sympathomimetic agents because of danger of pressor response • Avoid halothane • Avoid pancuronium, and use muscle relaxant with minimal cardiovascular effects
MAO inhibitors (eg, phenelzine, pargyline, iproniazid, and nialamide)	• Interact with sympathomimetic amines to produce dangerous hypertension • Hypertensive crises during anesthesia; hypotension • Unpredictable response to pressor amines • Interact with meperidine to produce excitation, coma, sweating, rigidity, hyperpyrexia, and hyper- or hypotension	• Discontinue MAO inhibitors 2 weeks before surgery, and substitute other medication • Treat hypertension with nitroprusside • Treat hypotension with fluids and direct-acting vasopressor • Avoid narcotics
NEUROLEPTIC AGENTS		
Phenothiazines (eg, chlorpromazine)	• Hypotension caused by α-adrenergic receptor blockade • Heat loss caused by vasodilation and direct effect on central temperature–regulating center	• Treat hypertension with α-adrenergic receptor agonist • Titrate inhalational anesthetic • Monitor fluid volume status
Butyrophenones (eg, haloperidol)	• α-Adrenergic receptor blockade and anticholinergic effects • Hypotension during anesthesia	• Treat hypotension with α-adrenergic receptor agonist • Monitor volume status. Titrate inhalational anesthetic with caution
LITHIUM	• Potentiates nondepolarizing and depolarizing muscle relaxants • Increases duration of pentobarbital narcosis in animals • May reduce anesthetic dose requirements • Intraoperative hypotension • Cardiac dysrhythmias	• Use peripheral nerve stimulator • >1.5 mEq/L toxic • Monitor volume status
MAGNESIUM	• Prolonged neuromuscular blockade with muscle relaxants • Central nervous system sedation	• Use peripheral nerve stimulator • Monitor serum magnesium (therapeutic range 4.0–6.0 mEq/L)
ANTICONVULSANT AGENTS		
Phenytoin, others	• See Table 45-6 • Hepatic enzyme induction	• Continue administration to the fasting time before surgery to minimize possibility of withdrawal seizures • More rapid clearance of muscle relaxants

continued

TABLE 45-5
Continued

PREVIOUS DRUG THERAPY	COMPLICATIONS	PREVENTION, TREATMENT, OR SIGNIFICANCE
Phenobarbital	• Hepatic enzyme induction	• Avoid enflurane • More rapid clearance of muscle relaxants
LEVODOPA	• Used in Parkinson's disease • Side effects are hypotension and cardiac dysrhythmias • Use cautiously if angina and cerebrovascular disease present • Interacts with inhalational anesthetics to produce cardiovascular instability and dysrhythmias	• Discontinue day of surgery but resume postoperatively as soon as possible • Avoid inhalational anesthetics • Avoid droperidol premedication which may worsen symptoms

depressant substituted. At least 2 weeks are required for the effects of these drugs to dissipate. If hypotension develops during anesthesia, a small dose of a directly acting vasopressor should be administered cautiously; hypertension may be controlled with nitroprusside. Regional anesthetic techniques have been used but are limited by the concern regarding administration of vasopressors should hypotension develop.

Tricyclic Antidepressants

Tricyclic antidepressant agents, such as imipramine, amitriptyline, nortriptyline, desipramine, and protriptyline, are used in the management of depression (see Table 45-5). They inhibit norepinephrine reuptake at the adrenergic nerve terminal and have anticholinergic and central nervous system effects, such as sedation and confusion.

The inhibition of norepinephrine reuptake by tricyclic antidepressants is thought to cause an adaptive decrease in central β-adrenergic receptors.[113] This effect may be responsible in part for their therapeutic efficacy.[113,114] The role of α-adrenergic receptors in tricyclic therapy is less clear.

The threshold for epinephrine-induced ventricular dysrhythmias during halothane anesthesia is diminished in dogs pretreated with imipramine for 1 to 2 weeks but not after 6 weeks of administration.[115,116] Orthostatic hypotension and cardiac dysrhythmias can occur in patients taking tricyclic

TABLE 45-6
Antidysrhythmic Drug Interactions

PREVIOUS DRUG THERAPY	COMPLICATIONS	PREVENTION, TREATMENT OR SIGNIFICANCE
Quinidine, phenytoin, disopyramide, lidocaine	• Potentiate myocardial depressant effects of inhalational anesthetics • Lidocaine decreases nitrous oxide and halothane requirements • Quinidine and procainamide can potentiate myasthenia gravis • Lidocaine concentrations higher during halothane anesthesia • Monitor for lidocaine toxicity during halothane anesthesia	• Monitor for lidocaine toxicity during halothane anesthesia
Bretylium	• Blocks norepinephrine reuptake • Intraoperative hypotension • Exaggerates response to catecholamines because of functional denervation hypersensitivity	• Treat hypotension with volume expansion • Avoid cathecholamines if possible
Amiodarone	• Bradycardia and pulmonary fibrosis • Discontinuation results in dysrhythmia recurrence only days or weeks later • Inhibits drug metabolism • Myocardial depression • Postoperative symptoms like adult respiratory distress syndrome	• Check preoperative pulmonary function • Titrate anesthetic dose cautiously • Monitor respiratory function in postoperative period • Limit inspired oxygen fraction if possible

TABLE 45-7
Chemotherapeutic Drug Interactions

PREVIOUS DRUG USE	COMPLICATIONS	PREVENTION, TREATMENT, OR SIGNIFICANCE
Polymixins, aminoglycosides (eg, streptomycin, neomycin, kanamycin, gentamicin)	• Alone, cause neuromuscular block • Interact with neuromuscular relaxants to cause prolonged neuromuscular blockade	• Monitor with peripheral nerve stimulator • Postoperative ventilation may be required
ANTICANCER DRUGS		
Alkylating agents	• See Table 45-8 • May cause or potentiate nondepolarizing neuromuscular blockade	• Monitor the effect of neuromuscular agents with nerve stimulator

agents, and severe dysrhythmias have been reported during halothane anesthesia.[117] If sympathomimetic amines are administered, an exaggerated response, with tachycardia and hypertension, may result.

CLINICAL RECOMMENDATIONS. Administration of tricyclic antidepressants should be tapered before surgery, if possible; if surgery is urgent, depression is severe, or therapy is chronic anesthesia may be administered with careful monitoring for cardiovascular instability and dysrhythmias. Pancuronium, a muscle relaxant with sympathomimetic-like effects, and halothane should be avoided.

Numerous other drugs affecting the central nervous system, including benzodiazepines,[118,119] phenothiazines,[120] lithium,[121-123] magnesium,[124] and L-dopa[125] are used both as adjuncts to anesthesia and for treatment of depression, anxiety, agitation, and delirium. Their effects in conjunction with anesthetic agents can be profound and often necessitate modification of technique (eg, reduction of anesthetic drug dosage; see Table 45-5).

Antidysrhythmic Drugs

Interactions with antidysrhythmic drugs are listed in Table 45-6.

Lidocaine

Lidocaine produces sedation; hence, concomitant lidocaine administration decreases anesthetic requirements.[126] Lidocaine also reduces myocardial contractility, especially in patients with reduced myocardial reserve. If a volatile anesthetic agent is administered to a patient receiving lidocaine antidysrhythmic therapy, the concentration of inhalation anesthetic should be titrated cautiously to the cardiovascular response.

Lidocaine should be used with care in the presence of β-adrenergic receptor blockade; bradycardia and hypotension can develop. Halothane reduces hepatic blood flow and inhibits drug metabolism, reducing lidocaine clearance.[22]

Quinidine and Similar Agents

Quinidine depresses myocardial automaticity, conduction, and contractility; hypotension can occur. Procainamide also can cause serious hypotension. Disopyramide has electrophysiologic properties similar to those of quinidine, and, like quinidine, can depress cardiac function.[127] Bretylium is an antidysrhythmic agent used in the treatment of ventricular tachycardia; the drug is concentrated in the postganglionic adrenergic neuron, displacing norepinephrine.[128] Hypotension can occur, especially in patients treated with tricyclic anti-

TABLE 45-8
Anticholinesterase Drug Interactions

PREVIOUS DRUG THERAPY	COMPLICATIONS	PREVENTION, TREATMENT, OR SIGNIFICANCE
Echothiophate (eye drops)	• Prolongs apnea with succinylcholine by inhibition of plasma pseudocholinesterase	• Avoid succinylcholine or change to other therapy at least 4 weeks before surgery
Organophosphate insecticide (eg, parathion) exposure	• See echothiophate	• Avoid succinylcholine • Monitor neuromuscular function with nerve stimulator • Administer atropine in large doses
Anticancer alkylating agents (eg, cyclophosphamide, mechlorethamine)	• See echothiophate	• Avoid succinylcholine • Monitor neuromuscular function with nerve stimulator
Diethylstilbesterol	• Prolongs succinylcholine paralysis by decreasing plasma cholinesterase	• Questionable clinical significance

TABLE 45-9
Histamine H_2-Receptor Blocking Agent Interactions

PREVIOUS DRUG THERAPY	COMPLICATIONS
Cimetidine	• Decreases clearance of warfarin • Inhibits drug metabolism • Increases concentrations of coadministered drugs, leading to possible toxicity (eg, postoperative somnolence) • Decreases hepatic blood flow
Ranitidine	• May increase plasma concentration of bupivacaine

depressants; these drugs appear to reverse bretylium's antiadrenergic effects by preventing its uptake into the adrenergic nerve endings.

When a patient is to undergo anesthesia and is receiving any of these antidysrhythmic drugs, particularly careful intraoperative monitoring of cardiovascular function is essential. The action of neuromuscular relaxants is enhanced by quinidine, phenytoin, propranolol, and lidocaine; neuromuscular function should be monitored with a nerve stimulator.[129,130]

AMIODARONE. This antidysrhythmic agent is used in the treatment of supraventricular and ventricular dysrhythmias.[131] It possesses an extremely long elimination half-life, measured in days, so withdrawal before anesthesia and surgery is impractical.[132] Amiodarone exerts definite but small negative inotropic effects that may be offset by its vasodilator actions. In addition, it may cause atropine-resistant bradycardia and hypotension during surgery and may potentiate the negative chronotropic and inotropic effects of the inhalation anesthetics.[133]

Amiodarone inhibits drug metabolism, and drug interactions have been reported with warfarin and digitalis.[132] It also has been shown to interact with other antidysrhythmic agents, such as quinidine and procainamide. Finally, amiodarone can cause pulmonary fibrosis; therefore, it is particularly important to assess respiratory function in patients to whom it has been administered, especially postoperatively. Its effect on lung function may be aggravated by an increased inspired oxygen fraction, which therefore should be limited if feasible. Use of amiodarone in the perioperative period should be considered especially carefully.

OTHER DRUGS. Newer antidysrhythmic drugs that may cause problems for the anesthesiologist include encainide, flecainide, lorcainide, and ethomozin.[127] Appropriate modifications of therapy before anesthesia and surgery remain to be defined.

OTHER CONSIDERATIONS

Several other classes of drugs can provoke potentially serious interactions of concern to anesthesiologists. These include chemotherapeutic agents for cancer (Table 45-7)[134–137] and antihypertensive,[138,139] diuretic,[140] and antibiotic[141] drugs, all of which potentially prolong neuromuscular blockade (see Table 45-2).

Antihypertensive agents may change the MAC requirement for inhalational agents.[142,143] Several agents affect cholinesterase concentrations, potentially altering the response to succinylcholine or mivacurium (Table 45-8).[24,134–136,144] Complications with histamine H_2 receptor–blocking agents have been discussed[15–19] and are summarized in Table 45-9. Anticoagulant agents present special problems, most of which are well known (Table 45-10).[145,146] Finally, drugs, legitimate or illicit, that are abused can be especially problematic (Table 45-11).[147–154]

The problem of drug abuse is worsening. The Office of Applied Studies at the Substance Abuse and Mental Health Services Administration recently reported an increase in emer-

TABLE 45-10
Anticoagulant Drug Interactions

PREVIOUS DRUG THERAPY	COMPLICATIONS	PREVENTION, TREATMENT, OR SIGNIFICANCE
Heparin	• Intraoperative bleeding	• Avoid regional anesthesia • Reverse heparin by protamine or delay surgery; elimination half-life 1–3 hours • Monitor partial thromboplastin time and whole-blood clotting time
Oral anticoagulant agents (eg, warfarin)	• Intraoperative bleeding • Interact with enzyme inducers (eg, phenobarbital to result in reduced anticoagulant effect and increased effect if barbiturates discontinued; increased risk of hemorrhage • Metabolism of warfarin inhibited by cimetidine to increase effect • Sensitivity to warfarin increased in elders	• Avoid regional anesthesia • Reversed by vitamin K, but may take 24 hours for prothrombin time to approach normal

TABLE 45-11
Interactions With Drugs of Abuse

DRUGS	COMPLICATIONS	SIGNIFICANCE
Alcohol	• Acute alcohol intoxication decreases anesthetic requirements • Chronic alcohol intoxication increases anesthetic requirements • In severe intoxication, interacts with barbiturates, phenothiazines, and anesthetics to produce increased central nervous system sedation in acutely intoxicated patients	• In chronic alcoholism, pathophysiologic states necessitate preoperative assessment (eg, cirrhosis, poor nutrition, or altered fluid and electrolyte balance) • Administer central nervous system hypnotic or sedative agents with caution • Administer antacid followed by rapid-sequence induction with cricoid pressure • All drugs require careful titration because of multiple factors that result in altered drug pharmacokinetics and pharmacodynamics
Disulfiram	• Blocks oxidation of acetaldehyde • Allows ethanol metabolite to accumulate in toxic amounts, resulting in nausea and vomiting if patient ingests alcohol • No serious interactions	
Street drugs (eg, narcotics, barbiturates, and phencyclidine derivatives)	• Withdrawal crisis • Hypertension or hypotension • Alter anesthetic requirements	• Examine for hepatitis and for poor nutrition, hydration • Titrate anesthetic drugs cautiously • Narcotic technique may prevent withdrawal symptoms • Establish dosage schedule postoperatively; do not attempt to taper or withdraw
CENTRAL NERVOUS SYSTEM SYMPATHOMIMETIC DRUGS		
Cocaine	• General problems of addiction • Halothane MAC increased • Sensitizes myocardium to halothane and exogenous catecholamines • Cardiovascular instability	• Monitor for cardiac dysrhythmias • Titrate anesthetic agents carefully • Monitor fluid volume status
Amphetamines	• Halothane MAC increased • Cardiovascular instability	• Monitor for cardiac dysrhythmias • Monitor fluid volume status • Titrate anesthetic dose
Cannabinoids	• Halothane MAC decreased • Cardiovascular effects include tachycardia and increase in systolic blood pressure • Chronic use associated with asthma and bronchitis • Chronic use may be associated with postoperative sedation	• Tachycardia can be blocked by propranolol • Acute episodic use is probably without clinical significance • Chronic use requires careful titration of anesthetic agent

MAC, minimum alveolar concentration.

gency department drug-related cases involving cocaine and heroin.[155] In 685 hospitals during the third quarter of 1992, 109,200 such cases were seen, compared with 106,000 in the preceding quarter. Of the total, 13,400 were heroin-related and 30,900 cocaine-related. In persons 35 years old or older, cases involving cocaine increased 30% and those involving heroin increased 42% compared with 1991. Thus anesthesiologists, particularly in major urban areas, are likely to see increasing numbers of drug abusers who require emergency surgery or intensive care.

REFERENCES

1. Jick H, Miettinen OS, Shapiro S, et al: Comprehensive drug surveillance. JAMA 213:1455, 1970
2. May FE, Stewart RB, Cluff LE: Drug interactions and multiple drug administration. Clin Pharmacol Ther 22:322, 1977
3. Miller RR: Boston Collaborative Drug Surveillance Program: drug surveillance utilizing epidemiologic methods. Am J Hosp Pharm 30:584, 1973
4. Rawlins MD: Drug interactions and anaesthesia. Br J Anaesth 50:689, 1978
5. Nimmo WS, Wilson J, Prescott LF: Narcotic analgesics and delayed gastric emptying during labour. Lancet 1:890, 1975
6. Todd JG, Nimmo WS: Effect of premedication on drug absorption and gastric emptying. Br J Anaesth 55:1189, 1983
7. Clarke JM, Seager SJ: Gastric emptying following premedication with glycopyrrolate or atropine. Br J Anaesth 55:1195, 1983
8. Cockshott WP, Thompson GT, Howlett LJ: Intramuscular or intralipomatous injection? N Engl J Med 307:356, 1982
9. Csogor SI, Kerek SF: Enhancement of thiopental anaesthesia by sulphafurazole. Br J Anaesth 42:988, 1970
10. Lasser EC, Elizondo-Martel G, Granke RC: Potentiation of pentobarbital anesthesia by competitive protein binding. Anesthesiology 24:665, 1963
11. McLain GE, Sipes IG, Brown BR: An animal model of halothane hepatotoxicity: roles of enzyme induction and hypoxia. Anesthesiology 51:321, 1979

12. Cousins MJ, Mazze RI, Kosek JC, et al: The etiology of methoxyflurane nephrotoxicity. J Pharmacol Exp Ther 190:530, 1974
13. Mazze RI, Hitt BA, Cousins MJ: Effect of enzyme induction with phenobarbital on the *in vivo* and *in vitro* defluorination of isoflurane and methoxyflurane. J Pharmacol Exp Ther 190: 523, 1974
14. Barr GA, Cousins MJ, Mazze RI, et al: A comparison of the renal effects and metabolism of enflurane and methoxyflurane in Fisher 344 rats. J Pharmacol Exp Ther 188:257, 1974
15. Feely J, Wilkinson GR, McAllister CB, et al: Increased toxicity and reduced clearance of lidocaine by cimetidine. Ann Intern Med 96:592, 1982
16. Somogyi A, Muirhead M: Pharmacokinetic interactions of cimetidine. Clin Pharmacokinet 12:321, 1987
17. Gray DRP, Meatherall RC, Chalmers JL, et al: Cimetidine alters pethidine disposition in man. Br J Clin Pharmacol 18:907, 1984
18. Lam AM, Parkin JA: Cimetidine and prolonged postoperative somnolence. Can Anaesth Soc J 28:450, 1981
19. Mitchard M, Harris A, Mullinger BM: Ranitidine drug interactions: a literature review. Pharmacol Ther 32:293, 1987
20. Reilly CS, Wood AJJ, Koshakji RP, et al: The effect of halothane on drug disposition: contribution of changes in intrinsic drug metabolizing capacity and hepatic blood flow. Anesthesiology 63:70, 1985
21. Borel JD, Bently JB, Nenadc RE, et al: The influence of halothane on fentanyl pharmacokinetics (abstract). Anesthesiology 57:A239, 1982
22. Bently JB, Glass S, Gandolfi AJ: The influence of halothane on lidocaine pharmacokinetics in man (abstract). Anesthesiology 59:A246, 1983
23. Chelly JE, Hysing ES, Abernethy D, et al: Effects of inhalational anesthetics on verapamil pharmacokinetics in dogs. Anesthesiology 65:266, 1986
24. Pantuck EJ: Ecothiophate iodide eye drops and prolonged response to suxamethonium. Br J Anaesth 38:406, 1966
25. Donati F, Bevan DR: Controlled succinylcholine infusion in a patient receiving echothiophate eye drops. Can Anaesth Soc J 28:488, 1981
26. Goldberg LI: Monoamine oxidase inhibitors: adverse reactions and possible mechanisms. JAMA 190:456, 1964
27. Hager WD, Fenster P, Mayersohn M, et al: Digoxin-quinidine interaction: pharmacokinetic evaluation. N Engl J Med 300: 1238, 1979
28. Ben-Shlomo I, Abd-El-Khalim, Ezry J, et al: Midazolam acts synergistically with fentanyl for induction of anaesthesia. Br J Anaesth 64:45, 1990
29. Pittinger C, Adamson R: Antibiotic blockade of neuromuscular function. Annu Rev Pharmacol 12:169, 1972
30. Vigran IM: Dangerous potentiation of meperidine hydrochloride by pargyline hydrochloride. JAMA 187:953, 1964
31. Clark B, Thompson JW: Analysis of the inhibition of pethidine N-demethylation by monoamine oxidase inhibitors and some other drugs with special reference to drug interactions in man. Br J Pharmacol 44:89, 1972
32. Rogers KJ, Thornton JA: The interactions between monoamine oxidase inhibitors and narcotic analgesics in mice. Br J Pharmacol 36:470, 1969
33. Fraser CG, Preuss FS, Bigford WD: Adrenal atrophy and irreversible shock associated with cortisone therapy. JAMA 149: 1542, 1952
34. Lewis L, Robinson RF, Tee J, et al: Fatal adrenocortical insufficiency precipitated by surgery during prolonged continuous cortisone treatment. Ann Intern Med 39:116, 1953
35. Salassa RM, Bennett WA, Keating FR, et al: Postoperative adrenal cortical insufficiency: occurrence in patients previously treated with cortisone. JAMA 152:1509, 1953
36. Winstone NE, Brooke BN: Effects of steroid treatment on patients undergoing operation. Lancet 1:937, 1961
37. Pooler HE: A planned approach to the surgical patient with iatrogenic adrenocortical insufficiency. Br J Anaesth 40:539, 1968
38. Plumpton S, Besser GM, Cole PV: Corticosteroid treatment and surgery: I. an investigation of the indications for steroid cover. Anaesthesia 24:3, 1969
39. Plumpton S, Besser GM, Cole PV: Corticosteroid treatment and surgery: II. the management of steroid cover. Anaesthesia 24:12, 1969
40. Salem M, Tairish RE, Bromberg J, et al: Perioperative glucocorticoid coverage: a reassessment 42 years after emergence of a problem. Ann Surg 219:416, 1994
41. Symreng T, Karlberg BE, Kagedal B, et al: Physiological cortisol substitution of long-term steroid-treated patients undergoing major surgery. Br J Anaesth 53:949, 1981
42. Kehlet H, Binder C: Adrenocortical function and clinical course during and after surgery in unsupplemental glucocorticoid-treated patients. Br J Anaesth 45:1043, 1973
43. Chernow B, Alexander HR, Thompson WR, et al: The hormonal response to surgical stress. Arch Intern Med 147:1273, 1987
44. Bromberg JS, Alfrey EJ, Barker CF, et al: Adrenal suppression and steriod supplementation in renal transplant recipients. J Transplantation 51:385, 1991
45. Stehling L: Hypoglycemic drugs. Clin Anesthesiol 10:233, 1973
46. Rossini AA: Why control blood glucose levels? Arch Surg 111: 229, 1976
47. Rossini AA, Hare JE: How to control the blood glucose in the surgical diabetic patients. Arch Surg 111:945, 1976
48. Schen RJ, Khazzam AS: Postoperative hypoglycemic coma associated with chlorpropamide. Br J Anaesth 47:899, 1975
49. Reves JG, Kissin I, Lell WA, et al: Calcium entry blockers: uses and implications for anesthesiologists. Anesthesiology 57: 504, 1982
50. Jenkins LC, Scoates PJ: Anaesthetic implications of calcium channel blockers. Can Anaesth Soc J 32:436, 1985
51. Stone PH, Antman EM, Muller JE, et al: Calcium channel blocking agents in the treatment of cardiovascular disorders: II. hemodynamic effects and clinical applications. Ann Intern Med 93:886, 1980
52. Reves JG: The relative hemodynamic effects of calcium entry blockers. Anesthesiology 61:3, 1984
53. Kates RA, Kaplan JA, Guyton RA, et al: Hemodynamic interactions of verapamil and isoflurane. Anesthesiology 59:132, 1983
54. Marshall AG, Kissin J, Reves JG, et al: Interaction between the negative inotropic effects of halothane and nifedipine in the isolated rat heart. J Cardiovasc Pharmacol 5:592, 1983
55. Kapur PA, Bloor BC, Blacke WE, et al: Comparison of cardiovascular responses to verapamil during enflurane, isoflurane or halothane anesthesia in the dog. Anesthesiology 61:156, 1984
56. Ramsay JG, Cutfield GR, Francis CM, et al: Halothane-verapamil causes regional myocardial dysfunction in the dog. Br J Anaesth 58:32, 1986
57. Chelly JE, Rogers K, Hysing ES, et al: Cardiovascular effects of and interaction between calcium channel blocking drugs and anesthetics in chronically instrumented dogs: I. verapamil and halothane. Anesthesiology 64:560, 1986
58. Kates RA, Zaggy AP, Norfleet NA, et al: Comparative cardiovascular effects of verapamil, nifedipine, and diltiazem during halothane anesthesia in swine. Anesthesiology 61:10, 1984
59. Brichard G, Zimmermann PE: Verapamil in cardiac dysrhythmias during anaesthesia. Br J Anaesth 42:1005, 1970
60. Shulte-Sasse V, Hess W, Markeschies-Hornung A, et al: Combined effects of halothane anesthesia and verapamil on systemic hemodynamics and left myocardial contractility in patients with ischemic heart disease. Anesth Analg 63:791, 1984
61. Kates RA, Kaplan JA: Cardiovascular responses to verapamil during coronary artery bypass graft surgery. Anesth Analg 62: 821, 1983
62. Maze M, Mason DM, Kates RE: Verapamil decreases MAC for halothane in dogs. Anesthesiology 59:327, 1983
63. Lawson NW, Kraynack BJ, Gintautas J: Neuromuscular and electrocardiographic responses to verapamil in dogs. Anesth Analg 62:50, 1983
64. Kraynack BJ, Lawson NW, Gintautas J, et al: Effects of vera-

pamil on indirect muscle twitch responses. Anesth Analg 62: 827, 1983
65. Durant NN, Nguyen N, Katz RL: Potentiation of neuromuscular blockade by verapamil. Anesthesiology 60:298, 1984
66. Van Poorten JF, Dhasmana KM, Kuypers RS, et al: Verapamil and reversal of vecuronium neuromuscular blockade. Anesth Analg 63:155, 1984
67. Pederson KE, Thaysen P, Klitgaard NA, et al: Influence of verapamil on the inotropism and pharmacokinetics of digoxin. Eur J Clin Pharmacol 25:199, 1983
68. Oesterle SN, Schroeder JS: Calcium entry blockade, beta-adrenergic blockade and the reflex control of circulation. Circulation 65:669, 1982
69. Green JA, Clement WA, Porter C, et al: Nifedipine-quinidine interaction. Clin Pharm 2:461, 1983
70. Burnakis TG, Seldon M, Czaplicki AD: Increased serum theophylline levels secondary to oral theophylline. Clin Pharm 2: 458, 1983
71. Raferty EB: Cardiovascular drug withdrawal syndromes: a potential problem with calcium antagonists. Drugs 28:371, 1984
72. Engelman RM, Hadj-Rousou IH, et al: Rebound vasospasm after coronary revascularization in association with calcium antagonist withdrawal. Ann Thorac Surg 37:469, 1984
73. Hirsch JA, Tomlinson DL, Slogoff S, et al: The overstated risk of preoperative hypokalemia. Anesth Analg 67:131, 1988
74. Wong KC, Schafer PG, Schultz JR: Hypokalemia and anesthetic implications. Anesth Analg 77:1238, 1993
75. Benotti JR, Grossman W, Braunwald E, et al: Hemodynamic assessment of amrinone. New Engl J Med 299:1373, 1987
76. Frishman WH: Beta-adrenoceptor antagonists: new drugs and new indications. N Engl J Med 305:500, 1981
77. Viljoen JF, Estafanous FG, Kellner GA: Propranolol and cardiac surgery. J Thorac Cardiovasc Surg 64:826, 1972
78. Kaplan JA, Dunbar RW, Bland JW, et al: Propranolol and cardiac surgery: a problem for the anesthetist? Anesth Analg 54: 571, 1975
79. Horan BF, Prys-Roberts C, Hamilton WK, et al: Haemodynamic responses to enflurane anesthesia and hypovolemia in the dog, and their modification by propranolol. Br J Anaesth 49:1189, 1977
80. Roberts JG, Foex P, Clarke TNS, et al: Haemodynamic interactions of high-dose propranolol pretreatment and anaesthesia in the dog: III. the effects of hemorrhage during halothane and trichloroethylene anaesthesia. Br J Anaesth 48:411, 1976
81. Roberts JG, Foex P, Clarke TNS, et al: Haemodynamic interactions of high-dose propranolol pretreatment and anaesthesia in the dog: I. halothane dose-response studies. Br J Anaesth 48:315, 1976
82. Horan BF, Prys-Roberts C, Roberts JG, et al: Haemodynamic responses to isoflurane anaesthesia and hypovolemia in the dog, and their modification by propranolol. Br J Anaesth 49: 1179, 1977
83. Slogoff S, Keats AS, Hibbs WC, et al: Failure of general anesthesia to potentiate propranolol activity. Anesthesiology 47: 504, 1977
84. Chung DA: Anaesthetic problems associated with the treatment of cardiovascular disease: II. beta-adrenergic antagonists. Can Anaesth Soc J 28:105, 1981
85. Shand DG, Wood AJJ: Propranolol withdrawal syndrome: why? Circulation 58:202, 1978
86. Wood AJJ: Beta-blocker withdrawal. Drugs 25(suppl 2):318, 1983
87. Slome R: Withdrawal of propranolol and myocardial infarction. Lancet 1:156, 1973
88. Myers MG, Freeman MR, Juma ZA, et al: Propranolol withdrawal in angina pectoris: a prospective study. Am Heart J 97: 298, 1979
89. Beta-Blocker Heart Attack Study Group: The beta-blocker heart attack trial. JAMA 246:2073, 1981
90. Norwegian Multi-Center Study Group: Timolol-induced reduction in mortality and reinfarction in patients surviving acute myocardial infarction. N Engl J Med 304:801, 1981
91. Sleight P: Beta-adrenergic blockade after myocardial infarction. N Engl J Med 304:837, 1981
92. Kopriva CJ, Brown ACD, Pappas G: Hemodynamics during general anesthesia in patients receiving propranolol. Anesthesiology 48:28, 1978
93. Roberts JG: Beta-adrenergic blockade and anaesthesia with reference to interactions with anaesthetic drugs and techniques. Anaesth Intensive Care 8:318, 1980
94. Taggart P, Carruthers M: Suppression by oxyprenolol of adrenergic response to stress. Lancet 2:256, 1972
95. McCammon RL, Hilgenberg JC, Stoelting RK: Effect of propranolol on circulatory responses to induction of diazepam-nitrous oxide anesthesia and to endotracheal intubation. Anesth Analg 60:579, 1981
96. Safwat AM, Reitan JA, Misle GR, et al: Use of propranolol to control rate-pressure product during cardiac anesthesia. Anesth Analg 60:732, 1981
97. Stanley TH, DeLange S, Boscoe MJ, et al: The influence of chronic preoperative propranolol therapy on cardiovascular dynamics and narcotic requirements during operation in patients with coronary artery disease. Can Anaesth Soc J 29:319, 1982
98. Hammon JW, Wood AJJ, Prager RL, et al: Perioperative beta blockade with propranolol: reduction in myocardial oxygen demands and the incidence of atrial and ventricular arrhythmias. Ann Thorac Surg 38:363, 1984
99. Foex P, Prys-Roberts C: Anaesthesia and the hypertensive patient. Br J Anaesth 46:575, 1974
100. Goldman L, Caldera DL: Risks of general anesthesia and elective operation in the hypertensive patient. Anesthesiology 50: 285, 1979
101. Lowenstein J: Clonidine. Ann Intern Med 92:74, 1980
102. Graham RM, Pettinger WA: Prazosin. N Engl J Med 300:232, 1979
103. Nielsen GD: Influence of various anaesthetics on the cardiovascular responses to noradrenaline in rats before and after guanethidine. Acta Pharmacol Toxicol 40:75, 1977
104. Alper MH, Flacke W, Krayer O: Pharmacology of reserpine and its implications for anesthesia. Anesthesiology 24:524, 1963
105. Katz RL, Weintraub HD, Papper EM: Anesthesia, surgery and rauwolfia. Anesthesiology 25:142, 1964
106. Ominsky AJ, Wollman H: Hazards of general anesthesia in reserpinized patients. Anesthesiology 30:443, 1969
107. Koch-Waser J: Hydralazine. N Engl J Med 295:320, 1976
108. Mitchell HC, Pettinger WA: Long-term treatment of refractory hypertensive patients with minoxidil. JAMA 239:2131, 1978
109. McDonald AJ, Smith G, Woods JW, et al: Intravenous diazoxide therapy in hypertensive crisis. Am J Cardiol 40:409, 1977
110. Woodside J Jr, Garner L, Bedford RF, et al: Captopril reduces the dose requirement for sodium nitroprusside–induced hypotension. Anesthesiology 60:413, 1984
111. Findlay JW, Butz RF, Williams BB, et al: Effect of monoamine oxidase inhibitors on codeine disposition and pentobarbitone sleep times in the rat. J Pharm Pharmacol 33:45, 1981
112. Eade NR, Renton KW: Effect of monoamine oxidase inhibitors on the N-demethylation and hydrolysis of meperidine. Biochem Pharmacol 19:2243, 1970
113. Banerjee SP, Kung LS, Riggi SJ, et al: Development of beta-adrenergic receptor subsensitivity by antidepressants. Nature 268:455, 1977
114. Creese I, Sibley DR: Receptor adaptations to centrally acting drugs. Annu Rev Pharmacol Toxicol 21:357, 1981
115. Wong KC, Puerto AY, Puerto BA, et al: Influence of imipramine and pargyline on the arrhythmogenicity of epinephrine during halothane, enflurane or methoxyflurane anesthesia in dogs. Life Sci 27:2675, 1980
116. Spiss CK, Smith CM, Maze M: Halothane-epinephrine arrhythmias and adrenergic responsiveness after chronic imipramine administration in dogs. Anesth Analg 63:825, 1984
117. Edwards RP, Miller RD, Roizen MF, et al: Cardiac response to imipramine and pancuronium during anesthesia with halothane or enflurane. Anesthesiology 50:421, 1979

118. Inagakiy, Sumikawa K, Yoshiya I: Anesthetic interaction between midazolam and halothane in humans. Anesth Analg 76: 613, 1993
119. Perisho JA, Buechel DR, Miller RD: The effect of diazepam on minimal alveolar anaesthetic requirements in man. Can Anaesth Soc J 18:536, 1971
120. Gold MI: Profound hypotension associated with preoperative use of phenothiazines. Anesth Analg 53:844, 1974
121. Hill GE, Wong KC, Hodges MR: Lithium carbonate and neuromuscular blocking agents. Anesthesiology 46:122, 1977
122. Mannisto PT, Saarnivarra L: Effect of lithium and rubidum on the sleeping time caused by various intravenous anaesthetics in the mouse. Br J Anaesth 48:185, 1976
123. Jephcott G, Kerry RJ: Lithium: an anaesthetic risk. Br J Anaesth 46:389, 1974
124. Krasner BS: Cardiac effects of magnesium with special reference to anaesthesia: a review. Can Anaesth Soc J 26:181, 1979
125. Goldbert KI: Anesthetic management of patients treated with antihypertensive agents or levodopa. Anesth Analg 51:625, 1972
126. Himes RS, DiFazio CA, Burney RG: Effects of lidocaine on the anesthetic requirements for nitrous oxide and halothane. Anesthesiology 47:437, 1977
127. Zipes DP, Troup PJ: New antiarrhythmic drugs: amiodarone, aprindine, disopyramide, ethmozin, mexiletine, tocainide, verapamil. Am J Cardiol 41:1005, 1978
128. Koch-Weser J: Drug therapy: bretylium. N Engl J Med 300: 473, 1979.
129. Harrah MD, Way WL, Katzung BG: The interaction of *d*-tubocurarine with antiarrhythmic drugs. Anesthesiology 33:406, 1970
130. Miller RD, Way WL, Katzung BG: The potentiation of neuromuscular blocking agents by quinidine. Anesthesiology 28: 1036, 1967
131. Heger JJ, Prystowsky EN, Miles WM, et al: Clinical use and pharmacology of amiodarone. Med Clin North Am 68:1339, 1984
132. Latini R, Tognoni G, Kates RE: Clinical pharmacokinetics of amiodarone. Clin Pharmacokinet 9:136, 1984
133. Gallagher JD, Lieberman RW, Meranze J, et al: Amiodarone-induced complications during coronary artery surgery. Anesthesiology 55:186, 1981
134. Gurman GM: Prolonged apnea after succinylcholine in a case treated with cytostatics for cancer. Anesth Analg 51:761, 1972
135. Zsigmond EK, Robins G: The effect of a series of anti-cancer drugs on plasma cholinesterase activity. Can Anesth Soc J 19: 75, 1972
136. Selvin BL: Cancer chemotherapy: implications for the anesthesiologist. Anesth Analg 60:425, 1981
137. Chung F: Cancer, chemotherapy, and anaesthesia. Can Anaesth Soc J 29:364, 1982
138. Glissen SN, El-Etr AA, Lim R: Prolongation of pancuronium-induced neuromuscular blockade by intravenous infusion of nitroglycerin. Anesthesiology 51:47, 1979
139. Wilson SL, Miller RN, Wright C, et al: Prolonged neuromuscular blockade associated with trimethaphan: a case report. Anesth Analg 55:353, 1976
140. Miller RD, Yung JS, Matteo RS: Enhancement of *d*-tubocurarine neuromuscular blockade by diuretics in man. Anesthesiology 45:442, 1976
141. Fogdall RP, Miller RD: Prolongation of a pancuronium-induced neuromuscular blockade by clindamycin. Anesthesiology 41: 407, 1974
142. Kaukinen S, Pyykko K: The potentiation of halothane anesthesia by clonidine. Acta Anaesthesiol Scand 23:107, 1979
143. Miller RD, Way WL, Eger EI II: The effects of alpha-methyldopa, reserpine, guanethidine and iproniazid on minimum alveolar anesthetic requirement (MAC). Anesthesiology 29:1153, 1968
144. Robertson GS: Serum cholinesterase deficiency: II. pregnancy. Br J Anaesth 38:361, 1966
145. Ellison N, Ominsky AJ: Clinical considerations for the anesthesiologist whose patient is on anticoagulant therapy. Anesthesiology 39:328, 1973
146. Tekkok IH, Cataltepe KT, Bertan V: Extradural haematoma after continuous extradural anaesthesia. Br J Anaesth 67:112, 1991
147. Johnstone RE, Kulp RA, Smith TC: Effects of acute and chronic ethanol administration on isoflurane requirement of mice. Anesth Analg 54:277, 1975
148. Rubin E, Gang H, Misra PS, et al: Inhibition of drug metabolism by acute ethanol intoxication. Am J Med 49:801, 1970
149. Keity SR: Anesthesia for the alcoholic patient. Anesth Analg 48:659, 1969
150. Wolfson B, Freed B: Influence of alcohol on anesthetic requirements and acute toxicity. Anesth Analg 59:826, 1980
151. Johnston RR, Way WL, Miller RD: Alteration of anesthetic requirement by amphetamine. Anesthesiology 36:357, 1972
152. Van Dyke C, Barash PG, Jatlow P, et al: Cocaine: plasma concentrations after intranasal application in man. Science 191: 859, 1976
153. Stoelting RK, Creasser CW, Martz RC: Effect of cocaine administration on halothane MAC in dogs. Anesth Analg 54:422, 1975
154. Stoelting RK, Mantz RC, Gartner J, et al: Effects of delta-9-tetrahydrocannabinol on halothane MAC in dogs. Anesthesiology 38:521, 1973
155. Office of Applied Studies at the Substance Abuse and Mental Health Services Administration: Heroin, cocaine incidents on rise in emergency rooms (Associated Press release). April 24, 1993

Complications in Anesthesiology, second edition,
edited by Nikolaus Gravenstein and Robert R. Kirby.
Lippincott-Raven Publishers, Philadelphia © 1996.

CHAPTER 46

Exacerbation of Inducible Porphyria

Fredrick K. Orkin

More than 40 years ago, anesthesiologists were exhorted never to use thiopental or other barbiturates in the anesthetic management of patients known or suspected to have porphyria.[1,2] The "dire" effects of barbiturate anesthesia in these patients included an acute neurologic syndrome consisting of abdominal pain, nausea and vomiting (among other autonomic dysfunctions), mental disturbances, and peripheral neuropathy, often leading to respiratory paralysis. Death occurred in as many as two thirds of those affected. Apart from an appreciation of an inheritable predisposition to this complication, its underlying pathogenesis was not understood, and no therapy was effective.

Porphyria is now recognized as a clinically heterogeneous group of diseases that may be acquired or inherited (Table 46-1). In these disorders, underlying disturbances involve the biosynthesis of heme, the prosthetic group in essential respiratory pigments such as hemoglobin and the cytochromes. Each of the porphyrias has a characteristic pattern of overproduction and accumulation of porphyrin precursors and porphyrins, tetrapyrrole pigments that are intermediates in the heme biosynthetic pathway.

Acute clinical episodes of three porphyrias, *acute intermittent porphyria*, *variegate porphyria*, and *hereditary coproporphyria*, may be precipitated by barbiturates and other drugs that, in experimental conditions, can induce porphyrin biosynthesis. Hence, these diseases may be termed *inducible*.[3] This chapter reviews the physical basis, symptoms, treatment, and prevention of life-threatening, though rare, acute episodes of these inducible porphyrias, which are of particular interest to the anesthesiologist.

CLASSIFICATION

Inborn Errors of Metabolism

Except for an acquired form, the porphyrias represent classic examples of disorders resulting from inborn errors of metabolism, first described by Garrod.[4] Hence, they are as much metabolic disorders as hematologic diseases. Because a mutant somatic gene is responsible for the metabolic derangement in each type, the porphyrias must be considered cellular diseases. Indeed, in a given form of porphyria, the accumulation of characteristic porphyrins and porphyrin precursors usually is found in all tissues studied. This observation is not surprising because all mammalian cells can synthesize the porphyrin required for essential heme-containing enzymes, such as the cytochromes, catalase, and peroxidase. Classification is based on the major site at which the error in metabolism occurs.[5]

Functional Characteristics

Functionally, the porphyrias also may be classified on the basis of symptoms. Acute intermittent porphyria, variegate porphyria, and hereditary coproporphyria are the only forms that have an acute neurologic syndrome induced by drugs, and therefore they are of principal interest to the anesthesiologist. Some patients with variegate porphyria and hereditary coproporphyria also have eruptions on areas of the skin exposed to sunlight.

Photosensitivity with dermatologic manifestations generally is characteristic of the *noninducible* porphyrias.[6,7] *Congenital erythropoietic porphyria* (Günther's disease), which expresses itself early in childhood and is associated with mutilating skin lesions, facial hirsutism, hemolytic anemia, port wine–colored urine, and early death is rare. *Erythropoietic coproporphyria* is a milder disorder that has been described in only one family. *Protoporphyria* begins early in life with skin rashes after exposure to sunlight and progresses to hepatic disease, with liver failure in some patients.

Porphyria cutanea tarda is probably the most common form of porphyria and is characterized by chronic lesions on areas of skin exposed to sunlight and by hepatic siderosis. Finally, several *cutaneous porphyrias* resemble porphyria cutanea tarda and are associated with lupus erythematosus, chronic

TABLE 46-1
Classification of Porphyrias

ERYTHROPOIETIC

- Congenital erythropoietic porphyria
- Erythropoietic coproporphyria

ERYTHROHEPATIC

- Photoporphyria

HEPATIC

- Acute intermittent porphyria
- Variegate porphyria
- Hereditary coproporphyria
- Porphyria cutanea tarda
- Cutaneous porphyrias

alcoholism, hepatic tumors, hemolytic anemias, and hexachlorobenzene poisoning. In addition to the major site of metabolic expression and the symptoms, the porphyrias may be differentiated on the basis of the mode of inheritance and on laboratory findings (Table 46-2).

PHYSICAL BASIS

Heme Biosynthesis

Figure 46-1 presents the heme biosynthetic pathway. Within the mitochondrion, succinate (from the metabolism of acetate in the Krebs tricarboxylic acid cycle) is converted to succinyl coenzyme A, which condenses with glycine in the presence of the enzyme δ-aminolevulinic acid synthetase (ALA-S) to form a five-carbon chain, δ-aminolevulinic acid (ALA).

The next several steps occur in the cytosol. Two chains condense to form the porphyrin precursor, porphobilinogen (PBG). Deamination and further condensation by uroporphyrinogen I synthetase (PBG deaminase) and uroporphyrinogen III cosynthetase (PBG isomerase) then form uroporphyrinogen III, which is converted to coproporphyrinogen III by uroporphyrinogen decarboxylase.

When it enters the mitochondrion, further oxidation and decarboxylation of coproporphyrinogen III by coproporphyrinogen oxidase results in the formation of protoporphyrinogen IX. The latter is converted to protoporphyrin IX by protoporphyrinogen oxidase before the insertion of ferrous iron by ferrochelatase to form heme, which by combining with four globin subunits in turn forms hemoglobin.

TABLE 46-2
Clinical and Laboratory Features of the Porphyrias

	ERYTHROPOIETIC	ERYTHROHEPATIC	HEPATIC						
	Congenital Erythropoietic Porphyria	*Protoporphyria*	*Acute Intermittent Porphyria*		*Variegate Porphyria*		*Hereditary Coproporphyria*		*Porphyria Cutanea Tarda*
CHARACTERISTICS									
Inheritance	Autosomal recessive	Autosomal dominant	Autosomal dominant		Autosomal dominant		Autosomal dominant		Autosomal dominant
Symptoms			*latent*	*acute*	*latent*	*acute*	*latent*	*acute*	
Photosensitivity (causing cutaneous lesions)	Yes	Yes	No	No	No	Yes or no	No	Yes or no	Yes
Neurologic syndrome	No	No	No	Yes	No	Yes	No	Yes	No
LABORATORY FINDINGS									
Red blood cells									
Uroporphyrin	↑↑↑	↑↑	N	N	N	N	N	N	N
Coproporphyrin	↑↑	↑↑	N	N	N	N	N	N	N
Protoporphyrin	N or ↑	↑↑↑	N	N	N	N	N	N	N
Urine									
Color*	Red	N	N	Red	N	N or red	N	N or red	Red
ALA	N	N	↑	↑↑	N	↑↑	↑	↑↑	N
PBG	N	N	↑↑	↑↑↑	N	↑↑	↑	↑↑	N
Uroporphyrin	↑↑↑	N	↑↑	↑↑	N	↑↑↑	N	↑↑	↑↑↑
Coproporphyrin	↑↑	N	↑↑	↑↑	N	↑↑↑	N or ↑	↑↑↑	↑↑
Feces									
Coproporphyrin	↑	N	N	↑	↑↑↑	↑↑	↑↑	↑↑↑	N
Protoporphyrin	↑	N or ↑	N	↑	↑↑↑	↑↑	N	↑	N

N, normal; ↑, increased to ↑↑↑, greatly increased.

* Freshly voided. On standing, the urine may become deep brownish red or black.

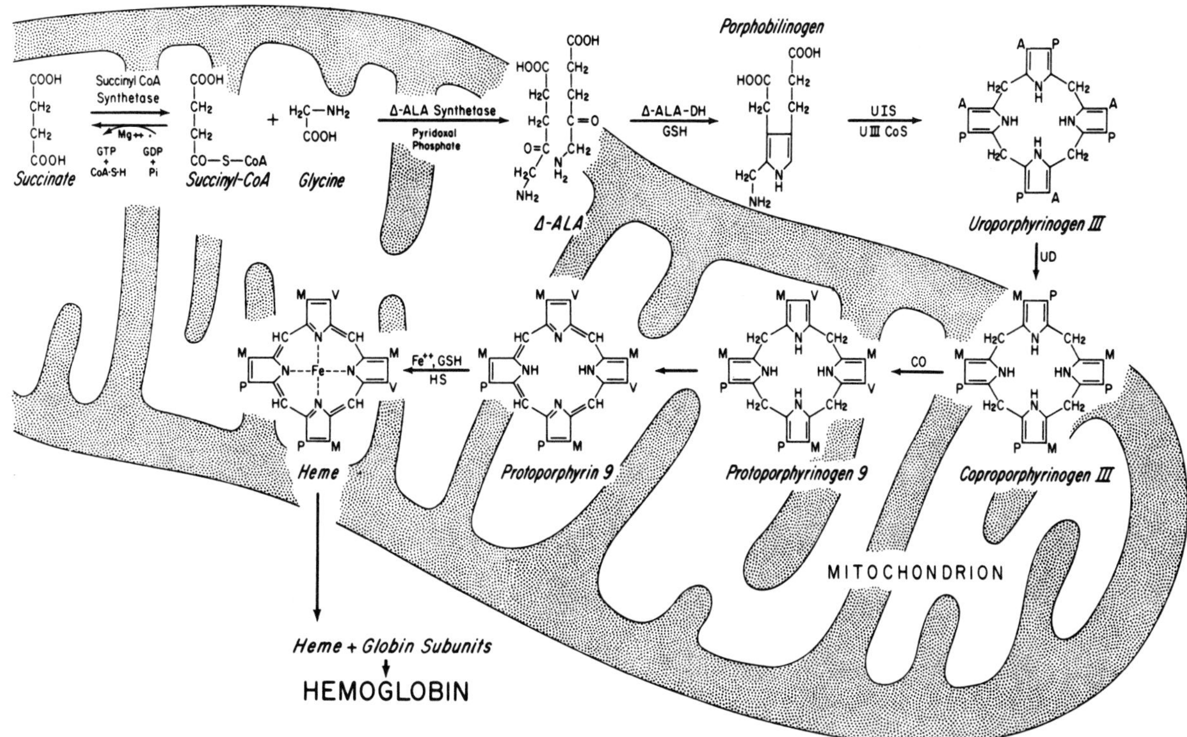

FIGURE 46-1. The biosynthesis of heme. *δ-ALA,* δ-aminolevulinic acid; *δ-ALA-DH,* δ-aminolevulinic acid dehydrase; *CO,* coproporphyrinogen oxidase; *CoA,* coenzyme A; *GDP,* guanosine diphosphate; *GSH,* glutathione; *GTP,* guanosine triphosphate; *HS,* heme synthetase; *UIII CoS,* uroporphyrinogen III cosynthetase; *UD,* uroporphyrinogen decarboxylase; *UIS,* uroporphyrinogen I synthetase. (Bunn HF: Pathophysiology of the anemias. In Braunwald E, Isselbacher KJ, Petersdorf RG, et al (eds): Harrison's principles of internal medicine, 11th ed. New York: McGraw-Hill, 1987: 1491)

Regulation

Many of the steps in heme biosynthesis are favored thermodynamically, and the degradation of heme, to bile pigments, proceeds along a different pathway. As a result, heme biosynthesis is unidirectional and irreversible. Control mechanisms for this type of pathway usually are located at the first enzymatic step uniquely involved in the synthesis of the end product.[8] In heme biosynthesis, this step is the formation of ALA. That ALA-S is the rate-limiting enzyme is suggested by its much lower activity than that of enzymes later in the pathway; the presence of abundant succinyl coenzyme A and glycine; and the presence of distal heme precursors in only trace quantities.[9]

Feedback Repression of δ-Aminolevulinic Acid Synthetase

In normal circumstances, heme biosynthesis is regulated to supply the heme required for the various hemoproteins efficiently. This regulation is accomplished, as shown in Figure 46-2, by the negative-feedback regulation of the end product, heme, on ALA-S.[10,11] Inhibition of ALA-S *activity,* as a result

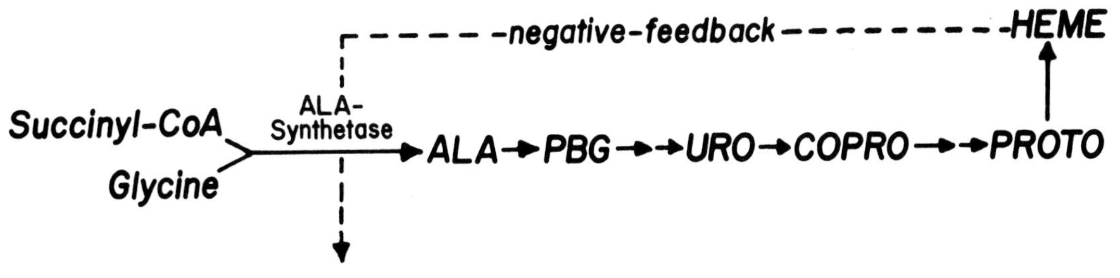

-negative-feedback- HEME

Succinyl-CoA / Glycine — ALA-Synthetase → ALA → PBG →→ URO → COPRO →→ PROTO

FIGURE 46-2. In heme biosynthesis, heme exerts negative-feedback regulation on ALA-S. *CoA,* coenzyme A; *COPRO,* coproporphyrinogen; *PROTO,* protoporphyrin; *URO,* uroporphyrinogen.

of conformational changes consequent to physical binding with heme, is a possible control mechanism[12]; however, this feedback inhibition has been demonstrated only with purified enzyme preparations. The principal mode of ALA-S regulation appears to be repression of enzyme *synthesis*.

Although the precise mechanism of this end-product inhibition is unclear, the data are consistent with the general model of protein synthesis regulation proposed by Jacob and Monod.[13] Applied to heme biosynthesis (Fig. 46-3), that model proposes that heme combines with a protein, termed an "aporepressor," whose synthesis is directed by a regulator gene.[14] The combination of heme, acting as a corepressor, and the aporepressor is termed a "repressor." The latter acts on the operator gene to repress the transcription of the structural gene responsible for synthesizing the messenger ribonucleic acid. The latter, in turn, controls the synthesis of ALA-S on the ribosome. Hence, the presence of excess heme serves to decrease the availability of ALA-S at the rate-limiting step, thereby diminishing the synthesis of heme itself.

Induction of δ-Aminolevulinic Acid Synthetase

In accordance with this scheme for the regulation of heme biosynthesis, increased heme utilization derepresses the operator gene, and more ALA-S is synthesized, providing more heme precursors to satisfy the demand for heme (see Fig. 46-3). In normal circumstances, most of the hepatic heme is used for the synthesis of cytochrome P-450, a group of microsomal enzymes that function as the terminal oxidase in drug metabolism. The administration of any of many diverse lipophilic chemicals and drugs induces increased synthesis of cytochrome P-450 and, in turn, ALA-S.[9] Although barbiturates

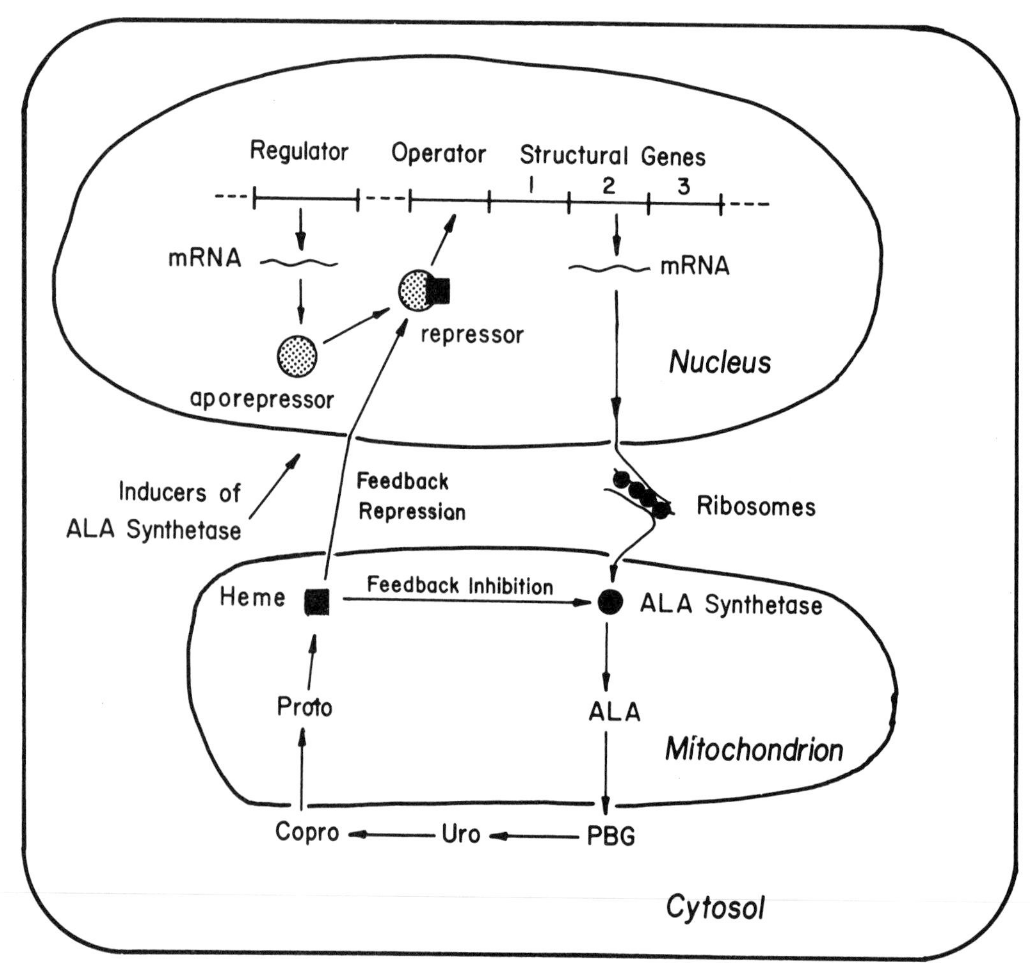

FIGURE 46-3. Regulatory mechanisms for heme biosynthesis. Heme, acting as a corepressor, combines with a repressor substance, the synthesis of which is directed by a regulator gene. The resultant repressor influences an operator gene to "turn off" the structural gene directing the synthesis of the messenger ribonucleic acid (*mRNA*) for the synthesis of ALA-S on the ribosomes. Decreased availability of mRNA and, in turn, ALA-S at the rate-limiting step results in diminished synthesis of heme precursors. Heme may also combine with ALA-S, changing the conformation of the enzyme and thereby inhibiting its activity. Less repressor is present when there is increased demand for heme, and the repressor may be inactivated when heme is displaced from its binding site by certain drugs, resulting in increased mRNA and ALA-S synthesis and permitting increased heme production. *Copro*, coproporphyrinogen; *Proto*, protoporphyrin; *Uro*, uroporphyrinogen.

are well-known inducers of the synthesis of drug-metabolizing enzymes, other inducing agents are insecticides, endogenous and exogenous steroids, and various therapeutic agents, principally antibiotic agents and nonbarbiturate hypnotic agents. Not unexpectedly, porphyria produced in the laboratory by chemicals that impair the regulatory mechanism and permit excessive ALA-S synthesis is termed *chemical* or *experimental porphyria*.[9,15,16]

Modification of δ-Aminolevulinic Acid Synthetase Induction

A variety of exogenous and endogenous factors, some having clinical relevance, can modify the induction of ALA-S synthesis.[17] Increased intake of carbohydrate or protein can block induction; the mechanism of this *glucose effect* is unknown.[15,18] On the other hand, fasting enhances induction of ALA-S synthesis, probably through increased breakdown of heme.[6,19] Chelated iron, in the form of ferric citrate or iron dextran, also results in loss of heme and marked increase in ALA-S synthesis as a secondary, expected event.[6] A diverse group of steroids, including metabolites of gonadal and adrenocortical hormones[20] and intermediates in bile acid degradation,[21] can induce ALA-S synthesis as well. In adrenalectomized animals, hydrocortisone exhibits a "permissive" effect on induction of ALA-S synthesis.[22]

Metabolic Defects

Given the regulatory interdependence between the availability of heme and the synthesis of ALA-S (see Fig. 46-2), any partial blockage in a biosynthetic step between ALA and heme should result in increased ALA-S synthesis and an accumulation of heme precursor immediately proximal to the defect. In fact, each of the inducible porphyrias is characterized by seemingly inappropriate increased ALA-S activity and a specific pattern of heme precursor accumulation and excretion (see Table 46-2; Fig. 46-4). In no case, however, is the enzymatic defect a complete blockage, for the absence of heme synthesis is incompatible with life.

Acute Intermittent Porphyria

In acute intermittent porphyria, there is deficiency of PBG deaminase (uroporphyrinogen I synthetase), resulting in the accumulation of ALA and PBG in the urine.[23,24] The pathogenic gene is located on autosome 11.[25] Immunologic analysis suggests four classes of defective PBG deaminase. This molecular genetic heterogeneity accounts at least partially for the highly varied clinical presentations of affected persons.[26]

Variegate Porphyria

The excretion pattern in variegate porphyria suggests that the enzyme defect is between protoporphyrinogen and heme; one study notes that the defect is a deficiency of protoporphyrinogen oxidase (ferrochelatase).[27] As a result, the excretion products consist of ALA and PBG in the urine and a variety of porphyrin compounds in the feces.

Hereditary Coproporphyria

The defect here is probably a deficiency of coproporphyrinogen oxidase.[28–30] Thus, ALA, PBG, and a variety of porphyrins also are excreted, as in variegate porphyria. Just as several forms of the genetic defect are present in acute intermittent porphyria, so also in this disease are there persons who exhibit slightly different genetic defects, leading to the coexistence of different porphyrias.[31,32] Albeit rare, this form of genetic heterogeneity also may account for the varied clinical presentations.

PATHOGENESIS

Whereas much is known about heme biosynthesis and the biochemical basis of porphyria, relatively little is understood about the relations between the enzymatic defects and the symptoms, particularly the neurologic syndrome. However, a superficial differentiation of the symptoms is possible on biochemical grounds.[33] Acute attacks of all of the inducible porphyrias are associated with a neurologic syndrome and the

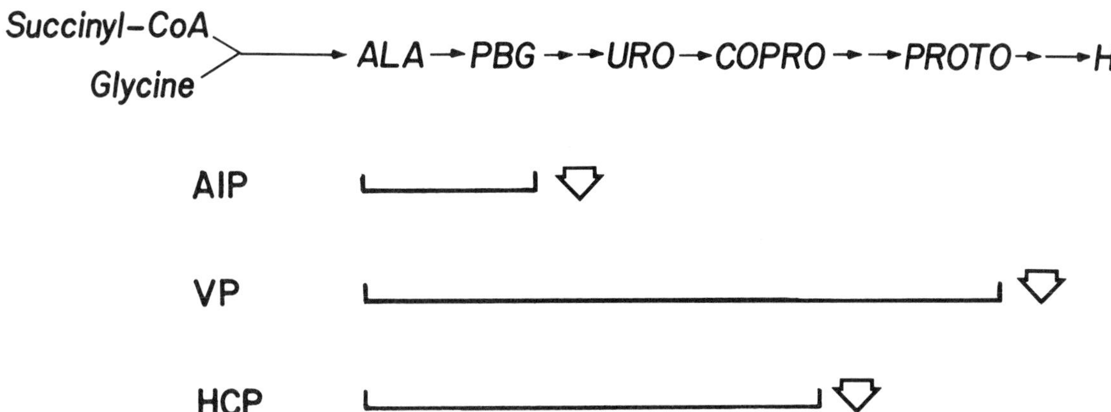

FIGURE 46-4. Postulated primary enzyme deficiencies (*outlined arrows*) and urinary excretion patterns (*brackets*) during acute attacks of the inducible porphyrias. *AIP*, acute intermittent porphyria; *CoA*, coenzyme A; *COPRO*, coproporphyrinogen; *HCP*, hereditary coproporphyria; *PROTO*, protoporphyrinogen; *URO*, uroporphyrinogen; *VP*, variegate porphyria.

excretion of ALA and PBG. Photosensitivity occurs in variegate porphyria and hereditary coproporphyria, both of which are associated with the additional accumulation of porphyrins, but not in acute intermittent porphyria, which is not associated with porphyrin excess.

Photosensitivity

Porphyrins fluoresce intensely in ultraviolet light at a wavelength of about 400 nm. Ultraviolet radiation in this band happens to evoke maximal cutaneous photosensitivity in experimental conditions.[6] Although the mechanism of formation of the dermatologic lesion is understood incompletely, porphyrins known to be capable of causing photosensitization are stored in lysosomes.[34] Absorption of light in the 400-nm band, in the presence of oxygen, may cause leakage of hydrolytic enzymes also stored in the lysosomes, with resultant disruption of the cell and the release of substances that give rise to the characteristic erythema, blistering, and subsequent scarring.

Neurologic Syndrome: Possible Causes

Accumulation of δ-Aminolevulinic Acid and Porphobilinogen

The ALA and PBG that accumulate in the blood during acute attacks of porphyria have been postulated to be neurotoxic. These compounds can cause presynaptic inhibition of neurotransmitter release, inhibition of adenosine triphosphatase in the brain, inhibition of monosynaptic reflexes in the spinal cord, and decrease in the resting membrane potential of muscle.[35] However, neither compound penetrates the blood–brain barrier sufficiently to achieve concentrations in nervous tissue approximating those required for these effects. Moreover, increasing blood concentrations of these compounds may not be associated with neurologic deterioration.[36]

Defect in Heme Biosynthesis

More plausible is the presence of a concomitant defect in *neural* heme biosynthesis, resulting in demyelination and secondary axonal degeneration.[35] Of interest, asymptomatic persons who have the biochemical defect but who have never had an acute attack demonstrate peripheral neuropathy on electromyography.[37] Thus, the latent genetic defect in neural cells, as in other somatic cells, likely is activated during acute episodes.

Impairment of Tryptophan Metabolism

Acutely impaired tryptophan metabolism may underlie the neurologic syndrome. In rats, chemically induced porphyria results in acute heme deficiency, with almost all available heme consumed by cytochrome P-450 synthesis and little heme left for the synthesis of other hemoproteins.

Of the latter, the most affected is tryptophan pyrrolase, which undergoes rapid degradation and, ordinarily, resynthesis. As the rate-limiting enzyme for tryptophan metabolism, it regulates tryptophan availability to the central nervous system and serotonergic tissues, such as the gastrointestinal tract. When its concentrations diminish, tryptophan concentrations increase, with a consequent increase in the urinary excretion of 5-hydroxyindoleacetic acid (the proximal metabolite of 5-hydroxytryptamine, or serotonin), whose concentrations in humans correlate well with abdominal symptoms.

The increased tryptophan concentration also results in blockage of hepatic gluconeogenesis, depriving neural tissue of glucose, its vital energy source. It may underlie the neurologic manifestations of acute attacks of the porphyrias. Of interest, starvation predisposes to attacks of human hepatic porphyria, and glucose administration is an important part of the acute therapy.

Finally, these events are reversed by the administration of heme, alleviated by administration of chlorophenylalanine (an inhibitor of 5-hydroxytyptamine synthesis), and worsened by administration of valine (which competes with tryptophan for central nervous system uptake).[38–40]

CLINICAL CORRELATES

Prevalence

The inducible porphyrias are transmitted genetically as autosomal dominant traits, with variable individual expressivity and with marked geographic and ethnic variability in prevalence. Because of this variable expressivity, some patients have frequent acute episodes of porphyria, and two thirds with the same enzymatic defect never have an attack. Therefore the presence of the disease cannot be identified in all affected persons without costly screening procedures. As a result, estimates of the prevalences of inducible porphyrias are imprecise. In turn, it is impossible to estimate accurately the incidence of acute episodes.

Acute Intermittent Porphyria

The most common type of inducible porphyria, acute intermittent porphyria accounts for three fourths of the cases encountered in unselected populations in the United States. In a study of hospital admissions in metropolitan Seattle during the period 1952 to 1962, when porphyria was beginning to attract widespread clinical interest, the hospital records of 66 patients with porphyrias of undetermined types were identified.[41] They accounted for 1 in 7088 admissions that usually were prompted for other medical problems. Although records of these patients were highly selected and incompletely characterized, this study represents the only such survey conducted in this country.

This disease is most common in Sweden, especially in Lapland, where its prevalence has been estimated to be greater than 1 in 1000.[42] Hence, it has been termed the "Swedish type" of porphyria. The prevalence is lower elsewhere: Northern Ireland, 1 in 5000; Ireland, 1 in 80,000; and Western Australia, 3 in 100,000.[41,43] In all of these series, the prevalence in women is higher than that in men, suggesting a hormonal cause in the acute episodes.[43]

Variegate Porphyria

Accounting for perhaps one fifth of the cases of inducible porphyria in the United States, variegate porphyria is most prevalent in South Africa; hence it is often termed the "South African type." The prevalence is as great as 3 in 1000 among Caucasians in South Africa, where the disorder was introduced by one of the original colonists from Holland in 1688.[43] The prevalence is considerably lower elsewhere.

Hereditary Coproporphyria

Hereditary coproporphyria accounts for the remaining 5% of cases of inducible porphyria seen in the United States. Because it is rare and because at least one half of affected patients are asymptomatic, no estimates of prevalence are available.

Causes of Acute Episodes

Largely accounting for the variable expressivity of the genetically determined tendency toward acute episodes of neurologic dysfunction is an interaction of the biochemical defect with any of several factors. These superimposed triggering factors include drugs, endogenous and exogenous steroids, infection, and starvation.[43]

Drugs

Barbiturates were among the earliest described triggering agents; with time, other therapeutic chemicals have been added to the growing list of drugs not to be given to susceptible persons[44] (Table 46-3).[45–62]

Originally, anecdotal case reports were the basis for adding drugs to the list of harmful agents. With understanding of the biochemical defects, screening of potentially porphyrinogenic drugs is possible prospectively in animals and in cell systems.[16,47,61–63] These screening procedures quantitate the accumulation of excess porphyrins and porphyrin precursors associated with the induction of ALA-S.[15,16,58,64] Thus, drugs found to be capable of inducing ALA-S, the rate-controlling enzyme in porphyrin metabolism, may be considered potentially porphyrinogenic. In addition, iron, lead, and other heavy metals can depress the activity of many of the enzymes in the heme biosynthetic pathway.[6]

Yet the sensitivities and specificities of screening procedures vary, and drugs that induce ALA-S synthesis in an experimental system are not necessarily porphyrinogenic in humans.[43] Moreover, an acute attack may not follow the administration of a known triggering agent to a susceptible person[6,43,46] or may occur after a variable and unpredictable time. The dose of the porphyrinogenic agent may be too small in some cases to produce an identifiable attack, whereas in others an erroneous diagnosis of an inducible porphyria may account for the absence of an attack. Finally, susceptibility is influenced by other superimposed factors, such as diet and hormonal status.

Compounding attempts to characterize drugs that are porphyrinogenic is the presence of more than one drug as well as other factors in the clinical setting. However, the high lipid

TABLE 46-3
Drugs and Other Stimuli Implicated in Acute Attacks of Porphyria

SEDATIVE AGENTS

Barbiturates[6,45–47]
- Thiopental
- Methohexital

Nonbarbiturate hypnotic agents[46–48]
- Chlordiazepoxide[49]
- Etomidate[47,62]
- Glutethimide
- Isopropylmeprobamate
- Meprobamate
- Methylprylon

ANALGESIC AGENTS

Pentazocine[47]*
Pyrazolone-derivative antipyretic agents[46]
Amidopyrine
Isopropylantipyrine
Dipyrone

INHALATION ANESTHETICS[47]

Enflurane*
Methoxyflurane*

LOCAL ANESTHETICS[47]

Lidocaine*

ANTICONVULSANT AGENTS[50,51]

Phenytoin[45,48]
Mephenyltoin[15]*
Methsuximide[48]
Phensuximide[15]*
Primidone

ANTIBIOTIC AGENTS

Chloramphenicol[15]*
Griseofulvin[6,46,52,53]
Sulfonamides[6,45,53]

STEROIDS[43]

Althesin[47]*
Alfathesin[54]
Hydroxydione
Estrogens[55,56]
Progesterone[56,57]
Metapyrone[58]*

HYPOGLYCEMIC SULFONYLUREAS[43]

Chlorpropamide
Tolbutamide[59]

TOXINS

Arsenic[6]
Ethanol[46,60]
Hexachlorobenzene[6]
Lead[6,61]

OTHER AGENTS

Amphetamine
Dichlorophenazone[46]
Ergot preparations[46]
Ferric chloride[6]
Imipramine[43]
Nikethamide[58]

solubility of these drugs facilitates their passage across membranes and their contact with microsomal enzymes in the cytosol.[43] Apart from anecdotal case reports and literature reviews,[1,2,65–78] few systematic studies of the ability of anesthetic drugs to induce ALA-S in vitro have been published.[47,54,62]

ULTRA–SHORT-ACTING BARBITURATES. Thiopental, the most commonly used induction agent, was highlighted in early case reports of acute porphyrias.[1,2,67,70] This drug is especially hazardous because it is administered intravenously in large dosages and often given to patients who already have symptoms; in this situation, their abdominal pain may simulate an acute appendicitis or other urgent abdominal disorder requiring surgery.[43]

The absence of an acute attack after thiopental administration has been reported in some patients who were found later to have an inducible porphyria.[41,45,74–76] The previously cited survey conducted among Seattle hospitals found that acute attacks were uncommon after barbiturate (usually thiopental) administration; only three attacks occurred after 36 thiopental inductions.[41] This survey, however, did not document the diagnosis of "porphyria" sufficiently to be certain that all patients had an inducible porphyria.

The diagnoses seem firmly established in other reports,[45,74–76] demonstrating that even in a given patient[45,74,76] an acute attack does not necessarily follow a thiopental induction. Of particular interest is the absence of an attack when the disease is in the latent phase at the time of the induction and the worsening of symptoms in most of those anesthetized during an acute attack.[76]

Methohexital also induces the synthesis of ALA-S,[47] although this drug has not been associated with acute attacks in humans, probably because it is used so infrequently.

OTHER INDUCTION AGENTS. Although no reports of acute porphyria are associated with etomidate, this imidazole derivative induces ALA-S synthesis in vitro.[47,62] One case report described etomidate's uneventful use in a woman known to have porphyria.[77] However, again, anecdotal reports are difficult to evaluate because susceptible persons may not have an attack when exposed to a triggering agent.

Ketamine, another induction agent, does not induce ALA-S synthesis in rat liver at a dose of 20 mg/kg,[47] twice the maximum recommended intramuscular dose for a single intramuscular administration in humans, or when administered clinically by intravenous infusion.[62] However, in the more sensitive chick embryo liver, slightly larger doses are porphyrinogenic.[79]

Ketamine has been used in a susceptible patient on two occasions without acute postoperative porphyria.[78] A report of the uneventful use of an induction dose of ketamine (75 mg) during an acute attack in a patient with known hereditary coproporphyria adds to the anecdotes suggesting that ketamine, at least in a small dose, is probably safe for use in patients with porphyria.[80] However, as with other drugs, extrapolations from experience with a single patient or small series can be misleading, given the unpredictability of the attacks. Further clinical experience is needed to determine whether, for example, prolonged ketamine anesthesia with larger doses might be porphyrinogenic.

Propofol has been used without evidence of disease exacerbation in cases of acute intermittent porphyria and variegate porphyria.[81,82]

INHALATIONAL ANESTHETICS. Enflurane and methoxyflurane induce ALA-S synthesis in vitro,[47] although they have not been implicated in causing clinical attacks. Curiously, halothane, which is metabolized to a greater degree than enflurane, has not been found to be porphyrinogenic. Given the ability of all inhalation agents, with the exception of cyclopropane, to stimulate microsomal enzymes nonspecifically,[83] the finding that only two of these drugs are potentially porphyrinogenic is surprising. However, the multiplicity of drugs used pre- and intraoperatively and the almost universal use of a barbiturate induction agent suggest that inhalation anesthetics cannot be implicated as causes of acute attacks.

LOCAL ANESTHETICS. Lidocaine is porphyrinogenic. Procaine decreases ALA-S synthesis in the rat liver model.[47] Whereas lidocaine is highly lipid soluble and is metabolized by microsomal enzymes, procaine has been reported to induce remission in acute porphyria.[84]

ANALGESICS. Pentazocine, capable of inducing ALA-S synthesis in vitro,[47] has an allyl group that is found in other porphyrinogenic drugs and that sterically hinders hydrolysis.[85]

ANTICHOLINESTERASES. Neostigmine and other anticholinesterases have been assumed to be porphyrinogenic because some insecticides (eg, chlordane and lindane) have anticholinesterase activity and can cause demyelination. However, axonal degeneration rather than demyelination occurs during acute porphyria; moreover, anticholinesterase agents have been used during attacks without aggravating the symptoms. Hence, no rational basis exists for considering anticholinesterases porphyrinogenic.

Steroids

Considerable circumstantial evidence implicates female sex hormones as triggering agents: the onset of biochemical and clinical manifestations after puberty; the predominance of women among those affected; the occurrence in many women of attacks just before menstruation; the activation of the disease during pregnancy; the precipitation of attacks by exogenous estrogens and oral contraceptive agents; and the weak porphyrinogenicity of estradiol, estrone, progesterone, and testosterone in the chick embryo liver model.[43] Yet in some patients, estrogens and oral contraceptive agents can prevent attacks. Exogenous and endogenous steroids having a 5β-H configuration, found in many steroid metabolites, are porphyrinogenic.

STEROIDAL ANESTHETIC INDUCTION AGENTS. Althesin, a mixture of two steroids, alphaxalone and alphadolone, induces ALA-S synthesis in vitro.[47] Alfathesin is a mixture of two steroids that differ in porphyrinogenicity: in a chick embryo liver cell preparation, alfadolone has low potency, whereas alfaxolone has about the same potency as standard porphyrin-inducing chemicals, such as thiopental. However, because alphaxolone's anesthetic potency is about three times that of thiopental, the investigators suggest that alfathesin is likely to be a safe induction agent in susceptible patients.[54]

Infection

Bacterial and viral infections seem to trigger acute porphyria. Whether the underlying mechanism relates to increased 5β-H steroid production (ie, increased catabolism) or decreased food intake (ie, starvation) is unknown.[43]

Starvation

Starvation has been identified as a triggering agent in experimental models.[86] Conversely, a diet rich in carbohydrates results in decreased porphyrin and porphyrin precursor excretion.[43,87,88]

Presentation of Acute Episodes

The features that characterize the acute attack are as diverse as the triggering factors. Although the variability in symptoms often is marked from patient to patient, usually a particular disease pattern recurs in a given patient. Taken collectively, however, the clinical features noted in one series of patients resemble those in others remarkably well (Table 46-4).[89–91]

Underlying the symptoms, but not well understood, is a polyneuropathy consisting of axonal degeneration. Although predominantly a motor neuropathy, almost any part of the nervous system can be involved, accounting for the diversity and unusual features of the presentations. Simulating so many other disorders, acute porphyria has been termed "the little imitator."[92] Compounding the difficulty in diagnosis is that the symptoms may not closely follow exposure to triggering agents. Although pain may be felt within hours of exposure, other neurologic symptoms may appear 1 month later; as a result, the precipitating agent may go unrecognized. This delay may explain, in part, how some patients appear to have tolerated thiopental without complications.

Autonomic Instability

Autonomic instability results in diffuse abnormalities. Imbalance in the innervation of the gut, with resultant spasm and relaxation, probably accounts for the severe abdominal pain that is felt by almost all affected persons. Although the pain simulates that caused by acute abdominal disorders, and fever and leukocytosis may be present, the patient should not be subjected to unnecessary laparotomy. Autonomic instability also manifests itself as tachycardia, labile hypertension, and postural hypotension, and incontinence or urinary retention.

Paralysis

Usually developing days to months after the abdominal pain, peripheral neuropathy often is manifested by pain in the back and extremities. Sometime flaccid paralysis appears within days; if concomitant involvement of bulbar cranial nerves is

TABLE 46-4
Clinical Features of Acute Attacks of Porphyria

FEATURES	MARKOWITZ,[89] 1954 (69 patients)	WALDENSTROM,[42] 1957 (233 patients)	GOLDBERG,[90] 1959 (50 patients)	EALES AND LINDER,[91] 1962 (80 patients)	STEIN AND TSCHUDY,[45] 1970 (46 patients)
Disorder	AIP	AIP	AIP	VP	AIP
Female gender	61%	60%	62%	70%	76%
Abdominal pain	95	85	94	90	95
Vomiting	52	59	78	80	43
Mental changes	80*	55	56	55	40
Constipation	46	48	74	80	48
Paralysis	72	42	68	53	32
Hypertension	49	40	56	55	40
Fever	36	37	14	38	9
Tachycardia	51	28	64	83	80
Cranial nerve involvement	51	?	29	9	?
Seizures	?	10	18	12	20
Sensory loss	24	9	38	15	26
Amaurosis	?	4	3	3	6
Diarrhea	11	9	12	8	5
Azotemia	67	9	6	69	32
Proteinuria	?	9	14	8	0
Leukocytosis	48	7	24	20	11
Electrocardiographic abnormalities	47	?	44	23	37

Values are numbers of patients except where otherwise indicated.
AIP, acute intermittent porphyria; *VP*, variegate porphyria.
* Includes seizures.

present, aphonia, dysphagia, and respiratory paralysis may occur. In particular, paralysis or paresis may be more common among patients who have received barbiturates[90] (Fig. 46-5). Unlike the Guillain-Barré syndrome, the paralysis generally progresses caudally, with the upper extremities more severely affected than the lower ones.[93]

Mental Changes

Often, these patients have insomnia and restlessness, prompting administration of barbiturates. The resultant mental changes are highly variable from one patient to another and range from a mild, acute confusional state to acute psychosis. In fact, "mad" King George III, against whom the American colonists fought for their independence, probably had acute intermittent porphyria.[94] He lost his throne after several episodes of madness associated with abdominal pain, constipation, limb weakness, hoarseness, tachycardia, and urine that darkened on sitting. During one attack, he passed the Stamp Act, one of the instigating factors in the American Revolution.

The familial acute bodily illness and mental disorder, including agitation, depression, abnormal behavior, and hallucinations, of Roderick and Madeline Usher in Poe's "The Fall of the House of Usher" also have been suggested to result from an inducible porphyria.[95]

Fluid and Electrolyte Imbalances

Vomiting and diarrhea occurring during acute attacks produce excessive fluid and electrolyte loss from the gastrointestinal tract. These problems result in sodium loss and hypovolemia. In most patients, however, retention of free water, failure of normal renal sodium conservation, and hyponatremia result from the inappropriate release of antidiuretic hormone.[96-98] Concomitantly, a metabolic encephalopathy often is present, heralded by seizures that may linger beyond restoration of fluid and electrolyte balance. Hypomagnesemia of a sufficient degree to produce tetany also may be present.[96,97] A syndrome of neurogenic hyperventilation, leading to marked alkalosis and secondary coma, has been described.[99]

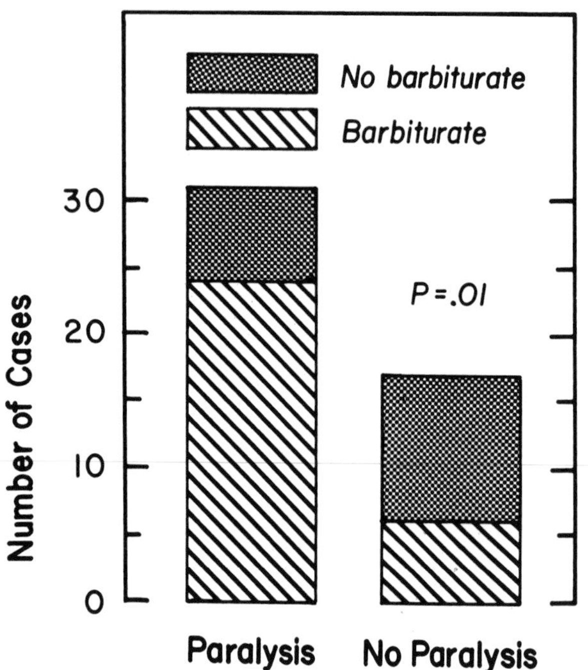

FIGURE 46-5. Barbiturate administration is overrepresented among patients with paralysis or paresis. (Data from Goldberg A: Acute intermittent porphyria: a study of 50 cases. Q J Med 28:183, 1959)

DIAGNOSIS

The detection of latent forms of inducible porphyria is extraordinarily difficult; routine laboratory studies do not screen for these disorders. In general, the diagnosis is suggested by unusual symptoms, perhaps related to an identifiable triggering agent. Once suggested, the diagnosis is established principally by chemical analysis of urine and, in some cases, blood and feces (see Table 46-2). Exposure to potential triggering agents should cease, and therapy should be instituted promptly while the laboratory tests are being performed to confirm the clinical diagnosis.

Acute Intermittent Porphyria

The diagnosis of acute intermittent porphyria is established during an attack by documentation of an increase in urinary ALA or PBG. In general, only PBG is assayed, because the analysis for ALA is very difficult; the concentrations of urine and stool porphyrins are normal. Several methods are available to determine whether the concentration of PBG is increased. Urine containing very high concentrations turns black on standing, particularly if it is acidified. Lesser concentrations of urinary PBG can be determined with the Watson-Schwartz test[100] or the simpler, and more specific, Hoesch test[101]; results of both of these tests usually are positive (urine turns red on addition of reagents) at PBG concentrations greater than 10 mg in a 24-hour period.[102] Chromatography also can be used.

During the latent phase between attacks and even during some attacks, however, the concentrations of ALA and PBG may be near normal (3 to 9 mg in a 24-hour period). A definitive diagnosis can be made by demonstrating a deficiency of PBG deaminase in red blood cells.[103] This test is also useful to screen relatives for the disorder.

Variegate Porphyria and Hereditary Coproporphyria

During acute attacks, urinary concentrations of ALA and PBG are increased as in acute intermittent porphyria, though not to the same degree. However, in the latent phase, the concentrations of ALA, PBG, and porphyrins in urine are normal. Fecal concentrations of coproporphyrin and protoporphyrin remain increased, even during the latent phase. The former compound is present in greater concentration in hereditary coproporphyria, whereas the concentration of the latter is greater in variegate porphyria.

TREATMENT

General Measures

For the most part, treatment is supportive, with correction of fluid and electrolyte imbalances, especially dehydration, hyponatremia, and hypomagnesemia. If hyponatremia coexists with normovolemia, the underlying syndrome of inappropriate secretion of antidiuretic hormone is treated with fluid restriction.

Excessive tachycardia and hypertension and, in some cases, anxiety and abdominal discomfort can be treated safely with β-adrenergic receptor blocking drugs (eg, propranolol).[104] Pain can be treated with commonly used narcotics (eg, meperidine or morphine); however, justifiable concern is expressed about the potential for narcotic addiction in these patients. Curiously, chlorpromazine, in doses of 25 to 100 mg, orally or parenterally, is often effective as an analgesic.[105]

Seizures may be treated with diazepam or clonazepam[106] as safe alternatives to barbiturates, hydantoins, and succinimides. All nonessential drugs should be discontinued. Of course, potential triggering agents (see Table 46-3), if present, should be withdrawn and assiduously avoided. Ventilatory support should be instituted for impending as well as frank respiratory failure.

Specific Measures

Pyridoxine

Some patients with porphyric neuropathy are deficient in pyridoxine (vitamin B_6), a neurologically active substance that is a cofactor for ALA-S activity, among other essential roles in intermediary metabolism.[107] Given its low toxicity, it should be administered, even though its efficacy has yet to be established.

Glucose

The intravenous infusion of glucose, 10 to 20 g/hour to approach 500 g/day, takes advantage of the "glucose effect," in which this simple carbohydrate blocks the induction of ALA-S.[43,87,88] However, for unknown reasons, the clinical response is often variable, and after the infusion is stopped, rebound increases in ALA-S activity and porphyrin precursor excretion occur.

Hematin

Should neurologic symptoms appear or any symptoms progress despite the use of glucose infusion and supportive care, an intravenous infusion of hematin, 4 mg/kg every 12 hours, should be started. Hematin is extracted from red cells and acts like heme in repressing ALA-S synthesis.[108] Like glucose and heme, hematin reduces porphyrin and porphyrin precursor excretion, producing a remission within 48 hours.[109–112] In general, neurologic improvement occurs within days, but the neuropathy can take months or even years to resolve; long-standing neurologic deficits do not respond to hematin.

After discontinuation of the hematin infusion, concentrations of ALA and PBG may increase, but the appearance of clinical illness does not necessarily coincide with these changes.[36] Although hematin infusion is usually reliable and effective therapy, it sometimes appears ineffective and may even have an anticoagulant effect. Use of decayed solutions is associated with treatment failure and an anticoagulation effect; only hematin that is freshly prepared should be infused.[113] Hematin also can cause acute renal failure, and its discontinuation results in a rebound increase in porphyrin and porphyrin precursor excretion.

PREVENTION

General Considerations

The most important element in prevention is education of susceptible persons about their disease and particularly about the need for strict avoidance of triggering agents (see Table 46-3) and avoidance of deliberate fasting. This approach, in turn, requires that susceptibility be identified by screening relatives of those known to have an inducible porphyria. Those found to be at risk should wear wrist bands or similar identification and take as few medications as possible.

Anesthetic Management

The preoperative evaluation should include a thorough neurologic assessment to document existing deficits, particularly those affecting respiratory and other bulbar functions. Existing fluid and electrolyte imbalances should be corrected.

Because regional anesthetic techniques introduce confounding considerations should an attack occur or become more severe, general anesthesia usually is chosen. However, a spinal anesthetic without consequence after bupivacaine has been reported.[114] Apart from strict avoidance of the drugs listed in Table 46-3, no general recommendation about the choice of anesthetic techniques and agents can be made. Given the large number of drugs that hospitalized patients often receive, and the diversity of potentially porphyrinogenic drugs, as few drugs as possible should be administered. For patients with variegate porphyria or hereditary coproporphyria with dermal lesions, special care should also be exercised during positioning and transporting.

REFERENCES

1. Dean G: Porphyria. Br Med J 2:1291, 1953
2. Dundee JW, Riding JE: Barbiturate narcosis in porphyria. Anaesthesia 10:55, 1955
3. Watson CJ, Pierach CA, Bossenmaier I, et al: Postulated deficiency of hepatic heme and repair by hematin infusions in the 'inducible' hepatic porphyrias. Proc Natl Acad Sci U S A 74: 2118, 1977
4. Garrod AE: Inborn errors of metabolism, 2nd ed. London: Frowde, Hodder, and Stoughton, 1923
5. Meyer UA: Hepatic porphyrias: new findings on the nature of metabolic defects. Prog Liver Dis 5:280, 1976
6. Meyer UA, Schmid R: The porphyrias. In Stanbury JB, Wyngaarden JB, Frederickson DS (eds): The metabolic basis of inherited disease, 4th ed. New York: McGraw-Hill, 1978: 1166
7. Elder GH, Gray CH, Nicholson DC: The porphyrias: a review. J Clin Pathol 25:1013, 1972
8. Kaplan BH: Synthesis of heme. In Williams WJ, Beutler E,

Erslev AJ, et al: Hematology, 2nd ed. New York: McGraw-Hill, 1977: 149

9. Granick S, Urata G: Increase in activity of δ-aminolevulinic acid synthetase in liver mitochondria induced by feeding of 3′5-dicarbethoxy-1,4-dihydrocollidine. J Biol Chem 238:821, 1963
10. Burnham BF, Lascelles J: Control of porphyrin biosynthesis through a negative-feedback mechanism: studies with preparations of δ-aminolevulinate synthetase and δ-aminolevulinate dehydrase from *Rhodopseudomonas* spheroids. Biochem J 87: 462, 1963
11. Granick S, Sassa S: δ-Aminolevulinic acid synthetase and the control of heme and chlorophyll synthesis. In Vogel HJ (ed): Metabolic regulation. New York: Academic Press, 1971: 77
12. Monod J, Changeux JB, Jacob F: Allosteric proteins and cellular control systems. J Mol Biol 6:306, 1963
13. Jacob F, Monod J: Genetic regulatory mechanisms in the synthesis of proteins. J Mol Biol 3:318, 1961
14. Granick S, Levere RD: Heme synthesis in erythroid cells. Progress in Hematology 4:1, 1964
15. Granick S: The induction *in vitro* of the synthesis of δ-aminolevulinate acid synthetase in chemical porphyria: a response to certain drugs, sex hormones and foreign chemicals. J Biol Chem 241:1359, 1966
16. Tschudy DP, Bonkowski HL: Experimental porphyria. Fed Proc 31:147, 1966
17. DeMatteis F: Drug interactions in experimental hepatic porphyria. Enzyme 16:266, 1973
18. Tschudy DP, Welland FH, Collins A, et al: The effect of carbohydrate feeding on the induction of aminolevulinic acid synthetase. Metabolism 13:396, 1964
19. Rose JA, Hellman ES, Tschudy DP: Effect of diet on the induction of experimental porphyria. Metabolism 10:514, 1961
20. Granick S, Kappas A: Steroid control of porphyrin and heme biosynthesis: a new biological function of steroid hormone metabolites. Proc Natl Acad Sci U S A 57:1463, 1967
21. Javitt NB, Rifkind A, Kappas A: Porphyrin-heme pathway: regulation by intermediates in bile acid synthesis. Science 182: 841, 1973
22. Marver HS, Collins A, Tschudy DP: The permissive effect of hydrocortisone on the induction of ALA-S. Biochem J 99:31C, 1966
23. Strand JL, Felsher BF, Redeker AG, et al: Heme biosynthesis in intermittent acute porphyria: decreased hepatic conversion of porphobilinogen and increased δ-aminolevulinic acid synthetase activity. Proc Natl Acad Sci U S A 67:1315, 1970
24. Meyer UA, Strand LJ, Doss M, et al: Intermittent acute porphyria: demonstration of a genetic defect in porphobilinogen metabolism. N Engl J Med 286:1277, 1972
25. McKusick VA: The anatomy of the human genome. Am J Med 69:267, 1980
26. Goldberg A: Molecular genetics of acute intermittent porphyria. Br Med J 291:499, 1985
27. Becker DM, Viljoien JD, Katz J, et al: Reduced ferrochelatase activity: a defect common to variegate porphyria and protoporphyria. Br J Haematol 36:171, 1977
28. Elder GH, Evans JD, Thomas N, et al: The primary enzyme defect in hereditary coproporphyria. Lancet 2:1217, 1976
29. Brodie MJ, Thompson GG, Moore MR, et al: Hereditary coproporphyria: demonstration of the abnormalities in heme biosynthesis in peripheral blood. Q J Med 46:229, 1977
30. Nordmann Y, Grandchamp B, Phung N, et al: Coproporphyrinogen-oxidase deficiency in hereditary coproporphyria. Lancet 1:140, 1977
31. Day RS, Eales L, Meissner D: Coexistent variegate porphyria and porphyria cutanea tarda. N Engl J Med 307:36, 1982
32. Qadiri MR, Church SE, McColl KEL, et al: Chester porphyria: a clinical study of a new form of acute porphyria. Br Med J 292:455, 1986
33. Brodie MJ, Moore MR, Goldberg A: Enzyme abnormalities in the porphyrias. Lancet 2:699, 1977
34. Allison AC, Magnus IA, Young MR: Role of lysosomes and of cell membranes on photosensitization. Nature 209:974, 1966
35. Shanley BC, Percy VA, Neethling AC: Pathogenesis of neural manifestations on acute porphyria. S Afr Med J 51:458, 1977
36. Watson CJ: Hematin and porphyria. N Engl J Med 293:605, 1975
37. Mustajoki P, Seppalainen AM: Neuropathy in latent hereditary hepatic porphyria. Br Med J 2:310, 1975
38. Litman DA, Correia MA: L-Tryptophan: a common denominator of biochemical and neurological events of acute hepatic porphyria? Science 222:1031, 1983
39. Litman DA, Correia MA: Elevated brain tryptophan and enhanced 5-hydroxytryptamine turnover in acute hepatic heme deficiency: clinical implications. J Pharmacol Exp Ther 232: 337, 1985
40. Correia MA, Litman DA, Lunetta JM: Drug-induced modulations of hepatic heme metabolism: neurologic consequences. Ann N Y Acad Sci 514:248, 1987
41. Ward RJ: Porphyria and its relation to anesthesia. Anesthesiology 26:212, 1965
42. Waldenstrom J: The porphyrias as inborn errors of metabolism. Am J Med 22:758, 1957
43. Tschudy DP, Valsamis M, Madnussen CR: Acute intermittent porphyria: clinical and selected research aspects. Ann Intern Med 83:851, 1975
44. Dean G, Barnes HD: Porphyria: a South African screening experiment. Br Med J 1:298, 1958
45. Stein JA, Tschudy DP: Acute intermittent porphyria: a clinical and biochemical study of 46 patients. Medicine 49:1, 1970
46. Eales L: Acute porphyria: the precipitating and aggravating factors. South African Journal of Laboratory and Clinical Medicine 17:120, 1971
47. Parikh RK, Moore MR: Effect of certain anaesthetic agents on the activity of rat hepatic δ-aminolaevulinate synthetase. Br J Anaesth 50:1099, 1978
48. Cowger ML, Labbe RF: Contraindications of biological oxidation inhibitors in the treatment of porphyria. Lancet 1:88, 1965
49. Goldberg A, Rimington C, Lockhead AC: Hereditary coproporphyria. Lancet 1:632, 1967
50. Birchfield RI, Cowger ML: Acute intermittent porphyria with seizures: anticonvulsant medication-induced metabolic changes. Am J Dis Child 112:561, 1966
51. Davidson R: Acute porphyria in an epileptic. Br J Clin Pract 17:33, 1963
52. Redeker AG, Sterling RE, Bronow RS: Effect of griseofulvin in acute intermittent porphyria. JAMA 188:466, 1964
53. Berman A, Franklin RL: Precipitation of acute intermittent porphyria by griseofulvin therapy. JAMA 192:1005, 1965
54. Fischer PWF, Ferizovic A, Neilson IR, et al: Porphyrin-inducing activity of alfaxolone and alfadolone acetate in chick embryo liver cells. Anesthesiology 50:350, 1979
55. Welland FH, Hellman ES, Collins A, et al: Factors affecting the excretion of porphyrin precursors by patients with acute intermittent porphyria: II. the effect of ethynyl estradiol. Metabolism 13:251, 1964
56. Wetterberg L: Oral contraceptives and acute intermittent porphyria. Lancet 2:1178, 1964
57. Levit EJ, Nodine JH, Perloff WH: Progesterone-induced porphyria. Lancet 2:1178, 1964
58. DeMatteis F: Disturbances of liver porphyrin metabolism caused by drugs. Pharmacol Rev 19:523, 1967
59. Schlesinger FG, Gastel C: Possible aggravation of abdominal symptoms by tolbutamide in a patient with diabetes and hepatic porphyria. Acta Medica Scandinavica 169:433, 1961
60. Goldberg A, McColl KEL, Moore MR, et al: Alcohol and porphyria. Lancet 2:925, 1981
61. Maxwell JD, Meyer UA: Drug sensitivity in hereditary hepatic porphyria. In Porphyrins in human disease: First International Porphyrin Meeting, Freiburg, 1975. Basel: Karger, 1976: 1
62. Harrison GG, Moore MR, Meissner PN: Porphyrinogenicity of etomidate and ketamine as continuous infusions: screening in the DDC-primed rat model. Br J Anaesth 57:420, 1985
63. Eales L: Porphyria and the dangerous life-threatening drugs. S Afr Med J 56:914, 1979

64. DeMatteis F: Drugs and porphyria. South African Journal of Laboratory and Clinical Medicine 17:126, 1971
65. Dundee JW, Riding JE: Barbiturate narcosis in porphyria. Anaesthesia 10:55, 1955
66. Norris W, Macnab GW: Anaesthesia in porphyria. Br J Anaesth 32:505, 1960
67. Dundee JW, McCleery WNC, McLoughlin G: The hazard of thiopental in porphyria. Anesth Analg 41:567, 1962
68. Lepinskie FF: Porphyria as a problem in anaesthesia. Can Anaesth Soc J 10:286, 1963
69. Murphy PC: Acute intermittent porphyria: the anaesthetic problem and its background. Br J Anaesth 36:801, 1964
70. Eales L: Porphyria and thiopentone. Anesthesiology 27:703, 1966
71. Mees DE Jr, Frederickson EL: Anesthesia and the porphyrias. South Med J 68:29, 1975
72. Sumner E: Porphyria in relation to surgery and anaesthesia. Ann R Coll Surg Eng 56:81, 1975
73. Silvay G, Miller R: Porphyrias. Anesthesiology Reviews 6:51, 1979
74. Slavin SA, Christoforides C: Thiopental administration in acute intermittent porphyria without adverse effect. Anesthesiology 44:77, 1976
75. Mustajoki P, Koskelo P: Hereditary hepatic porphyrias in Finland. Acta Medica Scandinavica 200:171, 1976
76. Mustajoki P, Heinonen J: General anesthesia in 'inducible' porphyrias. Anesthesiology 53:12, 1980
77. Famewo CE: Induction of anaesthesia with etomidate in a patient with acute intermittent porphyria. Can Anaesth Soc J 32: 171, 1985
78. Rizk SF, Jacobson JH II, Silvay G: Ketamine as an induction agent for acute intermittent porphyria. Anesthesiology 46:305, 1977
79. Kostrzewskaa E, Gregor A, Lipinska D: Ketamine in an acute intermittent porphyria: dangerous or safe? Anesthesiology 49: 376, 1978
80. Capouet V, Dernovoi B, Azagra JS: Induction of anaesthesia with ketamine during an acute crisis of hereditary coproporphyria. Can J Anaesth 34:388, 1987
81. Meissner PN, Harrison GG, Hift RJ: Propofol as an I.V. anesthetic agent in variegate porphyria. Br J Anaesth 66:60, 1991
82. Kantor G, Robin SH: Acute intermittent porphyria and Caesarean delivery. Can J Anaesth 39:282, 1992
83. Linde HW, Berman ML: Nonspecific stimulation of drug-metabolizing enzymes by inhalation anesthetic agents. Anesth Analg 50:656, 1971
84. Grubschmidt HA: A case of acute porphyria remissions induced with procaine intravenously. Calf Med 77:243, 1950
85. Racz WJ, Moffat JA: Drug metabolism in cell cultures: I. importance of steric factors for activity in porphyrin inducing drugs. Biochem Pharmacol 23:215, 1974
86. Rose JA, Hellman ES, Tschudy DP: Effect of diet on the induction of experimental porphyria. Metabolism 10:514, 1961
87. Welland FH, Hellman ES, Collins A, et al: Factors affecting the excretion of porphyrin precursors by patients with acute intermittent porphyria: I. the effect of diet. Metabolism 13: 232, 1964
88. Perlroth MG, Tschudy DP, Ratner A, et al: The effect of diet in variegate (South African genetic) porphyria. Metabolism 17:571, 1968
89. Markowitz M: Acute intermittent porphyria: a report of five cases and a review of the literature. Ann Intern Med 41:1170, 1954
90. Goldberg A: Acute intermittent porphyria: a study of 50 cases. Q J Med 28:183, 1959
91. Eales L, Linder GC: Porphyria: the acute attack—an analysis of 80 cases. S Afr Med J 367:284, 1962
92. Waldenstrom J: Neurological symptoms caused by so-called acute porphyria. Acta Psychiatr Scand 14:375, 1939
93. Sergay SM: Management of neurologic exacerbations of hepatic porphyria. Med Clin North Am 63:453, 1979
94. Macalpine I, Hunter R: Porphyria and King George III. Sci Am 221:38, July 1969
95. Rickman LS, Kim CR: 'Poe-phyria,' madness, and *The Fall of the House of Usher*. JAMA 261:863, 1989
96. Hellman ES, Tschudy DP, Bartter FC: Abnormal electrolyte and water metabolism in acute intermittent porphyria: the transient inappropriate secretion of antidiuretic hormone. Am J Med 32:734, 1962
97. Nielsen B, Thorn NA: Transient excess urinary excretion of antidiuretic material in acute intermittent porphyria with hyponatremia and hypomagnesemia. Am J Med 38:345, 1965
98. Lipshutz DE, Reiter JM: Acute intermittent porphyria with inappropriately elevated ADH secretion. JAMA 230:716, 1974
99. Baker NH, Messert B: Acute intermittent porphyria with central neurogenic hyperventilation. Neurology 17:559, 1967
100. Watson CJ, Taddeini L, Bossenmaier I: Present status of the Erhlich aldehyde reaction for urinary porphobilinogen. JAMA 190:501, 1964
101. Lamon J, With TK, Redeker AG: The Hoesch test: beside screening for urinary porphobilinogen in patients with suspected porphyria. Clin Chem 20:1438, 1974
102. Lamon JM, Frykholm BC, Tschcudy DP: Screening tests in acute porphyria. Arch Neurol 34:709, 1977
103. Pierach C, Weimer MK, Cardinal RA, et al: Red blood cell porphobilinogen deaminase in the evaluation of acute intermittent porphyria. JAMA 257:60, 1987
104. Atsmon A, Blum I, Fischl J: Treatment of acute attack of porphyria variegata with propranolol. S Afr Med J 46:311, 1972
105. Monaco RN, Leeper RD, Robbins JJ, et al: Intermittent acute porphyria treated with chlorpromazine. N Engl J Med 256: 309, 1957
106. Larson AW, Wasserstrom WR, Felsher BR, et al: Posttraumatic epilepsy and acute intermittent porphyria: effects of phenytoin, carbamazepine, and clonazepam. Neurology 28:824, 1978
107. Elder TD, Mengel CE: Effect of pyridoxine deficiency on porphyrin precursor excretion in acute intermittent porphyria. Am J Med 41:369, 1966
108. Waxman AD, Collins A, Tschudy DP: Oscillations of hepatic δ-aminolevulinic acid synthesis produced in vivo by heme. Biochem Biophys Res Commun 24:675, 1966
109. Bonkowsky HL, Tschudy DP, Collins A, et al: Repression of the overproduction of porphyrin precursors in acute intermittent porphyria by intravenous infusions of hematin. Proc Natl Acad Sci U S A 68:2725, 1971
110. Peterson A, Bossenmaier I, Cardinal R, et al: Hematin treatment of acute porphyria: early remission of an almost fatal relapse. JAMA 235:520, 1976
111. Lamon JM, Frykholm BC, Bennett M, et al: Prevention of acute porphyric attacks by intravenous haematin. Lancet 2:492, 1978
112. McColl KEL, Thompson GT, Moore MR, et al: Haematin therapy and leucocyte δ-aminolevulinic acid synthase activity in prolonged attack of acute porphyria. Lancet 1:133, 1979
113. Goetsch CA, Bissell DM: Instability of hematin used in the treatment of acute hepatic porphyria. N Engl J Med 315:235, 1986
114. McNeill MJ, Bennet A: Use of regional anesthesia in a patient with acute porphyria. Br J Anaesth 64:371, 1990

FURTHER READING

Jensen NF, Fiddler DS, Striepe V: Anesthetic considerations in porphyrias. Anesthesiology 80:591, 1995

London IM: Iron and heme: Crucial carriers and catalysts. In Wintrobe MM (ed): Blood, Pure and Eloquent. New York, McGraw-Hill, 1980: 170

Complications in Anesthesiology, second edition,
edited by Nikolaus Gravenstein and Robert R. Kirby.
Lippincott-Raven Publishers, Philadelphia © 1996.

CHAPTER 47

Acquired Methemoglobinemia and Sulfhemoglobinemia

Fredrick K. Orkin

The sudden appearance of cyanosis usually suggests cardiorespiratory catastrophes such as airway obstruction, pneumothorax, cardiac dysrhythmia, and cardiac arrest. Typically, cyanosis is a manifestation of hypoxia. Rarely, however, cyanosis results because the hemoglobin structure has been altered to form methemoglobin or sulfhemoglobin, substances that impair oxygen transport. This chapter reviews how such alterations in hemoglobin structure are produced by drugs administered during or shortly before or after anesthesia.

PHYSICAL BASIS

The respiratory molecule hemoglobin consists of four subunits, each an iron-containing porphyrin heme united with a globin polypeptide chain (Fig. 47-1). Iron contained in heme is in the reduced, or ferrous, state. Each iron atom binds to four pyrrole rings; a fifth bond of the iron attaches to a histidine residue of globin, leaving a sixth valence bond to combine reversibly with one molecule of oxygen.

The binding of oxygen to hemoglobin is a complex, sequential, *cooperative* process. As oxygen binds to each heme, the affinity of the remaining hemes for oxygen increases. Hence, the oxyhemoglobin dissociation curve at first rises slowly and then more steeply. Finally, once an oxygen molecule has combined with each of the four hemes, the curve flattens again.

To account for heme–heme interactions, Perutz has proposed that hemoglobin shifts back and forth between two alternate structures.[1] In the tense (T) structure, the heme "pockets" in the hemoglobin subunits are so narrow that oxygen cannot enter, whereas in the relaxed (R) structure the heme pockets are wide enough to permit oxygen to bind easily with heme (Fig. 47-2A).

Binding of oxygen to heme in the lungs is associated with breakage of the salt bridges that link the subunits tightly in the T structure (see Fig. 47-2B). Breakage of the salt bridges, in turn, causes conformational changes in hemoglobin that increase the affinity of hemes elsewhere in the molecule, now in the R state, for oxygen (in what is called an allosteric effect). Loss of oxygen molecules in the capillary allows the salt bridges to reestablish, with resultant narrowing of the heme pockets and return to the T structure. According to this theory, any alteration in hemoglobin structure that prevents transition between the R and T structures impairs oxygen transport by hemoglobin.

Methemoglobinemia

In normal circumstances, a very small fraction of hemoglobin in living erythrocytes spontaneously undergoes oxidation. As a result, some of the heme iron is in the ferric state, forming methemoglobin ($HbFe^{3+}$) that exists in equilibrium with hemoglobin ($HbFe^{2+}$):

$$HbFe^{2+} + H_2O \rightleftharpoons HHbFe^{3+} + OH^-$$

In the oxidized state, the sixth valence bond combines with a hydroxyl group (in the alkaline form, as in Fig. 49-2) or a water molecule (in the acid form) and can no longer combine with oxygen.[2] In terms of Perutz's model, methemoglobin is stabilized in the R structure and cannot shift between the T and R structures.[1]

Methemoglobinemia exists when more than 1% of hemoglobin is methemoglobin. This small but relatively constant concentration of methemoglobin reflects the difference between the rate at which methemoglobin is formed spontaneously and the rate at which it is reduced to hemoglobin. Infants are especially susceptible to methemoglobinemia; their capacity for methemoglobin reduction is compromised at birth and for several months thereafter. For example, the enzymatic activity of reduced nicotinamide adenine dinucleotide (NADH)–dependent cytochrome B_5 reductase in umbilical

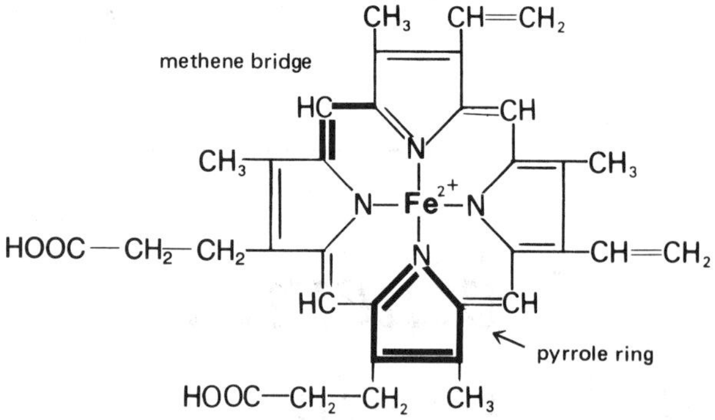

FIGURE 47-1. The structure of the iron-containing porphyrin heme (ferroprotoporphyrin). Heme consists of an iron atom in the ferrous state bound to four pyrrole rings joined in a plane by methene bridges. For clarity, the carbon atoms of the pyrrole ring are represented as the corners of the pentagons, and the hydrogen atoms are omitted. On one side of this plane the iron binds with a globin polypeptide chain and on the other, oxygen. Four heme–polypeptide subunits constitute hemoglobin, with each heme nestled at the surface of the molecule.

cord red blood cells is about 60% of that in adult red blood cells.[3]

Four intraerythrocytic mechanisms reduce methemoglobin to hemoglobin (Fig. 47-3). About 80% of the methemoglobin-reducing capacity of the red cell involves NADH, which is generated during the oxidation of glucose. The previously mentioned NADH-dependent cytochrome B_5 reductase, also called NADH dehydrogenase or methemoglobin reductase, reduces cytochrome B_5, using NADH as a hydrogen donor; the reduced cytochrome B_5 then reduces methemoglobin.[4]

A second enzymatic reducing mechanism involves reduced nicotinamide adenine dinucleotide phosphate, which is generated in the hexose monophosphate shunt during the conversion of glucose-6-phosphate to 6-phosphoglucose.[5] If reduced nicotinamide adenine dinucleotide phosphate is present, a methemoglobin reductase that is dependent on it reduces methemoglobin; however, this mechanism functions only when a cofactor or an artificial electron carrier, such as methylene blue, is present. In fact, administration of methylene blue causes methemoglobin reduction to occur at a rate much

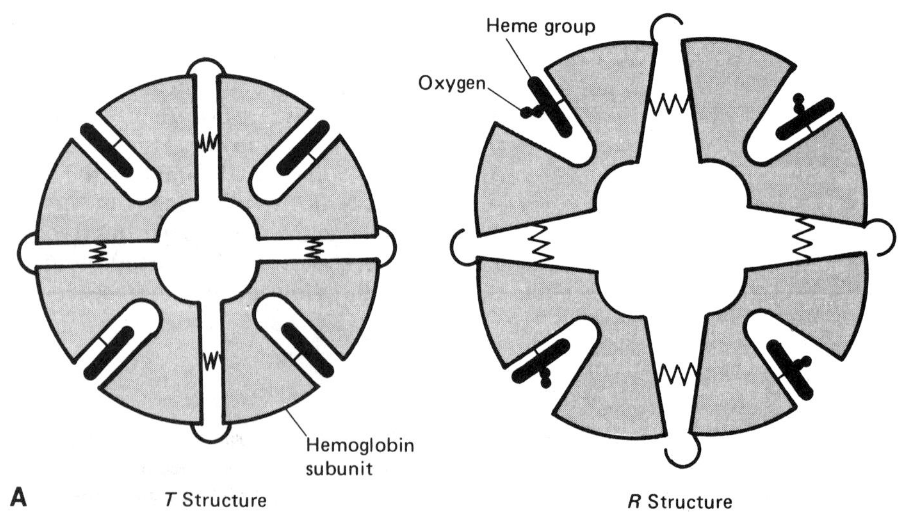

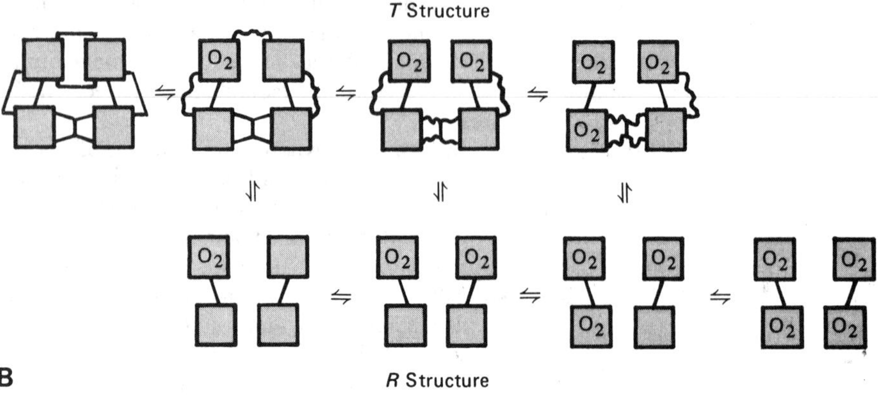

FIGURE 47-2. The transport of oxygen by hemoglobin is postulated to involve a transition between two structures. (**A**) In the T structure, the subunits are clamped tightly by salt bridges against springs, narrowing the heme pockets; in the R structures, the salt bridges have ruptured, allowing the heme pockets to open wide enough to admit oxygen easily. (**B**) The transition from the T structure to the R structure involves the progressive rupture of salt bridges as oxygen is bound. Simultaneous weakening of salt bridges (*wavy lines*) occurs elsewhere in the molecule (in an allosteric effect), enhancing the likelihood of further oxygen binding. (Perutz MF: Hemoglobin structure and respiratory transport. Sci Am 239:92, 1978)

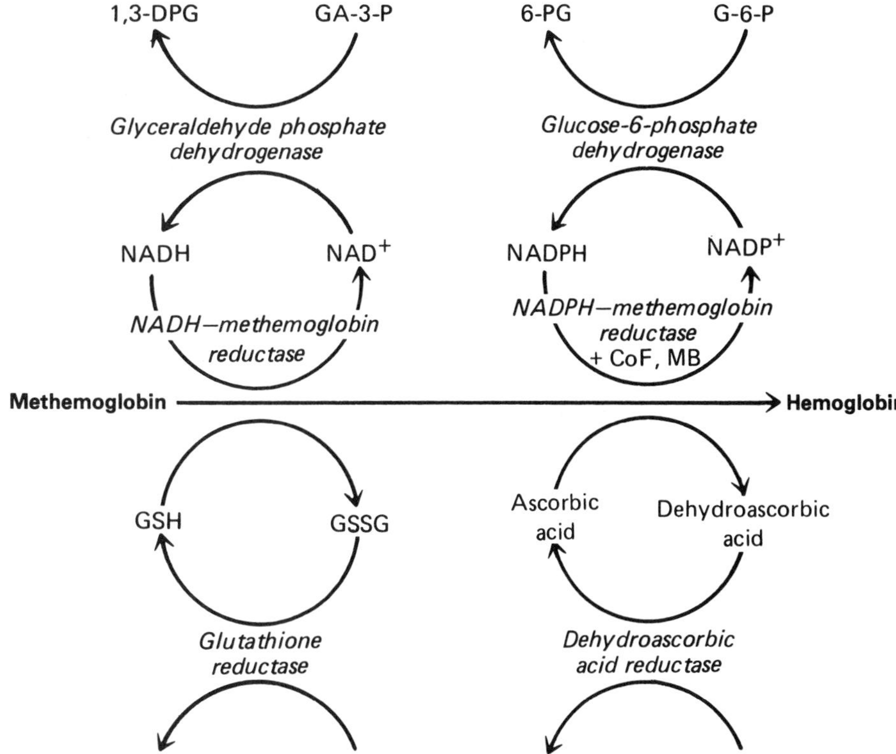

FIGURE 47-3. The metabolic mechanisms for the reduction of methemoglobin to hemoglobin in the red blood cell and the regeneration of the reducing agents. *CoF*, cofactor; *1,3-DPG*, 1,3-diphosphoglucose; *G-6-P*, glucose-6-phosphate; *GA-3-P*, glyceraldehyde-3-phosphate; *GSH*, reduced glutathione; *GSSG*, oxidized glutathione; *MB*, methylene blue; *NAD+*, nicotinamide adenine dinucleotide; *NADP+*, nicotinamide adenine dinucleotide phosphate; *NADPH*, reduced nicotinamide adenine dinucleotide phosphate; *6-PG*, 6-phosphoglucose.

greater than the rate during normal red cell metabolism[6,7] (Fig. 47-4). Nonenzymatic reduction of small amounts of methemoglobin also occurs after the administration of glutathione,[8] ascorbic acid,[9] or riboflavin.

Sulfhemoglobinemia

Unlike methemoglobin, sulfhemoglobin has not been characterized structurally. Moreover, sulfhemoglobin is formed in normal conditions. Exposure to any of the chemical agents that induce the formation of methemoglobin may also cause formation of sulfhemoglobin. Once formed, however, sulfhemoglobin cannot be converted back to hemoglobin. Instead, sulfhemoglobin is removed from the circulation only when the affected red blood cells reach the end of their life span.

CAUSES

Methemoglobinemia may be inherited or acquired. Sulfhemoglobinemia, except for a single report of a possibly congenital case, occurs only in the acquired form. The inherited forms are rarely encountered in anesthetic practice; in this chapter they are discussed only briefly.

Inherited Methemoglobinemia

Deficiency of Reduced Nicotinamide Adenine Dinucleotide-Dependent Cytochrome B_5 Reductase

This disorder is rare; only a few hundred cases have been reported. Approximately 15 variants may be caused by actual deficiency of the enzyme[10] or by synthesis of an abnormal enzyme, resulting in reduced activity. About half of the hemoglobin of persons homozygous for the disorder exists as methemoglobin. Although they are cyanotic from birth, they are otherwise well, and treatment with methylene blue or

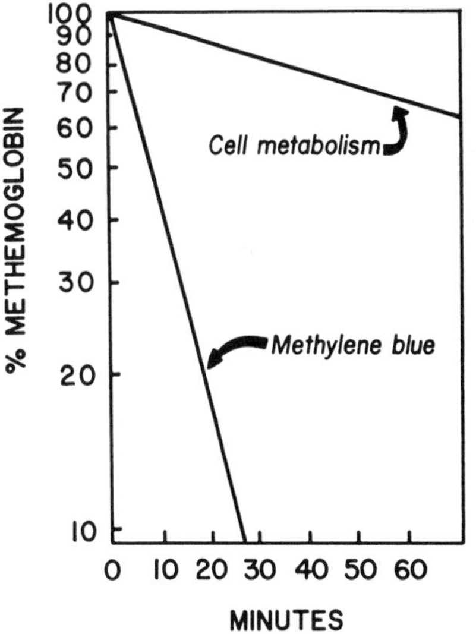

FIGURE 47-4. The rate of methemoglobin reduction with normal red cell metabolism and with the addition of methylene blue. The ordinate represents the percentage of the initial concentration of methemoglobin, which was 2 to 5 g/dL in the patients studied (Modified from Finch CA: Methemoglobinemia and sulfhemoglobinemia. N Engl J Med 239:470, 1948)

ascorbic acid is undertaken for cosmetic reasons only. In general, persons who are heterozygous for the disorder are not cyanotic but are highly susceptible to drugs and chemicals that produce the acquired form of methemoglobinemia. Only in exceedingly rare instances does this disorder account for cyanosis during anesthesia.[11]

Hemoglobin M Disease

Five variants of this rare disorder exist. In each, an amino acid substitution occurs in the globin polypeptide chain close to heme, and the resulting altered molecule coexists with normal hemoglobin (hemoglobin A). Once formed by spontaneous oxidation, hemoglobin M becomes an unsuitable substrate for enzymatic reduction because of the abnormal structure. No homozygous cases have been described, presumably because such a disorder would be incompatible with life.

In persons with the heterozygous disorder, as much as one third of the hemoglobin is hemoglobin M, the specific amount depending on the quantities of hemoglobin M and hemoglobin A present. Methylene blue and ascorbic acid are ineffective in treating the cyanosis. No reports of this disorder in association with anesthesia have been published.

Acquired Methemoglobinemia and Sulfhemoglobinemia

Acquired or toxic methemoglobinemia is far more common than the hereditary forms. It results from any of a variety of drugs and chemicals that cause the rate of hemoglobin oxidation to exceed the erythrocyte's reductive capacity. Except for nitrates and nitrites, the same oxidants that cause methemoglobinemia may cause sulfhemoglobinemia.

Exposure to industrial chemicals capable of oxidizing hemoglobin (chlorates, nitrobenzenes, and quinones)[12] has decreased as a result of improved occupational health standards.[13,14] Methemoglobinemia may still occur because oxidants are present in many therapeutic agents that patients may be given during or near the time of anesthesia.

In general, no widely used drug given in clinical doses produces methemoglobinemia or sulfhemoglobinemia. Most of the case reports involve uncommonly used drugs given in excessive dose or, more rarely, drugs given to patients having NADH-dependent cytochrome B_5 reductase deficiency. The oxidant in most cases is a metabolite rather than the drug itself, and the amount of methemoglobinemia is dose related.

Analgesic-Antipyretic Agents

These drugs, as well as less commonly used *p*-aminophenol derivatives (eg, acetanilide and *p*-aminosalicylic acid), cause dose-related methemoglobinemia,[14] though usually only when taken in excess. Phenacetin abuse has been especially prevalent in Great Britain, where one report associated the drug with nine of ten cases of methemoglobinemia occurring in surgical patients in one hospital during a 3-year period.[15] The drug has been implicated in cases of methemoglobinemia[16] and sulfhemoglobinemia[17] occurring during anesthesia in the United States, where it is no longer approved.

Although therapeutic doses of phenacetin usually do not cause methemoglobin production sufficient to cause cyanosis, some patients have a heightened sensitivity because they metabolize a greater proportion of the drug to an oxidizing product.[18] Newborns are particularly sensitive to these drugs because the hepatic glucuronide conjugation enzymes that detoxify *p*-aminophenol are as immature at birth[19] as is their NADH-dependent cytochrome B_5 reductase.[9]

Antimicrobial and Antiseptic Agents

Methemoglobinemia after administration of the antimalarial agents chloroquine and dapsone,[20] other sulfonamide derivatives, the urinary tract antiseptic agent phenazopyridine, and other, less commonly used drugs has been reported.[14]

Vasodilators

AMYL NITRITE AND NITROGLYCERIN. These drugs are potent oxidants; glyceryl trinitrate is converted to a nitrite by intestinal bacteria and may cause methemoglobinemia if used continually. Nitrates and nitrites used as meat preservatives[13] and condiments also have been implicated in production of the disorder. Methemoglobinemia has been documented in a person with NADH-dependent cytochrome B_5 reductase deficiency who sniffed butyl nitrite as an aphrodisiac.[21] In other cases it has followed accidental overdosage,[22] high dosages (7 μg/kg/min),[23,24] and even customary clinical dosages[25–28] of nitroglycerin and nitrates, usually in dose-related fashion. One patient who received 30 μg/kg/min of nitroglycerin for 6 days before coronary revascularization had dark blood intraoperatively, but the methemoglobin level was only 9.6% and arterial blood gas values were normal.[23]

SODIUM NITROPRUSSIDE. In one patient with a massive acute myocardial infarction, methemoglobinemia developed after 4 days of therapy.[29] During bed rest and while receiving supplemental oxygen, he was asymptomatic with a methemoglobin level of 16%, probably because he also had 10.5 g/dL of normal hemoglobin. Another vasodilator was substituted, perhaps with transient loss of hemodynamic stability, and his infarction extended fatally that day. Others have shown that production of methemoglobin is an intermediate state in the production of cyanmethemoglobin and cyanide that occurs after administration of nitroprusside.[30]

THERAPEUTIC IMPLICATIONS. Therapeutic dosages of vasodilators can produce mild methemoglobinemia that usually does not appear to be clinically important. However, the clinical importance of these observations remains uncertain in the presence of anemia or severe coronary artery disease associated with anemia.

Local Anesthetics

PRILOCAINE. A toluidine derivative, prilocaine is an anesthetic drug infamous for its ability to produce methemoglobin.[31–48] Introduced in the early 1960s as an alternative to other local anesthetics (because of its longer clinical duration and reduced central nervous system toxicity), prilocaine never achieved wide popularity because of this problem. As with other drugs that may cause methemoglobinemia, a metabolite of prilocaine, probably *o*-toluidine, rather than prilocaine itself, is the oxidant.[33,34]

Cyanosis occasionally appears after administration of doses as small as 400 mg following nerve blocks or epidural anesthesia[31,34,36–38]; however, it usually occurs after administration of considerably larger doses (eg, 600 to 1600 mg), that might be administered during prolonged continuous epidural anesthesia.[31,34–40] Although the likelihood that cyanosis will appear is dose related,[34] the correlation between dose and methemoglobin production is weak enough to suggest that other pharmacokinetic considerations, such as the injection site, the patient's metabolic rate,[48] and vasoconstrictor use, are critical factors.

Cyanosis appears 90 minutes to 6 hours after administration, depending on the type of block used and the presence of vasoconstrictor; it usually disappears within 24 hours if untreated. None of the published reports describes tachycardia, hypertension, or clinical symptoms of hypoxia accompanying the cyanosis. Concern about use of prilocaine during a prolonged epidural block for labor is justified, however, because the drug affects the fetus to the same extent as it does the mother.[41–43] As mentioned, the drug-metabolizing system[19] and the NADH-dependent cytochrome B_5 reductase[9] of a fetus are immature.

BENZOCAINE. A *p*-aminobenzoic acid derivative, benzocaine has been implicated in cases of cyanosis occurring in infants after topical oropharyngeal,[49,50] esophageal,[50,51] and rectal[52–55] administration. Older children have become cyanotic after topical administration of benzocaine[56] and after tracheal intubation with a lubricant containing benzocaine.[57] A commonly available benzocaine-containing anesthetic spray preparation is involved in most of the cases that occur after topical administration.[46,49,50,58–62]

LIDOCAINE. Lidocaine bears a structural similarity to prilocaine and is listed in standard reference works[63,64] among the agents causing methemoglobinemia, apparently on the basis of three case reports. One, an obstetric case, involved a woman who had received a total of 1.8 g of lidocaine during a period of about 8 hours and who appeared cyanotic 9 hours after delivery.[65] Methemoglobinemia was confirmed spectrophotometrically, and the cyanosis disappeared after administration of methylene blue. This patient also had received phenacetin after the delivery, however, making it impossible to be sure that the methemoglobinemia was caused solely by lidocaine; in addition, after clinical doses of lidocaine, methemoglobinemia sufficient to cause cyanosis does not occur.[37,46] Furthermore, the response to methylene blue required "a few hours" rather than several minutes, suggesting that the patient may have had glucose-6-phosphate deficiency (see Fig. 47-3).[66]

Another case involved a young man who had full-mouth dental extractions with 300 mg of lidocaine.[67] After the procedure he received codeine and remained hospitalized overnight; 4 hours after returning home the next morning, he suddenly became dizzy and lost consciousness. He was readmitted to the hospital, where he was observed to be cyanotic. The cyanosis disappeared after methylene blue administration but, as in the case above, more slowly than expected. The acute problem occurred almost 24 hours after the nerve blocks, at a time when lidocaine would have been almost entirely cleared from the body. Perhaps the patient also received an analgesic agent containing phenacetin, such as aspirin–phenacetin–caffeine (APC) or even another, unmentioned, drug rather than codeine alone.

In a third patient, methemoglobinemia developed after the administration of an unreported volume of 4% lidocaine to the posterior pharynx twice in 1 hour, less than 1 day after the occurrence of methemoglobinemia with benzocaine.[62] Although no predisposing hematologic defect was found, one must question whether the normal reductive mechanisms had returned to normal after the first episode of cyanosis. In short, insufficient evidence implicates lidocaine as a cause of methemoglobinemia.

Surface-acting Agents

MAFENIDE ACETATE. This sulfonamide derivative, used as a topical agent in the treatment of burns, caused severe methemoglobinemia in two children who had burns over about half of their body surface.[68] The agent is absorbed rapidly through the burned surface and reaches a peak plasma concentration within a few hours. The two children came from communities in which intermarriage was common, raising the possibility of an inherited metabolic defect (eg, NADH-dependent cytochrome B_5 reductase deficiency) that would have made them more sensitive to the oxidant.

SILVER NITRATE. Silver nitrate therapy for burns also has been implicated in a few cases of methemoglobinemia.[69,70] Bacterial infection probably converts the nitrate to nitrite, which acts as the oxidant. Cyanosis and the possibility of anaerobic metabolism in patients treated with mafenide acetate or silver nitrate suggest methemoglobinemia and the need for co-oximeter evaluation.[71]

ANILINE DYES. When used for laundry marking of diapers, aniline dyes have been associated with nursery epidemics of methemoglobinemia.[72] Dyes used on shoes and in crayons also have been implicated.

CLINICAL SIGNIFICANCE

Whereas 5 g/dL of reduced hemoglobin must be present before cyanosis is evident, cyanosis of equal severity can be caused by as little as 1.5 g/dL of methemoglobin or 0.5 g/dL of sulfhemoglobin. The cyanosis reflects diminished oxygen-carrying capacity of the blood and greater affinity of the remaining hemoglobin for oxygen. The oxyhemoglobin dissociation curve shifts to the left, with decreased release of oxygen to the tissues at low partial pressures of oxygen.[73]

Symptoms

Clinical symptoms reflect not only the amount of methemoglobin or sulfhemoglobin present but also the ability of the patient's cardiorespiratory system to compensate. For example, 600 mg of prilocaine, the maximum recommended dose for a single administration, causes a loss of about 5% of the blood's oxygen-carrying capacity, a deficit that is offset easily by an increase in cardiac output. Even the deficits imposed by much larger prilocaine doses (eg, a 20% deficit after 1200 to 1600 mg) pose little challenge; during exercise, cardiac output in a healthy adult can increase by about 300%.

Difficulty arises, however, when the loss in oxygen-carrying capacity is greater, especially in persons with limited cardiac reserve. With a methemoglobinemia level greater than 25%, which is not uncommon after the ingestion of nitrates and nitrites, weakness, fatigue, headache, dizziness, and tachycardia appear. A methemoglobinemia level of more than 50% causes methemoglobinemic stupor. A level of more than 60% to 70% causes coma and death. Sulfhemoglobinemia produces cyanosis at lower levels.

The clinical manifestations of methemoglobinemia and sulfhemoglobinemia in a given patient vary depending on other factors that also reduce oxygen delivery to the tissues (eg, anemia, reduced cardiac output, and hypoxemia). Thus, symptoms appearing in the postoperative period, when oxygen delivery may be impaired by anemia and shivering, should be interpreted with caution.

DIAGNOSIS

In general, cyanosis unresponsive to oxygen therapy suggests the presence of acquired methemoglobinemia or sulfhemoglobinemia, particularly in the absence of cardiorespiratory disease. The venous blood of patients with methemoglobinemia has been described as reddish brown, and of those with sulfhemoglobinemia, as mauve brown. The color persists after the blood sample has been mixed with air, whereas reduced hemoglobin (eg, from a patient with a large right-to-left shunt) turns bright red.

A pulse oximeter indicates the hemoglobin saturation as relatively low for a given partial pressure of arterial oxygen, but the measured saturation corresponds to the color of the blood and the degree of the patient's cyanosis. Moreover, because the oximeter's computer program assumes that only oxyhemoglobin, deoxyhemoglobin, and carboxyhemoglobin are present in the sample,[43] this device calculates a falsely low value for hemoglobin and a negative value for carboxyhemoglobin.

For definitive diagnosis, wider range spectrophotometry is used. Methemoglobin absorbs maximally at 502 and 632 nm, whereas sulfhemoglobin has its peak absorption at 620 to 630 nm. Identification of sulfhemoglobin in a sample also containing methemoglobin requires comparison of the spectrums of air- and carbon dioxide–equilibrated samples and subsequent confirmatory procedures.

The diagnosis of sulfhemoglobinemia is sufficiently complicated that in many patients this disorder is diagnosed as methemoglobinemia.[74] Hemoglobin M variants are identified by hemoglobin electrophoresis. Finally, addition of a few drops of a 10% cyanide solution to a sample of brown blood produces a bright red pigment (cyanmethemoglobin) and removes the peaks from the methemoglobin spectrum but not from that of sulfhemoglobin.

TREATMENT

Therapy usually is undertaken for cosmetic reasons and not because of medical necessity. Intravenous administration of methylene blue, 1 mg/kg, promptly relieves cyanosis caused by methemoglobinemia (see Fig. 47-4). The dose should be given over a period of 5 minutes to avoid symptoms of toxicity, such as restlessness, apprehension, tremor, and precordial pain, which also occur after very large doses (⩾500 mg).[75]

Severe methemoglobinemia in infants has been treated with exchange transfusion.[51] Methylene blue should not be given to patients with glucose-6-phosphate deficiency because acute hemolysis could result.[66] Hemolysis also is possible after repeated injections of methylene blue.[76] No specific therapy exists for sulfhemoglobinemia; of course, the administration of the offending agent should be discontinued.

REFERENCES

1. Perutz MF: Stereochemistry of cooperative effects in haemoglobin (haem-haem interaction and the problem of allostery). Nature 228:726, 1970
2. Jaffe ER, Heller P: Methemoglobinemia in man. Progress in Hematology 4:48, 1964
3. Ross JD: Deficient activity of DPNH-dependent methemoglobin diaphorase in cord blood erythrocytes. Blood 21:51, 1963
4. Hultquish DE, Passon PG: Catalysis of methaemoglobin reduction by erythrocyte cytochrome B5 and cytochrome B5 reductase. Nature (New Biol) 229:252, 1971
5. Gibson QH: The reduction of methaemoglobin in red blood cells and studies on the cause of idiopathic methaemoglobinaemia. Biochem J 42:13, 1948
6. Wendel WB: Control of methemoglobinemia with methylene blue. J Clin Invest 18:179, 1939
7. Bodansky O, Gutmann H: Treatment of methemoglobinemia. J Pharmacol Exp Ther 89:46, 1947
8. Morrison DB, Williams EF: Methemoglobin reduction by glutathionone or cysteine. Science 87:15, 1938
9. Gibson QH: Reduction of methaemoglobin by ascorbic acid. Biochem J 37:615, 1943
10. Hegesh E, Hegesh J, Kaftory A: Congenital methemoglobinemia with a deficiency of cytochrome b_5. N Engl J Med 314:757, 1986
11. Gabel RA, Bunn HF: Hereditary methemoglobinemia as a cause of cyanosis during anesthesia. Anesthesiology 40:516, 1974
12. Hooper RR, Husted SR, Smith EL: Hydroquinone poisoning aboard a navy ship. Morb Mortal Wkly Rep 27:237, 1978
13. Bodansky O: Methemoglobinemia and methemoglobin-producing compounds. Pharmacol Rev 3:144, 1951
14. Smith RP, Olson MV: Drug-induced methemoglobinemia. Semin Hematol 10:253, 1973
15. Joseph D: Methaemoglobinaemia and anaesthesia. Br J Anaesth 34:309, 1963
16. Easley JE, Condon BF: Phenacetin-induced methemoglobinemia and renal failure. Anesthesiology 41:99, 1974
17. Schmitter CR Jr: Sulfhemoglobinemia and methemoglobinemia: uncommon causes of cyanosis. Anesthesiology 43:586, 1975
18. Shahidi NT, Hemaidan A: Acetophenetidin-induced methemoglobinemia and its relation to the excretion of diazotizable amines. J Lab Clin Med 74:581, 1969
19. Vest MF, Streiff RR: Studies on glucoronide formation in newborn infants and older children. Am J Dis Child 98:688, 1959
20. Mayo W, Leighton K, Robertson B, et al: Intraoperative cyanosis: a case of dapsone-induced methaemoglobinaemia. Can J Anaesth 34:79, 1987

21. Horne MK, Waterman RR, Simon LM, et al: Methemoglobinemia from sniffing butyl nitrite. Ann Intern Med 91:417, 1979
22. Marshall JB, Ecklund RE: Methemoglobinemia from overdose of nitroglycerin. JAMA 24 244:330, 1980
23. Gibson GR, Hunter JB, Raabe DS Jr, et al: Methemoglobinemia produced by high-dose intravenous nitroglycerin. Ann Intern Med 96:615, 1982
24. Pasch T, Hoppelshauser G: Methaemoglobin levels during nitroglycerin infusion for the intraoperative induction of controlled hypotension. Arzneimittelforschung 33:879, 1983
25. Fibuch EE, Cecil WT, Reed WA: Methemoglobinemia associated with organic nitrate therapy. Anesth Analg 58:521, 1979
26. Saxon SA, Silverman MR: Effects of continuous infusion of intravenous nitroglycerin on methemoglobin levels. Am J Cardiol 56:461, 1985
27. Kaplan KJ, Taber M, Teagarden JR, et al: Association of methemoglobinemia and intravenous nitroglycerin administration. Am J Cardiol 55:181, 1985
28. Arsura E, Lichstein E, Guadagnino V, et al: Methemoglobin levels produced by organic nitrates in patients with coronary artery disease. J Clin Pharmacol 24:160, 1984
29. Bower PJ, Peterson JN: Methemoglobinemia after sodium nitroprusside therapy. N Engl J Med 293:865, 1975
30. Smith R, Kruszyna H: Nitroprusside produces cyanide poisoning via a reaction with hemoglobin. J Pharmacol Exp Ther 191:557, 1975
31. Daly DJ, Davenport J, Newland MC: Methaemoglobinaemia following the use of prilocaine ('Citanest'). Br J Anaesth 36: 737, 1964
32. Sadove MS, Rosenberg R, Heller FN, et al: Citanest, a new local anesthetic agent. Anesth Analg 43:527, 1964
33. Onji Y, Tyuma I: Methemoglobin formation by a local anesthetic and some related compounds. Acta Anaesthiol Scand Suppl 16: 151, 1965
34. Crawford OB, Hollis RW, Covino BG: Clinical tolerance and effectiveness of propitocaine, a new local anesthetic agent. Journal of New Drugs 5:162, 1965
35. Lund PC, Cwik JC: Citanest, a clinical and laboratory study: II. Anesth Analg 44:712, 1965
36. Hjelm M, Holmdahl MH: Clinical chemistry of prilocaine and clinical evaluation of methaemoglobinaemia induced by this agent. Acta Anaesthesiol Scand Suppl 16:161, 1965
37. Hjelm M, Holmdahl MH: Biochemical effects of aromatic amines: II. cyanosis, methaemoglobinaemia and heinz-body formation induced by a local anaesthetic agent (prilocaine). Acta Anaesthesiol Scand 9:99, 1965
38. Sadove MS, Jobgen EA, Heller FN, et al: Methemoglobinemia: an effect of a new local anesthetic, L-67 (prilocaine). Acta Anaesthesiol Scand Suppl 16:175, 1965
39. Lund PC, Cwik JC: Propitocaine (Citanest) and methemoglobinemia. Anesthesiology 26:569, 1965
40. Scott DB: Toxicity and clinical use of prilocaine. Proc R Soc Med 58:420, 1965
41. Poppers PJ, Vosburgh GJ, Finster M: Methemoglobinemia following epidural analgesia during labor: a case report and literature review. Am J Obstet Gynecol 95:630, 1966
42. Climie CR, McLean S, Starmer GA, et al: Methaemoglobinaemia in mother and foetus following continuous epidural analgesia with prilocaine: clinical and experimental data. Br J Anaesth 39:155, 1967
43. Marx GF: Fetal arrhythmia during caudal block with prilocaine. Anesthesiology 28:222, 1967
44. Mazze RI: Methemoglobin concentrations following intravenous regional anesthesia. Anesth Analg 47:122, 1968
45. Harris WH, Cole DW, Mital M, et al: Methemoglobin formation and oxygen transport following intravenous regional anesthesia using prilocaine. Anesthesiology 29:65, 1968
46. Bridenbaugh PO, Bridenbaugh LD, Moore DC: Methemoglobinemia and infant response to lidocaine and prilocaine in continuous caudal anesthesia: a double-blind study. Anesth Analg 48: 824, 1969
47. Arens JF, Carrera AE: Methemoglobin levels following peridural anesthesia with prilocaine for vaginal deliveries. Anesth Analg 49:219, 1970
48. Duncan PC, Kobrinsky N: Prilocaine-induced methemoglobinemia in a newborn infant. Anesthesiology 59:75, 1983
49. Haggerty RJ: Blue baby due to methemoglobinemia. N Engl J Med 267:1303, 1962
50. Seibert RW, Siebert JJ: Infantile methemoglobinemia induced by a topical anesthetic, Cetacaine. Laryngoscope 94:816, 1984
51. Kellett PB, Copeland CS: Methemoglobinemia associated with benzocaine-containing lubricant. Anesthesiology 59:463, 1983
52. Bhatt DN, Bifano EM, Stark DC: Postoperative methemoglobinemia in a neonate. Anesthesiology 62:210, 1985
53. Peterson H DeC: Acquired methemoglobinemia in an infant due to benzocaine suppository. N Engl J Med 263:454, 1960
54. Hughes JR: Infantile methemoglobinemia due to benzocaine suppository. J Pediatr 66:797, 1965
55. Bloch A: More on infantile methemoglobinemia due to benzocaine suppository. J Pediatr 67:509, 1965
56. Klein SL, Nustad RA, Feinberg SE, et al: Acute toxic methemoglobinemia caused by a topical anesthetic. Pediatric Dentistry 5:107, 1983
57. Steinberg JB, Zepemick RG: Methemoglobinemia during anesthesia. J Pediatr 67:885, 1962
58. Douglas WW, Fairbanks VF: Methemoglobinemia induced by topical anesthetic spray (Cetacaine). Chest 71:587, 1977
59. Spielman FJ, Anderson JA, Terry WC: Benzocaine-induced methemoglobinemia during general anesthesia. J Oral Maxillofac Surg 42:740, 1984
60. Sandza JG Jr, Roberts RW, Shaw RC, et al: Symptomatic methemoglobinemia with a commonly used topical anesthetic, Cetacaine. Ann Thorac Surg 30:187, 1980
61. Olson ML, McEvoy GK: Methemoglobinemia induced by local anesthetics. Am J Hosp Pharm 38:89, 1981
62. O'Donohue WJ Jr, Moss LM, Angelillo VA: Acute methemoglobinemia induced by topical benzocaine and lidocaine. Arch Intern Med 140:1508, 1980
63. Beutler E: Methemoglobinemia and sulfhemoglobinemia. In Williams WJ, Beutler E, Erslev AJ, et al (eds): Hematology, 3rd ed. New York: McGraw-Hill, 1983: 704
64. Bunn HF: Disorders of hemoglobin. In Braunwald E, Isselbacher KJ, Petersdorf RG, et al (eds): Principles of internal medicine, 11th ed. New York: McGraw-Hill, 1987: 1518
65. Burne D, Doughty A: Methaemoglobinaemia following lignocaine. Lancet 2:971, 1964
66. Rosen PJ, Johnson C, McGehee WG, et al: Failure of methylene blue treatment in toxic methemoglobinemia: association with glucose-6-phosphate deficiency. Ann Intern Med 75:83, 1971
67. Deas TC: Severe methemoglobinemia following dental extractions under lidocaine anesthesia. Anesthesiology 17:204, 1956
68. Ohlgisser M, Adler M, Ben-Dov D, et al: Methaemoglobinaemia induced by mafenide acetate in children: a report of two cases. Br J Anaesth 50:299, 1978
69. Ternberg JL, Luce E: Methemoglobinemia: a complication of the silver nitrate treatment of burns. Surgery 63:328, 1968
70. Cushing AH, Smith S: Methemoglobinemia with silver nitrate therapy of burns: report of a case. Pediatrics 74:613, 1969
71. Deppe SA: Co-oximetry and its application in critical care medicine. Problems in Critical Care 5:82, 1991
72. Graubarth J, Bloom CJ, Coleman FC, et al: Dye poisoning in the nursery: a review of seventeen cases. JAMA 128:1155, 1945
73. Darling RC, Roughton FJW: Effect of methemoglobin on equilibrium between oxygen and hemoglobin. Am J Physiol 137:56, 1942
74. Park CM, Nagel RL: Sulfhemoglobinemia: clinical and molecular aspects. N Engl J Med 310:1579, 1984
75. Finch CA: Methemoglobinemia and sulfhemoglobinemia. N Engl J Med 239:470, 1948
76. Harvey JW, Keitt AS: Studies of the efficacy and potential hazards of methylene blue in aniline-induced methaemoglobinaemia. Br J Haematol 54:29, 1983

Complications in Anesthesiology, second edition, edited by Nikolaus Gravenstein and Robert R. Kirby. Lippincott-Raven Publishers, Philadelphia © 1996.

CHAPTER 48

Complications Associated With Muscle Relaxants

Richard R. Bartkowski
Jan Charles Horrow

Neuromuscular blocking agents are among the safest drugs available as long as ventilation is controlled. When administered to spontaneously breathing patients, however, they lead to respiratory acidosis, hypoxemia, and death if ventilation is not supported. In their classic study of deaths associated with anesthesia in the early 1950s, Beecher and Todd highlighted the role of muscle relaxants, which were just coming into widespread anesthesia practice. They attributed the cause of death to hypoxemia in 63% of patients whose perioperative demise was thought to have been caused by misuse of a muscle relaxant.[1] The therapeutic index (the ratio of the median lethal dose to the median effective dose) of these drugs is meaningless in these conditions. However, with controlled ventilation and adequate sedation, even overdosage is well tolerated.

This discussion of muscle relaxant complications begins with respiratory depression from residual paralysis in the absence of controlled ventilation. We then discuss the cardiovascular effects and potential for overdosage resulting from alterations in the pharmacokinetic and pharmacodynamic properties of nondepolarizing relaxant drugs. Next we deal with problems relating to pharmacologic antagonism of relaxants and conclude with a discussion of complications relating to the depolarizing relaxant, succinylcholine.

RESPIRATORY IMPAIRMENT

Muscle relaxant overdosage is harmful when it is unrecognized, the trachea is extubated prematurely, and ventilation is not properly supported. Many situations can lead to prolonged or excessive relaxant effects: the drug frequently may be given in overly generous doses; synergism with other drugs can potentiate its effect; patient disease can alter muscle relaxant pharmacokinetics leading to prolonged effect; pharmacologic antagonism may have been inadequate; or insufficient time may have elapsed since antagonist drugs were administered. Whatever the cause of relaxant overdosage, morbidity can be avoided by continuing ventilatory support and adequate sedation until neuromuscular function returns.

Diagnosis

If awake enough and able to speak, the patient may complain of air hunger. Writhing, uncoordinated movements of the extremities ("fish out of water") and spasmodic paradoxical abdominal motion are hallmarks of partial paralysis. Hypertension, tachycardia, and pupillary dilatation are common in the unsedated patient. In a completely paralyzed, awake patient, these may be the only signs. Respiratory measurements alone cannot diagnose relaxant-induced paralysis specifically, because many drugs and conditions affect ventilation.

Peripheral Nerve Stimulation

Confirmation of residual paralysis is obtained by peripheral nerve stimulation. In clinical practice, a force transducer is usually not available; as a substitute, the practitioner should feel, rather than observe, the force of adduction of the thumb on stimulation of the ulnar nerve with one of the available nerve stimulators. If both stimulating electrodes are located at the wrist, polarity is unimportant. Otherwise, place the positive electrode proximally.[2]

TRAIN-OF-FOUR. Train-of-four stimulation has been adopted widely because it facilitates quantitation of the neuromuscular response to muscle relaxants without the need for comparison with a control response. This technique consists of a short train of supramaximal stimuli at a relatively low frequency of 2 Hz for 2 seconds; each train is repeated no more frequently than once every 10 to 12 seconds.[3] Use of four stimuli in 2 seconds is described by the term "train-of-four."

Thumb adduction is the response that is evaluated. The ratio of the amplitude of the fourth evoked response to the first in the train provides a clinically adequate and convenient assessment of the magnitude of neuromuscular block present.[4,5] The fourth response is eliminated when the first is depressed about 75%; the third response disappears at 80% suppression of the first.[5] The second response disappears when the first is depressed about 90%.

For clinical purposes, counting the number of thumb adduction responses in a train grades the extent of neuromuscular block (Fig. 48-1). The presence of less than three responses correlates with adequate clinical muscle relaxation. Perhaps not unexpectedly, train-of-four stimulation is also valuable in assessing lesser degrees of residual neuromuscular blockade; in particular, the fourth response to train-of-four stimulation correlates with the patient's ability to sustain a normal tidal volume (Table 48-1).[6]

Unrecognized, incomplete antagonism of neuromuscular blockade occurs frequently when monitoring of neuromuscular function is not performed routinely. Train-of-four ratios of less than 70% occurred in 25% to 42% of patients in the postanesthetic care unit.[7,8] Presumably, routine use of peripheral nerve stimulators would lead to a decreased incidence of this problem.

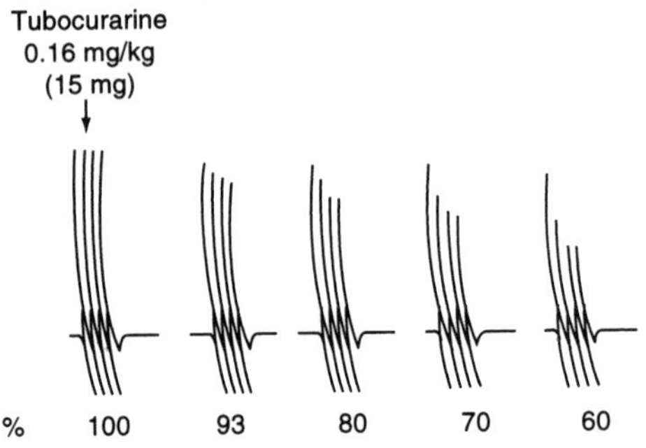

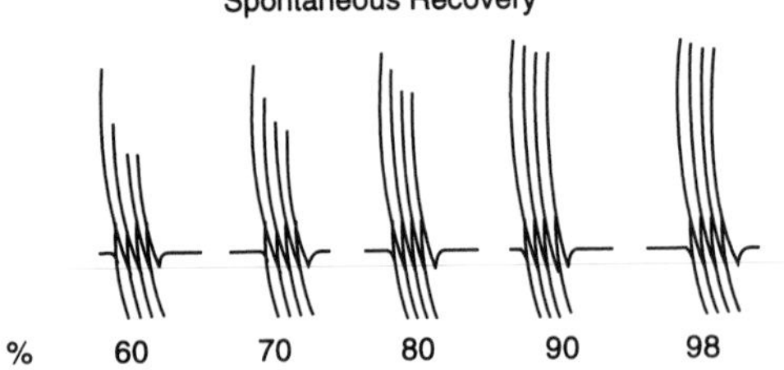

FIGURE 48-1. Correlations of responses (thumb adduction) to train-of-four stimulation (2 Hz) of the ulnar nerve of volunteers receiving d-tubocurarine. There are clinically important changes only when the train-of-four response is less than or equal to 70%. (Modified) from Ali HH, Utting JE, Gray TC: The effect of tubocurarine on indirectly elicited train-of-four muscle response and respiratory measurements in humans. Br J Anaesth 47:572, 1975

CLINICAL FEATURES OF PARTIAL PARALYSIS

Respiratory Muscle Weakness

Claude Bernard reported in 1851 that curare killed animals by paralyzing the muscles of respiration.[9] Table 48-1 shows how increased doses of relaxant correlate with progressively decreased twitch, train-of-four, respiratory function, and improved surgical relaxation.

Awake, trained, unmedicated volunteers can generate a negative (subambient) inspiratory pressure ("inspiratory force") of -120 cmH_2O and a vital capacity of 6 L. Respiratory volumes, but not pressures, can be maintained during partial paralysis despite a loss of muscular strength. The lungs are noncompliant at the extremes of volume that are reached when a vital capacity maneuver is performed: large decrements in attainable peak pressure diminish volume minimally. Thus, head lift for 5 seconds is barely possible, and inspiratory pressure is halved when the train-of-four ratio is 60%, while vital capacity is 85% of normal and tidal volume remains unaffected. These conditions can occur with about 0.15 mg/kg of d-tubocurarine (see Table 48-1).[10] This discussion uses doses of d-tubocurarine for comparison because most investigative work has used that relaxant. Fractions of its intubating dose, 0.6 mg/kg, are generally comparable to those of pancuronium (0.1 mg/kg) and of other relaxants.

When the fourth response to train-of-four stimulation is barely visible, vital capacity is markedly compromised. Tidal volume, however, is still normal, and surgical relaxation is "fair." Good surgical relaxation requires only one visible twitch of the train-of-four, corresponding to 90% receptor occupancy. In this case, tidal volume is markedly diminished, necessitating controlled ventilation. The association of d-tubocurarine dose and respiratory measurements is quite crude; interpatient variation precludes applying these rules strictly.

Skeletal Muscle Weakness

Whereas respiratory volumes can be maintained despite significant respiratory muscle weakness,[10] the nonrespiratory muscular weakness accompanying partial paralysis is of great concern. Dysphagia, implying weakness of the pharyngeal sphincter, and impaired cough occur when vital capacity is 66% of normal,[10] a capacity much greater than the 20 mL/kg that denotes adequate respiratory function in patients. Thus, passive regurgitation of stomach contents is possible even when pulmonary ventilation is adequate. As a result, significant partial paralysis in a patient demands intervention by the anesthesiologist or constant attendance by qualified personnel.

CLINICAL ASSESSMENT OF REVERSAL

From the foregoing discussion, one can appreciate the modalities used to diagnose reversal of neuromuscular blockade. Postoperative patients because of sedation and pain cannot achieve the inspiratory pressures or vital capacities of trained

TABLE 48-1
Clinical Correlations With Nondepolarizing Neuromuscular Blockade

					RESPIRATORY PARAMETERS			
d-TUBOCURARINE DOSE (mg/kg)	TWITCH HEIGHT (%)	TRAIN-OF-FOUR RESPONSE	RECEPTORS OCCUPIED (%)	CLINICAL RELAXATION	*Tidal Volume*	*Vital Capacity (%)*	*Maximum Inspiratory Pressure (%)*	COMMENTS
0.05	100	Normal	<50		Normal	100	86	Fade at 100 Hz
0.10	90	4th = 75% 1st	75	Poor	Normal	97	71	Head lift possible for 5 seconds
0.15	80	4th = 60% 1st			Normal	85	58	
0.20	75	4th = 40% 1st	80		Normal	66	39	
0.25	50	4th = 15% 1st	85	Fair	Normal	↓↓		
0.29	25	3 of 4 visible			↓			
	20	2 of 4 visible						3–14 minutes reversal
0.33	10	1 of 4 visible	90	Good	↓↓			
0.40	5	Absent		Very good				
0.60	0	Absent	100	Excellent	0			

volunteers. Thus, modest values for these measurements are used to designate the return of neuromuscular function. Evaluation of muscular strength commonly is performed with head lift or hand grip, because these sites are usually removed from the site of surgery. Responses to train-of-four stimulation diagnose residual paralysis adequately. In pediatric patients, spontaneous leg lift correlates with adequate reversal.[11] This technique is useful, because infants do not maintain resting tension in the thenar muscles for 2-second periods, thus precluding train-of-four measurement.

COMPLICATIONS RELATED TO NONDEPOLARIZING RELAXANTS

Cardiovascular Effects

Beecher and Todd attribute the cause of death to "cardiovascular failure notwithstanding artificial respiration" in 37% of those patients whose deaths were judged to be caused by the misuse of muscle relaxants.[1] Untoward cardiovascular effects of muscle relaxants can be predicted by a knowledge of their underlying pharmacologic mechanisms. Because these drugs produce a block at one type of cholinergic receptor, the neuromuscular junction, they are likely to bind somewhat to other cholinergic receptors, such as those at autonomic ganglia and at muscarinic sites. This section discusses the resultant hypotension, hypertension, tachycardia, and dysrhythmias attributed to nondepolarizing muscle relaxant drugs.

Hypotension

Mechanisms by which muscle relaxants decrease blood pressure include anaphylaxis, histamine release, and ganglionic blockade. Although anaphylactic reactions to these drugs have been documented,[12] they are rare. In these cases, skin testing can be valuable in diagnosis.[13]

HISTAMINE RELEASE. Pharmacologic histamine release, unrelated to anaphylaxis, occurs with many positively charged compounds.[14] All muscle relaxants contain at least one positively charged quaternary nitrogen group, but only d-tubocurarine, metocurine, and atracurium have been associated with clinically important histamine release. d-Tubocurarine was implicated in histamine release as early as 1939, before its first clinical use in 1942.[15]

Drug doses that cause hypotension and tachycardia from histamine release, expressed as a multiple of the dose to achieve 95% twitch reduction (ED_{95}), are one time for ED_{95} d-tubocurarine, two times ED_{95} for metocurine, and three times ED_{95} for atracurium.[16,17] d-Tubocurarine-induced hypotension lasts less than 5 minutes, in accordance with the rapid plasma half-life of histamine.[18] Whereas hypotension from exogenous histamine occurs with plasma concentrations about 2.5 times normal, intubating doses of d-tubocurarine (0.6 mg/kg) increase the histamine concentration fourfold.[18]

BLOCKADE OF AUTONOMIC GANGLIA. Blockade of autonomic ganglia has been demonstrated with large doses of relaxants given to animals. For example, a dose 3.9 times the ED_{95} for neuromuscular block of d-tubocurarine produces ganglionic block in 50% of cats. The comparable dose of metocurine is 176 times the ED_{95} for neuromuscular block (five times the median effective dose for histamine release) in the cat.[19]

In humans, histamine release alone accounts for only part of the hypotension seen after d-tubocurarine.[18] Antihistamines prevent the decrease in systemic vascular resistance, but not the decrease in blood pressure after curare in humans.[20] Because of great disparities in the response of different species to relaxants,[21,22] additional work is needed to clarify the contributions of histamine release and ganglionic blockade to hypotension.

PREVENTION. Prevention of relaxant-induced hypotension requires choosing a drug not associated with histamine release. Administration of antihistamines before the relaxant is also helpful, but both histamine H_1 and H_2 blockers must be given.[23] Finally, administer the muscle relaxant slowly. As with other drugs sharing the property of pharmacologic histamine release, more rapid administration produces more histamine release.[14] What rate is too fast? When a large dose of metocurine (0.4 mg/kg) was given over a 2-minute period to patients with aortic stenosis, blood pressure was unchanged and heart rate increased slightly.[24] An experimental relaxant that releases histamine was tolerated better when given over a 30-second period than when given over a 5-second period.[25] Thus, the hypotension commonly seen with muscle relaxants is due mostly to histamine release. It is a function of the drug chosen, the rate of administration, and the dose of drug administered.

Hypertension

Pancuronium can increase systemic blood pressure by stimulating sympathetic ganglia and by inducing tachycardia. Three mechanisms account for ganglionic stimulation; in each case the drug causes a blockade. First, block of muscarinic feedback receptors on adrenergic nerve terminals results in augmented catecholamine release. Second, reuptake of catecholamines is blocked. Third, inhibitory muscarinic pathways to sympathetic ganglia are blocked, permitting unbalanced stimulatory activity.[26]

The first of these mechanisms may have been responsible for a dramatic pressor response to pancuronium in a patient with pheochromocytoma.[27] Gallamine, which may share these mechanisms and effects, caused a similar response in a patient with preeclampsia.[28]

The net effect on blood pressure of pancuronium in the presence of a general anesthetic agent and other drugs is complex. The drug has no effect on systemic blood pressure when it is administered during opioid anesthesia (fentanyl or morphine) to patients taking β-adrenergic receptor blocking drugs.[29-31] Blood pressure is also unchanged when it is given with volatile anesthetics to healthy patients.[32] In one investigation, mean arterial pressure increased 24% when pancuronium was administered to patients who were receiving halothane anesthesia for coronary artery surgery.[33] In general, pancuronium has a tendency to increase blood pressure, but the effect is inconsistent, of small magnitude, and of minimal clinical importance. Of greater concern is the drug's effect on heart rate.

Tachycardia

HISTAMINE RELEASE. In patients receiving an insufficient depth of anesthesia, tachycardia may develop from the terror of paralysis. This fact aside, muscle relaxants increase heart rate either directly or by histamine release. In the latter case, hypotension triggers a baroreceptor-mediated increase in heart rate, that may climb from 80 to 120 beats/min with intubating doses of d-tubocurarine. When patients with aortic stenosis received metocurine, 0.4 mg/kg over a 2-minute period, a mild histamine-releasing challenge, heart rate increased slightly.[24] Large doses of atracurium, a weak histamine releasing agent, increased heart rate by only eight percent.[16]

DIRECT STIMULATION. Gallamine and pancuronium can directly increase heart rate. The mechanism, probably the same for each, is a combination of vagal block and sympathetic stimulation.[34] With gallamine, even a defasciculating dose (20 mg for a 70-kg person) increased the mean heart rate for 10 patients from 78 to 95 beats/min.[27] Although similar doses of pancuronium (0.5 mg for a 70-kg person) had no such effect, intubating doses (0.1 mg/kg) given to healthy patients during inhalational anesthesia increased heart rate by 33% with halothane and by 16% with enflurane.[32]

Tachycardia increases myocardial oxygen demand, a circumstance that leads easily to ischemia in patients with coronary artery disease. The choice of muscle relaxant in these patients remains complex, however, because of drug interactions. During halothane anesthesia in one study, pancuronium increased heart rate by 22%.[33] However, when combined with a high-dose fentanyl technique, pancuronium antagonizes the opioid-induced bradycardia: heart rate is restored to its pre-fentanyl level[35] or to a level minimally greater than control.[29] Coexistence of β-adrenergic receptor blockade tends to prevent an overall change in heart rate,[30] but cannot be relied on in individual cases.[31]

COMPARATIVE EFFECTS. The effect of other muscle relaxants on heart rate has been compared with that of pancuronium. Vecuronium had no effect in two studies in which pancuronium increased heart rate. In one using halothane anesthesia, pancuronium increased heart rate 22%.[33] In the other study, vecuronium had no effect on heart rate in patients receiving halothane or enflurane, whereas pancuronium induced increases of 16% to 33%.[32]

Metocurine, alone or in combination with pancuronium, is purported to be superior to pancuronium alone in avoidance of tachycardia. When combined with fentanyl, pancuronium had the same effect as metocurine or a combination of metocurine and pancuronium in one study,[30] but caused a significantly greater heart rate in another.[31] Several patients in the latter investigation had electrocardiographic evidence of ischemia; all had received pancuronium.

Dysrhythmias

Pancuronium can elicit ventricular dysrhythmias in patients and in dogs that receive tricyclic antidepressant medication and are anesthetized with halothane.[36] However, the dysrhythmogenic dose of epinephrine in dogs during halothane anesthesia is unaffected by pancuronium or d-tubocurarine,[37] suggesting that the tricyclic antidepressant is a necessary part of the drug interaction. The combination of pancuronium and halothane should be avoided in patients taking tricyclic antidepressant medication.

Postparalysis Myopathy

Following prolonged infusions of relaxants, nearly entirely restricted to patients in intensive care settings, atrophy of skeletal muscles may result in a prolonged state of weakness or paralysis.[38]

Pathologic studies reveal a denervation-like pattern, including up-regulation of postsynaptic receptors. Factors that may contribute to the development of this syndrome include administration of other medications such as corticosteroids and antibiotics, multiple organ failure with concomitant decrement in relaxant elimination, and sepsis. Reported cases frequently feature doses of relaxant administered over a week that are hundreds of times those given during an anesthetic.[39]

Although most reports of this syndrome mention pancuronium and vecuronium, this preponderance probably obtains from the popularity of these agents for paralysis in the intensive care setting.[40] However, accumulation of active steroidal metabolites of these drugs and exacerbation by high dose corticosteroid administration suggest a relaxant-specific effect.

Because weakness, paralysis, and myopathic changes occur in some intensive care unit patients who have not received skeletal muscle relaxant infusions, the role of relaxants in this syndrome remains controversial.[41] Until further clarification occurs, prudent clinicians will provide prolonged paralysis only when necessary, employ techniques such as neuromuscular blockade monitoring to limit total relaxant dose, and take additional precautions in patients with sepsis or those receiving high dose corticosteroids.

ABNORMAL RESPONSES TO NONDEPOLARIZING RELAXANTS

Abnormal Pharmacokinetic Parameters

Various disease states or other factors can modify the response to nondepolarizing relaxants. This section deals with those circumstances in which the plasma concentrations associated with usual dosages of muscle relaxant are modified, often risking overdosage.

A full discussion of relaxant pharmacokinetics is not appropriate here,[42] so attention will be restricted to two parameters, the volume of distribution and the plasma clearance. A change in the volume of distribution alters the appropriate loading dose of drug; more drug is needed to obtain similar plasma concentrations when the volume of distribution is increased.

A change in the plasma clearance of a drug alters the amount or frequency of repeat ("top-up") doses; when clearance is increased, the drug must be given in greater amounts or more frequently to maintain similar plasma concentrations. Relaxant pharmacokinetics are abnormal in renal failure, hepatic disorders, hypothermia, and with extremes of age.

Renal Failure

Table 48-2 displays the volume of distribution and plasma clearances measured by various investigators[43–46] for several relaxants in the presence of renal failure.

VOLUME OF DISTRIBUTION. The volumes of distribution of relaxant drugs are unchanged or slightly increased compared with those in patients with normal renal function. Thus, the initial relaxant dose should not be reduced if the usual plasma concentrations are desired.

PLASMA CLEARANCE. A marked disparity in plasma clearances occurs among relaxants. Other factors being the same, the choice of drug would proceed in the following order: mivacurium or atracurium, vecuronium, d-tubocurarine, pancuronium or metocurine, and gallamine. For prompt recovery from neuromuscular block, only mivacurium, atracurium, or vecuronium should be considered among nondepolarizing drugs.[47] Renal failure has no effect on the pharmacodynamics (dose-response) of relaxant drugs.

Hepatic Disorders

Cirrhosis is known to increase the proportion of globulin to albumin plasma proteins. Reports of cirrhotic patients with resistance to d-tubocurarine originally attributed this alteration to binding of the drug to γ-globulin proteins. More recent work on relaxant-protein binding shows that albumin is the major binding site of d-tubocurarine. The proportion bound to albumin, about 50%, is not modified by renal or hepatic diseases.[48]

VOLUME OF DISTRIBUTION. A pathophysiologic alteration in cirrhosis that more likely explains relaxant resistance is an increase in circulating blood volume and volume of distribution.

The volume of distribution of pancuronium is increased by almost 50% in cirrhosis (Table 48-3[48–54]). Cirrhotic patients who have received vecuronium, however, show no such increase when compared with normal patients.[49] This observation may result from two competing factors: an increase in circulating blood volume, which would increase the volume of distribution; and diminished hepatocyte uptake of vecu-

TABLE 48-2
Effect of Renal Failure on Pharmacokinetics of Nondepolarizing Neuromuscular Blocking Drugs

DRUG	VOLUME OF DISTRIBUTION* (%†)	PLASMA CLEARANCE (%†)	REFERENCE
Pancuronium	170	27	42
d-Tubocurarine	>100	50	43
Vecuronium	126	83	44
Atracurium	123	100	45

* Volume of distribution in the central compartment.

† Percentage of the value in patients with normal renal function.

TABLE 48-3
Effect of Hepatic Disorders on Pharmacokinetics of Nondepolarizing Neuromuscular Blocking Drugs

DISORDER	DRUG	VOLUME OF DISTRIBUTION* (%†)	PLASMA CLEARANCE (%†)	REFERENCE
Cirrhosis	Pancuronium	149	78	47
	Vecuronium	100	64	48
Cholestasis	Gallamine	100	100	49
	Pancuronium	100	48	50
	Vecuronium	100	58	51
Hepatitis	Pancuronium	100	40	52
	Atracurium	131‡	100	53

* Volume of distribution in the central compartment.
† Percentage of the value in healthy patients.
‡ Measurements in patients with both hepatic and renal failure.

ronium, which would decrease the effective volume of distribution.[55] Data to support this theory are not yet available.

Cholestasis and hepatitis do not alter the volume of distribution of muscle relaxants. Although Ward and Neill measured an expanded volume of distribution of atracurium in patients with hepatitis,[54] these patients also had renal failure, which, as discussed previously, also produces this alteration.

PLASMA CLEARANCE. The excretion of gallamine and atracurium does not depend on hepatic processes. Plasma clearances of these drugs is unaffected by liver disease (see Table 48-3). The liver eliminates other relaxants by metabolism, secretion into bile or both. Plasma clearance of pancuronium is decreased by cholestasis,[51] cirrhosis[53] or hepatitis.[53] A similar decrease in plasma clearance occurs with vecuronium.[49,52] No data are available for d-tubocurarine. Do these decreased clearances result in prolonged duration of paralysis? The answer is yes, by a factor of at most two.[55] Even this difference is enough to justify consideration of even vecuronium, an intermediate-acting muscle relaxant.

Hypothermia

Studies in cats document delayed excretion and metabolism[56] of relaxants at 28°C versus at 36°C. A study of patients with esophageal temperatures of 32°C or 37°C revealed no effect of hypothermia on d-tubocurarine pharmacokinetics,[57] probably owing to the narrow temperature range. For temperatures encountered in clinical practice, changes in excretory and metabolic activity probably play a minor role in relaxant duration. However, this consideration may not hold for temperatures reached during cardiopulmonary bypass. One study showed that atracurium infusion rates halved during cardiopulmonary bypass and hypothermia to 26°C; however, the investigators did not measure plasma concentrations.[58]

Age

Compared with adults, infants have a larger volume of distribution and lower plasma clearance of d-tubocurarine.[59] Thus, they have the same unfortunate combination of pharmacokinetic parameters as patients with chronic renal failure; larger doses of relaxant are required for initial effects but prolong the duration of the paralysis so obtained.

In geriatric patients, the volume of distribution of relaxants is unchanged, whereas the plasma clearance decreases linearly with age. Patients aged 80 to 89 years have a plasma clearance of pancuronium half that of patients aged 20 to 29 years.[60] Duvaldestin and colleagues measured a 35% decrease in plasma clearance of pancuronium in elderly patients (mean age, 81 years) versus a control group (44 years).[61] These changes were associated with approximately 60% increases in the duration of paralysis measured as time to 25% recovery of control twitch response.

Abnormal Pharmacodynamic Parameters

The pharmacodynamic parameter we shall consider is the plasma concentration associated with a given degree on neuromuscular blockade, usually 50% ($Cp_{ss(50)}$). Interestingly, the mode of assessing the degree of neuromuscular block may affect the value obtained for $Cp_{ss(50)}$. For example, with stable plasma concentration, twitch tension decreases with hypothermia, whereas the electromyogram remains unchanged. Thus, during hypothermia the $Cp_{ss(50)}$ measured by twitch depression is less than that measured by electromyography.[57] Twitch tension reflects effects on both the neuromuscular junction and the muscle, whereas the electromyogram is affected only by neuromuscular transmission.

Thermal Burns

Patients with thermal injury exhibit a resistance to all nondepolarizing relaxants tested, including relaxant combinations.[62–66] Pharmacokinetics of muscle relaxants are unchanged, but the $Cp_{ss(50)}$ is increased (Table 48-4). A part of the increase in d-tubocurarine requirement has been explained by increased protein binding in burned patients.[67] Resistance to nondepolarizing relaxants begins about 6 days after the burn and persists for 6 weeks. It gradually decreases but still

TABLE 48-4
Pharmacokinetics of Nondepolarizing Neuromuscular Blocking Drugs in Patients With Burns

DRUG	$Cp_{ss(50)}$ (%*)	ED_{50} (%*)	$Cp_{ss(95)}$ (%*)	ED_{95} (%*)	MEASUREMENT	REFERENCE
d-Tubocurarine	575	—	471	—	Serum concentration	62
Metocurarine	433	—	676	—	Plasma concentration	63
Pancuronium	—	258	—	240	Drug dose (intravenous)	64
Metocurarine–pancuronium combination	—	—	—	312	Drug dose (intravenous)	65
Atracurium	—	178	—	204	Drug dose (intravenous)	66

* Percentage of the value in patients without burns.

is present 1 year after injury.[63,66] The magnitude of relaxant resistance increases with the severity of burn.[64]

Motor Neuron Disease

Patients with upper motor neuron disease behave in a fashion similar to patients with thermal burns.[68] The $Cp_{ss(50)}$ for block in the paretic arms of these patients is more than four-fold that in neurologically intact patients. Supposedly, burn injury or upper motor neuron disease causes resistance to nondepolarizing relaxants by the spread of extrajunctional cholinergic receptors. Patients with lower motor neuron diseases (eg, poliomyelitis, amyotrophic lateral sclerosis) may be overly sensitive to nondepolarizing neuromuscular blocking drugs.[69]

Myasthenic States

Myasthenia gravis and myasthenic (Eaton-Lambert) syndrome are associated with an increased sensitivity to nondepolarizing relaxants. In myasthenia gravis, weakness progresses with activity and dissipates with anticholinesterase drugs; with myasthenic syndrome, activity yields increased strength, and weakness responds poorly to anticholinesterase drugs. These distinctions reflect the postulated disease mechanisms. Antibodies to muscle acetylcholine receptors in myasthenia gravis reduce the ability of acetylcholine to bind to receptors. In myasthenic syndrome, the number of quanta released by the prejunctional cell is reduced.[70]

Drug Interactions

Potentiation of neuromuscular blockade by the potent inhalational anesthetics is well known. Halothane decreases the $Cp_{ss(50)}$ of d-tubocurarine in a dose-dependent fashion.[71] The effects of enflurane are more complex: $Cp_{ss(50)}$, though decreased compared with that in patients receiving nitrous oxide anesthesia, is initially greater than the $Cp_{ss(50)}$ for halothane but decreases over a period of several hours to a value less than that for halothane.[72]

Other drugs that potentiate nondepolarizing relaxants include antidysrhythmic agents, ganglionic blockers, antibiotics,[73] and anticonvulsants. Drugs that result in resistance to blockade with nondepolarizers include aminophylline, some cytotoxic agents, and possibly furosemide.[69]

Clinical Implications

Patients with renal failure or hepatic disorders and those hypothermic or at the extremes of age are subject to changed relaxant kinetics. Complications that might result from these pharmacokinetic alterations include, at most, an unexpected resistance to an initial dose of drug (as a result of increased volume of distribution), an unexpected prolonged duration of paralysis (as a result of decreased plasma clearance), or both.

Likewise, altered sensitivity of the neuromuscular junction to muscle relaxants (a change in pharmacodynamic response) can result in poor muscle relaxation (increased $Cp_{ss(50)}$) or prolonged paralysis (decreased $Cp_{ss(50)}$).

The magnitude of these effects may be overshadowed by the variability in response to relaxants seen in any clinical population. Nevertheless, the best guess at relaxant dose can be refined by knowing the effects of these conditions on relaxant kinetics. In certain circumstances, such as the need to establish rapid relaxation in a burn patient, these considerations are essential to avoid complications.

COMPLICATIONS OF NEUROMUSCULAR BLOCK REVERSAL

Three drugs are available for antagonism of a nondepolarizing neuromuscular block: neostigmine, pyridostigmine and edrophonium. These drugs inhibit acetylcholinesterase, the enzyme that metabolizes acetylcholine at the nerve terminal. This inhibition leads to an increase in acetylcholine concentration, which in turn can overcome the competitive block.

Complications can arise in several ways. The drugs can fail to antagonize the block, leaving a partially paralyzed patient. They also can have activity at other sites, leading to cholinergic excess and undesirable side effects. All of these problems can and do occur in the clinical setting, leading to potentially serious complications.

Failure to Reverse Neuromuscular Blockade

A commonly encountered and discussed problem of reversal agents is a failure to reverse completely an established neuromuscular block. Although a first impression may be that any competitive block can be reversed by giving enough drug, further consideration shows that this is not the case. The nondepolarizing relaxants are thought to act by competing with acetylcholine for binding sites at active acetylcholine receptors. This competitive antagonism can be overcome by increasing the concentration of acetylcholine. Reversal agents accomplish this goal by inhibiting acetylcholinesterase, allowing the acetylcholine concentration to increase and to remain high for a longer time. Both increased concentration and duration can overcome the competitive block.

This reversal action, however, is limited. Once the enzyme acetylcholinesterase is totally inhibited, further injections of reversal agents fail to increase acetylcholine concentration and, thus, are ineffective. A maximal or ceiling effect exists for reversal.[74] The dose for this maximal effect appears to be in the clinical range for these drugs, so that if this amount is ineffective in providing adequate reversal, the residual block is prolonged.[75,77] Prolonged, irreversible block can occur because of external interfering factors but is also seen in apparently normal patients who appear to have a relative or absolute overdose of muscle relaxant.[76]

Factors Inhibiting Reversal

Several factors inhibit reversal of neuromuscular blockade (Table 48-5). They include drugs that augment the block, leading to a different noncompetitive or more profound blockade that cannot be reversed. Physiologic factors such as metabolic disturbances that interfere with reversal, can also be important.

TABLE 48-5
Inhibition of Reversal of Neuromuscular Blockade

INTERACTION WITH ANTIBIOTIC AGENTS
Polymyxins A and B
Neomycin
Streptomycin
Gentamicin
Kanamycin
Colistin
Tetracycline
Clindamycin
INTERACTION WITH POTENT INHALATIONAL ANESTHETICS
Especially enflurane and isoflurane
RESPIRATORY ACIDOSIS
METABOLIC ALKALOSIS
Questionable
ELECTROLYTE DISORDERS
Hypocalcemia
Hypomagnesemia
Hypokalemia
HYPOTHERMIA
May cause slow elimination

Antibiotic Interactions

A large number of antibiotics have been implicated in interactions with nondepolarizing neuromuscular blocking drugs.[77,78] Several are frequently mentioned: polymyxin A and B, neomycin, streptomycin, gentamicin, kanamycin, colistin, tetracycline, and clindamycin. Their effects do not follow a single pattern and are not always profound.

In spite of the increasing use of prophylactic antibiotic therapy, problems from this interaction do not appear more frequent. This observation may be related to greater awareness, with resultant closer monitoring of neuromuscular blockade. Interactions do occur, however, and may lead to inadequate antagonism by the anticholinesterases. In these cases, calcium chloride, 1 g intravenously, has been recommended, because it has been effective in some cases.[78]

General Anesthetic Interactions

Interactions with general anesthetics are known to potentiate the action of nondepolarizing muscle relaxants. Enflurane and isoflurane are particularly potent synergists. Study of this interaction has shown impaired reversal of neuromuscular blockade during enflurane anesthesia as compared with halothane or narcotic-supplemented nitrous oxide anesthesia.[79] In this study, spontaneous recovery from a single pancuronium dose was markedly prolonged in the presence of enflurane. Moreover, reversal of blockade at 10% twitch height by neostigmine, 36 μg/kg, was adequate within 10 minutes in the halothane and narcotic group, but still inadequate (train-of-four ratio 61%) in the enflurane group 30 minutes after reversal.

Drugs such as enflurane and antibiotics may augment neuromuscular block by pathways other than the competitive block at the cholinergic receptor. These other mechanisms may not be susceptible to the antagonistic action of an anticholinesterase, leading to a loss in our ability to reverse completely an established block.

Local Anesthetics/Calcium Channel Blockers

Whereas local anesthetics and calcium channel blocking drugs have been proposed as enhancers of neuromuscular blockade, clear evidence to conclude that they constitute a clinically important problem does not exist.

Acid-Base Imbalance

RESPIRATORY ACIDOSIS. Respiratory acidosis (arterial carbon dioxide partial pressure >50 mm Hg) is the disturbance best correlated with inadequate reversal.[80] In cats, an arterial carbon dioxide partial pressure of 66 mm Hg was associated with slight augmentation of d-tubocurarine blockade and failure of antagonism by neostigmine at degrees of blockade that normally are fully reversible. This failure to reverse continued until the arterial carbon dioxide partial pressure was decreased to the normal range (35 to 45 mm Hg).

This phenomenon poses a particular hazard in the clinical setting. If ventilation is inadequate because of residual neuromuscular blockade, reversal agents may be ineffective, leading to a self-perpetuating cycle of block, respiratory insufficiency, respiratory acidosis, and continuing blockade. Only assisted ventilation and monitoring of neuromuscular blockade reversal can interrupt the downward spiral.

METABOLIC ALKALOSIS. Metabolic alkalosis also inhibits reversal of nondepolarizing neuromuscular block.[80] However, investigators are hesitant to extend this observation to the clinical setting because the alkalosis studied was acute, induced by infusion of sodium bicarbonate. This situation, which is not often seen in the operating room, can lead to acute disturbance of intracellular pH and ion concentrations. In contrast, the chronic alkalosis seen clinically is usually accompanied by compensatory changes.

Electrolyte Imbalance

Ions particularly important in neuromuscular transmission are calcium, magnesium, and potassium. Hypocalcemia has been associated with augmented neuromuscular block and difficult reversal.[81] It is also a proposed mechanism for antibiotic potentiation of neuromuscular block. Hypomagnesemia sensitizes the neuromuscular junction to the effects of depolarizing and nondepolarizing relaxants in a manner similar to that noted in hypocalcemia.[82] Potassium is important in maintaining membrane potentials at the neuromuscular junction. Hypokalemia also has a small but definite sensitizing effect. These electrolyte disturbances usually are responsible for only a part of the overall sensitivity of an patient to muscle relaxants.[83] If the relaxant is administered slowly to avoid overdosage in patients with these disturbances, blockade and reversal often proceed in a normal manner.

Hypothermia

The effects of temperature on neuromuscular block are varied, depending on the conditions of measurement and the particular relaxant administered. The importance of hypothermia in the clinical setting is controversial. Over the range of temperatures seen clinically (31°C to 38°C), slight changes in the intensity of block are noted that are of questionable importance. A postulated effect, however, is the increase in the duration of block as a result of slower elimination of drug during hypothermia.[84] This alteration can lead to overdosage if the drug is given by schedule rather than assessment of the degree of the block. Hypothermia also leads to slower recovery if profound blockade is reached. Hypothermia, per se, does not lead to difficult reversal if the degree of block was in a reversible range.[84]

Problems at Other Sites of Action

Cardiovascular

The anticholinesterases have pharmacologic activity at sites other than the neuromuscular junction. Of particular importance are cholinergic pathways in the heart. Administration of these agents can lead to cholinergic excess with resultant dysrhythmia or bradycardia, even to asystole. They should be administered along with a vagolytic agent to suppress the cardiac side effects. When 2.5 mg of neostigmine is used, a dose of 1.0 mg of atropine or 0.4 mg of glycopyrrolate is needed to minimize cardiac effects. The relation of anticholinesterase, vagolytic administration, and dysrhythmia, such as junctional rhythm, premature contraction or conduction abnormalities, is often unclear.[85] These drugs are given at a time of changing anesthetic level, increasing awareness and excitement, and the potential for respiratory difficulty with some degree of hypoxia or hypercarbia.

Cholinergic Excess

BOWEL. Anticholinesterases augment gastrointestinal tone through their stimulation of parasympathetic and vagal sites in the bowel. Cramping is a clinical problem in patients with myasthenia gravis treated with neostigmine (less so with pyridostigmine). This increase in bowel tension was proposed as a cause of disruption of ileorectal anastomoses.[86] Those authors found a greater anastomotic leakage in patients receiving intraoperative neostigmine compared with patients receiving only cyclopropane anesthesia. They suggested that the increased peristalsis and tone led to disruption of the suture line. Subsequent investigation in animal models and in clinical practice failed to find any association of neostigmine with bowel anastomotic leakage.[87,88]

SALIVARY. Other vagally innervated sites stimulated by neostigmine are the salivary glands. Profuse salivation is a consequence of anticholinesterase treatment and cholinergic excess. This effect, however, seldom leads to severe complications. The widespread use of vagolytic drugs (atropine or glycopyrrolate) has reduced salivation to a point where coughing is occasional and laryngospasm rare.

Recurarization

A reported complication is recurrence of the block after apparently successful reversal.[89,90] To investigate the occurrence of recurarization, large doses of d-tubocurarine were given to well-monitored patients while the block was reversed normally or with small doses of edrophonium. In no cases was recurrence of block seen.[75] Significantly, this investigation did provide insight into the "recurarization" phenomenon. An observer viewing only clinical signs often reported recurrence of block, whereas the investigator documented by neuromuscular monitoring that reversal was inadequate from the onset.

A further report of recurarization proposed that this phenomenon could occur in patients with renal failure, a pathophysiologic state in which relaxant elimination is impaired.[91] Unfortunately, the investigator did not document reversal and recurrence by neuromuscular monitoring. In another study recurrence of block in organ failure was tested in well monitored patients who demonstrated prolonged block in another study. Even though reversal was slow, in no case did a block recur.[92]

COMPLICATIONS ASSOCIATED WITH SUCCINYLCHOLINE

Neuromuscular Depolarization

Succinylcholine is the only depolarizing neuromuscular blocking drug in current use. Many complications arise from its unique mode of action. Administration is associated with stimulation of neuromuscular transmission followed in short order by neuromuscular block. The stimulating effect of this drug leads to complications not seen with nondepolarizing competitive neuromuscular blocking drugs (Table 48-6). These complications in pediatric patients are now considered to be sufficiently extreme that some investigators believe the drug should be avoided, unless an emergency full-stomach rapid-sequence induction is planned.[93,94] Others strongly disagree,[95,96] advising only that a warning be inserted into the product labeling.

Fasciculations

Random contractures of muscle fibers follow succinylcholine administration in a majority of patients. These fasciculations are usually considered harmless but can lead to significant limb and body movements. Although patient injury can occur as a result of this movement, precautionary restraint appears capable of providing safety. Whereas fasciculations are not intrinsically harmful, associated phenomena, such as muscle pain or increased pressure in confined spaces such as the stomach and eye, have been proposed as complications.

TABLE 48-6
Complications With Succinylcholine

FASCICULATIONS

MUSCLE PAIN

INCREASED PRESSURE
Intraocular
Intragastric
Intracranial

ACUTE HYPERKALEMIA
Nerve injury and disease
Muscle injury and disease
Burns
Irradiation

INFECTION

RENAL FAILURE

RHABDOMYOLYSIS
Myoglobinemia and renal failure

MASSETER SPASM AND MALIGNANT HYPERTHERMIA

DYSRHYTHMIAS

HYPERTENSION OR HYPOTENSION

PROLONGED PARALYSIS
Overdose (phase II block)
Abnormality in cholinesterase
Insufficient cholinesterase

Postoperative Muscle Pain

Muscle pain after the administration of succinylcholine can be an important problem because of its frequency and potential severity. The most common complaint on the 1st or 2nd day after surgery from persons having minor surgery on an ambulatory basis often is severe muscle pain when succinylcholine has been used. This pain may be sufficient to limit normal activities.

Incidence

Myalgia occurring after administration of succinylcholine was recognized soon after the introduction of this drug.[97] Churchill-Davidson reported in 1954 that 66% of ambulatory patients had muscle pain on the day after surgery.[98] Of these, 62% had generalized myalgias, and 67% described these as severe. The muscle pain lasted 3 to 4 days in 48% of patients. Inpatients, on the other hand, had a 14% incidence of myalgia that occurred only in those who were mobile on the day of surgery. Attempts to prevent muscle pains by pretreatment with gallamine produced results that were equivocal.

Two decades later, other investigators reexamined succinylcholine myalgia to determine more accurately their frequency, locus, and prevention. The incidence in these more recent studies varies widely from near zero to about 90%. This finding is not surprising, because these myalgias have been shown to be influenced by age, gender, and previous drug administration. The young (less than 15 years) appear to have a lower, but clinically noticeable, incidence of fasciculation and pain: 3% (5 to 9 years) and 23% (10 to 15 years).[98] The incidence may also decrease at age 50 years and after.[98,99] It is greater in women than men.[99,100] The suggestion has been advanced that athletes and laborers who are more fit have a lower incidence of pain,[100] because the pain and stiffness is often likened to that occurring after strenuous exercise.

Prevention

DEFASCICULATION. Much interest has been directed toward "defasciculation" by pretreatment with a variety of drugs administered intravenously. Although Churchill-Davidson's results with gallamine pretreatment were not striking, pretreatment with gallamine[101] (20 to 40 mg) and d-tubocurarine[102,103] (3 to 5 mg) have been shown in controlled series of ambulatory patients to reduce pain incidence by approximately one-half.

Timing of the dose is important. In the studies demonstrating effectiveness of pretreatment, several minutes (unspecified to 4 minutes) were allowed between pretreatment and succinylcholine; administration of the defasciculating drug immediately before succinylcholine appears ineffective.[104] A recent study found that 3 minutes is the minimum time to reduce fasciculation intensity, but myalgia incidence was the same when d-tubocurarine was administered 0 to 7 minutes before succinylcholine.[105] Although d-tubocurarine is generally superior to other nondepolarizing neuromuscular blocking drugs in terms of defasciculation, it is not necessarily the optimal drug for prevention of postoperative myalgia. For example, whereas d-tubocurarine, 0.05 mg/kg, was more effective in reducing the incidence of fasciculations than atracurium, 0.025 mg/kg, the latter was far more effective in preventing postoperative myalgia.[106]

Pretreatment with gallamine, 20 mg, or d-tubocurarine, 3 mg, delays onset of neuromuscular block and results in poorer intubating conditions, in turn necessitating an increase in succinylcholine dosage from 1.0 to 1.5 mg/kg.[107] Pancuronium, in a dosage of 0.5 to 1.0 mg, is ineffective in blocking fasciculation, but does delay the onset of block.[107,108] A similar study using twitch rather than clinical criteria did not find decreased potency for succinylcholine after pretreatment with gallamine or curare, indicating differences in methods and results.[109]

SLOW INFUSION OF SUCCINYLCHOLINE. A slow infusion of a 0.2% succinylcholine solution over a 20-minute period also reduces the incidence of pain about one-half,[102] but less prolonged administration (eg, 10 mg over a 30-second period) does not. Most studies have not found a good correlation between fasciculations or their intensity and muscle pains.

LIDOCAINE AND PROCAINE. Lidocaine[103,110] and procaine, also decrease the incidence of succinylcholine-induced muscle pain, but their use for this purpose is not common. One study noted that pretreatment with lidocaine, 1.5 mg/kg, administered just before succinylcholine markedly augmented the effect of d-tubocurarine, 0.06 mg/kg, administered 3 minutes before the depolarizing relaxant.[103] Whereas d-tubocurarine pretreatment was associated with a reduction in the incidence of muscle pain from 43% to 24%; the addition of lidocaine reduced the incidence to 8.3%.

OTHER DRUGS. Diazepam, 0.05 mg/kg to 10 mg, given 5 minutes before succinylcholine, 1 mg/kg, is remarkably effective at reducing fasciculations, postoperative muscle pain, and cardiovascular and humoral side effects associated with this muscle relaxant.[111,112] A variety of other drugs have been shown to modify succinylcholine-induced fasciculations, muscle pain, or both: dantrolene, 150 mg (100 mg if body weight is <45 kg)[113]; thiopental, 5.2 mg/kg[114]; fentanyl, 1 to 2 μg/kg[115]; and calcium gluconate, 10 mL of 10% solution.[116]

STRETCH EXERCISES. A series of stretch exercises undertaken 1 hour before induction of anesthesia in a group of ambulatory patients was associated with a reduction in muscle pain from 52% to 12%.[117]

Clinical Implications

Although the optimum technique to reduce succinylcholine-induced muscle pain has not been identified, some effort to reduce postoperative discomfort can be used. This approach ranges from pretreatment before succinylcholine in one or more of the ways discussed to the avoidance of succinylcholine altogether. The intermediate-acting, nondepolarizing drugs, atracurium, vecuronium, and possibly mivacurium, can be employed. The introduction of rocuronium, which has an onset of action near 60 seconds, has proved to be a suitable alternative in many, but not all situations.

The currently available alternative relaxants (except rocuronium) require at least 1 minute longer than succinylcholine to achieve acceptable conditions for tracheal intubation. In certain critical situations such as emergency cesarean sections, succinylcholine remains the drug of choice for rapid intubation.

Pressure Increase

Intraocular

Succinylcholine long has been known to produce an increase in intraocular pressure of 4 to 10 mm Hg from contracture of the extraocular muscles.[118,119] These muscles appear to have two types of fibers, one of which responds to succinylcholine with sustained contraction rather than the usual brief twitch. Soon after the introduction of succinylcholine into clinical anesthesia, concern was expressed that the increase in pressure may be detrimental in ophthalmologic surgery. The area of particular attention was the loss of vitreous in cases involving an open eye. Dillon reported one early case where this complication may have occurred,[119] whereas Lincoff implicated succinylcholine in other cases.[120] This concern has led during the past three decades to a reconsideration of succinylcholine use in eye surgery and to investigations into ways of preventing the pressure increase.

MECHANISMS. Contraction of extraocular muscles is not the only mechanism by which intraocular pressure is increased acutely. Another relevant factor is vascular congestion in the orbit, caused by coughing, straining or body movement, all of which may be prevented by rapid, profound relaxation. The trauma patient is often at increased risk for pulmonary aspiration of gastric contents unless tracheal intubation is performed promptly after induction of general anesthesia.

A series of investigations studied the effect on intraocular pressure of pretreatment with d-tubocurarine, 3 mg, or gallamine, 20 mg, administered 3 minutes or more before succinylcholine, 1 mg/kg. No significant increase in intraocular pressure (measured by tonometry) occurred in volunteers, patients with glaucoma, or cats (measured directly).[121] This technique has been used with apparent success in many institutions. Controversy was interjected when a subsequent study reported no blunting of the succinylcholine-induced intraocular pressure increase by d-tubocurarine or gallamine.[122]

CLINICAL IMPLICATIONS. Stimulated by this controversy and the apparent safety of pretreatment with a nondepolarizing relaxant before succinylcholine administration, one large ophthalmologic center reviewed its clinical experience with 228 patients presenting with an open eye injury.[123] Their customary practice included pretreatment with gallamine, 10 to 15 mg, or d-tubocurarine, 3 to 6 mg, 3 to 3.5 minutes before a rapid induction with thiopental and succinylcholine, 60 to 160 mg. Their chart review identified no cases of vitreous loss. Further, the investigators found no cases of succinylcholine related vitreous loss in their institution in the previous 10 years, during which time similar techniques were used. Although chart review is inherently biased in the direction of underreporting, this large experience argues rather cogently for the overall safety of succinylcholine after nondepolarizer pretreatment when rapid induction and relaxation are required.

Intragastric

An increase in intragastric pressure carries the risk of forcing gastric contents retrograde through the esophagus to the posterior pharynx from which they can be aspirated. Regurgitation of gastric contents is more likely when the stomach is not empty because of bowel obstruction, recent food ingestion, blood, or poor emptying caused by illness, anxiety, drugs or obesity. Regurgitation occurs with gastric pressures as low as 28 cmH_2O.[124] However, it can occur at even lower pressure in pregnant and obese patients with an incompetent lower esophageal sphincter. Because the fasciculations induced by succinylcholine can increase intragastric pressure,[125,126] interest in preventing intragastric pressure evaluation has been widespread.

PREVENTION. The succinylcholine-induced increase in intragastric pressure ranges from zero to 41 mm Hg and correlates with the intensity of fasciculations.[127] As expected from the discussion of succinylcholine induced muscle pain and increased intraocular pressure, increased intragastric pressure is also prevented by the administration of d-tubocurarine, 3 mg, before the succinylcholine dose. Lidocaine, 6 mg/kg, also may prevent this increase.

A subsequent study verified the relation between fasciculation and pressure increase by quantitative abdominal muscle electromyography.[128] Children (3 weeks to 12 years) apparently do not have a clinically important increase in intragastric pressure after succinylcholine.[129] This observation has been attributed to the lack of strong fasciculations in this age group; thus, the investigators consider pretreatment with a nondepolarizing relaxant unnecessary in this population.

In patients especially at risk for regurgitation and pulmonary aspiration, several techniques are recommended. These include pretreatment with d-tubocurarine, 3 mg, 3 minutes before succinylcholine administration. Additionally, atropine, 0.5 mg, is often given because it increases lower esophageal sphincter tone and the pressure required for reflux.[130] Interestingly, succinylcholine also increases lower esophageal sphincter tone.[131] This increase offsets the intra-abdominal pressure increase and thus the barrier pressure gradient is preserved. Finally, pressure on the esophagus transmitted from direct manual pressure on the cricoid cartilage (Sellick's maneuver) is effective at sealing the esophagus and preventing regurgitation.[131]

Intracranial

Perhaps not unexpectedly after the foregoing discussion, succinylcholine use also has been associated with an increase in intracranial pressure. As a result, caution has been expressed regarding its use in patients who have space-occupying cerebral lesions lest the intracranial pressure increase to the point at which cerebral circulation would be compromised or undue pressure applied to the brain.[132]

This caution was repeated after controlled experiments in cats showed a consistent increase in intracranial pressure after succinylcholine administration.[133] A brief report of eight patients showed that the intracranial pressure increase after succinylcholine is not large if the relaxant is incorporated into an induction using thiopental, 4 mg/kg, and assisted ventilation.[134] Complete neuromuscular blockade with vecuronium, 0.14 mg/kg administered 3 minutes before succinylcholine, also prevents the intracranial pressure increase associated with the latter relaxant.[135]

Acute Hyperkalemia

Succinylcholine administration has been associated with severe and even life-threatening hyperkalemia in certain groups of susceptible persons.[94] The conditions leading to a high incidence of reported hyperkalemic response involve nerve and muscle injury or disease and burn injury. Conditions with a weaker association include closed head injury, intra-abdominal infection, and renal failure.

Nerve Injury and Disease

Denervation leads to supersensitivity of the involved muscle to subsequently administered succinylcholine.[136] Although major denervation is not a common clinical occurrence, peripheral nerve injury has been associated with a clinically important increase in serum potassium arising principally from the denervated limb. The increase in mean serum venous potassium is less than 2 mEq/L in those patients,[137] possibly reflecting the relatively limited muscle mass involved.

More problematic and common are the upper motor neuron lesions, such as spinal cord injuries, tetanus, and cerebral motor deficiencies resulting from multiple sclerosis, encephalitis, or closed head injury. After several case reports described cardiac arrest following succinylcholine administration, Cooperman prospectively studied the serum potassium concentration in 32 patients with a variety of upper motor neuron lesions during the induction of anesthesia.[138] Of the 15 patients with acute increases in potassium concentration of 1 mEq/L or more, nine had neuromuscular diseases for less than 1 year and four of the others had progressive disease. Patients within 2 weeks of their disease onset did not show abnormal responses. A correlation of the increase in potassium concentration with the degree and extent of the involved muscle was noted. A similar syndrome of acute hyperkalemic cardiac arrest has been reported in a patient with head injury.[139] This type of patient is considered at risk either because of the upper nervous system lesion or prolonged immobility.[136]

Muscle Disease and Injury

Duchenne muscular dystrophy, even before the onset of clinical symptoms, also has been associated with acute hyperkalemia and even cardiac arrest after the administration of succinylcholine.[138,140] Warner and Wedel, in a population-based study, have noted that the risk of an anesthesiologist encountering a child older than 9 years of age with undiagnosed Duchenne muscular dystrophy is very low.[141] In their series spanning 37 years, all cases had been diagnosed by age 9. Muscle may also respond abnormally to succinylcholine because of direct traumatic injury. Among severely traumatized patients receiving multiple sequential anesthetics, the largest acute increase in serum potassium occurs 20 to 50 days after injury; responses return to normal as the patient heals. d-Tubocurarine, 6 mg, offers protection from acute hyperkalemia in these patients.[142,143]

Irradiation

A cardiac arrest after succinylcholine, 100 mg, in a healthy, 65-kg teenager receiving therapeutic irradiation led to laboratory investigation of the effects of radiation-induced muscle injury as a cause of acute hyperkalemia.[144] The results were similar to those in patients with burns and trauma. One week after radiation no effect was seen. In rats 3 weeks after irradiation of only the hind leg, the plasma potassium increased from 3.6 to 7.7 mEq/L after succinylcholine. Thus major muscle radiation should be considered one of the factors predisposing muscle to potassium release after succinylcholine.

Thermal Burns

Patients with severe burns can also be susceptible to hyperkalemic cardiac arrest in a manner similar to that of patients with neuromuscular disorders. The increased susceptibility to succinylcholine-induced hyperkalemia appears about 20 days after the burn injury and persists for about 2 months.[145] Severe cases of thermal burn are more likely to provoke symptoms, but occasional patients with burns of only small areas of the body also have had an exaggerated response. In general, burn patients should be considered at risk for succinylcholine-induced hyperkalemia 20 to 60 days after injury, during which period another relaxant should be chosen.

Infection

Many of the patients with trauma or burns who have had acute hyperkalemia after succinylcholine administration also had concurrent infection. Infection alone, particularly intra-abdominal infection, has been associated with cardiovascular collapse and hyperkalemia in patients without other predisposing factors.[146] Even in patients pretreated with pancuronium, 2 mg, serum potassium has increased to near 8 mEq/L. The patients with an increase of serum potassium >1.5 mEq/L all had severe intra-abdominal infection lasting 24 to 71 days. Patients with recent infection (4 to 9 days) did not show this increase. In a series of 21 patients with severe, but generally nonabdominal infections, the increase in serum potassium averaged 1.7 mEq/L in those most severely infected.[147]

Renal Failure

After reports of several patients with renal failure who had cardiac arrest or hyperkalemia associated with electrocardiographic changes after succinylcholine administration,[148,149] this drug was believed to be contraindicated in that type of case. Two prospective controlled studies, however, dispelled this notion.[150,151] Patients with renal failure who were maintained on hemodialysis (10 in one, 34 in the other) were found to behave similarly to matched patients with normal renal function. The investigators speculate that in some of the previous adverse reports other factors, such as uremic neuropathy, may have contributed to the reported hyperkalemia.

Rhabdomyolysis, Myoglobinemia, and Renal Failure

The use of succinylcholine has resulted in muscle injury, reflected by myoglobin release into the blood and eventually into the urine. In a group of 40 children as old as 10 years who received a single dose of succinylcholine, 1 mg/kg intravenously, 16 had myoglobinemia as determined from venous blood samples 15 and 60 minutes after drug administration.[152] Thirty-one received halothane anesthesia; this group included 14 cases of myoglobinemia. Of the nine other children having a variety of anesthetics, only two had measurable myoglobinemia. No myoglobinemia was detected in 12 children receiving intramuscular administration of succinylcholine, 1 mg/kg. In the same study, only 1 of 30 adults showed detectable myoglobin. No further complications of myoglobin were noted in this group.

Succinylcholine-induced myoglobinemia also occurs in children receiving isoflurane; however, the degree of myoglobinemia is considerably lower.[153] Although the presence of visible fasciculations did not correlate with the serum myoglobin concentration, another study noted that pretreatment with d-tubocurarine, 0.05 mg/kg, or pancuronium, 0.02 mg/kg, reduced the incidence of both fasciculations and the occurence of detectable myoglobinemia.[154] Rhabdomyolysis with visible and measurable myoglobinemia has been reported after succinylcholine in children[155] and an adult.[156] In the adult and several of the children, renal failure accompanied the muscle injury. Although reports of renal failure are well documented, the incidence is unknown.

Abnormal Muscle Contracture

Myotonia

Myotonia is a clinical sign of a group of neuromuscular diseases in which the affected muscles show a delayed relaxation after contraction. Two of the better categorized myotonic syndromes are myotonia dystrophica, which begins in mid- or late life, and myotonia congenita, a congenital and lifelong disorder. Generalized, severe muscle spasm induced by succinylcholine has been noted in these patients.[156,157] Spasm can be severe enough to interfere with airway management and ventilation.[158] The musculature of other patients having a diagnosis of myotonia, however, reportedly responds normally with muscle relaxation after succinylcholine.[159,160] Because the response to succinylcholine in the myotonic disorders is unpredictable, it should be avoided.[161]

Masseter Spasm

Rigidity, particularly that of the jaw (masseter spasm) is an occasional consequence of succinylcholine use. Although this condition may be a prelude to malignant hyperthermia, it can occur after succinylcholine in patients with myotonic syndromes, those with other muscle disorders, and even in apparently normal persons. When faced with this problem, some experts believe that a presumptive diagnosis of malignant hyperthermia should be made, the anesthetic terminated, and the patient referred for evaluation and possible muscle biopsy.[162] Masseter muscle rigidity when associated with a peak creatine kinase measurement of more than 20,000 IU in children is believed to be virtually pathognomonic.[163] However, recent data suggest that 1 in 20 patients may have increased masseter tone sufficient to be interpreted as spasm without any evidence for a hypermetabolic disorder.[164]

Cardiovascular Complications

Dysrhythmias

BRADYCARDIA. Bradycardia is the most common cardiovascular problem noted after succinylcholine administration. Two distinct circumstances commonly elicit bradycardia. A single intravenous injection of succinylcholine can produce heart rate slowing. This effect is common in children[165] and less so in adults. Intramuscularly administered atropine, 6 μg/kg, given either 60 to 90 minutes or 15 to 20 minutes before induction does not change the incidence of heart rate slowing.[166] Intravenously administered atropine, 0.4 to 0.6 mg, given 5 to 10 minutes before succinylcholine, prevents the bradycardia.[167]

More profound bradycardia can occur with repeated doses of succinylcholine. This is a different effect in that it occurs commonly both in adults and children, even those not affected by the initial dose. The extent of heart rate slowing depends on the circumstances in which the drug is given. It is more pronounced with halothane anesthesia and is blunted by previous administration of thiopental.[168] The time course is also important, for a lower incidence of bradycardia is reported when the doses are separated by 2 minutes, and a higher incidence at 5 minutes.

Asystole has been reported as a rare complication of succinylcholine infusion.[169] Pretreatment with d-tubocurarine, 0.05 mg/kg, is also effective in blocking the bradycardia after repeat doses of succinylcholine.[170]

Evidence suggests that succinylcholine causes the cardiac slowing.[168] Often when the sinus node slows sufficiently, another lower pacemaker can dominate. If another autonomic pacemaker does not take over, asystole can supervene. The lack of rapid pacemaker activity can also predispose to ventricular ectopy, especially if other sympathetic stimuli, such as laryngoscopy, take place during this vulnerable period.

TACHYCARDIA AND HYPERTENSION. Tachycardia and hypertension are sometimes observed after succinylcholine administration, particularly after thiopental induction.[167] Again, the previous course of the patient appears important in determining whether tachycardia and stimulation, or bradycardia and depression occur.

Hypotension

Hypotension, histamine release, and anaphylaxis are more rarely reported complications of succinylcholine administration. The presentation is the same as that with other drugs. Signs include wheezing, bronchospasms, and hypotension.[171,172] The respiratory components can be masked by potent inhalational agents, leaving cardiovascular collapse as the first indication.

PROLONGED PARALYSIS

Abnormal Pseudocholinesterase

Abnormal metabolism of succinylcholine can result in slower recovery from neuromuscular block. The breakdown of succinylcholine proceeds by enzymatic hydrolysis in the blood. The enzyme responsible for this metabolism is plasma pseudocholinesterase, a circulating enzyme produced in the liver. This enzyme normally is so efficient that only a fraction of the initial dose of succinylcholine is active when it reaches the motor endplate. Continuous metabolism of succinylcholine in the plasma to succinylmonocholine, and eventually to choline and succinic acid, leads to a rapid termination of action. Many reported cases of prolonged paralysis after succinylcholine involve some abnormality of pseudocholinesterase.

Genetic Variants

The more severe cases of low activity involve genetic variants of atypical pseudocholinesterase that are unable to metabolize succinylcholine, even though they metabolize acetylcholine normally. The most common variant is the dibucaine-resistant enzyme with an incidence of homozygosity of about 1 in 2500 in European and American populations.[173] Other genetic variants of lesser frequency are known and are easily determined by plasma testing.[174] In general, the response to a customary single dose of succinylcholine in patients with a genetic variant enzyme is markedly prolonged, with paralysis lasting many hours.

Normal Pseudocholinesterase

Even with normal pseudocholinesterase, variability in the metabolism of succinylcholine occurs. Patients heterozygous for the abnormal variant enzyme constitute 3% to 5% of the population and have a lower than normal plasma concentration of normal enzyme.[173] Pregnancy is associated with a 20% to 30% decrease in enzyme concentrations, beginning in the first trimester and continuing into the early postpartum period.[175,176] Liver disease also can lead to decreased concentration.[177] Several drugs have affinity for pseudocholinesterase and lower its activity, including hexafluorenium,[178] echothiophate,[179] phenelzine,[179] cholinesterase inhibitors,[180,181] and neuromuscular blockers, particularly pancuronium.[182] Plasmapheresis can produce a marked decrease in circulating enzyme.[183]

Although these factors can reduce enzyme activity to a clinically important extent, the potential for producing prolonged apnea is less. When pseudocholinesterase activity is 20% of normal, apnea is prolonged from a normal 3 to 9 minutes.[178] A clinical study in 70 patients with normal enzyme found that muscle recovery after succinylcholine varied from 6 to 22 minutes, whereas cholinesterase activity varied from 2200 to 200 U/L (normal 620 to 1470).[184]

Although variation in pseudocholinesterase activity can produce variability in response, some variability may be intrinsic, as seen in the wide range of response of persons with normal measured activity.[184] In patients tested by a range of single-dose and infusion techniques, recovery time varied by a factor of four for single doses, whereas a 10-fold difference was noted in the infusion rate required to maintain a constant block.[185] The investigators noted that persons with a history of prolonged neuromuscular block who subsequently were tested were more sensitive to succinylcholine. They required one half to one third the normal dose for a normal effect. This sensitivity can lead to overdosage if normal rates of infusion are given over a prolonged period without adequate monitoring.

Phase II Block

This condition also is mentioned as a cause of prolonged blockade after succinylcholine. Patients exhibiting prolonged blockade are often labeled with this diagnosis if they demonstrate some characteristics of nondepolarizing block such as tetanic fade.[186] In a study using repeated single doses of succinylcholine, phase II blockade occurred after 3 to 5 mg/kg. This transition was marked by train-of-four fade (train-of-four ratio less than 0.3) and often by tachyphylaxis necessitating increased drug administration to maintain blockade.[187] The transition from phase I to phase II block is variable and affected by dosage regimen and concurrent anesthesia.[188] Whether phase II block delays recovery from succinylcholine block or is just a change in block characteristic associated with prolonged block and larger doses is still debated. Recovery times from phase II block in these well monitored patients, however, were not excessive.

Hypermagnesemia

Magnesium is also known to increase the sensitivity to succinylcholine. Patients receiving magnesium sulfate therapy for toxemia of pregnancy require succinylcholine at a dose of only 4.7 mg/kg/h to maintain the same degree of block that requires 9.4 mg/kg/h in healthy women.[189]

REFERENCES

1. Beecher HK, Todd DP: A study of the deaths associated with anesthesia and surgery. Ann Surg 140:2, 1954
2. Berger JJ, Gravenstein JS, Munson ES: Electrode polarity and peripheral nerve stimulation. Anesthesiology 56:402, 1982
3. Ali HH, Utting JE, Gray TC: Stimulus frequency in the detection of neuromuscular block in humans. Br J Anaesth 42: 967, 1970
4. Ali HH, Utting JE, Gray TC: Quantitative assessment of residual antidepolarizing block: I. Br J Anaesth 43:473, 1971
5. Ali HH, Utting JE, Gray TC: Quantitative assessment of residual antidepolarizing block: II. Br J Anaesth 43:478, 1971
6. Ali HH, Wilson RS, Savarese JJ, et al: The effect of tubocurarine on indirectly elicited train-of-four muscle response and respiratory measurements in humans. Br J Anaesth 47:570, 1975
7. Lennmarken C, Lofstrom JB: Partial curarization in the postoperative period. Acta Anaesthesiol Scand 28:260, 1984
8. Viby-Mogensen J, Jogenson BC, Ording H: Residual curarization in the recovery room. Anesthesiology 50:539, 1979
9. Feldman SA: Muscle relaxants, 2nd ed. Philadelphia: WB Saunders, 1979: 1
10. Gal TJ, Goldberg SK: Relationship between respiratory muscle strength and vital capacity during partial curarization in awake subjects. Anesthesiology 54:141, 1981
11. Mason LJ, Betts EK: Leg lift and maximum inspiratory force: clinical signs of neuromuscular blockade reversal in neonates and infants. Anesthesiology 52:441, 1980
12. Fisher McD, Munro I: Life-threatening anaphylactoid reactions to muscle relaxants. Anesth Analg 6:559, 1983
13. Vervloet D, Nizankowska E, Arnaud A, et al: Adverse reactions to suxamethonium and other muscle relaxants under general anesthesia. J Allergy Clin Immunol 71:552, 1983
14. Garrison JC: Histamine, bradykinin, 5-hydroxytryptamine and their antagonists. In Gilman AG, Rall TW, Nies AS, Taylor P, (eds): The pharmacological basis of therapeutics, 8th ed. New York: Macmillan, 1990: 575
15. Alam M, Anrep GV, Baroum GS, et al: Liberation of histamine from the skeletal muscle by curare. J Physiol (Lond) 95:148, 1939
16. Basta SJ, Ali HH, Savarese JJ, et al: Clinical pharmacology of atracurium besylate (BW 33A): a new nondepolarizing muscle relaxant. Anesth Analg 61:723, 1982
17. Basta SJ, Savarese JJ, Ali HH, et al: Histamine-releasing potencies of atracurium, dimethyl tubocurarine and tubocurarine. Br J Anaesth 55:105S, 1983
18. Moss J, Rosow CE, Savarese JJ, et al: Role of histamine in the hypotensive action of *d*-tubocurarine in humans. Anesthesiology 55:19, 1981
19. Savarese JJ: The autonomic margins of safety of metocurine and *d*-tubocurarine in the cat. Anesthesiology 50:40, 1979
20. Inada E, Philbin DM, D'ambra M, et al: Protective effects of H_1 and H_2 histamine antagonists with *d*-tubocurarine administration: a double blind study. Proceedings of the 7th annual meeting of the Society of Cardiovascular Anesthesiologists. Phoenix, AZ. Richmond, VA: Society of Cardiovascular Anesthesiologists, 1985: 59
21. Drane SE, Evans MH: The relative vagolytic potencies of six muscle relaxants in the rabbit. J Pharm Pharmacol 31:384, 1979
22. Maclagan J: Competitive neuromuscular blocking drugs. In Zaimis E (ed): Neuromuscular junction. The handbook of experimental pharmacology, vol 4. New York: Springer-Verlag, 1976: 421
23. Philbin DM, Moss J, Akins CW, et al: The use of H_1 and H_2 histamine antagonists with morphine anesthesia: a double-blind study. Anesthesiology 55:292, 1981
24. Zaidan JR, Kaplan JA: Cardiovascular effects of metocurine in patients with aortic stenosis. Anesthesiology 56:395, 1982
25. Moss J, Rosow CE: Histamine release by narcotics and muscle relaxants in humans. Anesthesiology 59:330, 1983
26. Savarese JJ, Lowenstein E: The name of the game: no anesthesia by cookbook. Anesthesiology 62:703, 1985
27. Jones RM, Hill AB: Severe hypertension associated with pancuronium in a patient with a pheochromocytoma. Can Anaesth Soc J 28:394, 1981
28. Kingsley BP, Vaughan S, Baughan RW: Cardiovascular effects of nondepolarizing relaxants employed for pretreatment prior to succinylcholine. Can Anaesth Soc J 31:13, 1984
29. Waller JL, Hug CC, Nagle DM, et al: Hemodynamic changes during fentanyl–oxygen anesthesia for aortocoronary bypass operation. Anesthesiology 55:212, 1981
30. McDonald DH, Zaidan JR: Hemodynamic effects of pancuronium and pancuronium plus metocurine in patients taking propranolol. Anesthesiology 60:359, 1984
31. Thomson IR, Putnins CL: Adverse effects of pancuronium during high-dose fentanyl anesthesia for coronary artery bypass grafting. Anesthesiology 62:708, 1985
32. Gregoretti SM, Sohn YJ, Sia RL: Heart rate and blood pressure changes after ORG NC45 (vecuronium) and pancuronium during halothane and enflurane anesthesia. Anesthesiology 56:392, 1982
33. Morris RB, Cahalan MK, Miller RD, et al: The cardiovascular effects of vecuronium (ORG NC45) and pancuronium in patients undergoing coronary artery bypass grafting. Anesthesiology 58:438, 1983

34. Miller RD, Savarese JJ: Pharmacology of muscle relaxants and their antagonists. In Miller RD: Anesthesia, 2nd ed. New York: Churchill Livingstone, 1986: 889
35. Salmenpera M, Peltola K, Takkunen O, et al: Cardiovascular effects of pancuronium and vecuronium during high-dose fentanyl anesthesia. Anesth Analg 62:1059, 1983
36. Edwards RP, Miller RD, Roizen MF, et al: Cardiac responses to imipramine with halothane or enflurane. Anesthesiology 50:421, 1979
37. Schick LM, Chapin JC, Munson ES, et al: Pancuronium-, *d*-tubocurarine-, and epinephrine-induced arrhythmias during halothane anesthesia in dogs. Anesthesiology 52:207, 1980
38. Hansen-Flaschen J, Cowen J, Raps EC: Neuromuscular blockade in the intensive care unit: more than we bargained for. Am Rev Respir Dis 147:234, 1993
39. Kupfer Y, Namba T, Kaldawi E, Tessler S: Prolonged weakness after long-term infusion of vecuronium bromide. Ann Intern Med 117:484, 1992
40. Klessig HT, Giger HJ, Murray MJ, Coursin DB: A national survey on the practical patterns of anesthesiologists/intensivists in the use of muscle relaxants. Crit Care Med 20:1341, 1992
41. Bolton CF: Neuromuscular abnormalities in critically ill patients. Intensive Care Med 19:309, 1993
42. Miller RD: Pharmacokinetics of muscle relaxants and their antagonists. In Prys-Roberts C, Hug CC (eds): Pharmacokinetics of anaesthesia. Oxford: Blackwell Scientific, 1984: 246
43. McLeod K, Watson MJ, Rawlins MD: Pharmacokinetics of pancuronium in patients with normal and impaired renal function. Br J Anaesth 48:341, 1976
44. Miller RD, Matteo RS, Benet LZ, et al: The pharmacokinetics of *d*-tubocurarine in man with and without renal failure. J Pharmacol Exp Ther 202:1, 1977
45. Fahey MR, Morris RB, Miller RD, et al: Pharmacokinetics of ORG NC45 (Norcuron) in patients with and without renal failure. Br J Anaesth 53:1049, 1981
46. Fahey MR, Rupp SM, Fisher DM, et al: The pharmacokinetics and pharmacodynamics of atracurium in patients with and without renal failure. Anesthesiology 61:699, 1984
47. Caldwell JE: Muscle relaxants and renal failure. Problems in Anesthesia 489, 1989
48. Walker JS, Shanks CA, Brown KF: Determinants of *d*-tubocurarine plasma protein binding in health and disease. Anesth Analg 62: 870, 1983
49. Lebrault C, Berger JL, D'Hollander A, et al: Pharmacokinetics and pharmacodynamics of vecuronium (ORG NC 45) in patients with cirrhosis. Anesthesiology 62:601, 1985
50. Ramzan IM, Shanks CA, Triggs EJ: Pharmacokinetics and pharmacodynamics of gallamine triethiodide in patients with total biliary obstruction. Anesth Analg 60:289, 1981
51. Somogyi AA, Shanks CA, Triggs EJ: Disposition kinetics of pancuronium bromide in patients with total biliary obstruction. Br J Anaesth 49:1103, 1977
52. Lebrault C, Strumza P, Henzel D, et al: Pharmacokinetics and pharmacodynamics of vecuronium in patients with cholestasis (abstract). Anesthesiology 63:A314, 1985
53. Ward S, Judge S. Corall I: Pharmacokinetics of pancuronium bromide in liver failure. Br J Anaesth 54:277, 1982
54. Ward S, Neill EAM: Pharmacokinetics of atracurium in acute hepatic failure (with acute renal failure). Br J Anaesth 55: 1169, 1983
55. Duvaldestin P, Lebrault C, Chauvin M: Pharmacokinetics of muscle relaxants in patients with liver disease. Clin Anaesthesiol 3:293, 1985
56. Miller RD, Agoston S, van der Pol F, et al: Hypothermia and the pharmacokinetics and pharmacodynamics of pancuronium in the cat. J Pharmacol Exp Ther 207:532, 1978
57. Ham J, Stanski DR, Newfield P, et al: Pharmacokinetics and dynamics of *d*-tubocurarine during hypothermia in humans. Anesthesiology 55:631, 1981
58. Flynn PJ, Hughes R, Walton B: Use of atracurium in cardiac surgery involving cardiopulmonary bypass with induced hypothermia. Br J Anaesth 56:967, 1984
59. Goudsouzian NG: Relaxants in paediatric anaesthesia. Clin Anaesthesiol 3:539, 1985
60. McLeod K, Hull CJ, Watson MJ: Effects of ageing on the pharmacokinetics of pancuronium. Br J Anaesth 51:435, 1979
61. Duvaldestin P, Saada J, Berger JL, et al: Pharmacokinetics, pharmacodynamics and dose-response relationships of pancuronium in control and elderly subjects. Anesthesiology 56: 36, 1982
62. Martyn JAJ, Szyfelbein SK, Ali HH, et al: Increased *d*-tubocurarine requirement following major thermal injury. Anesthesiology 52:352, 1980
63. Martyn JAJ, Matteo RS, Szyfelbein SK, et al: Unprecedented resistance to neuromuscular blocking effects of metocurine with persistence after complete recovery in a burned patient. Anesth Analg 61:614, 1982
64. Martyn JAJ, Liu LMP, Szyfelbein SK, et al: The neuromuscular effects of pancuronium in burned children. Anesthesiology 56:561, 1983
65. Satwicz PR, Martyn JAJ, Szyfelbein SK, et al: Potentiation of neuromuscular blockade using a combination of pancuronium and dimethyltubocurarine: studies in children following acute burn injury or during reconstructive surgery. Br J Anaesth 56:479, 1984
66. Mills A, Martyn JAJ, Szyfelbein SK: Evaluation of atracurium neuromuscular blockage in patients with thermal injury (abstract). Anesthesiology 63:A339, 1985
67. Leibel WS, Martyn JAJ, Szyfelbein SK, et al: Elevated plasma binding cannot account for the burn-related *d*-tubocurarine hyposensitivity. Anesthesiology 54:378, 1981
68. Silverberg PA, Matteo RS, Diaz J: Decreased sensitivity to *d*-tubocurarine in patients with upper motor neuron disease (abstract). Anesthesiology 63:A343, 1985
69. Ali HH: Monitoring of neuromuscular function and clinical interaction. Clin Anaesthesiol 3:447, 1985
70. Miller J, Lee C: Muscle diseases. In Katz J, Benumof J, Kadis LB (eds): Anesthesia and uncommon diseases, 2nd ed. Philadelphia: WB Saunders, 1981: 530
71. Stanski DR, Ham J, Miller RD, et al: Pharmacokinetics and pharmacodynamics of *d*-tubocurarine during nitrous oxide–narcotic and halothane anesthesia in man. Anesthesiology 51: 235, 1979
72. Stanski DR, Ham J, Miller RD, et al: Time-dependent increase in sensitivity to *d*-tubocurarine during enflurane anesthesia in man. Anesthesiology 52:483, 1980
73. Sokoll MD, Gergis SD: Antibiotics and neuromuscular function. Anesthesiology 55:148, 1981
74. Bartkowski RB: Incomplete reversal of pancuronium neuromuscular blockade by neostigmine, pyridostigmine, and edrophonium. Anesth Analg 66:594, 1987
75. Miller RD, Larson CP Jr, Way WL: Comparative antagonism of *d*-tubocurarine, gallamine, and pancuronium induced neuromuscular blockades by neostigmine. Anesthesiology 37:503, 1972
76. Katz RL: Neuromuscular effect of *d*-tubocurarine, edrophonium and neostigmine in man. Anesthesiology 38: 327, 1967
77. Pittinger CB, Eryasa Y, Adamson R: Antibiotic induced paralysis. Anesth Analg 49:487, 1970
78. Miller RD: Antagonism of neuromuscular blockade. Anesthesiology 44:293, 1976
79. Delisle S, Bevan DR: Impaired neostigmine antagonism of pancuronium during enflurane anaesthesia in man. Br J Anaesth 54:441, 1982
80. Miller RD, Van Nyhuis LS, Eger EI, et al: The effect of acid–base balance on neostigmine antagonism of *d*-tubocurarine–induced neuromuscular blockade. Anesthesiology 42:377, 1975
81. Feldman SA: Effect of changes in electrolytes, hydration and pH upon the reactions to muscle relaxants. Br J Anaesth 35: 546, 1963
82. Ghoneim MM, Long JP: The interaction between magnesium and other neuromuscular blocking agents. Anesthesiology 32: 13, 1970
83. Miller RD, Roderick L: Diuretic induced hypokalemia, pan-

curonium neuromuscular blockade, and its antagonism by neostigmine. Br J Anaesth 50:541, 1978
84. Miller RD, Van Nyhuis LS, Eger EI: The effect of temperature on a *d*-tubocurarine neuromuscular blockade and its antagonism by neostigmine. J Pharmacol Exp Ther 195:237, 1975
85. Cronnelly R, Morris RB: Antagonism of neuromuscular blockade. Br J Anaesth 54:183, 1982
86. Bell CM, Leura CB: Effects of neostigmine on integrity of ileorectal anastomoses. Br Med J 3:587, 1968
87. Wilkins JL, Hardcastle JD, Mann CV, et al: Effects of neostigmine and atropine on motor activity of ileum, colon, and rectum of anaesthetized subjects. Br Med J 1:793, 1970
88. Coter TW Jr, Ray JE, Gathright JB Jr: Does neostigmine cause disruption of large intestinal anastomoses? A negative answer. Dis Colon Rectum 17:235, 1974
89. Jenkins IR: Three cases of apparent recurarization. Br J Anaesth 33:314, 1961
90. Hershey WN, Wahrenbrock EA, DeJong RH: Residual curarization. Anesthesiology 26:834, 1965
91. Miller RD, Cullen DJ: Renal failure and postoperative respiratory failure: recurarization? Br J Anaesth 48:253, 1976
92. Lee C, Mok MS, Barnes A, et al: Absence of 'recurarization' in patients with demonstrated prolonged neuromuscular block. Br J Anaesth 49:485, 1977
93. Fisher DM: Should succinylcholine continue to be used routinely in pediatric anesthesia? Problems in Anesthesia 3:394, 1989
94. Anectine® (succinylcholine chloride) injection, USP Anectine® (succinylcholine chloride) sterile powder Flo-Pack® (package insert). Research Triangle Park, NC: Burroughs Wellcome, 1995
95. Morell RC, Berman JM, Royster RI, et al: Revised label regarding use of succinylcholine in children and adolescents: I (letter). Anesthesiology 80:242, 1994
96. Badgwell JM, Hall SC, Lockhart C: Revised label regarding use of succinylcholine in children and adolescents: II (letter). Anesthesiology 80:243, 1994
97. Bourne JB, Collier HOJ, Somers GF: Succinylcholine: muscle relaxant of short action. Lancet 1:1225, 1952
98. Churchill-Davidson HC: Suxamethonium (succinylcholine) chloride and muscle pains. Br Med J 1:74, 1954
99. Burtles R: Muscle pains after suxamethonium and suxethonium. Br J Anaesth 33:147, 1961
100. Newman PTF, Loudno JM: Muscle pain following administration of suxamethonium: the etiological role of muscular fitness. Br J Anaesth 38:533, 1966
101. Foster CA: Muscle pains that follow administration of suxamethonium. Br Med J 2:24, 1960
102. Larmoreaux LF, Urbach KF: Incidence and prevention of muscle pain following the administration of succinylcholine. Anesthesiology 21:394, 1960
103. Melnick B, Chalasani, Lim Uy NT, et al: Decreasing post-succinylcholine myalgia in outpatients. Can J Anaesth 34: 238, 1987
104. White DC: Observations on the prevention of muscle pain after suxamethonium. Br J Anaesth 34:332, 1962
105. Horrow JC, Lambert DH: The search for an optimal interval between pretreatment dose of *d*-tubocurarine and succinylcholine. Can Anaesth Soc J 31:528, 1984
106. Sosis M, Broad T, Larijani GE, et al: Comparison of atracurium and *d*-tubocurarine for prevention of succinylcholine myalgia. Anesth Analg 66:657, 1987
107. Cullen DJ: The effect of pretreatment with nondepolarizing muscle relaxants on the neuromuscular blocking action of succinylcholine. Anesthesiology 35:572, 1971
108. Miller RD, Way WL: The interaction between succinylcholine and subparalyzing doses of *d*-tubocurarine and gallamine in man. Anesthesiology 35:567, 1971
109. Brodsky JB, Brock-Utne JG, Samuels SI: Pancuronium pretreatment and post-succinylcholine myalgias. Anesthesiology 51:259, 1979
110. Haldia KN, Chatterji S, Kackar SN: Intravenous lignocaine for prevention of muscle pain after succinylcholine. Anesth Analg 52:849, 1973
111. Verma RS, Chatterji S, Mathur N: Diazepam and succinylcholine induced muscle pains. Anesth Analg 57:295, 1978
112. Fahmy RN, Malek NS, Lappas DG: Diazepam prevents some adverse effects of succinylcholine. Clin Pharmacol Ther 26: 395, 1979
113. Collier CB: Dantrolene and suxamethonium. The effect of preoperative dantrolene on the action of suxamethonium. Anaesthesia 34:152, 1979
114. Manani G, Valenti S, Segatto A, et al: The influence of thiopentone and alfathesin on succinylcholine induced fasciculations and myalgias. Can Anaesth Soc J 28:253, 1981
115. Lindgren L. Saarnivaara L: Effect of competitive myoneural blockade and fentanyl on muscle fasciculations caused by suxamethonium in children. Br J Anaesth 55:747, 1983
116. Shrivastava OP, Chatterji S, Kachhawa S, et al: Calcium gluconate pretreatment for prevention of succinylcholine induced myalgia. Anesth Analg 62:59, 1983
117. Magee DA, Robinson RJS: Effect of stretch exercises on suxamethonium induced fasciculations and myalgia. Br J Anaesth 59:596, 1987
118. Lincoff HA, Ellis CH, DeVoe AG, et al: The effect of succinylcholine on intraocular pressure. Am J Ophthalmol 40:501, 1955
119. Dillon JB, Sabawala P, Taylor DB, et al: Action of succinylcholine on extraocular muscles and intraocular pressure. Anesthesiology 18:44, 1957
120. Lincoff HA, Breinen GM, DeVoe AG: The effect of succinylcholine on the extraocular muscles. Am J Ophthalmol 43:44, 1957
121. Miller RD, Way WL, Hickey RF: Inhibition of succinylcholine-induced increased intraocular pressure by nondepolarizing muscle relaxants. Anesthesiology 29:123, 1968
122. Meyers EF, Krupin T, Johnson M, et al: Failure of nondepolarizing neuromuscular blockers to inhibit succinylcholine-induced increased intraocular pressure: a controlled study. Anesthesiology 48:149, 1978
123. Libonati MM, Leahy JJ, Ellison NE: The use of succinylcholine in open eye surgery. Anesthesiology 62:637, 1985
124. Marchand P: The gastro-oesophageal 'sphincter' and the mechanism of regurgitation. Br J Surg 42:504, 1955
125. Anderson N: changes in intragastric pressure following the administration of suxamethonium: preliminary report. Br J Anaesth 34:363, 1962
126. Roe RB: The effect of suxamethonium on intragastric pressure. Anaesthesia 17:179, 1962
127. Miller RD, Way WL: Inhibition of succinylcholine induced increased intragastric pressure by nondepolarizing muscle relaxants and lidocaine. Anesthesiology 34:185, 1971
128. Muravchick S, Burkett L, Gold MI: Succinylcholine-induced fasciculations and intragastric pressure during induction of anesthesia. Anesthesiology 55:180, 1981
129. Salem MR, Wong AY, Li YH: The effect of suxamethonium on the intragastric pressure in infants and children. Br J Anaesth 44:166, 1972
130. Clark GG, Riddock ME: Observations on the human cardia at operation. Br J Anaesth 34:875, 1962
131. Sellick BA: Cricoid pressure to control regurgitation of stomach contents during induction of anesthesia. Lancet 2:402, 1961
132. Cotton BR, Smith G: The lower oesophageal sphincter and anaesthesia. Br J Anaesth 56:38, 1984
133. Cottrell JE, Hartung J, Griffin JP, et al: Intracranial and hemodynamic changes after succinylcholine administration in cats. Anesth Analg 62:1006, 1983
134. Marsh ML, Dunlap BJ, Shapiro HM, et al: Succinylcholine: intracranial pressure effects in neurological patients. Anesth Analg 59:550, 1980
135. Minton MD, Grosslight K, Stirt JA, et al: Increases in intracranial pressure from succinylcholine: prevention by prior nondepolarizing blockade. Anesthesiology 65:165, 1986

136. Gronert GA, Theye RA: Pathophysiology of hyperkalemia induced by succinylcholine. Anesthesiology 43:89, 1975
137. Tobey RE, Jacobsen PM, Kahle CT, et al: The serum potassium response to muscle relaxants in neural injury. Anesthesiology 37:332, 1972
138. Cooperman LH: Succinylcholine induced hyperkalemia in neuromuscular disease. JAMA 213:1867, 1970
139. Steizner J, Eberlin HJ, Schumucker I, et al: Anaesthesia–induced cardiac arrest in two infants with unsuspected muscular dystrophy. Anaesthesist 42:44, 1993
140. Henderson WA: Succinylcholine induced cardiac arrest in unsuspected Duchenne muscular dystrophy. Can Anaesth Soc J 31:444, 1984
141. Warner MA, Wedel DJ: Prevalence of undiagnosed Duchenne's muscular dystrophy. Anesth Analg 80:S540, 1995
142. Birch AA, Mitchell GD, Playford GA, et al: Changes in serum potassium response to succinylcholine following trauma. JAMA 210:490, 1969
143. Mazze RI, Escue HM, Houston JB: Hyperkalemia and cardiovascular collapse following administration of succinylcholine to the traumatized patient. Anesthesiology 31:540, 1969
144. Cairoli VJ, Ivankovich AD, Vucicevic D, et al: Succinylcholine induced hyperkalemia in the rat following radiation injury to muscle. Anesth Analg 61:83, 1982
145. Schaner PJ, Brown RL, Kirksey ED, et al: Succinylcholine induced hyperkalemia in burned patients. Anesth Analg 48: 764, 1969
146. Kihlschuetter B, Baur H, Roth F: Suxamethonium induced hyperkalemia in patients with severe intra-abdominal infections. Br J Anaesth 48:557, 1976
147. Khan TZ, Khan RM: Changes in serum potassium following succinylcholine in patients with infections. Anesth Analg 62: 327, 1983
148. Roth F, Wuthrich H: The clinical importance of hyperkalemia following suxamethonium administration. Br J Anaesth 41: 311, 1969
149. Powell JN: Suxamethonium induced hyperkalemia in a uremic patient. Br J Anaesth 42:806, 1970
150. Miller RD, Way WL, Hamilton WK, et al: Succinylcholine-induced hyperkalemia in patients with renal failure? Anesthesiology 36:138, 1972
151. Koide M, Waud BE: Serum potassium concentrations after succinylcholine in patients with renal failure. Anesthesiology 36:142, 1972
152. Ryan JF, Kagen LJ, Hyman AJ: Myoglobinemia after a single dose of succinylcholine. N Engl J Med 285:824, 1971
153. Harrington JF, Ford DJ: Myoglobinemia after succinylcholine in children undergoing isoflurane anesthesia. Anesthesiology 65:S69, 1986
154. Blanc VF, Vaillancourt GV, Brisson G: Succinylcholine, fasciculations and myoglobinemia. Can Anaesth Soc J 33:178, 1986
155. Schaer H, Steinmann B, Jerusalem S, et al: Rhabdomyolysis induced by anaesthesia with intra-operative cardiac arrests. Br J Anaesth 49:495, 1977
156. Hool GJ, Lawrence PJ, Sivaneswaram N: Acute rhabdomyolytic renal failure due to suxamethonium. Anaesth Intensive Care 6:141, 1978
157. Cody JR: Muscle rigidity following administration of succinylcholine. Anesthesiology 29:159, 1968
158. Thiel RE: The myotonic response to suxamethonium. Br J Anaesth 39:815, 1967
159. Haley FC: Anesthesia in dystrophic myotonia. Can Anaesth Soc J 9:270, 1962
160. Talmage EA, McKechnie RB: Anesthetic management of a patient with myotonia dystrophica. Anesthesiology 20:717, 1959
161. Azar I: The response of patients with neuromuscular disorders to muscle relaxants: a review. Anesthesiology 61:173, 1984
162. Ellis FR, Halsall PJ: Suxamethonium spasm: a differential diagnostic conundrum. Br J Anaesth 56:381, 1984
163. Larach MG, Rosenberg H, Larach DR, et al: Prediction of malignant hyperthermia susceptibility by clinical signs. Anesthesiology 66:547, 1987
164. Leary NP, Ellis FR: Masseteric muscle spasm as a normal response to suxamethonium. Br J Anaesth 64:488, 1990
165. Leith MD, McCoy DD, Belton MK, et al: Bradycardia following intravenous administration of succinylcholine chloride to infants and children. Anesthesiology 18:698, 1957
166. Stoelting RK, Peterson C: Heart rate slowing and junctional rhythm following intravenous succinylcholine with and without intramuscular atropine preanesthetic medication. Anesth Analg 54:705, 1975
167. Stoelting RK: Comparison of gallamine and atropine as pretreatment before anesthetic induction and succinylcholine administration. Anesth Analg 56:493, 1977
168. Yasudo I, Hirano T, Amaha K, et al: Chlorotropic effects of succinylcholine and succinylmonocholine on the sinoatrial node. Anesthesiology 57:289, 1982
169. Greenfeld AL, Rosenberg H: Succinylcholine infusion may cause asystole. Anesthesiology 52:378, 1980
170. Magee DA, Sweet PT, Holland AJC: Effect of atropine on bradydysrhythmias induced by succinylcholine following pretreatment with *d*-tubocurarine. Can Anaesth Soc J 29:573, 1982
171. Smith NL: Histamine release by suxamethonium. Anaesthesia 12:293, 1957
172. Katz AM, Mulligan PG: Bronchospasm induced by suxamethonium. Br J Anaesth 44:1097, 1972
173. Lubin AH, Garry PG, Owen GM: Sex and population difference in the incidence of a plasma cholinesterase variant. Science 173:161, 1971
174. Viby-Mogensen J, Hand HK: Prolonged apnea after suxamethonium. Acta Anaesthesiol Scand 22:371, 1977
175. Robertson GS: Serum cholinesterase deficiency: II. pregnancy. Br J Anaesth 38:361, 1966
176. Hazel B, Monier D: Human serum cholinesterase: variations during pregnancy and postpartum. Can Anaesth Soc J 18: 272, 1971
177. Foldes FF, Rendell-Baker L, Birch JH: Causes and prevention of prolonged apnea with succinylcholine. Anesth Analg 35: 609, 1956
178. Foldes FF, Molloy FE, Zsigmond EK, et al: Hexafluorenium: its anticholinesterase and neuromuscular activity. J Pharmacol Exp Ther 129:400, 1960
179. Pantuck EJ, Pantuck CB: Cholinesterases and anticholinesterases. In Katz RL (ed): Muscle relaxants. Amsterdam: Excerpta Medica, 1975: 143
180. Kopman AF, Strachovsky G, Lichtenstein L: Prolonged response to succinylcholine following physostigmine. Anesthesiology 49:142, 1978
181. Bentz EW, Stoelting RK: Prolonged response to succinylcholine following pancuronium reversed with pyridostigmine. Anesthesiology 44:258, 1976
182. Stovner J, Oftendel N, Holmboe J: The inhibition of cholinesterases by pancuronium. Br J Anaesth 47:949, 1975
183. Evans RT, MacDonald R, Robinson A: Suxamethonium apnoea associated with plasmapheresis. Anaesthesia 35:198, 1980
184. Viby-Mogensen J: Correlation of succinylcholine duration of action with plasma cholinesterase activity in subjects with the genotypically normal enzyme. Anesthesiology 53:517, 1980
185. Katz RL, Ryan JF: The neuromuscular effects of suxamethonium in man. Br J Anaesth 41:381, 1969
186. Churchill-Davidson HC, Katz RL: Dual, phase II or desensitization block? Anesthesiology 27:53, 1968
187. Lee C: Dose relationships of phase II, tachyphylaxis and train-of-four fade in suxamethonium induced block in man. Br J Anaesth 47:841, 1975
188. Durant NN, Katz RL: Suxamethonium. Br J Anaesth 54:195, 1982
189. Morris R, Giesecke AH Jr: Potentiation of muscle relaxants by magnesium sulfate therapy in toxemia of pregnancy. South Med J 61:25, 1968

Complications in Anesthesiology, second edition, edited by Nikolaus Gravenstein and Robert R. Kirby. Lippincott-Raven Publishers, Philadelphia © 1996.

CHAPTER 49

Teratogenicity

Bradley E. Smith

Allegations of the toxic potential of surgical anesthesia to the human reproductive process began even before the thalidomide disaster.[1,2] These concerns are clinically important, because 2% of all pregnant women may receive an anesthetic for surgery during pregnancy.[3] About 29% of young women presenting for elective surgery possibly are pregnant, and 5% may not inform the anesthesiologist of possible pregnancy.[4]

Sterility, abortion, stillbirth, premature delivery, perinatal mortality, congenital abnormalities, and postnatal functional defects have been alleged to occur more frequently than normal after surgical anesthesia.[5,6] In addition, chronic inhalation of anesthetics in the operating room has been said to result in similar human reproductive malfunction.[7,8] Therefore, anesthesiologists should be familiar with the basic principles of reproductive toxicology.

TERATOLOGY

Teratology is the science of the causes, mechanisms, and manifestations of structural or functional developmental deviations.[9] About 200,000 infants with birth defects are born in the United States each year. These defects may be associated with 17% of fetal deaths and 29% of neonatal deaths.[10] However, only about 3% of birth defects are attributed to drugs or chemicals,[11] and an exact cause can be determined in less than half of cases.[12]

Research in this area probably is more difficult than in any other area of human biology because of a multitude of epidemiologic and biologic variables. For example, even the "normal" incidence of human reproductive malfunction is not generally agreed on, leading to misconceptions when abortion or congenital anomaly data are reported after exposure to drugs. In fact, normal human abortion rates may be as great as 11%, and the congenital anomaly rate may be 7.4%.[10]

Teratogens in Humans

Known

Consider that the characteristic congenital abnormality caused by thalidomide, shortened limbs (phocomelia), occurs naturally only once in 100,000 births. Even though thalidomide increased this incidence more than 50,000-fold, 5 years passed and more than 10,000 phocomelic babies were born before the problem was identified.[13,14] More than a quarter century later, the list of drugs shown conclusively to be teratogenic in humans is still very short (Table 49-1).[14–17]

Alleged

Other substances alleged to be teratogenic in humans, such as lithium carbonate, kanamycin, and streptomycin, are not accepted as such by all authorities.[18] Tetracycline, which certainly causes mottling of teeth in children who were exposed to it in utero, is defined as *embryotoxic* rather than *teratogenic*.[19] Even in the few cases where adequate human epidemiologic data can exonerate a substance (eg, Bendectin), the public and even the courts sometimes seem unable to grasp the intricacies of the scientific process, to their own ultimate disservice.[20] Bendectin was removed from the marketplace in 1983.

Teratogens in Animals

In contrast to the very short list of substances proven to be teratogenic in humans is the seemingly endless list of proven teratogens in animals. Anesthetics are not exceptions. Nearly every inhalation anesthetic now available has been alleged to be teratogenic to some species in specific conditions. However, as in other fields, a great deal of research in the teratogenicity of anesthetic drugs can be criticized for its methods or conclusions.

TABLE 49-1
Teratogens in Humans

KNOWN
Thalidomide
Hydantoins
Isoretinoin
Alcohol
Androgens (some)
Progestins (some)
Folic acid antagonists
Methotrexate
Cyclophosphamide
Diethylstilbestrol
Dihydrostreptomycin
Quinine
Radioactive iodine
Valproic acid
Coumarin
POSSIBLE
Lithium carbonate
Kanamycin
Streptomycin
Tetracycline

Problems of Study

United States Food and Drug Administration guidelines require separate teratologic studies in at least two species. The Food and Drug Administration assumes that animal testing is of value in making decisions concerning the relative dangers to humans of potential teratogens. However, several difficulties exist in the extrapolation of animal teratogenicity data to humans (Table 49-2).[21]

In 1985, the Food and Drug Administration listed 38 compounds as "suspicious" potential teratogens in humans. More than 80% of these compounds were associated with teratogenicity in multiple species. A positive response was exhibited 85% of the time in the mouse, 80% in the rat, 60% in the rabbit, and most surprising, only 30% in the monkey. However, of the 165 compounds that the Food and Drug Administration believes probably are not teratogenic in humans, 41% exhibited false-positive teratogenicity in more than one animal species.[21]

Variability of Response

The apparent variability in response to teratogenic agents among animal species is caused by several factors. The terms teratogenicity, embryotoxicity, fetotoxicity, malformations, and deviations have been used to describe similar fetal drug effects. Classic defects such as hydrocephalus, micrognathia, and anophthalmia are easily agreed to be teratogenic ("terata" from Greek for "monster"). Some have sought to attach the term embryotoxicity instead of teratogenicity to a wide variety of less notable defects, including supernumerary ribs, enlarged renal pelves, reduced fetal weight, edema, or death. Regardless of semantics, these induced defects represent important toxicity in the fetus. Currently, these distinctions have been found impossible to defend scientifically. That any given observed morphologic derangement is not detrimental to postnatal life or function is impossible to prove unless function has been tested.[8,22]

Morphologic Changes Versus Changes in Function

An example of the importance of this distinction is pertinent. One study revealed an increased incidence of enlarged renal pelves after exposure of mice to isoflurane.[23] The authors concluded that the defect was (morphologically) reversible and therefore of no teratogenic significance. However, they did not examine kidney function of the offspring.[23]

An analogy can be made with the insecticide nitrofen. The routine observance of enlarged renal pelves after exposure to nitrofen revealed that most exposed pups, including those appearing morphologically normal, display diminished renal function.[24] This defect would have been dismissed as "not teratogenic" had it been assumed to have been a reversible, induced effect without testing of renal function.[24]

Similarly, behavioral teratology is extremely pertinent to anesthesiology. Permanent behavioral defects may be induced by diazepam[25] and some anesthetics[26] at dosages that frequently produce only minor or reversible morphologic deviations in tested offspring or no *dysmorphogenesis* at all. Therefore, the inadequacy of classic morphologic test procedures to exclude teratogenicity is clear.

Dose-related Factors

Teratogenic effects of drugs are almost always dose-related. They almost always exhibit a threshold exposure dose below which no teratogenic effects are found, despite chronic exposure to subthreshold doses, and they rarely exhibit stochastic phenomena or phenomena not related to dose.[27] Most teratogenic drugs are embryocidal at some dose. Usually, the dose necessary for a *litter* LD_{50} is much less than half the maternal LD_{50}. The dose range that produces the greatest number of anomalous fetal survivors is usually in the litter LD_{50} range. Most often no observable toxic effects are present in embryos at one half or less of the litter LD_{50}. Research in which the exposure exceeds or does not approach this range may give a totally erroneous impression of the danger or safety of the test substance.[28]

Some potential teratogens administered to the mother may accumulate to very high concentrations in the fetus because of fetal inability to degrade and excrete some drugs. For example, fetal hepatic glucuronyltransferase has very low activity, resulting in difficulty with conjugation and excretion of bilirubin, sulfobromophthalein, lidocaine, mepivacaine, and

TABLE 49-2
Problems in Determining Teratogenicity

Response variability
Morphologic changes vs changes in function
Dose-related factors
Stage of gestation
Species variability

meprobamate. Fetal liver microsomal enzymes also degrade some drugs slowly, and renal clearance of some (eg, penicillin) is markedly depressed. Thus, similar defects might lead to disproportionately high blood concentrations of teratogens in the fetus and could also prolong the exposure of the fetus, heightening the teratogenic effects.[6,28]

Stage of Development

Maternal exposure to teratogens at one stage of gestation can result in anomalies totally different from those produced at other stages. For example, embryonic mice risk little danger of teratogenicity after repeated exposure to methoxyflurane on days 6 through 11. However, similar exposure on days 12 and 13 results in a high incidence of congenital anomalies.[6] Without a systematic search at all stages of development, this prominent effect would have been overlooked. However, several reports of supposedly negative results on tests for anesthetic teratogenicity have examined only one or two stages of gestation.

Species Differences

Susceptibility to a teratogen varies with genetic susceptibility not only between species, but even among different strains. For example, cortisone, which causes cleft palate in 100% of A-Jax mice, leads to this anomaly with the same drug dose in only 12% of C57BL mice.[29] Other differences in species responses may be caused by diversity in drug uptake and distribution or detoxification pathways. In one strain of mice, 5-fluorouracil is destroyed by hepatic enzymes, thereby affording protection against the teratogenicity demonstrated in another strain lacking this enzyme system.[28]

MECHANISMS

Direct

Numerous factors may contribute to teratogenicity (Table 49-3).

TABLE 49-3
Potential Mechanisms of Teratogenicity

DIRECT
Genetic damage
Energy substrate interference
Antimitosis
INDIRECT: MATERNAL TOXICITY
Hypoxemia
Hypercapnia
Impaired uterine blood flow
Hyperoxia (possible)

Genetic Damage

Many potent teratogens, including several cancer chemotherapeutic agents, have the ability to damage deoxyribonucleic acid (DNA) or messenger ribonucleic acid (RNA). For example, the antibiotic actinomycin D forms a stable complex with DNA, thereby preventing the formation of messenger RNA and ultimately leading to complete breakdown of cellular protein synthesis.[30] Although several anesthetics depress formation of DNA and RNA,[31] the common anesthetics probably are not mutagenic at clinically relevant concentrations.[32–36]

Energy Substrate Interference

Teratogens can cause disruption of development by interference with an essential metabolic pathway. General energy requirements and use of specific substrates increase abruptly in specific organs as they enter their period of rapid development. During this phase an organ is more susceptible to shortages of energy or specific substrates that might be caused by inhibition or competition from a teratogen. This deficit may lead to deformity of the rapidly developing organ, although the fetus survives.[37]

Antimycin, a cytochrome C antagonist, causes widespread death of myoblasts in the chick embryo when administered at a specific time in development. However, if it is administered earlier or later, no effect is seen. Therefore, one can assume that the myoblasts have a high requirement for the substrate acted on by cytochrome C (succinate) or have a deficiency of cytochrome C relative to metabolic needs at that time.[37]

Of interest in this regard is the depression of electron transfer and oxidative phosphorylation caused by inhalation anesthetics.[38] This mechanism of organ damage and cell death is similar to the induction of anomalies in chick embryos by exposure to diethyl ether. When examined 24 hours after exposure, the eye cells appear to have died and are necrotic. The rest of the embryo, however, continues to develop normally.[39]

Antimitosis

Antimitotic effects of drugs (eg, colchicine) are shared by the inhalation anesthetics and are discussed later.

Indirect: Maternal Toxicity

Maternal toxicity may lead to embryonic or fetal damage. Hypoxemia, hypercapnia, and impaired uterine blood flow caused by complications of anesthesia are of concern in this regard. Although hypoxemia and hypercapnia are incontrovertibly teratogenic, their danger possibly was exaggerated in the past.[40] Protective mechanisms are used effectively by the mammalian embryo during a variety of maternal stresses including hypoxemia and hypercapnia. Human fetuses, for example, appear surprisingly often to survive maternal cyanotic heart disease and prolonged artificial circulation during cardiac surgery.[6] However, endogenous and exogenous catecholamines cause a marked decrease in uterine blood flow and have teratogenic effects in mammals.[40] In the human, teratogenicity from prolonged exposure to hyperoxia, such as may also be encountered during anesthesia, has not been demonstrated, but exposure to high oxygen partial pressure in other species can be teratogenic.[41]

HUMAN REPRODUCTIVE OUTCOME AFTER SURGICAL ANESTHESIA

Anesthetic Agents

From a study population of 18,248 pregnant women, I described the reproductive outcome of 67 women who underwent surgery with general or major regional anesthesia (but not infiltration of local anesthesia) for procedures other than obstetric delivery. An overall 15% perinatal mortality was noted, but no congenital anomalies occurred.[2]

Another study of 9073 births reported 147 in which the mother had surgical anesthesia during pregnancy, including local anesthesia. The incidence of congenital birth defects in babies of operated women was 9.3% compared with 6% in the control group; perinatal mortality rate was 7.5% versus 2.1% in the control group. However, the investigators identified a 33.3% perinatal mortality in a subset of 18 women having cerclage procedures.[5]

The same report cited sketchy statistics from 60,912 women gathered by the Obstetrical Statistical Cooperative. The incidence of birth defects was 5% and perinatal mortality was 2% in nonsurgical pregnancy compared with 6% birth defects and 3.3% perinatal mortality in 50 pregnant women who underwent appendectomy.[5]

Still another study reviewed the reproductive outcomes among dental personnel: birth and other health data from 12,929 pregnancies were reported, but the types of anesthesia were unknown.[42] Spontaneous abortions occurred in 7.9% of pregnant women who experienced surgery and who had no occupational exposure to anesthesia versus 6.4% in 8210 controls. The congenital anomaly rate was 3.9% after surgery compared to 4.5% in controls.[37]

In a series of 77 pregnant women receiving surgical anesthesia with thiopental, cyclopropane, ether, and ethylene (but not local anesthesia),[43] the incidence of congenital malformations was 5.2%. This rate is not significantly different from the overall rate of human anomalies, 7.4%, noted by that investigator in a prospective study of 10,259 pregnancies.[10] Another study examined the possible influence of a 30-minute exposure to nitrous oxide given to 175 women having cervical cerclage and noted an incidence of congenital anomalies similar to that in the local population not undergoing an operation (6%).[44]

In 1989 Mazze and Källén reported no increase in congenital malformations or stillbirths in pregnant surgical patients.[45] However, in their registry series of 5405 the incidences of low- and very-low-birthweight infants and death within the first 168 hours of life were increased. The low-birthweight infants were the consequence of both prematurity and intrauterine growth retardation. Mazze and Källén concluded that no specific type of anesthesia or surgical procedure was associated with an increased incidence of adverse reproductive outcome (ie, congenital anomalies), but that low birth weight and death within the first week of life were more common.[45]

Subsequently Källén and Mazze reported in 1990 that there was an increased risk of neural tube defects among the offspring of women who underwent surgery during the first trimester of pregnancy. They observed six such cases where the expected number was only 2.5.[46] Sylvester and colleagues report a related observation from a series of 694 mothers of infants with central nervous system defects studied in Atlanta, Georgia.[47] In that study, 12 of 694 cases of central nervous system defects reported first-trimester anesthesia exposure, compared with 34 of 2984 control mothers, for an odds ratio of 1.7. In particular, a striking association was noted between first trimester anesthesia exposure and hydrocephalus with another major defect (odds ratio 9.6), especially eye defects (odds ratio 39.6) and specifically cataracts.[47] No association with single defects was noted. Thus, the question of possible teratogenicity of general anesthesia exposure continues to merit and receive attention.

Stress of Surgery and Trauma

In a review of government health records in Manitoba, Duncan and associates[3] described the reproductive experience of pregnant women, who had surgery or nonsurgical trauma, and matched pairs of pregnant women with nontrauma, nonsurgical illnesses. They identified 2568 surgical procedures during pregnancy. The incidence of congenital anomalies after surgery was 1.7%, similar to 1.3% in the nonoperated group.

The spontaneous abortion rate was 7.1% after surgery, again similar to 6.5% in controls. Although the risk of abortion after general anesthesia was estimated as 1.58 times that among matched controls, even the matched controls for this general anesthesia group displayed a twofold increase in abortion compared with the local anesthesia control and a threefold increase over "nil anesthesia" control groups.

This observation suggests the possibility that the slightly increased risk of abortion attributed to general anesthesia may reflect only the stress effects of more serious trauma or surgical conditions. In general, procedures performed with local or no anesthesia are not as major as those requiring general anesthesia.[3]

Another illustration that maternal and fetal mortality rates are directly related to the severity of the surgical illness is found in a study of appendectomy in pregnancy.[48] Maternal mortality in simple appendicitis without perforation was almost nonexistent. However, it still was a problem when perforation of the appendix occurred. Fetal mortality, too, was almost nonexistent in operated cases of appendicitis without perforation but averaged 33% to 43% in cases of perforated appendicitis.[48]

In Vitro Fertilization

Anesthetics received by the mother during in vitro fertilization have not been shown to exert any toxic or inhibiting effect on fertilization or teratogenic effects in the subsequent pregnancy. A prospective, randomized study found similar success in achieving pregnancy and reproductive outcome with isoflurane, with and without nitrous oxide.[49] Nonetheless, the apparent increased incidence of spontaneous abortion (27% in one report)[49a] and of preterm births (threefold increase) and current knowledge of the antimitotic effects of anesthetics necessitate careful examination of all aspects of the procedure.

REPRODUCTIVE TOXICOLOGIC EFFECTS OF ANESTHETIC AGENTS

Anesthetic agents potentially can affect several factors critical to reproduction (Table 49-4).

Mitosis

Inhibition of mitosis and cell division is a universal effect of inhalation anesthetics but is reversible when the anesthetic is dissipated.[50] Halothane inhibits microtubule assembly or depolymerizes preassembled tubules in the developing aster formation. Therefore, halothane impairs both spindle and aster growth early in metaphase in both sea urchin and mammalian cell cultures. However, halothane has no effect on the cleavage process if applied later than metaphase, in which case cell division continues to completion. Halothane has no direct effect on the structure of microfilaments or the actomyosin-like interaction that develops the contractile force for cleavage. Instead it inhibits the process that initiates the formation and assembly of the contractile ring.[51] Whereas 1.25 mM halothane causes 96% abnormal cleavage in developing sea urchin eggs, no effect is associated with 2.5 mM enflurane nor with 1.25 mM methoxyflurane, suggesting that this process is not directly proportional to anesthetic potency.[52]

Cell cleavage may be defective when Chinese hamster cell cultures are exposed to 2% halothane. Nitrous oxide in 75% concentration has no effect in the same preparation but has a markedly synergistic effect with halothane.[50] Fentanyl, in clinically relevant concentrations, does not inhibit fertilization or early development of sea urchin eggs, but morphine has an adverse effect on in vitro fertilization in a similar model.[53]

Rodier and colleagues[54] exposed pregnant mice to 75% nitrous oxide, 0.5% (5000 ppm) halothane, or a mixture of 75% nitrogen and 25% oxygen for 6 hours on the 14th day of gestation or for 4 hours on the 2nd day after birth. Cellular studies of fetal cerebellar cortex made 12, 24, or 48 hours after exposure showed significant deviations from normal mitosis in all test groups; only the postnatally exposed nitrous oxide group showed characteristics of an antimitotic teratogen. Therefore, nitrous oxide did appear to be antimitotic to the late-forming cells of the cerebellar cortex in mice.[54]

Mutagenesis

Sturrock, using mammalian cell cultures, found no mutagenic effects with halothane, chloroform, or enflurane.[32,33] Baden and Simmon, using the Ames test (which uses *Escherichia coli* cultures), also reported no mutagenicity with halothane, enflurane, isoflurane, methoxyflurane, nitrous oxide, or cyclopropane. Mutagenicity resulted from exposure to fluroxene and divinyl ether, but results were equivocal with trichloroethylene.[34]

In fruit flies, exposures to enflurane, isoflurane, halothane, fluroxene, or nitrous oxide at various concentrations produced dose-dependent increases in the duration of metamorphosis and a decrease in the number of flies but no effects on development or morphologic features.[35] However, in another mutagenicity study using fruit flies, results were negative with nitrous oxide and halothane.[36]

TABLE 49-4
Possible Toxicologic Effects of Anesthetics

Inhibition of mitosis
Mutagenesis
Chromosomal damage
Changes in fertility
Changes in spermatogenesis

Chromosomal Damage

Chromosomal damage occurred in bone marrow and spermatogonial cells of rats chronically exposed to subanesthetic concentrations of halothane (1 ppm) and nitrous oxide (50 ppm).[55] No sister chromatid exchanges were noted after exposure of Chinese hamster ovarian cell cultures to anesthetizing concentrations of isoflurane, methoxyflurane, chloroform, diethyl ether, enflurane, halothane, nitrous oxide, or trichlorethylene. However, exchanges were observed after exposure to fluroxene, ethylvinyl ether, and divinyl ether.[56] Several concentrations of halothane administered to hamsters and mice did not have mutagenic effects in yet another study.[57]

An early study of human leukocyte cultures found no chromosomal damage after exposure to halothane in clinically significant concentrations.[58] More recent studies of human lymphocytes after patient exposure to halothane, enflurane, fluroxene, isoflurane, or nitrous oxide have failed to reveal any sister chromatid exchange.

Fertility

No studies in humans, even if retrospective, discuss fertility after anesthetic exposure. However, extensive data concerning chronic exposure of animals to various inhalation anesthetics exist. In one study, exposure of male and female adult rats to subanesthetic concentrations of halothane (10 ppm) or enflurane (20 ppm) for as long as 64 days before mating and subsequently throughout the entire pregnancy had no abortifacient or fertility effects. Some minor ossification disturbances, but no major teratologic effect or organ damage after chronic exposure were noted.[59]

Bruce reported no adverse effects on reproduction or fertility in three strains of mice exposed to 0.0016% (16 ppm) halothane for 7 hours per day, 5 days a week for 6 weeks before mating.[60] Exposure to enflurane at 0.01% (100 ppm), 0.1% (1000 ppm), 0.5% (5000 ppm), or 1.0% (10,000 ppm) for 4 hours per day, 7 days a week for 3 weeks before mating and throughout pregnancy resulted in no adverse effect on fertility.[61] Another study of mice exposed to 0.1% (1000 ppm) or 0.4% (4000 ppm) of isoflurane, 4 hours per day for 2 weeks before and during pregnancy, also found no adverse reproductive effects. Offspring delivered spontaneously displayed no differences from control animals in survival or weight gain.[62]

Exposure of male mice to 0.3% (3000 ppm) halothane 4 hours per day for 17 weeks had no effects on reproduction and copulation or the litters of untreated female mates.[63] Exposure of male and female mice to halothane 0.05% (500 ppm), 0.5 or 2 hours per day, or 0.1% (1000 ppm), 0.3% (3000 ppm), or 1.0% (10,000 ppm), 4 hours per day for 9 weeks before mating and throughout pregnancy, was studied. At 0.025 and 0.1 minimum alveolar concentration (MAC)-hour per day no observable effects were present, but at 0.4 MAC-hour some inhibition of maternal weight gain and fetal size occurred. At 1.2 MAC-hours the pregnancy rate decreased by one third, and implantation and litter size were depressed. At 1.0% halothane, 4 hours per day (4 MAC-hours), most males and females died before the end of the experiment.[63]

Male mice were exposed to 0.01% (100 ppm) or 0.1% (1000 ppm) enflurane 4 hours per day, 5 days a week for 11 weeks before mating with unexposed females. Fertility and reproductive indexes for the resulting matings were all normal.[61] Female mice were exposed to 0.01% (100 ppm), 0.1% (1000 ppm), or 0.5% (5000 ppm) enflurane, 4 hours per day, 7 days a week for 3 weeks before and throughout pregnancy. No effects on fertility or reproductive indexes, except some abnormalities of ossification and renal development at the highest concentration, were seen.[61]

Male mice inhaled 0.1% (1000 ppm) or 0.4% (4000 ppm) isoflurane, 4 hours per day 3 weeks before and during the mating period with no observable effects on reproduction.[62] Male and female mice were exposed to 0.1% (1000 ppm) or 0.4% (4000 ppm) isoflurane, 4 hours per day 2 weeks before mating and throughout pregnancy; a light anesthetic state was induced by 0.4% isoflurane. No adverse effects on fertility indexes, fetal weights, or growth of pups observed to 28 days postnatal age were found; however, no internal morphologic examinations were made.[62]

Spermatogenesis and Sperm

Halogenated Anesthetics

Male mice were exposed 4 hours per day to 0.1% (1000 ppm) or 0.4% (4000 ppm) isoflurane for 8 weeks before and during mating with unexposed females. No adverse reproductive effects were noted, either on mating performance or in the resulting pups.[62]

In a dose-dependent manner, and at clinically relevant concentrations, halothane, enflurane, isoflurane, and methoxyflurane appear to induce an acrosomal reaction in sea urchin sperm, that is not blocked by addition of the calcium channel blocking agents verapamil, diltiazem, or nitrendipene. This process facilitates the interaction of the sperm and the egg. However, diethyl ether is only about half as effective, and trichlorethylene only about 10% to 15% as effective in initiating this reaction.[64]

Nitrous Oxide

After 4-hour per day exposures to 10%–80% nitrous oxide for 5 days, young male mice did not undergo change in the amount of DNA present in the epididymis compared with control animals. Neither was there increase in the incidence of abnormal sperm after the exposure to any concentration of nitrous oxide.[65] In another experiment, male mice were exposed to various concentrations, up to 50%, of nitrous oxide for 4 hours per day for 10 weeks before and during mating to untreated females, without any decreased ability of males to impregnate females and without effect on litter size, fetal wastage, or fetal weight.[66]

Young male and female mice were exposed to nitrous oxide from 0.5% to 50% for 4 hours per day, 5 days a week for 14 weeks, without significant effect on testes weight, percentage of abnormally shaped sperm, sperm count, histologic characteristics of the testes, or incidence of abnormal sperm. Similarly, nitrous oxide produced no significant effect on the mean number of oocytes in the female mice.[67]

Male mice breathed 80% nitrous oxide, 4 hours per day for 5 days, with no increase in the incidence of abnormal sperm. An increase in abnormal sperm was reported after 0.08% chloroform, 0.2% trichloroethylene, or 1.0% enflurane.[68] Exposure to halothane 0.6% in 50% nitrous oxide resulted in an increase in abnormal sperm in another study.[69]

Male rats exposed to 0.5% (5000 ppm) nitrous oxide for 30 days were mated immediately and at 6 months after the last nitrous oxide exposure. A significant reduction in mean litter size and individual fetal weight occurred among offspring of the first mating after exposure. These changes did not occur in those conceived 6 months after the last exposure.[70]

Atrophy of seminiferous tubules, decreased testicular weight, a decrease in the number of spermatozoa, and an increased incidence of abnormal spermatozoa occurred in rats after exposure to 20% nitrous oxide, continuously or for 8 hours per day for 35 days. Adverse effects were noted as early as 2 days after the beginning of the 8-hour per day exposures but were reversible when nitrous oxide was discontinued.[70] Similar findings have been reported in rats by others.[71] In another study, chromosomal abnormalities occurred in the spermatogonia of rats exposed to a combination of 50 ppm nitrous oxide and 1 ppm halothane, 7 hours per day, 5 days a week for 52 weeks. However, the offspring resulting from mating these rats with unexposed females were entirely normal.[55]

Studies in Humans

Among 46 anesthetists, spermatogenesis was reduced only if preexisting testicular abnormalities were present. However, a subgroup who had one or more confounding factors, in addition to exposure to anesthesia, were more likely to have sperm abnormalities after 1 year of work in the operating room than a control group of men with an occupational exposure to trace concentrations.[72]

TERATOGENIC EFFECTS OF ANESTHETICS DURING AND AFTER ORGANOGENESIS

Nitrous Oxide

In one study, rats inhaled nitrous oxide, 250 or 1000 ppm, throughout pregnancy. After 250 ppm no effects were noted. However, pups of rats exposed to 1000 ppm exhibited smaller litter size, increased incidence of fetal resorption, and smaller crown-to-rump measurements; organ anomalies were not significantly more frequent in either group.[73] Exposure of mice

4 hours per day on days 6 to 15 of pregnancy to 0.5%, 5.0%, or 50% nitrous oxide resulted in no adverse effect on any measured parameter. Exposure to 50% nitrous oxide caused no apparent sedative or anesthetic effect.[66]

In a landmark study,[74] pregnant female rats were exposed to 70% to 75% nitrous oxide or 75% xenon for 24 hours on day 9 of pregnancy. Only rats exposed to nitrous oxide exhibited an increased incidence of soft tissue resorptions and skeletal anomalies in the resulting fetuses. This study demonstrates that toxicity of nitrous oxide and not the state of anesthesia, which was of a level similar to that of xenon, was responsible for the teratogenic effects.[74]

In another study,[31] rats breathed subanesthetic (0.75% and 25%) and anesthetic (75%) concentrations of nitrous oxide for 24 hours on day 9 of gestation. Adverse reproductive effects did not occur at 0.75% and 25% exposures, but 75% nitrous oxide caused significant increases in resorptions; decreases in the number of live fetuses; and increases in the numbers of runts, ocular malformations, limb deformities, and rib abnormalities.[31] Fink and colleagues exposed pregnant rats continuously to 50% nitrous oxide from days 8 to 10, 8 to 12, or 8 to 14 of pregnancy and found a direct relation between exposure time and increasing fetal resorption rate, fetal skeletal malformations, and a selective male fetal lethality.[75]

Fujinaga and Bader suggested that decreased methionine plays the major role in nitrous oxide–induced teratogenicity in rats.[76] Administration of supplemental methionine to a rat whole embryo culture system exposed to 75% nitrous oxide for the first 24 hours of culture prevented almost all induced malformations and growth retardation.

Halogenated Anesthetics

Basford and Fink found no effect on the offspring of pregnant rats exposed to 0.8% (8000 ppm) halothane at several 12-hour periods during pregnancy.[77] Smith and associates found that only one 3-hour exposure to 1.5% halothane on either day 13, 14, or 15 in C57BL mice results in a 35% incidence of cleft palate and 27% limb anomalies without maternal lethality. Similar defects were not found in unexposed fetuses, and blood halothane concentration was similar to those used for clinical anesthesia in humans.[78]

After inhaling a mixture of 60% nitrous oxide and 0.6% halothane for 3 hours on day 9, 10, or 11 of gestation, the offspring of pregnant hamsters exhibited definite fetotoxicity.[79] However, the internal structure and function of the offspring was not examined.[79] In another study,[80] pregnant rats inhaled 1.0%, 10%, and 50% nitrous oxide, 0.16% of 0.32% halothane, or 0.01% or 0.08% methoxyflurane, 8 hours per day throughout gestation. Offspring of mothers exposed to the larger subanesthetic doses exhibited slight developmental retardation but no increase in congenital anomalies. This finding was thought to represent indirect effects from the prolonged maternal sedative effect of the larger doses.[80] Mild hypoxia, in itself insufficient to affect the developing embryo, can enhance the teratogenicity of nitrous oxide but has not been investigated with other anesthetics.[81]

Pregnant mice inhaled 0.05% (500 ppm) or 0.75% (7500 ppm) enflurane for 1 hour per day, days 7 through 12 of pregnancy. In addition, pregnant rats inhaled 0.05% or 1.25% (12500 ppm) enflurane for 1 hour per day on days 9 through 14 of pregnancy. There were no observed effects on reproductive toxicity or teratogenesis.[82]

Mice exposed to 0.01%, 0.1%, or 1.0% enflurane on day 6 through 15 of pregnancy for 4 hours per day displayed a significant incidence of congenital anomalies. These included cleft palate, a 67% incidence of renal pelvic cavitation and other variants, and a 21% incidence of enlarged brain ventricles.[61] Exposure of seven pregnant rabbits to oxygen, 1.6% halothane, or 2.6% enflurane for 2 hours per day on days 14 through 18 revealed few effects after oxygen or halothane. However, 35% of surviving kits displayed enlarged kidneys after enflurane. A second study revealed a 22.2% incidence of enlarged fetal kidneys.[83] Yet inhalation by rats of 0.0011% (11 ppm) or 0.0064% (64 ppm) enflurane for 8 hours per day throughout pregnancy resulted in no toxic reproductive effects on the offspring[84]; neither did inhalation of 0.32% (3200 ppm) enflurane for 8 hours per day throughout pregnancy.[80]

Mazze and colleagues exposed pregnant mice to 0.006% (60 ppm), 0.06% (600 ppm), or 0.6% (6000 ppm) isoflurane, 4 hours per day on days 6 through 15 of pregnancy. This revealed no adverse effects at 60 or 600 ppm, but 6000 ppm resulted in significantly decreased fetal weight, decreased skeletal ossification, increased renal pelvic cavitation, an increased incidence of cleft palate (48% of all litters and 12.1% of all pups versus 0.6% in controls), and a fourfold increase in external anomalies.[85]

Pregnant rats inhaled 75% nitrous oxide, 0.8% halothane, 1.05% isoflurane, or 1.65% enflurane for 6 h/day on 3 consecutive days on either gestational days 8 to 10, 11 to 13, or 14 to 16. On days 14 to 16, nitrous oxide resulted in a threefold increase in fetal resorptions. After enflurane, a 2.5-fold increase in skeletal abnormalities, a threefold increase in so-called developmental variants, and a 2.5-fold increase in rib anomalies. Halothane-treated pups had no skeletal anomalies, but developmental variants were found in 47% of fetuses, with none in controls or in other anesthetic-treated fetuses.[23]

Inhalation of 0.01% (100 ppm) trichloroethylene by pregnant rats resulted in minor fetal toxicity but no teratogenesis.[86] Diethyl ether in clinically relevant conditions increased the death rate in chick embryos and anomalies in 21% of the survivors.[39] A fragmentary study of pregnant rats and mice exposed to concentrations of ether that led to much maternal mortality reported little teratogenicity.[87] Cyclopropane caused a dose-related increase in death and abnormality in surviving chick embryos[88] but not in 32 briefly exposed humans.[89] Exposure of C57BL mice on days 11 through 13 of gestation to 0.3% methoxyflurane resulted in an exceedingly high incidence of minor bony developmental anomalies but no increase in fetal or maternal death.[6]

Narcotic Analgesics

In dosages small enough to avoid serious respiratory depression, fentanyl, sufentanil, and alfentanil are not teratogenic in rats.[90,91] Fetotoxicity at greater dosages is thought to be related to respiratory depression. In addition, morphine, meperidine, and methadone usually display adverse reproductive effects only at dosages sufficient to depress respiration.[90] Experience gained from human addicts suggests little teratogenicity with morphine and heroin.[92]

Barbiturates and Other Adjuvants

The potential teratogenicity of barbiturates is disputed, but studies in humans and a consensus of experts suggests they are probably not teratogenic.[93] Meprobamate is associated with impairment of learning in pups of pregnant rats.[40] Chlorpromazine, prochlorperazine, trifluoperazine, promethazine, and imipramine are teratogenic in animals, but apparently not in humans.[40] Early reports alleged that diazepam caused cleft palate, but this relation is now considered to be highly unlikely in humans.[94] Ketamine[95] and lidocaine[96] do not appear to be teratogenic in rats. Developmental abnormalities in cultured rat embryos did not occur with d-tubocurarine, pancuronium, atracurium, and vecuronium until doses thirty times those used clinically were administered.[97]

BEHAVIORAL TERATOLOGY

Anesthetic Agents

Rats exposed to 0.00125% (12.5 ppm) halothane from day 2 of conception through 30 or 60 days after birth were tested at 1 year of age.[98] Both groups showed significant deficits in neurologic function and learning. Before 55 days of age, spontaneous alternation (the tendency to explore new places) was depressed significantly in both groups, but was normal thereafter. The 60-day exposure group, but not the 30-day group, showed deficits in learning light–dark discrimination, indicating that continuing trace concentration exposure to halothane during postnatal days 30 to 60 is necessary for inducing this noticeable long-term learning deficit.[98] Mice whose mothers had been exposed to 0% to 10% halothane or 0% to 4% enflurane for only 30 minutes during days 6 and 10 or days 14 and 17 of gestation showed long-lasting deficits in spatial maze learning.[99] Enflurane-treated pups recovered learning more rapidly than the halothane-treated pups.[99]

After chronic inhalation by rats of 0.001% (10 ppm) halothane, 8 hours per day, 5 days a week throughout pregnancy and until 60 days after birth, another group demonstrated a long-lasting learning deficit when the pups reached adulthood. These deficits included retarded acquisition of light–dark discrimination and a low threshold for motor responses. However, other rats exposed to halothane only after reaching adulthood (days 60 to 150) did not exhibit these findings. They found histologic evidence of impaired development of the synaptic web and postsynaptic apparatus in 30% of the cortical synapses of halothane exposed offspring.[100]

Pregnant rats were exposed to 0.0025% (25 ppm) or 0.01% (100 ppm) halothane, 8 hours per day, 5 days a week from day 2 of gestation until day 60 after birth, or 0.0025% (25 ppm), 24 hours per day, 7 days a week for the same period. After 100 ppm, but not after 25 ppm, development of spontaneous alternation was retarded. Histologic examination revealed retarded synaptogenesis and impaired dendritic growth in the brains of treated pups.[26,101,102]

In another study, rats were exposed to 0.001% (10 ppm) halothane for 8 hours per day, 5 days a week throughout pregnancy. The pups displayed significant ultrastructural damage of the cortical pyramidal cells, which persisted at least beyond 100 days of life.[103] After their dams had been anesthetized with 1.2% halothane for 2 hours on day 3, 10, or 17 of gestation, grown male offspring required 39% and 41% more error trials and altered foot shock threshold than controls to learn the maze task. However, male offspring of dams exposed in the third trimester revealed no significant difference from control to the neurologic tests administered.[104]

Nonanesthetic Agents

A variety of sedatives and depressants other than anesthetics, including diazepam, chlorpromazine, meprobamate, bromides, barbiturates, and salicylates,[25,40] have been found in the offspring of rats and mice to cause behavioral or functional impairment that persists through adulthood. Though not verified in humans, remarkable and permanent defects of learning and memory in pups have been demonstrated clearly to occur after short-term administration of clinically relevant dosages of diazepam to pregnant rats. These defects can be prevented by the concurrent administration of the benzodiazepine receptor antagonist flumazenil. Apparently, that receptor activity is permanently affected by benzodiazepine administered during the developmental phase of the brain; this observation has important implications for humans.[25]

CLINICAL IMPLICATIONS AND RECOMMENDATIONS

As is apparent from the foregoing discussion, the implications of teratologic research are notoriously difficult to synthesize. Epidemiologic studies of the dangers of surgical anesthesia to pregnant women are meager, but they suggest that the risk from anesthesia is reasonably low. However, no neurologic testing of humans has been carried out. A wealth of animal data makes it clear that chronic inhalation of anesthetics at concentrations likely to be encountered in a modern, well-ventilated operating suite has no effect on fertility, spontaneous abortion, or development in animals. However, evidence of potential neurologic damage to animals treated for extremely long periods at very high exposures and fetuses exposed to clinical anesthesia should not be dismissed.

Although most inhaled anesthetics have antimitotic effects in tissue preparations, the implications of these findings for humans are unclear. Apparently, no important mutagenic activity occurs. However, chronic exposure to low concentrations, or shorter exposures to anesthetic concentrations, of most inhaled anesthetics during organogenesis in rats, mice, hamsters, and rabbits certainly results in a wide array of abnormal responses in the fetus. Authorities disagree on the interpretation of these findings.

For example, one group stated that "the order of reproductive toxicity of the inhaled anesthetics in Swiss/Webster mice is isoflurane > enflurane > halothane > methoxyflurane > nitrous oxide" and recommended avoidance of isoflurane in pregnant humans.[85] However, the following year, after studying isoflurane in rats, the same authors reached a different conclusion. Cleft palate was the only significant teratogenic finding in their study in mice, but was not seen in their rat study. The incidence of cleft palate did not appear to them to be increased in pregnant women after surgery. Thus, neither isoflurane nor any of the other inhaled anesthetics, when administered in the usual clinical conditions, appear to cause teratogenic effects in the human.[23]

This reversal in conclusions may be explained by the myriad confusing variables already noted but deserves discussion. An attempt to characterize the rat as a more reliable indicator of drug teratogenicity in humans than the mouse has been discussed earlier and has been demonstrated to be questionable.[18] The tendency to disregard fetal abnormalities such as renal pelvic cavitation and dilated brain ventricles, also discussed earlier, is likewise questionable.[9]

Although induction of cleft palate in Swiss/Webster mice may be easier than in rats, evidence does not show that rats are more resistant than humans to induction of cleft palate. The suggestion that cleft palate has not been observed after human anesthesia and therefore is not a problem after anesthesia during pregnancy, rests on a worldwide reports of only 219 documented first-trimester exposures and only 3082 reported cases in all trimesters. Furthermore, the types of anomalies encountered in these reported cases have been incomplete. To reveal a doubled incidence of an anomaly such as cleft palate, which occurs once in 1000 births,[105] would require study of 23,000 pregnant women, all treated identically with regard to agent and time of gestation, among other parameters, with complete follow-up records.[13]

The complacency with which some authorities view well-demonstrated fetotoxic, embryotoxic, or teratogenic effects of inhalation anesthetics in animals has been questioned here. The commonly accepted animal screening criteria for teratogenicity, which require evidence of effect in two or more species in clinically analogous situations, has been met at least for nitrous oxide and halothane but less clearly for enflurane and isoflurane. For these and other reasons, statements concerning either the safety or danger of anesthesia to humans during pregnancy should be considered very carefully before they are accepted.

Most authorities agree that some caution is advised in offering anesthesia to the pregnant woman for elective procedures at any time during pregnancy and not just during the first trimester. Authorities disagree greatly regarding translation of these principles into specific drugs and doses.

I believe that anesthesia and surgery during pregnancy should be avoided if possible. If anesthesia during pregnancy is required, anesthetic techniques using the least toxic drugs, in the lowest possible concentration, for the shortest possible time, should be chosen. For example, spinal anesthesia (avoiding hypotension, of course) is preferable when it is as applicable as general anesthesia, because very little drug reaches the fetus. I also believe barbiturates, narcotics, and muscle relaxants are less toxic to the reproductive system than other current drugs used during general anesthesia. The evidence for the dose-related teratogenicity of nitrous oxide is very clear; it should be avoided when possible. If an inhalation agent is absolutely required, I replace nitrous oxide with comparable MAC levels of isoflurane but never in concentrations greater than 0.5 MAC.

If anesthesia becomes necessary during gestation at any time after the detection of fetal heart sounds, attempts should be made to monitor the fetal heart rate during surgery. Doing so, however, has very limited application, because labor is absent and anesthesia seems to interfere with patterns of heart rate variability.[106]

REFERENCES

1. Ingalls TH, Philbrook FR: Monstrosities induced by hypoxia. N Engl J Med 259:558, 1958
2. Smith BE: Fetal prognosis after anesthesia during gestation. Anesth Analg 42:521, 1963
3. Duncan PG, Pope WDB, Cohen MM, et al: Fetal risk of anesthesia and surgery during pregnancy. Anesthesiology 64:790, 1986
4. Strunin L, Knights K, Strunin JM, et al: General anaesthesia during early pregnancy. Br J Surg 62:471, 1975
5. Shnider SM, Webster GM: Maternal and fetal hazards of surgery during pregnancy. Am J Obstet Gynecol 92:891, 1965
6. Smith BE: Teratology in anesthesia. Clin Obstet Gynecol 17:145, 1974
7. Cohen EN, Brown BW Jr, Bruce DL: Occupational disease among operating room personnel: a national study. Anesthesiology 41:21, 1974
8. Tannenbaum TN, Goldberg RJ: Exposure to anesthetic gases and reproductive outcome: a review of the epidemiologic literature. J Occup Med 27:659, 1985
9. Chernoff N: The science of teratology in a regulatory setting. Basic Life Sci 34:285, 1985
10. Mellin GW: The fetal life study of the Columbia-Presbyterian medical center: a prospective epidemiological study of prenatal influences on fetal development and survival. In Chipman SS (eds): Research methodology and needs in perinatal studies. Springfield, IL: Charles C Thomas, 1966: 88
11. Council on Scientific Affairs: Effects of toxic chemicals on the reproductive system. JAMA 253:3431, 1985
12. Larsen JW Jr, Greendale K: ACOG Technical Bulletin Number 84—February 1985: Teratology. Teratology 32:493, 1985
13. Sullivan FM: quoted in Miller RW: How environmental effects on child health are recognized. Pediatrics 53:798, 1974
14. Newman CG: Teratogen update: clinical aspects of thalidomide embryopathy—a continuing preoccupation. Teratology 32:133, 1985
15. Lum JT, Wells PG: Pharmacological studies on the potentiation of phenytoin teratogenicity by acetaminophen. Teratology 33:53, 1986
16. Rosa FW, Wilk AL, Kelsey FO: Teratogen update: vitamin A congeners. Teratology 33:355, 1986
17. Pauli RM, Feldman PF: Major limb malformations following intrauterine exposure to ethanol: two additional cases and literature review. Teratology 33:273, 1986
18. Schardein JL: Current status of drugs as teratogens in man. Prog Clin Biol Res 163:181, 1985
19. Beckman DA, Brent RL: Mechanisms of teratogenesis. Annu Rev Pharmacol Toxicol 24:483, 1984
20. Holmes LB: Teratogen update: Bendectin. Teratology 27:277, 1983
21. Frankos VH: FDA perspectives on the use of teratology data for human risk assessment. Fundam Appl Toxicol 5:615, 1985
22. Manson JM, Murphy M, Richdale N, et al: Effects of oral exposure to trichloroethylene on female reproductive function. Toxicology 32:229, 1984
23. Mazze RI, Fujinaga M, Rice SA, et al: Reproductive and teratogenic effects of nitrous oxide, halothane, isoflurane, and enflurane in Sprague-Dawley rats. Anesthesiology 64:339, 1986
24. Kavlock RJ, Gray JA: Morphometric, biochemical, and physiological assessment of perinatally induced renal dysfunction. J Toxicol Environ Health 11:1, 1983
25. Simmons RD, Kellogg CK, Miller RK: Prenatal diazepam ex-

posure in rats: long-lasting, receptor-mediated effects on hypothalamic norepinephrine-containing neurons. Brain Res 293:73, 1984

26. Uemura E, Levin ED, Bowman RE: Effects of halothane on synaptogenesis and learning behavior in rats. Exp Neurol 89: 520, 1985
27. Brent RL: Definition of a teratogen and the relationship of teratogenicity to carcinogenicity. Teratology 34:359, 1986
28. Runner MN: Comparative pharmacology in relation to teratogenesis. Fed Proc 26(4):1131, 1967
29. Kalter H: Interplay of intrinsic and extrinsic factors. In Wilson JG, Warkany J (eds): Teratology: principles and techniques. Chicago: University of Chicago Press, 1965: 57
30. Wilson JG: General principles and mechanisms derived from animal studies. In Wilson JG, Fraser FC (eds): Handbook of teratology, vol 1. New York: Plenum Press, 1977: 47
31. Mazze RI, Wilson AI, Rice SA, et al: Reproduction and fetal development in rats exposed to nitrous oxide. Teratology 30: 259, 1984
32. Sturrock JE: No mutagenic effect of enflurane on cultured cells. Br J Anaesth 49:777, 1977
33. Sturrock JE: Lack of mutagenic effect of halothane or chloroform on cultured cells using the azaguanine test system. Br J Anaesth 49:207, 1977
34. Baden JM, Simmon VF: Mutagenic effects of inhalational anesthetics. Mutat Res 75:169, 1980
35. Kundomal YR, Baden JM: Toxicity and teratogenicity of inhaled anesthetics in drosophila melanogaster. Toxicol Lett 25:287, 1985
36. Kramer PG, Burm GL: Mutagenicity studies with halothane in drosophila melanogaster. Anesthesiology 50:510, 1979
37. Ritter EJ: Altered biosynthesis. In Wilson JG, Fraser FC (eds): Handbook of teratology, vol 2. New York: Plenum Press, 1977: 99
38. Cohen PJ, Marshall BE: Effects of halothane on respiratory control and oxygen consumption of rat liver mitochondria. In Fink BR (ed): Toxicity of anesthetics. Baltimore: Williams & Wilkins, 1968: 24
39. Smith BE, Gaub ML, Usubiaga L: Teratogenic effects of diethylether. In Fink BR (ed): Toxicity of anesthetics. Baltimore: Williams & Wilkins, 1968: 269
40. Smith BE: Teratogenic capabilities of surgical anaesthesia. In Woollam DHM (ed): Advances in teratology, vol 3. London: Logos Press, 1968: 127
41. Smith BE, Lehrer S, Usubiaga L, et al: Toxic effect of oxygen: developmental age dependence. Pharmacologist 9:206, 1967
42. Brodsky JB, Cohen EN, Brown BW Jr, et al: Surgery during pregnancy and fetal outcome. Am J Obstet Gynecol 138:1165, 1980
43. Mellin GW: Fetal life study: maternal surgical anesthesia as a complication of pregnancy in relation to fetal survival and malformation. Proceedings of The American Pediatric Society 78th annual meeting, May 1968. 53
44. Aldridge LM, Tunstall ME: Nitrous oxide and the fetus: a review and the results of a retrospective study of 175 cases of anaesthesia for insertion of Shirodkar suture. Br J Anaesth 58:1348, 1986
45. Mazze RI, Källén B: Reproductive outcome after anesthesia and operation during pregnancy: A registry study of 5,405 cases. Am J Gynecol 161:1178, 1989
46. Källén B, Mazze RI: Neural tube defects and first trimester operations. Teratology 41:717, 1990
47. Sylvester G, Khoury MJ, Lu X, et al: First-trimester Anesthesia exposure and the risk of central nervous system defects: A population-based case-control study. American Journal of Public Health 84:1757, 1994
48. Horowitz MD, Gomez GA, Santiesteban R, et al: Acute appendicitis during pregnancy. Arch Surg 120:1362, 1985
49. Rosen MA, Roizen MF, Eger EI II, et al: The effect of nitrous oxide on in vitro fertilization success rate. Anesthesiology 67: 42, 1987

49a. Australian In Vitro Fertilisation Group. High incidence of preterm births and early losses in pregnancy after in vitro fertilisation. Br Med J 291:1160, 1985

50. Nunn JF: Faulty cell replication: abortion, congenital abnormalities. Int Anesthesiol Clin 19:77, 1981
51. Hinkley RE, Chambers EL: Structural changes in dividing sea-urchin eggs induced by the volatile anaesthetic halothane. J Cell Sci 55:327, 1982
52. Hinkley RE Jr, Wright BD: Comparative effects of halothane, enflurane, and methoxyflurane on the incidence of abnormal development using sea urchin gametes as an in vitro model system. Anesth Analg 64:1005, 1985
53. Bruce DL, Hinkley R, Norman PF: Fentanyl does not inhibit fertilization or early development of sea urchin eggs. Anesth Analg 64:495, 1985
54. Rodier PM, Aschner M, Lewis LS, et al: Cell proliferation in developing brain after brief exposure to nitrous oxide or halothane. Anesthesiology 64:680, 1986
55. Coate WB, Kapp RW, Lewis TR: Chronic exposure to low concentrations of halothane–nitrous oxide: reproductive and cytogenetic effects in the rat. Anesthesiology 50:310, 1979
56. White AE, Takehisa S, Eger EI II, et al: Sister chromatid exchanges induced by inhaled anesthetics. Anesthesiology 50: 426, 1979
57. Basler A, Rohrborn G: Lack of mutagenic effects of halothane in mammals in vivo. Anesthesiology 55:143, 1981
58. Usubiaga LE, Smith BE: Studies of the effects of halothane on chromosomes in human leukocyte cultures. In Advances in anaesthesiology and resuscitation. Hoder J, Jedlička R, Pokorný J, (eds) Avicenum, Czechoslovak Medical Press Prague, 1972: 1019
59. Halsey MJ, Green CJ, Monk SJ, et al: Maternal and paternal chronic exposure to enflurane and halothane: fetal and histological changes in the rat. Br J Anaesth 53:203, 1981
60. Bruce DL: Murine fertility unaffected by traces of halothane. Anesthesiology 38:473, 1973
61. Wharton RS, Mazze RI, Wilson AI: Reproduction and fetal development in mice chronically exposed to enflurane. Anesthesiology 54:505, 1981
62. Mazze RI: Fertility, reproduction, and postnatal survival in mice chronically exposed to isoflurane. Anesthesiology 63: 663, 1985
63. Wharton RS, Mazze RI, Baden JM, et al: Fertility, reproduction and postnatal survival in mice chronically exposed to halothane. Anesthesiology 48:167, 1978
64. Hinkley RE, Wright BD, Greenberg CA: Induction of the acrosome reaction in sea urchin spermatozoa by the volatile anesthetic halothane. Biol Reprod 34:119, 1986
65. Land PC, Owen EL, Linde HW: Morphologic changes in mouse spermatozoa after exposure to inhalational anesthetics during early spermatogenesis. Anesthesiology 54:47, 1981
66. Mazze RI, Wilson AI, Rice SA, et al: Reproduction and fetal development in mice chronically exposed to nitrous oxide. Teratology 26:11, 1982
67. Mazze RI, Rice SA, Wyrobek AJ, et al: Germ cell studies in mice after prolonged exposure to nitrous oxide. Toxicol Appl Pharmacol 67:370, 1983
68. Land PC, Owen EL, Linde HW: Morphologic changes in mouse spermatozoa after exposure to inhalational anesthetics during early spermatogenesis. Anesthesiology 54:53, 1981
69. Land PC, Owen EL: Halothane plus N_2O:O_2 increases sperm abnormalities in mice (abstract). Anesthesiology 55:A196, 1981
70. Kripke BJ, Kelman AD, Shah NK, et al: Testicular reaction to prolonged exposure to nitrous oxide. Anesthesiology 44: 104, 1976
71. Vieira E, Cleaton-Jones P, Moyes D: Effects of low intermittent concentrations of nitrous oxide on the developing rat fetus. Br J Anaesth 55:67, 1983
72. Wyrobek AJ, Brodsky J, Gordon L, et al: Sperm studies in anesthesiologists. Anesthesiology 55:527, 1981
73. Vieira E, Cleaton-Jones P, Austin JC, et al: Effects of low concentrations of nitrous oxide on rat fetuses. Anesth Analg 59:175, 1980

74. Lane GA, Nahrwold ML, Tait AR, et al: Anesthetics as teratogens: nitrous oxide is fetotoxic, xenon is not. Science 210: 899, 1980
75. Fink BR, Shepard TH, Blandau RJ: Teratogenic activity of nitrous oxide. Nature 214:146, 1967
76. Fujinaga M, Bader J: Methionine prevents nitrous oxide–induced teratogenicity in rat embryos grown in culture. Anesthesiology 81:184, 1994
77. Basford AB, Fink BR: Teratogenicity of halothane in the rat. Anesthesiology 29:1167, 1968
78. Smith BE, Usubiaga LE, Lehrer SB: Cleft palate induced by halothane anesthesia in C-57 black mice. Teratology 4:242, 1971
79. Bussard DA, Stoelting RK, Peterson C, et al: Fetal changes in hamsters anesthetized with nitrous oxide and halothane. Anesthesiology 41:275, 1974
80. Pope WDB, Halsey MJ, Phil D, et al: Fetotoxicity in rats following chronic exposure to halothane, nitrous oxide, or methoxyflurane. Anesthesiology 48:11, 1978
81. Smith BE, Gaub ML, Moya F: Teratogenic effects of anesthetic agents: nitrous oxide. Anesth Analg 44:726, 1965
82. Saito N, Urakawa M, Ito R: Influence of enflurane on fetus and growth after birth in mice and rats. Pharmacometrics 8: 1269, 1974
83. Smith BE, Lehrer SB, Usubiaga LE: Reproductive effects of Ohio-347. Unpublished report to Ohio Medical Products (Madison, WI), 1970
84. Strout CD, Nahrwold ML, Taylor MD, et al: Effects of subanesthetic concentrations of enflurane on rat pregnancy and early development. Environ Health Perspect 21:211, 1977
85. Mazze RI, Wilson AI, Rice SA, et al: Fetal development in mice exposed to isoflurane. Teratology 32:339, 1985
86. Healy TEJ, Poole TR, Hopper A: Rat fetal development and maternal exposure to trichloroethylene 100 ppm. Br J Anaesth 54:337, 1982
87. Schwetz BA, Becker BA: Embryotoxicity and fetal malformations of rats and mice due to maternally administered ether. Toxicol Appl Pharmacol 17:275, 1970
88. Andersen NB: The teratogenicity of cyclopropane in the chicken. Anesthesiology 10:113, 1968
89. Mellin GW: Comparative teratology. Anesthesiology 29:1, 1968
90. Fujinaga M, Stevenson JB, Mazze RI: Reproductive and teratogenic effects of fentanyl in Sprague-Dawley rats. Teratology 34:51, 1986
91. Fujinaga M, Bader JM, Mazze RI: Reproductive and teratogenic effects of sufentanil and alfentanil in Sprague-Dawley rats. Anesth Analg 67:166, 1988
92. Wilson JG: Embryotoxicity of drugs in man. In Wilson JG, Fraser FC (eds): Handbook of teratology: general principles and etiology. New York: Plenum Press, 1977: 340
93. In Shepard TH: Catalog of teratogenic agents, 4th ed. Baltimore: Johns Hopkins University Press, 1983: 144
94. Shiono PH, Mills JL: Oral clefts and diazepam use during pregnancy. N Engl J Med 311: 919, 1984
95. In Shepard TH: Catalog of teratogenic agents, 4th ed. Baltimore: Johns Hopkins University Press, 1983: 751
96. Fujinaga M, Mazze RI: Reproductive and teratogenic effects of lidocaine in Sprague-Dawley rats. Anesthesiology 65:626, 1986
97. Fujinaga M, Bader JM, Mazze RI: Developmental toxicity of nondepolarizing muscle relaxants in cultured rat embryos. Anesthesiology 76:999, 1992
98. Levin ED, Bowman RE: Behavioral effects of chronic exposure to low concentrations of halothane during development in rats. Anesth Analg 65:653, 1986
99. Chalon J, Tank C-K, Ramanathan S, et al: Exposure to halothane and enflurane affects learning function of murine progeny. Anesth Anal 60:794, 1981
100. Quimby KL, Katz J, Bowman RE: Behavioral consequences in rats from chronic exposure to 10 ppm halothane during early development. Anesth Analg 54:628, 1975
101. Uemura E, Bowman RE: Effects of halothane on cerebral synaptic density. Exp Neurol 69:135, 1980
102. Uemura E, Ireland WP, Levin ED, et al: Effects of halothane on the development of rat brain: a Golgi study of dendritic growth. Exp Neurol 89:503, 1985
103. Chang LW, Dudley AW Jr, Lee YK, et al: Ultrastructural studies on the pathological changes in the neonatal kidney following in utero exposure to halothane. Environ Res 10:174, 1975
104. Smith RF, Bowman RE, Katz J: Behavioral effects of exposure to halothane during early development in the rat: sensitive period during pregnancy. Anesthesiology 49:319, 1978
105. Safra MJ, Oakley GP Jr: Association between cleft lip with or without cleft palate and prenatal exposure to diazepam. Lancet 2:478, 1975
106. Liu PL, Warren TM, Ostheimer GW, et al: Foetal monitoring in parturients undergoing surgery unrelated to pregnancy. Can Anaesth Soc J 32:525, 1985

FURTHER READING

Baden JM: Teratogenicity of inhaled anesthetics. In Baden JM, Brodsky JB (ed): The pregnant surgical patient. Mt. Kisco, NY: Futura, 1985: 29

Friedman JM: Teratogen update: anesthetic agents. Teratology 37: 69, 1988

Rice SA, Pellegrini M: Basic principles of teratology. In Baden JM, Brodsky JB (eds): The pregnant surgical patient. Mt. Kisco, NY: Futura, 1985: 1

Rice SA, Pellegrini M: Teratogenicity of fixed agents. In Baden JM, Brodsky JB (eds): The pregnant surgical patient. Mt. Kisco, NY: Futura, 1985: 53

Tannenbaum TN, Goldberg RJ: Exposure to anesthetic gases and reproductive outcome. J Occup Med 27:659, 1985

Complications in Anesthesiology, second edition,
edited by Nikolaus Gravenstein and Robert R. Kirby.
Lippincott-Raven Publishers, Philadelphia © 1996.

CHAPTER 50

Postoperative Nausea and Vomiting

Fredrick K. Orkin

Although nausea and vomiting are associated with significant morbidity in virtually any practice of anesthesia, they are discussed infrequently, even though they constitute the most memorable distress for many patients who have an otherwise uncomplicated anesthetic and surgical course. Even when other complications occur, nausea and vomiting may stand out as uniquely unpleasant.

Nausea is the vague sensation, difficult to describe or localize, that often is a prodrome to vomiting. *Vomiting* is a complex physiologic reflex involving coordinated activity of many skeletal muscles and of the autonomic nervous system, resulting in the forceful expulsion of gastric and even intestinal contents. This chapter reviews the physical basis of nausea and vomiting and their incidence, treatment, and prevention.

ANATOMIC FEATURES AND PHYSIOLOGIC MECHANISMS

Neural Connections

Like other reflexes, nausea and vomiting have afferent pathways, a central integrator, and efferent pathways.[1,2] Much of our knowledge of the mechanism of nausea and vomiting derives from the work of Borison and Wang, who identified a vomiting center located bilaterally in the dorsolateral border of the lateral reticular formation in the medulla at the level of the olivary nuclei.[3] The vomiting center is situated in the midst of the nuclei and centers that regulate the visceral and somatic responses involved in vomiting. These regulatory structures include the spasmodic respiratory center, inspiratory and expiratory respiratory centers, vasomotor center, salivary nuclei, and bulbar facilitory and inhibitory systems.

Stimuli arise from various sites throughout the gastrointestinal tract through vagal and sympathetic afferents, higher cerebral centers, and a chemoreceptor trigger zone (CTZ) located on the floor of the fourth ventricle (Fig. 50-1). Additional stimuli include distention of the uterus, renal pelvis, or urinary bladder; rotation or unequal stimulation of the vestibular labyrinths (transmitted by way of the cerebellum and the CTZ); increased intracranial pressure; and pain.[2]

Efferent impulses leave the vomiting center by way of cranial nerves V, VII, IX, X, and XII to the upper gastrointestinal tract and through the spinal nerves to the diaphragm and abdominal muscles.

The Act of Vomiting

Often, as a prodrome to vomiting, the awake person experiences nausea, a feeling of imminent desire to vomit. Accompanying vasomotor and autonomic disturbances include a feeling of faintness, weakness, anorexia, and emptiness, with simultaneous pallor, pupillary dilatation, diaphoresis, and tachycardia or, sometimes, bradycardia with hypotension. Salivation increases, breathing becomes deep, rapid, and irregular, and retching begins. The latter consists of simultaneous and poorly coordinated spasmodic contractions of the chest and abdominal muscles, with descent and sudden spasm of the diaphragm.[4] Contraction of abdominal musculature forces gastric contents up into the esophagus; relaxation after each contraction allows refilling of the stomach from the esophagus.

Nausea gives rise to vomiting when retching becomes a coordinated and forceful expulsion of gastric contents through the mouth. Vomiting begins with a deep breath, followed immediately by the ascent of the hyoid bone and larynx, a movement that opens the cricoesophageal sphincter. The glottis closes and remains shut until expulsion has occurred, thereby preventing pulmonary aspiration of vomitus. Similarly, the soft palate rises, closing the posterior nares (a not always successful defense mechanism, to which many can attest). Then the diaphragm moves caudally as the abdominal muscles contract forcefully, squeezing the stomach and thereby raising intragastric pressure. The gastroesophageal sphincter and

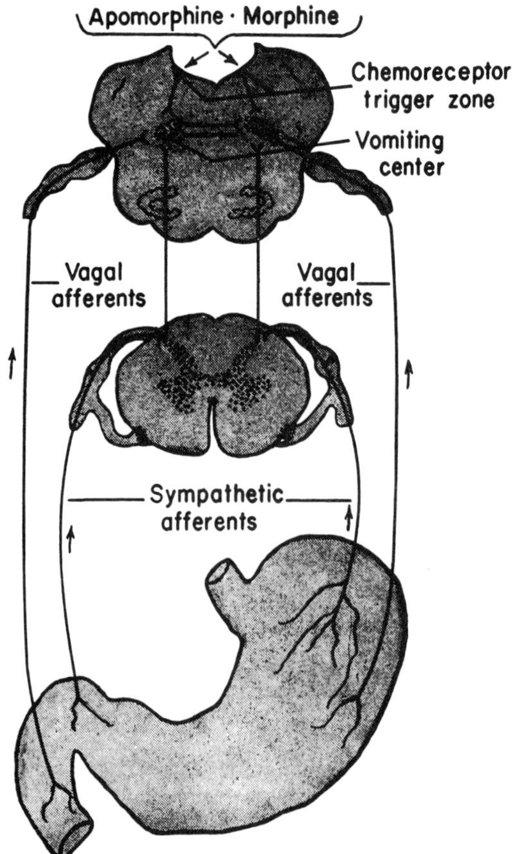

FIGURE 50-1. The vomiting center and some of its afferent pathways. (Guyton AC: Textbook of medical physiology, 7th ed. Philadelphia: WB Saunders, 1986: 803)

esophagus relax, and gastric contents are expelled up the esophagus.[4] The more forceful or prolonged the vomiting, the more likely it is that bile-stained duodenal contents or even material from lower intestinal levels will be forced into the stomach and then expelled.

Regurgitation

Frequently confused with vomiting, *regurgitation* is a passive event. Loss of the sphincter-like activity of the lower esophagus and of the pharyngoesophageal musculature, loss of esophageal peristalsis, and reversal of normal pressure gradients in the upper gastrointestinal tract allow the passive transfer of gastric contents into the pharynx. All of these changes may occur in anesthetized patients. Indeed, *silent regurgitation* is a common occurrence in patients who receive uneventful anesthesia by mask but in whom pulmonary aspiration of small volumes of gastric contents occurs.

CAUSES AND THEIR ASSOCIATED NEURAL PATHWAYS

The diverse afferent pathways to the vomiting center permit an equally diverse set of stimuli to cause nausea and vomiting (Fig. 50-2). Although various (and arbitrary) etiologic classifications can be used, these stimuli are discussed here according to neural pathways, insofar as they are known.[5]

Cortical

Emotional responses that are themselves manifestations of stress, fear, or depression may result in nausea and vomiting. Similar stimuli include sights (such as blood), odors, tastes, associations particular to the individual person, and even neuroses and psychoses. Organic disturbances such as pain, severe hypotension, vascular headache (migraine), hypoxia, and increased intracranial pressure are also subserved by cortical pathways.

Visceral Afferent

Abdominal visceral stimuli subserved by vagal and sympathetic afferents include visceral traction, intestinal obstruction, acute inflammation (such as appendicitis), acute inflammation of nonintestinal viscera accompanied by ileus (such as pancreatitis, cholecystitis), visceral pain, functional gastrointestinal disorders (such as aerophagia), irritation of gastrointestinal mucosa (such as that caused by gastric acid, aminophylline, salicylate, antibiotics, chemotherapeutic agents, endotoxin), and heart disease (acute myocardial infarction or congestive heart failure).

A common factor in many of these situations is delayed gastric emptying with resultant gastric distention, which not only is a stimulus for vomiting but also predisposes to regurgitation and aspiration. Other causes of delayed gastric emptying include narcotic analgesic administration, intra-abdominal masses (such as the gravid uterus), increased intracranial pressure, pain, and anxiety.

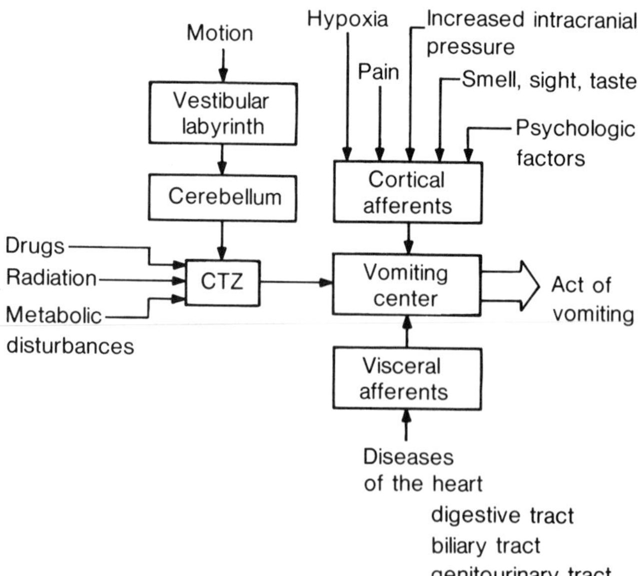

FIGURE 50-2. Some of the stimuli causing nausea and vomiting, shown organized by their afferent pathways.

Vestibular

Motion, otitis media, and tumors and vascular changes of the labyrinth are stimuli subserved by the vestibular impulses that pass by way of the auditory nerve to the cerebellum and then the CTZ en route to the vomiting center. Opiates can sensitize the vestibular apparatus to motion. Motion sickness is also enhanced by visual, psychic, olfactory, and proprioceptive stimuli that are subserved by the cortical pathways.

Chemoreceptor Trigger Zone Afferent

A variety of drugs, including apomorphine, morphine (and other narcotic analgesics), cardiac glycosides, amphetamines, ergot derivatives, and nitrogen mustard act directly on the CTZ to cause nausea and vomiting. Very likely, the nausea and vomiting associated with deficiency states (such as hypovitaminosis, hypothyroidism, and hypoadrenalism), electrolyte imbalance (such as ketoacidosis), ionizing radiation, and uremia are caused by an effect on the CTZ or nearby hypothalamic and medullary centers.

INCIDENCE

Postoperative sickness is a very common problem, with an incidence of 3.6% to 85% reported during the past 5 to 6 decades. With newer anesthetics and other improvements in surgical care, the overall incidence is now about 30%, although recent studies have documented an incidence of 12% to 67%, depending on the clinical circumstances. What precludes an accurate prediction in a given patient is the multitude of predisposing factors, the relative importance of which and interrelations among which have not been evaluated systematically.

TABLE 50-1
Risk Factors for Nausea and Vomiting

PATIENT

1. Obesity
2. Female gender
3. Young age
4. History of motion sickness or postanesthetic vomiting
5. Uncontrolled pain
6. Ambulation

TYPE OF SURGERY

1. Intraabdominal
2. Intracranial
3. Middle ear
4. Laparoscopic
5. Abdominal hysterectomy
6. Eye (especially strabismus)
7. Testicular

DRUGS

1. Narcotics
2. Anticholinesterases
3. Etomidate > pentothal > propofol (by incidence)
4. Isoflurane
5. Regional anesthetic level above T5
6. Nitrous oxide?

OTHER

1. Hypotension
2. Hypoglycemia
3. Bowel obstruction
4. Swallowed blood

Guyton AC: Oral, nasopharyngeal, and gastrointestinal systems. In Gravenstein N (ed): Manual of complications during anesthesia. Philadelphia: JB Lippincott, 1991: 638.

Predisposing Factors

Factors predisposing to postoperative nausea and vomiting are summarized in Table 50-1.

Age

The incidence of postoperative nausea and vomiting is greatest in children, especially the preadolescent 11- to 14-year-old group; at ages greater than 20 years, the incidence decreases.[6–14] Although some believe that the higher incidence reported in children results from the deep level of ether anesthesia formerly given for procedures common in that age group (ie, tonsillectomy),[6] the association has been noted more recently with the newer anesthetics and even in institutions in which light halothane anesthesia is used.[10,13]

Gender

Women are two to four times more prone to nausea and vomiting than are men.[6,8,10,14–16] Bellville and colleagues noted that the incidence is particularly high for women in the 3rd or 4th week of the menstrual cycle and suggested that a high gonadotropin concentration is responsible for this increased susceptibility.[1,8] Additional evidence that they cited includes the nausea that follows orally administered estrogens; the nausea and high gonadotropin concentrations associated with hyperemesis gravidarum; and the persistence of a high incidence of nausea and vomiting (and high gonadotropin concentrations) in postmenopausal and oophorectomized women but its decrease in women older than 70 years (when gonadotropin concentrations decrease).[8] Nausea and vomiting also occurs more frequently when laparoscopy is performed during the menses.[16]

Body Habitus

Obese patients have a higher incidence of nausea and vomiting,[8] possibly because their larger fat compartment serves as a reservoir for slow and prolonged release of larger amounts of anesthetic. In effect, the body is exposed to the anesthetic for a longer period, and increasing exposure is associated with a higher incidence of nausea and vomiting. Obese patients also have a higher resting gastric volume and are more prone to gastric insufflation during airway management.

Individual Predisposition

Patients with a history of motion sickness or postanesthetic vomiting are about three times more likely to have nausea and vomiting than are other patients.[10] Similarly, those with diseases associated with nausea and vomiting (such as renal failure or intestinal obstruction) also have these symptoms more often postoperatively.[18]

Preanesthetic Medication

Narcotics

Patients receiving narcotic analgesic agents preoperatively are about three times more likely to have postoperative nausea and vomiting than are those not receiving these drugs.[18–22] A close relation exists between movement and sickness after morphine administration[22]; the onset may be delayed for hours,[23] and the effect can last as long as 18 hours.[24] Whether morphine is associated with more postoperative sickness than meperidine is controversial.[1,6,11,25–27]

Parasympatholytic Agents

Administration of a parasympatholytic agent such as atropine or scopolamine with the narcotic diminishes the latter's effect,[28,29] whereas parasympatholytics given alone are antiemetic agents.[20] An especially well-designed study demonstrated these relations in a group of patients having minor gynecologic surgery with the use of a standard general anesthetic technique: for women who had received 10 mg morphine, 0.6 mg atropine decreased the incidence of nausea and vomiting from 66.7% to 35.2%; in those not receiving other preanesthetic medication, however, this dose of atropine reduced the incidence of postoperative emetic symptoms from 22.4% to 11.5%.[20]

Barbiturates and Other Agents

Similarly, barbiturates[15] (pentobarbital), antihistamines[15,30,31] (diphenhydramine), and especially phenothiazines[14,15,32,33] (chlorpromazine and promethazine), butyrophenones[16,34–37] (droperidol), and serotonin antagonists (ondansetron)[38,39] can decrease the incidence of nausea and vomiting to as low as 5% to 12%.

Although the data are contradictory, metoclopramide, which is efficacious in preventing regurgitation and thereby decreasing the risk of pulmonary aspiration, also may be effective as an antiemetic agent.[5,33,40] Inconsistency in results with metoclopramide may reflect its relatively short duration of action; although not shown to be efficacious after ambulatory surgery, its use is associated with a lower incidence of postoperative dizziness.[41]

Anesthetic Adjunctive Agents

Multiple factors relating to the anesthetic technique and agents affect the incidence of postoperative emetic symptoms.

Intravenous Agents

The incidence is lower (eg, 0% to 20%) when an intravenously administered induction agent such as thiopental, methohexital, midazolam, or propofol is used rather than an inhalation agent[11,29,42,43]; however, a higher incidence is associated with ketamine and etomidate.[43] The use of thiopental[11,45] or propofol[45–47] for maintenance of anesthesia also is associated with a lower incidence of emetic symptoms than are inhalation agents.

Inhalation Agents

Inhalation agents differ greatly in their association with postoperative emetic symptoms: the flammable agents (diethyl either, cyclopropane, and fluroxene)[1,6,7,10,11,29,31,48,49] used in early practice are associated with the highest incidence, reaching 80%, whereas the modern halogenated agents have a lower incidence than nitrous oxide supplemented with a narcotic.[10,11,50]

Nitrous oxide probably does not increase the incidence of nausea and vomiting in customary clinical circumstances[51–59]; however, emetic symptoms may be associated with high concentrations[51–54] or with the increased sympathetic stimulation that is a pharmacologic characteristic of nitrous oxide.[54] Differences among anesthetic agents are less pronounced or are absent after the first few postoperative hours.[10,29,60–62]

Neostigmine

Antagonism of neuromuscular blockade with neostigmine is associated with a higher incidence of postoperative emetic symptoms, possibly related to the drug's muscarinic effects on the bowel, resulting in increased peristalsis and spasm[63]; this effect may partially account for the increased incidence noted in some studies after nitrous oxide with muscle relaxants, compared with the volatile inhalation anesthetics.[55–58]

Regional Techniques and Agents

The incidence of sickness after regional anesthesia is relatively unstudied but is probably one third that with general anesthesia.[31,64] The same stimuli that may cause emetic symptoms after general anesthesia—hypotension, hypoxia, anxiety, reflux esophagitis, and visceral traction reflex—are operative with regional techniques.

Duration of Anesthesia

The longer the anesthetic, the higher the incidence of postoperative nausea and vomiting,[6–8,11,21,65] an observation that has been explained on a dose–response basis.[1]

Site of Operation

Intra-abdominal, particularly gynecologic, procedures are associated with the highest incidence of emetic symptoms[10,11,31,66]; head and neck, especially ophthalmologic and otolaryngologic, procedures are also more likely to be followed by sickness.[6,7,11,66–68] Surgical care on an outpatient basis also probably is independently associated with a higher incidence than care of inpatients, because the outpatient setting necessarily involves earlier movement and ambulation.

Recognizing the multifactorial etiology of postoperative emetic symptoms, investigators evaluating potential antiemetics conduct their studies in clinical circumstances associated with a high incidence of postoperative sickness: in young children having orchiopexy, strabismus repair, or myringotomy, and in women having pelvic laparoscopy, especially with carbon dioxide rather than nitrous oxide as the insufflating gas.

PREVENTION

As with other anesthetic complications, prevention of postoperative emetic symptoms is often easier and more satisfactory than treatment. Although a variety of antiemetic drugs may be given, more general considerations should not be overlooked.

General Considerations

Numerous, often overlooked, aspects of patient preparation and anesthetic technique should be considered. Particular care should be used to avoid inflating the stomach while ventilating the lungs, because this process leads to gastric distention with a greater likelihood not only of emetic symptoms but also of regurgitation and pulmonary aspiration.[69] Patients who are likely to have delayed gastric emptying with resultant gastric distention benefit postoperatively from gentle suction through an oral or nasogastric tube intraoperatively.[6-8,15,70]

Because visceral pain can cause nausea and vomiting[11,71] and because narcotics are associated in a dose-related fashion with emetic symptoms,[1,10,11,20] especially careful dosing perioperatively is necessary for patients predisposed to postoperative sickness. When possible, propofol or regional anesthesia should be selected, especially for patients at higher risk for emetic symptoms.

After anesthesia, regardless of the technique, the patient should be transported gently, and frequent and abrupt changes in position should be avoided. Another nonpharmacologic approach to prophylaxis that has undergone favorable evaluation is acupuncture with a 24- to 48-G needle inserted without local anesthesia to a depth of 1 cm at acupuncture point P6; several minutes' stimulation is applied to a point proximal to the distal wrist crease by two widths of the intraphalyngeal joint of the thumb.[72]

Prophylactic Antiemetic Drugs

The efficacy of many drugs in treating postoperative emetic symptoms has encouraged many practitioners to use antiemetic drugs prophylactically, especially in the care of outpatients.[73,74] However, as was noted earlier, the incidence may be reduced by nonpharmacologic means. Furthermore, the overall incidence of the problems that they seek to prevent is only about 30%, and in many cases the symptoms are mild and transient. Thus, few patients, perhaps only 5% to 10%, actually need antiemetics.

Side Effects

Not to be overlooked are the side effects of antiemetic drugs, which can be more problematic than the symptoms for which they are administered (Table 50-2). The more effective antiemetic drugs are sedatives and tranquilizers; however, these agents can interact synergistically with residual general anesthesia and narcotics to result in prolonged emergence, a complication that in the ambulatory setting may delay discharge or require hospital admission.

Drug-specific problems can occur. For example, the prophylactic use of chlorpromazine, an aliphatic phenothiazine, which had proved to be an excellent sedative and antiemetic agent, is associated with marked hypotension at induction of anesthesia; it now has been abandoned for antiemesis.[75]

Transdermally administered scopolamine, especially efficacious in motion sickness, may be associated with visual problems and hallucinations; even in the absence of treatment complications, the efficacy of scopolamine skin patches is controversial.[76-81]

The long-acting antiemetic agent droperidol, 1.25 mg intravenously, administered to adults undergoing ambulatory surgery has been associated with restlessness or anxiety the evening after surgery[82]; whether the more commonly used dose of 0.625 mg in adults is associated with dysphoria is unknown. Odansetron, though expensive, has shown promise as a prophylactic antiemetic agent without significant side effects in patients at high risk for postoperative vomiting.[38,39] Thus, the longstanding recommendation that antiemetics not be used prophylactically in all patients continues to be valid.[83]

Beneficial Effects

Although the indiscriminate use of antiemetics prophylactically is not justified, specific clinical circumstances arise in which patients are likely to benefit from prophylactic therapy: a strong history of motion sickness or postoperative sickness; intraocular surgery, with possible interruption of sutures and resultant loss of vitreous and vision; outpatient procedures associated with a high incidence of sickness (eg, strabismus repair, orchiopexy, pelvic laparoscopy); oral surgery with wiring of the jaw; and cases in which retching and vomiting might especially threaten esophageal laceration with hemorrhage (Mallory-Weiss syndrome) or mediastinitis.

Drugs useful prophylactically are described in the following section on therapeutic agents. In some cases, an effective dose may be relatively large; for example, children undergoing strabismus repair may require droperidol in a dose of 50 to 75 μg/kg intravenously, five to eight times the dose given to an adult.[66]

TREATMENT

General Measures

As with other complications, the underlying problems should be identified and treated as early as possible, before any immediate consideration of antiemetic drug therapy. Correction of hypotension, hypovolemia, hypoxia, and pain can relieve emetic symptoms. Nausea and vomiting occurring during regional anesthesia can be treated with 0.5 to 1.0 mg atropine intravenously, 10- to 25-mg increments of ephedrine intravenously (if hypotension is present), oxygen by mask, judicious sedation, and skilled psychologic support.

Antiemetic Therapy

A wide variety of drugs from different pharmacologic classes have antiemetic effects with efficacy in treating postoperative

TABLE 50-2
Receptor Site Affinity of Antiemetic Drugs

PHARMACOLOGIC GROUP AND DRUG	DOPAMINE D_2	MUSCARINE CHOLINERGIC	HISTAMINE	SEROTONIN
Phenothiazines				
Fluphenazine	++++	+	++	−
Chlorpromazine	++++	++	++++	+
Prochlorperazine	++++			
Butyrophenones				
Droperidol	++++	−	+	+
Haloperidol	++++	−	+	−
Domperidone	++++			
Antihistamines				
Diphenyhdramine	+	++	++++	−
Promethazine	++	++	++++	−
Anticholinergic				
Scopolamine	+	++++	+	−
Benzamides				
Metoclopramide	+++	−	+	++
Antiserotonin				
Ondansetron	−	−	−	++++
Granisetron (BRL 43694)	−	−	−	++++
Zacopride	−	−	−	++++
RG 12915	−	−	−	++++
Tricyclic antidepressants				
Amitriptyline	+++	++	+++	−
Nortriptyline	+++	++	+++	−

The number of positive signs (+) indicates degree of activity at receptor; the negative sign (−) indicates no activity.

Watcha MF, White PF: Postoperative nausea and vomiting: its etiology, treatment and prevention. Anesthesiology 77:173, 1992.

Modified from Peroutka SJ, Snyder SH: Antiemetics: Neurotransmitter receptor binding predicts therapeutic action. Lancet 1:658, 1982. Hamik A, Peroutka SJ: Differential interactions of traditional and novel antiemetics with D_2 and 5-hydroxytryptamine 3 receptors. Cancer Chemother Pharmacol 24:307, 1989.

emetic symptoms. However, not all antiemetic agents are effective in surgical patients; some antiemetics are more efficacious in other clinical settings (eg, cancer chemotherapy, radiation therapy, motion sickness, vertigo, or pregnancy). The following sections describe only the more effective drugs; general drug groups are defined by the site of drug action (see Table 50-2).

Anticholinergic Drugs

Anticholinergic drugs seem to reduce the excitability of labyrinth receptors, thus decreasing nerve conduction in the vestibular cerebellar pathways or perhaps reducing the recruitment of impulses in the CTZ in the medulla. Although scopolamine is superior to atropine and glycopyrrolate as a prophylactic antiemetic agent,[11,20,28,29,73] its efficacy is inconsistent, as was noted earlier.[76–81]

Recent interest in this drug stems from its efficacy in reducing motion sickness, especially when it is combined with *d*-amphetamine. To enhance its efficacy and to reduce side effects (eg, blurred vision, dry mouth, and hallucinations) and abuse potential, scopolamine has been combined with other drugs (eg, promethazine or ephedrine).[84,85] Building on this work in the aerospace field, one study of patients at high risk for postoperative emetic symptoms suggests the efficacy of the prophylactic use of a combination of 25 mg of the antihistamine hydroxyzine and 25 mg ephedrine, both intramuscularly administered at the end of the anesthetic.[86] Others have noted inconsistent results with ephedrine alone.[87,88]

Histamine H_1-Receptor Antagonists

These antihistamines seem to affect neural pathways in the vestibular labyrinth. In addition to hydroxyzine, use of diphenhydramine, promethazine, and especially cyclizine is efficacious in treating postoperative sickness. Although their side effects are less problematic than those of other antiemetics, their sedative effects may prolong emergence. The antiemetic effect lasts only a few hours.[73] Thus, they are not drugs of choice.

Antidopaminergic Drugs

These antiemetics act primarily at dopaminergic D_2 receptors by depressing the CTZ and secondarily by inhibiting afferent autonomic impulse conduction along the vagus nerve to the vomiting center. This group, especially diverse in terms of chemical structure, efficacy, and side effects, includes two potent antiemetic drugs: droperidol, a butyrophenone, and triethylperazine, a piperazine phenothiazine.

As mentioned earlier, droperidol has a long duration of action (eg, 18 h), which partially accounts for its efficacy and distinguishes this most commonly used antiemetic agent from a similar butyrophenone, haloperidol.[73] Although droperidol can synergize with residual general anesthesia to prolong emergence, this potent antiemetic is effective at intravenous doses as small as 10 μg/kg, which do not contribute materially to somnolence.

Side effects include idiosyncratic extrapyramidal reactions resembling Parkinsonism and dose-related problems, such as dysphoria[82] and potentiation of anesthetic-related respiratory and cardiovascular depression. With the exception of dysphoria, the efficacy and side effects of 0.07 mg/kg intramuscular triethylperazine resemble those of droperidol.

Other Drugs

This residual category includes dissimilar drugs that also are efficacious in treating postoperative emetic symptoms.

BENZQUINAMIDE. Benzquinamide, a derivative unrelated to the phenothiazines, inhibits the CTZ and is the only antiemetic that is effective at a dose (0.2 to 0.4 mg/kg intravenously or 0.5 to 1.0 mg/kg intramuscularly) that does not synergize with general anesthetics in causing respiratory depression and prolonged emergence.[89] Nonetheless, its principal side effect is drowsiness. Sympathetic stimulation (eg, tachycardia, increased cardiac output, hyper- and hypotension, and dysrhythmias) occurs, especially with rapid intravenous administration. Benzquinamide also has mild central anticholinergic actions that may manifest as hallucinations, disorientation, or confusion.

DIPHENIDOL. Diphenidol, structurally not related to other antiemetics, acts at the vestibular apparatus, making it especially well suited for use in patients who have had surgery of the middle and inner ear or who have Ménière's disease. This antiemetic is available only for oral use (25 mg), and its principal side effects are mental disturbances related to its similar central anticholinergic action.

ONDANSETRON. Ondansetron, a serotonin type-3 receptor antagonist, has no effect on cholinergic, adrenergic, histaminic, or dopaminergic receptors and does not appear to synergize with central nervous system depressants. It is increasingly popular and is one of the most effective antiemetics currently available but is very expensive compared with other agents.[90–92] Some[90,91] but not all[38] evidence suggests that the antiemetic action of this drug is greater than its prevention of nausea.

PROPOFOL. This increasingly popular anesthetic already has been noted to be associated with a decreased incidence of nausea and vomiting.[46–48,94,95] Recent limited work suggests that when it is administered prophylactically in very small dosages (an initial bolus of 0.1 mg/kg followed by a continuous infusion of 1 mg/kg/h), nausea and vomiting also are decreased in patients with cancer.[96] What application this therapy might have to anesthetized patients remains to be seen.

REFERENCES

1. Bellville JW: Postanesthetic nausea and vomiting. Anesthesiology 22:773, 1961
2. Brown HG: The applied anatomy of vomiting. Br J Anaesth 35: 136, 1963
3. Borison HL, Wang SCP: Physiology and pharmacology of vomiting. Pharmacol Rev 5:193, 1953
4. McCarthy LE, Borison HL, Spiegel PK, et al: Vomiting: radiological and oscillographic correlates in the decerebrate cat. Pharmacol Rev 5:193, 1953
5. Gibbs D: Diseases of the alimentary system: nausea and vomiting. Br Med J 2:1489, 1976
6. Burtles R, Peckett BW: Postoperative vomiting. Br J Anaesth 29:114, 1957
7. Smessaert A, Schehr CA, Artusio JF: Nausea and vomiting in the immediate postanesthetic period. JAMA 170:2072, 1959
8. Bellville JW, Bross IDJ, Howland WS: Postoperative nausea and vomiting: IV. factors related to postoperative nausea and vomiting. Anesthesiology 21:186, 1960
9. Cohen MM, Cameron CB, Duncan PG: Pediatric anesthesia morbidity and mortality in the perioperative period. Anesth Analg 70:160, 1990
10. Purkis IE: Factors that influence postoperative vomiting. Can Anaesth Soc J 11:335, 1964
11. Palazzo MGA, Strunin L: Anaesthesia and emesis: I. etiology. Can Anaesth Soc J 31:178, 1984
12. Cookson RF: Mechanisms and treatment of postoperative nausea and vomiting. In Davis CJ, Lake-Bakaar GV, Grahame-Smith DG (eds): Nausea and vomiting: mechanisms and treatment. Berlin: Springer-Verlag, 1986
13. Rowley MP, Brown TCK: Postoperative vomiting in children. Anaesth Intensive Care 10:309, 1982
14. Boulton TB: Oral chlorpromazine hydrochloride: a clinical trial in thoracic surgery. Anaesthesia 10:233, 1955
15. Knapp MR, Beecher HK: Postanesthetic nausea, vomiting, and retching: evaluation of the antiemetic drugs dimenhydrinate (Dramamine), chlorpromazine, and pentobarbital sodium. JAMA 10:373, 1956
16. Beattie WS, Lindblad T, Buckley DN, et al: The incidence of postoperative nausea and vomiting in women undergoing laparoscopy is influenced by the day of the menstrual cycle. Can J Anaesth 38:298, 1991
17. Dundee JW, Nicholl RM, Moore J: Studies of drugs given before anaesthesia: III. a method for the studying of their effects on postoperative vomiting and nausea. Br J Anaesth 34:572, 1962
18. Phillips OC, Nelson AJ, Lyons WB, et al: The effect of Trilafon on postanesthetic nausea, retching and vomiting: a controlled study. Anesth Analg 37:341, 1958
19. Phillips OC, Nelson AC, Lyons WB, et al: The effect of Trilafon on postanesthetic nausea, retching and vomiting: continued study. Anesth Analg 39:38, 1960
20. Riding JE: Postanesthetic vomiting. Proc R Soc Med 53:671, 1960
21. Morrison JD, Hill GB, Dundee JW: Studies of drugs given before anaesthesia: XV. evaluation of the method of study after 10,000 observations. Br J Anaesth 40:890, 1968
22. Riding JE: Minor complications of general anaesthesia. Br J Anaesth 47:91, 1975
23. Comroe JH, Dripps RD: Reactions to morphine in ambulatory and bed patients. Surg Gynecol Obstet 89:221, 1948
24. Wangeman CP, Hawk MH: The effects of morphine, atropine and scopolamine on human subjects. Anesthesiology 3:24, 1942
25. Robbie DS: Postanesthetic vomiting and antiemetic drugs. Anaesthesia 14:349, 1959
26. Dundee JW, Loan WB, Morrison JD: Studies of drugs given before anaesthesia: XIX. the opiates. Br J Anaesth 42:54, 1970
27. Feldman SA: A comparative study of four premedications. Anaesthesia 18:169, 1963
28. Dundee JW, Moore J, Clarke RSJ: Studies of drugs given before anaesthesia: V. pethidine 100 mg alone and with atropine or hyoscine before anaesthesia. Br J Anaesth 36:703, 1964

29. Gold MI: Postoperative vomiting in the recovery room. Br J Anaesth 41:143, 1969
30. Armer AL: The control of postoperative nausea with the use of dimenhydrinate. Journal of Oral Surgery 10:225, 1952
31. Dent SJ, Ramachandra V, Stephen CR: Postoperative vomiting: incidence, analysis and therapeutic measures in 3,000 patients. Anesthesiology 16:564, 1955
32. Bellville JW, Bross IDJ, Howland WS: Postoperative nausea and vomiting: V. antiemetic efficacy of trimethobenzamide and perphenazine. Clin Pharmacol Ther 1:590, 1960
33. Lind B, Breivik H: Metoclopramide and perphenazine in the prevention of postoperative nausea and vomiting. Br J Anaesth 42:614, 1970
34. Patton CM Jr, Moon MR, Dannemiller FJ: The prophylactic antiemetic effect of droperidol. Anesth Analg 53:361, 1974
35. Wetchler BV, Collins IS, Jacob L: Antiemetic effects of droperidol on the ambulatory surgery patient. Anesthesiol Rev 9:23, 1982
36. Korttila K, Kauste A, Tuominen M, et al: Droperidol prevents and treats nausea and vomiting after enflurane anesthesia. Eur J Anaesth 2:379, 1985
37. Wheaton NE: Comparison of benzquinamide hydrochloride and droperidol in preventing postoperative nausea and vomiting following general outpatient anesthesia. J AANA 54:322, 1985
38. Leeser J, Lip H: Prevention of postoperative nausea and vomiting using ondansetron, a new, selective, 5-HT_3 receptor antagonist. Anesth Analg 72:751, 1991
39. Larijani GE, Gratz I, Afshar M, et al: Treatment of postoperative nausea and vomiting using ondansetron: a randomized double-blind comparison with placebo. Anesth Analg 73:246, 1991
40. Breivik H, Lind B: Antiemetic and propulsive peristaltic properties of metoclopramide. Br J Anaesth 43:400, 1971
41. Cohen SE, Woods WA, Wyner J: Antiemetic efficacy of droperidol and metoclopramide. Anesthesiology 60:67, 1984
42. Tracey JA, Holland AJC, Unger L: Morbidity in minor gynaecological surgery: a comparison of halothane, enflurane, and isoflurane. Br J Anaesth 54:1213, 1982
43. Clarke RSJ: Nausea and vomiting. Br J Anaesth 56:19, 1984
44. Dundee JW, Kirwan MJ, Clarke RSJ: Anaesthesia and premedication as factors in postoperative vomiting. Acta Anaesthesiol Scand 9:223, 1965
45. Doze V, Shafer A, White PF: Propofol–nitrous oxide versus thiopental–isoflurane–nitrous oxide for general anesthesia. Anesthesiology 69:63, 1988
46. Gunawardene RD, White DC: Propofol and emesis. Anaesthesia 43:65, 1988
47. Korttila K, Faure E, Apfelbaum J, et al: Recovery from propofol versus thiopental–isoflurane in patients undergoing outpatient anesthesia (abstract). Anesthesiology 69:A564, 1988
48. Moore DC, Bridenbaugh LD, VanAckeren EG, et al: Control of postoperative vomiting with perphenazine (Trilafon): a double-blind study. Anesthesiology 19:72, 1958
49. Bonica JJ, Crepps W, Monk B, et al: Postoperative nausea and vomiting. West J Surg Obstet Gynecol 67:332, 1959
50. Rising S, Dodgson MS, Steen PA: Isoflurane v fentanyl for outpatient laparoscopy. Acta Anaesthesiol Scand 29:251, 1985
51. Parkhouse J, Henrie JR, Duncan GM, et al: Nitrous oxide analgesia in relation to mental performance. J Pharmacol Exp Ther 128:44, 1960
52. Steubner EA: Nitrous oxide: analgesia or anesthesia. Dent Clin North Am 17:51, 1973
53. Cook TL, Smith M, Starkweather JA, et al: Behavioral effects of trace and subanesthetic halothane and nitrous oxide in man. Anesthesiology 49:419, 1978
54. Hornbein TF, Eger EI II, Winter PM, et al: The minimum alveolar concentration of nitrous oxide in man. Anesth Analg 61: 553, 1982
55. Alexander GD, Skupski JN, Brown EM: The role of nitrous oxide in postoperative nausea and vomiting. Anesth Analg 63:A175, 1984
56. Lonie DS, Harper NJN: Nitrous oxide anaesthesia and vomiting: the effect of nitrous oxide anaesthesia on the incidence of vomiting following gynaecological laparoscopy. Anaesthesia 41:703, 1986
57. Muir JJ, Warner MA, Buck CF, et al: The role of nitrous oxide in producing postoperative nausea and vomiting: a randomized and blinded prospective study. Anesthesiology 66:513, 1987
58. Korttila K, Hovorka J, Erkola O: Nitrous oxide does not increase the incidence of nausea and vomiting after isoflurane anesthesia. Anesth Analg 66:761, 1987
59. Melnick BM, Johnson LS: Effects of eliminating nitrous oxide in outpatient anesthesia. Anesthesiology 67:982, 1987
60. Dhamee MS, Gandhi SK, Callen KM, et al: Morbidity after outpatient anesthesia: a comparison of different endotracheal anesthetic techniques for laparoscopy (abstract). Anesthesiology 57:A375, 1982
61. Hovorka J, Kortilla K, Erkola O: Nausea and vomiting after general anesthesia with isoflurane, enflurane or fentanyl in combination with nitrous oxide and oxygen. Eur J Anaesthesiol 5: 177, 1988
62. Bloomfield E, Hilberman M, Brown P, et al: Postoperative nausea and vomiting: a comparison of sufentanil, nitrous oxide, and isoflurane. Cleve Clin J Med 55:549, 1988
63. King MJ, Milazkiewicz R, Carli F, et al: Influence of neostigmine on postoperative vomiting. Br J Anaesth 61:403, 1988
64. Ratra CK, Badola RP, Bhargava KP: A study of factors concerned in emesis during spinal anaesthesia. Br J Anaesth 44:1208, 1972
65. Smith JM: Postoperative vomiting in relation to anaesthetic time. Br Med J 2:217, 1945
66. Lonie DS, Harper NJN: Nitrous oxide anaesthesia and vomiting: the effect of nitrous oxide anaesthesia on the incidence of vomiting following gynaecological laparoscopy. Anaesthesia 41:703, 1986
67. Abramowitz MD, Oh TH, Epstein BS, et al: The antiemetic effect of droperidol following outpatient strabismus surgery in children. Anesthesiology 59:579, 1983
68. Hardy J-F, Charest J, Giroouard G, et al: Nausea and vomiting after strabismus surgery in preschool children. Can Anaesth Soc J 33:57, 1986
69. Olsson GL, Hallen B, Hambraeus-Johnzon K: Aspiration during anaesthesia: a computer-aided study of 185,358 anaesthetics. Acta Anaesthesiol Scand 30:84, 1986
70. McCarroll SM, Mori S, Bras S, et al: The effect of gastric intubation and removal of gastric contents on the incidence of postoperative nausea and vomiting. Anesth Analg 70:S262, 1990
71. Andersen R, Krohg K: Pain as a major cause of postoperative nausea. Can Anaesth Soc J 23:366, 1976
72. Dundee JW, Ghaly RG, Bill KM, et al: Effect of stimulation of the P6 antiemetic point on postoperative nausea and vomiting. Br J Anaesth 63:612, 1989
73. Palazzo MGA, Strunin L: Anaesthesia and emesis: II. management and treatment. Can Anaesth Soc J 31:407, 1984
74. White PF, Shafer A: Nausea and vomiting: causes and prophylaxis. Semin Anesth 6:300, 1987
75. Dripps RD, Vandam LD, Pierce EC: The use of chlorpromazine in anesthesia and surgery. Arch Surg 142:774, 1955
76. Jackson SH, Schmitt MN, McGuire J, et al: Transdermal scopolamine as a preanesthetic drug and postoperative antinauseant and antiemetic (abstract). Anesthesiology 57:A330, 1982
77. Gibbons PA, Nicolson SC, Betts EK, et al: Scopolamine does not prevent postoperative emesis after pediatric eye surgery (abstract). Anesthesiology 61:A435, 1984
78. Uppington J, Dunnet J, Blogg CE: Transdermal hyoscine and postoperative nausea and vomiting. Anaesthesia 41:16, 1986
79. Tigerstedt I, Salmela L, Aroma U: Double-blind comparison of transdermal scopolamine, droperidol and placebo against postoperative nausea and vomiting. Acta Anaesthesiol Scand 32:454, 1988
80. Loper KA, Ready LB, Dorman BH: Prophylactic transdermal scopolamine patches reduce nausea in postoperative patients receiving epidural morphine. Anesth Analg 68:144, 1989
81. Koski EMJ, Mattila MAK, Knapik S, et al: Double blind comparison of transdermal hyoscine and placebo for the prevention of postoperative nausea. Br J Anaesth 64:16, 1990
82. Melnick B, Sawyer R, Karambelkar D, et al: Delayed side effects of droperidol after ambulatory general anesthesia. Anesth Analg 69:748, 1989

83. Adriani J, Summers FW, Antony SO: Is the prophylactic use of antiemetics in surgical patients justified? JAMA 175:661, 1961
84. Wood CD, Graybiel A: theory of antimotion sickness drug mechanisms. Aerospace Med 43:249, 1972
85. Wood CD: Antimotion sickness and antiemetic drugs. Drugs 17: 471, 1979
86. Freeman LA: Ephedrine and hydroxyzine as treatment for postoperative nausea and vomiting: a study of 40 problem patients (abstract). Presented at the annual meeting of the Society for Ambulatory Anesthesia, April 1989
87. Rothenberg S, Parnass S, Newman L, et al: Ephedrine minimizes postoperative nausea and vomiting in outpatients (abstract). Anesthesiology 71:A322, 1989
88. Poler SM, White PF: Does ephedrine decrease nausea and vomiting after outpatient anesthesia? (abstract). Anesthesiology 71: A995, 1989
89. Mull TD, Smith TC: Comparison of the ventilatory effects of two antiemetics, benzquinamide and prochlorperazine. Anesthesiology 40:581, 1974
90. Alon E, Himmelseher S: Ondansetron in the treatment of postoperative vomiting: a randomized, double-blind comparison with droperidol and metoclopramide. Anesth Analg 75:561, 1992
91. Dundee JW, McMillan CM: Antiemetic or antinauseant effect of ondansetron? Anesth Analg 74:467, 1992
92. Bodner M, White PF: Antiemetic efficacy of ondansetron after outpatient laparoscopy. Anesth Analg 73:250, 1991
93. Watcha MF, Simeon RM, White PW, et al: Effect of propofol on the incidence of postoperative vomiting after strabismus surgery in pediatric outpatients. Anesthesiology 75:204, 1991
94. Weir PM, Munroe HM, Reynolds PI, et al: Propofol infusion and the incidence of emesis in pediatric outpatients. Anesth Analg 76:760, 1993
95. Scher CS, Amar D, McDowall RH, et al: Use of propofol for the prevention of chemotherapy-induced nausea and emesis in oncology patients. Can J Anaesth 39:170, 1992

FURTHER READING

Cookson RF: Mechanisms and treatment of postoperative nausea and vomiting. In Davis CJ, Lake-Bakaar GV, Grahame-Smith DG (eds): Nausea and vomiting: mechanisms and treatment. Berlin: Springer-Verlag, 1986

Haigh CG, Kaplan JA, Durham JM, et al: Nausea and vomiting after gynaecological surgery: a meta-analysis of factors affecting their incidence. Br J Anaesth 71:517, 1993

Palazzo MGA, Strunin L: Anaesthesia and emesis: I. etiology. Can Anaesth Soc J 31:178, 1984

Palazzo MGA, Strunin L: Anaesthesia and emesis: II. management and treatment. Can Anaesth Soc J 31:407, 1984

Watcha MF, White PF: Postoperative nausea and vomiting: its etiology, treatment, and prevention. Anesthesiology 77:162, 1992

Complications in Anesthesiology, second edition, edited by Nikolaus Gravenstein and Robert R. Kirby. Lippincott-Raven Publishers, Philadelphia © 1996.

CHAPTER 51

Inhalation Anesthesia and Hepatic Injury

Burnell R. Brown

A wide variety of physiologic variations occur during the course of inhalation anesthesia. Examples are loss of consciousness, depression of myocardial contractibility, decreases in blood pressure, and altered renal function. These changes, strictly speaking, are pathologic, but they may be accepted by the anesthesiologist because they usually are ephemeral and controllable and cause no lasting detrimental effects.

In a similar manner, numerous functions of the liver are transiently decreased during clinical anesthesia. A partial list includes inhibition of mitochondrial oxidation, urea synthesis, bilirubin formation, and drug biotransformation.[1,2] Temporary perturbations in standard liver function tests (such as bromsulphalein retention) result, not unexpectedly, when enzymatic processes are interrupted by potent anesthetic drugs.

Liver blood flow via the portal vein and hepatic artery is reduced during anesthesia and is further compromised by surgical tools such as retractors and pads. All of these changes, however, are fully reversible. Akin to unconsciousness and negative cardiac inotropic effects, they are not only temporary but also are pharmacologically dose-related, diminishing in magnitude with decreasing concentrations of anesthetics.

This chapter is concerned with immutable pathologic changes in the liver occurring after general inhalation anesthesia. In broad terms, hepatic injury that follows an anesthetic can be ascribed to an unpredictable problem directly caused by the anesthetic or to other reasons. The causes of postoperative jaundice are legion.

THE HAZARDS OF PREEXISTING LIVER DISEASE

Because of the lack of sensitivity of tests that specifically indict halogenated anesthetics as vectors for hepatic necrosis, preexisting liver disease is often overlooked as a cause of postoperative jaundice. This omission is of concern because previous liver disease is unequivocally the most common event precipitating severe postoperative hepatic failure.

Schemel[3] found unrecognized parenchymal liver disease in a series of patients who had routine liver function tests performed on the day of admission for elective surgery. The incidence of abnormal values was approximately 1 in 700 routine admissions. Surgery was canceled in these patients pending further evaluation. In 30% jaundice developed.

Mortality Rates

Viral Hepatitis

Mortality rates for surgical patients with unrecognized viral hepatitis can only be estimated because ethical consideration preclude detailed prospective studies. However, the additional stresses of anesthesia and surgery may readily lead to worsening of viral hepatitis. Hepatitis A, common infectious hepatitis, has a low mortality rate, less than 0.1%, in patients not undergoing surgery. Hepatitis B and non-A, non-B hepatitis (including hepatitis C) have higher mortality rates. A study published in 1963 indicated that surgery and anesthesia in patients with viral hepatitis caused a mortality rate of 10%.[4] A later study of unrecognized viral hepatitis after exploratory laparotomy yielded an incredible 100% mortality rate in a small series.[5]

Cirrhosis

The patient with recognized or unrecognized cirrhosis is unquestionably at risk of complications after surgery and anesthesia. A review of surgical risk for the cirrhotic published in 1962 revealed an appalling overall mortality rate of 25%.[6] Aranha and colleagues[7] reviewed mortality and morbidity rates of 429 known cirrhotics operated on for cholecystectomy. Even for mild to moderate cirrhotics (defined by prothrombin times < 2.5 seconds greater than control) the mortality rate was 9%.

Implications

Studies such as these emphasize that diagnosis of parenchymal liver disease can be overlooked preoperatively and that the results of these mistakes on postoperative mortality are grave. Rather than indictment of an anesthetic as a cause of postoperative jaundice, a far more common scenario is subjection of the patient to surgical intervention without previous knowledge that he or she had liver disease. This important fact must be appreciated before discussions of the much rarer postoperative anesthetic-induced hepatic necrosis.

ANESTHESIA AS A CAUSE OF LIVER NECROSIS

Chloroform

Reports of jaundice and hepatic necrosis after the administration of inhalation anesthetics have appeared for more than 80 years. The early clinical and experimental work on the association of chloroform with fatal liver injury, which led to condemnation of the anesthetic by the Committee on Anesthesia of the American Medical Association in 1912, has been reviewed by Dykes.[8] Although *delayed chloroform poisoning* (or "hepatic necrosis") after chloroform was anecdotally recognized as a true entity, neither incidence nor absolute cause–effect relation was proven after anesthesia in humans during the seven decades of its popularity. In fact, Sykes stated the death rate with chloroform anesthesia was 1 in 3000, comparable to statistics of modern times, and the majority of these deaths resulted from cardiac, not hepatic, complications.[9]

Halothane

Because of the association of halogenated hydrocarbons with hepatic necrosis, the effects of halothane on liver function were studied extensively in the 1950s in animals and humans before its release for widespread clinical use. Minor morphologic changes, primarily fatty infiltration without necrosis, were observed in some animals after exposure.[10] The likelihood of hepatic necrosis in humans was considered to be no greater with halothane than with other inhalation anesthetics; the only abnormality was a transient increase in bromsulphalein retention,[11,12] which is also observed with nonhalogenated inhalation anesthetics.

All currently used halogenated anesthetics have been associated, at least anecdotally, with liver damage after surgery. Throughout this chapter, reference is frequently made to halothane. This particular halogenated anesthetic is selected because of its widespread (though diminishing) use and because it has been the subject of extensive toxicologic study.

Early Reports of Hepatotoxicity

Shortly after the clinical introduction of halothane in 1958, isolated case reports appeared suggesting a link between it and postanesthetic hepatic necrosis.[13–15] In 1963, three series of cases of severe hepatic dysfunction after halothane anesthesia were reported.[16–18] Of the 15 patients studied, 6 died of massive hepatic necrosis, and in 6, liver injury developed after a second halothane anesthetic.

Clinical Presentation

These and other early case reports indicated that liver injury associated with halothane administration strongly resembled viral hepatitis. Clinical features included fever, anorexia, nausea, vomiting, malaise, lethargy, and pain in the right upper quadrant, which appeared before clinical jaundice. Physical findings included minimal to moderate liver enlargement with tenderness. Laboratory findings were consistent with nonspecific hepatocellular dysfunction: increases in serum bilirubin concentration, serum transaminase concentrations, prothrombin time, and bromsulphalein retention.

Pathologic findings at autopsy included massive hepatic centrilobular and midzonal necrosis that frequently extended to entire hepatic lobules. Vacuolar cytoplasmic degeneration was present in cells peripheral to the central necrosis. These observations were so nonspecific that they engendered (and still do) debate regarding whether an entity such as *halothane-related jaundice* or *halothane hepatotoxicity* exists.

Proposed Mechanisms

Two interesting corollaries that subsequently would receive a great deal of attention emerged from these early clinical reports: the association of hepatic necrosis with the administration of a second halothane anesthetic; and Lindenbaum and Lieffer's observation of leukopenia and eosinophilia in several patients,[17] suggesting an allergic process. Thus, *halothane sensitization*, by way of an immunologic process leading to liver damage on subsequent exposure was hypothesized.[18] This hypothesis received support by Tygstrup, who reported that a patient became jaundiced after a second and third halothane anesthetic.[19] Liver biopsies on both occasions did not confirm a specific histologic pattern but rather revealed changes similar to viral hepatitis.

Publication of these early reports stimulated investigation to determine the etiologic role of halothane in postanesthetic liver dysfunction and the incidence of this problem. Perhaps because of abysmal failure to reproduce this hepatic dysfunction in the laboratory, early efforts used epidemiologic methods, principally large-scale retrospective case analysis. Later, intense laboratory immunologic and biochemical studies were used.

THE NATIONAL HALOTHANE STUDY

Shortly after the first isolated case reports of massive hepatic necrosis after halothane anesthesia, the Committee on Anesthesia of the National Academy of Science–National Research Council appointed a group to study clinical aspects of halothane anesthesia, with special attention to the association of postanesthetic hepatic necrosis. Initially, a prospective, randomized clinical trial was planned. After publication of several new case reports, however, the prospective study was abandoned in favor of a retrospective survey, with the hope that this approach would quickly clarify the issue and obviate extensive clinical trials.

Epidemiologic Features

The National Halothane Study surveyed 856,515 general anesthetic administrations in 34 hospitals during the period from 1959 to 1962. It had two major goals. The first was to compare halothane with other general anesthetics with respect to the incidence of fatal hepatic necrosis within 6 weeks after surgery. The second was to compare halothane with other general anesthetics with regard to hospital mortality. A total of 16,840 deaths, with 10,171 autopsies were in the series. A panel of pathologists examined microscopic liver sections from cases of possible hepatic necrosis and independently rated the extent of the necrosis.

Findings

Eighty-two of the autopsied cases had massive hepatic necrosis (1 in 10,000 anesthetic administrations) including an incidence of 1.7 in 10,000 with cyclopropane, 0.69 in 10,000 with nitrous oxide–barbiturate, and 0.49 in 10,000 with ether. Many of these cases were definitely of nonanesthetic cause. Seven of the 82 cases had received a previous halothane anesthetic within 6 weeks. The clinical course of these unexplained cases of massive hepatic necrosis included fever, followed in rapid progression by jaundice, confusion, and hepatic coma. Clinical signs appeared within 2 to 3 days after surgery. The course was rapid and similar to fulminant viral hepatitis. Histologic appearance was similar to viral or drug-induced hepatitis in 6 of the 7 cases. Although the overall incidence of explained jaundice was higher with cyclopropane, a definite association of unexplained massive hepatic necrosis after exposure to halothane was noted.

Conclusions

The conclusions of the National Halothane Study were that fatal postoperative hepatic necrosis after single or multiple administrations of halothane could not be excluded. Of interest, halothane had a strong record of safety, with an overall mortality of 1.87%, compared with the average mortality of 1.93% for other general anesthetics based on standardized patient populations for the entire study.

This large study was not conclusive, however. It can be interpreted to verify or contradict the existence of halothane hepatitis depending on the views of the reader. Its retrospective nature and its volunteer bias were salient deficiencies. That is, before initiation of the National Halothane Study, four of the seven cases of unexplained fatal necrosis had been published, and two more were known to be a stimulus for the study.

MULTIPLE ADMINISTRATIONS OF HALOTHANE

Many of the early case reports indicated a higher incidence of unexplained jaundice after second administrations of halothane. Dykes and associates specifically looked for this relation in a retrospective study of 47,000 general anesthetics.[20] In eight patients clinical and laboratory evidence of hepatic disease developed after halothane. Four of these eight had been anesthetized previously with halothane, without evidence of liver problems.

Little reviewed the literature before 1968 and found 404 cases of liver dysfunctions after halothane anesthesia.[21] Data concerning the number of administrations were available for 346 patients. Forty-nine percent had two or more exposures. Klatskin reported 41 cases of "well-documented" halothane-associated hepatitis from the literature and another nine from personal records.[22] In 68%, jaundice followed a second exposure to the anesthetic.

Fulminant Hepatic Failure Surveillance Study

The Fulminant Hepatic Failure Surveillance Study was established to collect and reviewed cases of liver failure to determine possible etiologic factors. This type of registry was one recommendation of the National Halothane Study. By 1970, 318 patients in all stages of hepatic coma had been reported.[23] Sixty-four (20%) of the 318 patients were assumed to have halothane-associated hepatic failure. Some of these patients, however, had blood transfusions, usually during operation. A history of multiple halothane exposures was present in 40 (77%) of the 64 cases.

Two major criticisms were directed at this study, and, indeed are applicable to all such series. First, significant and indeterminate bias is introduced when cases are reported with the presumptive diagnosis made by the reporting physician. In fact, McPeek and Gilvert stated, "In voluntary case reporting, persons report what they want. There is no control over bias nor even any good way of knowing what the bias is towards."[24] Second, the lack of a known sample group or patient population makes a determination of incidence impossible.

Other Reports

Sharpstone and Colleagues

Sharpstone and colleagues reported 11 cases of hepatic dysfunction after two or more halothane anesthetics at two hospitals over a 4-year period.[25]

Six deaths in this series resulted from massive liver necrosis of the hepatocellular type, but many of these patients had other disorders that could have resulted in liver damage, such as blood transfusion and sepsis.[26]

Moult and Sherlock

Moult and Sherlock reviewed the clinical and laboratory findings of 26 patients among those referred to their hepatology department whose illness was attributed to halothane and in whom no other cause for liver disease could be found.[27] All had the onset of jaundice within 15 days of a halothane anesthetic, and none had perioperative hypotension or severe congestive failure before development of hepatic problems. Eight had received a blood transfusion within the month before the onset of jaundice. Twenty-four of these 26 patients had multiple halothane anesthetics, including 18 who had halothane twice within 28 days.

Two other findings of importance in this study were the lack of positive immunologic correlates using lymphocyte transformation and antimitochondrial antibodies, and an inability to exclude viral hepatitis histologically. Interesting, Sherlock, who previously hypothesized that the so-called syndrome of halothane hepatitis was an immunologic phenomenon, suggested other etiologic factors after the publication of this report.

Carney and Van Dyke

Carney and Van Dyke reviewed nearly 600 cases, from the literature and from their own institution, of jaundice or hepatitis occurring within 4 weeks after exposure to halothane.[28] To reduce bias, they selected cases for analysis based on certain criteria, rather than on the reporting author's diagnosis. Cases were eliminated when a cause other than halothane was demonstrated convincingly; when postoperative jaundice was present, but no histologic or biochemical evidence of hepatocellular damage could be found; when minimal abnormalities of liver function (serum glutamic-oxaloacetic transaminase <100 IU) were unaccompanied by clinical findings; when minimal focal hepatic necrosis was found incidentally in autopsies; when cases were reported in groups without individual details; when the patient was less than 13 years old; and when circumstances of occupational exposure were present.

Using these criteria, they developed a series of 234 cases. Of these, 120 were from the National Halothane Study, 102 were published subsequent to that study, and 12 were from the investigator's own institution, collected over a 3-year period. The number of halothane exposures and the interval between them were analyzed in all 234 cases. The incidence of postoperative liver dysfunction after repeated halothane exposure within a 3-month period was 50%.

Mushin and Colleagues

Mushin and colleagues analyzed 67 cases of jaundice after halothane anesthesia reported at the Committee of Safety of Drugs of England and Wales between 1964 and 1970.[29] Of these, 68% had two halothane anesthetics within a 4-week period. They then reviewed 74 patients who had jaundice after a second halothane anesthetic and found that in 85% halothane had been administered twice within 1 month. Subsequently, they extrapolated a 10-year analysis of anesthetic practice in their own institution to the total surgical population in England and Wales for 1964 to 1967. Based on these data, they estimated the incidence of jaundice after two halothane anesthetics within 1 month to be between 1 in 11,000 and 1 in 38,000. This study, however, was criticized because, similar to the National Halothane Study, a causal relation between halothane and postanesthetic jaundice in each case that they reported was deemed highly unlikely.

Trowell and Colleagues

An article that created considerable resurgence of interest in this problem was that of Trowell and associates.[30] In a series of 39 patients with carcinoma of the cervix treated with radium and requiring repeated general anesthetics, they found that the group anesthetized with halothane had a far greater increase in serum glutamic-pyruvic transaminase concentrations than a control group whose primary anesthetic was nitrous oxide. None of the 21 patients in the group treated with nitrous oxide had serum glutamic-pyruvic transaminase concentrations increasing to more than 100 IU. However, in none of the patients in this series did overt liver disease develop; they merely showed serum glutamic-pyruvic transaminase increases.

Allen and Downing

In direct contrast to Trowell's report, Allen and Downing studied 400 African women with multiple exposure to both halothane and enflurane anesthesia.[31] They found no changes in the concentrations of serum glutamic-oxaloacetic transaminase and serum glutamic-pyruvic transaminase, or serum lactate dehydrogenase, alkaline phosphatase, or bilirubin.

Questions and Interpretations

The differences in these studies have yet to be resolved. The following question comes to mind: is a genetic predisposition to development of this syndrome present among Caucasian women, or are environmental or drug-related differences prevalent? Certainly the issue of heredity and susceptibility to the entity "halothane hepatitis" is an extremely attractive one. Hoft and coworkers[32] described three pairs of closely related Mexican-American women with a putative genetic susceptibility to hepatic damage after halothane. Farrell and associates published results linking phenytoin-induced lymphocyte epoxide formation with adverse liver reactions to halothane.[33] This study implies that a genetically determined metabolic disease is the cause of the syndrome. Certainly animal studies indicate varying susceptibilities depending on species and strain.[34]

POSSIBLE FACTORS CONTRIBUTING TO HEPATIC INJURY

Middle Age, Female Sex, and Obesity

Several possible contributing factors have been associated with halothane-related liver injury (Table 51-1). Obesity was pres-

TABLE 51-1
Possible Factors Contributing to Halothane-related Liver Injury

- Obesity
- Multiple procedures
- Female gender
- Middle age
- History of hepatic dysfunction after halothane
- Preexisting liver disease
- Mexican-American ethnicity
- Major surgery
- Hepatic enzyme induction

ent in 56% and 40% of patients in two series.[29,35] Another report stated that female sex and middle age are common findings and cause the most concern, when present, of the possible factors contributing to halothane liver injury.[36] Carney and van Dyke stated that unexplained jaundice after the administration of halothane anesthesia occurred more frequently in obese, middle-aged persons.[28] In fact, all but one of the 26 patients reported by Moult and Sherlock were older than 40 years.[27] Thus, from an epidemiologic point of view, middle-aged, obese women appear to be at greatest risk for development of jaundice after the administration of halothane. Mexican-American ethnicity may add another risk factor.

TABLE 51-2
Proposed Etiologic Factors in Halothane Hepatitis

- Viral hepatitis (indistinguishable anatomically and clinically)
- Allergic reactions
- Liver hypoxia
- Liver ischemia
- Biotransformation
  - Oxidative
  - Reductive
- Haptene formation (after biotransformation)

Concurrent Liver Disease

Early in its clinical use, halothane was restricted for patients with concurrent liver disease or a past history of liver disease. The scientific evidence indicating that halothane administration per se may have an adverse effect on patients with cirrhosis or patients who have had viral hepatitis in the past is tenuous to say the least. The National Halothane Study did not find an increased incidence of massive hepatic necrosis after biliary tract surgery. A review of a large series of patients with cirrhosis of the liver and clinical and laboratory evidence of liver dysfunction who were also undergoing portocaval shunting procedures found no difference in mortality or in postoperative hepatic failure between halothane and nonhalothane anesthetics.[37] Recall also that overall mortality rates are always high in liver disease patients undergoing surgery, whatever the anesthetic.

The present consensus is that preexisting liver disease, such as hepatitis or cirrhosis, does not enhance the susceptibility of the liver to injury by halothane.[38,39] In fact, the United States Food and Drug Administration lifted any restrictions to halothane use in patients with a past history of liver disease. Remember that the results that have been discussed come from retrospective surveys, usually based on a report of a small personal series and often enlarged by cases collected from the literature. In only a relatively few of these cases were new serologic tests used to exclude viral hepatitis. Unexplained postoperative fever does not contraindicate the use of halothane for subsequent anesthetics.[40]

PROPOSED ETIOLOGIES

A multitude of factors have been proposed to play a role in the development of halothane hepatitis (Table 51-2).

Viral Hepatitis

The inability to distinguish viral hepatitis from halothane-associated hepatitis, clinically and histologically, has generated considerable controversy.[26] The stress of anesthesia and surgery has been suggested to unmask incubating or subclinical viral hepatitis, result in a fulminant course of the disease, and culminate in massive, fatal hepatic necrosis as discussed earlier in this chapter. This type of fulminant course has been described after laparotomy in patients with jaundice and possible extrahepatic biliary obstruction, in whom viral hepatitis was eventually found to be the etiologic agent.[41] Indeed, many cases of hepatic necrosis routinely ascribed to halothane anesthesia are probably caused by viral hepatitis.

Although investigators have reported histologic and electron microscopic features that differentiate viral and halothane-associated hepatitis, the consensus is that the two diseases cannot be separated on a morphologic basis.[42] Sherlock stated that although some cases occur in which interesting differences are shown by light and electron microscopy, between halothane and viral hepatitis, the detection depends on the experience of the pathologist. Absolutely no diagnostic characteristics distinguish one from the other.[27,43]

Infectious hepatitis, characterized by a relatively short incubation period after fecal–oral transmission, is categorized as hepatitis A. Serum hepatitis with a longer incubation period and transmitted by parenteral exposure to human blood or blood products is known as hepatitis B. However, the overlap of incubation periods, 31 to 53 days for hepatitis A and 41 to 69 days for hepatitis B, is too great to make the differentiation useful clinically.[44]

Current hepatitis antigen testing methods in widespread use have yielded significant information concerning the prevalence of hepatitis B in its carrier state. Approximately 0.1% of the general population has B antigen when tested. Endemic hepatitis among an urban adult population may be caused by the hepatitis B virus, transmitted by a route other than parenteral.[45] Although incubation periods may be useful in differentiating viral from halothane-associated hepatitis, the incubation period may be less than 1 month in nearly 5% of hepatitis cases.[30]

Presence of hepatitis B antigen is of diagnostic value only if seroconversion can be documented. A lack of hepatitis B antigen is of little value, however, because the antigen may be present for only several days.[44] An early report described 22 patients with hepatitis associated with transfusion in whom no serologic evidence of hepatitis A, hepatitis B, or cytomegalic virus could be found.[46] Currently, about 90% of transfusion-associated hepatitis is caused by non-A, non-B hepatitis, including hepatitis C, with an incubation period and clinical course similar to those of hepatitis B.[47]

A death from massive hepatic necrosis after enflurane anesthesia eventually was found to be caused by a type of herpes virus, although the initial diagnosis had implicated the anesthetic as the cause.[48] Thus, the distinction between viral hepatitis and the syndrome of halothane hepatitis is certainly not clear.

Enflurane Hepatotoxicity

Although halothane has the longest use of modern anesthetics and has received the greatest amount of publicity and research with respect to hepatitis, several case reports of putative enflurane hepatotoxicity have been published.[49,50] In general, indictments against enflurane, and, in particular, isoflurane, have been weak and few. At the time that Lewis[50] collected his 24 possible cases of enflurane hepatitis, an estimated 13,000,000 administrations of the anesthetic had been given. This incidence of liver dysfunction (0.0002%) is astronomically lower than the incidence of unrecognized liver function abnormalities in surgical patients demonstrated by Schemel[3] (0.15%) and lower than the spontaneous attack rates of hepatitis A.

Because enflurane could not be incriminated except by exclusion, the cause–effect relation is not concrete. Dykes has commented that the case against enflurane is very weak indeed, particularly because it is predicated solely on a temporal association and exclusion of other (but not all) factors.[51] Eger and colleagues conclude that the case for enflurane hepatotoxicity is not supported by all available evidence (Fig. 51-1).[52]

Allergic Reactions

After the early case reports of death from massive liver necrosis associated with halothane anesthesia, investigators attempted to reproduce this syndrome in animals. They were universally unsuccessful in these studies and postulated that halothane hepatitis was an allergic phenomenon specific only to humans. The supporting evidence for this theory included the higher incidence of liver necrosis after second administrations of the anesthetic, although many cases were reported in which only one anesthetic had been given. Several other features that suggested an immunologic or allergic basis for halothane-associated hepatitis included arthralgias, eosinophilia, and skin rashes.

This theory of halothane-associated allergic liver damage predominated throughout the 1960s. It was reinforced by two clinical studies. In the first, that of Paronetto and Popper,[53] lymphocytes from patients with suspected halothane hepatitis were harvested and incubated with halothane in the presence of tritiated thymidine. An increased incorporation of this nucleic acid, a test for allergy, was detected. The other evidence suggesting an allergic mechanism was that reported by Klatskin and Kimberg.[54] A subanesthetic concentration of halothane had been administered to an anesthesiologist who was known to have liver disease, possibly connected with occupational exposures. Shortly after this challenge, serum enzyme and other parameters indicating abnormal liver function were increased.

Critique

The difficulty with these studies is now apparent. The nonspecificity of the lymphocyte stimulation test has been documented.[55] Moreover, an idiosyncratic reaction that follows administration of a drug does not indicate the mechanism but merely that a drug reaction has occurred. When alterations in liver function follow administration of a small dose of halothane, an allergic reaction is not necessarily the cause. Many other mechanisms may be operant. Animal studies have failed

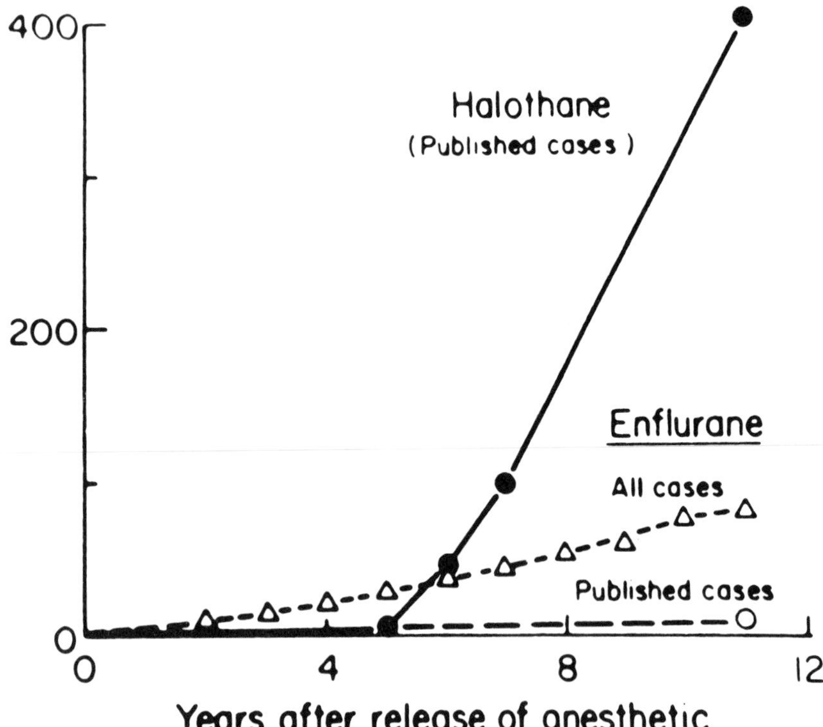

FIGURE 51-1. Total reported cases of liver injury or jaundice occurring after halothane or enflurane since the introduction of these anesthetics. The number of published reports of hepatic injury after halothane anesthesia dramatically increased about 5 years after the introduction of halothane (*solid circles*) into clinical practice. No such increase has appeared in the 11-year period since the release of enflurane, for all cases (*triangles*) or for published cases (*open circles*). (Eger SI, Smuckler EA, Ferrell LD, et al: Is enflurane hepatotoxic? Anesth Analg 65:21, 1986)

to substantiate an allergic basis with either halothane or its primary metabolite, trifluoroacetic acid.[56] Moreover, the syndrome is almost (<1 in 82,000) unknown among infants and children, who constitute the largest group at risk for allergic diseases.[57]

Nonetheless, given this theory of allergy, safe intervals between halothane exposures were postulated. Various investigators stated that halothane anesthesia should not be given for 3 to 12 months after a previous administration. These intervals were based on theoretic considerations, however, rather than on actual data. In fact, Bruce[58] stated that, given the absence of a reaction, the subsequent choices of anesthesia for the patient should be made by the anesthesiologist, based on experience and the requirements for surgery. He also noted that halothane may be the agent of choice in patients with chronic liver disease; if overall liver function is poor, mechanisms that produce liver damage also probably function poorly.

Currently, then, pure allergic origin is theoretic at best. However, if an allergy to halothane should be proven, once sensitization has occurred the patient should not be given halothane again, irrespective of the interval.

Liver Hypoxia

The blood supply of the liver is unusual in that more than 50% of oxygen used by the organ is derived from a low-pressure venous source, the portal vein. The regulation of total blood flow to the liver is interesting. The hepatic artery contains a muscular coat and sympathetic nerves so that it is capable of increasing or decreasing resistance to flow. The portal vein is not similarly endowed. When portal venous blood flow decreases, hepatic arterial resistance decreases and arterial inflow increases; conversely, when portal flow increases, hepatic arterial resistance increases and arterial inflow decreases. This is the major mechanism governing total hepatic blood supply.[59]

A multitude of factors can decrease hepatic blood flow, including hemorrhage, mechanical ventilation, laparotomy, position, and anesthetic drugs.[60,61] Severe hypoxia can produce hepatic damage. Potent inhalation anesthetics decrease hepatic blood flow; of the commonly used agents, the effect of halothane is greatest in this respect.[61] Shingu and others suggested that hypoxia coupled with states of low flow produced by anesthesia-induced circulatory depression are the cause of hepatic necrosis ascribed to the halogenated anesthetics.[62,63]

Hypoxia as a common unifying mechanism must however implicate all anesthetics including narcotics, barbiturates, and the nonhalogenated inhalation drugs. This relation does not seem likely. For example, the central nervous system is far more sensitive to hypoxia than is the liver. In fact animal experiments counter to the work of these investigators have been conducted to demonstrate that hypoxic damage and halothane induced injury are distinct entities.[64] In addition, patients with cyanotic congenital heart disease, who are more dependent on reductive metabolism have no differences in postoperative hepatic function compared with acyanotic patients.[65]

Biotransformation

Hepatotoxins

Hepatotoxicity of alkyl halides such as carbon tetrachloride and chloroform is attributed to interaction of highly reactive intermediates with liver cell macromolecules. The reactive intermediates are of an ephemeral nature and are produced by biotransformation of the parent molecules by the hepatic microsomal enzymes. This bioactivation of relativity inert substance into toxic intermediates is well documented as a major mechanism of chemical toxicity.[65–69] Little interest in biotransformation as a cause of anesthetic hepatotoxicity was apparent until the demonstration that clinically used halogenated inhalation anesthetics are biotransformed in animals[71] and humans.[72,73]

Halogenated Anesthetics

That hepatotoxicity caused by the "classic" hepatotoxins such as carbon tetrachloride and chloroform was predicated on biotransformation of these substances to reactive intermediates led to the theoretic conclusion that perhaps this was the ultimate mechanism of halogenated anesthetic hepatic toxicity. Stier and colleagues,[73] Rehder and colleagues,[74] and Cohen and colleagues[75] studied biotransformation of halothane in humans, initially concentrating on the oxidative metabolism of the anesthetic.

Certainly, oxidation is a most common type of biotransformation reaction, and it was not conceived that the trifluorocarbon bond could be broken by hepatic microsomal enzymes. However, Uehleke and associates[76] demonstrated in vivo that more covalent bonding of halothane metabolites occurred in nitrogen than in oxygen. The implications of this landmark paper were considerable. First, halothane can be biotransformed by a non–oxygen-dependent route ("reductive") as well as by classic oxidation; second, the metabolites formed during reduced oxygen biotransformation of halothane were reactive species, bonding avidly to contiguous hepatocyte proteins and lipoproteins, and producing micromolecular damage. This work was confirmed in vitro by Widger and coworkers.[77]

As a result of these studies, two animal models of hepatic destruction after clinically relevant inhaled concentration of halothane were generated. Previous experiments with animals failed to produce consistent hepatic lesions attributable to halothane and had been a source of great frustration. The first of these reliable hepatotoxicity models was produced by a "shotgun" induction of P-450 species responsible for reductive biotransformation using polychlorobiphenyls (Arochlor) as the inducing agent.[78]

ENZYME INDUCTION AND REDUCTIVE METABOLISM. Because polychlorobiphenyls may themselves originate abnormalities of liver function tests, a better animal model was developed. This model became known as the halothane–hypoxia model. Rats were induced with phenobarbital for several days, and then administered 1% halothane in a reduced oxygen environment (fraction of inspired oxygen 0.14). In this fashion, not only was the biotransformation of halothane induced (phenobarbital) but it was forced into a reductive mode by decreasing oxygen availability to the hepatic microsomal P-450 enzyme system.[79,80]

This model is specific: in rats adulthood and female sex is required. Various strains are more sensitive than others. In addition, exquisite species differences exist. Lesions can be produced in rats, cats, and guinea pigs, but not in mice and dogs. No degree of hepatic damage seems to parallel conversion of halothane to reductive metabolites (primarily 1,1,1-trifluoroethane and 1,1-difluoro-2-chloroethylene), and covalent binding. Metabolites of reductive biotransformation of halothane have been found in humans. However, real difficulties accrue to ascribing the human entity, halothane hepatitis, solely to increased reductive metabolism paralleling these animal models. In essence, the damage seen in animals is not nearly as severe as the massive hepatic necrosis that causes death in humans.

Biotransformation and Hapten Formation: A Unifying Concept

The pure allergy and the pure biotransformation theories of halothane toxicity are not, in all probability, directly applicable to the human situation of massive hepatic necrosis. Vergani and colleagues[81] demonstrated an in vitro sensitization of leukocytes from patients with putative halothane hepatitis to rabbit liver cells previously exposed to the anesthetic. This work was continued by the discovery, from patients with possible halothane hepatitis, of circulatory antibodies that bound to the cell surface of rabbit presensitized hepatocytes.

First, these investigations implicate a biotransformation of halothane as an initiating factor of hepatitis. Metabolites of halothane bind to liver protein and lipoprotein macromolecules to produce haptens that then supposedly act as antigens.[82] Thus speculation holds that the initiating process is biotransformation followed by antibody production to attack the liver. The interesting point is that oxidative, not reductive, metabolites apparently are responsible. The second point of interest is that it may be possible in specialized centers to differentiate "halothane hepatitis" by an antibody test, a diagnosis that until now has been impossible.

CLINICAL IMPLICATIONS

Prevention

The subject of direct, lasting hepatic complications from inhalation anesthetics is a sea of mystery, with some islands of knowledge, but generally pervaded by clouds of speculation, misinformation, and ignorance. Thus, hard and fast clinical guidelines insofar as prevention, diagnosis, and therapy are fraught with difficulty. At the present time, the recommendations in Table 51-3 are favored.

Although isolated case reports of children with hepatic necrosis have appeared, in general, the drug can be used liberally in these patients. A history of liver disease (unless caused by halothane, of course) definitely is not a contradiction to use of halothane, nor is use of any halogenated modern anesthetic.

TABLE 51-3
Prevention of Halothane Hepatitis

An ultraconservative user of halothane will avoid the drug in the following circumstances:

- History of undiagnosed jaundice after routine halothane anesthesia
- Closely spaced administrations. The ideal time between administrations cannot be defined because of lack of adequate knowledge. I recommend 6 months except in prepubertal patients, for whom more closely spaced anesthetics appear to be safe.
- Obesity. Halothane and other inhalation anesthetics undergo far more biotransformation per minimum alveolar concentration–hour administration in obese patients than in those of normal body mass.[84]
- Middle age in women
- Mexican-American ethnicity, particularly of female patients

Diagnosis

Halothane hepatitis probably is overdiagnosed. Anecdotal stories abound concerning the hepatologist who diagnoses halothane hepatitis in the jaundiced patient postoperatively when review of the anesthetic record shows the drug was not even used.

Transient Dysfunction

Conceivably, two forms of liver damage can be ascribed to halothane. The first of these is the common mild disturbance of liver function frequently observed after halothane anesthesia.[83,84] Speculation is that this entity is caused strictly by enhanced reductive biotransformation. It implies a short latency to onset (<24 hours), transient depression of liver function (<1 week), no permanent sequelae, and common occurrence.

Modification and enhancement might occur with drug-produced enzyme induction, obesity, and alterations of hepatic blood flow.[85] This cause would be consistent with the "challenge tests" that have been reported.[86] Absolute diagnosis is difficult, but early increased blood concentrations of reductive metabolites are a possibility. Therapy is not necessary because the problem should be self-limiting.

Halothane Hepatitis

The second form of halothane damage is the severe entity customarily termed halothane hepatitis. In light of present knowledge, this is in all likelihood a true antibody–antigen hepatocyte destruction initiated by a metabolite–hapten immunologic interaction. The disease carries with it a high lethality, approaching 50%. Diagnosis can be based on detection of the trifluorocetate antibody 8 to 10 days after the anesthetic. This type of halothane–liver interaction develops later than the pure biotransformation effect. Incidence of this complication is perhaps 1 in 9000 administrations. Therapy is conservative and generally fruitless. Orthotopic liver transplantation might be a consideration.

Enflurane, Isoflurane, and Desflurane

Currently available information indicates that enflurane, isoflurane, and desflurane do not share the magnitude or incidence of hepatic necrosis ascribed to halothane. Data are insufficient to preclude the use of these agents in most circumstances. Lessened degrees of biotransformation, more inherent stability of the molecules, and diminished partition coefficients are certainly responsible for the greater safety of enflurane and isoflurane in this regard. Again, previous liver disease does not prohibit their use. In fact, patients with severe liver disease handle the halogenated inhalation anesthetics far better than they do fixed, intravenously administered drugs that depend primarily on hepatic elimination for termination of action. Thus, they are unquestionably safer for the cirrhotic than numerous intravenously administered drugs.

SUMMARY

Although unproven, a substantial body of evidence suggests that on rare occasions, the anesthetic halothane can produce severe hepatic necrosis. Guidelines for use of halothane to reduce this danger have been discussed. The cause of this damage is probably a constellation of events initiated by biotransformation and followed by antigen formation.[87] Liver disease (unless caused by halothane) does not prohibit use of halogenated inhalation anesthetics.

Enflurane and isoflurane most likely have far less probability of generating severe hepatic necrosis and thus have fewer clinical sanctions imposed at this time.[88-90] Of the two, only enflurane is remotely likely to be a factor of importance, perhaps because it produces covalently bound liver antigens that react with antibodies in patients with halothane-induced hepatitis.[91] No clinical significance of this relation is known, but another technique may be advisable for subsequent anesthetics in a sensitized person. This approach may reduce, but probably will not eliminate postoperative hepatitis.[89]

REFERENCES

1. Biebuyck JF: Anesthesia and hepatic metabolism: current concepts of carbohydrate homeostasis. Anesthesiology 39:188, 1973
2. Brown BR Jr: The diphasic action of halothane on the oxidative metabolism of drugs by the liver: an *in vitro* study in the rat. Anesthesiology 35;241, 1971
3. Schemel WH: Unexpected hepatic dysfunction found by multiple laboratory screening. Anesth Analg 45:810, 1976
4. Harville DD, Summerskill WHJ: Surgery in acute hepatitis. JAMA 184:257, 1963
5. Powell-Jackson P, Greenway B, William R: Adverse effects of exploratory laparotomy in patients with unsuspected liver disease. Br J Surg 69:449, 1982
6. Lindemuth WW, Eisenberg MM: The surgical risk in cirrhosis of the liver. Arch Surg 86:77, 1962
7. Aranha GV, Sontag SJ, Greenlee HB: Cholecystectomy in cirrhotic patients: a formidable operation. Am J Surg 143:55, 1982
8. Dykes MHM: The early years: 1846-1912. Int Anesthesiol Clin 8:175, 1970
9. Sykes WS: Essays on the first hundred years of anesthesia, vol 2. Edinburgh: Churchill Livingstone, 1961: 87
10. Jones WM, Margolis G, Stephen CR: Hepatotoxicity of inhalation of anesthetic drugs. Anesthesiology 19:715, 1958
11. Little DM Jr, Barbour CM: Hepatic function following Fluothane anesthesia. Anesthesiology 19:105, 1958
12. Little DM Jr, Barbour, Given JB: Effects of Fluothane, cyclopropane, and either anesthesia on liver function. Surg Gynecol Obstet 197:712, 1958
13. Burnap TK, Galla SJ, Vandam LD: Anesthetic, circulatory, and respiratory effects of Fluothane. Anesthesiology 19:307, 1958
14. Virtue RW, Payne KW: Postoperative death after Fluothane. Anesthesiology 19:562, 1958
15. Temple RL, Cote RA, Gorens SW: Massive hepatic necrosis following general anesthesia. Anesth Analg 41:586, 1962
16. Brody GL, Sweet RB: Halothane anesthesia as a possible cause of massive hepatic necrosis. Anesthesiology 24:29, 1963
17. Lindenbaum J, Leiffer E: Hepatic necrosis associated with halothane anesthesia. N Engl J Med 268:525, 1963
18. Bunker JP, Blumenfeld CM: Liver necrosis after halothane anesthesia. N Engl J Med 28:531, 1963
19. Tygstrup M: Halothane hepatitis. Lancet 2:466, 1963
20. Dykes MHM, Wolzer SG, Slater EM, et al: Acute parenchymatous hepatic disease following general anesthesia. JAMA 193: 89, 1965
21. Little DM: Effect of halothane on hepatic function. In Greene NM (ed): Halothane. Philadelphia: FA Davis, 1968:134
22. Klatskin G: Mechanisms of toxic and drug induced hepatic injury. In Fink BR (ed): Toxicity of anesthetics. Baltimore: Williams & Wilkins, 1968: 159
23. Trey O: Case records of the Massachusetts General Hospital: case 10-1970. N Engl J Med 282:558, 1970
24. McPeek B, Gilvert JP: Onset of postoperative jaundice related to anesthetic history. Br Med J 3:615, 1974
25. Sharpstone P, Medley DRK, Williams SR: Halothane hepatitis: a preventable disease. Br Med J 50:448, 1971
26. Simpson BR, Strunin L, Walton B: The halothane dilemma: a case for the defense. Br Med J 4:96, 1971
27. Moult PGA, Sherlock S: Halothane related hepatitis. Q J Med 44:99, 1975
28. Carney FMT, Van Dyke RA: Halothane hepatitis: a critical review. Anesth Analg 51:135, 1972
29. Mushin WW, Rosen M, Jones EB: Posthalothane jaundice in relation to previous administration of halothane. Br Med J 3: 18, 1971
30. Trowell J, Peto R, Crampton-Smith A, et al: Controlled trial of repeated halothane anesthetics in patients with carcinoma of the uterine cervix treated with radium. Lancet 1:821, 1975
31. Allen PJ, Downing JW: A prospective study of hepatocellular function after repeated exposures to halothane or enflurane in women undergoing radium therapy for cervical cancer. Br J Anaesth 49:1035, 1977
32. Hoft RH, Bunker JP, Goodman IE, et al: Halothane hepatitis in three pairs of closely related women. N Engl J Med 304:1023, 1981
33. Farrell G, Prendergast D, Murray M: Halothane hepatitis: detection of a constitutional susceptibility factor. N Engl J Med 313:1310, 1985
34. Brown BR Jr: Pharmacogenetics and the halothane hepatitis mystery. Anesthesiology 55:93, 1981
35. Peters RL, Edmondson HA, Reynolds TB, et al: Hepatic necrosis associated with halothane anesthesia. Am J Med 47:748, 1976
36. Bottinger LE, Dalen E, Hallen B: Halothane induced liver damage: an analysis of the material reported to the Swedish Adverse Reaction Committee 1966-1973. Acta Anaesthesiol Scand 20: 40, 1976
37. Jones RR, Dawson B, Adson M, et al: Halothane and non-halogenated anesthetic agents in patients with cirrhosis of the liver: mortality and morbidity following porto-systemic venous anastomoses. Surg Clin North Am 45:983, 1965
38. La Mont JT, Isselbacher KJ: Postoperative jaundice. N Engl J Med 288:305, 1973
39. Brown BR Jr: General anesthetics and hepatic toxicity. Arizona Medicine 34:5, 1977
40. Dykes MHM: Unexplained post-operative fever; its value as a sign of halothane sensitization. JAMA 216:641, 1971

41. Morley TJ: Halothane hepatitis. JAMA 225:1659, 1973
42. Summary of the National Halothane Study. JAMA 197:775, 1966
43. Sherlock S: Progress report: halothane hepatitis. Gut 12:324, 1971
44. Blumberg BS, Sutnick AI, London WT, et al: Australia antigen and hepatitis. N Engl J Med 283:349, 1970
45. Prince AN, Hargrove RL, Sznuness W, et al: Immunologic distinction between infectious and serum hepatitis. N Engl J Med 282:987, 1970
46. Feinstone SM, Kapikian AZ, Purcell RH, et al: Transfusion associated hepatitis not due to viral hepatitis A or B. N Engl J Med 292:767, 1975
47. Feinstone SM, Purcell RH: Non-A, non-B hepatitis. Annu Rev Med 29:359, 1978
48. Douglas HJ, Eger EI II, Biava CG, et al: Halothane hepatic necrosis associated with viral infection after enflurane anesthesia. N Engl J Med 296:553, 1977
49. Kline MM: Enflurane associated hepatitis. Gastroenterology 79: 126, 1980
50. Lewis JH, Zimmerman JH, Ishak KG, et al: Enflurane hepatotoxicity: a clinicopathologic study of 24 cases. Ann Intern Med 98:984, 1983
51. Dykes MHM: Is enflurane hepatotoxic? (editorial). Anesthesiology 61:235, 1984
52. Eger EI, Smuckler EA, Ferrell LD, et al: Is enflurane hepatotoxic? Anesth Analg 65:21, 1986
53. Paronetto F, Popper N: Lymphocyte stimulation induced by halothane in patients with hepatitis following exposure to halothane. N Engl J Med 283:277, 1970
54. Klatskin G, Kimberg DV: Recurrent hepatitis attributable to halothane sensitization in an anesthetist. N Engl J Med 280: 515, 1969
55. Tong MJ, Wallace AM, Peters RL, et al: Lymphocytes stimulation of hepatitis B infections. N Engl J Med 293:318, 1975
56. McCracken LE: Failure to induce halothane hepatic pathology in animals sensitized to halothane metabolites and subsequently challenged with halothane. Anesth Analg 55:235, 1976
57. Wark HJ: Postoperative jaundice in children. Anaesthesia 38: 237, 1983
58. Bruce DL: What is the safe interval between halothane exposures? JAMA 221:1140, 1972
59. Hanson KM, Johnson PC: Local control of hepatic and portal venous flows in the dog. Am J Physiol 211:712, 1966
60. Gelman SI: Disturbances in hepatic blood flow during anesthesia and surgery. Arch Surg III:881, 1976
61. Gelman S: General anesthesia and hepatic circulation. Can J Physiol Pharmacol 65:1762, 1987
62. Shingu K, Eger EI II, Johnson BH: Hypoxia may be more important than reductive metabolism in halothane-induced hepatic injury. Anesth Analg 61:824, 1982
63. Shingu K, Eger EI II, Johnson BH, et al: Hepatic injury induced by anesthetic agents in rats. Anesth Analg 62:140, 1983
64. Lind RC, Gandolfi AJ, Sipes IG, et al: Comparison of the requirements for hepatic injury with halothane and enflurane in rats. Anesth Analg 64:955, 1985
65. Moore RA, McNicholas KW, Gallagher JD, et al: Halothane metabolism in acyanotic and cyanotic patients undergoing open heart surgery. Anesth Analg 65:1257, 1986
66. Slater TE: Necrogenic action of carbon tetrachloride in the rat: a speculative mechanism based on activation. Nature 209:36, 1966
67. Recknagel RO: Carbon tetrachloride hepatotoxicity. Pharmacol Rev 19:145, 1967
68. Castro JA, Sasame H, Sussman H, et al: Diverse effects of SKF 525-A and antioxidants on carbon tetrachloride-induced changes in liver microsomal P-450 content and ethylmorphine metabolism. Life Sci 7:129, 1968
69. Scholler KL: Modification of the effects of chloroform in the rat liver. Br J Anaesth 42:602, 1970
70. Van Dyke RA, Chenoweth MB, Van Poznak A: Metabolism of volatile anesthetics: I. conversion in vivo of several anesthetics to C^{14}, O_2 and chloride. Biochem Pharmacol 13:1239, 1964
71. Stier A, Altre H, Hessler O, et al: Urinary excretion of bromide in halothane anesthesia. Anesth Analg 43:723, 1964
72. Holaday DA, Rudofsky S, Treuhaft PS: The metabolic degradation of methoxyflurane in man. Anesthesiology 33:579, 1970
73. Stier A, Alter H, Hessler O, et al: Urinary excretion of bromide in halothane anesthesia. Anesth Analg 43:723, 1964
74. Rehder K, Fobes J, Alter H, et al: Halothane biotransformation in man: a quantitative study. Anesthesiology 28:711, 1967
75. Cohen EN, Trudell GR Jr, Edwards HN, et al: Urinary metabolites of halothane in man. Anesthesiology 43:392, 1975
76. Uehleke H, Hillmer KH, Tabarelli-Poplawski S: Metabolic activation of halothane and its covalent binding to liver endoplasmic proteins in vitro. Naunyn Schmiedebergs Arch Pharmacol 279:39, 1973
77. Widger LA, Gandolfi AJ, Van Dyke RA: Hypoxia and halothane metabolism in vivo: release of inorganic fluoride and halothane metabolite binding to cellular constituents. Anesthesiology 44: 197, 1976
78. Sipes IG, Brown BR Jr: An animal model of hepatotoxicity associated with halothane anesthesia. Anesthesiology 45:622, 1976
79. Brown BR Jr, Sipes IG: Biotransformation and hepatotoxicity of halothane. Biochem Pharmacol 26:2091, 1977
80. Mclain GE, Sipes IG, Brown BR Jr: An animal model of halothane hepatotoxicity: roles of enzyme induction and hypoxia. Anesthesiology 51:321, 1979
81. Vergani D, Tsantoulas D, Eddleston ALWF, et al: Sensitization to halothane altered liver component in severe hepatic necrosis after halothane anesthesia. Lancet 2:801, 1978
82. Hubbard AK, Poth TP, Gandolfi AS, et al: Halothane hepatitis patients generate an antibody response toward a covalently bound metabolite of halothane. Anesthesiology 68:792, 1988
83. Trowell J, Peto R, Crampton-Smith A: Controlled trial of repeated halothane anesthetics in patients with carcinoma of the uterine cervix treated with radium. Lancet 1:821, 1975
84. Fee JPH, Black GW, Dundee JW, et al: A prospective study of liver enzyme and other changes following repeat administration of halothane and enflurane. Br J Anaesth 51:1133, 1979
85. Benumof JL, Bookstein JJ, Saidman LJ, et al: Diminished hepatic arterial flow during halothane administration. Anesthesiology 45:545, 1976
86. Bentley JB, Vaughan RW, Gandolfi AJ, et al: Halothane biotransformation in obese and non-obese patients. Anesthesiology 57:94, 1982
87. Halsey MJ: Drug interactions in anaesthesia. Br J Anaesth 59: 112, 1987
88. Brown BR Jr: Hepatotoxicity and inhalation agents: views in the era of isoflurane. J Clin Anesth 1:368, 1989
89. Stoelting RK, Blitt CD, Cohen PJ, et al: Hepatic dysfunction after isoflurane anesthesia. Anesth Analg 66:147, 1987
90. Carpenter RL, Eger EI, Johnson BH, et al: The extent of metabolism of inhaled anesthetics in humans. Anesthesiology 65: 201, 1986
91. Christ DD, Kenra JG, Kammerer W, et al: Enflurane metabolism produces covalently bound liver adducts recognized by antibodies from patients with halothane hepatitis. Anesthesiology 69:838, 1988

Complications in Anesthesiology, second edition,
edited by Nikolaus Gravenstein and Robert R. Kirby.
Lippincott-Raven Publishers, Philadelphia © 1996.

CHAPTER 52

Uteroplacental Perfusion and Aortocaval Compression

Catherine O. Hunt
Gerard W. Ostheimer

The pregnant patient challenges the anesthesiologist to provide analgesia that is safe for both mother and fetus. The anesthesiologist must understand the physiologic adaptations that the patient has undergone and, in particular, the dynamics of uteroplacental perfusion. Aortocaval compression threatens systemic hypotension (supine hypotensive syndrome) with resultant decreased uteroplacental perfusion when the gravid uterus is permitted to rest on the great vessels of the abdomen. This chapter surveys this common problem after reviewing the determinants of uteroplacental perfusion.

UTEROPLACENTAL PERFUSION

To meet the demands of the growing uterus and fetus, the mother makes several physiologic adaptations during pregnancy. These include increases in blood volume, cardiac output, and pulmonary minute ventilation. At term, the uterus has grown to 6000 g from a nongravid weight of 45 to 80 g. Uterine blood flow is approximately 700 mL/min, representing 10% of the cardiac output. Eighty percent of the blood flows through the placenta to the fetus and 20% to the myometrium and endometrium.

Uterine Hemodynamics

In normal pregnancy, the uterine vasculature is maximally dilated and does not exhibit autoregulation.[1] Uterine perfusion is proportional to the difference between the uterine arterial venous pressures and inversely proportional to uterine vascular resistance. Thus, uterine perfusion can be diminished by increased venous pressure and vascular resistance or decreased arterial pressure.

Uterine Arterial Resistance

The uterine vascular bed has α- and β-adrenergic receptors in the myometrial vessels,[2,3] whereas the intervillous vasculature appears to contain only α-adrenergic receptors. The release of endogenous catecholamines that occurs during maternal stress, during anxiety, and during severe hypoxia, hypocarbia, or hypercapnia is associated with increased uterine vascular resistance and decreased placental perfusion.[4–7] Exogenous catecholamines produce a similar reduction in uterine perfusion. In sheep, uterine blood flow decreases in a dose-related fashion after the administration of 5 to 20 μg epinephrine intravenously.[8] These doses approximate the amounts used as a test dose in humans when epidural anesthesia is administered. Uterine vascular resistance also increases during myometrial contractions, which reduce the caliber of arcuate and spiral arteries and increase uterine venous tone.[9]

Uterine Venous Tone

Uterine venous pressure increases during each contraction, and at intra-amniotic pressures of 60 to 70 mm Hg, uterine perfusion ceases.[9]

Placental Insufficiency

Placental insufficiency results in late decelerations of the fetal heart rate pattern. Similarly, uterine perfusion ceases during uterine hypertonus, which can result from high concentrations of local anesthetics,[10,11] overstimulation with oxytocin, ketamine in doses greater than 1.5 mg/kg,[12] abruptio placentae, and tetanic contractions. Whenever uteroplacental perfusion is impaired, fetal distress can develop rapidly, with fetal acidosis and generalized CNS depression (as evidenced by low Apgar scores) in the infant at delivery.

Effect of Anesthesia and Technique

Anesthetic management can influence uteroplacental perfusion both favorably and unfavorably. The ultimate effect of anesthesia on uterine blood flow reflects the balance between its effects on uterine vascular resistance and perfusion pressure.

Regional Anesthesia

The beneficial aspects of epidural and spinal analgesia during labor include elimination of pain-induced hyperventilation and a decrease in maternal circulating catecholamines.[13,14] Studies with radioactive clearance techniques in humans confirm these beneficial effects: intervillous blood flow increases 35% in normotensive parturients and 77% in parturients with severe preeclampsia after lumbar epidural analgesia for labor.[15,16]

EPINEPHRINE-CONTAINING LOCAL ANESTHETICS. The effect of epinephrine-containing local anesthetic solutions used for epidural analgesia remains controversial. As noted earlier, even the amount of epinephrine used in an epidural test dose can cause a decrease in uterine blood flow. Wallis and colleagues reported a 14% decrease in uterine blood flow in sheep when epinephrine, 1:100,000, was added to 2-chloroprocaine for epidural anesthesia.[17] Albright and associates, however, did not find a significant decrease in intervillous blood flow when they used radioactive xenon in humans with normal pregnancies.[18] However, their conclusion must be examined cautiously because of the reproducibility of the technique, the inclusion in the data analysis of two patients with very large increases in intervillous blood flow, and the lack of data on maternal heart rate, which may be influenced by epinephrine.

In a more recent study, Skjöldebrand and colleagues demonstrated a significant decrease in uteroplacental blood flow in nine of ten parturients undergoing cesarean section.[19] Epidural bupivacaine, 0.5%, with epinephrine, 2.5 μg/mL, was used. However, fetal heart rate was not affected, and Apgar scores at 1 and 5 minutes were normal. Also, maternal blood pressure changes did not correlate with changes in uteroplacental flow. The effect of epinephrine-containing solutions in patients with compromised placental blood flow, such as those with diabetes or preeclampsia, remains to be examined.

Uterine vasoconstriction also can occur with the high concentrations of local anesthetics that result from unintentional intravascular injection or paracervical block. This response appears to be a direct effect of the drugs on uterine vasculature and myometrium.[10,11,20]

General Anesthesia

Just as improvement in uterine perfusion occurs with regional anesthesia because of reductions in uterine vascular resistance, so too can the inhalation agents, halothane and isoflurane, improve uterine blood flow.[21] With deep inhalation anesthesia, the improvement is offset, however, by the decrease in perfusion pressure that occurs with hypotension.

Thiopental decreases uterine blood flow in association with a decrease in maternal blood pressure, but diazepam and propofol do not affect uterine perfusion unless hypotension occurs.[22] However, administration of these agents usually is followed by administration of succinylcholine, laryngoscopy, and tracheal intubation. The accompanying maternal catecholamine release is believed to be responsible for a subsequent decrease in uterine blood flow.[23] Positive-pressure ventilation can also increase uterine vascular resistance by impeding venous return to the heart and eliciting a compensatory increase in sympathetic tone.[6]

AORTOCAVAL COMPRESSION

Historical Background

The influence of the gravid uterus on maternal cardiovascular stability was first examined by McLennan in 1943.[24] He described an increase in mean femoral venous pressure from 9.1 cmH_2O during the first trimester to 24 cmH_2O at term (Fig. 52-1). After delivery, the pressure decreased to its level before pregnancy. No changes in the mean antecubital venous pressures occurred during pregnancy.

Although McLennan attributed this effect to the pressure exerted by the gravid uterus, the clinical significance was not appreciated until 1951, when McRoberts reported a syndrome of "postural shock" during pregnancy.[25] He described six term parturients who became severely hypotensive when placed in the supine position but who were normotensive when they were placed on their side. He also noted that several patients reported nausea, shortness of breath, faintness, sweating, and pain and numbness in their arms when they were placed in the supine position. McRoberts postulated that this hypotension resulted from obstruction of the venous return from the pelvis and lower extremities by pressure from the gravid uterus.[25]

This hypothesis was confirmed by Howard and colleagues in 1953.[26] They documented a 30-mm Hg depression in systolic blood pressure in 11% of term parturients when they lay supine. This effect took 5 to 10 minutes to develop in some patients. They confirmed this possibility by ligating the vena cava in pregnant dogs and producing hypotension (Fig. 52-2). Howard's group also examined the effect of uterine contractions on blood pressure and found that contractions counteracted the supine hypotensive effect (Fig. 52-3). They postulated that during contractions, the uterus tilted upward on the vertebral column, and pressure on the vena cava was removed.[26]

Subsequently, in the late 1960s, Bieniarz and associates demonstrated compression of the aorta[27] and of the vena cava[28] (Fig. 52-4) with maintenance of blood pressure in the brachial artery but not the femoral artery. The clinical importance of decreased aortic perfusion was recognized by the depression of the fetal heart rate and what we would now interpret as late decelerations on fetal heart rate monitoring, or uteroplacental insufficiency.

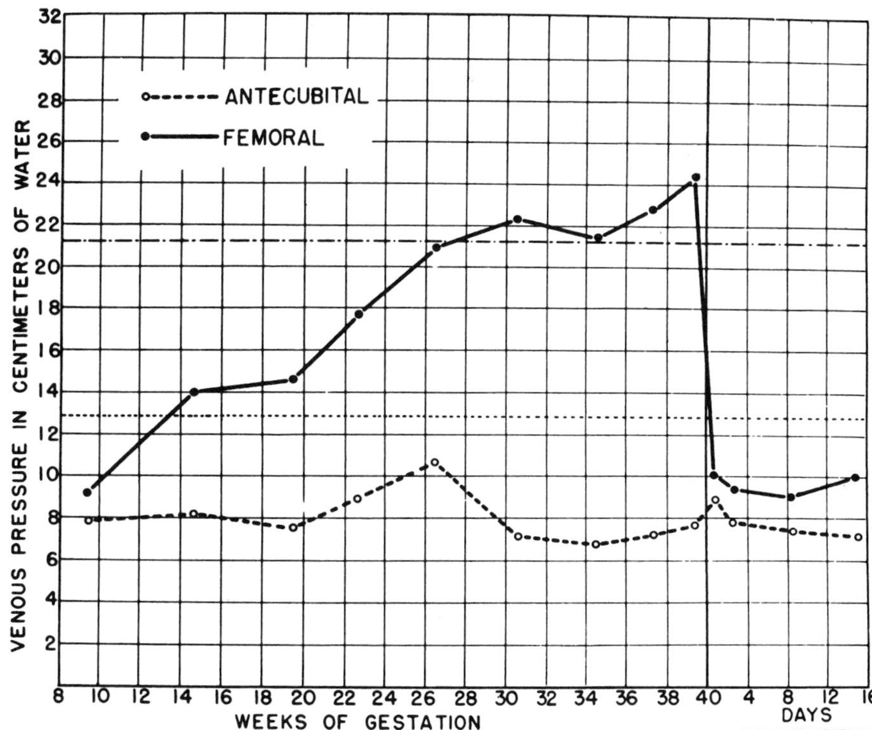

FIGURE 52-1. Femoral and antecubital venous pressures during pregnancy. (McLennan CE: Antecubital and femoral venous pressure in normal and toxemic pregnancy. Am J Obstet Gynecol 45:568, 1943)

A Current View

Additional studies have highlighted the importance of maternal position on cardiac output at term.[29–31] Formerly, cardiac output was believed to increase during pregnancy until about gestational week 32 and thereafter to decrease to levels found in the nonpregnant state. However, invasive methods have shown that the apparent reduction in cardiac output during the last 8 weeks of pregnancy is observed only when the measurements are made with patients in the supine position. In that position, vena caval occlusion occurs in almost all parturients at term, with venous return from the lower half of the body largely dependent on a long, narrow, tortuous diversion through paravertebral and azygos veins. Thus, the venous return is impaired, and cardiac output may decrease by as much as 50%.[30–32]

The markedly impaired cardiac output, especially with a superimposed bradycardia, results in the supine hypotensive syndrome. The reduction in systemic vascular resistance caused by general and regional anesthesia augments the decrease in cardiac output, leading to severe hypotension, which threatens to cause fetal distress. Even a small amount of left

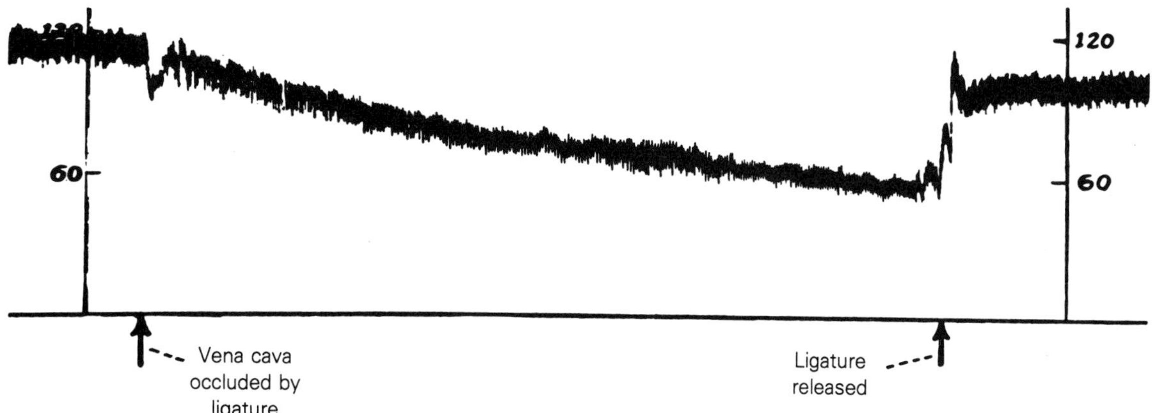

FIGURE 52-2. Change in systolic blood pressure consequent to vena caval occlusion in a pregnant dog. (Howard BK, Goodson JH, Mengert WF: Supine hypotensive syndrome in late pregnancy. Obstet Gynecol 1:371, 1953)

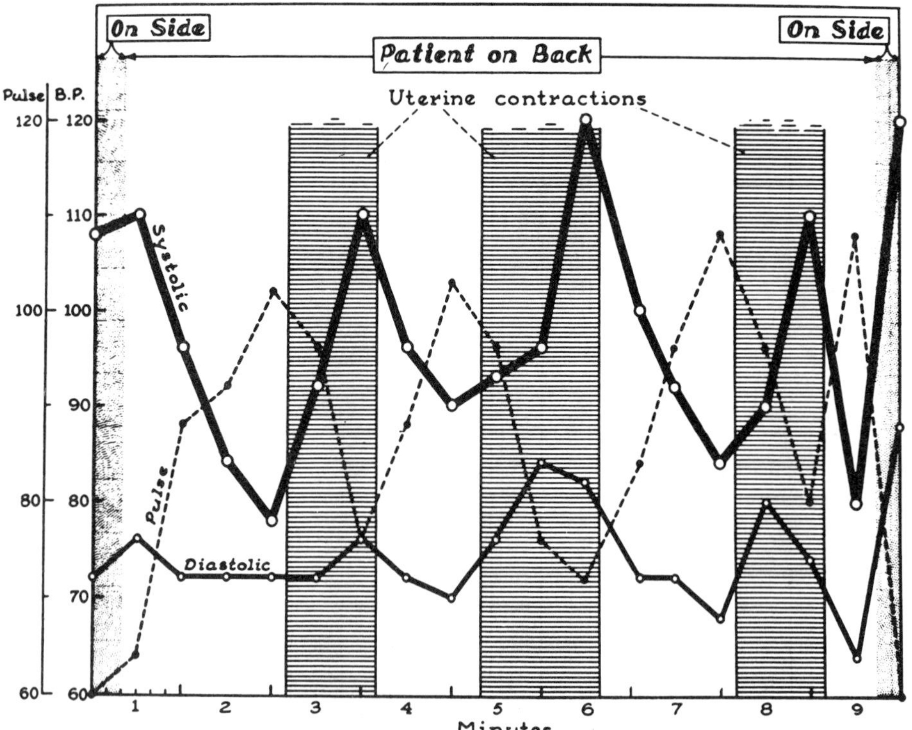

FIGURE 52-3. Changes in blood pressure (*B.P.*) (millimeters mercury) and pulse (beats per minute) in supine hypotensive syndrome during labor. (Howard BK, Goodson JH, Mengert WF: Supine hypotensive syndrome in late pregnancy. Obstet Gynecol 1:371, 1953)

lateral tilt (eg, 10°) substantially relieves the supine hypotensive syndrome.[33–35]

Treatment

Most patients compensate for the decrease in venous return and cardiac output by an increase in systemic vascular resistance and heart rate, produced by increases in sympathetic activity.[31,35] However, this compensatory mechanism is blocked by epidural and spinal anesthesia, necessitating displacement of the gravid uterus off the great vessels.

Left Lateral Uterine Displacement

Left lateral uterine displacement can be accomplished easily by placing a wedge under the patient's right hip (Figs. 52-4

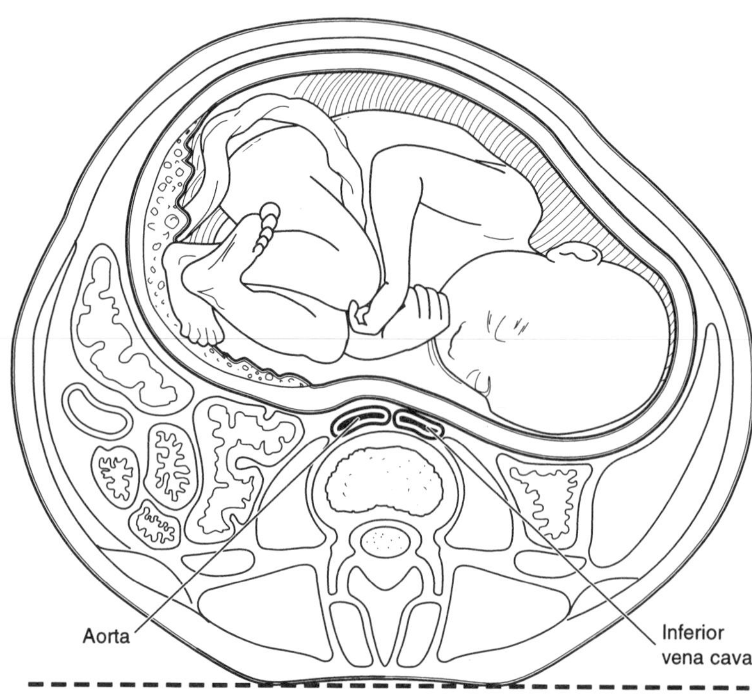

FIGURE 52-4. The pregnant uterus compresses the aorta and inferior vena cava (aortocaval compression) when the patient is supine. (Adapted from Ostheimer GW: Regional anesthesia techniques in obstetrics. New York: Breon Laboratories, 1980)

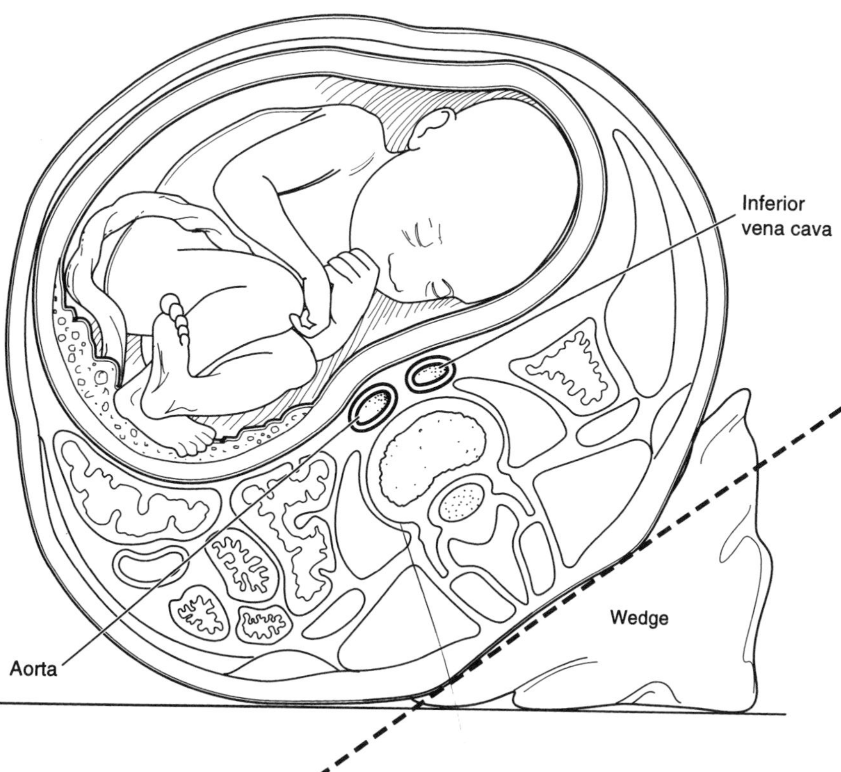

FIGURE 52-5. Uterine displacement with a wedge under the right hip relieves aortocaval compression. (Adapted from Ostheimer GW: Regional anesthesia techniques in obstetrics. New York: Breon Laboratories, 1980)

and 52-5). Treatment of hypotension with vasopressors without alleviation of aortocaval compression has been recognized as futile for more than 30 years.[27]

Increased Intravenous Hydration

A balanced salt solution (eg, lactated Ringer's solution or normal saline) partially compensates for the impaired venous return and anesthetic-induced peripheral dilatation.

Vasopressors

Vasopressors should be administered if the foregoing measures are ineffective; prompt treatment of hypotension is critical for uterine perfusion and fetal well-being. Ephedrine is regarded as the vasopressor of choice for the parturient.[36]

A vasopressor may be chosen properly according to its effects on the uterine vascular resistance. Drugs that act primarily through α-adrenergic receptor stimulation and vasoconstriction restore maternal blood pressure but further compromise uterine perfusion by increasing uterine vascular resistance.[37,38] In general, therefore, drugs such as methoxamine and metaraminol should be avoided. Short-term use of phenylephrine has not caused any problem for the fetus.[39,40]

Pure α-adrenergic agonists may have a place when peripheral vascular resistance must be maintained, as in the parturient with severe cardiac disease. Despite stimulation of β-adrenergic and dopaminergic receptors, stimulation of uterine α-adrenergic receptors predominates over the action of dopamine and cannot be used to restore uterine perfusion.[41]

Alternatively, vasopressors such as ephedrine, which acts primarily through β-adrenergic stimulation, do not have detrimental effects on uterine perfusion. Blood pressure is restored by enhanced cardiac output. Ephedrine, administered intravenously in 5- to 10-mg doses at the first decrease in blood pressure, is effective in maintaining uterine blood flow even with high sympathetic blockade (T2 to T4) during regional anesthesia for cesarean delivery. Intervillous blood flow is maintained and neonatal acid–base status is improved when hypotension is promptly treated in this manner.[42–44]

Other Measures

Prompt treatment of other causes of decreased uteroplacental perfusion must be undertaken. For example, tetanic uterine contractions can be treated with β-adrenergic agonists, which relax the myometrium.[45] The same effect can be obtained with inhalation agents.[46]

Prevention

As in so many other clinical situations, prevention is much easier (and better) than treatment. The beneficial effects of regional anesthesia require that maternal hypotension be avoided.

Left lateral uterine displacement, as mentioned previously, should be instituted throughout labor and delivery. During labor, the patient can assume a comfortable lateral position. After she has been moved to the delivery table, left lateral uterine displacement should be maintained. The lateral position does not impair satisfactory spread of local anesthetic solutions for epidural anesthesia.[47]

Short-term hydration before anesthesia is also important in reducing the incidence of hypotension.[48,49] A minimum of 1 L of balanced electrolyte solution should be infused before induction of the anesthetic. Solutions without dextrose should be used because dextrose can result in neonatal hypoglycemia.[50]

REFERENCES

1. Greiss FC: Pressure-flow relationship in the gravid uterine vascular bed. Am J Obstet Gynecol 96:41, 1966
2. Greiss FC: Differential reactivity of the myometrial and placental vasculatures: adrenergic responses. Anesthesiology 29:374, 1968
3. Kauppila A, Kuibba J, Tuimela R: Effect of fenoterol and isoxsuprine on myometrial and uterine blood flow during late pregnancy. Obstet Gynecol 52:558, 1978
4. Shnider SM, Wright RG, Levinson G, et al: Uterine blood flow and plasma norepinephrine changes during maternal stress in the pregnant ewe. Anesthesiology 50:524, 1979
5. Dilts PV, Brinkman CR, Kirschbaum TH, et al: Uterine and systemic hemodynamic interrelationships and their response to hypoxia. Am J Obstet Gynecol 103:138, 1969
6. Levinson G, Shnider SM, deLorimier AA, et al: Effects of maternal hyperventilation on uterine blood flow and fetal oxygenation and acid–base status. Anesthesiology 40:340, 1974
7. Walker AM, Oakes GK, Ehrenkranz R, et al: Effect of hypercapnia on uterine and umbilical circulations in conscious pregnant sheep. J Appl Physiol 41:727, 1976
8. Hood DD, Dewan DM, James FM: Maternal and fetal effects of epinephrine in gravid ewes. Anesthesiology 64:610, 1986
9. Wheeler AS, Harris BA: The uterus, placenta and fetus. Seminars in Anesthesia 1:101, 1982
10. Greiss FC, Still JG, Anderson SG: Effects of local anesthetic agents on uterine vasculatures and myometrium. Am J Obstet Gynecol 124:899, 1976
11. Morishima HO, Covino BG, Yeh M, et al: Bradycardia in the fetal baboon following paracervical block anesthesia. Am J Obstet Gynecol 140:775, 1981
12. Galloon S: Ketamine for obstetric delivery. Anesthesiology 44: 522, 1976
13. Abboud TK, Artal R, Henriksen EH, et al: Effects of spinal anesthetics on maternal circulating catecholamines. Am J Obstet Gynecol 142:252, 1982
14. Shnider SM, Abboud TK, Artal R, et al: Maternal catecholamines decrease during labor after lumbar epidural anesthesia. Am J Obstet Gynecol 147:13, 1983
15. Hollmen AI, Jouppila R, Jouppila P, et al: Effect of extradural analgesia during labor on intervillous blood flow during normal labor. Br J Anaesth 54:837, 1982
16. Jouppila P, Jouppila R, Hollmen A, et al: Lumbar epidural analgesia to improve intervillous blood flow during labor in severe preeclampsia. Obstet Gynecol 39:158, 1982
17. Wallis KL, Shnider SM, Hicks JS, et al: Epidural anesthesia in the normotensive pregnant ewe: effects on uterine blood flow and fetal acid–base status. Anesthesiology 44:481, 1976
18. Albright GA, Jouppila R, Hollmen AI, et al: Epinephrine does not alter human intervillous blood flow during epidural anesthesia. Anesthesiology 54:131, 1981
19. Skjöldebrand A, Eklund J, Lunell N-O, et al: The effect on uteroplacental blood flow of epidural anaesthesia containing adrenaline for caesarean section. Acta Anaesthesiol Scand 34:85, 1990
20. Gibbs CP, Noel SC: Human uterine artery response to lidocaine. Am J Obstet Gynecol 126:313, 1976
21. Palakniuk RJ, Shnider SM: Maternal and fetal cardiovascular and acid–base changes during halothane and isoflurane anesthesia in the pregnant ewe. Anesthesiology 41:462, 1974
22. Shnider SM, Levinson G, Cosmi EV: Obstetric anesthesia and uterine blood flow. In Shnider SM, Levinson G (eds): Anesthesia for obstetrics, 2nd ed. Baltimore: Williams & Wilkins, 1993: 29
23. Jouppila R, Jouppila P, Hollmer A, et al: Effect of anesthetic method, epidural and general anesthesia, on intervillous blood flow in cesarean sections. Reg Anesth 2:4, 1977
24. McLennan CE: Antecubital and femoral venous pressure in normal and toxemic pregnancy. Am J Obstet Gynecol 45:568, 1943
25. McRoberts WA: Postural shock in pregnancy. Am J Obstet Gynecol 62:627, 1951
26. Howard BK, Goodson JH, Mengert WF: Supine hypotensive syndrome in late pregnancy. Obstet Gynecol 1:371, 1953
27. Bieniarz J, Maqueda E, Caldeyro-Barcia R: Compression of the aorta by the uterus in late human pregnancy. Am J Obstet Gynecol 95:795, 1966
28. Bieniarz J, Crottogini JJ, Curachet E, et al: Aortocaval compression by the uterus in late human pregnancy. Am J Obstet Gynecol 100:203, 1968
29. Lees MM, Scott DB, Kerr MG, et al: The circulatory effects of recumbent postural change in late pregnancy. Clin Sci (Colch) 32:453, 1967
30. Lees MM, Taylor SH, Scott DB, et al: A study of cardiac output at rest throughout pregnancy. Journal of Obstetrics and Gynaecology of the British Commonwealth 74:319, 1967
31. Weaver JB, Pearson JF, Rosen M: Posture and epidural block in pregnant women at term. Anaesthesia 30:752, 1975
32. Ueland K, Gills RE, Hansen JM: Maternal cardiovascular dynamics. Am J Obstet Gynecol 100:42, 1968
33. Vorys N, Ullery JC, Hanusek GE: The cardiac output changes in various positions. Am J Obstet Gynecol 82:1312, 1961
34. Newman B, Derrington C, Dore C: Cardiac output and the recumbent position in late pregnancy. Anaesthesia 34:332, 1983
35. Eckstein KL, Marx GF: Aortocaval compression and uterine displacement. Anesthesiology 40:92, 1974
36. Ralston DH, Shnider SM: The fetal and neonatal effects of regional anesthesia in obstetrics. Anesthesiology 48:34, 1978
37. James FM, Greiss FC, Kemp RA: An evaluation of vasopressor therapy for maternal hypotension during spinal anesthesia. Anesthesiology 33:25, 1970
38. Ralston DH, Shnider SM, deLorimier AA: Effects of equipotent ephedrine, metaraminol, mephenteramine, and methoxamine on uterine blood flow in the pregnant ewe. Anesthesiology 40: 354, 1974
39. Ramanathan S, Grant GJ: Vasopressor therapy for hypotension due to epidural anesthesia for cesarean section. Acta Anesthesiol Scand 32:559, 1988
40. Moran DH, Perillo M, LaPorta RF, et al: Phenylephrine in the prevention of hypotension following spinal anesthesia for cesarean delivery. J Clin Anesth 3:301,1991
41. Rolbin SH, Levinson G, Shnider SM, et al: Dopamine treatment of spinal hypotension decreases uterine blood flow in the pregnant ewe. Anesthesiology 51:36, 1979
42. Jouppila R, Jouppila P, Kuikka J, et al: Placental blood flow during cesarean section under lumbar extradural analgesia. Br J Anaesth 50:275, 1978
43. Jouppila P, Jouppila R, Barinoff T, et al: Placental blood flow during caesarean section performed under subarachnoid blockade. Br J Anaesth 56:1379, 1984
44. Datta S, Alper MH, Ostheimer GW, et al: Method of ephedrine administration and nausea and hypotension during spinal anesthesia for cesarean section. Anesthesiology 56:68, 1982
45. Anderson KE, Bengtsson LPH, Gustafson I, et al: The relaxing effect of terbutaline on the human uterus during term labor. Am J Obstet Gynecol 121:602, 1974
46. Phillips JM, Evans JA: Acute anesthetic and obstetric management of patients with severe abruptio placenta. Anesth Analg 49:998, 1970
47. Norris MC, Leighton BL, DeSimone CA, et al: Lateral position and epidural anesthesia for cesarean section. Anesth Analg 67: 788, 1988
48. Wollman SB, Marx GF: Acute hydration for prevention of hypotension of spinal anesthesia in parturients. Anesthesiology 29:374, 1968
49. Clark RB, Thompson PS, Thompson CH: Prevention of spinal hypotension associated with cesarean section. Anesthesiology 45:670, 1976
50. Kenepp NB, Shelley WC, Gabbe SG et al: Fetal and neonatal hazards of maternal hydration with 5% dextrose before Caesarean section. Lancet 1:1150, 1982

FURTHER READING

Bonica JJ: Maternal anatomic and physiologic alterations during pregnancy and parturition. In: Bonica JJ, McDonald JS (eds): Principles and practice of obstetric analgesia and Anesthesia. Baltimore: Williams and Wilkins, 1995:66

Complications in Anesthesiology, second edition,
edited by Nikolaus Gravenstein and Robert R. Kirby.
Lippincott-Raven Publishers, Philadelphia © 1996.

CHAPTER 53

Postpartum Hemorrhage and Uterine Atony

Ronald Hurley
Gerard W. Ostheimer

Hemorrhage is one of the leading causes of maternal death during and following labor and delivery.[1–3] From 1954 to 1975 in the United States, the estimated maternal mortality rate associated with hemorrhage was 2 to 10 deaths per 100,000 live births.[4–8] In rural areas and developing countries such as India, maternal mortality is often eight to ten times that in urban communities, and hemorrhage accounts for 29% to 57% of maternal deaths.[9,10] Experts agree that nearly all of these deaths are preventable with good medical care. In Massachusetts, for example, with increased attention to reducing the incidence of preventable maternal death, the maternal mortality rate associated with hemorrhage decreased from 3.8 deaths per 100,000 live births from 1954 to 1957 to 0.3 per 100,000 live births from 1982 to 1985.[8]

This chapter surveys the causes, pathophysiologic features, and treatment of postpartum hemorrhage, with special emphasis on the role of anesthetic care in cases of this disorder.

POSTPARTUM HEMORRHAGE

Postpartum hemorrhage has been defined as blood loss exceeding 500 mL during the first 24 hours after the infant's birth,[3] and in some countries statutory obligation requires the reporting of all postpartum blood losses greater than 500 mL. However, this definition makes little sense. First, the average postpartum blood loss after normal vaginal delivery is at least 500 mL and is even greater after cesarean section. More importantly, the blood loss in both vaginal and abdominal deliveries is notoriously difficult to measure. Postpartum hemorrhage is better defined as any blood loss after birth that threatens the hemodynamic stability of the mother and, thus, the mother's health and survival.[11] Comparative blood losses after vaginal delivery, cesarean section, and cesarean hysterectomy are shown in Figure 53-1.

Causes

As part of normal parturition, the uterus contracts when the placenta separates, resulting in mechanical control of uterine bleeding during the third stage of labor. Impairment of uterine contractility results in increased bleeding and has many possible causes.[11]

Uterine Atony

Uterine atony is the primary cause of postpartum hemorrhage, accounting for as many as 90% of all cases.[12] Causes are listed in Table 53-1.

UTERINE OVERDISTENTION. In this condition, uterine smooth muscle is maintained at full fiber length, resulting in poor contractility. Among the causes of overdistention are a large fetus, multiple fetuses, polyhydramnios, and prolonged labor, especially with oxytocin stimulation.

HYPOTENSION. Any cause of hypotension (eg, regional anesthesia or cardiac failure) can lead to underperfusion of the myometrium, which then is unable to contract adequately as a result of ischemia, hypoxia, or both.

VOLATILE GENERAL ANESTHETICS. Halothane, enflurane, isoflurane, and desflurane can almost completely abolish uterine contractions at surgical planes of anesthesia. At 0.5, 1.0, and 1.5 minimum alveolar concentration, the halogenated volatile agents are equipotent in producing dose-dependent depression of uterine contractility.[13] The resultant uterine relaxation is not counteracted by oxytocin stimulation and dissipates only slowly after the anesthetic is discontinued. In contrast, nitrous oxide has no effect on uterine contractility.[14]

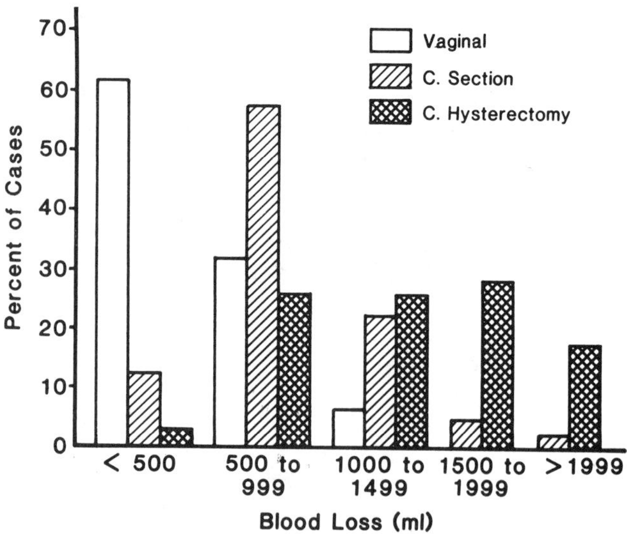

FIGURE 53-1. Blood loss after vaginal delivery, cesarean (C.) section, and cesarean hysterectomy. (Pritchard JA: Am J Obstet Gynecol 84:1271, 1962)

TOCOLYSIS. Tocolytic agents used intentionally to arrest uterine contractions antepartum are associated, not unexpectedly, with an increased incidence of uterine atony postpartum, if they have been administered recently. The commonly used tocolytic agents include the β-sympathomimetic agents, ritodrine, terbutaline, and isoxsuprine. In addition, the parturient woman may have received any of a variety of drugs with tocolytic action, such as magnesium sulfate, ethyl alcohol, calcium channel blocking agents, and prostaglandin inhibitors.

OTHER FACTORS. Multiparity, previous hemorrhage from uterine atony, and rapid labor are associated with a higher incidence of uterine atony.

Trauma to the Lower Genital Tract

Lacerations to the cervix, vagina, and perineum are the second most common cause of excessive maternal hemorrhage. These tears occur usually in instrumented deliveries. Associated factors include a large fetus, attendance by an inexperienced obstetrician, and inadequate anesthesia.

Retained Placenta

Retained placental fragments prevent the uterus from contracting effectively and thus from controlling blood loss mechanically. Retained placenta is the third most common cause of postpartum hemorrhage, occurring in about 1% of all vaginal deliveries. Retained placenta usually consists of fragments of normal placenta that can be removed easily by curettage or by the obstetrician's hand. However, abnormally adherent placenta (placenta accreta, increta, or percreta) occasionally is the cause and often leads to intractable blood loss unless hysterectomy is performed.

Occasionally the obstetrician requests relaxation of the uterus for manual exploration. General anesthesia with halogenated agents will relax the uterus and provide anesthesia, though with the attendant risks. Nitroglycerine administered as 50–100 μg intravenous boluses may provide the necessary relaxation.[15,16]

Lower-segment Implantation

Placental implantation in the lower uterine segment, a site that does not contract well, can lead to hemorrhage that is not controlled by fundal massage and oxytocin, as in placenta previa (Fig. 53-2). Similarly, excessive bleeding can occur when the placenta has implanted at the site of an old scar. Surgical control of the bleeding may be necessary with a figure-of-eight suture or, if bleeding is intractable, with hysterectomy.

Uterine Inversion

Uterine inversion is a rare but potentially fatal complication of the third stage of labor, in which the uterus turns inside out and protrudes to some degree, into or out of the vagina. This obstetric complication is associated with fundal pressure on the inadequately contracting uterus or from premature traction on the umbilical cord. Early recognition and rapid reduction of the inversion by the obstetrician are essential. The reduction may require general anesthesia.

Uterine Rupture

Rupture of the uterus is a rare but much feared complication of labor that usually occurs antepartum. Risk factors are listed in Table 53-2. Uterine rupture is mentioned here because it is more common in patients with a classical vertical uterine cesarean section scar. Vaginal birth after a previous cesarean delivery is increasingly common, and obstetric anesthesiologists need to be aware of the potential risk.

Epidural anesthesia for labor and delivery may mask early signs of rupture. Vaginal bleeding is uncommon, because the blood enters the peritoneal cavity or the retroperitoneum. Unexplained abdominal pain or excessive hypotension in the patient giving vaginal birth after a previous cesarean delivery should not be discounted. Fetal distress may be the presenting sign of uterine rupture.

TABLE 53-1
Causes of Uterine Atony

- Uterine overdistention
- Hypotension
- Volatile anesthetic agents
- Tocolytic agents
- Multiparity
- Previous hemorrhage from uterine atony
- Rapid labor
- Prolonged labor

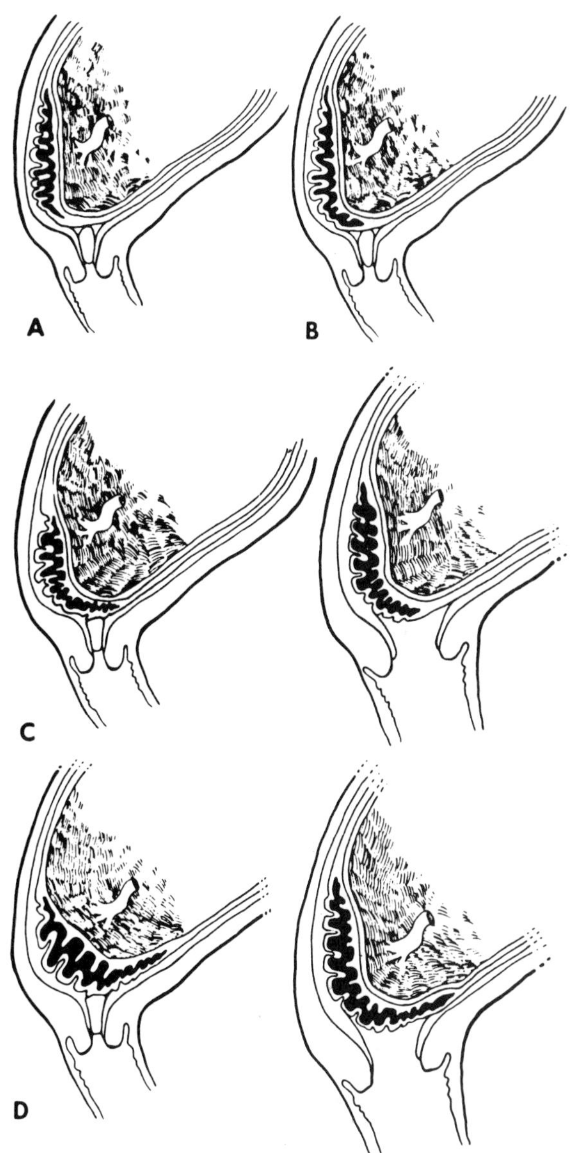

FIGURE 53-2. Classification of placenta previa. (**A**) Class I. (**B**) Class II. (**C**) Class III with closed (*left*) and partially open (*right*) cervix. (**D**) Class IV with closed (*left*) and partially open (*right*) cervix. (Hayoshi RH, Castillo MS: Bleeding in pregnancy. In: Knoeppel R, Drukker J (eds): High-rish pregnancy: a team approach. Philadelphia: WB Saunders, 1986: 426)

Abruptio Placentae

At cesarean section or after vaginal delivery, patients may continue to bleed because of uterine atony or coagulopathy. Hemorrhage can be severe, sometimes necessitating hysterectomy. The classification of abruptio placentae is summarized in Table 53-3.

Coagulation Defects

Excessive bleeding can result from acquired or inherited coagulation defects.[11,17] These defects may be caused by the pregnancy (eg, toxemia, abruptio placentae, amniotic fluid embolism, or fetal death) and may lead to defects in the coagulation cascade and in platelet function. Iatrogenic causes include warfarin and heparin therapy and use of antiplatelet aggregation drugs (eg, aspirin). In rare cases, the patient may have a congenital coagulation disorder, such as von Willebrand's disease.

TABLE 53-2
Factors Predisposing to Uterine Rupture

- Previous cesarean section
- Previous myometrial resection or other gynecologic surgery
- Grand multiparity
- Injudicious use of oxytocin
- Internal version
- Busch extraction
- Midforceps delivery
- Overly vigorous fundal pressure to facilitate vaginal delivery

Taylor CE: Hemorrhagic disorders of the obstetric patient. In Civetta JM, Taylor RW, Kirby RR (eds): Critical care, 2nd ed. Philadelphia: JB Lippincott, 1992: 865.

TREATMENT OF UTERINE ATONY

Considerations for treatment are listed in Table 53-4.

General Considerations

Normally, the uterus contracts after placental separation, and palpation reveals a firm, well-contracted fundus. Fundal massage and oxytocin infusion are used to help the natural process. Adherence to fundamental principles of good obstetric anesthetic care are also important.

TABLE 53-3
Grading System for Abruptio Placentae

GRADE	SYMPTOMS
0	The patient is asymptomatic, and there is no evidence of hemorrhage. However, at delivery, the abruption is obvious when the placenta is examined, and an adherent clot is found on its surface.
1	Vaginal bleeding is present but not excessive. Uterine tetany and tenderness may be present. The fetus is not affected.
2	Vaginal bleeding is present and may or may not be external. Uterine tenderness and tetany usually are evident, as are signs of fetal distress. Maternal cardiovascular symptoms are minimal.
3	Vaginal bleeding may or may not occur, and there is obvious uterine tetany with marked tenderness of the uterus. Maternal hypotension is common, and the fetus may have died. Clotting abnormalities also are common.

Gibbs CP: Hemorrhagic disorders in the obstetric patient. In Civetta JM, Taylor RW, Kirby RR (eds): Critical care. Philadelphia, JB Lippincott, 1988: 1360.

TABLE 53-4
Treatment of Uterine Atony

GENERAL MEASURES

- Establish large-bore intravenous cannulas
- Infuse fluids with pressurized systems as necessary
- Maintain left uterine displacement
- Administer clear antacid
- Have typed and screened blood immediately available
- Consider placement of central venous catheter

SPECIFIC MEASURES

- Discontinue uterine relaxants (including volatile anesthetic agents)
- Perform fundal massage, and give oxytocin
- Consider ergot derivatives if bleeding continues
- Consider 15-methylprostaglandin $F_{2\alpha}$, carboprost
- Consider surgery, including hysterectomy

The obstetric anesthesiologist must be able to infuse intravenous fluids rapidly; thus a large-bore intravenous cannula, preferably 16-G or greater, is essential. Pressurized infusion systems should be immediately available. Adequate intravenous volume expansion before regional anesthesia also is fundamental. Maintenance of left uterine displacement and therefore avoidance of the supine hypotensive syndrome before delivery should be standard practice. All laboring patients should receive a clear antacid before any major anesthesia technique is induced, because the hazard of pulmonary aspiration of gastric contents has been well documented (see Chap. 14).

The obstetric anesthesiologist must be aware of the normal blood losses associated with vaginal and cesarean delivery and should realize that these losses are often underestimated. Rapid availability of typed and screened blood is essential for all major obstetric procedures. Minimal delay in the administration of oxytocin after delivery of the infant by cesarean section and of the placenta in vaginal delivery can prevent many cases of uterine atony. Placement of a central venous catheter for accurate monitoring of volume replacement may be necessary.

Specific Therapy

Discontinuation of Uterine Relaxants

As soon as excessive bleeding is apparent, all drugs implicated in causing uterine atony, such as the volatile anesthetics, should be discontinued. These anesthetics are often used in conjunction with nitrous oxide during cesarean delivery; however, halogenated agents should be discontinued immediately after birth of the infant.

Stimulation or Augmentation of Uterine Contractions

OXYTOCIN. The fundus should be massaged vigorously. An intravenous infusion of synthetic oxytocin, 10 to 20 U in 500 to 1000 mL of lactated Ringer's solution, is appropriate to augment endogenous hormone production. Care should be exercised when administering single doses of oxytocin, to avoid cardiovascular problems: intravenously administered oxytocin, in doses of 5 to 10 U, can cause profound vasodilation and resultant hypotension, particularly in the anesthetized patient.[18,21]

In our practice at the Brigham and Women's Hospital (Boston, Massachusetts), intravenous doses of 2 or 3 U of oxytocin are administered after the placenta has been removed, without the development of hypotension. The half-life of oxytocin ranges from 12 to 17 minutes[22]; it is removed from the plasma largely by the kidneys and liver.

ERGOT DERIVATIVES. In 1824, Hosach recommended that ergot be used to control postpartum hemorrhage, and since then ergot derivatives have been used to produce tetanic uterine contractions. If oxytocin and massage fail to produce the desired degree of uterine contraction, methylergonovine should be considered. Normally, a dose of 0.2 to 0.3 mg administered intramuscularly is sufficient; however, some obstetricians advocate the use of as much as 0.2 mg intravenously, but with extreme caution to avoid severe hypertension.

Methylergonovine can produce marked systemic vasoconstriction when used parenterally in patients with increased blood pressure. This drug should not be given when the systolic blood pressure exceeds 140 to 150 mm Hg; when the patient has preexisting hypertension or pregnancy-related hypertension; or if she has recently received a parenteral vasopressor. Given this danger, we administer this drug intramuscularly rather than intravenously.

15-METHYLPROSTAGLANDIN $F_{2\alpha}$. Recently introduced to aid in uterine contraction is 15-methylprostaglandin $F_{2\alpha}$ (carboprost), a synthetic derivative of natural prostaglandin $F_{2\alpha}$. During the last two trimesters of pregnancy, the administration of 15-methylprostaglandin $F_{2\alpha}$ causes strong uterine contraction and can induce delivery. It also is used in inducing therapeutic abortion.

15-Methylprostaglandin $F_{2\alpha}$ also is indicated for the treatment of postpartum hemorrhage resulting from uterine atony that has not responded to conventional management. An initial dose of 250 μg is given by deep intramuscular injection, either in uterine or in somatic muscle. Additional injections at intervals of 15 to 90 minutes have been necessary in a minority of cases.

Of special interest to the obstetric anesthesiologist is the incidence of particular adverse reactions. Two thirds of the treated patients vomit and have diarrhea, and one in eight has a temperature increase greater than 1°C. This pyrexia usually occurs within the first 6 hours after the first injection. Maternal oxygen desaturation 5 to 10 minutes after administration, presumably resulting from increased pulmonary venous admixture, has been reported.[24] 15-Methylprostaglandin $F_{2\alpha}$ should be used with caution in the patient with a history of bronchospasm.

Surgery

When all of the foregoing pharmacologic interventions fail, surgery occasionally is necessary. Too much time cannot be lost before opting for a surgical method of controlling the bleeding, because prolonged bleeding makes the patient susceptible to a superimposed coagulation defect. Final attempts at therapy may include manual examination of the uterine cavity for placental fragments, uterine curettage, figure-of-eight sutures at a low uterine implant site, ligation of the internal iliac (hypogastric arteries), and, when all else fails, gravid hysterectomy. Packing the uterine cavity is no longer an accepted procedure, because the intrauterine contents deter firm and continuous contraction of the uterus, and thus, uterine bleeding may increase rather than decrease.

REFERENCES

1. Phillips OC, Davis GH, Frazier TM, et al: The role of anesthesia in obstetric mortality. Anesth Analg 40:557, 1961
2. Gibb D: Confidential inquiry into maternal death. Br J Obstet Gynaecol 97:97, 1990
3. Abnormalities of the third stage of labor. In Williams' obstetrics, 19th ed. New York: Appleton & Lange, 1993: 615
4. Hughes EC, Cochrane NE, Czyz PL: Maternal mortality study: I. New York State Journal of Medicine 76:2206, 1976
5. Jimerson SD, Crosby WM: Maternal mortality in Oklahoma: hemorrhage remains a problem. J Okla State Med Assoc 71: 197, 1978
6. Gibbs CE, Locke WE: Maternal deaths in Texas, 1969 to 1973: a report of 501 consecutive maternal deaths from the Texas Medical Association's Committee on Maternal Health. Am J Obstet Gynecol 126:687, 1976
7. Coppes JB, Messer RH: Maternal deaths in California from 1967: the need for mortality review. Am J Obstet Gynecol 125:393, 1976
8. Sachs BP, Brown DAJ, Driscoll SG, et al: Maternal mortality in Massachusetts: trends and prevention. N Engl J Med 316:667, 1987
9. Chowdhury NNR: Maternal deaths due to haemorrhage. J Indian Med Assoc 67:157, 1976
10. Rao KB: Maternal mortality in a teaching hospital in southern India. Obstet Gynecol 46:397, 1975
11. Plumer MH: Bleeding problems. In James FM III, Wheeler AS (eds): Obstetric anesthesia: the complicated patient. Philadelphia: FA Davis, 1982: 185
12. Phillips OC: Uterine atony. In Orkin FK, Cooperman LH (eds): Complications in anesthesiology. Philadelphia: JB Lippincott, 1983: 538
13. Munson ES, Embro WJ: Enflurane, isoflurane, and halothane on isolated human uterine muscle. Anesthesiology 46:11, 1977
14. Munson ES, Maier WR, Caton D: Effects of halothane, cyclopropane and nitrous oxide on isolated human uterine muscle. Journal of Obstetrics and Gynaecology of the British Commonwealth 76:27, 1969
15. Peng ATC, Gorman RS, Shulman SM, et al. Intravenous nitroglycerin for uterine relaxation in the postpartum patient with retained placenta (letter). Anesthesiology 71:172, 1989
16. DeSimone CA, Norris MC, Leighton BL. Intravenous nitroglycerin aids manual extraction of a retained placenta (letter). Anesthesiology 73:787, 1990
17. Laros RK Jr: Coagulation disorders and hemoglobinopathies in the obstetric and surgical patient. In Shnider SM, Levinson G (eds): Anesthesia for obstetrics, 2nd ed. Baltimore: Williams & Wilkins, 1987: 263
18. Nakano J: Cardiovascular actions of oxytocin. Obstet Gynecol Surv 28:75, 1973
19. Weis FR Jr, Peak J: Effects of oxytocin on blood pressure during anesthesia. Anesthesiology 40:189, 1974
20. Johnstone M: The cardiovascular effects of oxytocic drugs. Br J Anaesth 44:826, 1972
21. Weiss RF Jr, Markello R, Benjamin MO, et al: Cardiovascular effects of oxytocin. Obstet Gynecol 46:2, 1975
22. Amico JA, Seitchik J, Robinson AG: Studies of oxytocin in plasma of women during hypocontractile labor. J Clin Endocrinol Metab 58:274, 1984
23. Oleen MA, Mariano JP: Controlling refractory atonic postpartum hemorrhage with Hemabate sterile solution. Am J Obstet Gynecol 162:205, 1990
24. Hankins GV, Berryman GK, Scott RT, et al: Maternal arterial desaturation with 15-methyl prostaglandin F_2 alpha for uterine atony. Obstet Gynecol 72:367, 1988

FURTHER READING

Cunningham FG, MacDonald PC, Gant NF (eds): Abnormalities of the third stage of labor. In: Williams obstetrics, 19th ed. Norwalk, CT: Appleton & Lange, 1993

Taylor CE: Hemorrhagic disorders in the obstetric patient. In: Civetta JM, Taylor RW, Kirby RR (eds): Critical care, 2nd ed. Philadelphia: JB Lippincott, 1992: 861

Complications in Anesthesiology, second edition,
edited by Nikolaus Gravenstein and Robert R. Kirby.
Lippincott-Raven Publishers, Philadelphia © 1996.

CHAPTER 54

Hypoventilation and Apnea in the Newborn

Charles J. Coté
Letty M. P. Liu

Neonates and preterm infants are more prone to hypoventilation and apnea after anesthesia than are older children and adults. When these very young patients undergo anesthesia and surgery, their special needs must be considered in planning anesthetic management. This chapter discusses the problems of hypoventilation and apnea in infants receiving anesthesia, with specific reference to developmental differences in the respiratory system. A review of the problems unique to former preterm infants scheduled for outpatient surgical procedures is presented.

DEVELOPMENTAL PREDISPOSITION TO APNEA

Respiratory System

Anatomy

As with all bodily systems, the respiratory system undergoes maturation beginning in intrauterine life and continuing well into the postnatal period. At birth, the upper airway is incompletely developed: the neonate's larynx is located higher in the neck than is the adult's. The tongue is relatively large in proportion to the rest of the oropharynx, and the distance between the tongue and the roof of the mouth is less in an infant than in an adult. These anatomic differences make the infant more prone to airway obstruction.[1]

AIRWAY OBSTRUCTION. Obstruction of the oral airway by the tongue and the other soft tissue structures of the larynx may account, in part, for the predominant nasal breathing pattern of infants.[2,3] When the nasal passages are obstructed, as by choanal atresia, infection, tumor, or a nasogastric tube, neonates, especially preterm neonates, are more likely to have respiratory failure, apnea, or both because of the added resistance to airflow through the nasal passages or the inability to convert to oral breathing.[4,5] Although infants are able to overcome nasal airway obstruction, to do so usually takes several respiratory efforts. In one study, an infant required 32 seconds to breathe successfully through the mouth.[6,7] The amount of time an infant with nasal airway obstruction can sustain mouth breathing because of the required increased effort is unknown.[2]

Resistance to Air Flow

The nasal passages account for 25% of the resistance to air flow in the infant compared with 60% in the adult; thus, in the infant and young child, the bronchi and small airways account for the majority of resistance to air flow.[8,9] Since the resistance to air flow is inversely proportional to the radius of the lumen to the fourth power for laminar flow and to the fifth power for turbulent flow, any factor that materially reduces the lumen of the airway(s), increases the infant's work of breathing with the same degree of airway obstruction. This increase in the work of breathing may be as much as two- to threefold compared with that in the adult.[1] Since crying causes turbulent flow, infants and children may suddenly deteriorate if they become upset and cry, thus causing turbulent air flow. This relation accounts for the high incidence of respiratory failure caused by fatigue in the infant or small child with upper airway infection which causes airway narrowing (croup, epiglottitis), bronchiolitis, pneumonia, or a foreign body in the trachea. In infants, nasal flaring is often a sign of respiratory distress. Nasal flaring has a physiologic function; it results in a marked reduction in the resistance to air entry into the larynx and thus serves to increase gas exchange.[10]

Airway Compliance

High compliance of the upper-airway structures is another factor that can contribute to respiratory compromise. During normal, quiet respiration, the pressure within the extrathoracic trachea is negative relative to atmospheric pressure; this gradient results in a slight collapse of the extrathoracic trachea during inspiration.[11] With upper-airway obstruction, the infant attempts to inspire against the obstruction and generates a greater negative pressure, which in turn leads to further collapse of the trachea. If the child is upset and crying, tracheal collapse increases; this fact may account for the sudden respiratory decompensation occasionally observed in the crying child with upper-airway obstruction.

With lower-airway obstruction, a similar physiologic response occurs but in reverse: during inspiration, the intrathoracic airways enlarge, whereas during expiration they tend to collapse. Thus, with intrathoracic airway obstruction (eg, bronchiolitis, pneumonia, secretions, congestive heart failure, or an intrathoracic tracheal foreign body), the child produces a forced exhalation, which increases intrathoracic pressure and collapses the intrathoracic airways.[11,12] This effect partially explains the sudden increase in wheezing in the crying infant or child. Therefore, respiratory failure and apnea may be precipitated entirely by mechanical factors.

Chest Wall Compliance

The rib cage of the infant is structurally different from that of the older child or adult: the diaphragm and ribs are oriented differently, such that contraction of the respiratory muscles is less efficient. This relative reduction in efficiency, combined with the highly elastic nature of the neonatal chest wall, results in a greater tendency for inward movement during respiration and airway closure with each breath.[13–15]

Developmental Changes

Respiratory Muscles

Developmental changes in respiratory muscle power can contribute to fatigue, hypoventilation, and apnea. In addition to reduced muscle mass, the composition of intercostal and diaphragmatic muscle fibers changes with age. Type 1 muscle fibers, which provide the capacity to perform sustained, repetitive exercise (respiration), are reduced substantially in number in the premature infant's diaphragm and intercostal muscles, are more developed in the full-term neonate, and are fully developed by 2 years of age.[16,17] Therefore, any factor that increases the work of breathing leads to fatigue more readily in the child less than 2 years of age. A direct relation thus exists between the infant's ability to compensate for an increased respiratory load and gestational age.[13,17–21]

Functional Residual Capacity

The functional residual capacity is smaller in the premature infant than in the full-term infant and is smaller in the full-term neonate compared with the older child or adult. These differences are attributable, in part, to the continued development of alveoli well after the 1st year of life; the bronchial system is far more developed than the alveoli at birth.[22] This discrepancy in balance between alveoli and bronchial development explains the inability of an infant to sustain life independently before 24 to 26 weeks gestation. Other factors that may be important include the production of surfactant and the development of the chest wall musculature and compliance.[23]

Chemoreceptors

The premature infant has normal peripheral chemoreceptors but incompletely developed central chemoreceptors. He or she may respond to hypoxemia by hypoventilating rather than hyperventilating like an adult. The response to hyperoxia is a transient decrease followed by an increase in minute ventilation.[24–26] The carbon dioxide response curve is flattened; this shift in the curve is increased by hypoxemia. As the infant matures, the normal adult response to carbon dioxide develops.

Apnea

The response of the premature infant larynx to chemical irritants is also undeveloped, so that rather than coughing in response to a noxious stimuli, the infant may simply exhibit reflex apnea. This response may partially explain the higher incidence of sudden infant death syndrome in infants with gastroesophageal reflux.[27–31]

Pulmonary Circulation

The pulmonary circulation is not completely developed in the neonate, particularly the premature neonate. At birth, the infant converts from the intrauterine parallel circulation (fetal) to a series circulation (adult).[32] This process, however, does not occur immediately and may require days to weeks for complete maturation. Closure of the ductus arteriosus is mediated through prostaglandins and exposure to oxygen, whereas closure of the patent foramen ovale results from a decrease in pulmonary artery pressure.

Thus, the neonate has a *transitional circulation*, with potential right-to-left shunts at the foramen ovale and the ductus arteriosus. During this very unstable period, any process which results in hypoxemia and hypercarbia increases pulmonary artery pressure, resulting in shunting. If right-to-left shunting occurs, hypoxemia increases, aggravates the severity of the initial problem, and creates a downward cycle. Thus, apnea is intimately related to the adequacy of ventilation and oxygenation.

Metabolism

Factors that increase the metabolic rate can lead to hypoxemia and hypercarbia; combined respiratory and metabolic acidosis may eventually lead to respiratory failure. Oxygen consumption and carbon dioxide production are normally two to three times greater per unit of body mass in the infant compared with the adult.[33] This is further increased with sepsis or fever. Oral feeding, thermal stress, rapid-eye-movement sleep, and increased physical activity (eg, increased respiratory load) also increase the metabolic rate.[34–36] In these conditions, the infant must be able to meet the need for more oxygen by increasing pulmonary ventilation.

NEONATAL APNEA

An infant's respiratory pattern can be related to postconceptual age (PCA), which is the sum of gestational age (GA) at birth and the postnatal age: eg, a 10-week-old infant born after 31 weeks gestation has a postconceptual age of 41 weeks. A normal premature infant exhibits a periodic pattern of respiration (periodic breathing) for a considerable time. This breathing pattern is more common in preterm and former preterm babies and less common in full-term infants.[23,37] Periods of apnea(<15 seconds) or apnea accompanied by bradycardia (apnea < 15 seconds + bradycardia [heart rate < 80 beats per minute]), are also more common in preterm and former preterm infants.

Incidence and Causes

Neonatal apnea may occur for numerous reasons, including hypothermia, hypoglycemia, hypocalcemia, seizures, mechanical obstruction of the airway, central nervous system abnormalities, sepsis, congestive heart failure, laryngeal dysfunction, and airway obstruction. Whenever apnea is diagnosed, the physician must consider the diverse possible causes (Fig. 54-1).

When the cause cannot be determined, it generally is attributed to prematurity; 20% to 30% of these infants exhibit apneic spells. Apnea of prematurity may be triggered by central nervous system immaturity, chest wall receptors, pulmonary receptors, laryngeal receptors, or any combination of these factors.[2,3,13,19,23,27,30,38–44] In preterm infants, even without these problems, apnea is of central origin approximately 70% of the time, of mixed origin 20% of the time, and of obstructive origin in 10% of cases.[45–47]

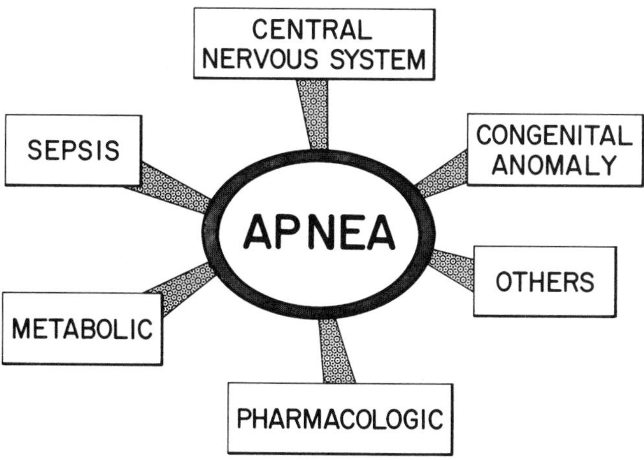

FIGURE 54-1. Common causes of apnea. (Reproduced with permission from Coté CJ, Todres ID, Ryan JF: Preoperative evaluation of pediatric patients. In Coté CJ, Ryan JF, Todres ID, Goudsouzian NG (eds): A practice of anesthesia for infants and children. Philadelphia: WB Saunders, 1992; 48)

Clinical Management

The frequency and severity of apnea can be better understood and followed with sleep studies, specifically examining the baby's respiratory and cardiac pattern, oxygen saturation, and expired carbon dioxide values. Management of patients with apnea of prematurity has focused on the use of respiratory stimulants, such as methylxanthines (eg, theophylline), and home apnea monitors.[43,48–61]

Theophylline

Theophylline dosage is determined by the baby's gestational, postnatal, and postconceptual ages.[62–64] Several different formulae have been used to estimate the dose of aminophylline required to produce a therapeutic level of 5 to 15 μg/kg. One formula appears to produce a more reliable therapeutic level:

$$0.2 \times \text{postnatal age in weeks} + 5 = \text{24-hour dose (mg/kg)}.^{62}$$

Serum theophylline concentrations should not exceed 10 μg/mL in neonates and 20 μg/mL in infants. Frequent monitoring of serum concentrations assists in maintaining the theophylline concentration in the therapeutic range. It appears that the level needed to prevent apnea is less than that required to treat bronchospastic disease.[62] Maintenance therapy should not be continued or dosages increased if toxic symptoms are present or if the drug effect is not beneficial. In general, with maturation, the severity and frequency of apneic periods decrease, and theophylline therapy can be discontinued.

Caffeine

Caffeine is another potent methylxanthine with respiratory and central nervous system stimulant effects but with fewer side effects than theophylline.[65,66] In a dosage of 5 to 10 mg/kg infused over a 2-minute period immediately after induction of anesthesia, caffeine was found effective in eliminating postoperative apneic episodes in former preterm infants between 37 and 44 weeks postconceptual age, compared with controls.[50,51] A dose of 10 mg/kg appears to be more effective than 5 mg/kg.[50] However, further evaluation of its overall effectiveness is needed since these studies had such a small population and because the kinetics of caffeine change so dramatically in the first few months of life (half-life 97 hours in preterm infants reduced to 6 hours by 60 weeks postconceptual age).[67,68]

ANESTHESIA AND NEONATAL APNEA

As discussed previously, many factors contribute to the development of apnea, some of which are preventable (Table 54-1).

General Considerations

When providing anesthetic care for a neonate or a former preterm infant, one must be careful to provide a stable and safe environment. The child must be kept warm on the way to the operating room by using a transport incubator, if indicated, and in the operating room by warming the room and

TABLE 54-1
Causes of Postoperative Apnea

- Upper-airway obstruction
  - Laryngospasm
- Pharmacologic causes
  - Narcotic overdose
  - Residual inhalation anesthesia
  - Residual neuromuscular block
- Metabolic imbalance
  - Hypocapnia
  - Acidosis
  - Hypoglycemia
  - Hypocalcemia
  - Hypothermia
- Pulmonary complication
  - Pulmonary aspiration
  - Pulmonary hemorrhage
  - Atelectasis
- Neurologic disorders
  - Seizures
  - Intracranial hemorrhage
- Anemia
- Dehydration
- Sepsis
- Idiopathic causes

by using warming blankets, radiant overhead heaters, heated humidified anesthetic gases, and warm surgical preparatory solutions. Equal attention must be paid to maintaining a stable temperature in the recovery period and during transport back to the ward.

Close attention is needed to maintain a stable thermal homeostasis. Normal thermal homeostasis will minimize oxygen consumption and therefore decrease metabolic demands. The increased respiration needed to meet these increased metabolic demands caused by hypothermia can increase the risk of hypoxia, apnea, or both. Similarly, close attention to glucose and calcium homeostasis will decrease the potential for apnea caused by hypocalcemia or hypoglycemia. Meticulous control of pulmonary ventilation will avoid hyper- or hypocarbia and resultant changes in cerebrospinal fluid pH. End-tidal carbon dioxide monitoring should ensure accurate measurement regardless of the circuit used.[69–71]

Anesthetic Management

The role of anesthetic management in the development of postoperative apnea in the neonate is complex and multifaceted. Although they may be discussed individually, the anesthetic-related factors are often linked (Fig. 54-2).

Effects on Hypoventilation and Apnea

Anesthetic agents contribute to hypoventilation and apnea through a variety of mechanisms. They act directly on the central respiratory center and depress the normal ventilatory responses to hypoxia and hypercapnia.[72,73] Anesthetic drugs, sedatives, narcotics, and barbiturates also decrease muscle tone, thus contributing to potential mechanical obstruction of the upper airway. They reduce functional residual capacity by altering skeletal muscle function and thus, decrease oxygen reserve.[74,75] A patient's propensity to apnea and hypoxia may increase as a result of decreasing normal chest wall reflexes mediated through the intercostal motor neurons.

Airway Obstruction

Airway obstruction is perhaps the most common cause of apnea in the perianesthetic period. It frequently results from a change in upper-airway muscle tone that is associated with tongue recession. The infant is more vulnerable to obstructive apnea due to a reduction in muscle tone because the hypopharynx is shallower than that of older patients, ie, the distance between the roof of the mouth and the tongue is shorter and the tongue is large relative to the oropharynx.[1] This type of apnea is easily treated by subluxing the jaw and lifting the mandible forward so the tongue is moved anteriorly, away from the posterior hypopharynx. Apnea in the immediate postoperative period especially after the effects of anesthetic agents have dissipated, may have an additional etiology, ie, obstruction at the level of the hypopharynx.[76–79]

Neuromuscular Blockade

If the neuromuscular junction is partially blocked by residual muscle relaxant effects, postanesthetic hypoventilation or apnea may occur. Premature and full-term neonates have minimal respiratory reserve and will not tolerate even slight changes in respiratory muscle function. Thus, even if an infant appears to be breathing adequately after receiving a neuromuscular blocking drug, neuromuscular blockade should be completely antagonized before allowing the child to breathe unassisted. It should be noted that vecuronium may last as long as pancuronium in neonates whereas atracurium has the same length of duration in both neonates and older patients.[80] Since atracurium is less dependent upon hepatic or renal ex-

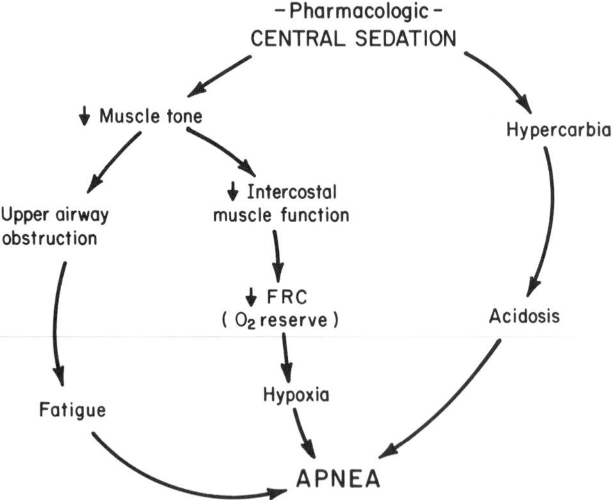

FIGURE 54-2. Possible sequences in the development of apnea in the neonate after general anesthesia. (Reproduced with permission from Coté CJ, Todres ID, Ryan JF: Preoperative evaluation of pediatric patients. In Coté CJ, Ryan JF, Todres ID, Goudsouzian NG (eds): A practice of anesthesia for infants and children. Philadelphia, WB Saunders, 1992; 48)

cretion than other relaxants, it would seem to offer advantage in the neonate and infant.[80]

Postconceptual Age

A number of studies have documented the increased incidence of perioperative respiratory complications in infants who are born before term (< 37 weeks gestational age [GA]).[50,51,81–92] The incidence of postoperative apnea is inversely related to GA and postconceptual age (PCA).[93] Other respiratory complications include atelectasis, pulmonary aspiration, and stridor.

Many of these infants appear to be completely normal before anesthesia and surgery, and the majority are free of apneic spells before anesthesia. Most postoperative apnea in former preterm infants occurs in the recovery room; however, apneic spells have been reported up to 12 hours after anesthesia.[93] Postoperative apnea has been recorded in infants as old as 60 weeks PCA.[84] Attempts to reduce this risk by the use of regional anesthesia appear to be somewhat effective, but apnea may still occur following spinal anesthesia as well as epidural anesthesia.[87,94–96] Apparently anesthesia and surgery can unmask a defect in the ventilatory control mechanism of young preterm infants. It should be noted however that postoperative apnea can occur in the absence of prematurity. At least three full-term infants have been reported to develop apnea in the immediate postoperative period.[33,97,98] Apnea has also been recently reported in full-term infants following pyloromyotomy.[99,100]

It is clearly difficult for the practitioner to determine when it is safe to perform a surgical procedure on former preterm infants. If one examines the papers that have attempted to answer this question the recommendations for postoperative monitoring range from 44 to 60 weeks PCA. One of the problems is that it is difficult to collect a large series at any one institution, particularly when one is attempting to study a relatively rare event. Since the incidence of apnea in former preterm infants is inversely related to GA and PCA, the actual number of patients in this older category is not very large. Furthermore, even if one has a series of 30 children without apnea does this rule out the potential for apnea? In order to feel comfortable that the risk is less than 5%, one would need to follow the rule of 3's,[101] which suggests that the risk is generally 3/N. For a population of 30 patients, even if none had demonstrated apnea, the risk would be 3/30 = 10%; for a population of 100 it would be about 3%. This analysis indicates that a very large series, particularly with children in the upper end of the age range, would be required to adequately examine this issue. Since most series contain 10 to 60 patients, it would be easy to fail to observe apnea in the upper age range in any one of the studies.

In order to gain some insight into this problem we obtained the original data from several investigators, all of whom obtained their data prospectively. These investigators provided their original data so that we could perform a detailed analysis.[50,51,77,84–87,89] Only prospective studies were included, and we focused on one operation, inguinal herniorrhaphy. We examined nine risk factors: GA, PCA, anemia (hematocrit < 30%), use of narcotics or muscle relaxants, history of apnea, necrotizing enterocolitis, history of respiratory distress syndrome or bronchopulmonary dysplasia, or ongoing apnea at home. We only included infants undergoing general anesthesia without special treatment such as caffeine.

A total of 384 infants were collected and 255 fulfilled study criteria. As expected, we found a very strong correlation with both GA and PCA (Fig. 54-3). This indicates that if one had two infants, one born at 28 weeks GA and another born at 32 weeks GA, and both were now 45 weeks PCA, the infant born at 28 weeks GA would have a greater risk for apnea.

We also found a relation with a history of ongoing apnea, but when the effects of GA and PCA were considered this relation was lost. *The only risk factor that was independent of both GA and PCA was anemia.* This means that the risk of apnea is the same in a 45-week PCA infant with anemia and in a 60-week PCA infant. Our analysis confirmed the studies performed by Welborn and coworkers.[86] Interestingly, small-for-gestational-age (SGA) infants seemed somewhat protected from apnea; none of the 18 SGA infants experienced postoperative apnea. We used logistic regression and determined significant institution-to-institution variability in the incidence of apnea. We also found that the two institutions that used computer monitoring[50,51,77,86,87,102] had a higher rate of apnea than those institutions that used standard impedance pneumography or nursing observation (Fig. 54-4).[85,89] Despite the apparently large number of infants in our analysis after combining the data from four institutions and eight studies, the data were still limited by the small number of patients in the upper age range, particularly those over 45 weeks PCA.

We constructed three different models:

A: the entire population
B: the entire population minus the infants with anemia
C: the entire population minus the infants with anemia or with apnea in the recovery room.[93]

With this narrowing of the population, the third model left us with 172 patients. Extrapolation of this model suggests that even if we exclude all anemic infants and those with

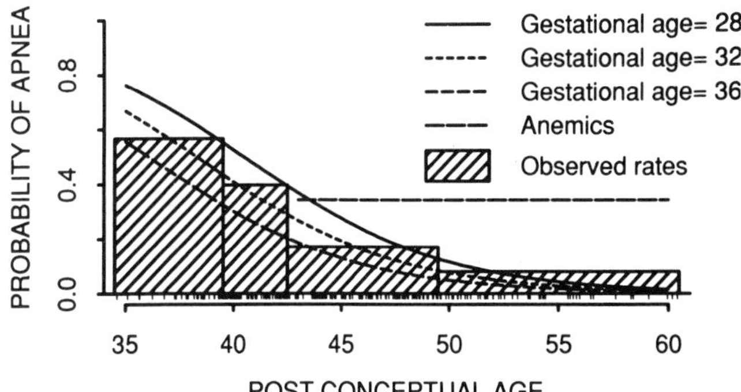

FIGURE 54-3. Predicted probability of apnea for all patients by gestational age and postconceptual age. Patients with anemia are shown as the horizontal hatched line. The shaded boxes represent the overall rates of apnea for infants within that gestational age range. The probability of apnea was the same regardless of postconceptual age or gestational age for infants with anemia (horizontal hatched line). (Reproduced with permission from Coté et al. Postoperative apnea in former preterm infants after inguinal herniorrhaphy: A combined analysis. Anesthesiology 82:809, 1995)

recovery room apnea (ie, admit the anemic patients and those with apnea in recovery room for postoperative monitoring), the risk for apnea after recovery room decreases to 5% (95% confidence) at postconceptual age 48 weeks with gestational age 35 weeks or at postconceptual age 50 weeks with gestational age 32 weeks. However, we would not have statistical confidence that the probability of apnea decreases to less than 1% (95% confidence) until postconceptual age 54 weeks with gestational age 35 weeks or postconceptual age 56 weeks with gestational age 32 weeks.

Apnea/bradycardia spells even of brief duration may have important clinical implications since cerebral blood flow is rapidly reduced when the heart rate falls to 80 beats/min (Fig. 54-5).[103] In addition, a decrease in cerebral surface oxygen concentrations has been demonstrated to occur within 5 seconds of beginning endotracheal suctioning; 15 seconds were required to return the values to baseline.[104] For these reasons even brief periods of apnea, particularly if associated with desaturation, should be considered clinically important.

Each practitioner and each institution must weigh the risks and the benefits of admission and monitoring. It should be obvious that if the hospital does not have the facilities and the skilled personnel to care for such infants they should be transferred to another institution that does have that capacity.

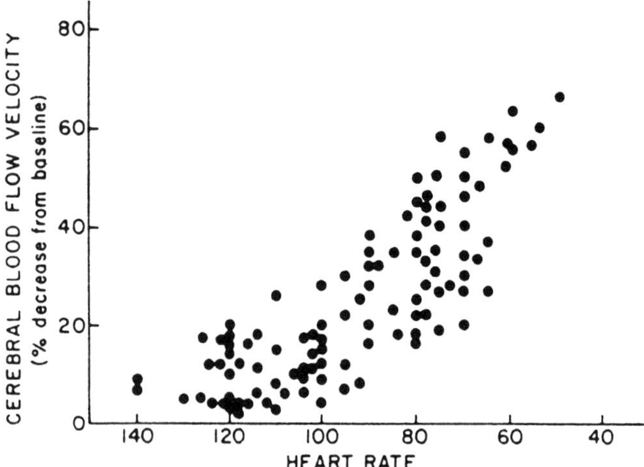

FIGURE 54-5. Relationship of change in heart rate with apnea to area under velocity curve. Individual values for 101 separate episodes of apnea and bradycardia are shown. (Reproduced with permission from: Perlman, JM, Volpe JJ: Episodes of apnea and bradycardia in the preterm newborn: Impact on cerebral circulation. Pediatrics 76: 333–338, 1985)

Clinical Recommendations

No ideal anesthetic agent or technique avoids idiopathic postanesthetic apnea in prematurely born infants. Regional anesthesia (without supplemental medications, eg, ketamine or midazolam) may reduce but not completely eliminate the risk of postoperative apnea. Careful monitoring of babies who are at risk for apnea during the postanesthetic period will reduce patient morbidity and mortality. Thus, whenever a former preterm infant is scheduled for a procedure requiring anesthesia, the anesthesiologist must obtain a thorough preoperative history and physical examination. Items of particular importance include the postnatal and gestational age, neonatal course, current medical problems, current medications, use of home apnea monitor, and a current hematocrit. All anemic former preterms should be admitted and monitored; we do not know how far out, ie, for how many weeks postconceptual age, this recommendation should be followed. Once this information has been obtained, an appropriate anesthetic prescription can be made.

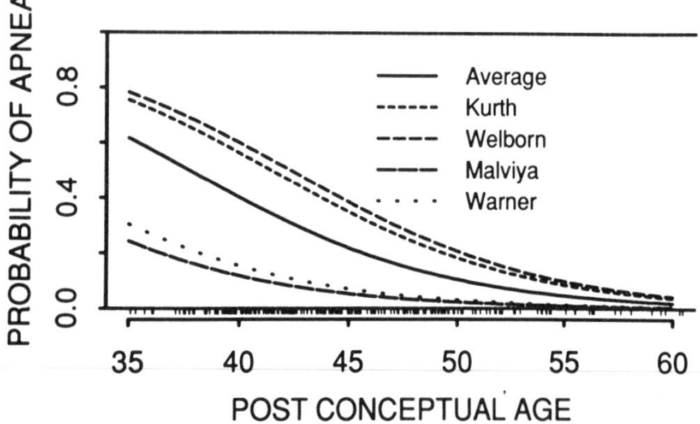

FIGURE 54-4. Predicted probability of apnea in recovery room and postrecovery room by weeks postconceptual age for all patients for each investigator. Bottom tick marks indicate the number of data points versus postconceptual age. Note that the curves for the Kurth and Welborn studies are nearly identical in the upper range and for the Malviya and Warner studies in the lower range; there was significant institution-to-institution variability. The reasons for this are unclear but may represent differences in monitoring technology as well as patient populations since the studies with the highest rate of apnea were also those which used continuous recording devices. (Reproduced with permission from Coté et al. Postoperative apnea in former preterm infants after inguinal herniorrhaphy: A combined analysis. Anesthesiology 82:809, 1995)

Infants who were born prematurely, especially those with ongoing apnea or anemia, and those less than 48 weeks postconceptual age, must be admitted and monitored. If one wants to keep the risk of apnea below 1%, this admission age should be increased to 55 weeks postconceptual age. Consideration should be given to delaying elective procedures until the infant is more mature if the surgeon agrees that this is reasonable.

When these patients receive anesthesia, theophylline should be continued throughout the perianesthetic period if they are receiving the drug to prevent apnea/bradycardia spells. Caffeine citrate 10 mg/kg should be considered as a prophylactic measure, but the data base that supports this is too small to be sure that it will prevent the apnea.

Infants at increased risk should be anesthetized in a facility that has the personnel and equipment to monitor at least the respiratory and electrocardiographic patterns and ideally the hemoglobin oxygen saturation by pulse oximetry continuously for at least 12 to 24 hours after anesthesia. In addition, personnel caring for these babies should be skilled in infant resuscitation. Despite many advances both in terms of pharmacology and anesthetic care, these children remain a special population with special needs.

REFERENCES

1. Eckenhoff JE: Some anatomic considerations of the infant larynx influencing endotracheal anesthesia. Anesthesiology 12: 401, 1951

2. Bosma JF: Introduction to the symposium: 5-49, 1974(Abstract)
3. Harding R: Nasal obstruction in infancy. [Review]. Aust Paediatr J 22 [Suppl 1]:59, 1986
4. Passy V, Newcron S, Snyder S: Rhinorrhea with airway obstruction. Laryngoscope 85:888, 1975
5. Stocks J: Effect of nasogastric tubes on nasal resistance during infancy. Arch Dis Child 55:17, 1980
6. Stark AR, Thach BT: Recovery of airway patency after obstruction in normal infants. Am Rev Respir Dis 123:691, 1981
7. Rodenstein DO, Perlmutter N, Stanescu DC: Infants are not obligatory nasal breathers. Am Rev Respir Dis 131:343, 1985
8. Lacourt G, Polgar G: Interaction between nasal and pulmonary resistance in newborn infants. J Appl Physiol 30:870, 1971
9. Polgar G, Kong GP: The nasal resistance of newborn infants. Journal of Pediatrics 67:557, 1965
10. Carlo WA, Martin RJ, Bruce EN, Strohl KP, Fanaroff AA: Alae nasi activation (nasal flaring) decreases nasal resistance in preterm infants. Pediatrics 72:338, 1983
11. Wittenborg MH, Gyepes MT, Crocker D: Tracheal dynamics in infants with respiratory distress, stridor, and collapsing trachea. Radiology 88:653, 1967
12. Coté CJ, Todres ID: The pediatric airway, a practice of anesthesia for infants and children. In: Coté CJ, Ryan JF, Todres ID, Goudsouzian NG (eds). Philadelphia: WB Saunders, 1992: 55
13. Muller NL, Bryan AC: Chest wall mechanics and respiratory muscles in infants. Pediatr Clin North Am 26:503, 1979
14. Mansell A, Bryan C, Levison H: Airway closure in children. J Appl Physiol 33:711, 1972
15. Anthonisen NR, Danson J, Robertson PC, Ross WR: Airway closure as a function of age. Respir Physiol 8:58, 1969
16. Keens TG, Bryan AC, Levison H, Ianuzzo CD: Developmental pattern of muscle fiber types in human ventilatory muscles. J Appl Physiol Resp Env Ex Physiol 44:909, 1978
17. Gerhardt T, Reifenberg L, Hehre D, Feller R, Bancalari E: Functional residual capacity in normal neonates and children up to 5 years of age determined by a N2 washout method. Pediatr Res 20:668, 1986
18. Muller N, Gulston G, Cade D, et al: Diaphragmatic muscle fatigue in the newborn. J Appl Physiol Resp Env Ex Physiol 46:688, 1979
19. Macklem PT: Respiratory muscles: the vital pump. Chest 78: 753, 1980
20. Macklem PT, Cohen C, Zagelbaum G, Roussos C: The pathophysiology of inspiratory muscle fatigue. Ciba Foundation Symposium 82:249, 1981
21. Roussos C, Macklem PT: The respiratory muscles. [Review]. N Engl J Med 307:786, 1982
22. Davies G, Reid L: Growth of the alveoli and pulmonary arteries in childhood. Thorax 25:669, 1970
23. Polgar G, Weng TR: The functional development of the respiratory system from the period of gestation to adulthood. [Review]. Am Rev Respir Dis 120:625, 1979
24. Rigatto H, Brady JP, De La Torre Verduzco R: Chemoreceptor reflexes in preterm infants: II. The effect of gestational and postnatal age on the ventilatory response to inhaled carbon dioxide. Pediatrics 55:614, 1975
25. Rigatto H, De La Torre Verduzco R, Gates DB: Effects of O_2 on the ventilatory response to CO_2 in preterm infants. J Appl Physiol 39:896, 1975
26. Rigatto H, Brady JP, De La Torre Verduzco R: Chemoreceptor reflexes in preterm infants: I. The effect of gestational and postnatal age on the ventilatory response to inhalation of 100% and 15% oxygen. Pediatrics 55:604, 1975
27. Downing SE, Lee JC: Laryngeal chemosensitivity: a possible mechanism for sudden infant death. Pediatrics 55:640, 1975
28. Byard RW, Moore L: Gastroesophageal reflux and sudden infant death syndrome. Pediatr Pathol 13:53, 1993
29. Reiterer F, Fox WW: Multichannel polysomnographic recording for evaluation of infant apnea. [Review]. Clin Perinatol 19: 871, 1992
30. Freed GE, Steinschneider A, Glassman M, Winn K: Sudden infant death syndrome prevention and an understanding of selected clinical issues. [Review]. Pediatr Clin North Am 41: 967, 1994
31. Krishnamoorthy M, Mintz A, Liem T, Applebaum H: Diagnosis and treatment of respiratory symptoms of initially unsuspected gastroesophageal reflux in infants. Am Surg 60:783, 1994
32. Rudolph AM: Developmental considerations in neonatal failure. Hospital Practice (Office Edition) 20:53, 1985
33. Tetzlaff JE, Annand DW, Pudimat MA, Nicodemus HF: Postoperative apnea in a full-term infant. Anesthesiology 69:426, 1988
34. Stothers JK, Warner RM: Oxygen consumption and neonatal sleep states. J Physiol 278:435, 1978
35. Rosen CL, Glaze DG, Frost JD Jr: Hypoxemia associated with feeding in the preterm infant and full-term neonate. Am J Dis Child 138:623, 1984
36. Silverman WA, Sinclair JC, Agate FJ Jr: The oxygen cost of minor changes in heat balance of small newborn infants. Acta Paediatr Scand 55:294, 1966
37. Ellingson RJ, Peters JF, Nelson B: Respiratory pauses and apnea during daytime sleep in normal infants during the first year of life: longitudinal observations. Electroenceph Clin Neurophysiol 53:48, 1982
38. Shannon DC, Kelly DH: SIDS and near-SIDS (first of two parts). [Review]. N Engl J Med 306:959, 1982
39. Shannon DC, Kelly DH: SIDS and near-SIDS (second of two parts). [Review]. N Engl J Med 306:1022, 1982
40. Gerhardt T, Bancalari E: Apnea of prematurity: I. Lung function and regulation of breathing. Pediatrics 74:58, 1984
41. Gerhardt T, Bancalari E: Apnea of prematurity: II. Respiratory reflexes. Pediatrics 74:63, 1984
42. Trippenbach T: Chest wall reflexes in newborns. Bull Eur Physiopathol Respir 21:115, 1985
43. Kelly DH, Shannon DC: Treatment of apnea and excessive periodic breathing in the full-term infant. Pediatrics 68:183, 1981
44. Henderson-Smart DJ, Pettigrew AG, Campbell DJ: Clinical apnea and brain-stem neural function in preterm infants. N Engl J Med 308:353, 1983
45. Finer NN, Barrington KJ, Hayes BJ, Hugh A: Obstructive, mixed, and central apnea in the neonate: physiologic correlates. J Pediatr 121:943, 1992
46. Ruggins NR, Milner AD: Site of upper airway obstruction in preterm infants with problematical apnoea. Arch Dis Child 66: 787, 1991
47. Upton CJ, Milner AD, Stokes GM: Upper airway patency during apnoea of prematurity. Arch Dis Child 67:419, 1992
48. Davi MJ, Sankaran K, Simons KJ, Simons FE, Seshia MM, Rigatto H: Physiologic changes induced by theophylline in the treatment of apnea in preterm infants. J Pediatr 92:91, 1978
49. Peliowski A, Finer NN: A blinded, randomized, placebo-controlled trial to compare theophylline and doxapram for the treatment of apnea of prematurity. J Pediatr 116:648, 1990
50. Welborn LG, Hannallah RS, Fink R, Ruttimann UE, Hicks JM: High-dose caffeine suppresses postoperative apnea in former preterm infants. Anesthesiology 71:347, 1989
51. Welborn LG, De Soto H, Hannallah RS, Fink R, Ruttimann UE, Boeckx R: The use of caffeine in the control of post-anesthetic apnea in former premature infants. Anesthesiology 68:796, 1988
52. Romagnoli C, De Carolis MP, Muzii U, et al: Effectiveness and side effects of two different doses of caffeine in preventing apnea in premature infants. Ther Drug Mon 14:14, 1992
53. Mulloy E, McNicholas WT: Theophylline in obstructive sleep apnea. A double-blind evaluation. Chest 101:753, 1992
54. Finer NN, Peters KL, Duffley LM, Coward JH: An evaluation of theophylline for idiopathic apnea of infancy. Dev Pharmacol Ther 7:73, 1984
55. Jamali F, Barrington KJ, Finer NN, Coutts RT, Torok-Both GA: Doxapram dosage regimen in apnea of prematurity based on pharmacokinetic data. Dev Pharmacol Ther 11:253, 1988
56. Moore ES, Faix RG, Banagale RC, Grasela TH: The population pharmacokinetics of theophylline in neonates and young infants. J Pharmacokin Biopharm 17:47, 1989
57. Kriter KE, Blanchard J: Management of apnea in infants. [Review]. Clin Pharm 8:577, 1989
58. Fuglsang G, Nielsen K, Kjaer Nielsen L, Sennels F, Jakobsen P, Thelle T: The effect of caffeine compared with theophylline

in the treatment of idiopathic apnea in premature infants. Acta Paediatr Scand 78:786, 1989
59. Bairam A, Boutroy MJ, Badonnel Y, Vert P: Theophylline versus caffeine: comparative effects in treatment of idiopathic apnea in the preterm infant. J Pediatr 110:636, 1987
60. Brouard C, Moriette G, Murat I, et al: Comparative efficacy of theophylline and caffeine in the treatment of idiopathic apnea in premature infants. American Journal of Diseases of Children 139:698, 1985
61. Muttitt SC, Tierney AJ, Finer NN: The dose response of theophylline in the treatment of apnea of prematurity. J Pediatr 112:115, 1988
62. Hogue SL, Phelps SJ: Evaluation of three theophylline dosing equations for use in infants up to one year of age [see comments]. J Pediatr 123:651, 1993
63. Kraus DM, Fischer JH, Reitz SJ, et al: Alterations in theophylline metabolism during the first year of life. Clin Pharmacol Ther 54:351, 1993
64. Nassif EG, Weinberger MM, Shannon D, et al: Theophylline disposition in infancy. J Pediatr 98:158, 1981
65. Murat I, Moriette G, Blin MC, et al: The efficacy of caffeine in the treatment of recurrent idiopathic apnea in premature infants. J Pediatr 99:984, 1981
66. Brouard C, Moriette G, Murat I, et al: Comparative efficacy of theophylline and caffeine in the treatment of idiopathic apnea in premature infants. Am J Dis Child 139:698, 1985
67. Pons G, Carrier O, Richard MO, et al: Developmental changes of caffeine elimination in infancy. Dev Pharmacol Ther 11: 258, 1988
68. Le Guennec JC, Billon B, Paré C: Maturational changes of caffeine concentrations and disposition in infancy during maintenance therapy for apnea of prematurity: influence of gestational age, hepatic disease, and breast-feeding. Pediatrics 76:834, 1985
69. Hillier SC, Badgwell JM, McLeod ME, Creighton RE, Lerman J: Accuracy of end-tidal P_{CO_2} measurements using a sidestream capnometer in infants and children ventilated with the Sechrist infant ventilator. Can J Anaesth 37:318, 1990
70. Badgwell JM, Heavner JE, May WS, Goldthorn JF, Lerman J: End-tidal P_{CO_2} monitoring in infants and children ventilated with either a partial rebreathing or a non-rebreathing circuit. Anesthesiology 66:405, 1987
71. Badgwell JM, McLeod ME, Lerman J, Creighton RE: End-tidal P_{CO_2} measurements sampled at the distal and proximal ends of the endotracheal tube in infants and children. Anesth Analg 66:959, 1987
72. Kafer ER, Marsh HM: The effects of anesthetic drugs and disease on the chemical regulation of ventilation. Int Anesthesiol Clin 15:1, 1977
73. Knill RL, Gelb AW: Ventilatory responses to hypoxia and hypercapnia during halothane sedation and anesthesia in man. Anesthesiology 49:244, 1978
74. Lopes J, Muller NL, Bryan MH, Bryan AC: Importance of inspiratory muscle tone in maintenance of FRC in the newborn. J Appl Physiol Resp Env Ex Physiol 51:830, 1981
75. Tusiewicz K, Bryan AC, Froese AB: Contributions of changing rib cage—diaphragm interactions to the ventilatory depression of halothane anesthesia. Anesthesiology 47:327, 1977
76. Mathew OP, Roberts JL, Thach BT: Pharyngeal airway obstruction in preterm infants during mixed and obstructive apnea. J Pediatr 100:964, 1982
77. Kurth CD, LeBard SE: Association of postoperative apnea, airway obstruction, and hypoxemia in former premature infants. Anesthesiology 75:22, 1991
78. Milner AD, Boon AW, Saunders RA, Hopkin IE: Upper airways obstruction and apnoea in preterm babies. Arch Dis Child 55: 22, 1980
79. Dransfield DA, Spitzer AR, Fox WW: Episodic airway obstruction in premature infants. Am J Dis Child 137:441, 1983
80. Gronert BJ, Brandom BW: Neuromuscular blocking drugs in infants and children. Pediatr Clin North Am 41:73, 1994
81. Steward DJ: Preterm infants are more prone to complications following minor surgery than are term infants. Anesthesiology 56:304, 1982
82. Gregory GA, Steward DJ: Life-threatening perioperative apnea in the ex-"premie" [editorial]. Anesthesiology 59:495, 1983
83. Liu LM, Coté CJ, Goudsouzian NG, et al: Life-threatening apnea in infants recovering from anesthesia. Anesthesiology 59:506, 1983
84. Kurth CD, Spitzer AR, Broennle AM, Downes JJ: Postoperative apnea in preterm infants. Anesthesiology 66:483, 1987
85. Malviya S, Swartz J, Lerman J: Are all preterm infants younger than 60 weeks postconceptual age at risk for postanesthetic apnea? Anesthesiology 78:1076, 1993
86. Welborn LG, Hannallah RS, Luban NLC, Fink R, Ruttimann UE: Anemia and postoperative apnea in former preterm infants. Anesthesiology 74:1003, 1991
87. Welborn LG, Rice LJ, Hannallah RS, Broadman LM, Ruttimann UE, Fink R: Postoperative apnea in former preterm infants: prospective comparison of spinal and general anesthesia. Anesthesiology 72:838, 1990
88. Welborn LG, Ramirez N, Oh TH, et al: Postanesthetic apnea and periodic breathing in infants. Anesthesiology 65:658, 1986
89. Warner LO, Teitelbaum DH, Caniano DA, Vanik PE, Martino JD, Servick JD: Inguinal herniorrhaphy in young infants: perianesthetic complications and associated preanesthetic risk factors. J Clin Anesth 4:455, 1992
90. Rescoria FJ, Grosfeld JL: Inguinal hernia repair in the perinatal period and early infancy: clinical considerations. J Pediatr Surg 19:832, 1984
91. Melone JH, Schwartz MZ, Tyson KRT, et al: Outpatient inguinal herniorrhaphy in premature infants: is it safe? J Pediatr Surg 27:203, 1992
92. Mayhew JF, Bourke DL, Guinee WS: Evaluation of the premature infant at risk for postoperative complications. Can J Anaesth 34:627, 1987
93. Coté CJ, Zaslavsky A, Downes JJ, et al: Postoperative apnea in former preterm infants after inguinal herniorrhaphy: A combined analysis. Anesthesiology 82:809, 1995
94. Harnik EV, Hoy GR, Potolicchio S, Stewart DR, Siegelman RE: Spinal anesthesia in premature infants recovering from respiratory distress syndrome. Anesthesiology 64:95, 1986
95. Gunter JB, Watcha MF, Forestner JE, et al: Caudal epidural anesthesia in conscious premature and high-risk infants. J Pediatr Surg 26:9, 1991
96. Watcha MF, Thach BT, Gunter JB: Postoperative apnea after caudal anesthesia in an ex-premature infant. Anesthesiology 71:613, 1989
97. Noseworthy J, Duran C, Khine HH: Postoperative apnea in a full-term infant [letter]. Anesthesiology 70:879, 1989
98. Cote CJ, Kelly DH: Postoperative apnea in a full-term infant with a demonstrable respiratory pattern abnormality [see comments]. Anesthesiology 72:559, 1990
99. Andropoulos DB, Heard MB, Johnson KL, Clarke JT, Rowe RW: Postanesthetic apnea in full-term infants after pyloromyotomy. Anesthesiology 80:216, 1994
100. Hannallah RS, Welborn LG, McGill WA: Postanesthetic apnea in full-term infants. Anesthesiology 81:264, 1994
101. Hanley JA, Lippman-Hand A: If nothing goes wrong, is everything all right? Interpreting zero numerators. JAMA 249:1743, 1983
102. Rolf N, Coté CJ: Persistent cardiac arrhythmias in pediatric patients: effects of age, expired carbon dioxide values, depth of anesthesia, and airway management [see comments]. Anesth Analg 73:720, 1991
103. Perlman JM, Volpe JJ: Episodes of apnea and bradycardia in the preterm newborn: impact on cerebral circulation. Pediatrics 76:333, 1985
104. Shah AR, Kurth CD, Gwiazdowski SG, Chance B, Delivoria-Papadopoulos M: Fluctuations in cerebral oxygenation and blood volume during endotracheal suctioning in premature infants [see comments]. J Pediatr 120:769, 1992

Complications in Anesthesiology, second edition,
edited by Nikolaus Gravenstein and Robert R. Kirby.
Lippincott-Raven Publishers, Philadelphia © 1996.

CHAPTER 55

Fetal and Neonatal Depression

John G. Shutack
Theodore G. Cheek
William W. Fox

After birth the neonate must rapidly initiate respiratory activity and alter cardiac and metabolic function. Thus, anesthesiologists who provide obstetric anesthetic care must understand the factors that may impair the neonate's ability to adapt. Drugs and other therapy that lead to fetal and neonatal depression predispose to neonatal asphyxia, airway obstruction, apnea, cyanosis, bradycardia, hypotonia, and hyporeflexia. These factors can be divided into five categories (Table 55-1). This chapter surveys the salient aspects of fetal and neonatal physiology, placental transport of drugs, the important role of fetal heart rate (FHR) monitoring during obstetric labor, and the special case of persisting pulmonary hypertension. It then considers the management of fetal and neonatal depression.

PHYSIOLOGIC FEATURES

Fetal Circulation

The placenta is the fetal organ of gas exchange, supplying a partial pressure of oxygen (P_{O_2}) of 30 mm Hg.[1] Oxygenated blood enters the fetus by way of the umbilical vein, from which it flows through the ductus venosus, mixing with desaturated blood from the inferior vena cava. Most of the blood entering the right atrium, directed by the crista dividens, flows into the left atrium through the foramen ovale. Some 10% to 20% of the blood from the inferior vena cava enters the right ventricle, mixing with desaturated blood from the superior vena cava, then flows into the pulmonary artery. Because of a high pulmonary vascular resistance (PVR), only 8% to 10% of blood enters the fluid-filled lungs; the remaining 90% shunts across the ductus arteriosus to the descending aorta. Oxygenated blood entering the left atrium from the right atrium flows to the left ventricle and out through the aortic arch, from which it supplies the brain by way of the carotid circulation.

Neonatal Circulation: Changes at Birth

Initiation of Breathing

At birth, multiple simultaneously occurring events result in conversion of fetal circulation to neonatal circulation, in which the lungs are the primary organ of gas exchange. During vaginal delivery the baby's thorax is squeezed by the birth canal, and fluid is expressed from its lungs. This lung fluid must overcome viscous forces in the trachea, surface forces in the bronchioles, and tissue forces in the alveoli during its passage from the lungs.[2] With the first breath an inspiratory pleural pressure of −60 to −70 cmH_2O may be required,[3] which decreases with subsequent breaths as a functional residual capacity of 30 to 35 mL/kg is established. Lung fluid not expressed by the trachea is removed by the pulmonary capillaries and lymphatics.

Lung Inflation and Pulmonary Vascular Resistance

Lung inflation, accompanied by a release of vasoactive substances such as prostaglandins and an increase in the alveolar P_{O_2} produces a decrease in PVR. Decreased PVR, which is most important to neonatal adaptation, is associated with an increase in pulmonary blood flow that, in conjunction with increased alveolar ventilation, causes an increase in arterial P_{O_2}. Normally, these changes result in closure of the ductus arteriosus and a further decrease in PVR. Pulmonary blood flow increases the pressure of the left atrium above that of the right atrium, in turn causing a closure of the foramen ovale. Decreased vena caval blood flow caused by clamping of the umbilical cord further decreases right atrial pressure. Because a decrease in PVR is so important during the transition to neonatal circulation, avoidance of factors that increase PVR such as hypercapnia, hypoxemia, and acidosis,[4] is paramount during resuscitation.

TABLE 55-1
Major Causes of Fetal and Neonatal Depression

MATERNAL AND PREGNANCY-INDUCED DISORDERS
- Hypertension
- Anemia
- Infection
- Thyroid disease
- Obesity
- Hypotension
- Diabetes mellitus
- Renal failure
- Cardiac disease

FETAL DISORDERS
- Pre- or postmaturity
- Congenital anomalies
- Meconium aspiration
- Growth retardation
- Rh sensitization

UTEROPLACENTAL MALFUNCTION
- Hyperactive or overstimulated labor
- Placental infarct
- Placenta previa
- Postmaturity
- Placental abruption

COMPLICATIONS OF LABOR AND DELIVERY
- Prolonged labor (especially second stage)
- Multiple gestation
- Sudden precipitous delivery
- Abnormal presentation (breech or transverse lie)
- Difficult or traumatic forceps delivery
- Umbilical cord compression or prolapse

DRUGS
- Direct depression
  - Prolonged or deep general anesthesia
  - Narcotics
  - Sedatives
  - Tranquilizers
- Indirect depression
  - Drugs causing maternal hypotension
  - Hypoxemia
  - Acidemia

Thermal Regulation

Neonates lose heat in the delivery room mainly by evaporation, although loss by conduction, convection, and radiation also plays a role. In response to this heat loss, the homeothermic neonate produces heat by metabolism of brown fat, so called nonshivering thermogenesis.[5] Brown fat accounts for 2% to 6% of body weight and is found at the nape of the neck, between the scapulae, in the mediastinum, and surrounding the kidneys and adrenal glands. The brown fat cells are rich in blood, sympathetic nerve supply, and mitochondria. With norepinephrine release during cold stress, triglycerides are hydrolyzed to glycerol and free fatty acids; these, in turn, are further oxidized to carbon dioxide and water, producing heat.[6]

As the environmental temperature decreases, neonatal oxygen consumption is increased above the basal level (4 to 6 mL/kg/min), which is twice that of the adult.[7] In this regard, the neonate's oxygen reserve is already reduced, for the functional residual capacity in 3-kg term neonates is only 90 mL. Of major importance is the maintenance of a neutral thermal environment (32° to 34°C for neonates).[8]

Cold stress in the neonate results in peripheral vasoconstriction. Subsequently, metabolic acidosis may result that can cause dysrhythmias and pulmonary vasoconstriction. An increased pulmonary artery pressure results in right-to-left shunting with reversion back to the fetal circulation and further hypoxemia.

PLACENTAL DRUG TRANSPORT

Placental transport and the effects of drugs on the fetus and neonate have been reviewed extensively[9,10]; thus, only the salient points will be cited here.

Simple Diffusion

Almost all drugs used in obstetrics cross the placenta by simple diffusion based on their concentration gradients. Additional mechanisms include active and facilitated enzymatic transport, and special processes such as leakage and pinocytosis. Important drugs used in obstetrics and obstetric anesthesia that cross the placenta include ritodrine, magnesium, narcotics, inhalation anesthetics, sedatives, tranquilizers, local anesthetics, and, to a lesser extent, muscle relaxants. These drugs cross the placenta at a rate defined by the Fick equation:[11]

$$Q/t = \frac{K \times A(C_m - C_f)}{D}$$

where Q/t = amount of substance Q transferred per time t; K = diffusion constant of a substance (at a given temperature, K depends on molecular weight, protein binding, lipid solubility, degree of ionization, and drug pK_a); A = placental surface area available for diffusion; C_m = concentration in maternal blood perfusing the placenta (uterine artery); C_f = concentration in fetal blood perfusing the placenta (umbilical artery); and D = thickness of placental membrane. Thus, the difference between the concentration in maternal blood perfusing the placenta and the concentration in fetal blood perfusing the placenta ($C_m - C_f$) constitutes the maternal–fetal concentration gradient of the drug, which serves as the motive force for simple diffusion.

The effect of maternal and fetal blood pH on transplacental diffusion of local anesthetics has been demonstrated by Biehl.[12] Lidocaine, for example, is a weak base with a pK_a (7.6) close to the pH of maternal blood. A simple representation of the equilibrium of lidocaine in the body is

$$(R{\equiv}NH)^+ \rightleftharpoons R{\equiv}NH + H^+$$

where R≡NH = base (here, lidocaine). As fetal acidosis occurs, the equilibrium of lidocaine in fetal blood shifts toward the ionized form $(R{\equiv}NH)^+$, drawing more un-ionized local anesthetic from the maternal circulation into the fetal blood. This phenomenon, known as "ion trapping," can lead to a vicious spiral if the trapped ion acts as a cardiac depressant.

However, this process can be reversed by normalization of fetal pH (Fig. 55-1).

Factors Influencing Placental Drug Transport

Maternal Drug Redistribution and Metabolism

Maternal drug redistribution and metabolism reduce the concentration available for transport (ie, reduce the concentration in maternal blood perfusing the placenta [uterine artery]) and, thus, the concentration gradient favoring diffusion across the placenta.

Although diffusion across the placenta is a major factor in the transport of drugs, other important variables must be considered.

Fetal Drug Distribution and Metabolism

Drug concentrations measured in the umbilical vein often do not reflect brain tissue concentrations, because blood is filtered through the fetal liver; drug-free blood from the extremities lowers the concentration further. These mechanisms serve to protect the brain from sudden high initial drug concentrations.[13] Microsomal drug metabolism is less active in the fetus than in the mother, however, resulting in prolonged duration of action.[14]

Drug Metabolites

Metabolites produced by the fetus and newborn can also result in central nervous system depression. An example is fetal production of normeperidine, a product of meperidine metabolism, which may result in greater respiratory depression than meperidine.[15]

Protein Binding

Highly protein-bound drugs in the mother are less available to pass the placenta. Conversely, if the drug binds in the fetus, prolonged drug effect results.

Other Effects

Drugs in the fetus can induce drug-metabolizing microsomal enzymes, as in the case of barbiturates; alternatively drugs can cause adverse reactions through competitive protein binding, as when diazepam administration results in hyperbilirubinemia.[16] In general adverse fetal–neonatal drug effects can be prevented by controlling dosage, timing of administration, and preferentially choosing rapidly distributed and metabolized drugs that are highly protein-bound.

CAUSATIVE AGENTS

Narcotics

Narcotics cause respiratory depression and shift the carbon dioxide response slope in neonates to the right in qualitatively the same fashion as in adults.[17] Thus, drugs associated with low blood and tissue concentrations at delivery are preferred. In general, meperidine, fentanyl, and alphaprodine, in maternal doses of 50 mg, 50 μg, and 20 mg, respectively, have only a slight effect on the fetus. Conversely, if total maternal dose and timing of these drugs are not restricted, narcotic-induced neonatal respiratory depression will occur.[18,19]

Infants born within 1 hour of maternal intramuscularly administered meperidine (up to 100 mg) do not appear more depressed than those from unmedicated mothers. In contrast, those infants whose mothers have received meperidine 2 to 3 hours before delivery have significantly lower Apgar scores when compared with infants from nonmedicated mothers.[20]

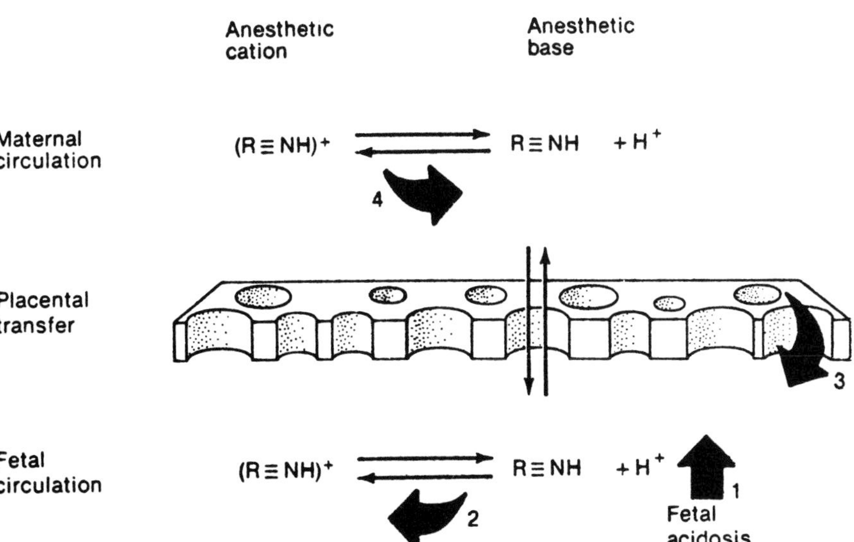

FIGURE 55-1. Fetal acidosis increases the transfer of local anesthetics across the placenta. The dissociation equilibrium of the local anesthetic in the fetus is driven to the left, reducing the amount of anesthetic base ($R \equiv NH$) available. As the dissociation equilibrium in the maternal circulation shifts to the right, more anesthetic base is transferred to the fetus. (Albright GA: Anesthesia in obstetrics: maternal, fetal, and neonatal aspects. Menlo Park, CA: Addison-Wesley, 1978: 116)

Metabolites of meperidine such as normeperidine are probably responsible for this depression.[15] Intravenous meperidine concentrations are much greater during the first 0.5 hour after injection, explaining the high incidence of depression in infants born soon after its administration by this route.

If a neonate is depressed and the mother has received meperidine intravenously within the preceding 0.5 hour, or intramuscularly within the last 2 to 4 hours, the effects on the infant can be reversed easily with naloxone, 10 μg/kg intravenously or intramuscularly. Because the half life of naloxone is about 1 hour, neonatal renarcotization may occur. Naloxone should not be given to the mother before delivery because it will have little effect on the fetus and will reverse maternal analgesia.

Though valuable, naloxone is not the drug of first choice for the depressed neonate and should be reserved until other causes of neonatal respiratory depression have been excluded. Narcotic mixed agonist-antagonists, such as butorphanol and nalbuphine, lack clinically important respiratory depression and have been recommended for labor analgesia.[21] However, these drugs produce limited analgesia and have no therapeutic or safety advantage over traditional opioid analgesics.

Inhalation Anesthetics

Contemporary inhalation drugs used during labor, delivery, or cesarean section include nitrous oxide, enflurane, halothane, and isoflurane. All of these agents have a low molecular weight and are highly lipid-soluble, predisposing them to placental transfer. Their most important effect on the neonate is respiratory depression manifested by a lowered carbon dioxide response slope. The degree of fetal–neonatal depression is directly proportional to the partial pressure of maternal anesthetic.[22]

When inhalation anesthetics are given in low concentrations, as for analgesia during labor or delivery, neonatal depression is not observed, even after prolonged administration.[23] Early studies of the newborn after cesarean section performed during nitrous oxide[24] and cyclopropane[25] noted an exposure- and time-related increase in neonatal depression. Subsequent investigations showed that restriction of nitrous oxide to 50% and maintenance of the supplemental volatile anesthetic agent at no more than 0.75 minimum alveolar concentration resulted in minimal neonatal depression, even if delivery occurred 20 to 30 minutes after induction of general anesthesia.[26,27] Should a neonate exhibit respiratory depression from maternal inhalation anesthesia, manual ventilation of the lungs accelerates drug excretion.

Sedatives and Induction Agents

Barbiturates, chloral hydrate, and scopolamine, commonly used in the past, are rarely used now during labor and vaginal delivery. These drugs are ineffective analgesics and may result in excitement when given to patients in severe pain. They are best reserved for the early stages of labor, when pain is minimal.

Thiopental

The prototype induction hypnotic agent for general anesthesia, thiopental, rarely is associated with neonatal depression, if the dose is restricted to 4 mg/kg.[28] Although fetal drug concentrations decrease with time, delaying delivery after thiopental induction does not result in an improved neonatal outcome, because fetal brain drug concentrations are low and the brain is protected in part by preferential liver uptake.[13] However, thiopental in high dose (eg, 8 mg/kg) is associated with significant neonatal depression.[28] If barbiturate-induced depression develops in a neonate, controlled ventilation should be maintained, until the drug effects subside. Analeptics are contraindicated because they further depress the cardiovascular system in the presence of barbiturates.

Ketamine

Ketamine is an alternative to thiopental for induction of general anesthesia and as an analgesic for delivery. Like thiopental, it gains rapid access to the fetal circulation. In a maternal dose greater than 2 mg/kg, ketamine is associated with neonatal respiratory depression and chest wall rigidity. If the maternal ketamine dose is restricted to 1 mg/kg or less, neonatal depression is unlikely. When given before delivery, ketamine and thiopental are associated with slight depression of neonatal neurobehavioral scores that may persist beyond 24 hours postpartum. This depression is slightly greater with thiopental than with ketamine.[29]

Propofol

Propofol is yet another alternative to thiopental. Its advantages include smooth induction, reduced cardiovascular response to tracheal intubation, prompt emergence without somnolence, and a lower incidence of other postoperative side effects. When used as an induction agent before cesarean section, in a dose of about 2.5 mg/kg, no apparent difference in neonatal well-being occurs, as assessed by Apgar score (see below) or umbilical cord blood analysis.[30–32] Similar results have been noted when propofol is continued by infusion at a rate of 5 mg/kg/h (83 μg/kg/min) for maintenance of anesthesia.[32]

Tranquilizers

Commonly given with narcotics to potentiate analgesia and sedation for labor, tranquilizers include the phenothiazines (eg, promethazine, propiomazine), benzodiazepines (eg, diazepam, midazolam), antihistamines (eg, hydroxyzine, diphenhydramine), and butyrophenones (eg, droperidol). Although these agents provide amnesia and sedation, they all possess long half-lives (eg, 6 to 12 hours) and may cause respiratory depression.[33,34] Other fetal–neonatal side effects include somnolence, vasodilation, hypotension, decreased muscle tone, poor feeding, and loss of temperature regulation. If required, hydroxyzine, 50 to 75 mg, propiomazine, 10 mg, or promethazine, 25 mg, may be given to the mother without adverse side effects in the neonate; there is no antidote for these agents.

Local Anesthetics

During the normal conduct of regional anesthesia for labor, delivery, or cesarean section, few if any adverse effects on the fetus or neonate are seen with the commonly used local anesthetics. Ester-type drugs such as tetracaine and 2-chloroprocaine, are metabolized rapidly by both mother and fetus. Amide derivatives, such as lidocaine, mepivacaine, bupivacaine, and etidocaine are metabolized by liver microsomal enzymes, and blood concentrations decrease more slowly. Peak maternal blood concentrations occur at 15 to 30 minutes after epidural injection, pudendal block, and local infiltration, with similar peaks occurring shortly afterward in the fetus. Repeated injections of these drugs during labor result in a gradual drug accumulation in mother and fetus.[35,36]

Fetal acidosis can result in ion trapping of local anesthetics from maternal blood, as was mentioned earlier (see Fig. 55-1). Previous studies suggested that epidural analgesia for labor resulted in neonates who were floppy but alert after lidocaine and mepivacaine; these effects were not noted after bupivacaine and 2-chloroprocaine.[37] Recent studies, using larger samples, have not corroborated differences in effects of neonatal neurobehavior between any of these drugs.[38,39]

Adverse fetal and neonatal effects of local anesthetics are typically indirect and result from adverse maternal responses. These include uterine tetany and maternal convulsions resulting from drug overdosage, either absolute (ie, excessive total dosage) or relative (ie, intravascular injection), and maternal respiratory depression, cardiovascular collapse, or both from high or total spinal anesthesia. If a fetus is delivered in a depressed condition in any of these circumstances, controlled ventilation, cardiovascular support, and acid–base correction should be instituted.[40]

Direct fetal and neonatal depression caused by local anesthetics is uncommon but can occur if maternal drug concentrations are excessive, if the drug is injected directly into the uterine artery during paracervical block,[41] or if it is injected directly into the fetus during caudal anesthesia.[42] Fetal and neonatal seizure activity has been reported after caudal block with mepivacaine, 1.5%, in volumes of 20 to 25 mL.[43] Resuscitation after this event includes treatment of seizures and maintenance of neonatal oxygenation. Some have recommended neonatal exchange transfusion if high neonatal blood concentrations of local anesthetics are documented.[43]

Muscle Relaxants

Placental transfer of muscle relaxants in usual clinical dosages is limited and of little importance in the context of neonatal respiratory depression, because these drugs are highly ionized and poorly lipid-soluble.

Succinylcholine

After administration of large doses (eg, 2 to 3 mg/kg) in the mother, succinylcholine does appear in the fetus[44]; however, it is metabolized rapidly by fetal pseudocholinesterase and rarely presents a problem. Treatment of a neonate who has atypical pseudocholinesterase or whose mother has received a very large succinylcholine dose is controlled ventilation until adequate respiratory effort has returned.

Nondepolarizing Muscle Relaxants

Drugs such as pancuronium or d-tubocurarine are metabolized slowly and excreted by the kidney. Large dosages of these drugs may cross the placenta and cause neonatal respiratory paralysis and airway obstruction, particularly if the induction-to-delivery time during cesarean section is prolonged. If neonatal respiratory paralysis is diagnosed after administration of a large dosage of nondepolarizing muscle relaxant to the mother, the effects are antagonized quickly by an anticholinesterase. Vecuronium and atracurium are metabolized rapidly in the mother and are safe for use during cesarean section before fetal delivery.[45,46]

Other Drugs

Several other drugs taken by the mother may result in neonatal respiratory depression, hyper- or hypoactivity, or poor feeding, among other signs.[47]

Magnesium

An important therapeutic agent for preeclampsia or eclampsia and premature labor, magnesium crosses the placenta rapidly and acts as a calcium competitor at the myoneural junction, thereby inhibiting depolarization. Magnesium is additive to all muscle relaxants.[48] In large dosage, it produces neonatal muscle weakness, airway obstruction, and respiratory depression. These problems are rare if normal maternal dosage recommendations are followed. Therapy for neonatal magnesium overdosage includes airway and ventilatory support. Calcium administered to the neonate may partially antagonize the depressant effect of magnesium.

Ritodrine

Widely used as a tocolytic agent in cases of preterm labor, ritodrine passes through the placenta and reaches peak fetal plasma concentrations (20% of maternal concentrations) 4 hours after infusion is begun.[49] Neonatal side effects include tachycardia, hypoglycemia, hyperbilirubinemia, and asphyxia after the administration of large doses to the mother. These effects result from maternal hypotension or increased uterine vascular resistance, producing decreased uterine blood flow. Other studies have shown no adverse fetal and neonatal effects after maternal tocolysis at recommended doses.[50]

Salicylates

Neonatal hemorrhage, acid–base disorders, and jaundice in the newborn may result from maternal salicylate use.

Alcohol

Maternal alcohol consumption during pregnancy may result in the fetal alcohol syndrome. Although alcohol is now rarely used as a tocolytic, it is associated acutely with neonatal hypoglycemia, acid–base disorders, irritability, and a decreased ability to suck.

Diuretics

These agents rarely are given during pregnancy; they can lead to electrolyte disorders and neonatal depression.

Antihypertensives

Reserpine taken by the mother may cause neonatal respiratory obstruction because of nasal stuffiness.

Antibiotics

Neonatal hematologic and coagulation abnormalities may result from antibiotic administration.

INDIRECT CAUSES

Depression of the fetus indirectly can result from insufficient placental oxygen delivery: maternal hypoventilation, hypoxia, hypotension, or uterine hypertonus. These maternal and fetal life-threatening adverse reactions can be caused by a variety of obstetric and anesthetic drugs.

Narcotics

In excessive dosage, particularly when combined with other respiratory depressants (eg, benzodiazepine or magnesium), narcotics can cause maternal hypoventilation, hypercapnia, hypoxia, and acidosis, which are rapidly transmitted to the fetus.

Regional Anesthesia

High spinal or epidural anesthesia without adequate fluid preload and left uterine displacement can result in dramatic maternal hypotension, uterine hypoperfusion, and fetal asphyxia. This problem can be minimized by prehydration with a dextrose-free electrolyte solution, in a volume of 20 mL/kg before regional block for cesarean section, and the maintenance of 10° to 15° left uterine tilt before delivery of the fetus. If these methods are insufficient, ephedrine in 5 mg intravenous increments may be used to maintain systolic blood pressure greater than 100 mm Hg.

Amide local anesthetics given intravenously instead of into the epidural space may result not only in maternal seizures or cardiopulmonary collapse, but also will cause intense uterine vasoconstriction with resulting fetal hypoxia. Use of an appropriate test dose with epinephrine and injection of the drug in fractionated increments, may avoid maternal toxicity.

Oxytocin

Oxytocin given to augment labor can cause an increase in uterine activity and tone producing decreased intervillous blood flow, fetal hypoxia, and acidosis. Uterine tetany during labor is a life-threatening emergency for the fetus that requires immediate tocolysis with β-adrenergic agents, amyl nitrate, or general anesthesia with a potent inhalation drug.

PATHOPHYSIOLOGIC FEATURES OF ASPHYXIA

Much of our knowledge of neonatal asphyxia comes from Dawes' work in rhesus monkeys.[51] The experimental model involved the near-term delivery of a normal fetal monkey without general anesthesia. After the umbilical cord was tied, the head was covered with a small bag of warm saline. A characteristic series of changes then ensued (Fig. 55-2). Within about 30 seconds of the development of asphyxia, respiratory efforts began with a profound decrease in heart rate and a slight increase in blood pressure. The animal became hypotonic and the skin cyanotic, blotchy, and finally, white, as intense vasoconstriction supervened. After primary apnea

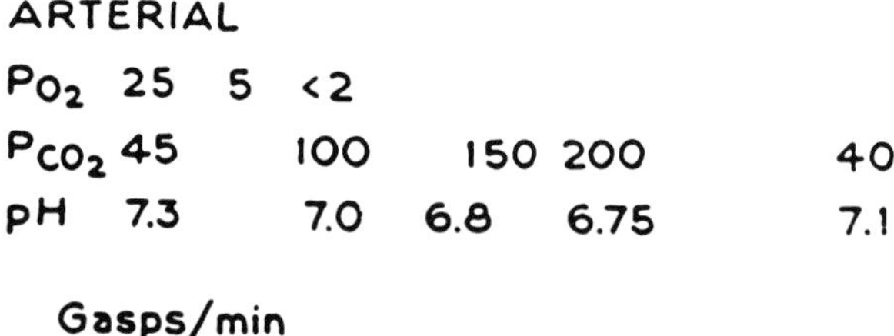

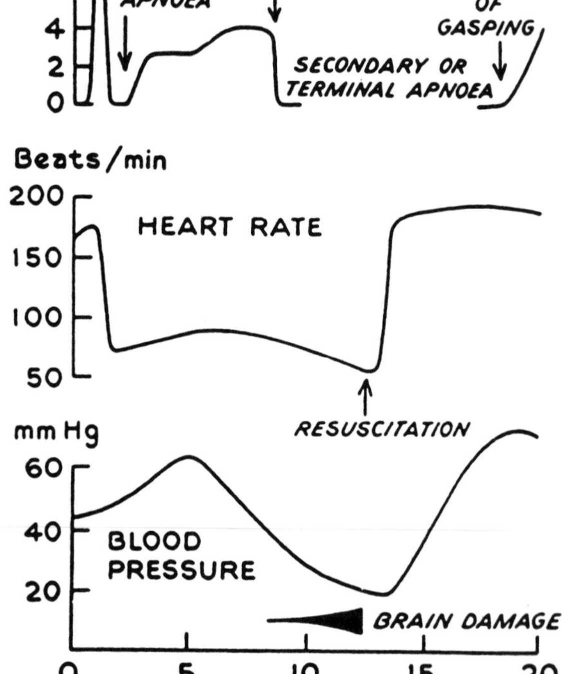

FIGURE 55-2. Schematic diagram of changes in rhesus monkeys during asphyxia and on resuscitation by positive pressure ventilation. Brain damage was assessed by histological examination some weeks or months later. (Dawes GS: Foetal and Neonatal Physiology. St. Louis: Mosby-Year Book, 1968.)

lasting for 30 to 60 seconds, the monkey began to gasp again. The respiratory effort increased 4 to 5 minutes after the development of asphyxia. Heart rate remained depressed, and blood pressure began to decrease. The gasps became weaker, and secondary or terminal apnea occurred. If resuscitation was not begun within a few minutes, death followed. Associated with this sequence were decreasing pH and arterial P_{O_2} and an increasing arterial carbon dioxide partial pressure (P_{CO_2}).

During the primary apneic period, tactile stimulation and oxygen-enriched positive-pressure ventilation causes the neonate to respond quickly. In the secondary (terminal) apnea stage, more vigorous resuscitation efforts, such as tracheal intubation, 100% oxygen administration, epinephrine and sodium bicarbonate are needed.

Overtreatment can occur if an apneic neonate is thought to be in a state of severe asphyxia (secondary apnea) when it really is in a state of primary apnea. Undertreatment can occur if one provides the secondary apneic neonate with only tactile stimulation. Clinical judgment to distinguish the two conditions may be difficult; therefore, proceeding from the least invasive to the most invasive therapy quickly and efficiently is the best approach. Pulse oximetry may have a very useful clinical application in this setting (Fig. 55-3).[52]

MONITORING OF FETAL HEART RATE

Intrapartum fetal heart rate (FHR) monitoring is an indispensable tool in modern obstetrics, because it reflects fetal oxygenation, perfusion (eg, umbilical blood flow), the metabolic state (ie, acidosis), and autonomic and humoral responses.[52,53] Obstetricians and anesthesiologists depend on this monitor to establish baseline fetal well-being, determine fetal response to the progress of labor, observe fetal response to pharmacologic agents (ie, oxytocin administration, narcotics, epidural anesthesia), and plan the management of labor and delivery. Because of its widespread use and despite its limitations, every anesthesiologist involved in obstetric care must have a basic understanding of the underlying principles, interpretation, and limitations (see Fig. 55-2). Anesthesiologists also should recognize that the overall value of this monitoring is increasingly challenged.[54]

The FHR can be assessed externally with Doppler ultrasound or internally with a fetal scalp-clip electrocardiogram. External monitoring does not require rupture of amniotic membranes and does not risk maternal or fetal trauma or infection. Its drawbacks include maternal movement artifact and inability to determine fetal beat-to-beat heart rate variability. Internal FHR monitoring is most accurate for rate-pattern diagnosis but requires rupture of amniotic membranes for application. It also carries a small risk of infection.

Four characteristics of the FHR tracing act as indicators of fetal oxygenation, perfusion, and metabolic state: (1) baseline value; (2) variability; (3) periodic changes (deceleration, acceleration, and their progression measured in relation to uterine contractions); and (4) prolonged changes.

Baseline Value

Normal FHR ranges between 120 and 160 beats/min. The natural stability of this rate recorded at the beginning of monitoring is a sign of well-being and, thus, is referred to as baseline rate. A slow FHR associated with decreased variability is a serious sign of fetal compromise and usually represents a terminal pattern. Fetal tachycardia is often an early sign of fetal hypoxia. Tachycardia is also associated with maternal fever, amnionitis, hyperthyroidism, maternal medications such as β-adrenergic agonists (eg, ritodrine, ephedrine) and anticholinergics, and fetal anemia or prematurity.

Variability

The natural irregularity in FHR is a most important indicator of fetal well-being. Short-term variability defines changes occurring in rate from one beat to the next. Long-term variability normally is observed as a variation in FHR by 10 to 15 beats, occurring three to four times during 1 minute of observation.

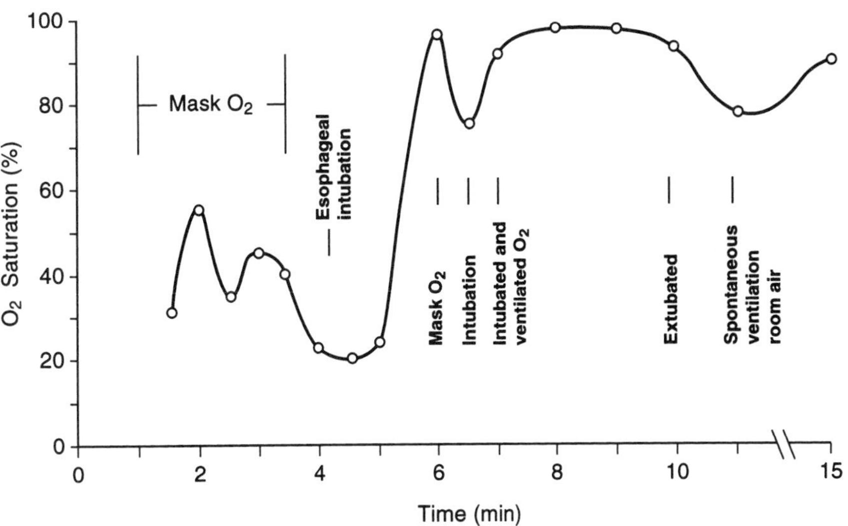

FIGURE 55-3. Record of hemoglobin oxygen saturation (by pulse oximetry) a 38.5-kg newborn with an Apgar score of 1 at 1 minute. Mask ventilation increased the hemoglobin oxygen saturation from 32% to 56%. Esophageal intubation caused it to decrease to 20%; it then improved with masking and then tracheal intubation.

FHR variability can be determined only by direct monitoring of the fetal electrocardiogram, by means of a clip attached to the fetal scalp.

FHR variability represents the healthy interplay of central autonomic control. Although loss of variability may be a sign of normal fetal sleep, it is also one of the first signs associated with fetal hypoxia and asphyxia. Common medications administered during obstetric care also can decrease variability. These drugs include central nervous system depressants, magnesium, tranquilizers, narcotics, anticholinergics, β-adrenergic agonists (tocolytics), and some local anesthetics (lidocaine).

Periodic Changes

The FHR normally increases and returns to baseline after fetal stimulation. These periodic accelerations usually are benign and represent a normal sympathetic response to uterine contractions, fetal movement, fetal wakening, or other stimulation. They also often occur preceding or after a variable FHR deceleration. Three categories of abnormal deceleration are described (Fig. 55-4).

Early Uniform Decelerations

These are mirror images of uterine contractions. Beginning with the contraction, they reach their lowest rate at the peak of the contraction and return to baseline at its end. The deceleration may present as moderate or severe bradycardia. This pattern is benign and represents a vagal reflex response to head compression, often occurring after rupture of membranes and during the late first and second stages of labor. Early decelerations require no therapy.

Late Decelerations

Late decelerations have a similar reciprocal relation with uterine contractions, offset as mirror images. A late deceleration begins well after the start of the uterine contraction, reaches the lowest rate after the peak of the contraction, and does not return to baseline until considerably after the conclusion of the contraction. FHR variability is often lost. Late uniform decelerations are ominous and represent uteroplacental insufficiency. Unless the pattern of early deceleration quickly disappears, prompt delivery is necessary.

Therapeutic measures for late decelerations include left uterine displacement, restoration of normal maternal blood pressure, and decreasing uterine hyperstimulation if present. A high inspired oxygen concentration should be given to the mother by face mask until the decelerations resolve or the fetus is delivered.

Variable Decelerations

These are the most common periodic rate slowing seen, occurring in more than 50% of labors. Variable decelerations are caused by umbilical cord compression. They are most often seen after rupture of membranes and just before the second stage of labor. They usually occur during a contraction, but

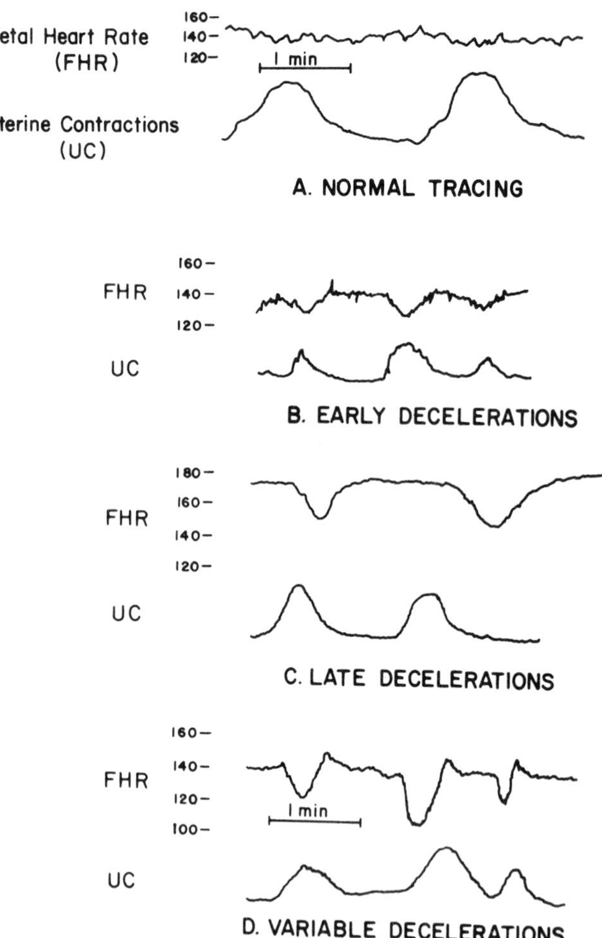

FIGURE 55-4. Bioelectronic monitoring of FHR and uterine contractions (*UC*). (Gutsche BB: Obstetric anesthesia and perinatology. In Dripps RD, Eckenhoff JE, Vandam LD (eds): Introduction to anesthesia: the principles of safe practice, 7th ed. Philadelphia: WB Saunders, 1987: 308)

their configuration and time relation to each contraction vary from one to the next. They are characterized by an abrupt onset and return to baseline FHR.

Variable decelerations are classified as mild, moderate, or severe according to the duration and the lowest FHR observed: mild variable decelerations last for less than 30 seconds, with the FHR remaining greater than 80 beats/min. Severe variable decelerations last longer than 60 seconds with a FHR nadir less than 70 beats/min. Mild variable decelerations accompanied by good beat-to-beat variability do not require treatment and are not a cause for concern. However, if variable decelerations become severe and demonstrate a loss of beat-to-beat variability, rebound tachycardia, or accelerations followed by decelerations, prompt evaluation of fetal pH and intervention is indicated. In addition to administration of a high inspired concentration of oxygen to the mother, maintenance of normal maternal blood pressure, and attenuation of uterine stimulation, therapy includes prompt change of maternal position to one in which decelerations are decreased. If improvement in FHR does not occur, prompt delivery is usually indicated.

Prolonged Changes

Prolonged fetal deceleration lasting longer than 90 seconds in conjunction with a loss of variability is an ominous sign that requires immediate evaluation and often indicates emergent delivery. This pattern may be associated with cord prolapse, maternal hypotension, uterine hypertonus, or paracervical block. Another serious FHR pattern is a sinusoidal rhythm in which rhythmical fluctuations in rate of 20 beats/min or greater occur four to eight times per minute. This alteration may represent a terminal pattern and is associated with severe fetal hypoxia or Rh isoimmunization anemia.

Although a divergence of medical opinion exists regarding the need for monitoring, some studies indicate that fetal heart monitoring, properly interpreted, is associated with a decreased cesarean section rate in the parturient patient at high risk[53] and with no significant change in cesarean section rate in unselected patients.[55]

Arguing against these conclusions is the progressive increase in the incidence of cesarean section during the past decade, suggesting that the studies are wrong or that many clinicians do not properly interpret the findings. Major conduction anesthesia, particularly in the presence of oxytocin augmentation, is a strong indication for fetal monitoring because the analgesia abolishes the mother's perception of the frequency, duration, and intensity of her contractions.

MANAGEMENT IN THE DELIVERY ROOM

The major complication of a depressed fetus in utero is a depressed, often asphyxiated neonate requiring immediate diagnosis and efficient resuscitation.

Examination

Initial evaluation of the neonate is made clinically by application of the Apgar score at 1 and 5 minutes postpartum (Table 55-2).[56] Whereas the 1-minute score correlates well with acidosis and survival,[57] the 5-minute score correlates with neurologic outcome.[58] Although five objective signs are assessed, heart rate and respiratory effort are particularly important for guiding treatment.[59]

Treatment of Asphyxia

Apgar Score

An Apgar score of 8 to 10 is indicative of neonatal well-being. Typically, the only interventions necessary are nasal and oral suctioning, drying of the skin, and maintenance of normal body temperature.

An Apgar score of 5 to 7 suggests mild asphyxia before birth. These neonates usually respond to vigorous stimulation and oxygen blown over the face. If they do not respond, oxygen should be administered by bag and mask.

An Apgar score of 3 or 4 indicates moderate depression, which usually responds to oxygen administration with a bag and mask. If the neonate has not breathed, tracheal intubation should be undertaken. Tracheal suctioning should precede ventilation if there has been meconium staining of the amniotic fluid or vaginal bleeding.

An Apgar score of 0 to 2 indicates severe asphyxia requiring immediate resuscitation, with tracheal intubation, cardiac massage, and correction of acidosis and hypovolemia.[40,59,60]

Head Positioning

Placement of a folded towel under the infant's head, in a manner similar to that used for adults and older children, may lead to airway obstruction. Similarly, extreme extension will also cause airway obstruction, although a 1-inch thick roll under the infant's shoulders may be helpful in maintaining head position for satisfactory airway control. Placement of the head and neck in the neutral position with a slight Trendelenburg position may be best for airway management, because the large, round occiput causes the head to be in the desired sniffing position.

Clearance of Secretions

Gentle suctioning should be performed with a bulb syringe, DeLee trap, or mechanical suction apparatus attached to an 8- or 10-French suction catheter, using pressures not exceeding −100 mm Hg (−136 cmH_2O).[60] Deep, vigorous suctioning of the nasopharynx and passage of a catheter into the stomach immediately after birth should be avoided, because vagally induced dysrhythmias and apnea may occur.[61] Suc-

TABLE 55-2
Apgar Scoring

	SCORE		
SIGN	*0*	*1*	2
Heart rate (beats/min)	Absent	<100	>100
Respiratory effort	Absent	Weak cry; hypoventilation	Good effort, strong cry
Muscle tone	Limp	Some flexion of extremities	Active motion; extremities well flexed
Reflex irritability	No response	Grimace	Cry
Color	Blue; pale	Body pink; extremities blue	Completely pink

Based on Apgar V: A proposal for a new method of evaluation of the newborn infant. Anesth Analg 32:260, 1953.

tioning of the mouth should continue for no longer than 10 seconds at a time, with allowance for interspersed ventilation with 100% oxygen, either spontaneously or mechanically. The heart rate must be monitored for possible bradycardia.

Tactile Stimulation

Drying the infant and gentle suctioning induce effective respirations in most infants. Two additional methods of tactile stimulation are rubbing the infant's back and slapping or flicking the soles of the feet. More vigorous methods such as spanking, cold water applications, milking the trachea, and dilation of the anal sphincter should be avoided.

Prevention of Meconium Aspiration

The passage of meconium in utero occurs in 12% of pregnancies and often is associated with fetal distress.[62] About 60% of neonates born in meconium-stained amniotic fluid have meconium in their tracheas at birth.[62] If this thick material is not suctioned from the trachea before or soon after the onset of breathing, it moves distally into the lungs, blocking small airways and threatening pneumonia, pneumothorax, and pneumomediastinum.

As soon as the head presents at the introitus, suctioning of the nasopharynx by the obstetrician before the infant's first breath is most important in preventing meconium aspiration syndrome.[60] A large bore (12- to 14-French) catheter is recommended, although a bulb syringe may be adequate.[63] After delivery, the baby's head should be maintained in a dependent position, turned to the side, and oral suctioning should continue. If meconium is thick or the baby is severely depressed with possible tracheal obstruction, immediate tracheal intubation and suctioning should be performed to allow adequate oxygenation and prevent aspiration pneumonia.[62,64]

Drug Therapy

SODIUM BICARBONATE. In the late 1970s sodium bicarbonate therapy was used in most resuscitations. Now it is used much less frequently, especially in premature infants, because the resultant sudden development of hyperosmolality and hypernatremia has been associated with intraventricular hemorrhage.[65,66] Most clinicians still use bicarbonate for treatment of extreme metabolic acidosis (base deficit 7 to 15 mEq/L) caused by asphyxia or shock. Even then, it is not the initial therapy for asphyxia and should be used only during prolonged cardiac arrest that does not respond to other therapy.[60]

ATROPINE. Bradycardia is primarily associated with hypoxemia, and the treatment of choice is oxygen, not atropine. If bradycardia persists after adequate oxygenation, atropine or epinephrine administration may be considered. Premature administration may cause tachycardia that could mask severe hypoxemia and, therefore, should be avoided.

CALCIUM. Although calcium has been recommended for electromechanical dissociation and asystole, objective evidence supporting its use is lacking.[67,68] In addition, intracellular calcium accumulation has been implicated in the final common pathway of cell death.[69,70] Calcium therapy, however, may be indicated to counteract the toxic effects of magnesium and potassium.

EPINEPHRINE. Epinephrine, an endogenous catecholamine with both α- and β-adrenergic receptor agonist properties, probably is the ideal agent for pediatric patients whose most common dysrhythmias are bradycardia and asystole. It also is a potent inotrope that can maintain blood pressure in the shock state while adequate fluid volume is administered. Intratracheal use of epinephrine is advocated when intravenous access is not possible.

PERSISTENT PULMONARY HYPERTENSION OF THE NEWBORN

Pathophysiologic Features

Important advances have occurred during the past 20 years in the understanding of the relation between asphyxia and pulmonary hypertension. A large number of infants, particularly at term, initially have perinatal depression, asphyxia, or both, with severe cyanosis that is refractory to standard resuscitation measures. Regardless of whether these infants have hypoventilation or a combination of acidosis and hypoxemia as the initial event, the cyanosis is caused by right-to-left shunting through the ductus arteriosus or foramen ovale; it results from pulmonary hypertension.

In the normal neonate immediately after birth, pulmonary arterial pressure is increased while the infant is still in transition from fetal to neonatal circulation. In newborn and adult animals, decreases in pH and arterial P_{O_2} are the major factors that increase PVR. In fetal animals increased arterial P_{CO_2} or decreased pulmonary ventilation also may increase PVR.[71]

Two forms of increased PVR occur in the asphyxiated neonate. In most delivery room conditions, asphyxia is brief, and a reactive pulmonary hypertension occurs. If acidosis is corrected and adequate alveolar ventilation is established, PVR decreases rapidly and the right-to-left shunt disappears.

The second type is termed persistent fetal circulation or persistent pulmonary hypertension. This condition frequently is associated with perinatal asphyxia but is also seen in the aspiration syndromes and diaphragmatic hernia. It progresses over a period of several hours or may begin acutely with asphyxia.

Typically, the infant is initially resuscitated and may transiently recover. Progressive hypoxemia, cyanosis, and respiratory distress usually follow. Anatomic studies of the pulmonary vascular bed indicate an extension or hypertrophy of pulmonary arteriolar musculature in these infants. In the case of diaphragmatic hernia, a decreased cross-sectional area of the pulmonary vascular bed is present. Subclinical perinatal asphyxia may predispose infants to this condition before birth because low-grade intrauterine hypoxemia may result in pulmonary periarteriolar muscular hypertrophy.

Treatment

When an asphyxiated infant is seen in the delivery room, immediate resuscitation with adequate ventilation and correction of respiratory acidosis should be initiated. If hypoxemia persists, a trial of hyperventilation should be attempted. Hyperventilation was established by Peckham and Fox to be a major factor in reversing pulmonary hypertension in this type of infant.[72] As shown in Figure 55-5, pulmonary arterial pressure can be markedly increased (100 mm Hg) in an infant with persistent pulmonary hypertension. Systemic arterial pressure in this infant initially was 70 mm Hg. As the infant was hyperventilated from an arterial P_{CO_2} of 80 to 25 mm Hg, the pulmonary artery pressure decreased to 55 mm Hg (a subsystemic level).

Infants with persistent pulmonary hypertension must be monitored closely and stabilized. Continuous monitoring of oxygen saturation will help the clinician decide how aggressive mechanical ventilation should be. In the delivery room, hand ventilation is most commonly used. If the infant is hyperventilated appropriately, a point usually is reached at which the right-to-left shunt is suddenly abolished and the infant becomes oxygenated. Hyperventilation is maintained at the pH and arterial P_{CO_2} levels necessary to maintain good oxygenation.[73] Subsequently, the infant can be transferred to an intensive care nursery. Another option soon to be more widely available is the use of inhaled nitric oxide, which works as an extremely potent pulmonary arteriolar vasodilator.[74] In the intensive care nursery, the decision can be be made whether to continue mechanical hyperventilation or whether to institute alternate therapies, such as nitric oxide inhalation, if available.

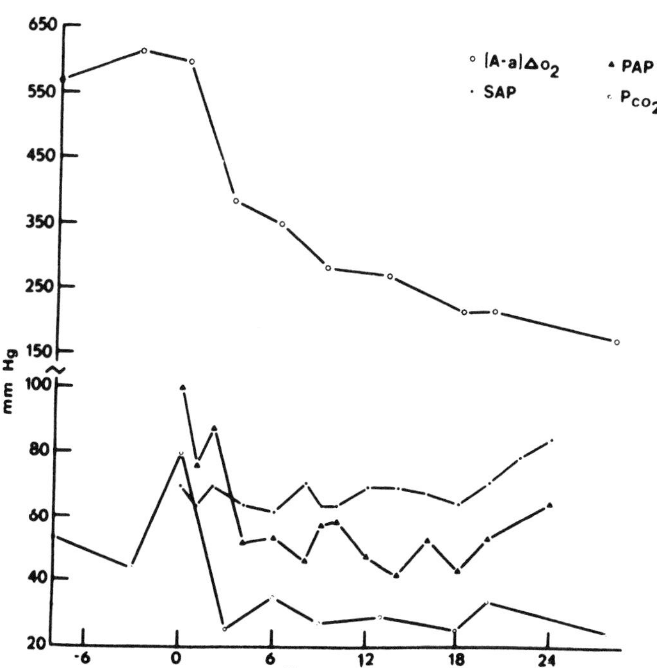

FIGURE 55-5. Continuous pulmonary artery pressure and other physiologic data from an infant with persistent pulmonary hypertension of the newborn. $[A\text{-}a]\Delta O_2$, alveolar–arterial difference in partial pressure of oxygen; *PAP*, pulmonary artery pressure; *SAP*, systemic artery pressure. (Duara S, Fox WW: Persistent pulmonary hypertension of the neonate. In Thibeault DW, Gregory GA: Neonatal pulmonary care, 2nd ed. Norwalk, CT: Appleton-Century-Crofts, 1986: 471)

REFERENCES

1. Levinson G, Shnider SM, Gregory GA: Resuscitation of the newborn. In Shnider SM, Levinson G (eds): Anesthesia for obstetrics, 3rd ed. Baltimore: Williams & Wilkins, 1993: 693
2. Avery ME, Fletcher BD, Williams RG: The lung and its disorders in the newborn infant. Philadelphia: WB Saunders, 1981: 29
3. Karlberg P, Koch G: Respiratory studies in newborn infants: III. development of mechanics of breathing during the first week of life—a longitudinal study. Acta Paediatr Suppl 51:121, 1962
4. Rudolph AN, Yuan S: Response of the pulmonary vasculature to hypoxia and H^+ ion concentration changes. J Clin Invest 45: 399, 1966
5. Klaus MH, Fanaroff AA, Martin RJ: The physical environment. In Klaus MH, Fanaroff AA (eds): Care of the high risk neonate, 3rd ed. Philadelphia: WB Saunders, 1986: 96
6. Dawkins M, Hull D: Brown adipose tissue and the response of newborn rabbits to cold. J Physiol (Lond) 172:216, 1964
7. Adamsons K Jr, Ganoy GM, James LS: The influence of thermal factors upon oxygen consumption of the newborn infant. J Pediatr 66:495, 1965
8. Hey E, Katz G: The optimum thermal environment for naked babies. Arch Dis Child 45:328, 1970
9. Ralston DH, Shnider SM: The fetal and neonatal effects of regional anesthetics in obstetrics. Anesthesiology 48:34, 1978
10. Moir DD, Thorburn J: Pharmacology of drugs used in labour. In Obstetric anaesthesia and analgesia, 3rd ed. London: Balliere Tindall, 1986: 50
11. Danielli JF: In Davson H, Danielli JF (eds): The permeability of natural membranes, 2nd ed. Cambridge: Cambridge University Press, 1952
12. Biehl D, Shnider SM, Levinson G, et al: Placental transfer of lidocaine: effects of fetal acidosis. Anesthesiology 48:409, 1978
13. Finster M, Morishima HO, Mark LC, et al: Tissue thiopental concentrations in the fetus and newborn. Anesthesiology 36: 155, 1972
14. DiFazio CA: Metabolism of local anesthetics in the fetus, newborn, and adult. Br J Anaesth 51:29S, 1979
15. Kuhnert B, Kuhnert P, Tu AL, et al: Meperidine and normeperidine levels following meperidine administration during labor (mother, fetus). Am J Obstet Gynecol 133:904, 1979
16. Schiff D, Chan G, Stern L: Fixed drug combinations and the displacement of bilirubin from albumin. Pediatrics 48:139, 1971
17. Way WL, Costley EC, Way EL: Respiratory sensitivity of the newborn infant to meperidine and morphine. Clin Pharmacol Ther 6:454, 1965
18. Roberts H, Kane KM, Percival N, et al: Effects of some analgesic drugs used in childbirth. Lancet 1:128, 1957
19. Refstad G, Lindbeck L: Ventilatory depression of the newborn from women receiving pethidine or pentazocine. Br J Anaesth 52:265, 1980
20. Shnider SM, Moya F: Effects of meperidine on the newborn infant. Am J Obstet Gynecol 89:1009, 1964
21. Maduska P: A double blind comparison of butorphanol and meperidine in labor: maternal pain relief and effect on the newborn. Can Anaesth Soc J 25:5, 1978
22. Moya F: Volatile inhalation agents and muscle relaxants in obstetrics. Anesthesiology 42:462, 1966
23. Shnider SM, Steffenson JL, Margolis AJ: Methoxyflurane analgesia in obstetrics. Obstet Gynecol 33:594, 1969
24. Finster M, Poppers PJ: Safety of thiopental used for induction of general anesthesia in elective cesarean section. Anesthesiology 29:190, 1968
25. Moya F: General anesthesia. In Shnider SM (ed): Obstetrical anesthesia: current concepts and practice. Baltimore: Williams & Wilkins, 1969: 88
26. Moir DD: Anesthesia for cesarean section: an evaluation of a method using low concentrations of halothane and 50% oxygen. Br J Anaesth 42:136, 1970
27. Galbert MW, Gardner AE: Use of halothane in a balanced technique for cesarean section. Anesth Analg 51:701, 1972
28. Kosaka Y, Takahaski T, Mark LC: Intravenous thiobarbiturate anesthesia for cesarean section. Anesthesiology 31:489, 1969

29. Hodgkinson R, Marx GF, Kim SS, et al: Neonatal neurobehavioral tests following vaginal delivery under ketamine, thiopental and extradural anesthesia. Anesth Analg 56:548, 1977
30. Moore J, Bill KM, Flynn RJ, et al: A comparison between propofol and thiopentone as induction agents in obstetric anesthesia. Anaesthesia 44:753, 1989
31. Valtonen M, Kanto J, Rosenberg P: Comparison of propofol and thiopentone for induction of anaesthesia for elective Caesarean section. Anaesthesia 44:758, 1989
32. Dailland P, Cockshott ID, Lirzin JD, et al: Intravenous propofol during cesarean section: placental transfer, concentrations in breast milk, and neonatal effects—a preliminary study. Anesthesiology 71:827, 1989
33. Matthews AE: Double blind trials of promazine in labor. Br Med J 2:423, 1963
34. Gross JB, Smith L, Smith TC: Time course of ventilatory response to carbon dioxide after intravenous diazepam. Anesthesiology 57:18, 1982
35. Finster M, Morishima HO, Mark LC, et al: The placental transfer of lidocaine and its uptake by fetal tissues. Anesthesiology 36: 159, 1972
36. Reynolds F, Taylor G: Maternal and neonatal blood concentrations of bupivacaine. Anaesthesia 25:14, 1970
37. Scanlon JW, Brown WU, Weiss JB, et al: Neurobehavioral response of newborn infants after maternal epidural anesthesia. Anesthesiology 40:121, 1974
38. Abboud TK, Sarkis F, Blikian A, et al: Lack of adverse neonatal neurobehavioral effects of lidocaine. Anesth Analg 62:473, 1983
39. Kileff M, James FM III, Dewan DM, et al: Neonatal neurobehavioral responses after epidural anesthesia for cesarean section using lidocaine and bupivacaine. Anesth Analg 63:413, 1984
40. Gregory GA: Resuscitation of the newborn. In Miller RD (ed): Anesthesia, 2nd ed. New York: Churchill Livingstone, 1986: 1729
41. Shnider SM, Asling JH, Holl JW, et al: Paracervical block anesthesia in obstetrics. Am J Obstet Gynecol 45:619, 1970
42. Finster M, Poppers PJ, Sinclair JC, et al: Accidental intoxication of the fetus with local anesthetic during caudal anesthesia. Am J Obstet Gynecol 92:922, 1965
43. Sinclair JC, Fox HA, Lentz JF, et al: Intoxication of the fetus by local anesthetic. N Engl J Med 273:1173, 1965
44. Drabkova J, Crul JF, Van de Kleijn E: Placental transfer of 14C labelled succinylcholine in near-term *Maccaca mulatta* monkeys. Br J Anaesth 45:1087, 1973
45. Flynn PJ, Frank M, Hughes R: Use of atracurium in caesarean section. Br J Anaesth 56:599, 1984
46. Dailey PA, Fisher DM, Shnider SM, et al: Pharmacokinetics, placental transfer, and neonatal effects of vecuronium and pancuronium administered during cesarean section. Anesthesiology 60:569, 1984
47. Mirkin BL: Perinatal pharmacology and therapeutics. New York: Academic Press, 1976
48. Ghoneim NN, Long JP: Interaction between magnesium and other neuromuscular blocking agents. Anesthesiology 32:23, 1970
49. Kleinhout J, Stolte LAM, Veth AFL: Passeert ritodrine de placenta? Med T Geneesk 118:1248, 1974
50. Hancock PJ, Setzer ES, Beydoun SN: Physiologic and biochemical effects of ritodrine therapy on mother and perinate. Am J Perinatol 2:1, 1985
51. Dawes GS: Foetal and neonatal physiology. Chicago: Yearbook Medical, 1968: 91
52. House JT, Schultetus RR, Gravenstein N: Continuous neonatal evaluation in the delivery room by pulse oximetry. J Clin Monit 3:96, 1987
53. Parer JT: Diagnosis and management of fetal asphyxia. In Shnider SM, Levinson G (eds): Anesthesia for obstetrics, 3rd ed. Baltimore: Williams & Wilkins, 1993: 657
54. Caton D: Fetal monitoring concerns. In Civetta JM, Taylor RW, Kirby RR (eds): Critical care, 2nd ed. Philadelphia: JB Lippincott, 1992: 889
55. Shy KK, Larson EB, Luthy DA: Evaluating a new technology: the effectiveness of electronic fetal heart rate monitoring. Ann Rev Public Health 8:165, 1987
56. Apgar V: A proposal for a new method of evaluation of the newborn infant. Anesth Analg 32:260, 1953
57. James LS, Weisbrot M, Prince CE, et al: The acid-base status of human infants in relation to birth asphyxia and onset of respiration. J Pediatr 52:379, 1958
58. Drage JS, Berendes H: Apgar scores and outcome of the newborn. Pediatr Clin North Am 13:635, 1966
59. McKlveen RE, Ostheimer GW: Neonatal resuscitation. Clinics in Anaesthesia 4:405, 1986
60. Guidelines for cardiopulmonary resuscitation and emergency cardiac care: neonatal resuscitation. JAMA 268:2276, 1992
61. Cordero L, Hon EH: Neonatal bradycardia following nasopharyngeal stimulation. J Pediatr 78:441, 1971
62. Wiswell TE, Tuggle JM, Turner BS: Meconium aspiration syndrome: have we made a difference? Pediatrics 85:715, 1990
63. Locus P, Yeomans E, Crosby U: Efficacy of bulb versus De Lee suction at deliveries complicated by meconium stained amniotic fluid. Am J Perinatol 7:87, 1990
64. Ting P, Brady JP: Tracheal suction in meconium aspiration. Am J Obstet Gynecol 122:767, 1975
65. Papile L, Burstein J, Burstein R, et al: Relationship of intravenous sodium bicarbonate infusions and cerebral hemorrhage. J Pediatr 93:834, 1978
66. Finberg L: The relationship of intravenous infusions and intracranial hemorrhage: a commentary. J Pediatr 91:777, 1977
67. Stevven HA, Thompson B, Aprahamian C, et al: The effectiveness of calcium chloride in refractory electromechanical dissociation. Ann Emerg Med 14:626, 1985
68. Stevven HA, Thompson B, Aprahamian C, et al: Lack of effectiveness of calcium chloride in refractory asystole. Ann Emerg Med 14:630, 1985
69. Katz A, Reuter M: Cellular calcium and cardiac cell death. Am J Cardiol 44:188, 1979
70. White BC, Winegar CO, Wilson RF, et al: Possible role of calcium blockers in cerebral resuscitation: a review of the literature and synthesis for future studies. Crit Care Med 11:202, 1983
71. Cassin S, Dawes GS, Mott JC, et al: The vascular resistance of the foetal and newly ventilated lung of the lamb. J Physiol 171: 61, 1964
72. Peckham GJ, Fox WW: Physiologic factors affecting pulmonary artery pressure in infants with persistent pulmonary hypertension. J Pediatr 93:1005, 1978
73. Fox WW, Duara S: Persistent pulmonary hypertension of the neonate: diagnosis and clinical management. J Pediatr 103:505, 1983
74. Roberts J, Polaner D, Todres D, et al: Inhaled nitric oxide (NO): A selective dilation of persistent pulmonary hypertension of the newborn (PPHN). Circulation 84(suppl):II-321, 1991

FURTHER READING

Gregory GA: Resuscitation of the newborn. In Miller RD (ed): Anesthesia, 4th ed. New York: Churchill Livingstone, 1994: 2077

Complications in Anesthesiology, second edition,
edited by Nikolaus Gravenstein and Robert R. Kirby.
Lippincott-Raven Publishers, Philadelphia © 1996.

CHAPTER 56

Chemical Dependency Among Physicians

H. Jerrel Fontenot
Marcia J. Howton
John H. Lecky

Young adults enter medical training with the goal of helping people to overcome physical affliction. Qualification for medical education, however, is a highly competitive process. Furthermore, once an applicant has been accepted, delayed gratification becomes a way of life. Out of necessity relationships are set aside in favor of reading, studying, performing, and facing evaluation. Because of the age at which medical training traditionally starts, many trainees enter marriage or begin families at the same time, and these situations also require significant expenditure of emotional energy and time. In addition, many finish medical school and enter residency training with substantial loan commitments, adding yet another stress. Thus, medical training, which is designed to condition young doctors to function for long hours, inadvertently works against the development and maturation of workable, harmonious relationships with significant others. Medical practice then continues the long hours for which doctors have been trained and so maintains the lifestyle to which they have been relegated.

Because of a lack of awareness concerning the importance of social support networks and a lack of formal training in relationships, many students and residents do not know how to access the support that might buffer the strain of years of training and of then maintaining a practice. Without that help and without the ability to respond appropriately to stress, physicians are at high risk for development of self-destructive means of coping with stress. *Denial* and poor coping mechanisms may precede alcohol or chemical *assistance*; eventually, chemical *addiction* is a strong possibility. Little attention has been dedicated to the occupational risk of chemical dependency during formal education in professional schools. This failing appears to be related in part to the limited fund of knowledge and to a global denial concerning the problem.

WORK-RELATED STRESS IN MEDICAL TRAINING

Humans have basic biologic needs, including rest and timely nourishment. If these needs are not adequately met, a stable social support network and healthy relationships may help with adjustment. Social support should guide a person to believe that he or she is cared for, esteemed, and belongs to a network of communication and mutual obligation (Table 56-1). During residency training, a person who believes that breaks from work are inadequate or that daily caseloads and call responsibilities are unreasonable is likely to feel overworked. If the time is taken to listen to these complaints and the problem is adequately addressed, the trainee's self-esteem will improve. Successful handling of stress promotes a sense of progress.

Conversely, the fact that stress has been inadequately managed inhibits personal growth and leads to an unbalanced lifestyle. The more a person accepts a state of sustained stress at the expense of basic human needs, the closer he or she edges toward deterioration and breakdown. Disregard of one's own well-being can never be a foundation for the longevity of professional excellence. Residents may receive encouragement as they progress through the learning process but frequently are criticized for not already knowing the answers or the procedures. The stress can be buffered by attending staff who use positive reinforcement or, conversely, can be

TABLE 56-1
Components of Healthy Social Support

- Nurturing
- Empathy
- Encouragement
- Information
- Material assistance
- Expressions of sharing

amplified by those who "teach" by intimidation, criticism, or negative reinforcement.

PREDISPOSING FACTORS

A trainee who responds to criticism by overcompensating, who has an unsatisfying personal life, and who does not have a healthy support system may be prone to drug abuse. Excessive work stress can produce intolerable anxiety, self-doubt, insomnia, and fatigue, all of which demand relief. Substance abuse often begins with experimental attempts at self-medication to relieve insomnia or anxiety. Substance abuse, or even suicide, may seem easier than reevaluation, changing dysfunctional relationships, or remedying an unhealthy lifestyle. The depleted person may not have the energy that change requires, and because the act of seeking help for emotional difficulties is viewed as further weakness, alternatives for coping become critically limited.

ADDICTION

The impairment of a physician by substance abuse is a gradual process. It follows a series of maladaptive choices made by a person trying to cope with a stressful, complicated life who may be genetically predisposed to addiction (Table 56-2). In the absence of healthy coping strategies, self-destructive behavior such as addiction may serve as protection against the emotional pain inevitable in life. Addiction is associated with compulsive and irresponsible use of drugs or alcohol and with continued use of the drug or alcohol despite the social and physical consequences. The disease is progressive, chronic, relapsing, and, if untreated, lethal. It often affects personal and family life for several years before it becomes evident in professional life.[1] Signs of chemical dependency are described in Table 56-3. According to the disease model, no cure for addiction is known; the result of successful treatment is called *recovery*.

Addiction to alcohol, sedatives, and other less potent drugs usually takes years to develop, during which time the signs are only gradually recognized. In time the addict will be "caught" when the volume of drug needed to function is so great that cover-up schemes fail, or the addiction will be discovered as a result of overdose or suicide. With potent narcotics, addiction manifests itself much sooner. The average time for a sufentanil abuser to become addicted is 1 to 6 months and for an abuser of fentanyl, 6 months to 1 year.[2] Clinical studies suggest that the order in which injury occurs is family, community, finances, spiritual and emotional health, physical health, and, finally, job performance.

TABLE 56-2
Factors in the Development of Chemical Dependence

- Genetic predisposition and environmental exposures
- Stress perceived as excessive and inadequate coping skills
- Lack of education regarding chemical dependence
- Absence of effective prevention and control strategies
- Drug availability in the context of a permissive professional and social environment
- Denial

TABLE 56-3
Signs of Chemical Dependency

LACK OF CONTROL OF CONSUMPTION OF THE DRUG

Inappropriate behavior
Illogical drug use
Denial and lack of recognition of problem
Irresponsible actions
Compulsive drug use

CHANGING TOLERANCE FOR QUANTITY OF THE DRUG

Early, high tolerance for drug
Later, significant decrease in tolerance

BLACKOUT

Not to be confused with "passing out." Continuing ability to function; later, totally inability to recall events or conversations. (Pilots have flown missions during a blackout; surgeons have done surgery during a blackout with no recall of having performed the surgery.)

WITHDRAWAL

Tremors, anxiety, sweating, increased blood pressure and pulse
Convulsions or seizures
Hallucinations
Delirium tremens

SERIOUS INTERFERENCE WITH HEALTH

Alcoholic cardiomyopathy
Blood disease
Neuropathy
Bone disease
Cirrhosis
Encephalopathy

DETERIORATION OF PSYCHOLOGICAL LIFE

Overwhelming anxiety
Inability to adjust
Exaggerated extremes of emotion
Deep depression
Extremes of anger

DESTRUCTION OF SOCIOCULTURAL AND ECONOMIC STATUS

Disintegration of family structure
Weakening or discarding of faith
Destruction of community life
Imminent or actual loss of job

Job Performance

Personality changes and changes in daily routine accompany the addictive process. Periods of euphoria alternate with periods of depression, anger, and irritability. Inappropriate ordering of large doses of narcotics or heavy wastage of drugs is an obvious sign of abuse. Sloppy charts and sloppy writing may occur late in the addiction process when the ability to hide the problem begins to falter. In the early stages, however, record-keeping may be meticulous to prevent suspicion. A desire to work alone, refusal of lunch relief, and the wearing of long-sleeved garments may be used to conceal on-the-job use. Frequent bathroom relief or frequent illness can indicate attempts to hide an addiction. Finally, a staff member who remains in the department for long periods when off duty may be acquiring drugs for personal use (Table 56-4).

Anesthesiologists are at significant risk for development of this disease, with residents being especially vulnerable.[3] The majority of those anesthesiologists who become addicted have performed in the top half of their medical class, and many are members of the Alpha Omega Alpha honor society into which medical students are elected, largely on the basis of their intellectual achievement rather than their capacity to recognize and deal with feelings and relationships. Most physicians overlook the personal changes that occur during their evolution from high school through residency. Little time is available for introspection, relaxation, recreation, and the development of effective family support. A tendency to discount the possibility of overwhelming stresses and addictive behaviors is almost always present. As a result, when addiction occurs, the physician is neither prepared to manage it competently nor aware of how to seek help.

Denial

All addicts, and particularly doctors, deny their addiction. *Denial* is the refusal to accept the reality of the disease and is the primary symptom of addiction among physicians. Addicts are simply incapable of recognizing their illness and seeking help. Because of a physician's specialized training, many people believe that he or she should "know better" than to abuse substances or become chemically dependent. Consequently, shame, embarrassment, fear, and guilt fuel the fires of denial in physicians and other health professionals.

TABLE 56-4
Events That Prompted Investigation for Possible Drug Abuse in 376 Incidents

- Changes in behavior
- Inappropriate drug response
- Mood swings
- Heavy wastage of drugs
- Remarkable preference for balanced anesthesia
- Frequent illness
- Unusual or strange anesthesia record
- Heavy use of adjuvant drugs
- Prominent desire to work alone and undisturbed
- Anesthesia mishaps (? "too frequent")
- Hostility from accused toward accusers

Ward CF, Ward GC, Saidman LJ: Drug abuse among anesthesiologists. JAMA 250:022, 1983.

Other physicians with little knowledge of the nature of addiction often harbor negative moralistic views of the addict and tend to ignore the poorly coping, stressed person until his or her inappropriate behavior has become so flagrant as to constitute a gross danger to others. Evidence of depression, substance abuse, or irrational behavior should not be ignored. Often, detection of chemical dependence in a health professional is delayed by the abuser's ability to protect job performance at the expense of every other dimension of his or her life.

Doctors usually make poor patients. They are reluctant to seek help early and fail to cooperate fully with treatment until the *massive denial* is acknowledged. *Malignant denial* in health professionals describes the situation of those who will die without intervention because they cannot spontaneously reach out for help. Physicians must overcome their reluctance to acknowledge vulnerability in themselves and in their colleagues. To do so may mean the difference between life and death.

Family Involvement

Early in the addiction process, family, neighbors, and friends may become involved in a conspiracy of denial to cover the early warning signs. When the problem is not acknowledged, the family begins to take on aspects of the disease, a condition characterized by codependency. Each family member adapts to the behavior of the chemically dependent person by developing behavior that causes the least amount of personal stress. Codependency requires treatment and a commitment to recovery if the family is to resume healthy internal functioning. Five roles have been described in the addicted family:

1. The *chief enabler's* job is to take responsibility as it is abdicated by the addict. Often the impaired person's spouse plays this role. Wives of medical students anticipate little difficulty in adjusting to their future role. By contrast, the wives of doctors say their husbands are professionally competent and successful, but distant, rigid, controlling, and uncomfortable with feelings in marital and family relationships.
2. The *hero* works constantly to improve the family situation, but because of the progressive nature of chemical dependence, always loses ground and feels inadequate. This role is frequently played by the eldest child, who deals with feelings of inadequacy by striving for and often achieving great success in school and in work. In the chemically impaired medical family, the hero is most likely to follow dad or mom into the medical profession.
3. The *scapegoat* withdraws from the dysfunctional family in destructive ways (running away, playing truant, or using drugs and alcohol), but by so doing provides distraction and focus to the family system.
4. The *lost child* learns not to make connections in the family, spends much time alone, and is ignored or neglected by the rest of the family.
5. Finally, the *mascot* is cute and fun to be around, using charm and humor to survive in a painful family system.

Other Physicians

In the past an impaired physician would be abandoned to fate by colleagues who ignored the problem until it was too late and then would be ostracized and isolated as the "drunk doctor." This behavior represented just one aspect of the great denial process that is characteristic of addiction. Denial is manifested not only by the addict but also by friends, family members, and colleagues. Every aspect of the impaired physician's life—marital, financial, professional, social, personal—begins falling apart, and he or she is powerless to pick up the pieces. Colleagues see this pattern and conclude that either the impaired physician is immoral, weak-willed, or selfish, or they fear the same problem in themselves and so remain silent.

In a large or bureaucratic organization, problematic performance often is ignored until it becomes catastrophic. The organization, like an individual person, may attempt to deny the problems of a poorly functioning physician with whom it does not wish to be identified.[4] Physicians often find difficulty in acknowledging personal difficulties and asking for help, largely because of the tremendous guilt they may feel for not being able to deal with it themselves. At the same time, other physicians often find it difficult to recognize and acknowledge maladaptive behavior in a friend or colleague and frequently fail to act.[5]

Urbach and colleagues found that chief residents were more perceptive concerning which residents were having difficulty managing stress in their lives, whereas program directors and department chairpersons estimated the number of residents having difficulties within the same department to be fewer.[6] Physicians are frequently high-functioning and can conceal their suffering from themselves and others until it reaches severe proportions.[7] However, the acceptance of chemical dependence as a disease, and not just as a lack of willpower, is crucial in dealing with the affliction in physicians and others.

TYPICAL CASES

Case 1. After excellent academic performance in college and medical school, a 29-year-old physician continued his successful career development during internship. After 6 months of anesthesia training, however, he became increasingly withdrawn. His knowledge of anesthesia remained superficial, and his personal appearance began to deteriorate. Patients began to complain about his conduct during preoperative visits, and fellow residents noted significant mood swings. Shortly after returning to the operating room from a "break," the circulating nurse noted that he was asleep and difficult to arouse.

Case 2. A highly regarded 47-year-old anesthesiologist began to refuse relief for lunch or during long cases. He offered to take additional call and preferred to work alone. Anesthetic records and narcotic sign-out sheets indicated the use of large doses of narcotics supplemented with potent inhalation agents. His personal appearance began to deteriorate, and colleagues regularly commented that he looked particularly tired on Monday mornings. Participation in departmental administrative activities and hospital committees virtually ceased. One evening while he was on call, this anesthesiologist was found unconscious in a men's room with a tourniquet around his arm and an empty 10-mL syringe next to him on the floor.

Possible Causes

These scenarios are not rare. The daily practice of anesthesia, which involves the personal administration of potent narcotics and sedatives, may place anesthesiologists at greater risks of addiction than other specialists, for whom occupational exposure to drugs is minimal.[7] Whereas the prevalence of addiction among all physicians appears to be at least 10%, about the same as the population at large,[8,9] anesthesiologists (3.6% of the physicians in the United States) represent 10% to 14% of physicians in addiction treatment programs.[10–12]

Self-medication, which increases drug exposure, is common among all physicians. For anesthesiologists, the temptation to "try" the drugs they use daily is an additional and far greater threat. For the majority of anesthesiologists treated in one program, addiction began with parenteral drug experimentation and progressed to severe disability in less than 2 years.[11] The data also indicate that the physicians most recently treated in that program have a long history of drug use and abuse, often predating medical school.

Drug dependence often starts with recreational use, especially among medical students and young physicians.[9] In fact, anecdotal reports suggest that medicine as a profession, and anesthesiology as a specialty, are chosen by some because of a perceived enhanced availability of drugs.[13] The danger of ready access to drugs is further underscored by the emergence of fentanyl as the drug most commonly abused by anesthesiologists.[14] Even its oral ingestion has been reported.[15] Propofol, a noncontrolled substance, reportedly also can cause chemical dependency,[16] suggesting that our classic interpretation of potentially addictive drugs needs revision.

THE DISEASE

Addiction is the net result of genetic, biologic, and environmental factors (see Table 56-2). In susceptible persons, if exposure to drugs occurs at a critical time, the chronic and progressive disease may develop.[17,18] In some cases (eg, alcohol abuse), a long period of chemical dependence may predate impairment. In others, minimal drug exposure, usually with parenteral agents such as fentanyl, may be sufficient to trigger addiction, characterized by compulsive use and rapid progression of the disease.[10] Although abuse of drugs interferes with health and social function, many abusers never become addicted.[18] Pharmacologic tolerance and withdrawal after cessation of long-term drug use can be produced in anyone by a variety of drugs; however, these physically dependent persons do not necessarily become addicted.

TREATMENT

Initiation

Denial, as has been noted, is a major component of the illness; thus, addicted physicians usually lack the insight and ability to help themselves. Treatment therefore depends on intervention and assistance by colleagues or family. In most cases, however, these persons are not trained to recognize or respond to the disease. Without education and guidance, well-meaning colleagues or family are unlikely to help and may aggravate the situation by "covering up" for the impaired physician.

Because the workplace usually is the location at which the advanced stages of chemical addiction are recognized, colleagues must be knowledgeable about the disease, and an intervention mechanism that takes effect before others are endangered must exist within the institution or department. This type of mechanism should permit prompt confrontation, admission to an inpatient unit for evaluation, and facilitation of long-term treatment.

Confrontation

When a colleague's health and patient safety are at issue, concern about addictive disease need not be proven beyond doubt before action is taken. During confrontation, persons close to the physician present the series of observations that concern them in a caring, nonjudgmental fashion. The observed constellation of signs necessitates removal of the addicted person from clinical activities for the sake of patient safety and for the person's own safety and reputation.

Dignified confrontation followed by referral for evaluation is an appropriate action in these circumstances. Regardless of whether denial is overcome, a structured treatment plan must be prepared in advance. This period is one of extreme emotional distress for the impaired physician. Thus, after confrontation, immediate inpatient admission for evaluation and prevention of withdrawal or overdose is both mandatory and humane.[19] A poorly planned confrontation is unlikely to lead to treatment and may even lead the confronters to join in the process of denial and concealment.

The American Society of Anesthesiologists has published guidelines for anesthesiology departments to help provide a formal framework for dealing with chemical dependence within the department and for facilitating a department member's subsequent reentry into the work force.[21]

Confidentiality

Requirements for reporting impairment in a physician vary greatly by state; however, physician impairment is not primarily a legal issue. Understandably, state and local committees relating to impaired physicians, whose activities require confidentiality, are greatly hampered by mandated reporting. New York has discontinued this type of reporting, and impaired physicians in California who have been reported to the state licensing agency can be diverted from disciplinary action into a statewide treatment program. The success of the California Diversion Program in assisting impaired physicians to obtain treatment and to return to practice underscores the value of treatment as an alternative to discipline for chemically dependent physicians.[12]

Liability

Most states provide immunity to professional societies and medical staff committees that review the quality of medical services. Persons providing information to these committees are also granted immunity if the information is believed to be correct and they are not acting with malice. Hospitals, medical staffs, and physicians, however, have been found negligent for failure to monitor or restrict the privileges of an incompetent physician. The major liability risk, then, is to be aware of and yet ignore chemical substance abuse. If an impairment in a physician is identified and the physician is treated and rehabilitated according to accepted medical principles, the risk of liability is virtually eliminated.

Therapeutic Regimens

Successful treatment of addiction requires detoxification and intensive therapy, usually in an inpatient setting. Abstinence, regular group psychotherapy, participation in fellowships such as Alcoholics Anonymous, and workplace monitoring are all part of a long-term recovery program.

Important in treatment are specific blocking drugs, such as disulfiram for alcohol ingestion. The opiate antagonist naltrexone is effective for more than 72 hours after oral administration. Naltrexone therapy is probably a prerequisite for return to a work place in cases in which opiates are the major drugs of abuse. Its use can negate a "slip" that might otherwise trigger a relapse and, more importantly, colleagues and administrators may be far more receptive to a recovering physician returning to work who is "protected" by naltrexone.[19]

PROGNOSIS

In general, the outcome of appropriate long-term treatment is good. Anesthesiologists aggressively treated for addictive disease appear to have the same favorable prognosis for recovery and professional rehabilitation as do other physicians. Physicians have higher rehabilitation rates than the general population if appropriate treatment, monitoring, and follow-up care are provided.[20] In a study of the first 334 chemically dependent physicians who completed a 4-month residential and 20-month "aftercare" program at the Medical Association of Georgia Impaired Physician Program, 93% were drug-free and practicing medicine 2.5 to 10 years after treatment. Eighty-two percent had reached 2 years of continuous sobriety, an important recovery landmark beyond which there appears to be a very low probability of relapse or need for additional treatment. The death rate from addictive disease was approximately 1%.[22] Arnold's survey of substance abuse in anesthesiology residency training programs estimates a relapse rate of 14% per year for the first 18 months after completion of formal treatment.[23]

The Medical Association of Georgia Impaired Physician Program is highly selective for physicians with advanced illness, most having had at least one previous unsuccessful treatment experience. Among the first 60 anesthesiologists who completed this program were equal numbers of anesthesia residents, academic faculty, and community practitioners. Comparison of anesthesiologists in treatment between 1980 and 1983 with those treated between 1977 and 1980 revealed the following differences: the average age decreased (52 to 34 years); alcohol abuse decreased (36% to 10%); and oral drug administration decreased (59% to 10%). Use of narcotics increased greatly (36% to 79%), as did parenteral drug administration (41% to 90%), with fentanyl replacing alcohol as the drug most often associated with addictive disease.

At the time of follow-up 55 of 56 (98%) of the anesthesiologists who completed treatment in the Medical Association of Georgia Impaired Physician Program had recovered and were practicing medicine. Of those who decided to return to anesthesia, 36 of 40 (90%) successfully did so; 4 of the 40 had switched to other specialties. Of 9 anesthesiologists who did not complete treatment, 4 died of their illness.* These results can be compared with the outcomes reported in a population of chemically dependent anesthesiologists surveyed by Ward and colleagues.[3] At a similar time of follow-up, 70% either were no longer practicing or could not be located, and at least 10% had died of complications related to addictive disease. Treatment in this group, however, was of variable quality and duration.

Return to medical practice is a powerful motivator. Physicians unable to practice because of treatment failure or employer resistance seem to be at greatly increased risk of suicide. Of 43 Oregon physicians on probation and not practicing in 1977, 8 committed suicide, and 2 made serious suicide attempts.[22]

RETURN TO PRACTICE

The decision to return to practice in anesthesia (or another specialty) should be based on the advice of the therapist. The history of drug abuse, particularly its duration and type, and the amount of time invested in the specialty (eg, 1st-year resident versus 20-year practitioner) may suggest that the person switch to a specialty in which drugs are less available for misappropriation than in anesthesia.

Ongoing communication and cooperation among the recovering physician, the treatment network, and the medical community are essential for successful return to practice.[21] The medical community must understand the need for this interaction and be willing to provide it. The key program elements should be detailed in a written agreement between the returning physician and the hospital or department. These guidelines structure the physician's return to practice and help to protect colleagues, patients, and the recovering physician from the consequences of an undetected and untreated relapse. Naltrexone therapy should also be considered in a specialty where fentanyl and other opioids are the major drugs of abuse.

Systems that dispense and account for controlled substances in the operating room limit exposure, provide meaningful audit help, and reduce, but do not eliminate, the risk to all operating room personnel.[24–27] Operating rooms should periodically review their dispensing practices for controlled drugs to ensure that the risk of misappropriation is minimized. Among proposed improvements in drug dispensing and auditing are unit-dose distribution[24] and use trend analysis.[25] Unfortunately, control and accountability are difficult to implement and to audit.[26,27]

Consequences of a Relapse

"Slips" after return to practice do not necessarily predict a poor treatment outcome.[28] One fourth of the anesthesiologists treated in the Medical Association of Georgia Impaired Physician Program relapsed.[22] Ninety percent of these relapses occurred in the 1st year, and 98% within the first 2 years. At the time of follow-up, 82% of the physicians who had relapsed and received additional treatment were practicing successfully.

This success rate is attributable to a highly structured support and monitoring system that ensures prompt identification and treatment. The possibility of relapse should not preclude return to practice if appropriate follow-up mechanisms exist. A recovering physician's colleagues should recognize that time is necessary to heal the personal and professional damage caused by addiction. Although addicted physicians are responsible for their own recovery, colleagues can provide the needed encouragement and support. A prompt return to practice in a supportive environment plays a very important role in recovery.[29]

Community Resources

At present, all state and most county medical societies have committees to assist impaired physicians, their colleagues, and their families. These committees provide confidential advice and referral to appropriate professional resources. Physician well-being committees of national medical societies, as well as regional referral centers for the treatment of chemically dependent physicians, are also available. These groups are valuable sources of educational information, expert advice, and assistance. In addition, the American Society of Anesthesiologists and the Association of Anesthesia Program Directors has been very responsive and supportive of efforts to educate anesthesiologists.[30]

At the local level, hospitals and departments must have policies addressing substance abuse.[21] A system should exist whereby concern about professional staff well-being can be referred to a medical staff or departmental impaired physician committee for confidential consideration. These committees can act as the impaired physician's advocate in obtaining advice, treatment, and a return to health. They should also educate the medical community regarding the causes, treatment, and prevention of addiction, and how colleagues can help the returning impaired health care professional.

* Farley WJ: Personal communication, 1991.

PREVENTION

Treatment of drug addiction has advanced considerably more than prevention. A variety of attempts have been made to define the population at risk for chemical abuse by searching for characteristics of the person in whom problems are likely to develop if drugs and alcohol are used.[31,32] Apart from studies of high familial rates of alcoholism and other types of chemical abuse, little progress has been made. However, alcohol and drug abuse among physicians has been found to be associated with psychologic maladaptations of physicians (and others) to a high level of stress at work.[33]

Only recently has much attention been directed to the problems discussed earlier: the stress experienced by physicians in training, particularly women in two-career families; the need for greater awareness and sensitivity to the effect of the stresses on social relationships; and the necessity to establish social support systems within residency programs.[34]

Until more is learned that will permit more effective prevention and earlier identification of particular risk for drug abuse, we must recognize that the anesthesiologist is faced with unique occupational drug exposure. The risks probably far exceed those purported to be related to chronic exposure to waste anesthetic gases and other occupational hazards. With appropriate treatment and follow-up, the prognosis for persons afflicted by this illness is good. Accordingly, anesthesiologists, anesthesia departments, and hospitals should become familiar with the signs of the illness and implement appropriate confrontation, treatment, and return-to-practice mechanisms so that the destructive consequences can be minimized.

REFERENCES

1. Jacyk W: Impaired physicians: they are not the only ones at risk. Can Med Assoc J 141:147, 1989
2. Arnold WP: Environmental safety including chemical dependency. In Miller RD (ed): Anesthesia, 3rd ed. New York, Churchill Livingstone, 1990: 2407
3. Ward CF, Ward GC, Saidman LJ: Drug abuse among anesthesiologists. JAMA 250:922, 1983
4. Swearingen C: The impaired psychiatrist. Psychiatr Clin North Am 13:1, 1990
5. Reuben DB: House officer responses to impaired physicians. JAMA 263:958, 1990
6. Urbach JR, Levenson JL, Harbison JW: Perceptions of housestaff stress and dysfunction within the academic medical center. Psychiatr Q 60:283, 1989
7. Martin CA, Julian RA: Causes of stress and burnout in physicians caring for the chronically and terminally ill. Hosp Journal 3: 121, 1987
8. Brewster JM: Prevalence of alcohol and other drug problems among physicians. JAMA 255:1913, 1986
9. McAuliffe WE, Rohman M, Santangelo S, et al: Psychoactive drug use among practicing physicians and medical students. N Engl J Med 315:805, 1986
10. Spiegelman WG, Saunders L, Mazze RI: Addiction and anesthesiology. Anesthesiology 60:335, 1984
11. Farley WJ, Talbott GD: Anesthesiology and addiction. Anesth Analg 62:465, 1983
12. Gualtieri AC, Consentino JJP, Becker JS: The California experience with a diversion program for impaired physicians. JAMA 249:226, 1984
13. Kleber DH: The impaired physician: changes from the traditional view. J Subst Abuse Treat 1:137, 1984
14. Silverstein JH, Silva DA, Iberti RJ: Opioid addiction in anesthesiology. Anesthesiology 79:354, 1993
15. Haye LR, Stillner V, Littrell R: Fentanyl dependence associated with oral ingestion. Anesthesiology 77:819, 1992
16. Follette JW, Farley WJ: Anesthesiologists addicted to propofol. Anesthesiology 77:817, 1992
17. Jellinek E: The disease concept of alcoholism. New Haven, CT: Kilbourne Press, 1960
18. Smith DE: Substance abuse disorders: drugs and alcohol. In Goldman H (ed): Clinical psychiatry. Los Altos, CA: Lange Medical Publications, 1983
19. Lecky JH, Aukburg SJ, Conahan TJ III, et al: A departmental policy addressing substance abuse. Anesthesiology 65:414, 1986
20. Morse RM, Martin MA, Swenson WM, et al: Prognosis of physicians treated for alcoholism and drug dependence. JAMA 251: 743, 1984
21. American Society of Anesthesiologists: ASA chemical dependence guidelines for departments of anesthesiology. Park Ridge, IL: American Society of Anesthesiologists, 1991
22. Talbott GD, Gallegos KV, Wilson PO, Porter TL: The Medical Association of Georgia's Impaired Physicians Program review of the first 1000 physicians: analysis of specialty. JAMA 257: 2927, 1987
23. American Society of Anesthesiologists: Survey of substance abuse in anesthesiology training programs: preliminary report of the third year. ASA Newsletter 57:21, 1993
24. Carmody G, Vogel D: Unit dose distribution of controlled substances for the operating room. Am J Hosp Pharm 43:413, 1986
25. Adler GR, Potts FE III, Kirby RR, et al: Narcotics control in anesthesia training. JAMA 253:3133, 1985
26. Klein RL, Stevens WC, Kingston HGG: Controlled substance dispensing and accountability in United States anesthesiology residency programs. Anesthesiology 77:806, 1992
27. Ward CF: Substance abuser: now and for some time to come. Anesthesiology 77:619, 1992
28. Herrington RE, Jacobson GR, Hauser RC: Substance abuse disorders: issues in returning to practice. Hosp Med Staff 2:13, 1982
29. Herrington RE, Benzer DG, Jacobson GR, et al: Treating substance use disorders among physicians. JAMA 247:2253, 1982
30. American Society of Anesthesiologists Committee on Occupational Health of Operating Room Personnel, Lecky JH (ed): Questions and answers about chemical dependence and physician impairment. Park Ridge, IL: American Society of Anesthesiologists, 1986
31. "Wearing masks": the potential for drug addiction in anesthesia [videotape]. Chicago, IL: Rainbow Productions Inc.
32. Vaillant GE, Sobavale NC, McArthur C: Some psychologic vulnerabilities of physicians. N Engl J Med 287:372, 1972
33. Vaillant GE, Brighton JR, McArthur C: Physicians' use of mood altering drugs. N Engl J Med 282:365, 1972
34. McCue JD: The effects of stress on physicians and their medical practice. N Engl J Med 306:458, 1982
35. Landau C, Hall S, Warman SA, et al: Stress in social and family relationships during the medical residency. Journal of Medical Education 61:654, 1986

FURTHER READING

Layon AJ, Lopalo S: Occupational hazards in the operating room. In: Kirby RR, Gravenstein N (eds): Clinical anesthesia practice. Philadelphia: WB Saunders, 1994:853

Complications in Anesthesiology, second edition,
edited by Nikolaus Gravenstein and Robert R. Kirby.
Lippincott-Raven Publishers, Philadelphia © 1996.

CHAPTER 57

Cardiac Arrest and Resuscitation

Burton A. Briggs
David J. Cullen
Robert R. Kirby

Hannah Greener, at the age of 15 years, died on January 28, 1848, during chloroform anesthesia for removal of a toenail.[1,2] Only 15 months before this event, Morton had first demonstrated that ether obliterated pain during surgery, and 2 months later, Simpson began using chloroform in his midwifery practice.[3] While Greener's death was being evaluated,[4] a second death occurred during chloroform anesthesia.[5] As other deaths followed, the mixed blessings of general anesthesia were discussed and analyzed by the French Academy of Medicine, Hyderabad Commissions, Royal Medical and Chirurgical Society, British Medical Association, and the Commission on Anesthesia of the American Medical Association.[3]

Since these inquiries and studies, the direct relation between cardiac arrest and anesthesia has continued to be the subject of many deliberations, including the following: Which anesthetic agents are safest? What is the effect of the patient's preoperative condition? What is the role of adjuvant drugs? How, if at all, do the skills of the surgeon and anesthesiologist influence mortality?

All anesthetic agents and techniques have been associated with cardiac arrests. These disasters have resulted directly or indirectly in many instances from errors in the examination of the patient, ignorance of anesthetic pharmacology and drug interactions, inattentiveness, and errors in technique. However, as has been noted repeatedly, sometimes even when the anesthesiologist is attentive and conscientious and cares for the patient seemingly according to recognized standards, the patient sustains cardiac arrest, permanent neurologic dysfunction, and death for no apparent reason.[6,7] This chapter discusses the factors contributing to cardiorespiratory arrest and methods for dealing with this crisis.

INCIDENCE OF INTRAOPERATIVE CARDIAC ARREST: RETROSPECTIVE STUDIES

In 1956, Briggs and colleagues reported a retrospective study of operating room deaths and cardiac arrests at the Massachusetts General Hospital from 1925 to 1954.[8] In the first 20 years of that period, the incidence of these catastrophes decreased steadily; this finding was attributed to improved patient selection, preoperative patient preparation, and improved surgical and anesthetic techniques. However, during the third decade, the incidence of cardiac arrest increased. Older and sicker patients, who previously would not have been candidates for some operations, were undergoing these procedures. During the 30-year period, the incidence of cardiac arrest was 1 in 1405 anesthetic administrations.

Memery reported that for a group of seven anesthesiologists in community practice, the incidence of cardiac arrest between 1955 and 1964 was 1 in 3149.[9] Pierce cited a 1957 incidence of 1 in 1025,[10] but the rate increased to 1 in 821 from 1963 to 1965. Again, the data suggested that despite improved monitoring and anesthetic techniques, increasing numbers of patients at high risk were being subjected to anesthesia and surgery. In 1970, Jude and coworkers reported an incidence of 1 in 1216.[11]

Data covering 190,000 anesthetics suggest an anesthetic mortality rate of only 1 in 10,000 for healthy (American Society of Anesthesiologists physical class 1 and 2) patients undergoing elective surgery, suggesting marked improvement in anesthetic risk.[12] Wherein lie the differences?

HISTORY OF CARDIOPULMONARY RESUSCITATION

Open Versus Closed Cardiac Compression

The first successful cardiopulmonary resuscitation (CPR) of a patient who had intraoperative cardiac arrest was performed in 1867 and included tracheostomy and the application of galvanism to the cardiac region.[13] In 1891, Maass successfully performed the first documented cardiac resuscitation with closed chest compression.[14] Approximately 10 years later, Igelsrud effectively performed the first open-chest cardiac massage.[15]

In the Massachusetts General Hospital study from 1925 to 1954, of 45 patients who underwent open-chest massage within 4 minutes of arrest, 26 (58%) recovered without neurologic deficit.[8] In Pierce's report, all successful resuscitations during 1957 and 1963 to 1965 were accomplished with open-chest cardiac massage.[10] However, the overall rate for successful resuscitation and recovery during both periods was only 35%.

Jude and coworkers reported in 1970 that resuscitation by the closed-chest technique was attempted in nine patients, of whom seven (78%) were resuscitated and five (56%) discharged.[11] Cardiac compression was used successfully in one of two patients whose chests were already open, and that patient subsequently also was discharged.

Outcome

Bedell and colleagues, reviewing 294 consecutive CPRs in a teaching hospital, noted that only 41 (14%) patients survived and were discharged.[16] In another series, comprising 1073 resuscitations in a community hospital, 56% of the patients were initially resuscitated, but only 24% survived to be discharged from the hospital.[17]

Factors apparently influencing the efficacy of CPR include time to initiation, associated disease(s), and the type of dysrhythmia (eg, ventricular fibrillation, asystole, or persistent ventricular bradycardia). Within the operating room, additional factors such as hypoxia, hemorrhage, acute myocardial infarction, or massive pulmonary embolism greatly influence outcome.[16–18]

PATHOPHYSIOLOGIC FEATURES OF CARDIAC ARREST

The Oxygen Cascade

The ultimate objective of cardiopulmonary function is to provide ample oxygen for mitochondrial respiration.[19] The oxygen cascade, from inspiration of gas to metabolism at the mitochondrial level, can be divided into several steps; the oxygen partial pressures (P_{O_2}) during some of these steps can be measured readily (Fig. 57-1).[20–22] At sea level, the inspired P_{O_2} is approximately 150 mm Hg; alveolar P_{O_2}, 100 mm Hg; arterial P_{O_2}, 90 to 95 mm Hg; and mixed venous P_{O_2}, 47 mm Hg.

Measurement of arterial P_{O_2} at a known fraction of inspired oxygen indicates only the efficiency of oxygenation by the lungs. During normal oxygen consumption, mean tissue P_{O_2} approximates 51 mm Hg.[20] Therefore, if mitochondria operate over a P_{O_2} range of 1.5 to 10 mm Hg, the P_{O_2} gradient from

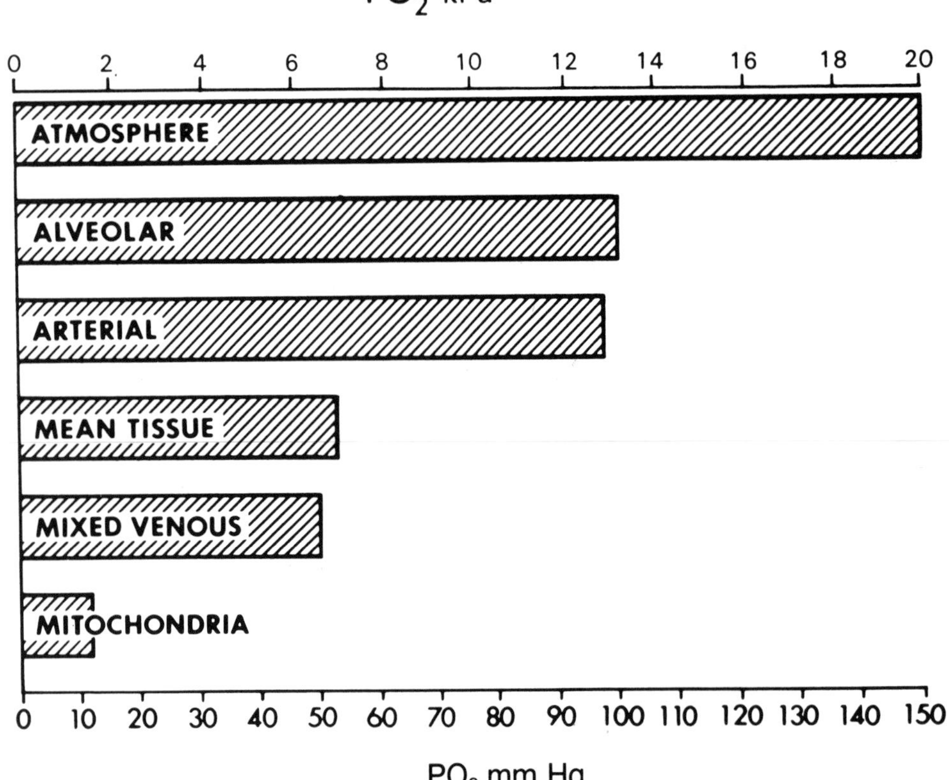

FIGURE 57-1. The oxygen cascade, in which PO_2 decreases from the level in ambient air to the level in mitochondria, the site of utilization.

tissue to mitochondria ranges from 41 to 49.5 mm Hg. The mixed venous P_{O_2} may indicate global adequacy of oxygen delivery to tissues but is influenced by hemoglobin concentration, cardiac output, metabolic rate, and distribution of blood flow.

Modifying Factors

The ability of hemoglobin to *unload* oxygen (as determined by 2,3-diphosphoglycerate concentration, pH, and temperature) influences the P_{O_2} gradient driving oxygen from the capillaries to the mitochondria. Increases in 2,3-diphosphoglycerate concentration or in temperature or a decrease in pH shift the hemoglobin oxygen dissociation curve to the right and increase the P_{O_2} gradient (Fig. 57-2). Because oxygen stores in the body are minimal at best,[21] any interruption in the normal oxygenation of hemoglobin within the lungs results in rapid depletion of the available oxygen.

Mitochondrial Oxygen Requirements

The mitochondria have been estimated to require a P_{O_2} of at least 1.5 mm Hg to produce adenosine triphosphate aerobically. Aerobic metabolism of one glucosyl unit of glycogen to carbon dioxide and water yields 38 molecules of adenosine triphosphate, whereas anaerobic metabolism produces only 2 molecules of adenosine triphosphate plus lactic acid.[19] Persistent hypoxia and reduced adenosine triphosphate production result in disruption of the intracellular lysosomal limiting membranes, enabling release of cellular lytic enzymes. These proteinases, esterases, hydrolases, and phosphatases not only destroy the cell but also form vasoactive and cytotoxic substances that initiate multiple organ failure and trigger disseminated intravascular coagulation.

Organ Failure

Ames and associates demonstrated that inadequate oxygenation of the brain produces capillary endothelial swelling and interstitial edema.[23] Flores and colleagues described the same process within the renal microcirculation.[24] This edema compresses the microvasculature and prevents restoration of tissue blood flow, even if circulation resumes; it is known as the *no-reflow phenomenon*. Thus, just as circulation and oxygenation must be maintained within narrow limits at the cellular level, whole-body circulation and oxygenation must be provided to maintain tissue blood flow. For this reason it is imperative to recognize and treat inadequate tissue perfusion to prevent the potentially irreversible sequelae of cardiac arrest.[25]

Clinical Implications

> If one does not see cardiac changes accompanying or occurring because of anesthesia, he or she just is not looking or listening. The specific actions of premedications, drugs, and anesthetic agents; the mechanical effects of surgery; and the patient's basic disease process may combine to alter rate, rhythm, and compliance of the heart.[26]

During anesthesia, the patient's ability to compensate and control circulatory changes is altered, and he or she becomes entirely dependent on the knowledge and skill of the anesthesiologist. For example, establishment of a safe and proper

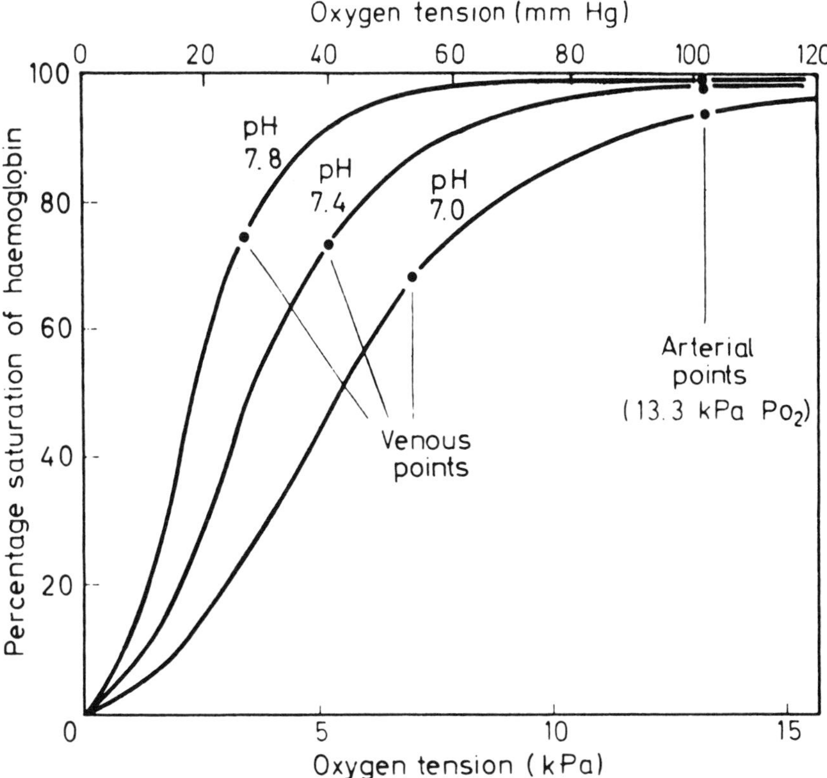

FIGURE 57-2. Normal hemoglobin oxygen dissociation curve (*center*) shifts to the right with acidosis and to the left with alkalosis, other factors remaining constant. (Nunn JF: Applied respiratory physiology, 2nd ed. London: Butterworth & Co, 1977: 354)

level of regional anesthesia in a patient with a full stomach may further aggravate intravascular volume deficits or cardiovascular disease. These and other considerations, such as the effects of potent inhalation and intravenous agents, the airway and circulatory reflexes that are present or abnormally active during light anesthesia, and the need to secure the airway rapidly must be kept in mind.

Dysrhythmias

Dysrhythmias occur in 60% to 90% of patients during anesthesia and surgery.[27–29] Most frequently they occur at the time of or immediately after intubation and usually are reflexive or ischemic in origin. Myocardial ischemia may be associated with hypotension or hypertension. Hypertension increases left ventricular afterload and may lead to myocardial ischemia. During some surgical procedures, vagal reflexes caused by visceral traction or the oculocardiac reflex may occur, usually during light or inadequate anesthesia. The following case reports illustrate these points.

Case 1 (Hypovolemia). A 21-year-old woman was 2 months pregnant. After she had eaten supper, acute left lower abdominal pain and signs of peritoneal irritation developed. She was brought to the operating room for an abdominal exploration, presumably for a ruptured ectopic pregnancy. Her blood pressure was 100/60 mm Hg, pulse 120 beats/min, respiration 30 breaths/min, height 168 cm, weight 55 kg, and hematocrit 30%; the chest radiograph was clear. Because she had recently eaten, spinal anesthesia (tetracaine 10 mg with epinephrine 0.2 mg) was selected and administered with the patient in the lateral position. When the patient was turned supine, a measurement of blood pressure could not be obtained.

Case 2 (Myocardial Ischemia). While mowing his lawn after supper, an active 63-year-old man sustained several lacerations of his left hand, requiring operative repair estimated to last 3 to 4 hours. His history included two myocardial infarctions, the last of which had occurred the previous year. Because he had a full stomach, anesthesia was induced rapidly with thiopental 300 mg and succinylcholine 80 mg. After intubation, systolic blood pressure was 70 mm Hg but during the next 2 minutes could not be measured. After successful resuscitation, additional history-taking revealed that the patient had been taking α-methyldopa and hydrochlorothiazide to control his hypertension and mild congestive heart failure.

Case 3 (Visceral Traction). A 57-year-old woman was undergoing an elective cholecystectomy performed with narcotic–nitrous oxide–relaxant anesthesia. During dissection of the gallbladder, traction was applied to the cystic duct. Bradycardia, from 88 to 40 beats/min, and decreasing systolic blood pressure, from 140 to 60 mm Hg, followed immediately. With release of traction, the pulse increased to 70 beats/min and systolic blood pressure to 110 mm Hg. Moments later, when the cystic duct was clamped, neither pulse nor blood pressure could be measured.

Causes and Prevention

In critically ill patients, blood gas and electrolyte or metabolic abnormalities plus anesthesia are most often responsible for potentially fatal dysrhythmias. This combination may be observed in the uremic patient, who may become more acidotic after being anesthetized and may have a hyperkalemic arrest. Respiratory compensation (respiratory alkalemia) for metabolic acidosis is prevented by the respiratory depressant effects of anesthesia or inadequately controlled ventilation. Respiratory acidemia superimposed on metabolic acidosis drives potassium from the cell, leading to hyperkalemia and arrest.

Prevention of dysrhythmias depends in part on adequate oxygenation and minimization of changes in pH.[30] "Normal" electrolyte values measured before anesthesia and surgery may not reflect electrolyte status during surgery. Extensive bowel preparations, diuretic agents, inanition, or recent administration of digitalis glycosides may predispose to significant changes. The administration of succinylcholine to patients with extensive burns,[31] uremia,[32] tetanus, massive trauma,[33,34] and denervation injuries[35] or neuromuscular disease also can produce hyperkalemic arrest. Cardiac arrests have been reported after anaphylactic and allergic reactions to drugs such as thiopental and succinylcholine,[36] to blood products, and even to latex.[37]

DIAGNOSIS OF CARDIAC ARREST

Monitoring

A precordial or esophageal stethoscope, electrocardiogram (ECG), temperature monitor, blood pressure cuff, pulse oximeter, and capnograph are basic and should be used routinely for all patients undergoing general anesthesia.[38] In addition, critically ill patients or those undergoing major operations may benefit from measurements of intra-arterial blood pressure and central venous pressure; serial arterial blood gas and electrolyte measurements; and, when appropriate, measurements of pulmonary artery and pulmonary artery occlusion pressure, measurement of cardiac output, and transesophageal echocardiography. Reliance on monitoring should add to but not replace careful and thoughtful personal attention to the patient. Continuous close observation and monitoring are mandatory for detecting any changes in vital signs.

Physical Signs

Cardiac arrest usually is diagnosed by the absence of a pulse or blood pressure. Occasionally, *false arrests* occur in the operating room if monitoring equipment malfunctions (eg,if the precordial or esophageal stethoscope disconnects; the blood pressure cuff slips; or an ECG lead detaches). However, the possibility of faulty monitoring should not blind the anesthesiologist to a true cardiac arrest. Other visual or tactile signs aid in making a rapid diagnosis. Inspection of the surgical field may reveal whether or not the patient's blood is well oxygenated, although cyanosis is difficult to recognize and is an often unreliable sign.[39] If the abdomen is open, palpation of the aorta or other major vessels by the surgeon will support or exclude a diagnosis of cardiac arrest.

Symmetrical chest expansion during inflation suggests that no major airway is obstructed, but ventilation should be verified by auscultation and capnographic observation.[38] Difficulties encountered while attempting to inflate the lungs may not be related to airway obstruction. The possibility of tension pneumothorax should always be considered when compliance worsens.

Equipment

A change in respiratory patterns should suggest the possibility of cardiovascular deterioration (in cases in which muscle relaxants are not used). Again, a thorough but quick check of the anesthesia apparatus for leaks or obstruction is imperative. The flowmeters should be scanned to exclude the possibility of delivery of a hypoxic gas mixture. Hypoxia normally stimulates respiration and cardiac activity. However, in dogs receiving surgical concentrations of halothane, hypoxia profoundly depresses circulatory and respiratory activity, leading swiftly to arrest.[40] The anesthesiologist also should check for excessive concentration of inhalation agents in the breathing circuit, which can result from spillage of liquid agents into the inspired gas line or a vaporizer left at a high setting.[41] These measures are aided by mass spectrometry or other means to detect specific end-exhaled concentrations.

TREATMENT

If a cardiac arrest is determined to be present, the steps listed in Table 57-1 should be followed in rapid sequence. Current guidelines for CPR have been established by the American Heart Association.[42] When external cardiac massage is unsuccessful in restoring circulation after 10 to 15 minutes, the chest should be opened,[43] particularly when tension pneumothorax, intrathoracic bleeding, or cardiac tamponade is possible. Direct cardiac massage often is ineffective when applied after more than 25 minutes of total arrest.[44]

After resuscitation efforts are begun, the size of the pupils should be noted. A marked change in pupillary size or reactivity may reflect the adequacy of circulation. Normal pupils dilate 10 to 15 seconds after the onset of cerebral anoxia. Dilation of the pupils may seem ominous but does not contraindicate CPR. When, after circulatory assistance, the pupils become smaller, cerebral circulation is at least marginally improved. Dilation of the pupils may also be influenced by the anesthetic. Narcotics may produce pupillary constriction; halothane and isoflurane do not cause pupillary dilation at normal anesthetic concentrations, but nitrous oxide will, either alone or in combination with other inhalation agents.[45]

The object of CPR is to prevent cerebral anoxia. If resuscitation is not attempted, irreversible changes begin approximately 3 to 4 minutes after cessation of cerebral perfusion, probably because of the no-reflow phenomenon. For CPR to be even partially successful, it must be initiated and performed adequately within the first 1 or 2 minutes of arrest, although even this measure does not ensure complete recovery.[6]

TABLE 57-1
Resuscitation of Patients in Cardiac Arrest

1. Discontinue administration of all anesthetic agents
2. Call for help
3. Flush the anesthetic circuit with oxygen, and administer 100% oxygen. Verify with O_2 analyzer.
4. Ensure patency of airway (preferably by intubation)
5. Check for excessive concentrations of anesthetic agents with an agent analyzer
6. Give a precordial thump (if an ECG monitor is being used), and then begin external cardiac massage
7. Obtain and charge the defibrillator
8. Obtain emergency drugs

The Airway

Basic Maneuvers

The upper airway of an unconscious person can become obstructed when supporting structures surrounding the airway relax. By extending the head and elevating the jaw of the patient, the clinician can establish a patent airway. In some "cardiac arrests," this maneuver is all that is necessary for resuscitation. One hand is positioned under the patient's neck, which is then lifted, while the other hand is placed on the forehead to extend the head. The tongue is thereby elevated away from the posterior pharynx, and the most common cause of airway obstruction is relieved.

If proper extension fails to clear the airway, the mandible may be displaced forward (even to the point of dislocating the temporomandibular joint). This maneuver sometimes opens the airway so that ventilation can continue. If obstruction persists, other causes must be sought, such as misplaced dentures or regurgitation of gastric contents into the oropharynx. Large items can be removed manually, but liquid and stomach contents must be suctioned.

Oxygen Delivery

After patency of the airway has been secured, oxygen should be administered. However, increased pressure may be required to ventilate the patient between cardiac compressions. This pressure may promote gastric distention, which raises the diaphragm and interferes with adequate inflation of the lung. Moreover, gastric distention promotes regurgitation and possible pulmonary aspiration. Hence, to protect the airway and permit the delivery of a high concentration of oxygen to the lungs, the trachea should be intubated as soon as is practical.

Tracheal Intubation

To facilitate intubation, the anesthesiologist must call "time out" from cardiac compression and swiftly insert the endotracheal tube. A belching or gurgling sound, associated with a rapidly enlarging abdominal mass and absence of breath sounds—signs of esophageal intubation, though not always obvious—demands immediate and proper replacement of the endotracheal tube. If esophageal intubation has been avoided, the chest wall moves well; breath sounds are present; and exhaled carbon dioxide can be detected (if cardiac massage is adequate to restore some cardiac output).

The position of the tube within the trachea must be checked to avoid bronchial intubation. Frequently, success at intubating the trachea overwhelms the operator, who is so relieved at accomplishing this technical feat in adverse conditions that he or she inserts the tube full length. The tip then enters the right mainstem bronchus, blocking ventilation to the left mainstem bronchus and often blocking ventilation to the right upper-lobe bronchus as well.

Adjuncts and Alternatives

Adjuncts to conventional intubation include oral or nasal pharyngeal airways. Alternatives may include esophageal obturator and esophageal gastric tube airways, pharyngeal lumen airways, combination esophageal–endotracheal tubes, laryngeal mask airways, transtracheal catheter ventilation, or surgical cricothyroidotomy.[42]

Breathing

In the operating room, ventilation usually is achieved with a mask or endotracheal tube attached to a semi-open or semiclosed system with a reservoir bag. Occasionally, mouth-to-mouth or mouth-to-tube ventilation may be necessitated by defective equipment, contamination of the anesthesia circuit from spilled inhalation agents, or respiratory arrest while the patient is in transit from the operating room to the recovery room. A self-inflating resuscitator bag should always be available for this circumstance. Respiratory assistance must be provided in all cases in which perfusion is inadequate. Manual positive-pressure ventilation should be used for patients undergoing external cardiac compression. Oxygen supplementation is required, and the patient should be ventilated with a tidal volume of 10 to 15 mL/kg, 10 to 12 times per minute during cardiac or respiratory arrest.[42]

Circulation

Precordial Thump

In well-oxygenated, well-monitored patients, a sharp blow to the midsternum (precordial thump) may reverse sudden ventricular tachycardia and, in rare cases, ventricular fibrillation, asystole, or ventricular tachycardia associated with inadequate circulation.[42] It is not effective for the patient with anoxic arrest. If the pulse and blood pressure do not return immediately, CPR should be instituted promptly. Application of successive precordial thumps, in the hope that the third or fourth blow will produce an effective cardiac rhythm, is discouraged.

External Cardiac Compression

For external cardiac compression to be effective, the patient must be horizontal on a hard surface[46]; the operating room table is ideal, although a board, tray, or floor serves well outside the operating room. The heel of one hand is placed parallel to and over the lower half of the sternum, and the heel of the second hand rests on top of the first. Application of pressure over the xyphoid is avoided because of danger to the liver or spleen from lacerations. The clinician's elbows should be extended and locked, and the weight of the shoulders should be directly perpendicular to the patient's chest. Rhythmic depression of the sternum, by 4 to 5 cm in adults, is accomplished by exerting a straight downward force. Compression should be smooth and firm, at a frequency of 80 to 100 compressions per minute. The compression duration should occupy approximately 50% of the cycle time.[42,47]

Studies comparing the effectiveness of standard CPR, interposed abdominal-compression CPR, and open-chest cardiac massage indicate that open-chest cardiac massage produces the best overall results.[42,48–50]

ERRORS IN TECHNIQUE. The most common errors in technique are the following: the heel of the hand is placed too low over the xyphoid; the elbows are flexed, thereby reducing the force generated by the trunk and shoulders; the fingers are not lifted off of the ribs, so that the ribs break or costochondral separations occur; the hands are removed from the sternum during relaxation, which leads to a tendency to "bounce" and to damage the thoracic cage when the compression is not applied directly over the sternum; and the sternum is not compressed at a regular and continuous rate.

The force required to depress the sternum varies, from mere finger pressure for the newborn, to hand and arm weight for the child, to full shoulder and trunk weight for the athletic adult. In older persons with arthritis and brittle ribs, extreme care should be exercised to avoid cracking or disarticulation of the ribs. The usual ratio for cardiac compression and ventilation is 5 to 1. Increasing the frequency of cardiac massage from 60 compressions per minute to 80 to 100 compressions per minute results in improvement in cardiac output.[42,51]

Defibrillation

If ventricular fibrillation is present, external defibrillation should be attempted with a direct-current defibrillator. Three sequential ("stacked") shocks of 200, 200 to 300, and 360 J should be provided, if necessary, for persistent ventricular tachycardia or fibrillation.[42] The power output of each defibrillator may vary, so the anesthesiologist must be acquainted with the characteristics of the equipment available. The defibrillator paddles should be covered well with electrode paste or with saline-soaked gauze pads. One paddle should be lateral to the left nipple in the midaxillary line, and the other should be placed to the right of the upper sternum, below the clavicle.[52]

After defibrillation is attempted, ventilation and external cardiac compression are continued until a functional rhythm has been restored. If an effective rhythm greater than 60 beats/min is obtained, the anesthesiologist may stop and palpate for carotid or femoral pulses. If both a pulse and adequate blood pressure are found, observation and assisted ventilation are indicated. Blood pressure should be measured frequently to evaluate cardiovascular trends and to help determine the need for catecholamine support. If pulses are not present, CPR is resumed immediately while additional attempts at defibrillation are made. If the chest is open, the defibrillator power should be 50 J.

Definitive Therapy

True cardiac arrest involves asystole or ventricular fibrillation. In asystole, the therapeutic objective is to initiate electric and contractile activity. Drugs, electric pacing, or both may be used. Appendix I provides algorithms for the treatment of ventricular fibrillation, pulseless ventricular tachycardia, sustained tachycardia, asystole, pulseless electric activity, bradycardia, and paroxysmal supraventricular tachycardia.[42]

Drugs

When only one ECG lead is monitored, a very fine ventricular fibrillation can appear as asystole. This observation may account for anecdotal reports of correction of asystole to normal cardiac activity after electric countershock. It also underlies the recommendation that prompt defibrillation of all patients with initial asystole may convert the rhythm of some patients to more organized cardiac electric activity.[53]

EPINEPHRINE. The drug of choice for asystolic cardiac arrest is 1.0 mg epinephrine, administered intravenously every 3 to 5 minutes during resuscitation.[54] Larger doses, as large as 0.2 mg/kg, may be used if the standard dose fails. However, published and unpublished studies to date have not shown improved outcome from this large-dose approach.[42,55]

ATROPINE. If severe bradycardia, heart block, or electric standstill is caused by a strong vagal stimulus, the intravenous administration of 0.5 to 1.0 mg atropine followed by subsequent doses as large as 0.04 mg/kg is indicated. However, atropine should not be given after epinephrine during a prolonged resuscitation.[56]

CALCIUM CHLORIDE. If the arrest is caused by hyperkalemia, hypocalcemia, or calcium channel–blocking agent toxicity, 2 to 4 mg/kg calcium chloride given at 10-minute intervals probably is helpful. Otherwise, it should not be used.[42]

SODIUM BICARBONATE. Sodium bicarbonate, once a mainstay of resuscitation, may actually worsen CPR outcome.[42] It should be considered only after other confirmed interventions such as defibrillation, cardiac compression, intubation, ventilation, and more than one trial of epinephrine have been attempted. If it is used, the initial dose should be 1 mEq/kg, followed by one half of that dose, as guided by arterial blood gas measurements, every 10 minutes thereafter.[42]

Emergency Pacemaker

The 1992 recommendations emphasize emergency transcutaneous pacemaking because of its ease of application and operability.[42] New, multifunctional electrodes allow "hands-off" defibrillation, pacing, and ECG monitoring. Transvenous pacing by specially modified pulmonary artery catheters also can be used effectively. When the chest is open, pacing wires may be attached directly to the epicardium.

Coronary Artery Perfusion

During resuscitation, efforts to improve coronary perfusion are necessary, particularly in the patient with a history of coronary vascular disease. This goal is best reached with epinephrine. Although defibrillation has been achieved, coronary perfusion must be maintained, even temporarily at the expense of other tissue, or fibrillation is likely to recur.

If ventricular fibrillation resumes despite adequate coronary perfusion, it probably is caused by an irritable focus within the heart. Ventricular irritability can usually be suppressed with lidocaine, 1 to 1.5 mg/kg administered in repeated intravenous boluses to a total dose of as much as 3 mg/kg. Bretylium tosylate, 5 mg/kg as an intravenous bolus and then 10 mg/kg every 5 minutes as needed to a total dose of as much as 30 to 35 mg/kg is a second choice.[42] When ventricular irritability persists after a reasonable cardiac output has been established, a continuous infusion of lidocaine, 2 to 4 mg/min, is indicated to suppress the irritable focus.

Local Anesthetic–Induced Cardiac Arrest

Cardiac arrest that occurs because of local anesthetics may require a slightly different resuscitation technique, given the profound myocardial depression that may be present. Kasten and Martin[57] reported that resuscitation of dogs in whom cardiac arrest had been produced by massive overdosage of bupivacaine required bretylium tosylate, 5 mg/kg every 30 seconds intravenously to a total dose of 30 mg/kg, for ventricular tachycardia. Epinephrine and atropine, 0.75 and 0.8 mg intravenously, respectively, followed by 0.5 and 0.4 mg, respectively, every 45 seconds also were used until the rhythm and blood pressure were stable.[57]

COMPLICATIONS

Even when CPR is performed properly, complications may occur.[58–63] These include costochondral separations, fracture of the sternum or ribs, pneumothorax or hemothorax, lung or cardiac contusions, gastroesophageal tear, gastric hemorrhage, lacerated liver or spleen, laceration of aorta, aspiration pneumonitis, hyperosmolality, hypercapnia, and fat or bone marrow embolism. Careful attention to detail will keep complications to a minimum.

EVALUATION OF RESUSCITATION

When cardiac arrest occurs during an anesthetic that includes the use of muscle relaxants, the usual signs of brain death (eg, areflexia and lack of respiratory effort) do not apply. In addition, pupillary signs may be modified, but to a lesser extent, by the anesthetic drugs.[45] If ventricular activity is inadequate after 30 to 60 minutes of maximal resuscitative effort, resuscitation should be stopped. When resuscitation has been successful, appropriate steps must be taken to monitor and support the patient's vital functions.

Postresuscitation Care

No current evidence supports the use of pharmacologic doses of corticosteroids in an attempt to prevent the sequelae of cardiovascular collapse, including "shock lung" and cerebral edema. Other measures, such as the administration of potent diuretic agents and controlled hyperventilation, may be used to reduce cerebral edema and to decrease cerebral metabolic demands[64]; they have no demonstrated positive effect on reducing mortality from global ischemia.

SUDDEN UNEXPECTED DEATH

Incidence

In 1964, Himmelhoch and colleagues reported the results of 65 resuscitations at the Peter Bent Brigham Hospital in Boston.[65] Only 3 cases occurred in the operating room; 9 occurred in the postanesthesia care unit. None of them was attributed to anesthetic-related problems. Only four (6%) patients survived to leave the hospital.

Meltzer, at the Presbyterian Hospital in Philadelphia, studied the incidence and cause of sudden hospital death.[66] In a 31-month period, 20,000 admissions and 1206 deaths occurred. Of these, 953 (79%) were expected, and 253 (21%) were unexpected. Ninety-six of the unexpected deaths were considered irreversible at the time of diagnosis; therefore, 157 (13%) of the 1206 deaths were unexpected but potentially reversible.

Onset and Therapy

Extrapolation of these data to the average hospital that admits 10,000 patients per year leads to the following conclusion: 78 patients per 10,000 hospital admissions may die unnecessarily each year. Approximately 35 million patients are admitted to hospitals in the United States annually. Thus 273,000 sudden and reversible deaths occur each year. Meltzer[66] asked the following question: "Is cardiopulmonary resuscitation an overall solution to the problem?"

In his study 38% of resuscitation efforts occurred in special care areas, with 18% survival. Sixty-two percent of resuscitations occurred in general ward areas, with a survival of only 4%. The results of resuscitation in Meltzer's study[66] were no better than those of Himmelhoch and colleagues.[65] This observation suggests that poor resuscitation in the general hospital setting is the result of an unacceptable lapse between the onset of cardiac arrest and the discovery and institution of appropriate therapy.

High-risk Categories

Meltzer's[66] recommendations included the recognition of high-risk categories. Of patients in whom sudden death occurred, in 90% the ECG on admission was abnormal; 92% were admitted for a medical illness; 69% had known heart disease; and 47% were older than 70 years. The better survival in patients given CPR in intensive care units suggests that their arrest was noted earlier and effective therapy was instituted sooner.

NEUROLOGIC RECOVERY

Goldberg emphasized that "the goal of CPR is to prevent irreversible cerebral anoxic damage after cardiac arrest."[51] Indeed, if resuscitation is accomplished efficiently and promptly, the overall neurologic outcome is remarkably good. However, prolongation of resuscitation efforts, whether because of delay in instituting CPR, poor technique, or patient disease, is associated with a poor neurologic outcome.[67]

Prognostic Signs

Particularly relevant is an evaluation of the neurologic recovery of 210 patients with nontraumatic coma, most of whom had cardiac arrest.[68] One fourth of this group lacked pupillary light reflexes at the time of the initial postresuscitation neurologic examination; none of these patients ever regained independent daily function. In contrast, presence of the pupillary light reflex, spontaneous eye movements that were at least conjugate, and motor response to pain at the time of the initial examination characterized 13% of the 210 patients, 41% of whom regained independent activities. One of 94 patients lacking motor responses to pain and roving conjugate or orienting spontaneous eye movements 24 hours after resuscitation regained independent activity. Overall, only 13% of the patients regained independent function at some time during the 1st year after arrest. These outcomes must be remembered when "heroic" measures are considered during the first few hours of coma.

Efforts to Improve Neurologic Recovery

The results with current therapy are so poor that aggressive measures, if applied early enough, are indicated in an attempt to improve neurologic recovery. In the postresuscitative period after cardiac arrest, four stages of cerebral impairment seem to be present (Table 57-2).[69–74]

Considerable research has established that, as expected, the neurologic insult produced by complete ischemia usually is greater than that produced by partial ischemia.[75–80] However, when hyperglycemia is present, partial ischemia is associated with a poorer outcome. A high concentration of glucose in the presence of incomplete ischemia provides substrate for continuation of the metabolic processes that increase the metabolic acidosis and the resultant sequelae.[81]

Reporting cases typical of the delayed deterioration that characterizes the third stage of cerebral impairment, White and coworkers described two children who at 24 and 48 hours

TABLE 57-2
Cerebral Impairment After Resuscitation From Cardiac Arrest

STAGE	
I	Multifocal no-reflow phenomenon[69,70]
II	Hyperemia[71–73]
III	Delayed prolonged postischemic hypoperfusion[71–73]
IV	Resolution, permanent disability, or recovery[69,74]

after resuscitation had good breathing patterns, reactive pupils, brisk corneal reflexes, and purposeful movements of all extremities. However, by about 72 hours their clinical condition had deteriorated to severe neurologic deficit.[82]

Calcium Channel Blockade

Several mechanisms proposed to account for delayed deterioration include excessive calcium ion flux, lipid perioxidation,[83] and direct injury to deoxyribonucleic acid or ribonucleic acid by hydroxyl radicals.[84] These events may lead to intracellular cascades of chemical reactions, followed by cell death and necrosis.[71,72] As a result of hypoxia and disruption of cellular metabolism, the intracellular calcium shifts cause the release of free fatty acids and the production of free oxygen radicals. This sequence is perhaps the cause of the no-reflow phenomenon. Studies have suggested that calcium channel–blocking agents may have a role in postresuscitation therapy.[85–88]

Modification of the No-reflow Phenomenon

Hypertension, heparinization, and hemodilution all are directed toward reversing the no-reflow phenomenon and restoring capillary flow in vessels that previously were obstructed. Much experimental work remains before this therapy can be recommended for humans. Of course, the therapeutic modalities used in experimental studies would be modified according to the cause of cardiac arrest. If ischemic heart disease is the basis for arrest, then severe hypertension is contraindicated because of the effect on afterload and increasing myocardial work. The administration of heparin depends on the clinical situation. However, in a young person who has an unexpected, sudden cardiac arrest and whose circulation and gas exchange can be restored rapidly, these maneuvers may be very useful. Neurologic recovery, infrequent in the past, may thereby be achieved.

TEAM APPROACH

Smooth, cooperative performance of CPR by a team does not happen by chance. Time must be devoted to education and practice so that each team member knows what is expected. The physicians and nurses in the operating room must be acquainted with the function and availability of equipment. After each resuscitation, the participants should discuss the procedure and ascertain errors in technique or diagnosis or account for the success of therapy. This approach may improve the quality of care provided for the next patient.[89] The responsibility for improving patient care belongs to both the anesthesiologist and the surgeon, who together must perfect the preoperative preparation of the patient and ensure that the anesthestic is administered skillfully and the operation performed carefully and efficiently.

REFERENCES

1. Fatal application of chloroform (editorial). Edinburgh Med Surg J 69:498, 1848
2. Sibson H: On death from chloroform. London Medical Gazette 42:108, 1848
3. Beecher HK: The first anesthesia death with some remarks suggested by it on the fields of the laboratory and the clinic in the appraisal of new anesthetic agents. Anesthesiology 2:443, 1941
4. Fatal application of chloroform (editorial). Lancet 1:161, 1848
5. Mussey RD: Chloroform in surgical operations. Boston Medical and Surgical Journal 38:194, 1848
6. Caplan RA, Ward RJ, Posner K, et al: Unexpected cardiac arrest during spinal anesthesia: a closed claims analysis of predisposing factors. Anesthesiology 68:5, 1988
7. Keats A: Anesthesia mortality: a new mechanism. Anesthesiology 68:2, 1988
8. Brigs BD, Sheldon DB, Beecher HK: Study of a thirty-year period of operating room deaths at the Massachusetts General Hospital, 1925-1954. JAMA 160:1439, 1956
9. Memery HN: Anesthesia mortality in private practice: a ten year study. JAMA 194:185, 1965
10. Pierce JA: Cardiac arrests and deaths associated with anesthesia. Anesth Analg 45:407, 1966
11. Jude JR, Bolooki H, Nagel E: Cardiac resuscitation in the operating room: current status. Ann Surg 171:948, 1970
12. Deaths during general anesthesia: technology-related, due to human error, or unavoidable? Technology for Anesthesia 5:1, 1985
13. Stetson JB: Resuscitation under anesthesia: some interesting early reports. Anesthesiology 20:62, 1959
14. Maass D: Die Methode der wiederbelebung der Herztod nach Chloroformeinatmung. Berliner Klinische Wochenschrift 12: 265, 1892
15. Keen WW: Case of total laryngectomy (unsuccessful) in which massage of the heart for chloroform collapse was employed with notes of 25 other cases of cardiac massage. Therapeutic Gazette 28:217, 1904
16. Bedell SE, Delbanco TL, Cook EF, et al: Survival after cardiopulmonary resuscitation in the hospital. N Engl J Med 309:569, 1983
17. DeBard ML: Cardiopulmonary resuscitation: analysis of six years' experience and review of the literature. Ann Emerg Med 10: 408, 1981
18. Davis DA: An analysis of anesthetic mishaps from medical liability claims. Int Anesthesiol Clin 22:31, 1984
19. Finch CA, Lenfant C: Oxygen transport in man. N Engl J Med 286:407, 1972
20. Flenley DC: The rationale of oxygen therapy. Lancet 1:270, 1967
21. Farhi LE: Gas stores of the body. In McDowell: Handbook of physiology, section 3, vol 1. Philadelphia: JB Lippincott, 1964: 873
22. Nunn JF: Applied respiratory physiology, 2nd ed. London: Butterworth, 1986: 232
23. Ames A III, Wright RL, Kowada N, et al: Cerebral ischemia: II. the no-reflow phenomenon. Am J Pathol 52:437, 1968
24. Flores J, DiBona DR, Beck CH, et al: The role of cell swelling in ischemic renal damage and the protective effect of hypertonic solute. J Clin Invest 51:118, 1972
25. Bass E: Cardiopulmonary arrest: pathophysiology and neurologic complications. Ann Intern Med 103:920, 1985
26. Jenkins MT: Editor's note. In Petty LD, Giesecke AH: Cardiac considerations in anesthesia. Clinical Anesthesiology 3:168, 1968
27. Bertrand CA, Steiner NV, Jameson AG, et al: Disturbances of cardiac rhythm during anesthesia and surgery. JAMA 216:1615, 1971
28. Kuner J: Cardiac arrhythmias during anesthesia. Dis Chest 52: 580, 1967
29. Berger JJ, Donchin M, Morgan LS: Perioperative changes in blood pressure and heart rate. Anesth Analg 63:647, 1984
30. Camarata SJ, Weil MH, Hanashiro PK, et al: Cardiac arrest in the critically ill. Circulation 44:688, 1971
31. Tolmie JD, Joyce TH, Mitchell GD: Succinylcholine danger in burned patients. Anesthesiology 28:467, 1967
32. Cook DR, Cosimi AB: Potassium release after succinylcholine in acutely uremic monkeys. Anesthesiology 36:297, 1972
33. Kopriva C, Ratliff J, Fletcher JR, et al: Serum potassium changes

after succinylcholine in patients with acute massive muscle trauma. Anesthesiology 34:246, 1971
34. Mazze RI, Escue HM, Houston JB: Hyperkalemia and cardiovascular collapse following administration of succinylcholine in traumatized patients. Anesthesiology 31:540, 1969
35. Smelt RB: Hyperkalemia following succinylcholine administration in neurological disorders: a review. Can Anaesth Soc J 18: 199, 1971
36. Jerums G, Whittingham S, Wilson P, et al: Anaphylaxis to suxamethonium: a case report. Br J Anaesth 39:73, 1967
37. Gold M, Swartz JS, Braude BM, et al: Intraoperative anaphylaxis: an association with latex sensitivity. J Allergy Clin Immunol 87: 662, 1991
38. American Society of Anesthesiologists: Standards for basic intraoperative monitoring. Approved by House of Delegates, October 2, 1986; last amended October 13, 1993
39. Comroe JH, Botelho S: The unreliability of cyanosis in the recognition of arterial anoxia. Am J Med Sci 214:1, 1947
40. Cullen DJ, Eger EI II: The effect of anesthetic depth on the respiratory response to hypoxia in dogs: a dose response study. Anesthesiology 33:487, 1970
41. Kopriva CJ, Lowenstein E: An anesthetic accident: cardiovascular collapse from liquid halothane delivery. Anesthesiology 30:246, 1969
42. Emergency Cardiac Care Committee and Subcommittees, American Heart Association. Guidelines for cardiopulmonary resuscitation and emergency cardiac care. JAMA 268:2171, 1992
43. Kern KB, Sanders AB, Badylak SF, et al: Long-term survival with open chest cardiac massage after ineffective closed chest compression in a canine model. Circulation 75:498, 1987
44. Geehr EC, Lewis FR, Auerbach PJ: Failure of open-heart massage to improve survival after prehospital nontraumatic cardiac arrest. N Engl J Med 314:1189, 1986
45. Cullen DJ, Eger EI II: Clinical signs of anesthesia. Anesthesiology 36:21, 1972
46. Kouwenhoven WB, Jude JP, Knickerbocker GG: Closed-chest massage. JAMA 173:1064, 1960
47. Taylor GJ, Tucker WM, Green HC: Importance of prolonged compression during CPR in man. N Engl J Med 296:1515, 1977
48. Jackson RE, Freeman SB: Hemodynamics of cardiac massage. Emerg Med Clin North Am 1:501, 1983
49. Jackson RE, Jayce K, Danasi S, et al: Blood flow in cerebral cortex during cardiac resuscitation in dogs. Ann Emerg Med 13: 657, 1984
50. Weisfeldt ML: Recent advances in cardiopulmonary resuscitation. Jpn Circ J 49:13:1985
51. Goldberg AH: Cardiopulmonary arrest. N Engl J Med 290:381, 1974
52. Kouwenhoven WB, Milnor WR, Knickerbocker GG, et al: Closed-chest defibrillation of the heart. Surgery 42:550, 1957
53. Thompson BM, Brooks RC, Pionkowski RS, et al: Immediate countershock treatment of asystole. Ann Emerg Med 13:827, 1984
54. Paradis NA, Martin GB, Rivers EP, et al: Coronary perfusion pressure and the return of spontaneous circulation in human cardiopulmonary resuscitation. JAMA 263:1106, 1990
55. Ditchey RU, Lindenfeld J: Failure of epinephrine to improve the balance between myocardial oxygen supply and demand during closed-chest resuscitation in dogs. Circulation 78:382, 1988
56. Stueven HA, Tonsfeldt DJ, Thompson BM, et al: Atropine in asystole: human studies. Ann Emerg Med 13:815, 1984
57. Kasten GW, Martin ST: Successful cardiovascular resuscitation after massive intravenous bupivacaine overdosage in anesthetized dogs. Anesth Analg 64:491, 1985
58. Bishop RL, Weisfeld ML: Sodium bicarbonate administration during cardiac arrest: effect on arterial pH, PCO_2 and osmolality. JAMA 235:506, 1976
59. Jackson CT, Greendyke RM: Pulmonary and cerebral fat embolism after closed chest massage. Surg Gynecol Obstet 120: 25, 1965
60. Mattar JA, Weil MH, Shubin H, et al: Cardiac arrest in the critically ill: II. hyperosmolal states following cardiac arrest. Am J Med 56:162, 1974
61. McIntyre KM, Parisi AF, Benfari R, et al: Pathophysiological syndromes of cardiopulmonary resuscitation. Arch Intern Med 138:1130, 1978
62. Bjork RJ, Snyder BD, Campton BC, et al: Medical complications of cardiopulmonary arrest. Arch Intern Med 142:500, 1982
63. Barrowcliffe MP: Visceral injuries following external cardiac massage. Anaesthesia 39:347, 1984
64. Marsh ML, Marshall LF, Shapiro HM: Neurosurgical intensive care. Anesthesiology 47:149, 1977
65. Himmelhoch SR, Dekker A, Gazzaniga AB, et al: Closed chest cardiac resuscitation: a prospective clinical and pathological study. N Engl J Med 270:118, 1964
66. Meltzer LE: The incidence of sudden unexpected death among hospitalized patients. Presented at the meeting of American Association for the Advancement of Science. Boston, 1976
67. Eisenberg M, Bergner L, Hallstrom A: Paramedic programs and out-of-hospital cardiac arrest: I. factors associated with successful resuscitation. Am J Public Health 69:30, 1979
68. Levy DE, Caronna JJ, Singer BH, et al: Predicting outcome from hypoxic-ischemic coma. JAMA 253:1420, 1985
69. Negovsky VA, Gurvitch AM, Kolotokrylina ES: Postresuscitation disease. Amsterdam: American Elsevier, 1984
70. Safar P: Resuscitation from clinical death: pathophysiologic limits and therapeutic potentials. Crit Care Med 16:923, 1988
71. Siesjo BK: Cell damage in the brain: a speculative synthesis. J Cereb Blood Flow Metab 1:155, 1981
72. Hossmann K-A: Treatment of experimental cerebral ischemia. J Cereb Blood Flow Metab 2:275, 1982
73. Snyder JV, Nemoto EM, Carroll RG, et al: Global ischemia in dogs: intracranial pressures, brain blood flow and metabolism. Stroke 6:21, 1975
74. Safar P, Vaagenes P: Systemic search for brain resuscitation potentials after total circulatory arrest. In Baethmann A, et al (eds): Mechanisms of secondary brain damage. NATO–Advanced Study Institute, Life Science Series. London: Plenum Press, 1984
75. Hossmann KA, Kleihues P: Reversibility of ischemic brain damage. Arch Neurol 29:375, 1973
76. Nordstrom CH, Rehncrona S, Siesjo BK: Effects of phenobarbital in cerebral ischemia: II. restitution of cerebral energy state as well as glycolytic metabolites, citric acid cycle intermediates, and associated amino acids after pronounced incomplete ischemia. Stroke 9:335, 1978
77. Rehncrona S, Rosen I, Siesjo BK: Excessive cellular acidosis: an important mechanism of neuronal damage in the brain. Acta Physiol Scand 110:435, 1980
78. Kalimo H, Rehncrona S, Soderfelt B: The role of lactic acidosis in the ischemic nerve cell injury. Acta Neuropathol (Berl) 7(suppl):20, 1981
79. Marshall LF, Durity F, Lounsbury R, et al: Experimental cerebral oligemia and ischemia produced by intracranial hypertension: I. Pathophysiology, electroenchalography, cerebral blood flow, blood brain barrier, and neurological function. J Neurosurg 43: 308, 1975
80. Steen PA, Michenfelder JD, Milde JH: Incomplete vs. complete cerebral ischemia: improved outcome with a minimal blood flow. Ann Neurol 6:389, 1979
81. Myers RE: A unitary theory of causation of anoxic and hypoxic brain pathology. Adv Neurol 26:195, 1979
82. White BC, Aust DS, Arfors KE, et al: Brain injury by ischemic anoxia: hypothesis extension—a tale of two ions? Ann Emerg Med 13:862, 1984
83. Anderson DK, Means ED: Lipid perioxidation in spinal cord: $FeCl_2$ induction and antioxidants. Neurochemical Pathology 1: 249, 1983
84. Brawn K, Fridovich I: Superoxide radical and superoxide dismutases: threat and defence. Acta Physiol Scand Suppl 492:9, 1980
85. Allen GS, Ahn HS, Preziosi TJ, et al: Cerebral arterial spasm: a controlled trial of nimodipine in patients with subarachnoid hemorrhage. N Engl J Med 308:619, 1983

86. White BC, Gadzinski DS, Hoehner PJ, et al: Correction of canine cerebral cortical blood flow and vascular resistance after cardiac arrest using flunarizine, a calcium antagonist. Ann Emerg Med 11:119, 1982
87. White BC, Winegar CD, Wilson RF, et al: Possible role of calcium blockers in cerebral resuscitation: a review of the literature and synthesis for future studies. Crit Care Med 11:202, 1983
88. Raichle ME: The pathophysiology of brain ischemia. Ann Neurol 13:2, 1983
89. Harley HRS: Reflections on cardiopulmonary resuscitation. Lancet 2:1, 1966

FURTHER READING

Melker RJ, Kirby RR, Marshall JR: Cardiopulmonary resuscitation. In: Kirby RR, Gravenstein N (eds): Clinical anesthesia practice. Philadelphia: WB Saunders, 1994: 835

APPENDIX
Resuscitation Algorithms

VENTRICULAR FIBRILLATION AND PULSELESS VENTRICULAR TACHYCARDIA

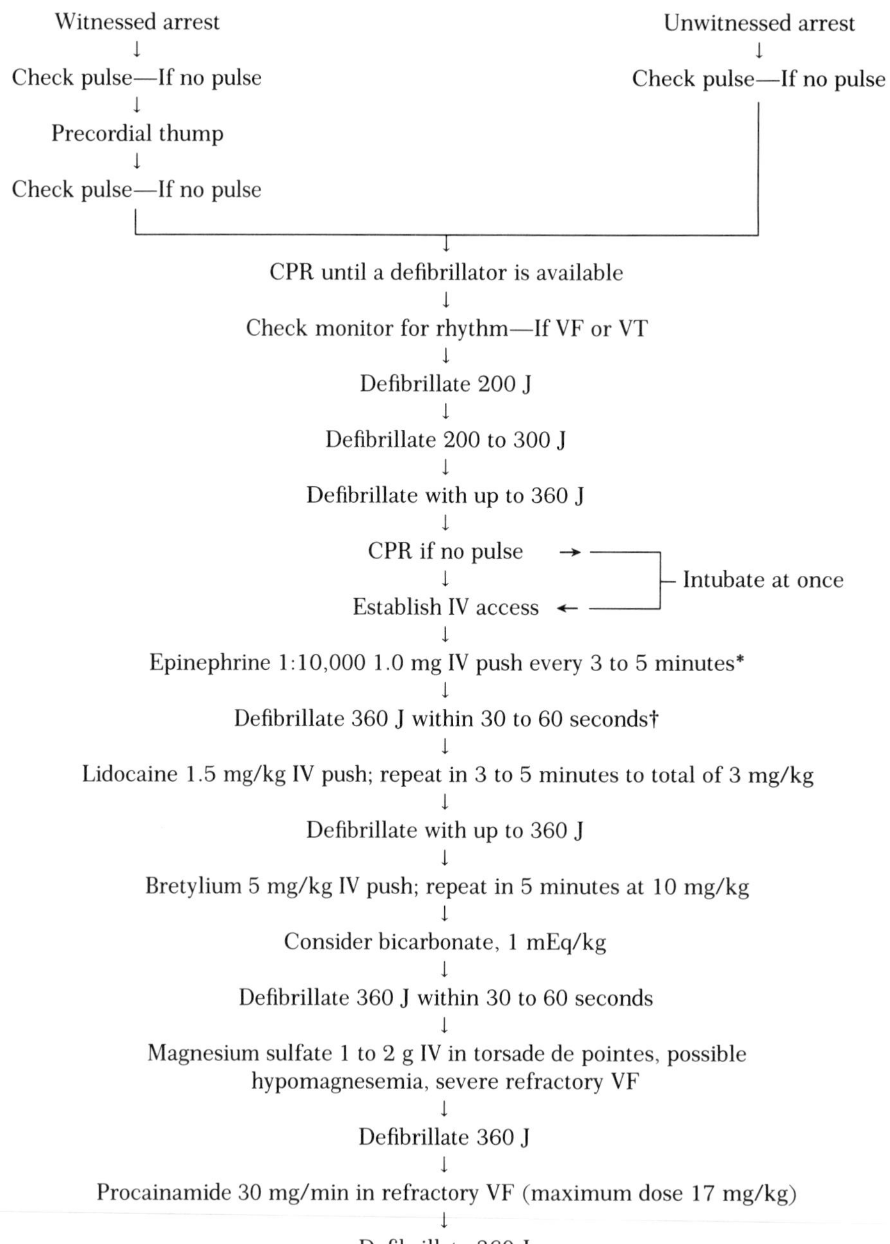

*Suggested treatment of ventricular fibrillation (*VF*) and pulseless ventricular tachycardia (*VT*). The algorithm presumes that VF or pulseless VT is continuing and represents suggested management only. Some patients may require care not specified here.* IV, *intravenous.*

* *Consider epinephrine 2 to 5 mg IV push every 3 to 5 minutes; or 1 to 3 to 5 mg IV push sequentially 3 minutes apart; or 0.1 mg/kg every 3 to 5 minutes if initial approach fails.*

† *Multiple sequential shocks (200, 200 to 300, 360 J acceptable).*

Modified from American Heart Association: Guidelines for cardiopulmonary resuscitation and emergency cardiac care. JAMA 268:2217, 1992.

SUSTAINED VENTRICULAR TACHYCARDIA

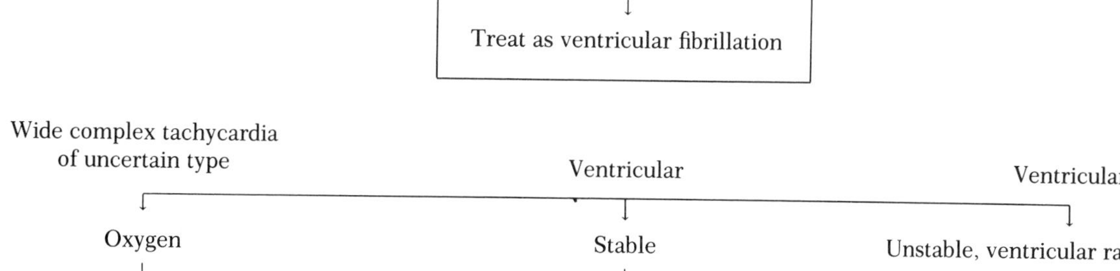

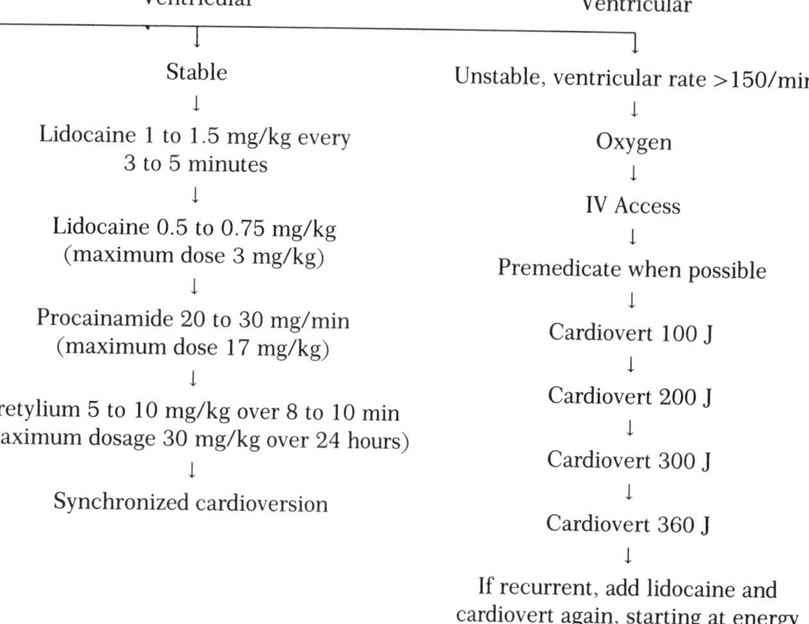

No Pulse
↓
Treat as ventricular fibrillation

Wide complex tachycardia of uncertain type
Oxygen
↓
IV access
↓
Lidocaine 1 to 1.5 mg/kg
↓
Lidocaine 0.5 to 0.75 mg/kg up to 3 mg/kg
↓
Procainamide 20 mg/min until VT resolves, or up to 1000 mg
↓
Adenosine 6 mg IV push over 1 to 3 seconds
↓ (1 to 2 minutes)
Adenosine 12 mg IV push over 1 to 2 seconds; repeat once in 1 to 2 minutes
↓
Procainamide 20 to 30 mg/min (maximum dose 17 mg/kg)
↓
Bretylium 5 to 10 mg/kg over 8 to 10 minutes (maximum dosage 30 mg/kg over 24 hours)
↓
Synchronized cardioversion

Ventricular
Stable
↓
Lidocaine 1 to 1.5 mg/kg every 3 to 5 minutes
↓
Lidocaine 0.5 to 0.75 mg/kg (maximum dose 3 mg/kg)
↓
Procainamide 20 to 30 mg/min (maximum dose 17 mg/kg)
↓
Bretylium 5 to 10 mg/kg over 8 to 10 min (maximum dosage 30 mg/kg over 24 hours)
↓
Synchronized cardioversion

Ventricular
Unstable, ventricular rate >150/min
↓
Oxygen
↓
IV Access
↓
Premedicate when possible
↓
Cardiovert 100 J
↓
Cardiovert 200 J
↓
Cardiovert 300 J
↓
Cardiovert 360 J
↓
If recurrent, add lidocaine and cardiovert again, starting at energy level previously successful; then procainamide or bretylium

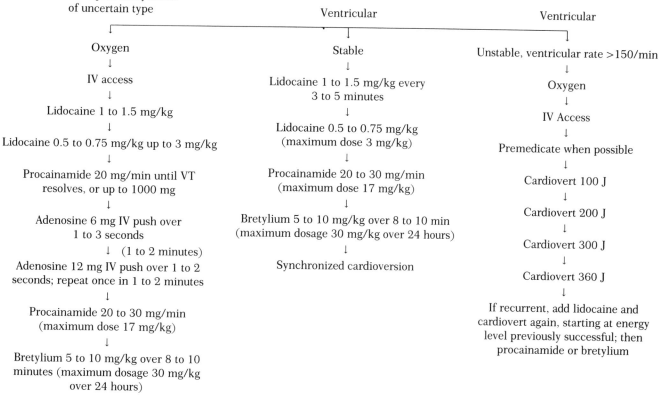

Suggested treatment of sustained ventricular tachycardia (VT). The algorithm presumes that VT is continuing. Unstable conditions include chest pain, dyspnea, hypotension (systolic blood pressure <90 mmHg), congestive heart failure, ischemia, or myocardial infarction. The algorithm represents suggested management only. Some patients may require care not specified here. IV, intravenous.

Modified from American Heart Association: Guidelines for cardiopulmonary resuscitation and emergency cardiac care. JAMA 268:2224, 1992.

ASYSTOLE

If rhythm is unclear and possibly ventricular fibrillation,
defibrillate as for ventricular fibrillation.

↓

If asystole is present continue CPR

↓ (Intubate at once)

Establish IV access

↓

Consider immediate transcutaneous pacing

↓

Epinephrine 1:10,000 1.0 mg IV push every 3 to 5 minutes*

↓

Atropine 1.0 mg IV push every 3 to 5 minutes up to 0.04 mg/kg

↓

Consider bicarbonate 1 mEq/kg

↓

Consider termination of efforts†

Suggested treatment of asystole. The algorithm presumes that asystole is continuing. The algorithm represents suggested management only. Some patients may require care not specified here. IV, *intravenous.*

* *Consider epinephrine 2 to 5 mg IV push every 3 to 5 minutes; or 1 mg to 3 mg to 5 mg IV push sequentially 3 minutes apart; or 0.1 mg/kg every 3 to 5 minutes if initial approach fails.*

† *If asystole persists or other agonal rhythm occurs after intubation and initial medications and no reversible cause identified.*

Modified from American Heart Association: Guidelines for cardiopulmonary resuscitation and emergency cardiac care. JAMA 268:2220, 1992.

PULSELESS ELECTRIC ACTIVITY

Electromechanical Dissociation, Pseudo-Electromechanical Dissociation, Idioventricular Rhythm, Ventricular Escape Rhythms, Bradysystolic Rhythms, and Postdefibrillation Idioventricular Rhythms

Continued CPR

↓ (Intubate at once)

Establish IV access

↓ (Assess blood flow with Doppler)

Consider hypovolemia, cardiac tamponade, tension pneumothorax, hypoxemia,
acidosis, pulmonary embolism

↓

Epinephrine 1.0 mg IV push (repeat every 3 to 5 minutes)*

↓

Consider bicarbonate 1 mEq/kg

↓

If absolute bradycardia (<60 beats/min)

↓

Atropine 1 mg IV push (repeat every 3 to 5 minutes to total of 0.04 mg/kg)

Suggested treatment of electromechanical dissociation. The algorithm presumes that EMD is continuing. The algorithm represents suggested management only. Some patients may require care not specified here. IV, *intravenous.*

* *Consider epinephrine 2 to 5 mg IV push every 3 to 5 minutes; or epinephrine 1 to 3 to 5 mg IV push sequentially 3 minutes apart; or 0.1 mg/kg IV push every 3 to 5 minutes if initial approach fails.*

Modified from American Heart Association: Guidelines for cardiopulmonary resuscitation and emergency cardiac care. JAMA 268:2219, 1992.

BRADYCARDIA

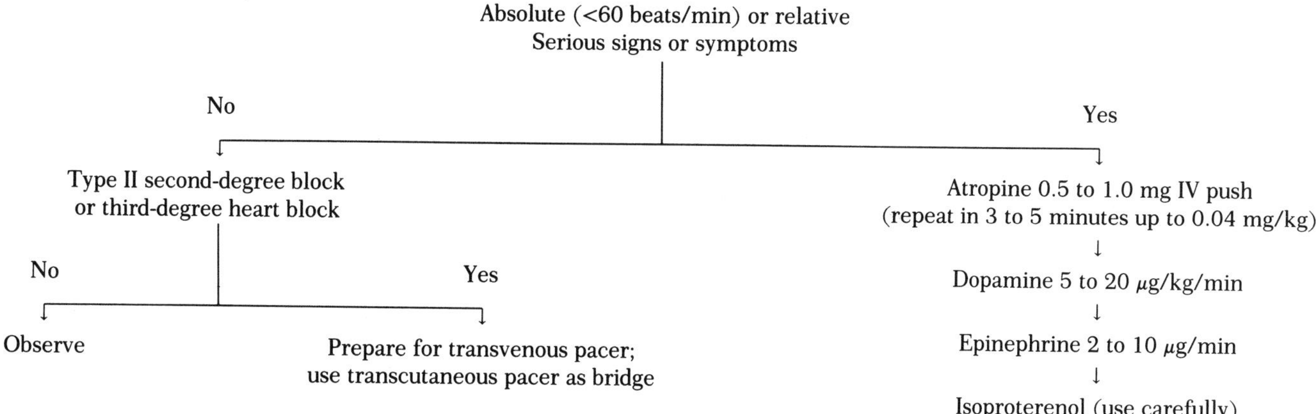

Suggested treatment of hemodynamically significant bradycardia. Significant symptoms include hypotension (systolic blood pressure <90 mm Hg), premature ventricular contractions, altered mental status, chest pain, dyspnea, ischemia, or myocardial infarction. The use of isoproterenol should be considered as temporizing therapy only. The algorithm represents suggested management only. Some patients may require care not specified here.

Modified from American Heart Association: Guidelines for cardiopulmonary resuscitation and emergency cardiac care. JAMA 268:1921, 1992.

PAROXYSMAL SUPRAVENTRICULAR TACHYCARDIA

Unstable

Synchronous cardioversion 100 J
↓
Synchronous cardioversion 200 J
↓
Synchronous cardioversion 300 J
↓
Synchronous cardioversion 360 J
↓
Correct underlying abnormalities
↓
Pharmacologic therapy and cardioversion

Stable

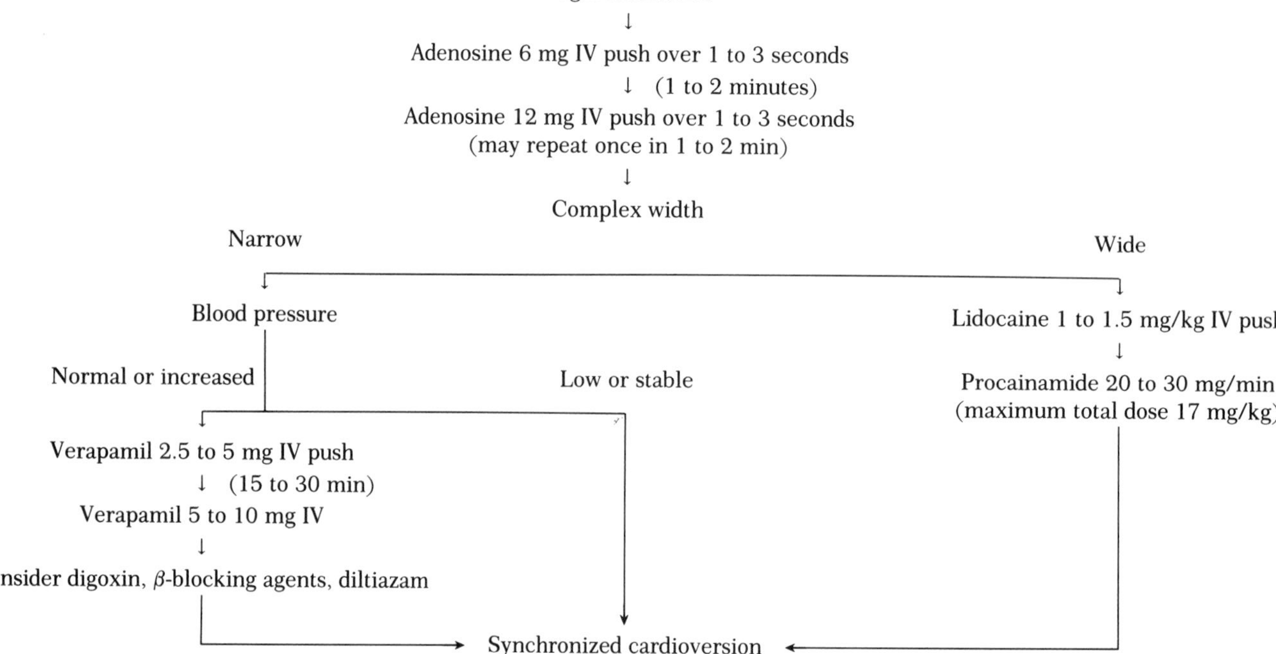

Suggested treatment of paroxysmal supraventricular tachycardia. The algorithm presumes that paroxysmal supraventricular tachycardia is continuing. The algorithm represents suggested management only. Some patients may require care not specified here.

Modified from American Heart Association: Guidelines for cardipulmonary resuscitation and emergency cardiac care. JAMA 268:2223, 2224, 1992.

Complications in Anesthesiology, second edition,
edited by Nikolaus Gravenstein and Robert R. Kirby.
Lippincott-Raven Publishers, Philadelphia © 1996.

CHAPTER 58

Complications of Hyperbaric Oxygenation

Christopher W. Dueker

The treatment of various disorders with increased atmospheric pressure has a complex history. In the 1920s, the popularity of compressed air therapy reached a peak, with the construction of entire hospitals designed for compression. These facilities mercifully became scrap iron, and hyperbaric therapy became less popular, except for decompression sickness and traumatic cerebral air embolism.

Early hyperbaric treatment used air. Even at five times normal atmospheric pressure, the oxygen thus supplied did not exceed that available by administering pure oxygen at normal atmospheric pressure. In the 1950s, a revival of hyperbaric therapy began, with the use of oxygen rather than air. It was widely recommended in radiation therapy and for a variety of disease states in addition to the more traditional applications.

Hyperbaric oxygen is, of course, different from compressed air and is a valuable contribution to our therapeutic armamentarium. However, many of the claims made for this therapy did not prove to be valid. Today, the popularity of hyperbaric oxygenation is again increasing (Table 58-1). Hyperbaric therapy is of great value in the treatment of decompression sickness, arterial air embolism, carbon monoxide poisoning, clostridial gas gangrene, and some problem wound infections. Intensive investigation is concentrated on expanding its range of usefulness and on minimizing the hazards associated with high-pressure environments.

Anesthesiologists may be involved in the care of patients undergoing surgery and receiving general anesthesia in hyperbaric chambers. More frequently, anesthesiologists provide respiratory support to critically ill patients treated with hyperbaric oxygenation. Even an elementary familiarity with hyperbaric therapy requires some knowledge of the environment in which this therapy is provided. Chambers range in size from one-person tanks to those large enough for surgery. Regardless of size, they are closed spaces with limited access. Rapid transfer of personnel is not possible because of the need for compression or decompression.

PRESSURE AND ITS MEASUREMENT

Increased gas pressure, which forms the basis of hyperbaric therapy, introduces several problems that dictate procedures for compression and decompression. Direct effects of pressure increase the risk of fire, cause barotrauma, and alter the performance of anesthetic equipment. Indirect effects lead to decompression sickness, inert gas narcosis, and oxygen poisoning. These effects interact to limit the tolerance of patients and health care providers to hyperbaric exposure.

Pressure within a chamber can be expressed in any of several, somewhat confusing ways (Table 58-2). At sea level, a pressure gauge reads zero, but the atmosphere actually exerts a force of 760 mm Hg, or 14.7 psi. This pressure is called 1 *atmosphere absolute* (ATA). Doubling the pressure creates 2 ATA, or 1 *atmosphere gauge*. Because of similarities to diving, the magnitude of pressurization is frequently stated as depth (in feet) of salt water. Descent through each 33 feet of salt water adds 14.7 psi to total pressure. Pressure expressed as depth of sea water can be converted to atmospheres gauge by dividing by 33 feet. To get atmospheres absolute, 1 must be added to this value. The absolute pressure is important; hence, pressures discussed in this chapter are expressed in terms of atmospheres absolute, unless otherwise noted.

FIRES AND EXPLOSIONS

Fire is a serious risk for all procedures performed in a hyperbaric chamber. Fire is dangerous in any small, closed space in which immediate evacuation is not possible. Furthermore, during therapy, not every person in the chamber has the freedom from other duties that is necessary to help fight a fire. Finally, an oxygen-enriched environment supports combustion vigorously.

TABLE 58-1
Indications for Hyperbaric Oxygen Therapy

- Air or gas embolization
- Carbon monoxide complicated by cyanide poisoning
- Crush injury or compartment syndrome
- Selected wound healing
- Necrotizing soft-tissue infections
- Refractory osteomyelitis
- Compromised skin grafts and flaps
- Carbon monoxide poisoning or smoke inhalation
- Gas gangrene
- Decompression sickness
- Severe anemia (exceptional blood loss)
- Progressive bacterial gangrene
- Osteoradionecrosis
- Thermal burns

Approved by Hyperbaric Oxygen Therapy Committee, Undersea and Hyperbaric Medicine Society, 1989.

Oxygen Percentage and Partial Pressure

A fire ignites more easily (because of a lower temperature of ignition) and then burns more rapidly in an oxygen-enriched environment. Chambers are therefore dangerous in two ways: they may contain a greater percentage of oxygen, and the increased total pressure raises the partial pressure of oxygen at a given percentage. Both percentage and partial pressure are important in determining fire hazard.

Total Pressure

In general, a given partial pressure of oxygen is more dangerous at lower total pressure than is the same amount of oxygen mixed with an inert gas at a higher total pressure. That is, pure oxygen at 2 ATA burns more rapidly than air at 10 ATA, which also contains 2 atm equivalents of oxygen. The inert gas dampens combustion.

Thermal Conductivity

Gases with higher thermal conductivity cause greater elevation of the threshold for ignition. More heat is necessary to ignite flammable material in helium and oxygen than in nitrogen and oxygen.

Prevention and Protection

Fire prevention requires stringent efforts to eliminate sources of ignition and fuel. Unless the gases are inherently flammable, sparking is a minor risk. However, electric arcs and local sources of heat are more difficult to eliminate. In addition, simply the presence of a human being provides fuel. The risk is minimized by using treated flameproof clothing, mattresses, blankets, and nonflammable paint. Nevertheless, materials that do not burn at sea level may burn in conditions of increased pressure.

The careful regulation of oxygen concentration in the chamber represents the best means for fire protection. Oxygen concentrations less than 5% do not support combustion, regardless of total pressure.[1] This concentration is useful at depths yielding pressures in excess of 4 ATA. Even at only 2 ATA, an oxygen concentration of 10% sustains life normally and markedly reduces combustibility, while the patient receives a higher partial pressure.

During most therapy, only the patient breathes pure oxygen; the chamber is filled with air. Exhalation from the patient, however, usually increases the oxygen concentration in the chamber to 25%. This small increment increases the burning rate by 25%. Therefore, the patient's exhalations should be vented outside the chamber.

Anesthetic Flammability

The flammability of anesthetic agents in hyperbaric conditions has not been evaluated thoroughly. Theoretically, potent flammable agents might not be dangerous: they would be used in very low concentrations because of the increased total pressure. However, the introduction of halogenated agents has obviated the use of flammable agents. Halothane is probably the most widely used inhalation anesthetic for hyperbaric anesthesia. Halothane in concentrations as great as 59 mm Hg (6.5% surface equivalent) does not burn in oxygen at a total pressure of 4 ATA,[2] whereas higher partial pressures of halothane burn at this pressure. However, halothane concentrations that are safe in oxygen alone may burn briskly in oxygen and nitrous oxide, which readily supplies its oxygen atom to combustion.

Fire Fighting

Rapid flame propagation frequently makes fire fighting in a hyperbaric chamber hopeless. In 1965, a chamber fire was caused by the overheating of a motor in an environment of 27% oxygen, 36.5% nitrogen, and 36.5% helium at 60 feet. Both occupants were killed almost immediately. The fire reached a temperature that raised the chamber pressure to 9 ATA within 1 minute.[3] The most efficient extinguishing system is an automatic deluge system operated through infrared emission or ultraviolet radiation detectors that distinguish between flame and background levels of radiation.

TABLE 58-2
Units of Pressure

DEPTH IN SEA WATER (FEET)	PSI ABSOLUTE	PSI GAUGE	mm Hg	ATA
Sea level	14.7	0	760	1
33	29.4	14.7	1520	2
66	44.1	29.4	2280	3
99	58.8	44.1	3040	4
132	73.5	58.8	3800	5
165	88.2	73.5	4560	6

BAROTRAUMA

The body's solid and liquid tissues freely transmit increased pressure in all directions. Thus, tissues are not affected by pressure changes. Joint pain may occur in rapid deep diving but not in the low-pressure ranges used in therapy. However, gas-filled spaces frequently are affected by pressure. Damage caused by pressure is called *barotrauma* or, descriptively, *squeeze*. Barotrauma may develop during either compression or decompression.

Compression

Middle Ear

By far the most common site of barotrauma during compression is the middle ear. Pressure increases linearly with depth, but the greatest relative changes are in shallow ranges. Pain typically begins in the first 10 feet of descent. During compression, the tympanic membrane bows inward, and the mucosa of the middle ear becomes engorged. Opening of the eustachian tube permits high-pressure air to enter the middle ear and equalize pressure, thus preventing tympanic membrane damage or mucosal transudation. Opening of the eustachian tube during compression usually requires a conscious act such as yawning, chewing, swallowing, moving the jaws, or performing a Valsalva's maneuver. Because of this problem, many physicians using hyperbaric therapy have myringotomies performed on unconscious patients.[4] Others have not found this procedure to be necessary.

Damage ranges from simple tympanic injection to actual rupture, which is preceded by severe pain. Of course, perforation eliminates pain by providing a pathway for equalization. A survey of submarine school candidates reported that 36% had clinical otic barotrauma after compression to 4 ATA.[5]

Slow compression with careful attention to clearing of the ears makes hyperbaric exposures tolerable for most patients. The most common mistake is failure to begin equalization early in the descent. Persons with allergic, infectious, or mechanical obstruction of the eustachian tubes should not be subjected to compression. Submarine school candidates with upper respiratory tract infections had a 61% incidence of barotrauma.[5] Systemic or topical decongestants may be useful.

Inner Ear

Much more rarely, barotrauma may affect the inner ear. The stapes can be dislodged from the oval window, causing hearing loss. Rupture of the round window, with subsequent vestibular disturbances, has been reported in divers.[6] The tympanic membrane may remain intact.

Sinuses

The sinuses are frequently affected by compression. When the ostia are obstructed, mucosal congestion and hemorrhage result. The signs of sinus squeeze are pain and epistaxis. No convenient way to equalize a blocked sinus is available, although decongestants may help. Similarly, repaired teeth sometimes have air spaces that can be squeezed. However, most of the pain felt in the teeth is probably caused by sinus barotrauma.

Lungs

Persons in a hyperbaric chamber do not have to worry about lung barotrauma during descent; the free breathing of pressurized gas eliminates this problem. Barotrauma may occur, however, in breath-hold diving, because air at high pressure is not available to counteract the inward thoracic pressure.

Decompression

Middle Ear

During decompression, otic barotrauma is uncommon but will occur if air in the expanding middle ear cannot be vented through the eustachian tube. In this condition, the tympanic membrane bulges outward. In general, the eustachian tube opens spontaneously to release air at positive pressure.

Sinuses and Teeth

Similarly, decompression may cause sinus and dental barotrauma. Gas in the gastrointestinal tract expands on ascent. This problem is not serious in healthy persons who are free of bowel obstruction and have normal volumes of bowel gas.

Lungs

One of the most serious of all hyperbaric complications, lung barotrauma, occurs during ascent. With decompression, the lungs begin to distend as ambient pressure decreases. As long as normal exhalation occurs, distention is immediately relieved as the gas escapes, and transthoracic pressure is equalized. However, even a brief failure to exhale can cause overdistention and rupture of the lungs. Divers using compressed air have died after ascending from depths as shallow as 10 feet while they are holding their breath.[7] Without exhalation, lung volume doubles during decompression from 33 feet. Lung barotrauma resulting from ascent is very rare in hyperbaric chambers because ascents are not rapid. Of course, a sudden failure in pressurization subjects all occupants of the chamber to the hazards of lung rupture.

Lung rupture also can occur in persons who exhale normally. Localized areas of trapped air may expand dangerously. Broncholiths, mucus plugs, or weakened airway walls may permit inspiration while impeding exhalation. Also, bullae may rupture more easily than areas of normal lung tissue. All candidates for treatment in hyperbaric chambers should be examined carefully for lung abnormalities. Patients with these abnormalities or with active respiratory infections should not be subjected to hyperbaric conditions.

Overdistention of the lungs may tear alveoli and release air into the interstitial tissue of the lung. Continued ascent after rupture results in expansion of this extra-alveolar air. Typically, the air passes along vascular sheaths to the mediastinum, resulting in pneumomediastinum. Having reached the hilum, air may dissect between the pleural layers and cause pneumothorax. Direct rupture into the pleural space is less common.[8] Air dissection upward into the neck results in subcutaneous emphysema.

Air Embolization

The ultimate disaster, air embolization, results from extrusion of alveolar air into the pulmonary blood vessels. Air carried directly to the left heart forms arterial emboli. With the body in the upright position, there is embolization to cerebral vessels, but coronary arteries also may be affected. Typically, air embolism becomes apparent by the immediate development of unconsciousness at the time of surfacing. Other manifestations of lung barotrauma usually have a slower onset.

Pressure changes can also affect the equipment used for hyperbaric therapy. Intravenous fluids should be administered from de-aired bags or air-space–vented bottles, so that the air space over the fluid is eliminated or cannot expand on decompression and force fluid and then air into veins. An air-filled endotracheal tube cuff shrinks on descent and expands on ascent. Cuffs should be emptied before ascent or filled with liquid. Anesthetic flowmeters also are affected by pressure.

Treatment

Most cases of air embolism occur during submarine escape training or, in scuba diving, during attempts to make *free ascents* (surfacing while exhaling continuously because of real or simulated failure of the breathing apparatus). Victims of air embolism must undergo recompression immediately; any delay markedly reduces the chances for survival. Most commonly, recompression is carried to 6 ATA, and slow decompression is begun when there is evidence of initial recovery. In many cases air embolization is fatal. For survivors, permanent central nervous system (CNS) sequelae are common. Pneumothorax, pneumomediastinum, and subcutaneous emphysema usually do not require recompression.

DECOMPRESSION SICKNESS

During general anesthesia, uptake of the anesthetic causes blood and tissue anesthetic concentrations to approach the inspired concentration. Many factors, including cardiac output, ventilation, inspired concentration, blood and tissue solubilities, and regional blood flow, affect the rate of uptake.

Nitrogen

Nitrogen in air undergoes a similar process during exposure to compressed air. As total gas pressure increases, the partial pressure of nitrogen correspondingly increases. Because of its low solubility (compared with anesthetics), nitrogen partial pressures equilibrate rapidly throughout the body. The total amount of anesthetic dissolved in a patient depends on the concentration administered and the duration of exposure. Similarly, during breathing of high-pressure air, total nitrogen uptake depends on the duration of exposure and the pressure.

With cessation of anesthetic inhalation, blood carries the anesthetic in solution to the lungs for excretion. During surfacing from a dive, nitrogen pressure begins to return to the lower, ambient partial pressure. Unlike the sudden cessation of anesthesia, however, a sudden decrease in pressure can overwhelm the pathway for elimination of inert gas. Instead of reaching the lungs in solution, the nitrogen may form bubbles within tissues and blood vessels. Through a variety of mechanisms, these bubbles cause the derangement known as *decompression sickness.* Decompression sickness includes skin rash, pruritus, fatigue, musculoskeletal pain, CNS and peripheral nervous system symptoms, respiratory distress, and shock.

Bubble Formation

Bubble formation is complex and is still incompletely understood. Tissues can hold gas at partial pressures greater than the ambient pressure. However, above a pressure threshold (varying from tissue to tissue and dependent on factors such as agitation and rate of ambient pressure change), bubbles form.

Ischemia

Bubbles have been considered the cause of decompression sickness; they produce ischemia by obstructing blood flow and cause direct tissue damage when present extravascularly. In 1938, End described red blood cell aggregation in decompression sickness and postulated that this phenomenon, rather than bubbles alone, impaired blood flow.[9] Not until many years later were End's findings confirmed and appreciated.[10]

Blood–Bubble Interface

Several other abnormalities have been identified. Although bubbles definitely cause mechanical disruption and remain the basic problem in decompression sickness, the interface between gas bubbles and blood is also important. Protein denaturation can occur at this interface and may account for the observed erythrocyte and platelet clumping and the activation of coagulation factors.[10] In severe decompression sickness, platelet counts are markedly depressed. Plasma loss occurs in decompression sickness and aggravates the sluggish blood flow. Lipid emboli also have been implicated. Evidence has been presented that spinal cord involvement results from obstruction of the epidural vertebral venous plexus rather than from generalized gaseous embolization.[10]

Physical Conditioning and Ar aptation

Factors that may vary from person to person are important. Old, obese divers in poor physical condition appear more susceptible to decompression sickness. Adaptation to hyperbaric work seems to occur in caisson and tunnel workers. Signs of decompression sickness vary somewhat between divers and caisson workers. No thorough evaluation has been made of decompression sickness occurring in hyperbaric therapy facilities.

Manifestations

Musculoskeletal Pain

Musculoskeletal pain, usually in a large joint, is the most common complaint. The popular term *the bends* applies only to this manifestation of decompression sickness. In 60% to 95% of affected military divers, it is the only symptom.[11] Typically, the deep, penetrating pain is not accompanied by local heat, tenderness, swelling, or discoloration.

Central Nervous System Involvement

CNS involvement is common. In recreational divers CNS injuries may be more frequent than musculoskeletal pain.[12] These injuries most commonly involve the spinal cord but may include cerebral centers. Usually spinal cord derangement begins with paresthesias in the legs and progresses to weakness, paralysis, and loss of autonomic function (eg, bladder and bowel control).

Respiratory Involvement

Respiratory involvement, *the chokes*, develops more rarely. Perhaps bubbles in the pulmonary circulation cause the dyspnea and chest pain.

Aseptic Bone Necrosis

Increased attention has been directed to aseptic bone necrosis in experienced divers. The incidence varies widely but is reported to be as great as 50%.[13] This avascular necrosis sometimes is juxta-articular. Eventually it may cause symptoms or, conversely, affect the bone shaft, which usually is asymptomatic. Often, affected divers have never had any other manifestation of decompression sickness.

Prevention

Prevention of decompression sickness depends on limiting the dose of inert gas and providing time for its orderly elimination. Because some overpressure is tolerable, decompression tables have been formulated to permit diving followed by immediate but gradual ascent (usually at a rate of 60 ft/min). As the depth of the dive increases, its duration must decrease to limit the total amount of nitrogen absorbed. In theory, a 2-atm exposure of any duration can be followed by immediate ascent, although very long dives to this depth may be followed by decompression sickness.[10]

When dives exceed the safe limits for direct ascent, decompression must be gradual. In staged decompression an initial ascent is followed by a pause to eliminate dissolved nitrogen before further ascent. Alternatively, a slower continuous ascent may be made. Because gas elimination, like uptake, is exponential, the pauses can be brief at deep levels but should lengthen as the excretion rate slows. Similarly, in continuous ascent, the rate can be faster initially but then must be slowed.

Decompression sickness sometimes occurs despite proper adherence to decompression standards. Furthermore, ultrasonic bubble detectors may demonstrate bubbling in the absence of clinical signs.[14] These *silent bubbles* are of undefined significance but may be responsible for chronic changes such as aseptic necrosis.

Treatment

Dive Tables

Basic treatment of decompression sickness requires recompression followed by gradual decompression. Because of the high incidence of failure of treatment based on early tables, treatment based on schedules that use oxygen breathing has been introduced (Figs. 58-1 to 58-4). Recompression to 60 feet is followed by alternating oxygen and air breathing (to reduce the risk of oxygen toxicity), with subsequent decompression to 30 feet; at this stage, oxygen–air cycles are continued. Recompression reduces bubble size, and oxygen breathing provides a steep partial pressure gradient for elimination of nitrogen.

Success depends on thorough examination and prompt treatment of patients. Fifty percent to 85% of decompression sickness develops within 1 hour after surfacing,[11] but delays of more than 24 hours are possible. Any person with symptoms compatible with decompression sickness should receive a trial of recompression therapy if a hyperbaric exposure has occurred within 24 to 36 hours. The choice of treatment tables depends on the symptoms; serious cases receive longer therapy. Careful examination is essential because severe joint pain may obscure early CNS signs. Delays in instituting treatment lessen the chance for complete recovery.

Ancillary Measures

Many therapists supplement recompression therapy. Hemoconcentration is sometimes treated with plasma. Low-molecular-weight dextran may relieve erythrocyte and platelet clumping; steroids frequently are used in cases involving the CNS.

Attendants (Tenders)

Decompression sickness should be uncommon in modern hyperbaric therapy. Because patients breathe oxygen rather than inert gases, they are not at risk. However, the low pressures used to avoid oxygen toxicity in the patient results in prolonged air exposure for the attendants. Because of the accumulation of inert gas, attendants ideally should be compressed for only one session each day. Many centers use oxygen during the last 30 feet of decompression to further speed nitrogen elimination by the attendants. If decompression sickness develops in an attendant, prompt treatment can be provided readily. Because decompression sickness may have a long latent period, all persons exposed to high pressure should remain near

1. Treatment of Type I decompression sickness when symptoms are relieved within 10 minutes at 60 feet and a complete neurological exam is normal.
2. Descent rate—25 ft/min.
3. Ascent rate—1 ft/min. Do not compensate for slower ascent rates. Compensate for faster rates by halting the ascent.
4. Time at 60 feet begins on arrival at 60 feet.
5. If oxygen breathing must be interrupted, allow 15 minutes after the reaction has entirely subsided and resume schedule at point of interruption (see Section 8.12.4.1).
6. If oxygen breathing must be interrupted at 60 feet, switch to Table 6 upon arrival at the 30 foot stop.
7. Tender breathes air throughout unless he has had a hyperbaric exposure within the past 12 hours in which case he breathes oxygen at 30 feet in accordance with Section 8.12.5.7.

Depth (feet)	Time (minutes)	Breathing Media	Total Elapsed Time (hrs:min.)
60	20	Oxygen	0:20
60	5	Air	0:25
60	20	Oxygen	0:45
60 to 30	30	Oxygen	1:15
30	5	Air	1:20
30	20	Oxygen	1:40
30	5	Air	1:45
30 to 0	30	Oxygen	2:15

Treatment Table 5: Depth/Time Profile

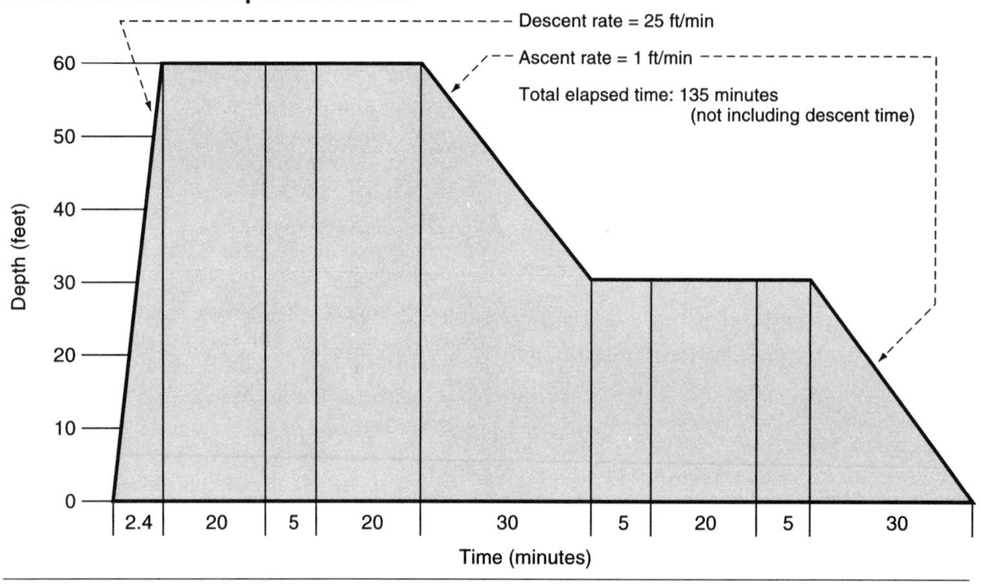

*Many diving physicians use Table 6 for Type I decompression sickness and exclude Table 5 from any initial therapy.

FIGURE 58-1. Treatment of type I decompression sickness (United States Navy oxygen treatment Table 5). In Bove AA, Davis JC (eds): Diving medicine, 2nd ed. Philadelphia: WB Saunders, 1990: 318

a chamber for several hours and should carry obvious identification of their pressure exposure.

Surgery and Anesthesia

In hyperbaric surgery, the anesthetic gas may cause decompression sickness. This is not a problem with the potent agents because the dose used is small. However, nitrous oxide can readily cause decompression sickness because large amounts are taken up. Nitrous oxide breathed after an air dive increases symptoms in mice, presumably by enlarging small air bubbles.[15] Dogs that have breathed large doses of nitrous oxide (eg, 80% at 3 ATA or 55% at 5 ATA) have a high incidence of fatal decompression sickness.[16] However, those exposed to 55% at pressures as great as 4 ATA have no fatalities or macroscopic bubbles.

The risk of decompression sickness and the limitation on oxygen concentration have led some investigators to conclude that nitrous oxide is inappropriate in hyperbaric therapy.[16] However, Faulconer and colleagues provided adequate anesthesia with 50% nitrous oxide at 2 ATA,[17] which agrees well with an independent determination of minimum alveolar concentration (MAC).[18] Because anesthesia depends on partial pressure and not on the concentration of anesthetic, surgery at 3 ATA can be performed with approximately 33% nitrous oxide. This dose probably does not represent a serious risk of decompression sickness, especially if the nitrous oxide is discontinued before decompression, thus providing maximum washout.

OXYGEN TOXICITY

The toxic effects of oxygen pose the most significant limitation to the use of hyperbaric oxygen therapy. Besides the lungs, oxygen toxicity affects the CNS and eyes and almost certainly

1. Treatment of Type II or Type I decompression sickness when symptoms are not relieved within 10 minutes at 60 feet.
2. Descent rate—25 ft/min.
3. Ascent rate—1 ft/min. Do not compensate for slower ascent rates. Compensate for faster rates by halting the ascent.
4. Time at 60 feet begins on arrival at 60 feet.
5. If oxygen breathing must be interrupted, allow 15 minutes after the reaction has entirely subsided and resume schedule at point of interruption.
6. Tender breathes air throughout unless he has had a hyperbaric exposure within the past 12 hours in which case he breathes oxygen at 30 feet in accordance with Section 8.12.5.7.
7. Table 6 can be lengthened up to 2 additional 25 minute oxygen breathing periods at 60 feet (20 minutes on oxygen and 5 minutes on air) or up to 2 additional 75 minute oxygen breathing periods at 30 feet (15 minutes on air and 60 minutes on oxygen), or both. If Table 6 is extended only once at either 60 or 30 feet, the tender breathes oxygen during the ascent from 30 feet to the surface. If more than one extension is done, the tender begins oxygen breathing for the last hour at 30 feet during ascent to the surface.

Depth (feet)	Time (minutes)	Breathing Media	Total Elapsed Time (hrs:min.)
60	20	Oxygen	0:20
60	5	Air	0:25
60	20	Oxygen	0:45
60	5	Air	0:50
60	20	Oxygen	1:10
60	5	Air	1:15
60 to 30	30	Oxygen	1:45
30	15	Air	2:00
30	60	Oxygen	3:00
30	16	Air	3:15
30	60	Oxygen	4:15
30 to 0	30	Oxygen	4:45

Treatment Table 6: Depth/Time Profile

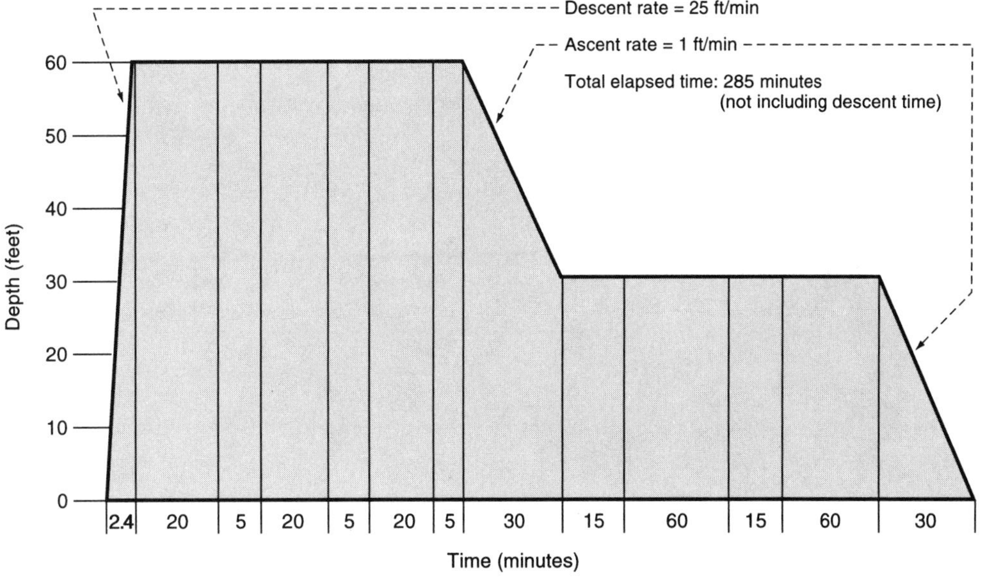

FIGURE 58-2. Treatment of type II decompression sickness (United States Navy oxygen treatment Table 6). In Bove AA, Davis JC (eds): Diving medicine, 2nd ed. Philadelphia: WB Saunders, 1990: 319

is toxic to other organs such as the liver, kidney, and heart, although data are limited. Oxygen toxicity is dose-dependent. The dose depends on the partial pressure of oxygen inspired and the length of exposure; an increase in either hastens the onset of toxicity.

Effects

Pulmonary

Pulmonary oxygen toxicity is clinically significant in the treatment of critically ill patients. Hyperbaric oxygen speeds the development of lung damage. Healthy volunteers breathing oxygen at 2 ATA have severe chest pain and dyspnea after 8 to 10 hours.[19] Vital capacity begins to decrease significantly within 4 hours of initiation of oxygen breathing; symptoms and changes in vital capacity persist hours after the exposure.

Eyes

Abnormalities in vision are associated with excessive oxygen in infants but generally are not a clinical problem in adults. However, in a 2-ATA exposure, 5 of 13 subjects had symptoms related to vision.[19] Only 1 subject, a man with a history of retrobulbar neuritis, had major signs, which included unilateral constriction of visual fields, scotoma, and decreased visual activity that necessitated termination of oxygen exposure.

1. Treatment of arterial gas embolism where complete relief obtained within 30 min. at 165 feet. Use also when unable to determine whether symptoms are caused by gas embolism or severe decompression sickness.
2. Descent rate—as fast as possible.
3. Ascent rate—1 ft/min. Do not compensate for slower ascent rates. Compensate for faster ascent rates by halting the ascent.
4. Time at 165 feet—includes time from the surface.
5. If oxygen breathing must be interrupted, allow 15 minutes after the reaction has entirely subsided and resume schedule at point of interruption (see Section 8.12.4.1).
6. Tender breathes oxygen during ascent from 30 feet to the surface unless he has had a hyperbaric exposure within the past 12 hours in which case he breathes oxygen at 30 feet in accordance with Section 8.12.5.7.
7. Table 6A can be lengthened up to 2 additional 25 minute oxygen breathing periods at 60 feet (20 minutes on oxygen and 5 minutes on air) or up to 2 additional 75 minute oxygen breathing periods at 30 feet (15 minutes on air and 60 minutes on oxygen), or both. If Table 6A is extended either at 60 or 30 feet the tender breathes oxygen during the last half at 30 feet and during ascent to the surface.
8. If complete relief not obtained within 30 min. at 165 feet, switch to Table 4. Consult with a Diving Medical Officer before switching if possible.

Depth (feet)	Time (minutes)	Breathing Media	Total Elapsed Time (hrs:min.)
165	30	Air	0:30
165 to 60	4	Air	0:34
60	20	Oxygen	0:54
60	5	Air	0:59
60	20	Oxygen	1:19
60	5	Air	1:29
60	20	Oxygen	1:44
60	5	Air	1:49
60 to 30	30	Oxygen	2:19
30	15	Air	2:34
30	60	Oxygen	3:34
30	15	Air	3:49
30	60	Oxygen	4:49
30 to 0	30	Oxygen	5:19

Treatment Table 6A: Depth/Time Profile

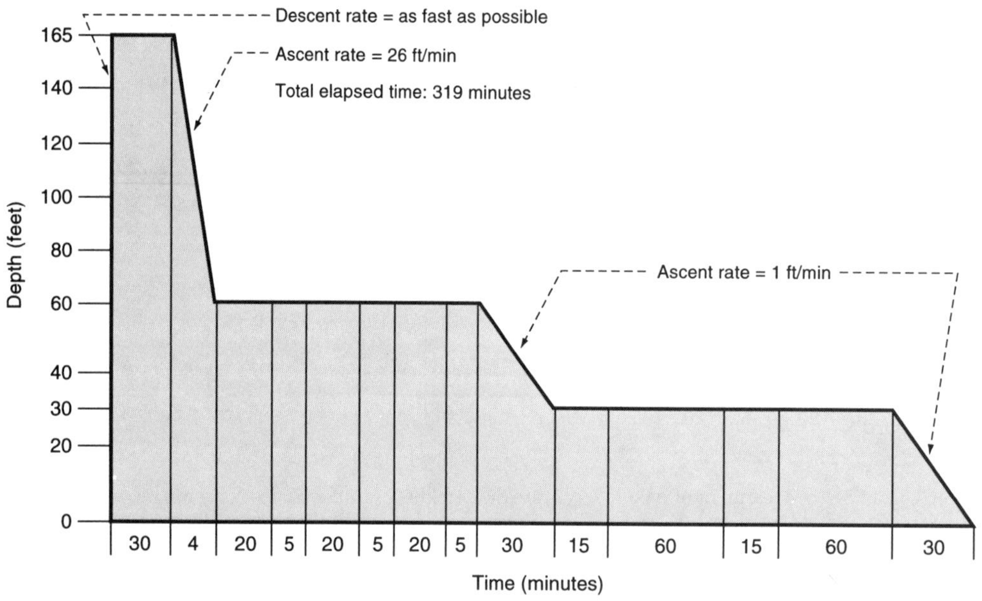

FIGURE 58-3. Initial air and oxygen treatment of arterial gas embolism (United States Navy oxygen treatment Table 6A). In Bove AA, Davis JC (eds): Diving medicine, 2nd ed. Philadelphia: WB Saunders, 1990: 320

Central Nervous System

At pressures exceeding 2 ATA, CNS toxicity limits tolerable oxygen exposure. Minor symptoms include nausea, muscle twitching (particularly facial), and numbness. Tonic-clonic seizures follow unless oxygen exposure is promptly terminated. Seizures may occur without warning or so rapidly that halting the administration of oxygen does not prevent them. No definite threshold can be established for CNS oxygen toxicity. Convulsions have been reported at only 2 ATA, although most persons can tolerate 2 hours of oxygen at 3 ATA while at rest.[20,21]

Latency

Because of the risk of oxygen toxicity, hyperbaric therapy with oxygen breathing is almost always limited to 3 ATA. Rather than seeking a threshold, the clinician should think

1. Used for treatment of unresolved life threatening symptoms after initial treatment on Table 6, 6A, or 4.
2. Use only under the direction of or in consultation with a Diving Medical Officer.
3. Table begins upon arrival at 60 feet. Arrival at 60 feet accomplished by initial treatment on Table 6, 6A, or 4. If initial treatment has progressed to a depth shallower than 60 feet, compress to 60 feet at 25 ft/min to begin Table 7.
4. Maximum duration at 60 feet unlimited. Remain at 60 feet a minimum of 12 hours unless overriding circumstances dictate earlier decompression.
5. Patient begins oxygen breathing periods at 60 feet. Tender need breathe only chamber atmosphere throughout. If oxygen breathing is interrupted no lengthening of the table is required.
6. Minimum chamber O_2 concentration 19%. Maximum CO_2 concentration 1.5% SEV (12 mmHg). Maximum chamber internal temperature 85°F (Section 8.12.5.4).
7. Decompression starts with a 2 foot upward excursion from 60 to 58 feet. Decompress with stops every 2 feet for times shown in profile below. Ascent time between stops approximately 30 sec. Stop time begins with ascent from deeper to next shallower step. Stop at 4 feet for 4 hours and then ascend to the surface at 1 ft/min.
8. Ensure chamber life support requirements can be met before committing to a Treatment Table 7.
9. See Section 8.12.3.5 for details.

Treatment Table 7: Depth/Time Profile

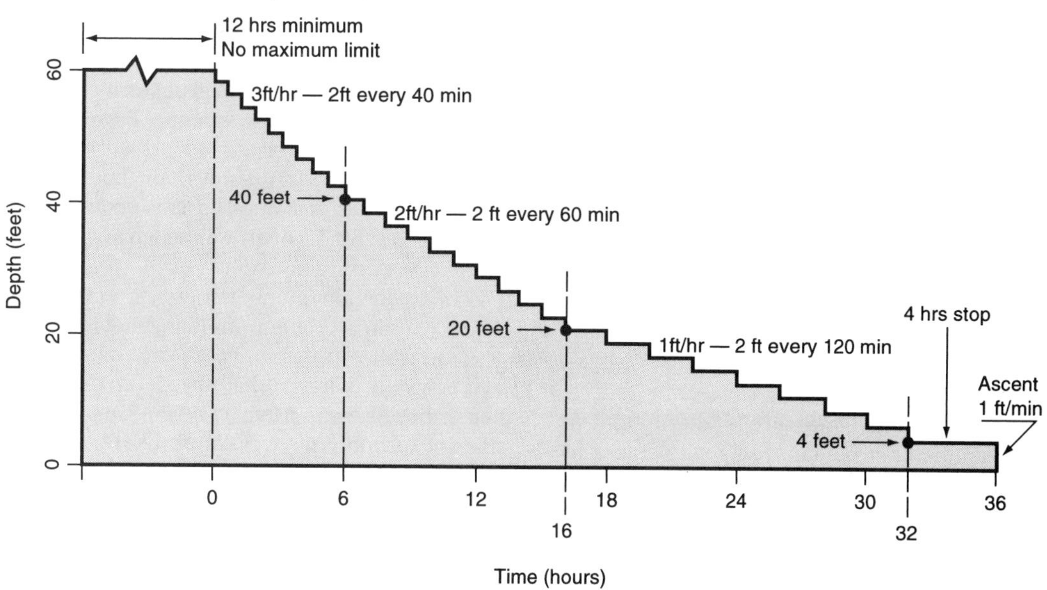

FIGURE 58-4. Oxygen-air treatment of unresolved or worsening symptoms of decompression sickness or arterial gas embolism (United States Navy oxygen treatment table 7). In Bove AA, Davis JC (eds): Diving medicine, 2nd ed. Philadelphia: WB Saunders, 1990: 321

in terms of latent periods before oxygen poisoning becomes manifest. In general, as pressure increases, the latent period decreases.

Carbon Dioxide Accumulation

Latency is also affected by other factors. Carbon dioxide accumulation hastens seizures, although moderately high carbon dioxide partial pressures may actually suppress oxygen convulsions.[22] The mechanism for the enhanced toxicity may be related to the increased cerebral blood flow associated with increased carbon dioxide partial pressures. Very high carbon dioxide partial pressure is itself convulsive but is not found with hyperbaric therapy. Exercise markedly decreases latency; whether this factor is primary or related to carbon dioxide retention is unknown. Of interest, underwater exposures seem to be tolerated less well than dry ones, even at comparable pressures. Navy experiments have demonstrated a lower oxygen tolerance in immersed, exercising divers.[23]

Incidence

Oxygen poisoning in hyperbaric therapy is affected by the physical condition of the patient and the treatment regimen that must be used. In a series of approximately 15,000 hyperbaric treatments, the overall incidence of oxygen toxicity symptoms was 1%.[24]

Mechanism

The mechanism of oxygen toxicity remains undefined; despite extensive investigation. Its universality suggests interference with very basic metabolic pathways, and several enzyme systems have been implicated. Hyperoxia increases the production of highly oxidative, partially reduced metabolites of oxygen, including hydrogen peroxide and free radicals.[25] In mice, oxygen tolerance is prolonged by the administration of catalase, which converts one of the metabolites (hydrogen peroxide) to water and oxygen.[26] Perhaps the syndrome results from interacting mechanisms rather than a single one.[27,28]

Treatment

Treatment of CNS toxicity is simple: the source of oxygen is removed. Patients breathing oxygen should begin receiving air instead. The chamber should not be decompressed during a seizure because apnea or airway obstruction may lead to lung rupture. If the exposure is terminated and the seizure managed properly, residual effects do not accompany oxygen-induced seizures. Apnea during the seizure is not a problem because the patient is well oxygenated. Presumably, prolonging oxygen exposure risks permanent damage.

Prevention

Prevention of toxicity requires limitations to exposure. Because the goal of hyperbaric therapy is to provide large amounts of oxygen, treatment schedules push the dose to toxic levels. Drugs may obtund the overt signs of poisoning. In dogs given halothane or barbiturates, seizures are delayed or absent, but the animals may manifest residual changes of severe oxygen poisoning.[29]

Intermittent Oxygen Breathing

The most promising preventive measure is intermittent oxygen breathing. In animals and humans, oxygen tolerance has been extended by the interposition of brief periods of air breathing between periods of oxygen inhalation.[30] Apparently, these intermissions provide time for partial recovery from oxygen toxicity. An initial evaluation of the effect of intermittent oxygen exposure in volunteers used a schedule of 20 minutes of oxygen followed by 5 minutes of air at 2 ATA.[31] Changes in vital capacity were delayed significantly by this regimen. Longer periods of air breathing might further reduce oxygen toxicity but at the expense of reducing the duration of oxygen administration or increasing the duration of treatment.

NITROGEN NARCOSIS

Another constraint in hyperbaric therapy is the narcotic effect of high-pressure nitrogen. Unlike oxygen toxicity, this problem affects the attendants in the chamber rather than the patient, who is protected when he or she breathes only oxygen.

Mechanism

Almost all inert gases can be narcotizing. However, narcosis has not been demonstrated with helium, although other CNS effects have been noted at very high pressures.[32] Probably inert gas narcosis results from the same mechanisms as those governing general inhalation anesthesia. The narcotic potency of the inert gases correlates well with their lipid solubility. In mice, the narcotic potency of nitrous oxide is 28 times that of nitrogen.[33] The oil–gas partition coefficient of nitrous oxide inhaled at sea level is 21 times that of nitrogen (1.4 versus 0.067). If lipid solubility is used as a determinant of the potency, air at 2.4 ATA (at which nitrogen partial pressure is 1400 mm Hg) should have the potency of 10% nitrous oxide inhaled at sea level,[34] which produces mild euphoria. Air at sea level, compared with a helium–oxygen mixture, contains enough nitrogen to impair cognitive performance slightly.[35]

Effects

Clinical effects of nitrogen narcosis are difficult to demonstrate in most people at pressures less than 4 ATA. However, performance tests show impairment at pressures as low as 3 ATA.[36] The choice of an appropriate test and the wide range of individual variability makes measurement difficult. Commonly, mood change, usually euphoria, is the first symptom. Decrements occur in conceptual reasoning (most affected), reaction time, and mechanical dexterity (least affected). Narcosis makes simple tasks complex. Performance continues to deteriorate with increasing air pressure until consciousness may be lost at depths greater than about 330 feet (11 ATA). Presumably, surgical anesthesia is obtained at about 20 ATA of nitrogen (25 ATA of air), although air at this pressure would cause severe oxygen toxicity.

Carbon dioxide retention intensifies inert gas narcosis. This effect can be a problem in diving suits but should not be an issue in well-ventilated hyperbaric chambers.

It is widely believed that nitrogen narcosis adaptation may occur, because experienced divers can often work at depths that incapacitate novices. More likely, these divers learn to work despite narcosis by narrowing their impaired attention to the task at hand.

Nitrogen narcosis limits air diving to depths of 125 feet; excursions to 200 feet should be undertaken only in emergencies. Many scuba divers have died in an attempt to establish a diving record. In modern deep diving, helium is used as a complete or partial substitute for nitrogen.

Even with the restricted pressures used for therapy, nitrogen narcosis occasionally may be a problem; effects can be demonstrated at 3 ATA. Therapy at 4 ATA would be expected to introduce observable problems of narcosis. As a result, all chamber operations are supervised by observers at sea-level pressure, whose decisions override those of the attendants in the chamber.

ANESTHETIC OVERDOSE

Minimum Alveolar Concentration

Administration of inhalation anesthetics on the basis of the percentage given at sea-level pressure can be fatal in a hyperbaric chamber. Doses must be expressed as partial pressure and not percentage concentration. For instance, 1 MAC of halothane (0.76%) is actually 0.76% of 760 mm Hg, or 6 mm Hg. At 2 ATA, this halothane pressure of 6 mm Hg is still equivalent to 1 MAC but constitutes only 0.4% of the total gas pressure. Conversely, if the sea level concentration of halothane (0.76%) were continued at 2 ATA, the patient would receive 2 MAC and, thus, an overdose.

Vaporizer Performance

With gaseous anesthetics, the main concern is reduction of inspired percentage as total pressure increases. Vaporization of volatile anesthetics does not depend on total ambient pressure. At 20°C, the partial pressure of halothane is 243 mm Hg, regardless of total pressure. Calibrated vaporizers, once set at sea-level pressure, compensate automatically for changes in ambient pressure. As total pressure increases, the pressure of emitted halothane stays constant and represents a smaller fraction of the effluent. However, the constant partial pressure maintains an unchanged anesthetic potency. Severinghaus found that changes in gas turbulence lead to small variations in anesthetic output.[34] McDowall found that the accuracy of this type of vaporizer is better when the anesthetic concentration is above 2% than in the lower ranges.[37]

Older vaporizers of the copper kettle type emit volatile anesthetics in accordance with the ratio of partial pressure of anesthetic to that of oxygen. As ambient pressure increases, the fraction represented by the anesthetic must decrease, because its pressure relative to total pressure decreases. For halothane at 2 ATA, each 100 mL of oxygen takes up 20 mL of halothane vapor. If diluent gas flows are unchanged, the percentage of halothane administered decreases. However, partial pressure of halothane is not changed.

Rotameter Flow

Rotameter flow depends on gas density, which increases directly with pressure. The following equation predicts the effect of hyperbaric conditions.[37]

$$F_1 = F_0 \times \frac{\rho_0}{\rho_1}$$

where F_1 = true flow; F_0 = rotameter flow reading; ρ_0 = density at normal pressure; and ρ_1 = density of gas at chamber pressure.

Because doubling the pressure doubles the gas density, at 2 ATA true flow should be 71% of indicated flow. Experiments support this approximation.[37] However, each facility performing hyperbaric therapy should calibrate its own flowmeters at various pressures.

Scavenging

Removal of anesthetic gaseous waste from the chamber is important to prevent anesthetic exposure of attendants, who are already at risk because of the narcotic properties of nitrogen. A bias valve must be incorporated in the scavenging system to maintain a safe differential pressure from inside to outside the chamber to avoid inadvertent exposure of the patient to this differential.

Mechanical Ventilation

Significant alterations in ventilator performance may occur at increasing pressures.[38] Drive pressures must be 50 psi gauge greater than the chamber atmospheric pressure. As gas density increases, movement through pneumatic cartridges changes, and the ventilators using them, which are calibrated at sea level, function poorly or not at all. The Penlon and prototype Emerson gas-driven ventilators continue to function in a satisfactory manner.[38] Exhaled gas from the patient and waste gas from the ventilator, high in oxygen content, must be scavenged.

REFERENCES

1. Schmidt TC, Dorr VA, Hamilton RW Jr: Chamber safety (technical memorandum UCRI-721). Tarrytown, NY: Ocean Systems, 1973
2. Gottlieb SF, Fegan FJ, Tieslink J: Flammability of halothane, methoxyflurane and fluroxene under hyperbaric oxygen conditions. Anesthesiology 27:195, 1966
3. Harter JV: Fire at high pressure. In Lambertsen CF (ed): Proceedings of the third symposium on underwater physiology. Baltimore: Williams & Wilkins, 1967: 55
4. Jacobson JH II, Pierce EC II: Hyperbaric oxygenation. In Norman JC (ed): Cardiac surgery, 2nd ed. New York: Appleton-Century-Crofts, 1972: 211
5. Alfandre HJ: Aerotitis media in submarine recruits. United States Navy Submarine Medical Center research report. Groton, CT, March, 1966
6. Edmonds C, Thomas RL: Medical aspects of diving: III. Med J Aust 2:1300, 1972
7. Cooperman EM, Hogg J, Thurlbeck WM: Mechanism of death in shallow-water scuba diving. Can Med Assoc J 99:1128, 1968
8. Schaefer KE, McNulty WP: Mechanism in development of interstitial emphysema and air embolism on decompression from depth. J Appl Physiol 13:15, 1958
9. End E: The use of new equipment and helium gas in a world record dive. Journal of Industrial Hygiene 20:511, 1938
10. Elliott DH, Hallenbeck JM, Bove AA: Acute decompression sickness. Lancet 2:1193, 1974
11. Rivera JC: Decompression sickness among divers: an analysis of 935 cases. Mil Med 129:314, 1964
12. Kizer K: Dysbarism in paradise. Hawaii Med J 39:106, 1980
13. Edmonds C, Thomas RL: Medical aspects of diving: IV. Med J Aust 2:1367, 1972
14. Evans A, Barnard EEP, Walder DN: Detection of gas bubbles in man at decompression. Aerospace Medicine 53:1095, 1972
15. Van Liew HE: Dissolved gas washout and bubble absorption in routine decompression. In Lambertsen CJ (ed): Underwater physiology. New York: Academic Press, 1971: 145
16. McIver RG, Fife WP, Ikels KG: Experimental decompression sickness from hyperbaric nitrous oxide anesthesia. United States Air Force School of Aerospace Medicine, San Antonio, TX, June, 1965
17. Faulconer A, Pender JW, Bickford RG: The influence of partial pressure of N_2O on the depth of anesthesia and the EEG in man. Anesthesiology 10:601, 1949
18. Winter PM, Hornbein TF, Smith G, et al: Hyperbaric nitrous oxide anesthesia in man: determination of anesthetic potency (MAC) and cardiorespiratory effects (abstract A103). American Society of Anesthesiologists, Annual Meeting, 1972
19. Clark JM, Lambertsen CJ: Rate of development of pulmonary O_2 toxicity in man during O_2 breathing at 2.0 ATA. J Appl Physiol 30:739, 1971
20. Donald KW: Oxygen poisoning in man: I and II. Br Med J 1:667 and 712, 1947
21. Yarbrough WW, Briton ES, Behnke AR: Symptoms of oxygen poisoning and limits of tolerance at rest and at work. Washington, DC: Experimental Diving Unit project X-337, subject 62. 1947
22. Lambertsen CJ: Effects of oxygen at high partial pressure. In Fenn WO, Rahn H (eds): Handbook of physiology, section 3, vol 2. Washington, DC: American Physiological Society, 1965: 1027
23. Butler FK, Thalmann ED: Central nervous oxygen toxicity in

closed circuit scuba divers: II. Undersea Biomed Res 13:192, 1986

24. Rettenmaier PA, Gresham B, Myers RAM: The incidence of acute oxygen toxicity in a clinical setting. Presented at the annual meeting of the Undersea Medical Society. Long Beach, CA, June 11 to 14, 1985
25. Jackson RM: Pulmonary oxygen toxicity. Chest 88:900, 1985
26. Hilton JC, Brown GL, Proctor P: Effects of superoxide dismutase and catalase on central nervous system toxicity of hyperbaric oxygen. Toxicol Appl Pharmacol 53:50, 1983
27. Clark JM, Lambertsen CJ: Pulmonary oxygen toxicity: a review. Pharmacol Rev 23:37, 1971
28. Haugaard N: The scope of oxygen poisoning. In Lambertsen CJ (ed): Underwater physiology. New York: Academic Press, 1971: 1
29. Harp JR, Gutsche BB, Stephen CR: Effect of anesthesia on central nervous system toxicity of hyperbaric oxygen. Anesthesiology 27:608, 1966
30. Clark JM: The toxicity of oxygen. Am Rev Respir Dis 110:40, 1974
31. Hendricks PL, Hall DA, Hunter WL Jr, et al: Extension of pulmonary oxygen tolerance in man at 2 ATA by intermittent oxygen exposure. J Appl Physiol 42:593, 1977
32. Brauer RW, Way RO: Relative narcotic potencies of hydrogen, helium, nitrogen, and their mixtures. J Appl Physiol 29:23, 1970
33. Brauer RW, Goldman SM, Beaver RW, et al: Nitrogen, hydrogen, and nitrous oxide antagonism of high pressure neurological syndrome in mice. Undersea Biomed Res 1:59, 1974
34. Severinghaus JW: Anesthesia and related drug effects. In Greenbaum L, Seeley S (eds): Fundamentals of hyperbaric medicine, publication 1298. Washington, DC: National Academy of Sciences, 1966: 115
35. Winter PM, Bruce DL, Bach MJ, et al: The anesthetic effect of air at atmospheric pressure. Anesthesiology 42:658, 1975
36. Kiesling FJ, Maay CH: Performance impairment as a function of nitrogen narcosis. Washington, DC: United States Navy Experimental Diving Unit research report, publication 3-60. 1960
37. McDowall DG: Anaesthesia in a pressure chamber. Anaesthesia 19:321, 1964
38. Blanch P, Desautels DA, Gallagher TJ: Deviations in function of mechanical ventilators during hyperbaric compression. Respiratory Care 36:803, 1991

FURTHER READING

Bennett PB, Elliot DH: Physiology and medicine of diving and compressed air work, 2nd ed. Baltimore: Williams & Wilkins, 1975

Bove AE, Davis JC (eds): Diving medicine. Philadelphia: WB Saunders, 1990: 1

Davis JC: Hyperbaric medicine: critical care aspects. In Shoemaker W (ed): Critical care: state of the art, vol 5. Fullerton, CA: Society of Critical Care Medicine, 1984 E1

Desautels D: Hyperbaric medicine. In Civetta JM, Taylor RW, Kirby RR (eds): Critical care, 2nd ed. Philadelphia: JB Lippincott, 1992: 1829

Complications in Anesthesiology, second edition,
edited by Nikolaus Gravenstein and Robert R. Kirby.
Lippincott-Raven Publishers, Philadelphia © 1996.

CHAPTER 59

Complications of Extracorporeal Circulation

James Scott
Allen K. Ream

Development of knowledge, techniques, and equipment for cardiopulmonary bypass (CPB), the most common clinical application of extracorporeal circulation, has facilitated great strides in cardiac surgery. The anesthesiologist caring for patients during these operations needs as much understanding of the underlying mechanisms and principles as possible. This chapter surveys the salient physical principles, pharmacology, physiologic alterations, and possible complications of extracorporeal circulation.

GENERAL CONSIDERATIONS

Historical Development

Although many believe that CPB was initiated by Carrel and Lindbergh in 1930, efforts began over 180 years ago.[1] LeGallois in 1812 seems to have been the first to predict that cardiopulmonary support could be provided by an externally manipulated perfusate.[2] However, actualization of his prediction awaited the discovery of heparin[3,4] and the development of the first film oxygenator during the period from 1910 to 1915.[5,6] The real contribution of Carrel and Lindbergh was their recognition of the need for bacterial filtering.[7]

Invention of the roller pump by DeBakey in 1934[8] was followed by Gibbon's CPB device in 1937,[9] the disk oxygenator in 1948,[10] and the bubble oxygenator, incorporating defoaming agents, in 1950.[11] An initial surgical application in 1951 failed because of an error in medical diagnosis rather than a fault in the equipment.[12] The first clinical success was one survivor among four having closure of atrial septal defects, reported by Gibbon in 1954.[13] Within 2 years, the disposable bubble oxygenator[14] was described and the first membrane oxygenator used.[15]

Critical in this sequence of events were the discovery of heparin, development of an adequate pump, identification of an acceptable antifoaming technique, appreciation of the dangers of sepsis, and identification and control of sources of blood trauma. Many complications reported during early clinical applications appeared to be related to the difficulty of distinguishing between the effects of sepsis and blood trauma. Several techniques for extracorporeal oxygenation were evaluated, including cross perfusion with another patient[16] and direct bubble injection.[17] The two techniques surviving today incorporate bubble or membrane oxygenators. Membrane oxygenators are believed to be physiologically superior; cost and complexity are their major limitations.

Apparatus and Monitoring

Major Circuit

Figure 59-1 shows a typical arrangement of the CPB apparatus, and Table 59-1 lists the primary components. In the major circuit, blood is accepted through a cannula or cannulae usually placed in the vena cavae, passed through the oxygenator, and returned by roller pump to the patient's arterial system. A filter is placed in the return limb to the patient to trap emboli (air and particulate matter). To remove shed particles and other material from the CPB apparatus, a filter also precedes the input to the oxygenator for closed circulation before the patient is perfused.[18] If a membrane oxygenator is used, a second pump may be required to raise the inlet pressure to the oxygenator. In some instances, this pump replaces the pump between the oxygenator and the return limb to the patient. Although pulsatile perfusion is beneficial,[19] controversy rages over its usefulness and the associated costs.[1,20–22]

Coronary Suction

A second circuit consists of the coronary or "clean" suction. It is used to remove blood from the surgical field. Blood is

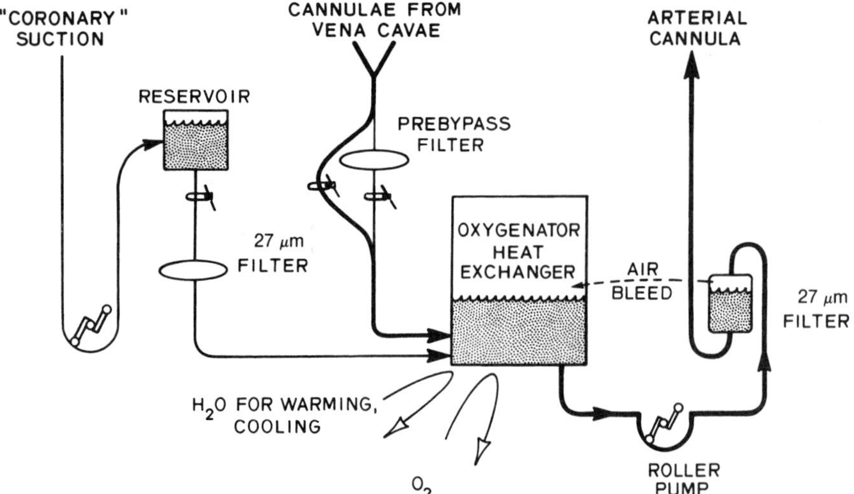

FIGURE 59-1. A typical arrangement of pump, filters, and oxygenator during cardiopulmonary bypass. (Modified from Ream AK: Cardiopulmonary bypass. In Ream AK, Fogdall RF (eds): Acute cardiovascular management: anesthesia and intensive care. Philadelphia: JB Lippincott, 1982: 422)

passed by a roller pump to a reservoir and then returned to the oxygenator through a filter. Sometimes this unit is replaced with a cell washer that passes the red cells through a washing cycle before returning only the cells to the oxygenator. Washing also permits the removal of cardioplegic solution, which also can be removed by ultrafiltration with equipment developed from experience with dialysis.

Heat Exchanger

All CPB systems include a heat exchanger that is usually integral to the oxygenator. A second heat exchanger, preferably one using countercurrent flow, may be required for recovery from deep hypothermia.

Other Equipment

Most CPB systems include some accessories for monitoring bypass flow rate, membrane oxygenator inlet pressure, oxygen saturation or partial pressure on the patient return limb, blood level in the oxygenator, and embolization.[23] An anesthesia vaporizer may be placed in the fresh gas flow line. It should be mounted securely to prevent accidental spills of volatile agents that might damage the plastic components of the circuit.[24]

TABLE 59-1
Components of a Typical Cardiopulmonary Bypass Circuit

- Venous drainage line
- Cardiotomy suction device
- Left ventricular vent
- Venous and arterial filters
- Oxygenator
- Heat exchanger
- Roller pumps
- Cardioplegia devices

Modified from Martin TJ: Cardiopulmonary bypass. In Kirby RR, Gravenstein N (eds): Clinical anesthesia practice. Philadelphia: WB Saunders, 1994: 320.

PHARMACOLOGY AND EXTRACORPOREAL CIRCULATION

The pharmacologic characteristics of many drugs are altered during cardiac surgery because extracorporeal circulation induces changes in organ blood flow, body fluid composition, binding protein concentrations, and temperature. Although alterations in blood concentrations or actions of various drugs by CPB have been described, our understanding in this area is incomplete. Only the basic pathophysiologic mechanisms responsible for alterations in pharmacologic characteristics during CPB are discussed here.

Distribution of Blood Flow

The normal distribution of blood flow is severely altered during CPB. Blood flow rates during CPB often are lower than those associated with normal cardiac output. This change, coupled with hypothermia, produces major changes in regional blood flow.[25] The major organs involved in intravenous drug elimination and metabolism (the kidneys and liver) may receive less blood, resulting in decreased metabolism and decreased elimination of many drugs. Hypothermia also directly contributes to decreased drug metabolism.[26,27]

Hemodilution

A second alteration accompanying CPB is hemodilution. Hemodilution with the priming solution of the CPB circuit (1–2 liters) decreases drug, protein, and cell concentrations in the vascular compartment shortly after the commencement of CPB.[28–31] Plasma proteins that bind many drugs also are diluted, increasing the concentrations of pharmacologically active, unbound drugs.[32] This change offsets the dilutional effect to some extent. Few studies have examined free drug concentrations[33]; the majority report only total drug concentrations.

Pulmonary Perfusion

The lungs can accumulate high concentrations of certain drugs, especially basic amines with moderate to high lipid solubility.[34-36] Most techniques of CPB significantly reduce pulmonary blood flow, causing some drugs (eg, fentanyl and propranolol) to be sequestered in the lungs.[37-39] With resumption of normal pulmonary perfusion, the stored drugs may be released, increasing the blood concentrations. Conversely, for certain drugs and biogenic amines (eg, norepinephrine), the lungs are the site of elimination or metabolism.[40] During CPB these processes are interrupted, leading to increased systemic concentrations.[41]

Circuit Absorption

The interaction of the extracorporeal circulation apparatus with various drugs has come under scrutiny. Many drugs (eg, fentanyl and benzodiazepines) adsorb to bubble and membrane oxygenator components.[42-45] Various plasticizers present in the apparatus tubing can alter drug–protein binding relations. Heparin, necessary for anticoagulation during CPB, affects drug–protein binding by increasing free fatty acids that competitively inhibit the binding of some drugs to plasma proteins.[32,46-48]

Termination of Cardiopulmonary Bypass

Whereas the pathophysiologic disturbances affecting drug action are greatest during CPB, termination of CPB does not reverse these disturbances entirely. The fluid shifts that have occurred resolve slowly, and drug distribution volumes are altered accordingly. Drug metabolism and elimination capabilities of the liver and kidneys also recover slowly. As a result, the effects of many classes of drugs are prolonged after CPB.[49-51] Abnormal plasma protein binding may evolve over a period of days as alpha 1-acid glycoprotein concentrations increase,[52] and the binding of commonly used drugs (eg, fentanyl, sufentanil, lidocaine, or propranolol) increases.[53] Albumin, to which many acidic drugs bind, can undergo major concentration fluctuations as well.

SPECIFIC COMPLICATIONS

The list of possible CPB complications is almost overwhelming, extending from death to occipital alopecia.[54] Mortenson and coworkers reviewed the world literature of nearly 400 reports,[55,56] and an edited summary is presented in Table 59-2. Until recently, in the vast majority of situations, an oxygenator could not be designed to be operated safely and reliably without a skilled user. In early applications of CPB, fully redundant monitoring systems would have been sufficiently complex to introduce significant unreliability. With modern technology, interest in fail-safe monitors is increasing. Proposed modifications should be evaluated in light of Mortenson and coworkers' list and the following discussion of specific complications.

Blood

Bleeding

Bleeding frequently occurs after CPB. Inadequate hemostasis is probably the most common cause and demands careful surgical technique. Occasionally, patients have a pre-bypass bleeding disorder that is congenital (eg, hemophilia or von Willebrand's disease) or acquired (eg, thrombocytopenia, vitamin K deficiency, or severe liver disease). Drug-related platelet defects are common in patients taking aspirin, nonsteroidal anti-inflammatory drugs, dipyridamole, and other platelet inhibitors.

A bleeding tendency usually can be detected by obtaining a careful drug and bleeding history and by looking for signs of easy bruising in the physical examination. If findings in the history or physical examination suggest such a tendency, a coagulation screen and bleeding time can be obtained before surgery. However, the predictive value of bleeding time has been challenged.[57,58]

Drug-induced platelet dysfunction can be prevented by withholding the offending drug for a sufficiently long period before surgery. Platelet transfusions can be administered before surgery if the bleeding time is excessive; otherwise, platelets may be required after CPB. Abnormal values for prothrombin time (PT) and partial thromboplastin time (PTT) can be corrected with vitamin K or fresh frozen plasma before surgery. Of course, if the surgery is elective and if the coagulation abnormality is likely to correct spontaneously with time (eg, with discontinuation of an offending drug), surgery may be postponed. An additional, uncommon cause of severe bleeding that must be considered is transfusion reaction.

ANTICOAGULATION AND ITS REVERSAL. Heparin is administered before CPB cannulation in a dose of approximately 300 U/kg. Before CPB is begun, the activated clotting time (ACT) should be greater than 400 seconds to ensure adequate anticoagulation during CPB. The ACT should be measured periodically throughout CPB, and heparin should be given if it is less than 400 seconds. Optimal ACT or heparin concentration for CPB has not been clearly established. Gravlee has written an excellent review concerning these issues.[59]

Inadequate neutralization of heparin after CPB can be a major cause of bleeding. Protamine sulfate is administered in a dose of 1 to 3 mg/100 U heparin, usually following the method described by Bull.[60] Additional protamine is given if the ACT remains greater than the control value. If additional protamine fails to shorten the ACT, a deficiency in coagulation factors or platelets may be present. Protamine in excess is a weak anticoagulant, but this effect probably is not clinically important in the setting of cardiac surgery.[61] Incremental administration of protamine guided by the ACT should permit administration of the appropriate dose without excess.

DIFFERENTIAL DIAGNOSIS. Identification of the cause is the key step in the treatment of post-CPB bleeding. The differential diagnosis often centers on the issue of coagulation abnormalities (coagulation factor deficiency, platelet abnormalities, fibrinolysis, or a combination thereof) versus surgical bleeding. If generalized oozing is present, adequate reversal of heparin should be ensured, and clotting studies (PT, PTT, thrombin time, and platelet count) performed. Other laboratory tests, such as thromboelastography, Sonoclot, fibrinogen, reptilase time, or fibrin degradation products) can be useful.

TABLE 59-2
Subjectively Rated Clinical Problems in Safety and Efficacy During Use of Blood Oxygenator

	FREQUENCY	SERIOUSNESS	AMENABILITY TO CORRECTION BY STANDARDS
MECHANICAL FAILURES OR ERRORS IN OXYGENATION			
Leaks or disruptions			
Gas lines, connections containers	+	+++	++
Blood lines, connections, containers	++	+++	++
Heat-exchanger water lines, connections, containers	++	++++	+++
Membranes, reservoirs	+++	++	++
Obstructions (resulting in impaired flow or increased pressure)	++	+	++
Gas lines			
Blood lines	+	++++	++
Heat-exchanger water or blood lines	++	+	++
Excessive foaming	+++	++	+
Water loss from blood	++	+	+
Into oxygenator spaces or membranes	++	+	+
Into effluent gases			
Water transfer to blood			
From gases	+++	++	+
From heat exchanger	+	++++	+++
Migration or slippage of membranes	+++	+++	+++
Errors in assembly or operation	+++	++	++++
CONTAMINATION OF BLOOD AT BLOOD-OXYGENATOR INTERFACES			
Viabile contaminants (bacteria, fungi, yeasts, or viruses)	++	++++	++
Chemical contaminants	++	++	+++
Toxic eluents			
Sterilizing agents	+	+++	+++
Anesthetic gases	+	+	+
Surface contaminants			
Sodium chloride	+	+++	+++
Antifoam agents: leached toxicants	+++	++	+++
Pyrogens	+	++	+++
Particulate debris	++++	+++	+++
ALTERATIONS IN BLOOD FLOWING THROUGH OXYGENATOR			
Hemolysis of red blood cells	++++	+++	+++
Destruction of platelets	++++	++	++
Alteration of platelet function	+++	++	++
Destruction of white blood cells	+++	+	++
Reduced phagocytosis	+++	+	++
Changes in blood viscosity	++	++	++
Formation of fibrin	+++	+	++
Loss of fibrinogen	+++	++	+
Denaturation of serum proteins	++++	++	+
Thrombosis (impaired gas transfer, obstruction to flow, or emboli)	++	++	++
Introduction of air bubbles (micro- or macroemboli or air leaks)	++	++	+++
Changes in blood pH	+++	+++	+
ALTERATIONS IN PHYSIOLOGIC STATE			
Anemia	+++	++	+
Pulmonary parenchymal injury	++	+++	+
Low flow (hemodynamic syndrome)	++	++	+
Systemic arterial hypotension	+++	++	+
Intravascular compartmentalization	++++	+	+
Sludging (impaired capillary flow, or increased blood viscosity)	++++	++	+
Hemorrhage	++	+++	+
Impaired renal function	++	++	++
Increased peripheral vascular resistance	++	++	+
Increased red cell fragility	++	++	+
Sepsis	+	+++	+++

continued

TABLE 59-2
Continued

	FREQUENCY	SERIOUSNESS	AMENABILITY TO CORRECTION BY STANDARDS
Impaired renal function	++	++	+
Unexplained death	+	++++	+
IMPROPER GAS TRANSFER			
Erratic or inadequate oxygen transfer	+++	++++	++
Erratic or inadequate carbon dioxide transfer	+++	+++	++
Excessive carbon dioxide transfer	++	+++	++
Introduction of air: micro- or macroemboli	++++	+++	++

+, minimal or least; ++++, maximal or most.

Ream AK: Cardiopulmonary bypass. In Ream AK, Fogdall RP (eds): Acute cardiovascular management: anesthesia and intensive care. Philadelphia: JB Lippincott, 1982: 422.

If, while awaiting the results of clotting studies, it is determined that therapy is urgently needed and the patient's history suggests a platelet defect (eg, previous aspirin therapy) or deficiencies in clotting factors (eg, congestive heart failure and liver congestion preoperatively), the appropriate replacement products can be ordered empirically. Blood product use should be guided by the observation of clinical, nonsurgical bleeding and laboratory clotting studies whenever possible.

If replacement products have been given and oozing continues, hyperfibrinolysis should be considered. Cryoprecipitate, epsilon-aminocaproic acid[62], aprotinin[63], or tranxemic acid may be useful in this setting. Knowledge of the expected hematologic abnormalities during CPB will allow detection of deviations from the norm.[64]

Cardiovascular Effects of Protamine

The effects of protamine on the cardiovascular system have generated much interest. In rare instances, protamine administration is associated with severe hypotension.[64–68] More commonly, a modest decrease in blood pressure is observed.[69–70]

Etiologic mechanisms are diverse.[71] Endogenously liberated vasoactive substances, including thromboxane, histamine, and complement have been implicated, as have anaphylactoid or anaphylactic reactions. Hypotension appears to develop as a result of decreased systemic vascular resistance (SVR), increased pulmonary artery pressures, and possibly a myocardial depressant action.[72,73] A test dose of protamine (eg, 5 to 10 mg) seems prudent. If severe hypotension occurs, some have advocated administering protamine into the left atrium or the aorta (with precautions taken to avoid air injection) to avoid further hypotension.[74–76] Otherwise, slow infusion over a period longer than 10 minutes usually suffices.

Patients with previous exposure to protamine (previous CPB, cardiac catheterization or dialysis with reversal of heparin, or use of protamine zinc insulin) fish allergy, or even vasectomy may be at increased risk for an anaphylactic response. This type of response is characterized by circulatory collapse, noncardiogenic pulmonary edema with a dramatic decrease in pulmonary compliance, and generalized urticaria.[77]

Trauma

Derangements of both formed and unformed elements in the blood are part of all CPB procedures, even short pump runs.[78–80]

RED BLOOD CELLS. Most perfusionists prime the system without blood during adult CPB, thereby hemodiluting the blood and decreasing its viscosity. Hematocrit values also may further decrease because of red cell destruction. Interaction with foreign surfaces can lead to hemolysis.[81] The most important cause of hemolysis during modern CPB procedures is suction with a high vacuum, which causes considerable shear stress.[82–84] Other causes are improperly adjusted roller pumps, contact with oxygenators, and turbulence. Bubble oxygenators appear to have higher hemolysis rates than membrane oxygenators.[79] With both types, the damage progresses with time.

The first evidence of injury is increased red cell fragility, reduced red cell survival time, and increased red cell clearance after CPB.[85] A 27% to 30% decrease in red blood cell deformability has been demonstrated during CPB.[86,87] Of interest, only 35% of red cell destruction occurs intravascularly; the remainder is extravascular, with removal of damaged erythrocytes by the reticuloendothelial system.[88]

With greater trauma or duration of perfusion, frank hemoglobinuria is observed and may continue after CPB; it is caused by the saturation of serum haptoglobin, followed by the presence of free hemoglobin. Caution is needed in interpreting free hemoglobin concentrations in plasma, because they represent a balance between production and removal. Free hemoglobin is bound by the alpha globulin haptoglobin. Hemoglobin-haptoglobin complexes are removed from the circulation very rapidly. If the amount of hemoglobin entering the plasma exceeds the haptoglobin binding capacity, free hemoglobin appears in the plasma and in the glomerular filtrate.

Hemoglobinuria occurs when the free hemoglobin concentration in the glomerular filtrate exceeds the renal clearance threshold (about 150 mg/dL).[89] The amount of free hemoglobin bound by haptoglobin in plasma is 40 to 200 mg/dL, but haptoglobin itself decreases during CPB. Very high concentrations of free hemoglobin can cause renal tubular damage; such high concentrations are rare, however, except after transfusion reactions from incompatible blood. Membrane oxygenators and limited cardiotomy suction at the lowest level necessary should limit shear stress and hemolysis to acceptable levels.

WHITE BLOOD CELLS. Hemodilution also decreases white blood cell counts, but a further mechanism has been postulated. Cardiopulmonary bypass activates complement, which in turn causes granulocytes to aggregate and marginate.[90,91] In general, white blood cell counts decrease to 25% to 50% of their pre-CPB count early in CPB and then increase to greater than the preoperative count, where they remain for several days postoperatively.[92] Whether steroids or complement activation inhibitors affect white blood cell counts is unknown.

PLATELETS. Platelets are the most severely affected formed blood element. The platelet count drops immediately after onset of CPB, reaching a nadir (50% to 70% of pre-CPB levels) within 15 to 20 minutes.[93] The count may recover slightly later or continue to decrease slowly. However, only about two thirds of the initial decrease is attributable to hemodilution. Other causes of thrombocytopenia are sequestration in the reticuloendothelial system, the liver, and the extracorporeal circuit, complement-induced platelet aggregation, and destruction resulting from shear stress.[94–96] Use of membrane oxygenators and avoidance of high vacuum levels in the suction lines decreases platelet damage.

Platelets also develop acquired qualitative defects, including an alpha-granule storage deficiency that can be prevented with prostacyclin and possibly other prostaglandin inhibitors.[97,98] Prostacyclin infusions during CPB increase platelet counts and preserve function but do not appear to decrease blood transfusion requirements materially or reduce morbidity.[99,100] Platelet counts can be monitored, but bleeding may not correlate well with these values.

As was noted previously, platelet function is also affected by many drugs, including preoperative use of aspirin and other nonsteroidal anti-inflammatory agents, dipyridamole, and possibly nitroprusside. Platelet transfusions may be required after long CPB runs but should not be given routinely.[101] Protamine-heparin interactions can decrease platelet counts and function.[77]

PLASMA PROTEINS. Clotting factors and other plasma proteins are also damaged by passage through the extracorporeal circuit and by suction.[102] Many of the proteins adsorb to foreign surfaces. Contact with an air–blood interface also causes denaturation. Adsorption of Hageman factor (factor XII), factor XI, and others can activate the intrinsic coagulation cascade.[103,104] Platelets adhere to fibrinogen, which causes consumption of platelets and clotting factors, and can lead to disseminated intravascular coagulation in rare cases. Concentrations of labile clotting factors, especially Factors V and VIII, can decrease appreciably,[63] leading to post-CPB bleeding. Clotting factors and plasma proteins are also washed out if a device such as the Haemonetics Cell Saver is used for blood salvage or hemoconcentration. Ideally clotting factors should be replaced with fresh frozen plasma, after clotting studies have demonstrated a need.

Complement Activation

Complement activation during and after CPB has been well documented.[90,105–107] Patients undergoing chronic hemodialysis or leukopheresis also have complement activation.[108,109] Contact of blood with foreign surfaces probably activates Hageman factor (factor XII), which initiates the complement cascade by the alternate (properdin) pathway. As was mentioned previously, the initial drop in white cell count on CPB is attributed to margination and complement-induced white blood cell aggregation.[97]

The lungs are a site of leukoembolization. Endothelial injury from the complement-activated white blood cells may occur. Chenoweth and others postulate that "postperfusion lung" may be caused in part by complement-mediated injury in some patients.[91,110–112] Many patients have evidence of complement activation during CPB, but clinically significant pulmonary dysfunction is uncommon. Perhaps complement-mediated damage is an important contributing factor in those patients with preoperative pulmonary dysfunction, long CPB times, and other added insults. The administration of protamine after CPB is associated with further complement activation.[113,114] Whether steroids or complement activation inhibitors can prevent pulmonary dysfunction is unknown.

Cold Hemagglutinins

Hemolysis and microvascular thrombosis (eg, intracoronary) are among the problems threatened during CPB in patients with cold hemagglutinin disease. The underlying problem is activation of immunoglobulin M autoantibodies directed against red blood cells at the levels of hypothermia used during CPB, rather than an alteration of serum proteins by CPB. Suggested approaches to avoid these problems include normothermic or slightly hypothermic bypass to avoid agglutination, preoperative plasmapheresis, warm crystalloid cardioplegia solutions, and postponement of non-urgent surgery if the cold agglutinins are present because of acute infection.[115,116]

Metabolic Concerns

Investigations of the metabolic derangements during and after CPB describe changes in vasoactive substances, endocrine hormones, and electrolytes. In most instances the changes are the result of interacting factors: hypothermia, altered blood flow patterns, anesthetic drugs, surgical intervention, and the CPB circuitry.

Electrolyte Alterations

HYPOKALEMIA. Before the era of frequent and liberal use of potassium-containing cardioplegia solutions, hypokalemia occurred commonly during and after CPB because of hemodilution; urinary loss; respiratory alkalosis, metabolic alkalosis, or both; activation of the renin-angiotensin-aldosterone system; increases in plasma catecholamine concentrations; and diuretic administration during CPB.[117,118] Many patients undergoing cardiac surgery have depressed serum potassium concentrations preoperatively, most commonly because of diuretic therapy.

In the absence of potassium cardioplegia, serum potassium concentrations fall during CPB. Simple dilution and renal excretion cannot account fully for the decrease in serum potassium. Progressive movement of potassium from the extracellular to the intracellular compartment appears to be a major factor.[119] Insulin-stimulated potassium uptake, particularly by the liver and muscle, is the major reason for the development of hypokalemia during rewarming and after discontinuation of bypass.[120]

Treatment. Priming solutions with physiologic potassium concentrations do not prevent the decrease in serum potassium during CPB; thus, additional potassium must be given to ensure therapeutic concentrations after discontinuation of CPB if potassium-containing cardioplegia solutions are not used. Typically, potassium chloride, 20 to 60 mEq, may need to be administered during CPB in adults. Avoidance of hypokalemia can prevent many cardiac dysrhythmias.[117,121,122] Frequent determinations of serum potassium may be necessary, especially in patients receiving digitalis therapy. Some have suggested use of triamterene to decrease the renal potassium loss during CPB.[123]

HYPERKALEMIA. Hyperkalemia occurs frequently, most commonly as a result of high volumes of potassium-containing cardioplegia solution. Other reasons are overzealous use of potassium replacement therapy in patients making little urine during CPB, renal failure and metabolic acidosis. Patients with diabetes mellitus may have a higher incidence of hyperkalemia because of difficulty moving glucose and potassium into cells.[124]

Hyperkalemia does not appear to result from the transfusion of old red blood cells.[125] The plasma concentration of potassium in stored blood does increase with time, because of leakage from the intracellular space, but the total potassium content is normal. With transfusion, a normal metabolic environment is restored within the transfused red cells, and potassium returns to the intracellular space.

Treatment. Treatment depends on the magnitude of the disturbance. For severe hyperkalemia during CPB, a glucose-insulin infusion (to drive potassium intracellularly), calcium chloride (to counteract the myocardial effects of the hyperkalemia), sodium bicarbonate (to ensure neutral or slightly alkaline pH), diuresis, and a low-dose epinephrine or isoproterenol infusion (0.01 to 0.02 μg/kg/min), if possible, generally will decrease potassium to an acceptable concentration. Cardiac pacing and a longer time on CPB may also be necessary.

The role of the liver in maintaining potassium homeostasis should not be underestimated. Patients with marginal hepatic function subjected to CPB are at risk for hyperkalemia. An adequate rewarming period prior to discontinuation of bypass and preservation of liver blood flow help to optimize liver function, so valuable for electrolyte, glucose and hemostatic homeostasis.

HYPOCALCEMIA. Lower total calcium and ionized calcium concentrations result from hemodilution produced by priming of the CPB system with solutions containing little or no calcium. The concentrations reached may not be clinically important.[126–128] Citrate-containing blood priming solutions produce marked decreases in serum ionized calcium concentrations that return to normal at the end of CPB.[129]

Treatment. Calcium-containing primes or cardioplegia solutions help to maintain normal ionized calcium concentrations during CPB. Controversy exists regarding whether hypocalcemia during CPB decreases myocardial oxygen requirements and, thus, may be advantageous. Hypercalcemia may increase the risk of myocardial injury. Hypocalcemia is common at termination of CPB.[130]

Administration of calcium chloride, 5 to 10 mg/kg, usually corrects the problem and may improve myocardial performance[131], although solid evidence for clinical efficacy has not been shown in controlled trials.[132,133] Reperfusion injury is worse if myocardial cells are exposed to a calcium-containing solution after the use of calcium-free cardioplegic solution. Calcium channel blocking agents and beta-adrenergic receptor blocking agents may be of value before or during the ischemic period but not during reperfusion.[134]

HYPOMAGNESEMIA. Hypomagnesemia may be associated with an increased incidence of spontaneous ventricular fibrillation and difficulty in defibrillation at the end of CPB.[135] The effect of hypomagnesemia on dysrhythmias has been well documented in patients having acute myocardial infarction.[136] Cardiac surgery patients commonly have low serum magnesium concentrations preoperatively. Factors contributing to abnormally low concentrations include preoperative dietary deficiency, diabetes, ethanol abuse, pancreatic disease, and diuretic use, as well as dilution by magnesium-deficient CPB fluids. Turnier and colleagues postulate that magnesium ion is exchanged for potassium ion.[137] Magnesium concentrations typically fall during CPB as a result of hemodilution and chelation by albumin that may be added to the priming solution.

Treatment. Some have suggested that replacement sufficient to eliminate the effects of dilution is sufficient in patients who have normal preoperative serum magnesium. However, not only is magnesium essential to a normal myocardial contractile response,[138] but it appears to offer the membrane stabilizing effects of potassium without the same risk of myocardial depression. Thus, it may be used for acute treatment of dysrhythmias, which may be associated with electrolyte deficiencies. We routinely administer it as a bolus injection during CPB if dysrhythmia is present.

HYPONATREMIA. A serum sodium concentration of less than 130 mEq/L can occur during or after CPB if excessive salt-poor solutions are used. Hyponatremia may be potentiated by increased antidiuretic hormone (ADH) secretion.[139] Unless the serum sodium concentration decreases to 120 mEq/L or less, hyponatremia usually is not clinically significant. However, the rate of decrease, as well as the absolute magnitude, also are important. Severe hyponatremia will cause neurologic symptoms, including a clouded sensorium, coma, and convulsions.

Treatment. Hyponatremia in most cases can be treated by administering isotonic saline solutions and limiting the amount of fluid infused.

Hypothermia

Cardiopulmonary bypass often is conducted with deliberate lowering of body temperature. Hypothermia per se is associated with important alterations of organ function and has its own inherent complications. The effects of rhythm and temperature on myocardial metabolism are summarized in Table 59-3. However, certain features are of particular importance during CPB.[140]

OXYGENATION. Studies at the cellular level suggest that the rate of oxygen consumption decreases by about 50% for each 9°C decrease in tissue temperature.[141] However, clinical experience suggests that the increase in time without blood flow before ischemic injury occurs is of greater importance than these data suggest. An important element in the difference is the increased availability of oxygen at the cellular level because of its increased solubility with decreasing temperature. These considerations, however, neglect the effect of temperature changes on the distribution of blood flow.

Some data, though only suggestive, support the need to use temperature gradients to improve tissue oxygenation.[142] Surface cooling appears to be desirable, because of the reduction of metabolic demand in advance of blood flow decrements. On the other hand, CPB warming appears to be preferable, because flow supports perfusion of warming tissue. Pulsatile perfusion enhances these processes.[143]

BLOOD VISCOSITY. Viscosity increases with decreasing temperature, and this effect is exaggerated at low flows (ie., blood is thixotropic).[144] The resistance to resuming flow increases dramatically as the hematocrit increases to greater than 50%[145] and is associated with sludging. Hemodilution originally was proposed to reverse these effects, but has other important advantages. If blood is withdrawn before CPB and reinfused later, it contains active clotting factors and can reduce the need for exogenously administered factors after CPB. A reduced hematocrit during CPB means reduced loss of red cells from the patient. The clinical cost of removal is low, because oxygen solubility is enhanced by the reduced temperatures during CPB.

CLOTTING. Abnormal clotting follows CPB and cooling but is largely corrected by restoring the normal body temperature.

HYPERTHERMIA. After surgery, most patients become hyperthermic to at least 38°C. Be sure to consider infection as a possible cause.[146] Hyperthermia during rewarming in the final stages of CPB is commonly seen. Modern heat exchangers can easily raise the temperature of the blood (and that of organs receiving high blood flow) to values in excess of 38°C. The effects of this hyperthermia on the brain and other organs are not well studied. Care should be taken not to raise the gradient between core body temperature and the perfusate above 10°C to avoid the formation of gaseous microemboli caused by rapidly decreasing gas solubility.[147] Blood temperatures above 42°C cause severe damage to blood elements and protein denaturation.[148]

Endocrine Changes

ANTIDIURETIC HORMONE. ADH secretion during anesthesia, surgery and CPB has been a subject of frequent investigation.[139,149-151] Despite the anesthetic regimen used, ADH concentrations in plasma increase markedly during CPB.[152,153] Several factors probably contribute. Decreased pressure or pulse pressure stimulates baroreceptors in the left atrium to increase secretion. Pain and visceral sensory stimulation can increase ADH concentrations.

Increased ADH may contribute to the observed increases in body water that occur during cardiac surgery. Very high concentrations (>50 pg/mL) reported during halothane and nitrous oxide anesthesia can lead to appreciable increases in blood pressure or to decreased organ function from vasocon-

TABLE 59-3
Myocardial Metabolism During Hypothermia

	37°C	32°C	28°C	22°C
Heart rate (beats/min)	164 ± 10	118 ± 10	77 ± 7	31 ± 3
$M\dot{V}_{O_2}$ per beat (mL/100 g/min)	0.033 ± 0.003	0.041 ± 0.005	0.051 ± 0.005	0.086 ± 0.12
$M\dot{V}_{O_2}$ per minute (mL/100 g/min)				
Beating empty	5.59 ± 1.95	4.93 ± 1.80	3.93 ± 1.10	2.87 ± 0.90
Fibrillating	6.50 ± 1.60	3.84 ± 0.51	2.93 ± 1.02	1.95 ± 0.86
Arrest	1.10 ± 0.41	0.83 ± 0.23	0.59 ± 0.30	0.31 ± 0.12

Values are means ± SD.

$M\dot{V}_{O_2}$, left ventricular myocardial oxygen consumption.

Buckberg GD, Brazier JR, Nelson RL, et al: Studies of the effects of hypothermia on regional myocardial blood flow and metabolism during cardiopulmonary bypass: I. the adequately perfused beating, fibrillating, and arrested heart. J Thorac Cardiovasc Surg 73:88, 1977.

striction and hypoperfusion.[154] High-dose narcotic techniques, but not those utilizing inhalation anesthetics, can block ADH secretion during surgery before CPB. However, in all regimens, ADH concentrations increase during CPB.[152] Fluid loading and decreases in plasma osmolality have no effect.

Prevention of ADH increases during CPB has not been reported, but pulsatile perfusion may attenuate the response, particularly after bypass.[155,156] The effect of increased ADH is to increase the minimum urine osmolality. For this reason, the typical intravenous solution and CPB prime should be a balanced-salt solution. Free-water administration (eg, dextrose 5% in water) only tends to increase fluid retention, promote hyponatremia, and predispose to water intoxication.

THYROID HORMONE. The effects of CPB on thyroid gland function, peripheral thyroid hormone metabolism and cardiovascular function have gained recent attention. Thyroid hormones interact with many organ systems and regulate numerous metabolic processes. For the cardiovascular system, they regulate the number and sensitivity of beta-adrenergic receptors and have adrenergic-like effects (increased metabolic rate, heat production, heart rate, cardiac output, motor activity and central nervous system excitation).

Positive inotropic effects are both indirect and direct. Thyroid hormone induces the myosin heavy chain alpha gene and represses the beta gene, thus increasing the velocity of myocardial contraction. The calcium-ATPase of the sarcolemmal reticulum is increased, which aids uptake of calcium from the cytoplasm during diastole and shortens relaxation time. Indirectly, thyroid hormone stimulates calcium uptake into the myocyte and enhances adenyl cyclase activity, which improves contractility.[157]

Administration of heparin increases free T_3 and T_4 concentrations by displacing them from binding proteins.[158] Although hemodilution acutely lowers total T_3 concentration, free T_3 falls much more slowly, reaching a nadir at 24 hours after surgery.[159] Although several studies suggest intravenous T_3 supplementation may be beneficial,[160,161] its efficacy in clinically euthyroid patients is unclear at this time.

RENIN-ANGIOTENSIN-ALDOSTERONE. Alterations have been reported in cardiac surgery patients.[162] Controversy exists regarding whether this system contributes substantially to intraoperative or postoperative hypertension. Roberts and colleagues noted high plasma renin activity in hypertensive coronary artery bypass patients;[163] others have reported high concentrations of angiotensin II during CPB and the immediate postoperative period.[153,164] In contrast, other investigators have not detected an increase in plasma renin activity in cardiac surgery patients, with or without hypertension.[165–167] Furthermore, saralasin, an angiotensin II inhibitor, fails to reduce increased blood pressure.

CATECHOLAMINES AND ENDORPHINS. Changes in plasma catecholamines during cardiac surgery have generated considerable interest,[168,169] as has the role of naturally occurring endorphins in cardiovascular control. Although most studies sample these very short-lived compounds only intermittently, thus providing an incomplete view of the fluctuations in plasma concentration with time, some generalizations can be made. Preanesthetic sedation, previous drug therapy, and even cessation of some drugs (eg, beta-adrenergic receptor blocking agents and clonidine) can influence catecholamine levels. The preoperative condition is important. Patients with valvular heart disease or congestive heart failure should be expected to have higher circulating catecholamine concentrations than those undergoing coronary artery bypass graft surgery.[170] Beta-endorphin concentration and stroke index are related inversely, and the relation has a greater correlation among patients having coronary artery bypass graft operations than among those having valvular procedures.[171]

ANESTHESIA. The type and level of anesthesia also can alter catecholamine concentrations. High-dose opioid techniques suppress increases in catecholamines and other endocrine changes before CPB.[172,173] Once CPB begins, a progressive increase in catecholamines occurs until the cross-clamp is removed, regardless of the type of anesthesia.[153,174–176] Epinephrine appears to be increased more than norepinephrine, suggesting an adrenomedullary source rather than sympathetic hyperactivity.

The potential of high circulating catecholamine concentrations to cause intra- and postoperative hypertension, dysrhythmias, systemic vasoconstriction, intra-organ blood shifts, and unfavorable myocardial oxygen supply-demand ratios, requires that adequate depth of anesthesia be insured.[177,178] Perioperative treatment of hypertension with appropriate vasodilator therapy or beta-adrenergic receptor blocking agents is important.

Pulsatile CPB results in lower norepinephrine and epinephrine concentrations during bypass and immediately postoperatively than nonpulsatile modes.[179,180] In fact, pulsatile bypass appears to attenuate many of the "stress responses" to bypass: increased ADH,[181] increased catecholamines, abnormal pituitary-adrenal axis responsiveness,[182] and hyperglycemia.[183] One study[184] showed pulsatile perfusion permitted cortisol concentrations to increase during CPB while during non-pulsatile perfusion, concentrations fell. Despite these observations, pulsatile bypass is not commonly used.

Carbohydrate Metabolism

Cardiac surgery, similar to most major surgical procedures, is associated with increases in serum glucose concentrations. The increase generally is slight and only of concern in patients with diabetes. It usually is ascribed to increases in *stress hormones*: catecholamines, cortisol, and growth hormone.

Cardiopulmonary bypass appears to cause even greater increases in serum glucose.[185,186] Insulin concentrations increase slowly but are ineffective in decreasing glucose concentrations to normal.[187] Use of glucose-containing primes can result in very high blood glucose concentrations and should be avoided. Deaths from hyperosmolar, hyperglycemic nonketotic coma after CPB using dextrose-containing primes have been reported.[188]

Among the reasons for depressed insulin secretion, despite high glucose concentrations, are alpha-adrenergic suppression of islet cells, hypothermia, and the possibility of decreased blood flow to the pancreas.[189] Pulsatile blood flow during CPB may preserve beta cell function.[190] Kuntschen and colleagues, in elegant glucose-clamp experiments during CPB, demonstrated insulin resistance as well as inadequate insulin response to hyperglycemia.[191]

DIABETES MELLITUS. Careful management of blood glucose concentrations in patients with diabetes mellitus is extremely important. A blood glucose determination should be obtained just before anesthesia and surgery. Only intravenously administered regular insulin should be used to decrease glucose; a glucose-insulin infusion may be used. In particular, subcutaneous administration of insulin should be avoided because the drug is subject to uncertain absorption.

Non–dextrose-containing solutions should be used for pump primes. Frequent determination of blood glucose and correction with insulin is necessary, but insulin resistance should be expected to decrease the effectiveness of a given dose. The serum potassium concentration decreases as glucose moves intracellularly. This alteration, as noted previously, may require potassium chloride supplementation.

Lipid Metabolism

Lipid metabolism is also perturbed during cardiac surgery.[192] Heparinization before CPB is associated with increases in free fatty acids and decreases in triglycerides. Concentrations of free fatty acids peak early during CPB and decrease substantially after protamine administration. The decrease during CPB may be attributable to peripheral utilization by cells unable to maintain normal glucose utilization in the presence of catecholamines and growth hormone.[191]

Myocardial Damage

An understanding of the purpose and mechanisms of CPB is essential to ensure adequate protection of the heart. Cardiopulmonary bypass is usually undertaken to interrupt the heart's pumping action while a repair is effected. In most instances perfusion to the heart must be interrupted. Adequate recovery after perfusion is reestablished depends on several factors, including good oxygenation and perfusion of the heart before circulatory arrest, adequate ventricular decompression, effective diastolic arrest by chemical cardioplegia, and myocardial hypothermia.[193] Cooling by external bathing or antegrade or retrograde cardioplegia extends the duration of arrest before unacceptable injury occurs (see Table 59-3). Several cardioplegic solutions have been investigated: the only certain finding is that low temperature is the critical primary ingredient.

Resuscitation

Successful resuscitation of the heart depends on several factors that do not always receive full consideration. Reperfusion and warming must occur before the heart can be expected to do useful work. The return of fibrillation, with a rapid rate, is usually evidence that successful defibrillation can be accomplished. Similarly favorable is the appearance of a circus rhythm, which indicates that the heart is sustaining a rate of repolarization close to that at normal temperature. Multiple shocks to a flaccid heart only increase the risk of injury.

Inotropic Agents

Inotropic agents should be avoided whenever possible because they always increase myocardial oxygen consumption. Their use is particularly hazardous immediately after the heart has begun to beat. Washout of the by-products of ischemia is not complete, and intracellular pH is undoubtedly low. A further reduction in intracellular pH, while aerobic energy consumption is resumed, increases the risk of injury. Inotropic stimulation should only follow a period of resuscitation, either to a point at which the heart is beating effectively and minimal support is required, or after the limit of improvement has been reached and weaning from CPB is not possible without inotropic stimulation. Use of inotropic agents to accelerate weaning from CPB is clearly injurious and should be avoided.[194]

Distention

Distention of the heart during CPB should be avoided because it overstretches the contractile fibers, resulting in disruption and failure. Thus, the heart usually is vented if distention is expected. Once distended, the heart requires several days to recover completely. The risk of distention continues during reperfusion.[195] Patient care subsequent to a period of distention must presume that myocardial contractility has been compromised.

Dysrhythmias

Dysrhythmias during resuscitation result from a variety of factors. Heart block is common if the surgical field has included the atrioventricular canal or adjacent areas (eg, during aortic valve replacement). Treatment is cardiac pacing, for as long as it is required. Premature ventricular contractions, or other dysrhythmias progressing to fibrillation, carry an ominous prognosis. The most common cause is ischemia, with acute injury, and depolarization of adjacent cells that otherwise might still contract effectively. Treatable causes, such as emboli, should be excluded or treated.

VASOPRESSORS. Controversy exists regarding whether aortic root pressure should be increased by administration of vasopressors after the aortic cross clamp is removed. Transient hypertension assists in expelling coronary air. Sustained vasopressor administration is unwise, however, because it reduces coronary collateral flow.[196] The administration of nitroprusside reduces the incidence of postoperative dysrhythmias,[197] presumably because of improved perfusion.

ANTIDYSRHYTHMIC DRUGS. Additional CPB time to permit further recovery in a seriously compromised heart can yield a satisfactory result in an otherwise intractable situation. Because the usual cause of the dysrhythmia is ischemia, antidysrhythmic agents usually are not helpful. However, if the patient is not responding to measures designed to improve perfusion, a trial of antidysrhythmic agents is indicated. Lidocaine, 1.5 to 3 mg/kg, and verapamil, in divided doses to a total of approximately 0.06 mg/kg acutely, or magnesium, 1 to 2 g, administered into the oxygenator seem to be particularly helpful.

Emboli

Meticulous attention should be given to avoiding particulate emboli from a valve resection, clot from previous injury, or air introduced by opening of the heart. Transesophageal echocardiography is very helpful in determining when the left heart has been completely "de-aired." Although sustained use of vasopressors is strongly discouraged, they may be helpful to achieve temporarily high aortic root pressures to flush air through the coronary vascular bed (overcoming the effects of surface tension) as was mentioned previously. The failure of a specific area of the heart to contract is often evidence of local embolization. In rare instances, acute embolectomy can salvage an otherwise unmanageable clinical situation. However, prevention is the most effective approach.

Damage to Blood Vessels

Cannulation of the femoral artery is associated with occasional subsequent dissection and aneurysm.[198,199] For these reasons, the ascending aorta is more commonly used unless the surgical approach is in question, as with acute aortic dissection or anatomic abnormalities.[200] Acute dissection caused by aortic cannulation is uncommon but is manifest by loss of monitored arterial pressure, associated with a high line pressure.

Pulmonary Damage

Atelectasis

Atelectasis following cardiac surgery is common. The lungs are generally allowed to collapse completely during bypass. After re-expansion and ventilation a variable degree of atelectasis remains. A higher incidence should be expected in heavy smokers, in obese patients, following prolonged CPB times, after entrance into the pleura as often occurs with internal mammary artery harvest, and in the presence of preexisting lung disease.

The consequences of atelectasis are an increased $P(A\text{-}a)O_2$ gradient and altered pulmonary mechanical properties. Treatment is usually accomplished by several Valsalva maneuvers at the end of CPB before beginning ventilation, use of positive-pressure ventilation with moderate levels of PEEP (5-8 cm H_2O), and large tidal volumes (10-12 mL/kg). Distention of the lungs during CPB might seem, intuitively, to prevent atelectasis, but Mandelbaum and Giammona reported decreased lung surfactant resulting from that approach.[201]

Pump Lung

Pulmonary injury long has been associated with CPB,[202,203] although some investigators have disputed its significance.[204] This injury was called the postperfusion pulmonary congestion syndrome or pump lung.[205] Lung compliance is reduced, and the $P(A\text{-}a)O_2$ gradient is increased. At autopsy, the lungs are dark red and congested with focal zones of collapse and parenchymal hemorrhage, essentially identical to their appearance in acute respiratory failure syndrome (ARDS).

Suggested causes include blood trauma, release of proteolytic enzymes,[206] and possible endotoxin injury. Dysfunction increases with time on CPB.[207] Cigarette smoking and other pulmonary trauma also predispose to injury.[208]

LEUKOCYTE EMBOLIZATION. The advent of blood filter use suggested a common cause: early lung biopsy in surviving patients demonstrated extensive occlusion of the capillary beds by aggregates of leukocytes. Filtration substantially reduced the incidence of these findings and the degree of pulmonary dysfunction.[209,210] Hypothermia also appears beneficial.[211]

EXTRAVASCULAR LUNG WATER. Early investigators suggested that an electrolyte prime solution increased lung water and impaired post-CPB gas exchange, but more recent studies propose that significant increases in lung water may not occur until after CPB and may not be related to the type of prime.[212]

HIGH OXYGEN PARTIAL PRESSURE. Exposure to high oxygen partial pressures during CPB, particularly with hypothermia, may lead to increased pulmonary dysfunction. However, this relation has yet to be documented. Nonpulsatile flow during CPB does not appear to affect postoperative gas exchange.[213]

CYTOKINE DAMAGE. The important remaining implication is that damage from complement activation and cytokine-mediated injury is a component of the pulmonary insult. Substitution of heparinized fresh blood for stored blood in the pump prime leads to increased pulmonary dysfunction,[214] suggesting that vasoactive factors are released from fully competent blood constituents. Large doses of heparin also accentuate pulmonary injury.

The increase in pulmonary dysfunction with time on CPB despite modern techniques suggests that blood trauma, complement activation, and other immunologic injury are important etiologic factors; their exact nature remains to be fully elucidated. The primary incentive for membrane oxygenator development is the reduction of pulmonary, renal, and cerebral injury produced by blood trauma.

PREVENTION AND TREATMENT. Acute lung injury seen after CPB can be prevented or attenuated by use of a membrane oxygenator,[215] blood filters (to remove aggregated platelets, leukocytes, or both), avoidance of airway distention, avoidance of pulmonary vascular distention,[216] and possibly by pharmacologic means. Prostaglandin E1 (prostacyclin) or Iloprost (a more stable, longer acting prostacyclin analog) inhibit platelet aggregation, maintain higher platelet counts on bypass, lower postoperative bleeding and inhibit thromboxane production. Another approach uses aprotinin, a serine protease inhibitor that lowers bradykinin concentrations during CPB, prevents platelet aggregation, decreases blood loss after bypass, inhibits fibrinolysis, and decreases kallikrein concentration.[217] Whether these drugs reduce lung injury remains to be clarified, although the rationale for their use appears sound.

Management of Lungs During Cardiopulmonary Bypass

In an attempt to determine whether there is a best way to manage the lungs with the goal of minimizing lung injury, Boldt and colleagues studied patients managed with one of six "lung" protocols during CPB.[218] Their groups included the following conditions:

1. Lungs collapsed
2. Static inflation with 5 cm H_2O and inspired oxygen fraction (FIO_2) 1.0
3. Static inflation with 5 cm H_2O and FIO_2 0.21
4. Static 15 cm H_2O and FIO_2 1.0
5. Static 15 cm H_2O and FIO_2 0.21; and,
6. Controlled ventilation (5 cm H_2O positive end-expired pressure and FIO_2 1.0).

They determined that extravascular lung water and shunt were highest in the high FIO_2 high-static inflation groups and recommended that static inflation with moderate positive end-expiratory pressure (5 cm H_2O) and air is the best way to optimize lung management during bypass.[218]

Brain Damage

Incidence

The brain is one of the organs most vulnerable to injury during extracorporeal circulation. Cerebral dysfunction after CPB procedures may be difficult to establish. The detected incidence depends on the sensitivity of the test used to measure dysfunction, the patient population studied, various technical factors, and the time of testing.

Types of dysfunction cover a spectrum from very subtle impairment (personality changes, memory loss, mild cognitive deficits, disorientation) through focal defects (paraplegia,[219] hemiplegia, visual deficits,[220] and hearing loss[221]), to coma and brain death. Sensitive psychometric tests early in the postoperative period may reveal an incidence of dysfunction as high as 50% to 70%.[222,223] If these patients are studied weeks to months later, most psychometric test results revert to normal.[224] Several studies report a 10% to 20% incidence of neurologic abnormalities.[225–228] Many patients have deficits that are transient; the incidence of permanent dysfunction is lower, probably less than 5% in major centers.

Causes

The cause of CPB-related cerebral dysfunction is almost always cerebral ischemia. Two major causes may be identified: inadequate cerebral perfusion and embolization to cerebral vessels (Table 59-4).

INADEQUATE CEREBRAL PERFUSION. The lower limits for adequate cerebral blood flow during CPB at a given temperature have not been defined. Earlier work suggested mean arterial pressures greater than 50 mm Hg were necessary to prevent cerebral ischemia,[229,230] but subsequent efforts have failed to identify 50 mm Hg as a reliable lower limit.[226,228] Apparently, low pressures are acceptable if flow is maintained.[231]

TABLE 59-4
Mechanisms of Central Nervous System Injury After Cardiac Surgery

MICROEMBOLIZATION
Air
Atherosclerotic plaque
Cellular aggregates
Silicone or fat
Fibrin
MACROEMBOLIZATION
Air
Atherosclerotic plaque
Calcium deposit
Intracardiac thrombus
REDUCED CEREBRAL PERFUSION
Decreased blood flow
Low perfusion pressure
Cerebrovascular disease
Technical problems with placement of aortic cannula
Inadequate venous drainage

Modified from Martin TJ: Cardiopulmonary bypass. In Kirby RR, Gravenstein N (eds): Clinical anesthesia practice. Philadelphia: WB Saunders, 1994: 327.

The composition of the pump prime and age and patency of cerebral vessels might be expected to be important factors in determining adequate cerebral blood flow; some data support this concept.[226,228,232]

Another potential source is increased cerebral venous pressure as a consequence of partial or complete obstruction to superior vena cava drainage. This complication is monitored by observing the central venous pressure monitored from a port within the superior vena cava, and inspecting the eyes and external jugular veins for engorgement. This observation is of particular importance during bicaval cannulation.

Care must be taken to ensure that the CVP measurement site is actually above the superior vena cava cannula and not within the atrium. More specifically, consider measuring CVP from the introducer side port rather than from the CVP lumen of the pulmonary artery catheter if one is in use.

EMBOLIZATION TO CEREBRAL VESSELS. The sources of emboli occurring on CPB are multiple: gas, silicone, fat, platelet aggregates, white blood cell aggregates, fibrin, and atherosclerotic plaque material. Emboli produce damage by obstructing blood flow in arterioles and possibly by liberation of harmful vasoactive substances.[233] Although arterial line filters should prevent much of the embolization, studies have not shown that their use improves neurologic outcome.[234,235]

Detection

Detection of brain ischemia or emboli during CPB is difficult. Accidental malposition of the aortic cannula with over- or underperfusion of the carotid arteries may result in unilateral facial edema, rhinorrhea and conjunctival edema, a unilateral cold neck, unilateral facial paleness,[236] or abnormalities in a radial artery pulse tracing.[237] Undoubtedly, the majority of insults are undetected at the time of occurrence and correlate poorly with routinely monitored variables (eg, temperature, blood pressure, and blood gas partial pressures).

One means to monitor regional brain function directly is with the electroencephalogram. Unfortunately, practical electroencephalographic monitoring in this clinical setting is in its infancy. Distinguishing between hypothermia, drug effects, and ischemic effects is difficult,[238] but asymmetric or regional electroencephalographic changes can be detected and causes sought. With more study and experience, electroencephalographic monitoring may become routine and more easily interpretable. In a second technique, transcranial Doppler ultrasound is used to monitor middle cerebral artery blood flow. Emboli are noted particularly during aortic root cannulation.[239]

Treatment

Treatment of neurologic dysfunction is mainly supportive. Adequate cerebral blood flow and oxygenation should be maintained. Pretreatment with thiopental may decrease the incidence of postoperative neuropsychiatric complications,[240] although this finding is not constant.[241] Avoidance of hyperglycemia has been recommended based on experimental results in animal models correlating cerebral damage to ischemia and reflow phenomena with pre-ischemia serum glucose concentrations[242] or brain glucose concentrations.[243]

Liver Damage

Although perfusion and pulse pressure in the viscera decrease during CPB, the frequency of clinically important injury to these organs is low. Little recognized is the incidence of mild injury to the liver, which can be detected by biochemical tests of hepatic function. Collins and colleagues noted overt jaundice within 2 days of CPB in 20% of 248 adults studied prospectively.[244] The jaundice was caused by an increased concentration of conjugated (direct) bilirubin. Of note is that 25% of the jaundiced patients died. The CPB-related cause in this study was not determined but may have been related to preoperative right heart failure, hepatic venous obstruction from the venous cannula, or valve procedures.

Others have noted a lower incidence of jaundice.[245,246] The incidence of hepatitis after the use of factor IX concentrates may be increased, but the etiology in most cases is multifactorial. In all studies, the appearance of jaundice carries a high morbidity and mortality. The treatment is mainly supportive and the diagnosis is made by liver function tests in the early postoperative period.

Pancreatic Dysfunction

Subclinical pancreatic injury has been documented in as many as 16% of autopsied patients dying of other causes after CPB. Two large studies noted an incidence of clinically evident pancreatic injury of about 0.1%.[247,248] A high incidence of increased serum and urinary amylases occurs after CPB,[249,250] but a recent study suggests that frequently the increased amylase is not of pancreatic origin.[251]

The cause of pancreatic injury is unknown, but presumably vascular compromise from hypoperfusion or venous stasis contributes. Other possible causes are atheromatous embolization, thromboembolism, or perioperative calcium administration.[252–255] Treatment includes nasogastric suction and drainage of pseudocysts or pancreatic abscesses, if necessary.

Gastrointestinal Dysfunction

Other abdominal complications reported after CPB are gastrointestinal bleeding, small bowel infarction, appendicitis, cholecystitis, diverticulitis, sigmoid volvulus and perforated gastroduodenal ulcers.[256–260] The incidence is about 1%.[261,262] A diagnosis of acute abdomen after CPB requires a high index of suspicion and early consultation with a general surgeon.

Renal Failure

Causes

Postoperative renal failure is a serious complication. It is secondary to morbidity directly related to cardiac failure as a major cause of morbidity associated with heart procedures requiring CPB and has been attributed to the effects of CPB,[263,264] and to post-CPB cardiac failure.[265,266] Urine output is severely depressed during CPB but usually recovers rapidly after cardiac function is restored.[267,268]

The pathogenesis of renal failure after CPB is generally multifactorial. Preoperative renal function,[264,269] duration of bypass,[270] hemolysis, microemboli, hypothermia,[271,272] and use of a bubble oxygenator have been implicated. Conversely, renal protection is offered by hemodilution (of both red blood cells and albumin),[273,274] furosemide,[275] mannitol,[276] low-dose dopamine, and membrane oxygenation. Some have suggested that high-flow CPB also is protective. Data are sparse, but animal studies suggest that higher bypass flows (100 mL/kg/min as opposed to 40 mL/kg/min) lead to less renal impairment.[277] Similarly, pulsatile perfusion results in less renal depression during CPB.[278]

The Stanford experience suggests that low, nonpulsatile flow in appropriate conditions does not increase morbidity and mortality relative to other procedures in clinical use.[268,277–279] Low-flow, low-pressure bypass usually provides satisfactory preservation of renal function during operative procedures. Severe depression of postoperative cardiac function with resultant renal ischemia is the critical common denominator. The development of acute renal failure depends on the sum of all insults to ischemic kidneys.

The aforementioned data were obtained in low-flow conditions in which vasopressors were not used to support the perfusion pressure during CPB. Although the use of vasopressors has been advanced to ensure improved perfusion of the brain and spinal cord, a prospective study failed to identify a benefit to central nervous system function.[228] We are similarly unaware of data showing vasopressor use enhances renal survival. Raising perfusion pressure does not improve postoperative renal function.[280,281] Furthermore, experience in the treatment of hypovolemic shock suggests that vasopressors increase morbidity and mortality. Thus, their use is discouraged in patients at risk of renal failure.

Treatment and Prevention

The general diagnosis and management of renal failure is discussed elsewhere. Considered here are practices associated with CPB that may reduce the incidence of failure or speed recovery. Acute ischemia is the most probable common pathway to renal injury.

VASOACTIVE DRUGS. In patients with congestive heart failure, nitroprusside infusion decreases left atrial pressure and arterial mean pressure, but increases renal perfusion. Similar changes have been noted in postoperative patients undergoing cardiac surgery.[282] Low-dose dopamine infusion (2 μg/kg/min) appears to enhance renal perfusion and urine output by inhibition of tubular reabsorption.[283] Dobutamine appears to be less effective.[284] Data for other inotropic agents are sparse, but an important effect appears to be enhanced perfusion produced by cardiac stimulation. However, secondary effects may provide clinically important differences between inotropic alternatives.

MANNITOL. The clinical effectiveness of mannitol has been suggested since the 1960s.[285] Mannitol blocks cell swelling after ischemia, which appears to be beneficial.[286,287] Thiazide diuretic agents, which increase renal vascular resistance and solute excretion, do not appear to be protective. Pretreatment with mannitol appears preferable, but an osmotic diuresis after the ischemic insult may still afford benefit. Many perfusionists add mannitol, 12.5 g, to the CPB prime solution. For patients at unusual risk, additional mannitol, as much as 12.5 g per 0.5 hour of CPB, may be added.

REFERENCES

1. Ream AK: Cardiopulmonary bypass. In Ream AK, Fogdall RF (eds): Acute cardiovascular management: anesthesia and intensive care. Philadelphia: JB Lippincott, 1982:420
2. Nelson RM: Era of extracorporeal respiration. Surgery 78:885, 1975
3. Howell WH, Hot E: Two new factors in blood coagulation: heparin and proantithrombin. Am J Physiol 47:328, 1918
4. McLean J: The discovery of heparin. Circulation 19:75, 1959
5. Hooker DR: The perfusion of the mammalian medulla: the effect of calcium and of potassium on the respiratory and cardiac centers. Am J Physiol 38:200, 1910
6. Richards AN, Drinker CK: An apparatus for the perfusion of isolated organs. J Pharmacol Exp Ther 7:467, 1915
7. Carrel A, Lindbergh CA: The culture of whole organs. Science 81:621, 1935
8. DeBakey M: A simple continuous flow blood transfusion instrument. N Orleans Med Surg J 87:386, 1934
9. Gibbon JH Jr: Artificial maintenance of circulation during experimental occlusion of pulmonary artery. Arch Surg 34:1105, 1937
10. Björk VO: Brain perfusion in dogs with artificially oxygenated blood. Acta Chirurgica Scandinavica Supplementum 96:1, 1948
11. Clark LC Jr, Gollan F, Gupta VB: The oxygenation of blood by gas dispersion. Science 111:85, 1950
12. Dennis C, Spreng DS Jr, Nelson GE, et al: Development of a pump oxygenator to replace the heart and lungs: an apparatus applicable to human patients and application to one case. Ann Surg 134:709, 1951
13. Gibbon JH Jr: Application of a mechanical heart and lung apparatus to cardiac surgery. Minn Med 37:171, 1954
14. DeWall RA, Warden HE, Read RC, et al: A simple expendable artificial oxygenator for open heart surgery. Surg Clin North Am 36: 1025, 1956
15. Clowes GHA Jr, Hopkins AL, Neville WE: An artificial lung dependent upon diffusion of oxygen and carbon dioxide through plastic membranes. J Thorac Cardiovasc Surg 32:630, 1956
16. Lillehei CW, Cohen M, Warden HE, et al: The direct vision intracardiac correction of congenital anomalies by controlled cross-circulation. Surgery 38:11, 1955
17. Dogliotti AM, Costantini A: Primo caso di applicazione all'uomo apparecchio di circolazione sanguinea extracorporea. Minerva Chir 6:657, 1951
18. Orenstein JM, Sato N, Aaron B: Microemboli observed following cardiopulmonary bypass surgery: silicone antifoam agents and polyvinyl chloride tubing as sources of emboli. Hum Pathol 13:1082, 1982
19. Taylor KM, Bain WH, Davidson KG, et al: Comparative clinical study of pulsatile and non pulsatile perfusion in 350 consecutive patients. Thorax 37:324, 1982
20. Ream AK, Portner PM: Cardiac assist devices and the artificial heart. In Ream AK, Fogdall RF (eds): Acute cardiovascular management: anesthesia and intensive care. Philadelphia: JB Lippincott, 1982:852
21. Philbin DM, Hickey PR, Buckley MJ: Should we pulse? J Thorac Cardiovasc Surg 84:805, 1982
22. Edmunds LH Jr: Pulseless cardiopulmonary bypass. J Thorac Cardiovasc Surg 84:800, 1982 23. Symposium on gaseous emboli. Med Instrum 19:52, 1985
23. Lake CL, Schwartz AJ, Campbell FW: Extracorporeal circulation. In: Lake CL (ed): Pediatric cardiac anesthesia. Norwalk, CT: Appleton and Lange, 1988:155.
24. Maltry DE, Eggers GWN: Isoflurane-induced failure of the Bentley-10 oxygenator. Anesthesiology 66:100, 1987
25. Stanley THE: Arterial pressure and deltoid muscle gas tensions during cardiopulmonary bypass in man. Can Anaesth Soc J 25: 286, 1978
26. Flynn PJ, Hughes R, Walton B: Use of atracurium in cardiac surgery involving cardiopulmonary bypass with induced hypothermia. Br J Anaesth 56:967, 1984
27. McAllister RG Jr, Bourne DW, Tau TG, et al: Effects of hypothermia on propranolol kinetics. Clin Pharmacol Ther 25: 1, 1979
28. d'Hollander M, Duvaldestin P, Henzel D, et al: Variations in pancuronium requirement, plasma concentration, and urinary excretion induced by cardiopulmonary bypass with hypothermia. Anesthesiology 58:505, 1983
29. Koska AJ, Romagnoli A. Kramer WG: Effect of cardiopulmonary bypass on fentanyl distribution and elimination. Clin Pharmacol Ther 29:100, 1981
30. Fischler M, Levron JC, Trang H, et al: Pharmacokinetics of phenoperidine in patients undergoing cardiopulmonary bypass. Br J Anaesth 57.877, 1985
31. Kanto J, Himberg JJ, Keikkila H, et al: Midazolam kinetics before, during and after cardiopulmonary bypass surgery. Int J Clin Pharmacol Res 5:123, 1985
32. Wood M, Shand DG, Wood AJJ: Propranolol binding in plasma during cardiopulmonary bypass. Anesthesiology 51:512, 1979
33. Morgan DJ, Crankshaw DP, Prideaux PR, et al: Thiopentone levels during cardiopulmonary bypass. Changes in plasma protein binding during continuous infusion. Anaesthesia 41:4, 1986
34. Roerig DL, Kotrly KJ, Vucins EJ, et al: First pass uptake of fentanyl, meperidine, and morphine in the human lung. Anesthesiology 67:466, 1987
35. Junod AF: Uptake, release and metabolism of drugs in the lungs. Pharmacol Ther B 2:511, 1976
36. Wilson AGE, Pickett RD, Eling TF, et al: Studies on the persistence of basic amines in the rabbit lung. Drug Metab Dispos 7:402, 1980
37. Roth RA, Wiersma DA: The role of the lung in total body clearance of circulating drugs. Clin Pharmacokinet 4:355, 1979

38. Bentley JB, Conahan TJ, Cork RC: Fentanyl sequestration in lung during cardiopulmonary bypass. Clin Pharmacol Ther 34: 703, 1983
39. Plachetka JR, Salomon NW, Copeland JG: Plasma propranolol before, during. and after cardiopulmonary bypass. Clin Pharmacol Ther 30:745, 1981
40. Pitt BR: Metabolic functions of the lung and systemic vasoregulation. Fed Proc 43:2574, 1984
41. Pitt BR, Gillis CN, Hammond GL: Depression of pulmonary metabolic function by cardiopulmonary bypass procedures increases levels of circulating norepinephrine. Ann Thorac Surg 38:508, 1984
42. Koren G, Crean P, Klein J, et al: Sequestration of fentanyl by the cardiopulmonary bypass. Eur J Clin Pharmacol 27:51, 1984
43. Dasta JF, Jacobi J, Wu LS, et al: Loss of nitroglycerin to cardiopulmonary bypass apparatus. Crit Care Med 11:50, 1983
44. Booth BP, Henderson M, Milne B, et al: Sequestration of glyceryl trinitrate (nitroglycerin) by cardiopulmonary bypass oxygenators. Anesth Analg 72:493, 1991
45. Skacel M, Knott C, Reynolds F, et al: Extracorporeal circuit sequestration of fentanyl and alfentanil. Br J Anaesth 58:947, 1986
46. Desmond PV, Robens RK, Wood AJJ, et al: Effects of heparin administration on plasma binding of benzodiazepines. Br J Clin Pharmacol 9: 171, 1980
47. Routhledge PA, Bjornsson TD, Kitchell BB, et al: Heparin administration increases plasma warfarin binding in man. Br J Clin Pharmacol 8:281, 1979
48. Storstern L, Janssen H. Studies on digitalis: VI. the effect of heparin on serum protein binding of digitoxin and digoxin. Clin Pharmacol Ther 20:16, 1976
49. Kramer WG, Romagnoli A: Papaverine disposition in cardiac surgery patients and the effect of cardiopulmonary bypass. Eur J Clin Pharmacol 27:127, 1984
50. Walker JS, Brown KF, Shanks CA: Alcuronium kinetics in patients undergoing cardiopulmonary bypass surgery. Br J Clin Pharmacol 16:237, 1983
51. Bovill JG, Sebel PS: Pharmacokinetics of high-dose fentanyl: a study in patients undergoing cardiac surgery. Br J Anaesth 52:795, 1980
52. Piafsky DM: Disease-induced changes in the plasma binding of basic drugs. Clin Pharmacokinet 5:246, 1980
53. Holley FO, Ponganis KV, Stanski DR: Effects of cardiac surgery with cardiopulmonary bypass on lidocaine disposition. Clin Pharmacol Ther 35:617, 1984
54. Lawson NW, Mills NL, Ockner JL: Occipital alopecia following cardiopulmonary bypass. J Thorac Cardiovasc Surg 71:342, 1976
55. Mortenson JD: Safety and efficacy of blood oxygenators, vol 1: summary; vol 2: report of testing; vol 3: literature review. Contract 223-74-5253, task order 10. Washington, DC: United States Food and Drug Administration, May 1976
56. Mortenson JD: Safety and efficacy of extracorporeal blood oxygenators: a review. Med Instrum 12:128, 1978
57. Rogers RPC, Levin JA: Critical reappraisal of the bleeding time. Semin Thromb Hemost 16:1, 1990
58. Glusko PR, Maring JK, Edmunds LH Jr: Bleeding time test [invited letter]. J Thorac Cardiovasc Surg 101:173, 1991
59. Gravlee GP: Anticoagulation for cardiopulmonary bypass. In Gravlee GP, Davis RF, Utley JR (eds): Cardiopulmonary bypass: principles and practice. Baltimore: Williams and Wilkins, 1993:340
60. Bull BS, Huse WM, Brauer FS, et al: Heparin therapy during extracorporeal circulation. II. The use of a dose-response curve to individualize heparin and protamine dosage. J Thorac Cardiovasc Surg 69:685, 1975
61. Ellison N, Ominsky AJ, Wollman H: Is protamine a clinically important anticoagulant? a negative answer. Anesthesiology 35:621, 1971
62. Hardy JF, Desroches J: Natural and synthetic antifibrinolytics in cardiac surgery. Can J Anaesth 39:353, 1992
63. Bidstrup BP, Royston D, Sapsford RN, et al: Reduction in blood loss and blood use after cardiopulmonary bypass with high dose aprotinin (Trasylol). J Thorac Cardiovasc Surg 97:364, 1989
64. Lowenstein E, Zapol WM: Protamine reactions, explosive mediator release, and pulmonary vasoconstriction [Editorial]. Anesthesiology 73:373, 1990
65. Lowenstein E, Johnston WE, Lappas DG, et al: Catastrophic pulmonary vasoconstriction associated with protamine reversal of heparin. Anesthesiology 59:470, 1983
66. Jackson DR: Sustained hypotension secondary to protamine sulfate. Angiology 21:295, 1970
67. Moorthy SS, Pond W, Rowland RG: Severe circulatory shock following protamine (an anaphylactic reaction). Anesth Analg 59:77, 1980
68. Nordstrom L, Fletcher R, Pavek K: Shock of anaphylactoid type induced by protamine: a continuous cardiorespiratory record. Acta Anaesthesiol Scand 22:195, 1978
69. Shapira N, Schlaff HV, Piehler JM, et al: Cardiovascular effects of protamine sulfate in man. J Thorac Cardiovasc Surg 84: 505, 1982
70. Jastrzebski J, Sykes MK, Wood DC: Cardiorespiratory effects of protamine after cardiopulmonary bypass in man. Thorax 29:534, 1974
71. Horrow JC: Protamine allergy. J Cardiothorac Anesth 2:225, 1988
72. Michaels IAL, Barash PG: Hemodynamic changes during protamine administration. Anesth Analg 62:831, 1983
73. Horrow JC: Protamine: a review of its toxicity. Anesth Analg 64:348, 1985
74. Frater RWM, Oka Y, Hong Y, et al: Protamine-induced circulatory changes. J Thorac Cardiovasc Surg 87:687, 1984
75. Sethna D, Gray R, Bussell J, et al: Further studies on the myocardial metabolic effect of protamine sulfate following cardiopulmonary bypass. Anesth Analg 61:476, 1982.
76. Aris A, Solanes H, Bonnin JO, et al: Intraaortic administration of protamine: method for heparin neutralization after cardiopulmonary bypass. Cardiovasc Dis Bull Texas Heart Inst 8:23, 1981
77. Horrow JC: Adverse reactions to protamine. Int Anesthesiol Clin 23:133, 1985
78. Hewitt WC Jr, Brown IW Jr, Eadie GS, et al: The ultimate in vivo survival of erythrocytes which have circulated through a pump-oxygenator. Surg Forum 7:271, 1956
79. de Jong JCF, ten Duis HJ, Smit SCT, et al: Hematologic aspects of cardiotomy suction in cardiac operations. J Thorac Cardiovasc Surg 79:227, 1980
80. Royston D: Blood cell activation. Semin Thorac Cardiovasc Surg 3:341, 1990
81. Forbes CD: Thrombosis and artificial surfaces. Clinical Haematology 10:653, 1981
82. Osborn JJ, Cohn K, Hait M, et al: Hemolysis during perfusion: sources and means of reduction. J Thorac Cardiovasc Surg 43: 459, 1962
83. Okies JE, Goodnight SH, Litchford B, et al: Effect of infusion of cardiotomy suction blood during extracorporeal circulation for coronary artery bypass surgery. J Thorac Cardiovasc Surg 74:440, 1977
84. Leverett LB, Hellums JD, Alfrey CP, et al: Red blood cell damage by shear stress. Biophys J 12:257, 1972
85. Blackshear PL, Dorman FD, Steinbach JH: Some mechanical effects that influence hemolysis. Trans Am Soc Artif Organs 11:112, 1965
86. Ekestrom S, Koul BL, Sonnenfeld T: Decreased red cell deformability following open-heart surgery. Scand J Thorac Cardiovasc Surg 17:41, 1983
87. Koul BL, Nordhas O, Sonnenfeld T, et al: The effect of pentoxifylline on impaired red cell deformability following openheart surgery. Scand J Thorac Cardiovasc Surg 18:129, 1984
88. Wallace HN, Blackmore WS: Intravascular and extravascular hemolysis accompanying extracorporeal circulation. Circulation 42:521, 1970
89. Clowes CHA: Extracorporeal maintenance of circulation and respiration. Physiol Rev 40:826, 1960
90. Hammerschmidt DE, Stroncek DF, Bower TK, et al: Complement activation and neutropenia occurring during cardiopulmonary bypass. J Thorac Cardiovasc Surg 81:370, 1981
91. Chenoweth DF, Cooper SW, Hugli TE, et al: Complement ac-

tivation during cardiopulmonary bypass. N Engl J Med 304: 497, 1981
92. Ryhanen P, Herva E, Hollman A, et al: Changes in peripheral blood leukocyte counts, lymphocyte subpopulations, and in vitro transformation after heart valve replacement. J Thorac Cardiovasc Surg 77:259, 1979
93. deLeval M, Hill JD, Mielke H, et al: Platelet kinetics during extracorporeal circulation. Trans Am Soc Artif Intern Organs 18:355, 1972
94. Tamari Y, Aledort L, Puszkin E, et al: Functional changes in platelets during extracorporeal circulation. Ann Thorac Surg 19:639, 1975
95. Peterson KA, Dewanjee MK, Kaye MP: Fate of indium 111-labeled platelets during cardiopulmonary bypass performed with membrane and bubble oxygenators. J Thorac Cardiovasc Surg 84:39, 1982
96. Hope AF, Heyns AD, Loltner MG, et al: Kinetics and sites of sequestration of indium 111-labeled human platelets during cardiopulmonary bypass. J Thorac Cardiovasc Surg 81:880, 1981
97. Rao AK, Walsh PN: Acquired qualitative platelet disorders. Clinical Haematology 12:201, 1983
98. Harker LA, Malpass TW, Branson HE, et al: Mechanism of abnormal bleeding in patients undergoing cardiopulmonary bypass: acquired transient platelet dysfunction associated with selective alpha-granule release. Blood 56:824, 1980
99. Addonizio VP, Smith JB, Strauss JF, et al: Thromboxane synthesis and platelet secretion during cardiopulmonary bypass with bubble oxygenator. Thorac Cardiovasc Surg 79:91, 1980
100. Plachetka JR, Salomon HW, Larson DF, et al: Platelet loss during experimental cardiopulmonary bypass and its prevention with prostacyclin. Ann Thorac Surg 30:58, 1979
101. Harding SA, Shakoor MA, Grindon AJ: Platelet support for cardiopulmonary bypass surgery. J Thorac Cardiovasc Surg 70: 350, 1975
102. Finlayson DC, Hunter RL, Check IJ, et al: Changes in serum and denatured proteins during CPB: evaluation by electrophoresis and biuret assay (abstract) In Abstracts of the 6th annual meeting of the Society of Cardiovascular Anesthesiologists. Boston, 1984: 241
103. Feijen J: Thrombosis caused by blood foreign surface interaction. In Kenedit RM, Courtney JM, Gaylor JCS, et al (eds): Artificial Organs. Baltimore: University Park Press, 1977: 235
104. Kalter RD, Saul CM, Wetstein L, et al: Cardiopulmonary bypass. Associated hemostatic abnormalities. J Thorac Cardiovasc Surg 77:427, 1979
105. Kirklin JK, Westaby S, Blackstone EH, et al: Complement and the damaging effects of cardiopulmonary bypass. J Thorac Cardiovasc Surg 86:845, 1983
106. Haslam PL, Townsend PJ, Branthwaite MA: Complement activation during cardiopulmonary bypass. Anaesthesia 35:22, 1980
107. Cavarocchi NC, Schaff HV, Orszulak TA, et al: Evidence for complement activation by protamine-heparin interaction after cardiopulmonary bypass. Surgery 98:525, 1985
108. Jacobs HS: Complement-mediated leukoembolization: a mechanism of tissue damage during extracorporeal perfusion, myocardial infarction and in shock. Q J Med 207:289, 1983
109. Hammerschmidt DE, Craddock PR, McCullough J, et al: Complement activation and pulmonary leukostasis during nylon filter filtration leukopheresis. Blood 51:721, 1978
110. Huttemeier PC, Berry D, Bloch KJ, et al: Pulmonary vasoconstriction and profound leukopenia in two sheep experimental models. Chest 83:24S, 1983
111. Flick MR, Perel A, Staub NC: Leukocytes are required for increased lung microvascular permeability after microembolization in sheep. Circ Res 48:344, 1981
112. Brande S, Nolop KB, Fleming JS, et al: Increased pulmonary transvascular protein flux after canine cardiopulmonary bypass. Am Rev Resp Dis 134:867, 1986
113. Rent R, Ertel N, Eisenstein R, et al: Complement activation by interactions of polyanions and polycations: heparin-protamine induced consumption of complement J Immunol 114:120, 1975
114. Best N, Sinosich MJ, Teisner B, et al: Complement activation during cardiopulmonary bypass by heparin-protamine interaction. Br J Anaesth 56:339, 1984
115. Park JV, Weiss CI: Cardiopulmonary bypass and myocardial protection: management problems in cardiac surgical patients with cold autoimmune disease. Anesth Analg 67:75, 1988
116. Diaz JH, Cooper ES, Ochsner JL: Cardiac surgery in patients with cold autoimmune disease. Anesth Analg 63:349, 1984
117. Dieter RA, Neville WE, Pifarre R: Hypokalemia following hemodilution cardiopulmonary bypass. Ann Surg 171:17, 1969
118. Henney PR, Riemenschneider TA, Deland EC, et al: Prevention of hypokalemic cardiac arrhythmias associated with cardiopulmonary bypass and hemodilution. Surg Forum 21:145, 1971
119. Abe T, Nagata Y, Yoshioka K, et al: Hypopotassemia following open heart surgery by cardiopulmonary bypass. J Cardiovasc Surg (Torino) 18:411, 1977
120. Rosa RM, Silva P, Young JB, et al: Adrenergic modulation of extrarenal potassium disposal. N Engl J Med 302:431, 1980
121. Ebert PL, Jude JR, Gaertner RA: Persistent hypokalemia following open-heart surgery. Circulation 31 (suppl 1):137, 1965
122. Shanahan EA, Anderson ST, Morris KN: Effect of modified preoperative, intraoperative, and postoperative potassium supplementation on the incidence of postoperative ventricular arrhythmias. J Thorac Cardiovasc Surg 57:413, 1969
123. Patrick J, Sivapragasam S: The prediction of postoperative potassium excretion after cardiopulmonary bypass. J Thorac Cardiovasc Surg 73:559, 1977
124. Weber DO, Yarnoz MD: Hyperkalemia complicating cardiopulmonary bypass: analysis of risk factors. Ann Thorac Surg 34:439, 1982
125. Horsey P: Blood transfusion. In Churchill-Davidson HC (ed): A practice of anaesthesia. 4th ed. Philadelphia: WB Saunders, 1978:705
126. Moffitt EA, Tarhan S, Goldsmith RS, et al: Patterns of total calcium and other electrolytes in plasma during and after cardiac surgery. J Thorac Cardiovasc Surg 65:751, 1973
127. Fuchs C, Brasche M, Spieckermann PG, et al: Divalent ions and myocardial function during cardiopulmonary bypass: changes of total calcium, calcium and magnesium in plasma. J Thorac Cardiovasc Surg 16:476, 1975
128. Hysing ES, Kofstad J, Lilleaasen P, et al: Ionized calcium in plasma during cardiopulmonary bypass. Scand J Clin Lab Invest 184:119, 1986
129. Abbott TR: Changes in serum calcium fractions and citrate concentrations during massive blood transfusions and cardiopulmonary bypass. Br J Anaesth 55:753, 1983
130. Auffant RA, Downs JB, Amick R: Ionized calcium concentration and cardiovascular function after cardiopulmonary bypass. Arch Surg 116:1072, 1981
131. Shapira N, Schaff HV, White RD, et al: Hemodynamic effects of chloride injection following cardiopulmonary bypass: response to bolus injection and continuous infusion. Ann Thorac Surg 37:133, 1984
132. Royster RL, Butterworth JF IV, Prielipp RC, et al: A randomized, blinded, placebo-controlled evaluation of calcium chloride and epinephrine for inotropic support after emergence from cardiopulmonary bypass. Anesth Analg 74:3, 1992
133. Johnston WE, Robertie PG, Butterworth JF IV, et al: Is calcium or ephedrine superior to placebo for emergence from cardiopulmonary bypass? J Cardiothorac Vasc Anesth 6:528, 1992
134. Opie LH: Reperfusion injury and its pharmacologic modification. Circulation 80:1049, 1989
135. Sala A, Ferrozzi G, Biglioli P, et al: Changes in the plasma magnesium content in patients subjected to cardiopulmonary bypass. Minerva Chir 30:513, 1975
136. Rasmussen HS, Svenson M, McNair P, et al: Magnesium infusion reduces the incidence of arrhythmias in acute myocardial infarction: a double-blind placebo-controlled study. Clin Cardiol 10:351, 1987
137. Turnier E, Osborn JJ, Gerbode F, et al: Magnesium and open heart surgery. J Thorac Cardiovasc Surg 64:694, 1972
138. Langer GA: Ionic movements and the control of contraction. In Langer GA, Brady AJ (eds): The mammalian myocardium. New York: John Wiley and Sons, 1974:193

139. Soliman MG, Brindle GF: Plasma levels of anti-diuretic hormone during and after heart surgery with extracorporeal circulation. Can Anaesth Soc J 21:195, 1974
140. Reitz BA, Ream AK: Uses of hypothermia in cardiovascular surgery. In Ream AK, Fogdall RP (eds): Acute cardiovascular management: anesthesia and intensive care. Philadelphia: JB Lippincott, 1982:830
141. Spurr GB, Hutt BK, Horvath SM: Responses of dogs to hypothermia. Am J Physiol 179:139, 1954
142. Baumgartner WA, Silverberg GD, Ream AK, et al: Reappraisal of cardiopulmonary bypass with deep hypothermia and circulatory arrest for complex neurosurgical operations. Surgery 94:242, 1983
143. Mori A, Sow J, Nakashima M: Application of pulsatile cardiopulmonary bypass for profound hypothermia in cardiac surgery. Jpn Circ J 45:315, 1981
144. Merrill EW, Gilliland ER, Cokelet G, et al: Rheology of human blood, near and at zero flow: effects of temperature and hematocrit level. Biophys J 3:199, 1963
145. Marty AT, Eraklis AJ, Pelletier GA, et al: The rheologic effects of hypothermia on blood with high hematocrit values. J Thorac Cardiovasc Surg 61:735, 1971
146. Mikaeloff P, Fleurette J, Louisgrand Y, et al: Factor analysis: fever in the early postoperative period following cardiopulmonary bypass surgery in adults. Arch Mal Coeur Vaiss 72: 1211, 1979
147. Clark RE, Dietz DR, Miller JG: Continuous detection of microemboli during cardiopulmonary bypass in animals and man. Circulation 54:74, 1975
148. Reed CC, Stafford TB: Cardiopulmonary bypass. Houston: Medical Press, 1985: 327
149. Wu W, Zbuzek VK, Bellevue C: Vasopressin release during cardiac operation. J Thorac Cardiovasc Surg 79:83, 1980
150. Oyama T, Sato K, Kimura K: Plasma levels of antidiuresis hormone in man during halothane anesthesia and surgery. Can Anaesth Soc J 18:614, 1971
151. Philbin DM, Coggins CH: Plasma vasopressin levels during cardiopulmonary bypass with and without profound hemodilution. Can Anaesth Soc J 25:282, 1978
152. Stanley THE, Philbin DM, Coggins CH: Fentanyl-oxygen anaesthesia for coronary artery surgery: cardiovascular and antidiuretic hormone responses. Can Anaesth Soc J 26: 168, 1979
153. Feddersen K, Aurell M, Delin K, et al: Effects of cardiopulmonary bypass and prostacyclin on plasma catecholamines, angiotensin II and arginine-vasopressin. Acta Anaesthesiol Scand 29:224, 1985
154. Philbin DM, Coggins CH: Plasma antidiuretic hormone levels in cardiac surgical patients during morphine and halothane anesthesia. Anesthesiology 49:95, 1978
155. Levine FN, Philbin DM, Konok K, et al: Plasma vasopressin levels and urinary sodium excretion during cardiopulmonary bypass with and without pulsatile flow. Ann Thorac Surg 32: 63, 1981
156. Kaul TK, Swaminathan R, Chatrath RR, et al: Vasoactive pressure hormones during and after cardiopulmonary bypass. Int J Artif Organs 13:293, 1990
157. Genuth SM: The thyroid gland. In Berne RM, Levy MN (eds): Physiology. St. Louis: Mosby-Year Book, 1993:943
158. Hershman JM, Jones CM, Bailey AL: Reciprocal changes in serum thyrotropin and free thyroxin produced by heparin. J Clin Endocrinol Metab 34:574, 1972
159. Holland FW II, Brown PS Jr, Weintraub BD, et al: Cardiopulmonary bypass and thyroid function: a "euthyroid sick syndrome." Ann Thorac Surg 52:46, 1991
160. Novitzky D, Cooper DKC, Barton CL, et al: Triiodothyronine (T3) as an inotropic agent after open heart surgery. J Thorac Cardiovasc Surg 98:972, 1989
161. Novitzky D, Human PA, Cooper DK: Effects of triiodothyronine (T3) on myocardial high energy phosphates and lactate after ischemia and cardiopulmonary bypass. An experimental study in baboons. J Thorac Cardiovasc Surg 96:600, 1988
162. Bailey DR, Miller ED, Kaplan JA, et al: The renin-angiotensin-aldosterone system during cardiac surgery with morphine nitrous oxide anesthesia. Anesthesiology 42:538, 1975
163. Roberts AJ, Niarchos AP, Subramanian VA, et al: Systemic hypertension associated with coronary artery bypass surgery: predisposing factors, hemodynamic characteristics, humoral profile and treatment. J Thorac Cardiovasc Surg 74:846, 1977
164. Taylor KM, Morton IJ, Brown JJ, et al: Hypertension and the renin-angiotensin system following open-heart surgery. J Thorac Cardiovasc Surg 74:840, 1977
165. Townsend GE, Wynands JE, Whalley DG, et al: Role of renin-angiotensin system in cardiopulmonary bypass hypertension. Can Anaesth Soc J 31: 160, 1984
166. Fouad EM, Estafanous FG, Bravo EL, et al: Possible role of cardioaortic reflexes in postcoronary bypass hypertension. Am J Cardiol 44:866, 1979
167. Wallach R, Karp RB, Reves JG, et al: Pathogenesis of paroxysmal hypertension developing during and after coronary bypass surgery: a study of hemodynamic and humoral factors. Am J Cardiol 46:559, 1980
168. Anton AH, Gravenstein JS, Wheat WM Jr: Extracorporeal circulation and endogenous epinephrine and norepinephrine in plasma, atrium and urine in man. Anesthesiology 25:262, 1964
169. Tan CK, Glisson SN, El-Etr AA, et al: Levels of circulating norepinephrine and epinephrine before. during, and after cardiopulmonary bypass in man. J Thorac Cardiovasc Surg 71: 928, 1976
170. Balasaraswathi K, Glisson SN, El-Etr M, et al: Serum epinephrine and norepinephrine during valve replacement and aorto-coronary bypass. Can Anaesth Soc J 25:198, 1978
171. Carr DB, Athanasiadis CG, Skourtis CT, et al: Quantitative relationships between plasma beta-endorphin immunoactivity and hemodynamic performance in preoperative cardiac surgical patients. Anesth Analg 68:77, 1989
172. Stanley THE, Berman L, Green O, et al: Fentanyl-oxygen anesthesia for coronary artery surgery: plasma catecholamine and cortisol responses (abstract). Anesthesiology 51:A139, 1979
173. Brandt MR, Korshin J, Prange Hansen A, et al: Influence of morphine on the endocrine-metabolic response to open heart surgery. Acta Anaesthesiol Scand 22:400, 1978
174. Roizen MF, Moss J, Henry DP, et al: Effects of halothane on plasma catecholamines. Anesthesiology 41:432, 1974
175. Reves JG, Karp RI, Buttner EE, et al: Neuronal and adrenomedullary catecholamine release in response to cardiopulmonary bypass in man. Circulation 66:49, 1982
176. Reves JG, Buttner E, Karp RB, et al: Elevated catecholamines during cardiac surgery: consequences of reperfusion of the postarrested heart. Am J Cardiol 53:722, 1984
177. Kehlet H: Surgical stress: the role of pain and analgesia. Br J Anaesth 63:189, 1989
178. Anand KJ, Hansen DD, Hickey PR: Hormonal-metabolic stress responses in neonates undergoing cardiac surgery. Anesthesiology 73:661, 1990
179. Minami K, Komer MM, Vyska K, et al: Effects of pulsatile perfusion on plasma catecholamine levels and hemodynamics during and after cardiac operations with cardiopulmonary bypass. J Thorac Cardiovasc Surg 99:82, 1990
180. Minami K, Koerner MM, Vyska K, et al: Effects of pulsatile perfusion on plasma catecholamine levels and hemodynamics during and after cardiac operations with cardiopulmonary bypass. J Thorac Cardiovasc Surg 99:82, 1990
181. Philbin DM, Levine EH, Emerson CW, et al: Plasma vasopressin levels and urinary flow during cardiopulmonary bypass in patients with valvular heart disease: the effect of pulsatile flow. J Thorac Cardiovasc Surg 78:779, 1979
182. Taylor KM, Wright GS, Bain WH, et al: Comparative studies of pulsatile flow during cardiopulmonary bypass: III. response of anterior pituitary gland to thyrotropin-releasing hormone. J Thorac Cardiovasc Surg 75:579, 1978
183. Ida Y: Experimental studies on carbohydrate metabolism during heart lung bypass, with special reference to a comparison of pulsatile flow with non-pulsatile flow. Nippon Geka Hokan 31: 181, 1962
184. Taylor KM, Wright GS, Reid JM, et al: Comparative studies of pulsatile and nonpulsatile flow during cardiopulmonary bypass:

II. The effects on adrenal secretion of cortisol. J Thorac Cardiovasc Surg 75:574, 1978
185. Stremmel W, Schlosser V. Koehnlein HE: Effect of open-heart surgery with hemodilution perfusion upon insulin secretion. J Thorac Cardiovasc Surg 64:263, 1972
186. Valentin NQ, Rasmussen SM: Plasma potassium and insulin during extracorporeal circulation using a glucose-containing prime. Scand J Thorac Cardiovasc Surg 9:169, 1975
187. Landymore RW, Murphy DA, Longley WJ: Effect of cardiopulmonary bypass and hypothermia on pancreatic endocrine function and peripheral utilization of glucose. Can J Surg 22: 248, 1979
188. Mills NL, Beaudet RL, Isom OW, et al: Hyperglycemia during cardiopulmonary bypass. Ann Surg 177:203, 1972
189. Yokita H, Kawashima Y, Takao TA, et al: Carbohydrate and lipid metabolism in open-heart surgery. J Thorac Cardiovasc Surg 73:543, 1977
190. Nagaoka H, Innami R, Watanabe M, et al: Preservation of pancreatic beta cell function with pulsatile cardiopulmonary bypass. Ann Thorac Surg 48:798, 1989
191. Kuntschen FR, Galletti PM, Hahn C, et al: Alterations of insulin and glucose metabolism during cardiopulmonary bypass under normothermia. J Thorac Cardiovasc Surg 89:97, 1985
192. Yokota H, Kawashima Y, Takao T, et al: Carbohydrate and lipid metabolism in open-heart surgery. J Thorac Cardiovasc Surg 73:543, 1977
193. Buckberg GD, Rosenkranz ER: Principles of cardioplegic myocardial protection. In Roberts AJ (ed): Myocardial protection in cardiac surgery. New York: Marcel Dekker, 1987:71
194. Lazar HL, Buckberg GD, Foglia RP: Detrimental effects of premature use of inotropic drugs to discontinue cardiopulmonary bypass. J Thorac Cardiovasc Surg 82:18, 1981
195. Lucas SK, Schaff HV, Flaherty JT, et al: The harmful effects of left ventricular distention during postischemic reperfusion. Ann Thorac Surg 32:486, 1981
196. Sink JD, Hill RC, Clintwood WE Jr, et al: Effects of phenylephrine on transmural distribution of myocardial blood flow in regions supplied by normal and collateral arteries during cardiopulmonary bypass. J Thorac Cardiovasc Surg 78:236, 1979
197. Arom KV, Angarin M, Lindsay WG, et al: Effect of sodium nitroprusside during the payback period of cardiopulmonary bypass on the incidence of postoperative arrhythmias. Ann Thorac Surg 34:307, 1982
198. Jones TW, Vetto RR, Winterscheid LC, et al: Arterial complications incident to cannulation in open heart surgery with special reference to the femoral artery. Ann Surg 152:969, 1960
199. Elliot DP, Roe BB: Aortic dissection during cardiopulmonary bypass. J Thorac Cardiovasc Surg 50:357, 1965
200. Salerno TA, Lince DP, White DN: Arch versus femoral artery perfusion during cardiopulmonary bypass. J Thorac Cardiovasc Surg 76:681, 1978
201. Mandelbaum I, Giammona S: Extracorporeal circulation, pulmonary compliance and pulmonary surfactants. J Thorac Cardiovasc Surg 48:881, 1964
202. McClenahan JB, Young WE, Sykes MK: Respiratory changes after open heart surgery. Thorax 20:454, 1965
203. Rea HH, Harris EA, Seelye ER, et al: The effects of cardiopulmonary bypass upon pulmonary gas exchange. J Thorac Cardiovasc Surg 75:104, 1978
204. Laver MB: Lung function following open heart surgery. In Litwack RS, Jurado RA (eds): Care of the cardiac surgical patient. New York: Appleton-Century-Crofts, 1982: 281
205. Baer DM, Osbom JJ: The postperfusion pulmonary congestion syndrome. Am J Clin Pathol 34:442, 1960
206. Massion WH, Downes P: Proteolytic enzyme levels during cardiopulmonary bypass. Adv Shock Res 8:129, 1982
207. Andersen NB, Ghia J: Pulmonary function, cardiac status, and postoperative course in relation to cardiopulmonary bypass. J Thorac Cardiovasc Surg 59:474, 1970
208. Llamas R, Forthman HJ: Respiratory distress syndrome in the adult after cardiopulmonary bypass. JAMA 225: 1183, 1973
209. Connell RS, Page VS, Bartley TD, et al: The effect on pulmonary ultrastructure of Dacron wool filtration during cardiopulmonary bypass. J Thorac Cardiovasc Surg 15:217, 1973
210. Reul GJ Jr, Greenberg SD, Lefrak EA, et al: Prevention of post-traumatic pulmonary insufficiency. Arch Surg 106:386, 1973
211. Barash PG, Berman MA, Stansel HC Jr, et al: Markedly improved pulmonary function after open heart surgery in infancy utilizing surface cooling, profound hypothermia, and circulatory arrest. Am J Surg 131:499, 1976
212. Byrick RJ, Kay C, Noble WH: Extravascular lung water accumulation in patients following coronary artery surgery. Can Anaesth Soc J 24:332, 1977
213. Clarke CP, Kahn DR, Dufek JH, et al: The effects of nonpulsatile blood flow on canine lungs. Ann Thorac Surg 6:450, 1968
214. Brismar B, Gullbring B, Olsson P: Effects of stored and fresh blood transfusions on postoperative pulmonary function: a clinical study on patients following extracorporeal circulation in association with aortic valve surgery. Eur Surg Res 10:153, 1978
215. VanOeveren W, Katatchkine M, Deschamps-Latscha B, et al: Deleterious effects of cardiopulmonary bypass. A prospective study of bubble versus membrane oxygenation. J Thorac Cardiovasc Surg 89:888, 1985
216. Byrick RJ, Finlayson DC, Noble WH: Pulmonary arterial pressure increases during cardiopulmonary bypass, a potential cause of pulmonary edema. Anesthesiology 46:433, 1977
217. Royston D: High-dose aprotinin therapy: a review of the first five years' experience. J Cardiothorac Vasc Anesth 6:76, 1992
218. Boldt J, King D, Scheld MD: Lung management during cardiopulmonary bypass: influence on extravascular lung water. J Cardiothorac Anesth 4:73, 1990
219. Gravlee GP, Hudspeth AS, Toole JF: Bilateral brachial paralysis from watershed infarction after coronary bypass surgery. J Thorac Cardiovasc Surg 88:742, 1984
220. Sweeney PJ, Breuer AC, Selhorst JB, et al: Ischemic optic neuropathy: a complication of cardiopulmonary bypass surgery. Neurology 32:560, 1982
221. Plasse HM, Spencer FC, Mittleman M, et al: Unilateral sudden loss of hearing, an unusual complication of cardiac operation. J Thorac Cardiovasc Surg 79:822, 1980
222. Tufo HM, Ostfield AM, Shekell R: Central nervous system dysfunction following open-heart surgery. JAMA 212:1333, 1970
223. Savageau JA, Stanton BA, Jenkins CD, et al: Neuropsychological dysfunction following elective cardiac operation: 1. early assessment. J Thorac Cardiovasc Surg 84:585, 1982
224. Savageau JA, Stanton BA, Jenkins CD, et al: Neuropsychological dysfunction following elective cardiac operation: II. a six-month reassessment. J Thorac Cardiovasc Surg 84:595, 1982
225. Garvey JW, Willner A, Wolpowitz A, et al: The effect of arterial filtration during open-heart surgery on cerebral function. Circulation 68(suppl 2):125, 1983
226. Slogoff S, Girgis KL, Keats AS: Etiologic factors in neuropsychiatric complications associated with cardiopulmonary bypass. Anesth Analg 61:903, 1982
227. Lee WH Jr, Brady MP: Central nervous system complications of extracorporeal circulation. In Cordell AR, Ellison RG (eds): Complications of cardiothoracic surgery. Boston: Little, Brown, 1979: 72
228. Kolkka R, Hilberman M: Neurological dysfunction following cardiac operation with low flow, low pressure cardiopulmonary bypass. J Thorac Cardiovasc Surg 79:432, 1980
229. Stockard JJ, Bickford RG, Schauble JF: Pressure dependent cerebral ischemia during cardiopulmonary bypass. Neurology 23:521, 1973
230. Branthwaite RA. Prevention of neurological damage during open-heart surgery. Thorax 30:258, 1975
231. Garman JK: Optimal pressures and flow during cardiopulmonary bypass: pro a low-flow, low-pressure technique is acceptable. J Thorac Cardiovasc Surg 5:399, 1991
232. Heller SS, Frank KA, Malin JR, et al: Psychiatric complications of open-heart surgery. N Engl J Med 283:1015, 1970
233. Wilson JW: Treatment or prevention of pulmonary cellular

damage with pharmacologic doses of corticosteroid. Surg Gynecol Obstet 134:675, 1972
234. Aris A, Solanes H, Camara ML, et al: Arterial line filtration during cardiopulmonary bypass: neurologic, neuropsychiatric, and hematologic studies. J Thorac Cardiovasc Surg 91:526, 1986
235. Nussmeier NA, Fish KJ: Neuropsychologic dysfunction after cardiopulmonary bypass: a comparison of two institutions. J Cardiothorac Vasc Anesth 5:584, 1991
236. Chapin JW, Nance P, Yarbough JW: Facial paleness. Anesth Analg 61:475, 1982
237. McLeskey CH, Cheney FW: A correctable complication of cardiopulmonary bypass. Anesthesiology 56:214, 1982
238. Levy WJ: Intraoperative EEG patterns: implications for EEG monitoring. Anesthesiology 60:430, 1984
239. Padayachee TS, Parsons S, Theobold R, et al: The detection of microemboli in the middle cerebral artery during cardiopulmonary bypass: a transcranial Doppler ultrasound investigation using membrane and bubble oxygenators. Ann Thorac Surg 44:298, 1987
240. Nussmeier NA, Arlund C, Slogoff S: Neuropsychiatric complications after cardiopulmonary bypass: cerebral protection by a barbiturate. Anesthesiology 64:165, 1986
241. Zaidan JR, Kochany A, Martin WM, et al: Effect of thiopental on neurologic outcome following coronary artery bypass grafting. Anesthesiology 74:406, 1991
242. LeMay DR, Gehua L, Zelenock GB, et al: Insulin administration protects neurologic function in cerebral ischemia in rats. Stroke 19:1411, 1988
243. Lanier WL, Stangland KJ, Scheithauer BW, et al: The effects of dextrose infusion and head position on neurologic outcome after complete cerebral ischemia in primates: examination of a model. Anesthesiology 66:39, 1987
244. Collins JD, Bassendine MF, Femer R, et al: Incidence and prognostic importance of jaundice after cardiopulmonary bypass surgery. Lancet 1:1119, 1983
245. Jenkins JG, Lynn AM, Wood AE, et al: Acute hepatic failure following cardiac operation in children. J Thorac Cardiovasc Surg 84:865, 1982
246. Lockey E, Mclntyre N, Ross DN, et al: Early jaundice after open-heart surgery. Thorax 22:165, 1967
247. Rose DM, Ranson JHC, Cunningham JN, et al: Patterns of severe pancreatic injury following cardiopulmonary bypass. Ann Surg 199:168, 1984
248. Hanks JB, Curtis SE, Hanks BB, et al: Gastrointestinal complications after cardiopulmonary bypass. Surgery 92:394, 1982
249. Moores WY, Cago O. Morris JD, et al: Serum and urinary amylase levels following pulsatile and continuous cardiopulmonary bypass. J Thorac Cardiovasc Surg 74:73, 1977
250. Murray WR, Mittra S. Mittra D, et al: The amylase-creatinine clearance ratio following cardiopulmonary bypass. J Thorac Cardiovasc Surg 82:248, 1981
251. Missavage AE, Weaver DW, Bouwman DL, et al: Hyperamylasemia after cardiopulmonary bypass. Am Surg 50:297, 1984
252. Probstein JG, Joshi RA, Blumenthal HT: Atheromatous embolization. An etiology of acute pancreatitis. Arch Surg 75:566, 1957
253. Feiner H: Pancreatitis after cardiac surgery. Am J Surg 131: 684, 1976
254. Fernandez-del Castillo C, Harringer W, Warshaw AL, et al: Risk factors for pancreatic cellular injury after cardiopulmonary bypass. N Engl J Med 325:382, 1991
255. Haas GS, Warshaw AL, Daggett WM, et al: Acute pancreatitis after cardiopulmonary bypass. Am J Surg 149:509, 1985
256. Harjola PT, Siltanen P, Appelqvist P, et al: Abdominal complications after open heart surgery. Ann Chir Gynaecol Fenn 57:272, 1968
257. Lawthorne TW, Davis JL, Smith GW: General surgical complications after cardiac surgery. Am J Surg 136:254, 1978
258. Long WB: Abdominal complications of cardiopulmonary bypass. In Utley JR (ed): Pathophysiology and techniques of cardiopulmonary bypass, vol 2. Baltimore: Williams & Wilkins, 1983: 175
259. Heikkinen LO, Ala-Kulju KV: Abdominal complications following cardiopulmonary in open-heart surgery. Scand J Thorac Cardiovasc Surg 21:1, 1987
260. Leitman IM, Paull DE, Barie PS, et al: Intra-abdominal complications of cardiopulmonary bypass operations. Surg Gynecol Obstet 165:251, 1987
261. Wallwork J, Davidson KG: The acute abdomen following cardiopulmonary bypass surgery. Br J Surg 67:410, 1980
262. Pinson GW, Alberty RE: General surgical complications after cardiopulmonary bypass surgery. Am J Surg 146:133, 1983
263. Bhat JG, Gluck M, Lowenstein J, et al: Renal failure after open heart surgery. Ann Intern Med 84:677, 1976
264. Abel RM, Buckley MJ, Austen WG, et al: Etiology, incidence and prognosis of renal failure following cardiac operations. Results of a prospective analysis of 500 consecutive patients. J Thorac Cardiovasc Surg 71:323, 1976
265. Porter GA, Kloster FE, Herr RJ, et al: Renal complications associated with valve replacement surgery. J Thorac Cardiovasc Surg 53:145, 1967
266. Hilberman M, Myers BD, Derby GC, et al: Sequential pathophysiological changes characterizing the progression from renal dysfunction to acute renal failure following cardiac surgery. J Thorac Cardiovasc Surg 79:838, 1980
267. Lundberg S: Renal function during anesthesia and open-heart surgery in man. Acta Anaesthesiol Scand Suppl 27:1, 1967
268. Hilberman M, Myers BD, Carrie QJ, et al: Acute renal failure following cardiac surgery. J Thorac Cardiovasc Surg 77:880, 1979
269. Yeboah ED, Petrie A, Pead JL: Acute renal failure and open heart surgery. Br Med J 1:415, 1972
270. Utley JR, Leyland SA, Johnson HD, et al: Correlation of preoperative factors, severity of disease, type of oxygenator and perfusion times with mortality and morbidity of coronary bypass. Perfusion 6:15, 1991
271. Kanter GS: Renal clearance of sodium and potassium in hypothermia. Can J Biochem Physiol 40:113, 1962
272. Karim F, Reza H: Effect of induced hypothermia and rewarming on renal hemodynamics in anesthetized dogs. Life Sci 9:1153, 1970
273. Utley JR, Wachtel C, Cain RB, et al: Effects of hypothermia, hemodilution, and pump oxygenation on organ water content, blood flow and oxygen delivery, and renal function. Ann Thorac Surg 31:121, 1981
274. Mielke JE, Hunt JC, Maher FT, et al: Renal performance during clinical cardiopulmonary bypass with and without hemodilution. J Thorac Cardiovasc Surg 51:229, 1966
275. Nuutinen L, Hollmen A: The effect of prophylactic use of furosemide on renal function during open heart surgery. An Chir Gynaecol 65:258, 1976
276. Kron IL, Joob AU, Meter CV: Acute renal failure in the cardiovascular surgical patient. Ann Thorac Surg 39:590, 1985
277. Senning A, Andres J, Bornstein P, et al: Renal function during extracorporeal circulation at high and low flow rates. Ann Surg 151:63, 1960
278. Jacobs LA, Klopp EH, Seamme W, et al: Improved organ function during cardiac bypass with a roller pump modified to deliver pulsatile flow. J Thorac Cardiovasc Surg 58:703, 1969
279. Hilberman M: The kidneys: function, failure and protection in the perioperative period. In Ream AK, Fogdall RP (eds): Acute cardiovascular management: anesthesia and intensive care. Philadelphia: JB Lippincott, 1982:806
280. Urzura J, Troncoso S, Bugedo G, et al: Renal function and cardiopulmonary bypass: effect of perfusion pressure. J Cardiothorac Vasc Anesth 6:299, 1992
281. Slogoff S, Reul GJ, Keats AS, et al: Role of perfusion pressure and flow in major organ dysfunction after cardiopulmonary bypass. Ann Thorac Surg 50:911, 1990
282. Maseda J, Hilberman M, Derby GC: The renal effects of sodium nitroprusside in postoperative cardiac surgical patients. Anesthesiology 54:284, 1981
283. Davis RF, Lappas DG, Kirklin JK, et al: Acute oliguria after cardiopulmonary bypass: renal functional improvement with low-dose dopamine infusion. Crit Care Med 10:852, 1982

284. Steen PA, Tinker JH, Pluth JR, et al: Efficacy of dopamine, dobutamine, and epinephrine during emergence from cardiopulmonary bypass in man. Circulation 57:378, 1978
285. Barry KG, Cohen A, Knochel JP, et al: Mannitol infusion: II. the prevention of acute functional renal failure during resection of an aneurysm of the abdominal aorta. N Engl J Med 264: 967, 1961
286. Flores J, DiBona DR, Beck CH, et al: The role of cell swelling in ischemic renal damage and the protective effect of hypertonic solute. J Clin Invest 51:118, 1972
287. Frega NS, DiBona DR, Leaf A: Enhancement of recovery from experimental ischemic acute renal failure. In Leaf A, Giebisch G, Bolis L, et al (eds): Renal pathophysiology: recent advances. New York: Raven Press, 1980

FURTHER READING

Casthely PA, Bregman D: Cardiopulmonary Bypass: Physiology, Related Complications, and Pharmacology. Mount Kisco, NY: Futura Publishing Company, 1991.

Gravlee GP, Davis RF, Utley JR: Cardiopulmonary Bypass: Principles and Practice. Baltimore: Williams & Wilkins, 1993

Hindman BJ, Lillehaug SL, Tinker JH: Cardiopulmonary bypass and the anesthesiologist. In Kaplan JA (ed): Cardiac Anesthesia. Philadelphia: WB Saunders. 1993: 919

Martin TJ: Cardiopulmonary bypass: In Kirby RR, Gravenstein N (eds): Clinical Anesthesia Practice. Philadelphia: WB Saunders, 1994: 320

Complications in Anesthesiology, second edition,
edited by Nikolaus Gravenstein and Robert R. Kirby.
Lippincott-Raven Publishers, Philadelphia © 1996.

INDEX

Page numbers followed by *f* indicate figures; page numbers followed by *t* indicate tabular material.

B

C

F

G

J

K